Textbook of the Neurogenic Bladder

Textbook of the Neurogenic Bladder

Adults and Children

Edited by

Jacques Corcos MD
Department of Urology
McGill University
Sir Mortimer B Davies-Jewish General Hospital
Montréal
Canada

Erik Schick MD
Department of Urology
University of Montreal
Maisonneuve-Rosemont Hospital
Montréal
Canada

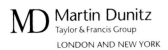

Martin Dunitz
Taylor & Francis Group

LONDON AND NEW YORK

© 2004 Martin Dunitz Ltd, a member of the Taylor & Francis group plc

First published in the United Kingdom in 2004
by Martin Dunitz, Taylor & Francis Group plc, 11 New Fetter Lane, London EC4P 4EE

Tel.:   +44 (0) 20 7583 9855
Fax.:   +44 (0) 20 7842 2298
E-mail: info@dunitz.co.uk
Website: http://www.dunitz.co.uk

Although every effort has been made to ensure that all owners of copyright material have been acknowledged in this publication, we would be glad to acknowledge in subsequent reprints or editions any omissions brought to our attention.

Although every effort has been made to ensure that drug doses and other information are presented accurately in this publication, the ultimate responsibility rests with the prescribing physician. Neither the publishers nor the authors can be held responsible for errors or for any consequences arising from the use of information contained herein. For detailed prescribing information or instructions on the use of any product or procedure discussed herein, please consult the prescribing information or instructional material issued by the manufacturer.

A CIP record for this book is available from the British Library.

ISBN 1 84184 206 0

Distributed in North and South America by
Taylor & Francis
2000 NW Corporate Blvd
Boca Raton, FL 33431, USA

Within Continental USA
Tel: 800 272 7737; Fax: 800 374 3401
Outside Continental USA
Tel: 561 994 0555; Fax: 561 361 6018
E-mail: orders@crcpress.com

Distributed in the rest of the world by
Thomson Publishing Services
Cheriton House
North Way
Andover, Hampshire SP10 5BE, UK
Tel.: +44 (0)1264 332424
E-mail: salesorder.tandf@thomsonpublishingservices.co.uk

Cover design by Catherine Schick

Composition by Newgen Imaging Systems (P) Ltd, Chennai, India
Printed and bound in Italy by Printer Trento

Contents

Contributors   ix
Foreword   xv
Introduction   xvii

Part I
The normal urinary tract   1

1.   Embryology of the lower urinary tract   3
    Hiep T Nguyen and Emil A Tanagho

2.   Simplified anatomy of the vesico–urethral functional unit   11
    Jacques Corcos

3.   Physiology of the smooth muscles of the bladder and urethra   17
    Marcus J Drake and William H Turner

4.   Physiology of the striated muscles   37
    John FB Morrison

5.   Pharmacology of the lower urinary tract   57
    Karl-Erik Andersson and Annette Schröder

6.   Integrated physiology of the lower urinary tract   73
    Naoki Yoshimura, Satoshi Seki, and Michael B Chancellor

Part II
Functional pathology of the lower urinary tract   89

7.   Epidemiology of the neurogenic bladder   91
    Patrick B Leu and Ananias C Diokno

8.   Ultrastructural pathology of neurogenic bladder   105
    Ahmad Elbadawi

9.   Pathophysiology of the overactive bladder   131
    Alison F Brading

10.   Pathophysiology of the areflexic bladder   143
    Katsumi Sasaki, Jun Nishiguchi, and Michael B Chancellor

11.   Pathophysiology of the low compliant bladder   157
    Emmanuel Chartier-Kastler, Jean-Marc Soler, and Pierre Denys

12.   Pathophysiology of the detrusor-sphincter dyssynergia   163
    Bertil FM Blok

13.   Pathophysiology of autonomic dysreflexia   169
    Waleed Altaweel and Jacques Corcos

14.   Pathophysiology of spinal cord injury   177
    Magdy Hassouna, Nader Elmayergi, and Mazen Abdelhady

Part III
Neurological pathologies responsible for the development of the neurogenic bladder   193

Developmental abnormalities

15.   Spina bifida in infancy and childhood   195
    Atsuo Kondo, Momokazu Gotoh, and Osamu Kamihira

16.   Spina bifida in adults   209
    JLH Ruud Bosch

17.   Syringomyelia and lower urinary tract dysfunction   215
    Marc Le Fort and Jean-Jacques Labat

Peripheral neuropathies

18.   Systemic illnesses: (diabetes mellitus, sarcoidosis, alcoholism and porphyrias)   221
    Ditlev Jensen and Bjørn Klevmark

19. Other peripheral neuropathies
     (lumbosacral zoster, genitourinary
     herpes, tabes dorsalis,
     Guillain–Barré syndrome)   229
     Vincent WM Tse and Anthony R Stone

20. Peripheral neuropathies of the lower urinary
     tract, following pelvic surgery and
     radiation therapy   235
     Richard T Kershen and Timothy B Boone

Hereditary and degenerative diseases

21. Dementia and lower urinary tract dysfunction 245
     Ryuji Sakakibara and Takamichi Hattori

22. Pathologies of the basal ganglia
     (Parkinson's disease and Huntington's disease) 259
     *Satoshi Seki, Naoki Yoshimura, and
     Osamu Nishizawa*

23. Urinary dysfunction in multiple
     system atrophy   265
     *Ryuji Sakakibara, Clare J Fowler, and
     Takamichi Hattori*

Demyelinating neuropathies

24. Multiple sclerosis   275
     Line Leboeuf and Angelo E Gousse

25. Other diseases (transverse myelitis,
     tropical spastic paraparesia, progressive
     multifocal leukoencephalopathy,
     Lyme disease)   293
     Tomáš Hanuš

*Vascular pathologies and tumors of
the brain*

26. Cerebrovascular accidents, intracranial
     tumors, and urologic consequences   305
     Adam J Flisser and Jerry G Blaivas

Disc prolapse and tumors of the spinal cord

27. Intervertebral disc prolapse   315
     Erik Schick and Pierre E Bertrand

28. Spinal and cord tumors   325
     Jacques Corcos and Rafael Glickstein

*Traumatic injuries of the central nervous
system*

29. Spinal cord injury and cerebral trauma 329
     Jerzy B Gajewski

*Other neurological pathologies responsible
for neurogenic bladder dysfunction*

30. Cerebral palsy, cerebellar ataxia, AIDS,
     phacomatosis, neuromuscular disorders,
     and epilepsy   345
     Mark W Kellett and Ling K Lee

Part IV
**Evaluation of neurogenic bladder
dysfunction**   **359**

31. Clinical evaluation: history and physical
     examination   361
     Gary E Lemack

32. Quality of life assessment in neurogenic
     bladder   365
     Patrick Marquis

33. The voiding diary   373
     Martine Jolivet-Tremblay and Pierre E Bertrand

34. The pad test   387
     Martine Jolivet-Tremblay and Erik Schick

35. Endoscopic evaluation of neurogenic
     bladder   393
     Jacques Corcos and Erik Schick

36. Imaging techniques in the evaluation of
     neurogenic bladder dysfunction   401
     Walter Artibani and Maria A Cerruto

37. Normal urodynamic parameters in children 409
     Steven P Lapointe and Diego Barrieras

38. Evaluation of neurogenic bladder dysfunction:
     basic urodynamics   415
     Christopher E Kelly and Victor W Nitti

39. Urodynamics in infants and children   425
     Kelm Hjälmås and Ulla Sillén

40. Electrophysiological evaluation: basic
     principles and clinical applications 441
     Simon Podnar and Clare J Fowler

41. Practical guide to diagnosis and follow-up of patients with neurogenic bladder dysfunction 463
Erik Schick and Jacques Corcos

Part V
Classification **467**

42. Classification of lower urinary tract dysfunction 469
Anders Mattiasson

Part VI
Treatment **481**

Non-surgical

43. Conservative treatment 483
Jean-Jacques Wyndaele

44. Systemic and intrathecal pharmacological treatment 495
Shing-Hwa Lu and Michael B Chancellor

45. Intravesical pharmacological treatment 507
Carlos Silva and Francisco Cruz

46. Transdermal oxybutynin administration 519
G Willy Davila

47. Management of autonomic dysreflexia 525
Waleed Altaweel and Jacques Corcos

Electrical

48. Peripheral electrical stimulation 529
Magnus Fall and Sivert Lindström

49. Emptying the neurogenic bladder by electrical stimulation 535
Graham H Creasey

50. Central neuromodulation 547
Philip EV Van Kerrebroeck

51. Intravesical electrical stimulation of the bladder 551
Helmut G Madersbacher

Surgical

52. Surgery to improve reservoir function 557
Manfred Stöhrer

53. Surgery to improve bladder outlet function 565
Gina Defreitas and Philippe Zimmern

54. Urinary diversion 599
Greg G Bailly and Sender Herschorn

Future developments

55. Tissue engineering applications for patients with neurogenic bladder 617
Anthony Atala

56. Restoration of complete bladder function by neurostimulation 625
Michael Craggs

57. Neuroprotection and repair after spinal cord injury 637
W Dalton Dietrich

Part VII
Synthesis of treatment **643**

58. Treatment alternatives for different types of neurogenic bladder dysfunction in adults 645
Erik Schick and Jacques Corcos

59. Treatment alternatives for different types of neurogenic bladder dysfunction in children 655
Roman Jednak and Joao Luiz Pippi Salle

60. The vesicourethral balance 667
Erik Schick and Jacques Corcos

Part VIII
Complications **673**

61. Complications related to neurogenic bladder dysfunction – I: infection, lithiasis and neoplasia 675
Andrew Z Buczynski

62. Complications related to neurogenic bladder dysfunction – II: reflux and renal insufficiency 683
Imre Romics, Antal Hamvas, and Attila Majoros

Part IX
Prognosis **693**

63. Evolution and follow-up of lower urinary tract dysfunction in spinal cord injury patients 695
Jean-Jacques Labat and Brigitte Perrouin-Verbe

Appendices **703**

Index *763*

Contributors

Mazen Abdelhady MD MSC
Department of Urology
Toronto Western Hospital
University of Toronto
Ontario
Canada

Waleed Altaweel MD
Resident in Urology
Department of Urology
McGill University
Montreal
Quebec
Canada

Karl-Erik Andersson MD PhD
Professor and Head
Department of Clinical Pharmacology
Lund University Hospital
Lund
Sweden

Walter Artibani MD
Professor and Chairman
Department of Urology
University of Verona
Verona
Italy

Anthony Atala MD
Associate Professor of Surgery
Director, Center for Genitourinary
Tissue Reconstruction
Children's Hospital and Harvard
Medical School
Boston MA
USA

Greg G Bailly MD FRCSC
Fellow in Urodynamics and Reconstruction
Sunnybrook and Women's College Health
Sciences Centre
University of Toronto
Ontario
Canada

Diego Barrieras MD FRCSC
Assistant Professor of Urology
Division of Urology
Hôpital Sainte-Justiné-University of Montréal
Montreal, PQ
Canada

Pierre E Bertrand MD FRCSC
Assistant Professor of Urology
University of Montreal
Maisonneuve-Rosemont Hospital
Montreal
Quebec
Canada

Jerry G Blaivas MD
Clinical Professor of Urology
Department of Urology
Joan and Sanford Weill College of Medicine
Cornell University and Director of
Urogynecology
Lenox Hill Hospital
New York, NY
USA

Bertil FM Blok MD PhD
Department of Urology
Academic Medical Center
University of Amsterdam
Amsterdam
The Netherlands

Timothy B Boone MD PhD
Professor and Chairman
Scott Department of Urology
Baylor College of Medicine
Houston, TX
USA

JLH Ruud Bosch MD PhD
Professor and Vice-Chairman
Department of Urology
Erasmus Medical Centre
Rotterdam
The Netherlands

Alison F Brading MA(oxon) PhD MSc
Oxford Continence Group
Professor, University Department of Pharmacology
Oxford University
Oxford
UK

Andrew Z Buczynski MD PhD
Urologist and Orthopedic Surgeon
Head, Department of Neurourology
Metropolitan Rehabilitation Center
Konstancin/Warsaw
Poland

Maria A Cerruto MD
Resident in Urology
University of Verona
Verona
Italy

Michael B Chancellor MD
Professor of Urology
Department of Urology
University of Pittsburgh Medical Center
Pittsburgh, PA
USA

Emmanuel Chartier-Kastler MD PhD
Professor of Urology
Department of Urology
Pitie-Salpetriere Hospital
Paris
France

Jacques Corcos MD FRCSC
Associate Professor of Urology
Department of Urology
Jewish General Hospital
McGill University
Montreal, Quebec
Canada

Michael Craggs
Professor, Spinal Research Centre
Royal National Orthopaedic Hospital
Stanmore, Middlesex
UK

Graham H Creasey MB ChB FRCSEd
Functional Electrical Stimulation Center
Case Western Reserve University
Cleveland, OH
USA

Francisco Cruz MD PhD
Professor of Urology, Faculty of Medicine of Porto
Vice-Chairman, Department of Urology
Hospital de S. João
Porto
Portugal

G Willy Davila MD
Chairman of the Department of Gynecology
Head of the Section of Urogynecology and
Reconstructive Pelvic Surgery
Cleveland Clinic Florida
Weston, FL
USA

Gina Defreitas MD
Fellow in Female Urology
Division of Urology
University of Texas Southwestern
Medicine School
Dallas, TX
USA

Pierre Denys MD
Professor of Physical Medicine and Rehabilitation
Department of Neurological Rehabilitation
Raymond-Poincaré Hospital
Garches
France

W Dalton Dietrich PhD
The Miami Project to Cure Paralysis
Department of Neurological Surgery
University of Miami School of Medicine
Miami, FL
USA

Ananias C Diokno MD
Chief, Department of Urology
William Beaumont Hospital
Royal Oak, MI
USA

Marcus J Drake DM MA FRCS
Clinical Lecturer
School of Surgical Sciences
The Medical School
University of Newcastle
Newcastle upon Tyne
UK

Ahmad Elbadawi MD
Professor Emeritus
Department of Pathology
SUNY, Upstate Medical University
Syracuse, NY
USA

Nader Elmayergi MD
Department of Urology
Toronto Western Hospital
University of Toronto
Toronto, Ontario
Canada

Magnus Fall MD PhD
Professor, Department of Urology
Institute of Surgical Sciences
Sahlgrenska University Hospital
University of Göteborg
Sweden

Adam J Flisser MD
Director
Division of Urogynecology
Mount Sinai Medical Center
New York, NY
USA

Clare J Fowler MBBS MSC FRCP
Reader and Consultant in Neuro-Urology
Department of Uro-Neurology
The National Hospital for Neurology and
Neurosurgery
London
UK

Jerzy B Gajewski MD FRCSC
Professor of Urology and Director of Research
Department of Urology
Associate Professor
Department of Pharmacology
Dalhousie University
Halifax, NS
Canada

Raphael Glickstein MD FRCPC
Assistant Professor of Radiology
McGill University
Department of Radiology
Jewish General Hospital
Montreal, Quebec
Canada

Momokazu Gotoh MD
Assistant Professor
Department of Urology
Nagoya University School of Medicine
Nagoya
Japan

Angelo E Gousse MD
Assistant Professor of Urology
Chief, Female Urology and Voiding Dysfunction
Miami Veterans Affairs Medical Center
Spinal Cord Injury Unit
University of Miami
Department of Urology
Miami, FL
USA

Antal Hamvas MD PhD
Associate Professor
Department of Urology
Semmelweis University
Budapest
Hungary

Tomáš Hanuš MD PhD
Associated Professor of Urology
Deputy of the Department of Urology
1st Medical School
Charles University
Prague
Czech Republic

Magdy Hassouna MD PhD FRCSC
Department of Urology
Toronto Western Hospital
University of Toronto
Toronto, Ontario
Canada

Takamichi Hattori MD
Professor, Department of Neurology
University of Chiba
Chiba
Japan

Sender Herschorn BSC MDCM FRCSC
Professor and Chairman, Division of Urology
University of Toronto
Director of Urodynamics and Attending Urologist
Sunnybrook and Women's College Health
Sciences Centre
Consultant Urologist Toronto Rehabilitation Institute
Toronto, Ontario
Canada

Kelm Hjälmås MD DMSC
Associate Professor of Pediatric Urology
Department of Pediatric Surgery/Urology
Göteborg University
Göteborg
Sweden

Roman Jednak MD FRCSC
Assistant Professor of Urology
Division of Pediatric Urology
The Montreal Children's Hospital/McGill University
Health Center
Montreal, Quebec
Canada

Ditlev Jensen MD PhD
Head, Out-Patient Department of Neurology
Head of the Laboratory of Neurourology
Assistant-Head of the Department of Neurology
Rikshospitalet (National Hospital)
University of Oslo
Oslo
Norway

Martine Jolivet-Tremblay MD FRCSC
Assistant Professor of Urology
University of Montreal
Division of Urology
Maisonneuve-Rosemont Hospital
Montreal, Quebec
Canada

Osamu Kamihira MD
Chief, Department of Urology
Komaki Shimin Hospital
Komaki
Japan

Mark W Kellett MD MRCP
Consultant Neurologist
Greater Manchester Neurosciences Centre
Hope Hospital
Salford
UK

Christopher E Kelly MD
Assistant Professor of Urology
Department of Urology
New York University School of Medicine
New York, NY
USA

Richard T Kershen MD
Assistant Professor, Division of Urology
University of Vermont/FAHC
Director, Female Urology & Voiding Dysfunction
South Burlington, Vermont
USA

Bjørn Klevmark MD PhD
Professor Emeritus
Department of Urology
Rikshospitalet University Hospital
Oslo
Norway

Atsuo Kondo MD PhD
Vice President
Department of Urology
Komaki Shimin Hospital
Komaki
Japan

Jean-Jacques Labat MD
Neurologist
Physical Medicine and Rehabilitation
Urological Clinic
University Hospital of Nantes
Nantes
France

Steven P Lapointe MD FRCSC
Assistant Professor of Urology
Division of Urology
Hôpital Sainte-Justiné-University of Montréal
Montreal, PQ
Canada

Marc Le Fort MD
Service de Rééducation Fonctionelle
Centre Hospitalo Universitaire
Nantes
France

Line Leboeuf MD FRCSC
Fellow, Department of Urology
Maisonneuve-Rosemont Hospital
University of Montreal
Montreal, Quebec
Canada

Ling K Lee MD FRCS(UROL)
Consultant Neurologist
Department of Urology
Royal Bolton Hospital
Bolton
UK

Gary E Lemack MD
Assistant Professor of Urology
Department of Urology
UT Southwestern Medical Center
Dallas, TX
USA

Patrick B Leu MD
Department of Urology
William Beaumont Hospital
Royal Oak, MI
USA

Sivert Lindström MD PhD
Professor, Department of Biomedicine
and Surgery
University of Health Sciences
Linköping
Sweden

Shing-Hwa Lu MD PhD
Department of Urology
National Yang-Ming University
School of Medicine and Taipei-Veterans
General Hospital
Taipei
Taiwan

Helmut G Madersbacher MD PhD
Associate Professor of Urology
Head of the Neurourology Unit
Landeskrankenhaus University Hospital
Innsbruck
Austria

Attila Majoros MD
Urologist
Department of Urology
Semmelweis University
Budapest
Hungary

Patrick Marquis MD MBA
Managing Director
Mapi Values
Boston, MA
USA

Anders Mattiasson MD PhD
Professor of Urology
Department of Urology
Lund University Hospital
Lund
Sweden

John FB Morrison MB ChB BSc PhD FRCSEd, FI Biol
Professor and Chairman
Department of Physiology
Faculty of Medicine and Health Sciences
United Arab Emirates University
Al Ain
UAE

Hiep T Nguyen MD
Assistant Professor of Urology and Pediatrics
Department of Urology
University of California
San Francisco, CA
USA

Jun Nishiguchi MD
Fellow, Department of Urology
University of Pittsburgh Medical Center
Pittsburgh, PA
USA

Osamu Nishizawa MD PhD
Professor of Urology
Shinshu University
School of Medicine
Matsumoto
Japan

Victor W Nitti MD
Associate Professor of Urology and
Vice-Chairman
Department of Urology
New York University School of Medicine
New York, NY
USA

Brigitte Perrouin-Verbe MD
Physical Medicine and Rehabilitation
Chief, Department of Rehabilitation
University of Nantes
Nantes
France

Joao Luiz Pippi Salle MD PhD
Associate Professor
The Hospital for Sick Children
Division of Urology
Toronto
Canada

Simon Podnar MD DSC
Institute of Clinical Neurophysiology
Division of Neurology
University Medical Center Ljubljana
Ljubljana
Slovenia

Imre Romics MD PhD DSC
Professor and Chairman
Department of Urology
Semmelweis University
Budapest
Hungary

Ryuji Sakakibara MD PhD
Lecturer, Neurology Department
Chiba University
Chiba
Japan

Katsumi Sasaki MD
Fellow, Department of Urology
University of Pittsburgh Medical Center
Pittsburgh, PA
USA

Erik Schick MD (LOUVAIN) LMCC FRCSC
Clinical Professor of Urology
University of Montreal
Maisonneuve-Rosemont Hospital
Consultant at Ste-Justine Hospital for Children
Montreal
Quebec
Canada

Annette Schröder MD DMSC
Department of Clinical Pharmacology
Lund University Hospital
Lund
Sweden

Satoshi Seki MD
Department of Urology
Shinshu University
School of Medicine
Matsumoto
Japan

Ulla Sillén MD DMSC
Professor of Pediatric Surgery/Urology
Göteborg University
Göteborg
Sweden

Carlos Silva MD
Department of Urology
Hospital de S. João
Porto, Portugal

Jean-Marc Soler MD
Physical Medicine and Rehabilitation
Centre Bouffard Vercelli Cerbère
Cap Peyrefitte
France

Manfred Stöhrer MD PhD
Professor and Chairman
Department of Urology
BG-Unfallklinik Murnau
Murnau
Germany

Anthony R Stone BSC MB FRCSEd
Professor of Urology
University of California Davis Medical Center
Sacramento, CA
USA

Emil A Tanagho MD
Professor of Urology
University of California
San Francisco, CA
USA

Vincent WM Tse MB BS MS Fracs(UROL)
Visiting Assistant Professor
Department of Urology
University of California Medical Center
Sacramento, CA
USA

William H Turner MD FRCS(UROL)
Consultant Urologist
Department of Urology
Addenbrooke's Hospital
Cambridge
UK

Philip EV Van Kerrebroeck MD PhD FELLOW EBU
Professor of Urology
Chairman
Department of Urology
University Hospital
Maastricht
The Netherlands

Jean-Jacques Wyndaele MD DSC PhD FELLOW EBU
Professor of Urology
University of Antwerpen
Fellow of the International Spinal Cord Society
Registered Rehabilitation Doctor and
Chairman, Department of Urology
University Hospital
Antwerpen
Belgium

Naoki Yoshimura MD PhD
Department of Urology
University of Pittsburgh
School of Medicine
Pittsburgh, PA
USA

Philippe Zimmern MD FACS
Professor of Urology
Holder of the Helen J and S Strauss Professorship
in Urology
Director of Bladder and Incontinence Center
UT Southwestern Medical Center
Dallas, TX
USA

Foreword

The publication of a new comprehensive textbook on "Neurogenic Bladder" is exciting news for anyone involved in the diagnosis and treatment of this disorder. The appearance of this book is very timely. There has been tremendous progress in understanding the function of the lower urinary tract during the last decade. New techniques have emerged, not least those relating to molecular biology. However, we have also seen breakthroughs in therapy. Nobody expects yet a complete cure for a number of patients with neurogenic bladder dysfunction, but every element of improvement is highly appreciated. And this is what has happened.

This book, edited by Jacques Corcos and Erik Schick with an impressive number of renowned contributors, is a natural sequel to the publications of Langworthy and Kolb (1940), Bors and Comarr (1971) and that of Bill Bradley and myself (1982). Looking back, there is a world of difference from then to the present time. When I made my debut in this field 40 years ago there were no effective drugs, no continent urostomy, no electrical manipulation, no artificial sphincter, not to mention bladder replacement. Seen in this light, one can surely be very satisfied of the progress accomplished in this field – and there is more to come!

I am convinced that this book should become standard reading for everyone involved in the care of neurogenic bladder patients and also for those with an interest in lower urinary tract physiology. Seen together this great number of contributors is in contrast to the situation 40 years ago when it was possible to know almost all by name. This is for a great part a tribute to the efforts of the International Continence Society and The Urodynamic Society.

Mainly because of the efforts of these Societies, neurourology and urodynamics have become well established subspecialities of Urology. In a way this book benefited from this and reflects this situation. It is very gratifying that ICS recommendations are included in the book.

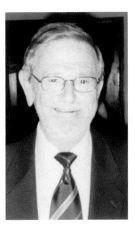

I cannot think of a single item in the overall topic that has not been carefully treated in depth. I congratulate the editors and all the contributors for the publication of this important text.

Tage Hald, Professor
Chairman of the
ICS Standard Committee

Introduction

"Men who are occupied with the restoration of health of other men, by the joint exercise of skill and humanity, are above all the noblest on earth. They even partake of divinity, since to preserve and renew is almost as noble as to create."

(Voltaire, 1694–1778)

As professors of urology, it is amazing to observe students and residents exceedingly interested in uro-oncology. Removing a prostate, or bladder, or kidney appears to be a noble task. They would like to "kill the disease", but their interest obviously declines when we speak to them about function, physiology, neuropharmacology, and neuromodulation. It seems obvious to them that there is less glamour, fewer lives to save, less fear to assuage, and probably less money too. But we are probably right to say, at least from the epidemiological point of view, that patients with voiding dysfunction, including those with neurogenic bladder dysfunction, are far more numerous than those suffering from urological cancers. Neurourology and, more specifically, neurogenic bladder care are fascinating aspects of our speciality because they relate to function. We operate for several hours, yet there are no surgical specimens, because we did not extirpate anything. We reconstruct. The real challenge lies in functional results.

To share our passion with the reader, we have attempted, in this book, to bring together some of the world's most distinguished experts in the field, assigning a difficult task to each of them. We asked them to summarize, synthesize, and simplify vast amounts of knowledge to make this book the reference source for students, residents, physicians, and health care professionals who want to have a precise, updated, well-documented and authoritative opinion on all aspects of the neurogenic bladder. We advised each author to try, according to our present level of comprehension, to explain all phenomena. We strongly believe that the readers will better remember pathophysiological events if they understand the nature of the underlying phenomena.

We structured this book into nine major parts.

After reviewing the normal embryology, anatomy, and physiology of the lower urinary tract in the first part, we devote a large segment of the second part to the epidemiology, pathology, and pathophysiology of different aspects of the neurogenic bladder. This essential part aims to clarify and explain the mechanisms underlying the different clinical entities developed in subsequent sections of the book.

We instructed the authors involved in the third part – dealing with different neurological pathologies responsible for neurogenic bladder dysfunction – to briefly describe the pathophysiology of this neurological disease and the ways it alters vesico–urethral function.

All patients with vesico–urethral dysfunction – regardless of the nature of the neurological process causing it – are investigated with the same diagnostic armamentarium. This constitutes the fourth part of the book. It includes an overview of quality of life instruments that help to determine the main outcome of our interventions in these patients. Imaging, electrophysiology, and, obviously, extensive urodynamic studies in adults as well as in infants and children are described in this part, which ends with a "practical guide to the diagnosis and follow-up of neurogenic bladders", a veritable handbook for medical students and residents.

Different classifications of neurogenic bladder dysfunction, based on symptoms, site of neurological lesions, and urodynamic findings, have been reported in the past. Recently, a new and highly original classification system has been proposed where structure and function are considered simultaneously. Professor Anders Mattiasson, former chairman of the Standardisation Committee of the International Continence Society, who presented this classification, accepted to develop it in the context of neurogenic bladder dysfunction. His chapter, on its own, constitutes the fifth part of the book.

Several new nonsurgical treatments, including new drugs and also new ways of administering them, have become standards in the last decade. The electrical treatments mentioned a few years ago already fill four chapters, and will most probably become future avenues to follow in this field.

After a description of the surgical treatments available, which are still widely used and necessary, we have three fascinating chapters showing us what we believe will happen in neurogenic bladder management in the next half century.

A large synthesis part follows, giving the reader an overview of the different available treatments that depend on patient age and the main dysfunction presented, but keeping in mind the principle of vesico–urethral balance.

The potential complications associated with neurogenic bladders and the prognosis of these clinical entities, in terms of evolution and follow-up, constitute the last two parts of the book.

As an addendum, we have reproduced *in extenso* three reports of the Standardisation Committee of the International Continence Society and the recently published Guidelines for the European Association of Urology on neurogenic lower urinary tract dysfunction. The first is the most recent update (2002) on the standardization of terminology in lower urinary tract function. The second report deals more specifically with neurogenic lower urinary tract dysfunction, including suggestions for diagnostic procedures. The third report is devoted to terminology and assessment of the functional characteristics of intestinal urinary reservoirs. We consider it important to include these reports because they represent a consensual view accepted by the international scientific community.

Medicine in general, and, more specifically, urology underwent tremendous evolution in the last few decades. This has radically modified our attitude toward neurogenic bladder dysfunction as well.

We felt it was imperative to summarize our present-day knowledge of the subject in a practical, but in-depth review of where we are today. We hope we have succeeded.

Our deepest gratitude goes to each and every author who accepted our invitation to take part in this venture – for readily sharing their expertise with us, and for the time they took to write their respective chapters.

We also thank Carole Goldberg for providing very capable secretarial support, much required in such an enterprise as well as Ovid DaSilva and his editorial team for correcting our grammar and vocabulary.

Last, but not least, our warmest gratitude goes to our wives, Sylvie and Micheline, who once again accepted to sacrifice part of the family life during the long months of intensive preparation of this book.

Jacques Corcos
Erik Schick
Montreal, February 2004

Part I

The normal urinary tract

1

Embryology of the lower urinary tract

Hiep T Nguyen and Emil A Tanagho

To better understand the diseases and congenital anomalies that affect the lower urinary tract, a thorough understanding of its embryology is essential. Our current understanding of lower urinary tract development is based upon observations derived from studies of fetal specimens and from clinical observations of congenital anomalies. However, these observations are only 'snap-shots' of a complex process that occurs during a brief period of time. Hence, much of what we know about the embryology of the lower urinary tract remains somewhat sketchy, and the exact details are filled by inferences and theories.

Development of germ layers

After fertilization of the ovum, the zygote undergoes cleavage and division to form a hollow sphere, the blastula. Some of the cells in the blastula aggregate to form an inner cell mass that will form the germ layers of the embryo (Figure 1.1). During the 2nd week of gestation, the inner cell mass flattens and forms two separate layers, the endoderm and ectoderm. A cleft develops within the ectoderm to form the amniotic cavity and within the endoderm to form the yolk sac. During the 3rd week of gestation, cells migrate from the endoderm and ectoderm to form a

middle layer, the mesoderm. On the caudal end of the germ layers, the mesoderm does not develop, and the endoderm remains apposed to the ectoderm without an intervening layer of mesoderm.[1]

Development of the cloaca

At the caudal end where the endoderm and ectoderm remain apposed, the cloacal membrane is formed. Differential growth of the mesenchyme near the cloacal membrane causes the caudal end of the embryo to fold onto itself, forming a chamber, the cloaca (Figure 1.2). The cloaca is lined primarily by endoderm. Further growth causes the caudal end to flex further, placing the cloacal membrane on the ventral surface of the embryo. Around the 4th week of gestation, the urorectal septum, also known as Tourneux's fold, expands caudally toward the cloacal membrane (Figure 1.3). Concurrently, the two folds from the lateral aspect of the cloaca, Rathke's plicae, migrate medially.[2] As a result, the cloaca is divided into the urogenital sinus anteriorly and the rectum posteriorly. Similarly, the cloacal membrane is divided into the urogenital membrane and the anal membrane. Rupture of these membranes allows the urogenital sinus and anal canal

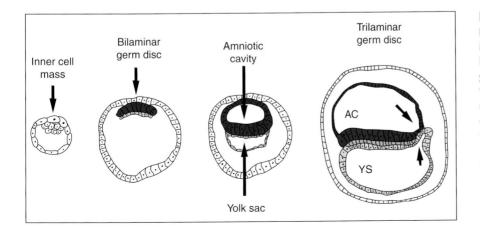

Figure 1.1
Development of the germ layers. An inner cell mass develops within the blastula. At the 2nd week of gestation, the cell mass differentiates to form two cell layers: ectoderm (blue) and endoderm (yellow). A cleft develops within each layer, forming the amniotic cavity (AC) and yolk sac (YS). During the 3rd week of gestation, a third layer, mesoderm (orange) develops in between the ectoderm and endoderm, except in the caudal region of the embryo (arrows).

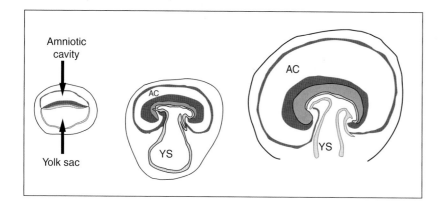

Figure 1.2
Creation of the cloaca. Differential growth of the mesenchyme in the cranial and caudal end of the embryo results in the infolding of yolk sac, creating the future GI and lower urinary tract. Rupture of the buccopharyngeal membrane (cranial) and the cloacal membrane (caudal) establishes communication between the amniotic cavity (AC) and the endoderm-lined yolk sac (YS).

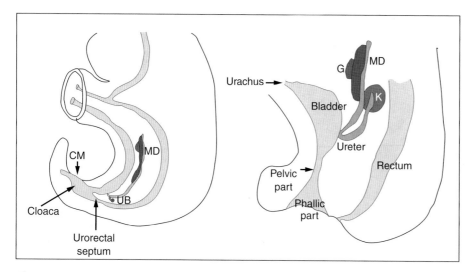

Figure 1.3
Differentiation of the cloaca. During the 4th week of gestation, the urorectal septum expands caudally to divide the cloaca into the urogenital sinus and the rectum. It also divides the cloacal membrane (CM) into the urogenital membrane and the anal membrane. The mesonephric duct (MD) develops adjacent to the primitive coelom. Cranially, it develops into the gonadal ductal system (G); caudally, it extends to join the urogenital sinus. A ureteric bud (UB) develops from each mesonephric duct and induces the surrounding mesenchyme to form the future kidney (K). After the 7th week of gestation, the urogenital sinus can be divided into three segments: the bladder, pelvic part, and phallic part.

to be in communication with the amniotic cavity. This process of cloacal division is completed by the 7th week of gestation.

After which, the urogenital sinus can be morphologically divided into three segments (Figure 1.3). The largest and most cranial segment will give rise to the urinary bladder. The second segment, the pelvic part of the urogenital sinus, is the narrowest portion of the urogenital sinus and will give rise to the prostatic and membranous urethra in males. The third segment, the phallic part of the urogenital sinus, is separated from the amniotic cavity by the urogenital membrane and will give rise to the urethra and external genitalia.[1] The cranial portion of the urogenital sinus, the urachus, maintains its connection to the amniotic cavity.

Development of the trigone

Around the middle of the 3rd week of gestation, the mesonephric duct develops from the mesoderm adjacent to the coelom, the primitive peritoneum (Figure 1.3). The mesonephric duct extends caudal and by the 4th week of gestation reaches the urogenital sinus. The endodermal lining of the urogenital sinus fuses with the mesodermal epithelium of the mesonephric duct, allowing the mesonephric duct to drain into the cloaca. At this time, a diverticulum develops from the posteromedial aspect of the mesonephric duct, forming the ureteric bud. By the 5th week of gestation, the segment of mesonephric duct caudal to the ureteric bud dilates to form the common excretory duct (Figure 1.4). The right and left common excretory

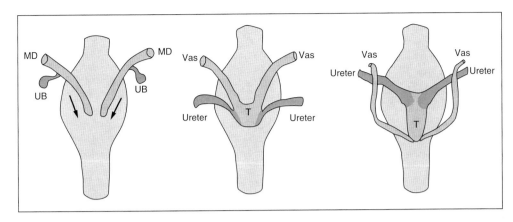

Figure 1.4
Development of the trigone. During the 5th week of gestation, the segment of the mesonephric ducts (MD) caudal to the ureteric bud (UB) is absorbed into the urogenital sinus. The right and left side merge midline to form the trigone (T). In midline, growth of the trigone and vas continues caudally, pulling the orifice of vas distally. Laterally, growth occurs laterally and superiorly, pulling the ureteral orifice superiorly.

ducts are then absorbed into the urogenital sinus. They fuse together medially to form the primitive trigone.[3] As the common excretory ducts are absorbed, the openings to the ureters move cranially, while those to the mesonephric ducts move caudally.[4] This pattern of development accounts for the contiguity of the musculature of the ureters with the trigone and the differential response of trigone musculature to pharmacological agents compared to the bladder musculature.

Development of the bladder

By the 6th week of gestation, the cranial portion of the urogenital sinus dilates to form the primitive bladder, presumably due to the production of fluid/urine from the mesonephros and subsequently by the metanephros. At this stage the bladder wall is composed primarily of connective tissue. At the 7th week of gestation, mesenchyme at the dome of the primitive bladder begins to differentiate to form detrusor muscles. This process extends caudally and, by the 8th week of gestation, muscle development is seen diffusely throughout the bladder wall. However, the muscle is neither organized nor abundant. By the 12th week of gestation, the urachus closes, becoming a fibrous cord, the median umbilical ligament. The emptying of the bladder becomes primarily dependent on the urethra. Concurrently, the bladder muscle fibers begin to be organized into circular, interlacing, and longitudinal bundles. Muscle formation is especially abundant at the bladder base and in the trigone, where it is five times thicker than elsewhere in the bladder.[5]

By the 17th week of gestation, there are three muscle layers in the bladder: inner and outer longitudinal layers and a middle circular layer (Figure 1.5). Muscle bundles from

the longitudinal layers interlace with the circular layer, making the distinction between the layers difficult, except around the bladder neck.[6] The outer layer forms a complete sheet of muscle bundles around the bladder to the level of the bladder neck. In the male fetuses, some of the muscle bundles from the outer layer extend into the prostate or loop around the proximal urethra. In the female fetuses, these bundles end in the vesicovaginal septum. In contrast, the inner muscular layer is only present on the anterior bladder wall and is deficient posteriorly except in the region of the trigone. In the trigone, the inner longitudinal muscle layer extends caudally to become contiguous with the longitudinal muscle layer of the urethra. At the level of the bladder neck, the middle muscular layer is quite prominent, since the muscle fibers in this area are quite closely packed together. The circularly oriented muscle bundles are complete anteriorly; they sweep through the sides of the bladder neck and fan outward as they travel posterior-cranially. The muscle bundles of the middle layer do not extend into the urethra but fuse to the lateral border of the trigone. As a result, by the 20th week of gestation, the bladder neck is bulky and pronounced. From the 20th week of gestation to term, there is continued increase in size of the muscles in the bladder, trigone, and urinary sphincter.

Development of the urethra

The phallic segment of the urogenital sinus differentiates to form the urethra. During the 3rd week of gestation, mesenchymal cells from the region of the primitive streak migrate around the cloacal membrane, forming the cloacal folds. Cranial to the cloacal membrane, the cloacal folds fuse to

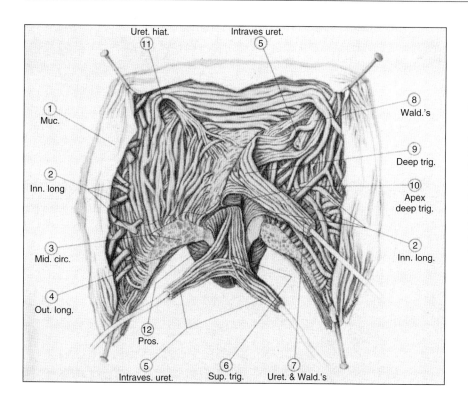

Figure 1.5
Muscle development of the bladder: (1) remaining edge of the bladder mucosa; (2) inner longitudinal muscle layer that extends toward the urethra (right side); (3) middle circular muscle layer that is most developed anteriorly; (4) outer longitudinal muscle layer; (5) intravesical ureter cut and reflected downward; (6) superficial trigone; (7) intramural ureter; (8) Waldeyer's sheath; (9) deep trigone; (10) apex of deep trigone extending toward the urethra; (11) ureteral hiatus; and (12) prostate. (Reproduced from Tanagho and Smith with permission.)[6]

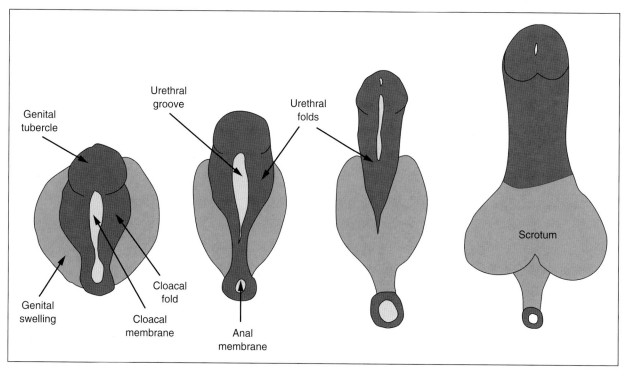

Figure 1.6
Development of the male urethra. Differentiation of the male urethra begins around the region of the cloacal membrane. Under the influence of androgens, the genital tubercle elongates and differentiates to form the glans and penis. Around the 12th week, the urethral folds fuse with primary luminization of the urethral groove. The genital swellings differentiate and fuse to form the scrotum.

form the genital tubercle. Concurrently, two protuberances, the genital swellings, develop lateral to the cloacal folds. During the 6th week of gestation with the descent of the urorectal septum, the cloacal folds become subdivided into the anal and the urethral folds.

In male fetuses, the development of the penile urethra occurs in concert with the masculinization of the genitalia during the 8th week of gestation. Under the influence of androgens produced by the fetal testis, there is a rapid elongation of the genital tubercle, forming the phallus (Figure 1.6). During this process, the phallus pulls the urethral folds forward to form the lateral wall of the urethral groove.[1] By the 12th week of gestation, the penile urethra arises from the fusion of the urethral folds with primary luminization of the urethral groove.[7] Fusion of the urethral folds lined by endoderm results in a continuous mesodermal compartment around the penile urethra.

Subsequent differentiation of this compartment forms the corpus spongiosum and cavernosum. During the 16th week of gestation, the glandular urethra develops. It is currently thought that, in the glans, the fused urethral folds undergo endodermal to ectodermal transformation with secondary luminization of the urethral folds.[8]

The process of urethral development in female fetuses is less well understood. It is not known whether the development of the female urethra is dependent on sex hormones (such as estrogen or progesterone) or is simply a default pathway when androgens are not present. In female fetuses, the genital tubercle only elongates slightly and forms the clitoris (Figure 1.7). The urethral folds do not fuse, as in male fetuses, but rather differentiate into labia minora.[3] The urogenital groove remains open to the surface and forms the vestibule. Rupture of the urogenital membrane allows the bladder to drain into the amniotic cavity.[9]

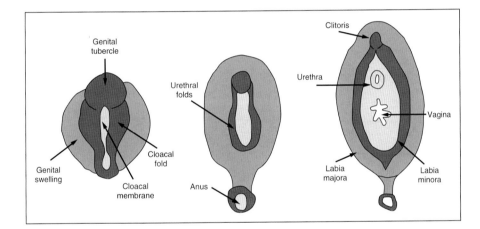

Figure 1.7
Development of the female urethra. The genital tubercle elongates slightly to form the clitoris. The urethral folds do not fuse and form the labia minora. The genital swellings differentiate to form the labia majora. Rupture of the urogenital membrane forms the opening of the female urethra.

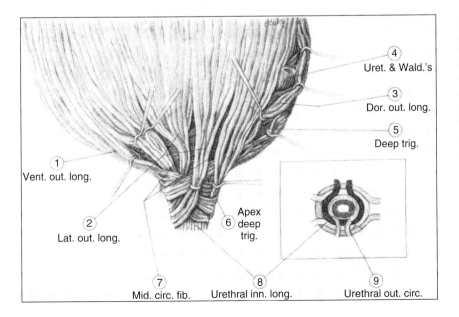

Figure 1.8
Arrangement of muscle around the female urethra: (1, 2, 3) the ventral, lateral, and dorsal outer longitudinal muscle layer of the bladder as they course downward to the urethra; (4) juxtavesical ureter surrounded by Waldeyer's sheath; (5) deep trigone; (6) apex of the deep trigone extending down toward the urethra; (7) middle circular muscle layer; (8) urethral inner longitudinal muscle layer; and (9) urethral outer circular layer. (Reproduced from Tanagho and Smith with permission.)[6]

Shortly after the formation of the urethra, the mesenchyme surrounding it begins to differentiate to form the two layers of the urethral musculature. They are present throughout the entire distance of the female urethra (Figure 1.8) and only in the proximal segment of the male urethra.[6] The inner layer is arranged longitudinally and is in continuity with the inner muscle layer of the bladder. This layer is relatively thick, since the muscle bundles are tightly packed and are held together by an abundance of collagen and elastic fibers. The outer layer consists of semicircular fibers, looping around the urethra. This layer is thick proximally but tapers off distally.

Development of the external urinary sphincter

Around the 9th week of gestation, mesenchyme near the urogenital membrane condenses around the future urethra. In the male fetuses, this primarily occurs in the area of the future membranous urethra and in the female fetuses, in the area of the mid-urethra. The mesenchyme develops into the external sphincter anteriorly and connective tissue with nerves and vessels posteriorly. By the 12th week of gestation, striated muscle fibers become apparent. Recent studies indicate that the external sphincter has an omega-shaped configuration in both the male and female fetuses, most developed anteriorly and incomplete posteriorly.[10]

Development of the innervation to the lower urinary tract

At the 3rd week of gestation, the ectoderm begins to thicken in the mid-dorsal region in front of the primitive pit, forming the neural plate (Figure 1.9). The lateral edges of the neural plates rapidly grow to form the neural folds. The neural folds migrate toward midline and fuse, forming a neural tube. In the wall of the recently closed neural tube, there are neuroepithelial cells. These cells rapidly proliferate and differentiate to form the spinal cord.[11] Due to the

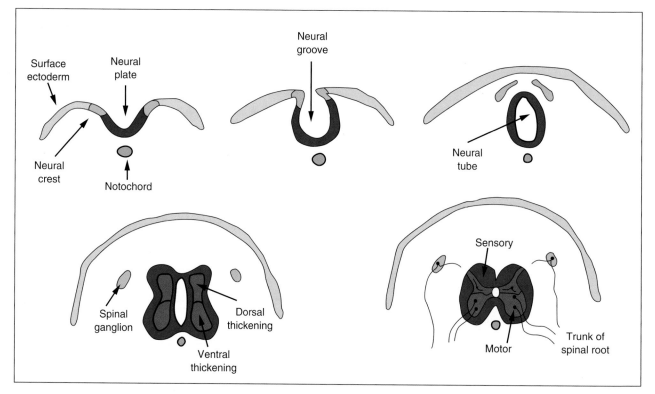

Figure 1.9

Development of motor and sensory innervation to the lower urinary tract. Around the 3rd week of gestation, a pit is developed on the ectoderm, forming the neural plate (blue). The lateral edges fuse midline to form a neural tube. Ventral (red) and dorsal (pink) thickening develops around the neural tube to form the spinal cord. Axons from the ventral thickening extend toward the pelvis to provide innervation to the lower urinary tract. In contrast, sensory innervation develops from neural crest cells (brown). They aggregate to form spinal ganglion. Neurons in the spinal ganglion develop two processes: one sent to the dorsal thickening to connect with the brain and spinal cord; and the second to the pelvic organs.

rapid growth of the neuroepithelial cells, a ventral and dorsal thickening develops on each side of the neural tube. The ventral thickening contains the ventral motor horn cells and forms the motor area of the spinal cord, while the dorsal thickening contains sensory neurons and forms the sensory area of the spinal cord.

During subsequent stages of development, the axons of neurons in the ventral thickening begin to extend out into the spinal cord and migrate to their designated organs, providing motor innervation[1] (Figure 1.9). The bladder and urethra receive motor innervation from two areas of the spinal cord – the sympathetic and parasympathetic system. Axons from neurons in the T11 to L2 region leave the spinal cord, forming the sympathetic nerve supply. These sympathetic fibers descend into the sympathetic trunk, then to the lumbar splanchnic nerves to reach the superior hypogastric plexus. This plexus then separates to form the right and left hypogastric nerves, which travel inferiorly to join the pelvic plexus (parasympathetic).[12] In the pelvic plexus, the axons from sympathetic nerves synapse, and postganglionic neurons are sent to the vesicle plexus. Axons from neurons in the S2–4 region form the parasympathetic system. They travel toward the bladder and form the pelvic plexus. After joining with the hypogastric nerves, they form the vesical plexus, whose branches ramify in the adventitia and penetrate throughout the muscular bladder wall. The parasympathetic axons synapse with their respective postganglionic neurons within the bladder wall. It is believed that the parasympathetic cholinergic nerve fibers are in a 1 : 1 ratio with each muscle fiber, while the sympathetic nerve fibers are more richly distributed in the trigone, bladder base, and proximal urethra.[12]

In contrast to the axons of the neurons in the ventral thickening, those in the dorsal thickening descend or ascend to a lower or higher level within the spinal cord to form association neurons (Figure 1.9). Sensory innervation to the lower urinary tract develops from neurons arising outside of the neural tube.[13] During the invagination of the neural plate, a group of cells (neural crest cells) develop along each edge of the neural groove. They migrate on each side to the dorsolateral aspect of the neural tube. With growth and differentiation, these cells form dorsal root ganglia. Neurons in the dorsal root ganglia develop two processes. One process penetrates the dorsal portion of the neural tube and synapses with association neurons or ascends to one of the higher brain centers. The second process extends peripherally and terminates in sensory receptor organs. When combined with the ventral motor root, the peripherally growing axons form the trunk of the spinal nerves. The sensory pathways then parallel that of the motor pathways. The sensations of stretch and fullness in the bladder are believed to be mediated along the pelvic parasympathetic pathways, while the sensations of pain, touch, and temperature are along the sympathetic pathways.

Innervation to the external urethral sphincter is mediated primarily by motor somatic fibers. Axons from motor neurons in S2–4 exit the spinal cord and travel as part of the pelvic nerve or the pudendal nerve to reach the sphincter. Sensation from the striated musculature of the external sphincter is mediated via the pudendal nerve to S2 and to a lesser extent S3.

The molecular biology of development

While we are beginning to understand the morphological events that occur during the development of the lower urinary tract, it remains largely unknown how this complex occur. Recent studies have begun to elucidate the mechanism of cellular interaction that leads to the formation of muscle in the bladder. In a rat model, it has been observed that smooth muscle develops from undifferentiated mesenchyme. The process occurs in an orderly sequence of differentiation defined by the temporal expression of smooth muscle (alpha-actin, myosin, vinculin, desmin, vimentin, and laminin) markers.[14] Smooth muscle differentiation begins in the periphery of the bladder mesenchyme subjacent to the serosa and continues toward the epithelium. Concurrently, the epithelium lining the bladder also undergoes differentiation as defined by the temporal expression of epithelial (cytokeratins 5, 7, 8, 14, 18, and 19) protein markers.[14] Interestingly, without the bladder epithelium, the bladder mesenchyme does not differentiate into smooth muscle.[15] Consequently, it is believed that mesenchymal–epithelial interactions with bladder epithelium (urothelium) are necessary for the differentiation of bladder smooth muscle. Peptide growth factors such as keratinocyte growth factor (KGF) and transforming growth factors (TGF) alpha and beta are likely candidates as mediators of these mesenchymal–epithelial interactions.[16] The smooth muscle-inducing property is not unique to the fetal bladder epithelium but is also present in adult bladder epithelium and in epithelia of other organs such as the bowel, cornea, and uterus (although the amount of smooth muscle induction varies with the type of epithelia).[17] Similarly, there appear to be signals originating from the induced mesenchyme that affect the growth and differentiation of the bladder epithelium.[18] Consequently, reciprocal communication and induction between epithelium and mesenchyme are needed for the proper formation of the bladder.

In-vivo and in-vitro studies are beginning to provide insights into the process of bladder development. Unfortunately, much of the molecular mechanisms that govern the development of the lower urinary tract still remain to be defined.

References

1. Sadler TW. Langman's medical embryology. Baltimore: Williams & Wilkins, 1985.

2. Stephens FD. Congenital malformations of the rectum, anus and genito-urinary tract. London, E & S Livingstone, 1963.

3. Hamilton WJ, Mossman HW. The urogenital system. In: Human embryology prenatal development of form and function. New York: Macmillan, 1976: 377.

4. Tejedo-Mateu A, Vilanova-Trias J, Ruano-Gil D. Contribution to the study of the development of the terminal portion of the Wolffian duct and the ureter. Eur Urol 1975; 1:41–45.

5. Droes JT. Observations on the musculature of the urinary bladder and the urethra in the human foetus. Br J Urol 1974; 46:179–185.

6. Tanagho EA, Smith DR. The anatomy and function of the bladder neck. Br J Urol 1966; 38:54.

7. van der Werff JF, Nievelstein RA, Brands E, et al. Normal development of the male anterior urethra. Teratology 2000; 61:172–183.

8. Baskin LS. Hypospadias and urethral development. J Urol 2000; 163: 951–956.

9. Gosling JA. The structure of the female lower urinary tract and pelvic floor. Urol Clin North Am 1985; 12:207–214.

10. Ludwikowski B, Oesch Hayward I, Brenner E, Fritsch H. The development of the external urethral sphincter in humans. BJU Int 2001; 87:565–568.

11. Fujita H, Fujita S. Electron microscopic studies on neuroblast differentiation in the central nervous system of domestic fowl. Z Zellforsch Mikrosk 1963; 60:463.

12. Fletcher TF, Bradley WE. Neuroanatomy of the bladder-urethra. J Urol 1978; 119:153–160.

13. Weston JA. The migration and differentiation of neural crest cells. In: Abercrombie M, Brachet J, King TJ, eds. Advances in morphogenesis. New York: Academic Press, 1970.

14. Baskin LS, Hayward SW, Young PF, Cunha GR. Ontogeny of the rat bladder: smooth muscle and epithelial differentiation. Acta Anat (Basel) 1996; 155:163–171.

15. Baskin LS, Hayward SW, Young P, Cunha GR. Role of mesenchymal–epithelial interactions in normal bladder development. J Urol 1996; 156:1820–1827.

16. Baskin LS, Sutherland RS, Thomson AA, et al. Growth factors and receptors in bladder development and obstruction. Lab Invest 1996; 75:157–166.

17. DiSandro MJ, Li Y, Baskin LS, et al. Mesenchymal–epithelial interactions in bladder smooth muscle development: epithelial specificity. J Urol 1998; 160:1040–1046; discussion 1079.

18. Li Y, Liu W, Hayward SW, et al. Plasticity of the urothelial phenotype: effects of gastro-intestinal mesenchyme/stroma and implications for urinary tract reconstruction. Differentiation 2000; 66:126–135.

2

Simplified anatomy of the vesico–urethral functional unit

Jacques Corcos

The bladder and the urethra should necessarily be described together. Functionally speaking, these two organs cannot be dissociated and, anatomically, their connections are too imbricated to distinguish them as two different organs. The pelvic floor, with its muscles, fascia, and ligaments, is a separate anatomical entity, but, functionally, it is also an important component of urethra–vesical physiology.

The bladder

The bladder (Figures 2.1a,b), located in the pelvis behind the pubic bone, can be divided into two portions. The dome, the upper part of the bladder is spherical, extensible, and mobile. The median umbilical ligament (urachus) ascends from its 'apex' behind the anterior abdominal wall to the umbilicus, and the peritoneum behind it creates the median umbilical fold. In males, the superior surface of the dome is completely covered by the peritoneum extending slightly to the base. It is in close contact with the sigmoid colon and the terminal coils of the ileum. In females, the difference arises from the posterior reflexion of the peritoneum on the anterior face of the uterus, forming the vesico–uterine pouch. In both sexes, the inferolateral part of the bladder is not covered by the peritoneum. In adults, the

bladder is completely retropubic and can be palpated only if it is in overdistention. In contrast, at birth, it is relatively high and is an abdominal organ. It descends progressively, reaching its adult position at puberty.

The base of the bladder, i.e. the lower part, is fixed. The trigone, the post part of the base, is triangular between three orifices – the two ureteral orifices and the urethral orifice or bladder neck.

At the level of the vesico–ureteral junction the ureters cross the bladder wall obliquely in a length of 1–2 cm. This type of path through the bladder wall creates a valve mechanism, preventing urine reflux toward the ureters when bladder pressure increases. Intramural ureter closure is completed by detrusor contraction.

At the level of the vesico–urethral junction or bladder neck, the original disposition of the muscle fibers allows closure during the bladder-filling phase (Figure 2.2).

The detrusor muscle

The detrusor muscle can be described as a sphere of smooth muscle bundles. It is a complex imbrication of smooth muscle fibers without a well-defined orientation, but is usually viewed as an external and internal longitudinal

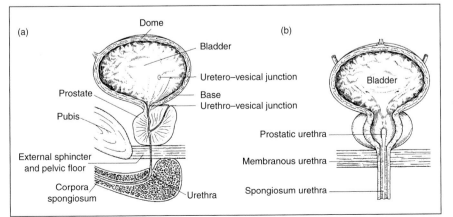

(a) Dome
Bladder
Uretero–vesical junction
Base
Urethro–vesical junction
Prostate
Pubis
External sphincter and pelvic floor
Corpora spongiosum
Urethra

(b)
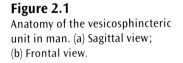
Bladder
Prostatic urethra
Membranous urethra
Spongiosum urethra

Figure 2.1
Anatomy of the vesicosphincteric unit in man. (a) Sagittal view; (b) Frontal view.

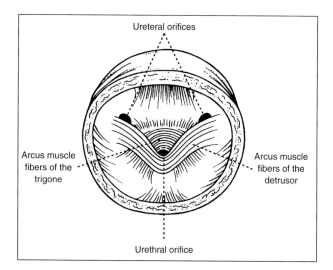

Figure 2.2
Trigone endovesical view.

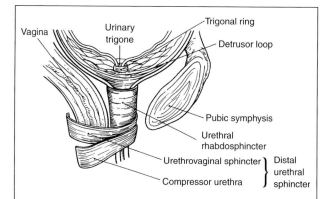

Figure 2.3
Architectural organization of the striated urethral sphincter. Location of its three components: the urethral rhabdosphincter, the compressor urethra, and the urethrovaginal sphincter.

layer with a circular intermediate layer. The muscle fibers of the inner layer extend down into the urethra in a funnel-shaped structure, allowing continence and emptying of the bladder. The muscle fibers from the two other layers arch toward and then away from the bladder neck to complete the sphincteric mechanism of this structure.

The bladder mucosa

The bladder mucosa, folded when the bladder is empty, is loosely adherent to the submucosal tissue and the detrusor. Over the trigone and all around the bladder neck it becomes much more adherent. The bladder mucosa is richly vascularized and very sensitive to pain, distention, temperature, etc.

The female urethra

The female urethra is 4 cm long and approximately 6 mm in diameter. It begins at the internal vesical orifice, extends downward and forward behind the symphysis pubis, and terminates at the external urethral meatus about 2 cm behind the glans clitoris. The urethral mucosa is surrounded by a rich, spongy, estrogen-dependent submucosal vascular plexus encased in fibroelastic and muscular tissue. The outer layer of the female urethra, covered two-thirds of its proximal length by a striated muscle, represents the external urinary sphincter. This sphincter has its largest diameter in the middle part of the urethra. The striated urogenital sphincter has two distinct portions: the upper sphincter portion, which is arranged circularly around the urethra, corresponds to the rhabdosphincter,

whereas the lower portion comprises arch-like muscular bands (Figure 2.3). Many small mucous glands open into the urethra, forming what are called the paraurethral ducts, which are usually located on the lateral margin of the external urethral orifice.

The male urethra

The male urethra (see Figures 2.1a,b) is 18–20 cm long and is usually divided into three portions: the proximal or prostatic urethra, the membranous urethra, and the penile or spongiose urethra.

- The first segment (3–4 cm) is mainly a thin tube of smooth muscle lined by mucosa and extending through the prostate from the bladder neck to the apex of the prostate. At the origin of the prostatic urethra, the smooth muscle surrounding the bladder neck is arranged in a distinct circular collar, which becomes continuous distally with the capsule of the prostate.
- The second segment, erroneously called the membranous urethra (there is nothing membranous at that level), is also known as the sphincteric urethra. The external sphincter has an omega shape and surrounds the urethra with a fibrotic segment in its posterior midline.
- The last segment, the spongiose urethra, is contained on the corpus spongiosum of the penis and extends from the previous segment to the urethral meatus. Its diameter is around 6 mm when passing urine. It is dilated at its commencement as the intrabulbar fossa and again within the glans penis, where it becomes the navicular fossa. All along the urethra, numerous small mucous glands (urethral glands) open into its lumen.

Vascular and lymphatic supply of the bladder and urethra

The superior and inferior vesical arteries are branches of the internal iliac arteries. The obturator and gluteal arteries also participate in bladder arterial supply. In females, an additional branch is derived from the uterine and vaginal arteries. Venous drainage forms a complex, extensive network around the bladder and into a plexus on its inferolateral face, ending in the internal iliac veins.

Lymphatic drainage originates from all layers of the bladder and ends in the external iliac nodes. Most urethral lymphatic drainage terminates in the external iliac nodes, except for the spongiose urethra and the glans penis where it goes to the deep inguinal nodes and from there to the external iliac nodes.

Urethro–vesical unit innervation

Three nerves provide an anatomic and somatic innervation to the bladder (Figure 2.4).

The hypogastric nerve

The hypogastric nerve has motor and sensitive fibers. It originates from preganglionic spinal neurons of the thoracolumbar intermediolateralis cord at the level of T10 to L1.

Preganglionic axons reach the paravertebral sympathetic ganglionic chain, where they synapse with ganglionic neurons. Postganglionic axons cross the superior hypogastric plexus to reach the vesical or interior hypogastric plexus. The vesical and urethral branches arise from this plexus.

The adrenergic innervations delivered by these nerves are B type at the level of the dome, and α_1 type at the level of the bladder base and neck (superficial trigone). The global effects of adrenergic bladder innervation are relaxation of the dome and contraction of the bladder neck. The hypogastric nerves are mainly adrenergic, but also have cholinergic as well as peptidergic contingents whose function is not well understood.

In contrast to the rich sympathetic innervation of the bladder neck in males, the bladder neck in females receives mainly cholinergic fibers and much less adrenergic innervation. This difference in nerve supply may relate to the main genital function attributed to the bladder neck in males and its lesser importance in females.

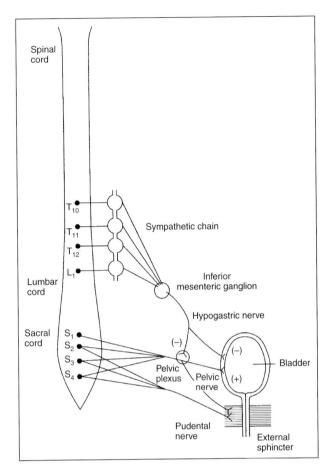

Figure 2.4
Spinal cord centers and nerves responsible for micturition.

The pelvic nerves

The pelvic nerves represent the parasympathetic component of bladder innervation. Their fibers arise from the 2nd to the 4th sacral segments of the spinal cord and merge at the level of the vesical plexus, from where branches reach the bladder. These fibers are cholinergic, but some noradrenergic fibers participate in the composition of the pelvic plexus.

The bladder, including the trigone, is profusely supplied by nerves from a dense plexus among the detrusor muscle fibers. The majority of these nerves are cholinergic and follow the vascular supply, only rarely extending among the nonstriated muscle components of the bladder and urethra.

Nonadrenergic noncholinergic innervation

Numerous neurotransmitters have been detected and studied in the intramural ganglia of the bladder: they include, among others, somatostatin, substance P, neurokinins, and bombesin. The anatomical and physiological relationships between nonadrenergic/noncholinergic innervations and cholinergic/adrenergic innervations are still being debated.

The pudendal nerves

The pudendal nerves convey both notoriety and sensitivity, arising from the spinal motoneurons of Onuf's nucleus located at the base of the anterior horn of S2–S4. Their axons cross the pudendal plexus composed of the 2nd, 3rd, and 4th sacral nerves and merge to constitute the pudendal nerves that are responsible for innervation of all the striated muscles of the pelvic floor, including the urethral and anal sphincters.

Afferent fibers

The origins of these sensory nerves incorporate different types of subepithelial receptors (simple or complex vesicles), capsulated or not, but with controversial distributions and functions (Figure 2.5). Present in sympathetic and adrenergic innervation, these sensory fibers transmit pain and awareness of distention to the central structures. Bladder afferents mainly follow the pelvic nerves. Urethral afferents follow the pelvic nerves for the proximal urethra, the hypogastric nerve for the mid-portion, and the pudendal nerves for the rest of the urethra and sphincter. However, their distribution is not clear-cut, and major overlapping exists.

The spinal sensory pathway (need to urinate, pain, temperature, urgency, sexual arousal) is found in the anterolateral white columns.

Fibers transmitting conscious sensitivity (bladder distention, ongoing micturition, tactile pressure) follow the posterior columns, synapsing in the gravelis nucleus and cuneatus of the brainstem before reaching the lateral ventral posterior nucleus of the thalamus and the cortex.

All these afferent pathways have important connections at the spinal cord and brainstem level with micturition motor fibers and the limbic system that explain the affective component of micturition.

Micturition integration centers

Micturition is not only an autonomic function, but is also a voluntary and emotional function under upper central nervous system control (Figures 2.5, 2.6, and 2.7).

Micturition centers at the level of the brain

Micturition is regulated voluntarily by cortical centers at the level of the frontal lobe and diffusively is the premotrice area (paracentral lobule).

The emotional control of micturition is complex and involves the limbic system with participation of the hypothalamus, the hippocampus, the callosal gyrus, the supraorbitrary cortex, the amygdala, and several nonspecific thalamic nuclei.

Locus caeruleus and subcaeruleus nucleus

At the level of the brainstem, particularly the pons and the medulla, stimulation of the locus caeruleus complex and

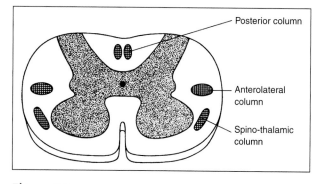

Figure 2.5
Transverse cut of the spinal cord showing the ascendent and descendent pathways of the vesico-sphincteric innervation.

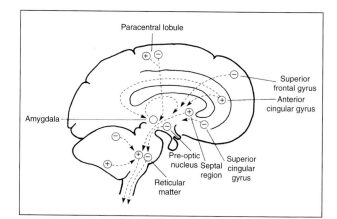

Figure 2.6
Micturition integration brain centers.

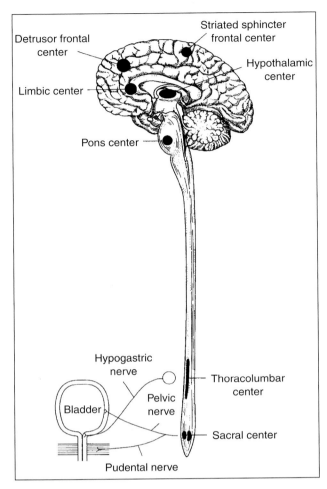

Figure 2.7
Micturition integration centers and nerves.

subcaeruleus nucleus complex (LCC) provokes contraction or relaxation of the vesicosphincteric units located in the anterior and dorsal parts of the pons and being a component of the Barrington center. Neurons of the LCC are mainly nonadrenergic, but all kinds of neurotransmitters are involved (cholinergic, serotoninergic, enkephalinergic, etc.).

The LCC influences micturition through ascending and descending fibers. The ascending fibers regulate emotional and voluntary decision processes. Descending connections arise from the ventral part of the LCC and innervate most of the cord. Two catecholaminergic pathways follow the intermediolateral column and reach the sympathetic thoracolumbar and the parasympathetic sacral neurons.

References

1. Galeano C, Corcos J, Schick E. Anatomie simplifiée de l'unité fonctionnelle vesico-urethrale. In: Corcos J, Schick E, eds. Les vessies neurogenes de l'adulte. France: Masson, 1996.

2. Haab F, Sebe P, Mondet F, Ciofu C. Functional anatomy of the bladder and urethra in females. In: Corcos J, Schick E, eds. The urinary sphincter. London: Marcel Dekker, 2001.

3. Meyers RP. The male striated urethral sphincter. In: Corcos J, Schick E, eds. The urinary sphincter. London: Marcel Dekker, 2001.

4. The urinary system. In: Gray's anatomy. Edinburgh: Churchill Livingstone, 1995.

3

Physiology of the smooth muscles of the bladder and urethra

Marcus J Drake and William H Turner

Introduction

The lower urinary tract (LUT) is a remarkably complex entity whose function remains incompletely understood. It is clear that the muscles of the bladder and urethra are crucial in normal function and that smooth muscle abnormalities play a major role in the pathophysiology of storage and voiding disorders.[1] In recent decades there has been a substantial increase in the knowledge base of LUT function, from the whole organ to the molecular level, acquired through the application of increasingly sophisticated experimental tools (reviewed in Turner[2]). This chapter will outline the present state of knowledge of detrusor and urethral smooth muscle physiology in the context of smooth muscle physiology in general.

Molecular cell biology of the detrusor

The biological behavior of a cell is determined by the proteins present in the cellular membrane, particularly the receptors and the ion channels, along with the components of the intracellular second messenger systems.

Receptors

Cellular response to hormones and neurotransmitters is determined by binding of ligands to specific membrane-bound receptors. This can result in either direct modification of ionic permeability of cell membranes (ionotropic action), or synthesis of intermediary substances known as second messengers (metabotropic action). Many different receptor types have been identified, reflecting the diverse array of endogenous ligands.

Adrenergic receptors

Adrenergic receptors are the best characterized receptors, mediating the response to the circulating hormone epinephrine (adrenaline) and the neurotransmitter norepinephrine (noradrenaline). They are classified as α adrenoceptors or β adrenoceptors, with further subclassification on the basis of structure and response to pharmacological agonists and antagonists into α_1 (α_{1A-D} and α_{1L}), α_2 (α_{2A-C}), and β_{1-3}.[3] In the bladder, subtype-selective ligand studies suggest the presence of β_2 receptors.[4] Nevertheless, functional responses are atypical for β_1 and β_2 adrenoceptors and the existence of β_3 receptors has been established.[5] The presence of mRNA responsible for encoding the α_{1D} receptor has also been documented.[6]

Cholinergic receptors

Tissue response to the neurotransmitter acetylcholine is mediated by muscarinic and nicotinic receptors, the former located in several cellular locations, the latter predominantly in the central nervous system, peripheral ganglia of the autonomic nervous system, and on skeletal muscle. Muscarinic receptors are classified on the basis of specific response to pharmacological agents (M_{1-5}) and molecular structure (m_{1-5}).[7] mRNA encoding m_2 and m_3 receptors, but not m_1, m_4, and m_5, is present in the human bladder.[8] M_3 receptors predominate on receptor binding studies,[9] although a 3:1 predominance of m_2 over m_3 has been reported using subtype-specific immunoprecipitation.[10] Nevertheless, the M_3 receptor appears to mediate contraction.[10,11] The role of the M_2 receptor is unclear, though it can cause contraction by opposing β-adrenoceptor-mediated relaxation.[12]

Purinergic receptors

Purinoceptors are present in the lower urinary tract, the agonists for which are extracellular adenosine, adenosine diphosphate (ADP), and adenosine triphosphate (ATP). The purinoceptors are predominantly ionotropic and have been classified as P_1 or P_2, which show differing affinity for the endogenous agonists. P_1 is further subclassified into A_1 and A_{2A-2B}, and P_2 into P_{2t}, P_{2u}, P_{2x-z}.[3] At least seven subtypes of the P_{2x} receptor are present in rat and human bladder.[13,14] The P_{2x1} receptor appears to predominate on smooth muscle cells,[15,16] but there is considerable plasticity in P_{2x} receptors according to physiological circumstances.[17]

Other receptors

Histamine H_1 receptors are present on smooth muscle cells.[18] Detrusor cells may also express the vanilloid receptor VR_1,[19] although its primary location appears to be on nerve fibers.[20,21]

Ion channels

The lipid bilayer of the cell membrane is relatively impermeable to the passage of charged ions. The presence of transmembrane protein channels allows ionic transfer into and out of the cytoplasm, the properties of the channels enabling tight control of the intracellular composition and membrane potentials.

Potassium channels

Several types of potassium (K^+) channels are recognized (reviewed in Quayle et al[22]). These fall into two main groups: voltage-sensitive channels, and inward rectifying channels, which conduct inward K^+ current much more readily than outward. There is substantial functional overlap between the two groups. Calcium-activated K^+ channels include the SK, BK, and maxi-K^+ channels. K_{ATP} channels are inward rectifying channels whose configuration is determined by the metabolic state of the cell. They are linked to sulfonylurea receptors and are sensitive to the action of glibenclamide. K^+ channel opening drugs, such as cromakalim, levcromakalim, pinacidil, and nicorandil, probably act by reducing the sensitivity of K^+ channels to inhibition by ATP.[22]

Current characteristics of several types of K^+ channel have been identified in detrusor myocytes, including voltage-sensitive delayed rectifier current,[23] Ca^{2+}-activated maxi-K^+ channels,[24–27] SK and BK channels,[28,29] and glibenclamide-sensitive K^+ channels.[30,31]. In the rat, an inwardly rectifying current, apparently carried by both Na^+ and K^+ ions, has been demonstrated.[32] K^+ channels appear to be fundamental both in determining the membrane potential and in repolarization following the action potential. K_{ATP} channels strongly influence the membrane potential in the bladder, since activation of only a small proportion of the channels present significantly inhibits action potentials.[33] Acetylcholine can inhibit K_{ATP} channels in the bladder through a muscarinic mechanism.[30] Potassium channel blocking drugs have varying effects on the membrane potential and they tend to increase spontaneous mechanical activity in isolated detrusor strips. Different K^+ channel blocking drugs affect the action potential in various ways, some blocking after-hyperpolarization, some slowing depolarization, and some doing both.[34]

Calcium channels

Several types of membrane channels allow the influx of calcium (Ca^{2+}), both specific and nonselective, but voltage-operated Ca^{2+} channels appear to predominate in smooth muscle.[35] Voltage-operated Ca^{2+} channels are classified according to the properties of the currents passing through them, comprising L-type (long lasting), T-type (transient), or N-type (neither L nor T).[3]

L-type Ca^{2+} channels are numerous in detrusor muscle, permitting high ion flux rates, which can result in a rapid rise in cytoplasmic Ca^{2+} levels. They only allow current flow in one of three possible channel states (open state), which is strongly regulated by the membrane potential. In guinea pig bladder they are inactivated by a rise in intracellular free Ca^{2+} ions,[36] but also show the unusual property of being switched into a long open state by depolarization, and having two open states, features that may have important implications for contractile function.[37,38] In detrusor strips from most animals studied, L-type Ca^{2+} channel blockers, such as nifedipine, reduce spontaneous contractile activity. Furthermore, the upstroke of the action potential is produced by current flowing through these channels. T-type channels, which are also present in the bladder, possibly have a role in replenishment of intracellular calcium stores.[39]

Nonspecific cation channels

Exogenously applied ATP elicits large inward currents in dispersed bladder smooth muscle cells from human and pig.[40] P_{2x} channels are ionotropic and following binding of ATP they permit Ca^{2+} flux, although Ca^{2+} may only carry 10% of the nonselective cation current.[35] In many smooth muscles, activation of M_2 receptors results in G-protein-mediated, nonselective, depolarizing cation current, facilitated by M_3-receptor-mediated release of Ca^{2+} from intracellular stores.[35] This acetylcholine response is biphasic in some smooth muscles, with a Ca^{2+}-activated inward chloride current preceding a sustained nonselective cation current.

Detrusor cells possess stretch-activated nonselective cation channels, which cause cell membrane depolarization. The degree of depolarization is modulated by secondary activation of Ca^{2+}-activated K^+ channels, which allow potassium to leave the cell.[41–43] As a result, the cellular response to stretch depends on the rate at which it is applied. Strips of detrusor muscle respond to rapid stretch with a rapid depolarization and increase in action potential frequency, leading to a nonsustained contraction. Slowly applied stretch does not activate this contractile response, presumably because K^+ channel activation keeps up with opening of the stretch-activated channels, preventing depolarization. The mechanisms of modulation of 'mechanogated' ion channels in smooth muscle have been reviewed elsewhere.[44]

Sodium channels

A family of sodium (Na^+) channels have been cloned and characterized pharmacologically, using Na^+ channel antagonists such as tetrodotoxin (TTX). Although many smooth muscles express Na^+ channels, their physiological role is uncertain.[3]

Chloride channels

Chloride channels permit passive transfer of Cl^- across the cell membrane and may regulate cell volume and membrane excitability in smooth muscles.[3] The calculated Cl^- equilibrium potential is -35 to -20 mV, while the measured intracellular Cl^- concentration is typically 40–50 mmol/L, indicating that an active transport system contributes to the accumulation of Cl^-.[3] Patch clamp studies have also revealed Ca^{2+}-dependent Cl^- currents in smooth muscle.

Second messenger systems

G proteins form a vast family of related proteins, each comprising several subunits. The binding of ligands to some cell surface receptors alters the subunit interactions within specific G-protein complexes, the precise nature of the response being determined by the type of G proteins related to the receptor. The G proteins in turn activate or inhibit enzymes such as phospholipase C (PLC), adenylate cyclase, or guanylate cyclase, changing the levels of soluble second messengers. Adenylate and guanylate cyclase synthesize cyclic adenosine monophosphate (cAMP) and cyclic guanine monophosphate (cGMP), respectively. PLC cleaves a membrane-bound phospholipid, phosphatidylinositol diphosphate (PIP_2) into diacylglycerol (DAG) and inositol triphosphate (IP_3). As a consequence, the phosphorylation state of diverse proteins throughout the cell is altered, affecting multiple aspects of cellular function.

The subtypes of muscarinic receptors have differing second messenger effects. M_1, M_3, and M_5 receptors link to the $G_{q/11}$ family of G proteins, which activate PLC. M_2 and M_4 receptors couple with the $G_{i/o}$ family and influence cAMP levels, along with K^+ and Ca^{2+} channel activity. The adrenoceptors also have various second messenger effects: α_1 adrenoceptors couple with $G_{q/11}$, whereas β adrenoceptors are linked to a G_s which activates adenylate cyclase.[3] The Ca^{2+} ion can be considered a second messenger, as it forms a complex with the cytoplasmic protein calmodulin, resulting in accelerated breakdown of cAMP and activation of the contractile apparatus.

Cellular physiology of the detrusor

Functionally, muscle cells alternate between states of active shortening and quiescence, determined by various stimuli, which serve to impose control over shortening and to maintain cell functionality.

Passive membrane properties and cell coupling

The degree to which the smooth muscle membrane will allow ions to pass between the intracellular and extracellular compartments varies, as the channels through which the ions pass change permeability according to various factors. At rest, the tendency of the ion to move down its concentration gradient is balanced by an electrical membrane potential (equilibrium potential). The overall membrane potential approximates to the membrane potential of the most permeant ion; at rest this is K^+, due to BK channels.[45] Resting membrane potential in detrusor is -40 to -45 mV in the guinea pig and -60 mV in the human.[46–48]

Electrical activity spreads between cells through specialized intercellular connections, characterized by the presence of proteins of the connexin family. Only a very small number of gap junctions are required to achieve effective coupling and a small increase in gap junction density could significantly influence tissue properties. The passive electrical behavior of nerve and smooth muscle cell membranes is quantified using two constants derived from analysis of the spread of injections of sub-excitation threshold current through microelectrodes. The space constant (λ) is an index of the decay of the injected current with distance, whereas the time constant (τ) describes the decay of current spread with time. Large values of λ indicate good intercellular coupling, exemplified by pregnant myometrium or cardiac muscle, whereas large values of τ indicate resistance to membrane charging. Measurement of current spread in guinea pig detrusor suggests that cells are coupled to their close neighbors, but that the tissue as a whole is poorly coupled[48,49] and electrical coupling between cells more than 40 μm apart axially only occurs rarely.[48] The detrusor also shows higher tissue impedance than other smooth muscles.[49,50] Furthermore, although double sucrose-gap recordings can be made in some small mammal detrusor strips, the electrical activity is not often resolved into clear spikes, and in the normal pig detrusor the technique does not work, probably because of insufficient electrical coupling.[51,52] This may explain the technical difficulties encountered during attempts to record electromyogram activity in the bladder.[53]

Poor coupling is consistent with the observation that gap junctions are infrequent in detrusor smooth muscle,[54–56] though recent evidence has emerged to indicate some communication across gap junctions between detrusor muscle cells in the guinea pig.[57] From a functional point of view, these features match well with the requirements that adjustments in the length of the smooth muscles can take place without the activity spreading to produce synchronous activation of the whole bladder wall.

Active membrane properties

Some smooth muscles show the facility to develop 'action potentials,' which are a transient change in the membrane potential as a result of temporary alterations in ionic fluxes across the cell membrane (Figure 3.1). Action potentials in detrusor muscle can be precipitated by various neuromuscular transmitters and by stretch. The phases of the action potential are the result of coordinated action of distinct membrane conductances and have been assessed using patch clamp studies on isolated myocytes from the guinea pig,[23,30,36] rat,[58] and human.[59–61] The upstroke results from Ca^{2+} entry through voltage-dependent Ca^{2+} channels, whereas the repolarization phase is attributed to voltage-dependent K^+ channels and Ca^{2+}-dependent K^+ channels.[23,45] Subsequently, the cell shows a prolonged after-hyperpolarization during which the membrane potential is more negative than the resting potential,[45,62] perhaps mediated by small conductance K_{Ca} (SK) channels.[34,62] BK and SK channels show a differential response to the Ca^{2+} source as a consequence of spatial relationships within the cell.[29]

Cell shortening
Contractile proteins

In both striated and smooth muscle, the contractile apparatus is made up of structural proteins arranged as

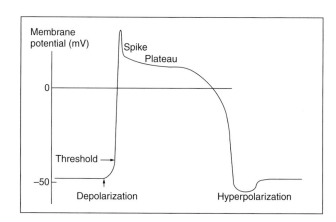

Figure 3.1
The phases of the action potential in the detrusor muscle cell. From the resting membrane potential, an extrinsic stimulus causes a slight depolarization. If this is sufficient to reach a threshold level, a transient reversal of the cell membrane potential occurs as a result of a rapid increase in the membrane permeability to calcium. This is followed by a plateau phase, before the cell repolarizes due to restoration of potassium as the most permeant ion. For a brief period, the membrane potential may become even more negative, 'after-hyperpolarization', rendering the cell less excitable, as a greater extrinsic stimulus will be required to bring the cell to its threshold potential.

thick (myosin) and thin (actin) filaments. The sliding filament theory of contraction, developed in skeletal muscle, suggests that muscle shortening occurs because overlapping fibers of fixed length (the thick and thin filaments) slide past each other in an energy-consuming process. Figure 3.2 illustrates the phases involved to achieve this. The configuration of the cytoskeleton is such that actin from all parts of the cell is drawn inwards towards the center, resulting in overall cell shortening. The process is powered by hydrolysis of ATP and regulated by the concentration of free calcium in the cytoplasm.

Myosin is the major component of the thick filaments in all tissues, smooth muscle myosin consisting of a heavy chain pair (MHC) and a light chain pair (MLC) (Figure 3.3). It has a globular head formed by folding of the N′-terminus of the MHC pair, whereas the C′-terminal parts intertwine to form an α-helix, which constitutes the thick filament. Smooth muscle myosin *in vivo* occurs in various isoforms, which influence assembly and function of the contractile apparatus, the types of MHC present in the muscle determining its biomechanical behavior. Two isoforms, SM1 and 2, differing in the C′-terminal portions, are generated by alternative splicing of the mRNA encoded by a single smooth muscle MHC gene.[63] Further isoforms are generated by alternative splicing at the 5′-end of the MHC mRNA, determining an insert that encodes seven amino acids in the N′-region, near the ATP-binding site. Non-inserted MHC (SM-A) predominates in tonically active

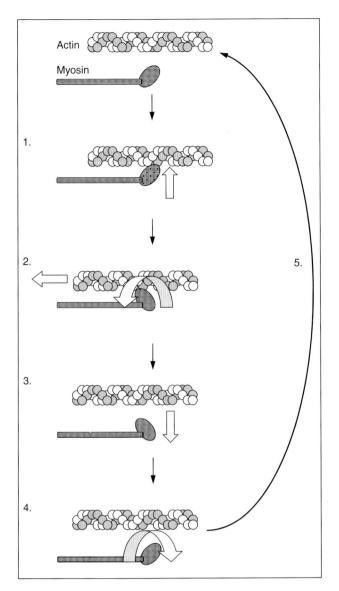

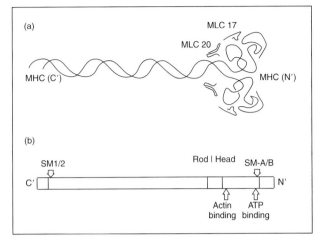

Figure 3.3
Smooth muscle myosin. (a) Smooth muscle myosin, showing the relationship between the two myosin heavy chain molecules (MHC) and the myosin light chains (MLC20 and MLC17). (b) The MHC, showing regions of actin and ATP binding and sites of isoform variation for SM1/2 and SM-A/B.

Figure 3.2
The phases in the sliding filament hypothesis of muscle contraction: (1) attachment of the myosin heads to actin filaments; (2) angulation of the attachment within the myosin molecule; (3) release of the binding; (4) straightening of the myosin angulation; and (5) repetition.

muscle, whereas the majority of MHC is inserted (SM-B) in phasic tissues, such as the bladder and visceral muscle in general.[64] SM-B has higher actin-induced ATPase activity and can move actin faster in an *in-vitro* motility assay.[65] MLCs are sited at the head–rod junction of the MHCs. They occur as a pair of 20 kDa chains (MLC20), and a 17 kDa pair (MLC17). The MLC20 is also known as the regulatory light chain because it regulates smooth muscle contraction according to its degree of phosphorylation. MLC17 extends close to the MHC ATP-binding site and is termed the essential light chain because its removal leads to loss of ATPase

activity. MLC isoforms are recognized which can influence shortening velocity in some smooth muscle types.[66]

Regulation of the contractile apparatus

The key event determining activation of smooth muscle cell contractile proteins is a sufficient rise in cytosolic Ca^{2+} concentration. Increased Ca^{2+} leads to the formation of a complex with the cytoplasmic protein calmodulin, resulting in activation of myosin light chain kinase (MLCK). Following phosphorylation of a specific site on the regulatory light chain by MLCK, using ATP as the phosphate donor, crossbridges form between myosin and actin. Angulation in the myosin molecule results in relative movement between the two types of fiber, which is the basis of cellular shortening. Once phosphorylated, repetitive cycles of attachment and angulation continue until MLC20 is dephosphorylated by myosin light chain phosphatase, which is usually bound tightly to myosin. This entire process can be modulated by intracellular factors. For example, MLCK is subject to phosphorylation by various kinases,[67] which influence its affinity for Ca^{2+}–calmodulin. One enzyme that can achieve this is phosphokinase A, which is activated by cAMP.[68]

Two sources of Ca^{2+} can generate the elevation in cytoplasmic levels that determine contraction:

1. Release of Ca^{2+} stored intracellularly in the sarcoplasmic reticulum (SR) through pharmacomechanical coupling, mediated by IP_3 and ryanodine receptors. Ryanodine

receptors trigger release of Ca^{2+} stores in response to an initial rise in intracellular Ca^{2+}; hence the term 'calcium-induced calcium release' (CICR).[69] CICR has been studied in cultured human detrusor cells[70] and guinea pig detrusor.[71] IP_3 receptors are also regulated by intracellular Ca^{2+}, with a marked increase in channel opening as the levels start to rise, followed by a reduction in activity at higher levels.[35] Muscarinic receptor activation appears primarily to work through generation of IP_3, but it can also cause a small degree of direct extracellular Ca^{2+} entry by activating nonselective cation channels and increasing the action potential frequency.

2. Influx of extracellular Ca^{2+} across the surface membrane, associated with altered cell membrane potential, through electromechanical coupling. The depolarization phase of the action potentials is associated with rapid entry of Ca^{2+} into the intracellular compartment, which is further enhanced as a consequence of CICR from intracellular stores.

The central role of Ca^{2+} in smooth muscle contraction is summarized in Figure 3.4.

At this stage, the relative importance of electromechanical and pharmacomechanical coupling, and of intracellular or

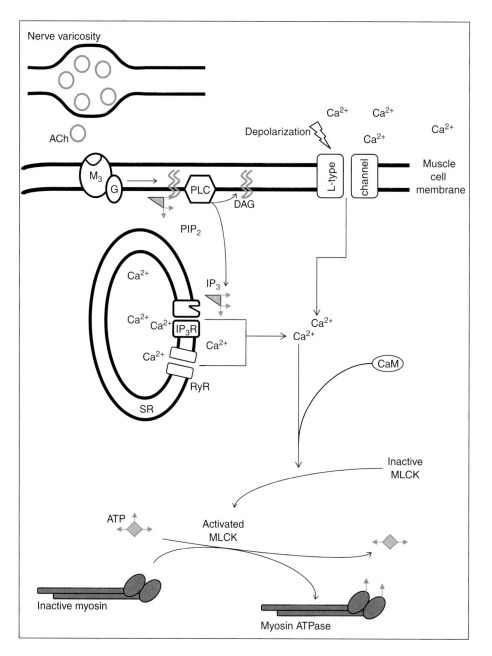

Figure 3.4
The role of calcium in detrusor muscle contraction. Cytosolic calcium increases rapidly as a result of release of intracellular stores, mainly in the sarcoplasmic reticulum, in response to second messenger signaling through the inositol triphosphate pathway and calcium-induced calcium release through ryanodine receptors. Extracellular calcium can also enter the cytoplasm through L-type calcium channels in the cell membrane in response to depolarization. The resulting generation of a calcium–calmodulin complex activates myosin light chain kinase, leading to binding of actin by myosin and cell shortening. ACh, acetylcholine; G, G protein; PLC, phospholipase C; PIP_2, phosphatidylinositol diphosphate; IP_3(R), inositol triphosphate (receptor); DAG, diacylglycerol; SR, sarcoplasmic reticulum; RyR, ryanodine receptor; CaM, calmodulin; MLCK, myosin light chain kinase.

extracellular Ca^{2+} sources in detrusor contraction, remain unclear[72] and may vary with the magnitude of stimulation.[73] The situation is highly complicated, as several further factors influence the ability of smooth muscle to generate phasic or tonic contraction. Shortening velocity is higher when intracellular Ca^{2+} and phosphorylation are high, whereas fairly low Ca^{2+} and phosphorylation support high levels of force generation. Myosin light chain dephosphorylation does not necessarily lead to relaxation: myosin may remain attached to actin for a period of time in what is known as a latch state, by mechanisms which are not fully understood. This allows maintenance of tension with minimal consumption of ATP. Some smooth muscles can maintain tone at low levels of LC_{20} phosphorylation, implying a different mechanism of regulation of contraction, directed at actin rather than myosin. Caldesmon inhibits actomyosin ATPase activity. When phosphorylated, caldesmon releases actin, allowing it to interact with myosin. Protein kinase C (PKC), activated by DAG, is also believed to play an important role in the regulation of sustained smooth muscle contraction in general, though its role in detrusor is not known.[74] Related to the PKC activation pathway may be other proteins, such as mitogen-activated protein kinase, caldesmon, small GTP-binding proteins, calponin, and others.[67]

Detrusor relaxation

The Ca^{2+} stores in the bladder are relatively labile: they can be readily depleted in Ca^{2+}-free solution, and rapidly filled from the extracellular source.[75] Studies of detrusor cell calcium handling have shown that in the guinea pig, the SR can buffer Ca^{2+} influx.[76] Relaxation occurs when Ca^{2+} is taken back into the intracellular stores through the sarcoplasmic/endoplasmic reticulum Ca^{2+} ATPase (SERCA) pump. Some Ca^{2+} is also lost across the cell membrane and has to be replenished between contractions to ensure a steady state for calcium balance. Mechanisms by which stores are replenished are uncertain, but could include action of a cellular membrane Ca^{2+}–Na^+ antiport, or a Ca^{2+}-ATPase.[74] A proportion of the calcium channels in the detrusor cell membrane are T-type,[39] which are active at a more negative membrane potential than L-type channels. Thus, at resting membrane potential, they may permit Ca^{2+} entry at a rate which will allow replenishment of stores, but not fast enough to precipitate contraction.

CICR does not only lead to contraction but may also promote activation of membrane-bound Ca^{2+}-activated channels. For example, CICR from ryanodine receptors appears to have a strong functional influence on BK channels in the surface membrane.[77] This may have a protective effect, as excessive accumulation of calcium activates Ca^{2+}-dependent enzymes such as proteases and lipases and can trigger apoptosis. Detailed discussion of the regulation of Ca^{2+} is given by Horowitz and colleagues.[67]

Metabolism

Relatively little is known about metabolic processes in normal detrusor muscle. The response of the bladder to various stimuli is biphasic,[78,79] comprising a rapid phasic rise in tension, followed by a prolonged period of force generation, the latter ensuring contraction is maintained until completion of voiding. The sustained phase is sensitive to depletion of glucose,[80] since glycogen stores in the detrusor are relatively small.[81] It is also acutely affected by removal of oxygen from the bathing medium, even though intracellular levels of ATP may be high.[82] This suggests that sustained tension is supported by high-energy phosphates derived directly from oxidative phosphorylation, rather than cytosolic ATP. However, the basal metabolic rate is high[80] and oxygen-consuming energy production accounts for only 60% of heat generated during contraction, so that bladder muscle produces lactate under aerobic conditions (aerobic glycolysis).[83]

Tissue physiology of the bladder

Spontaneous activity

Spontaneous contractions occur in isolated detrusor strips, although the proportion of strips showing activity and the frequency of the contractions shows marked species variation.[84–86] Individual contractions in isolated detrusor strips generally occur on a baseline of nearly zero tension, rising briefly to a variable amplitude and then falling back to baseline (Figure 3.5). This contrasts with intestinal smooth muscle, where contractions often fuse into a sustained high-tension tetanus. Fused tetanic contractions occur very infrequently in normal detrusor strips, a further indicator that electrical coupling is relatively poor.

Spontaneous activity appears to have a myogenic basis, as it is not abolished by various receptor antagonists or nerve blockade. In most species, L-type Ca^{2+} channel blockers reduce spontaneous mechanical activity, whereas K^+ channel blocking drugs have the opposite effect. Some smooth muscles show spontaneous changes in membrane potential, in the form of action potentials or oscillations ('slow waves'). Quantal release of neurotransmitter from nearby nerve fibers also leads to fluctuations in the membrane potential, manifesting as excitatory junction potentials (EJPs) or inhibitory junction potentials (IJPs). EJPs are depolarizations below the threshold, but if enough transmitter reaches a muscle cell in a limited time period, summation of the EJPs may depolarize sufficiently to initiate an action potential, resulting in contraction of the cell. The extent to which the action potential will be propagated through the tissue depends on the degree of intercellular coupling. In poorly coupled tissues, the rate of EJPs greatly exceeds the level of

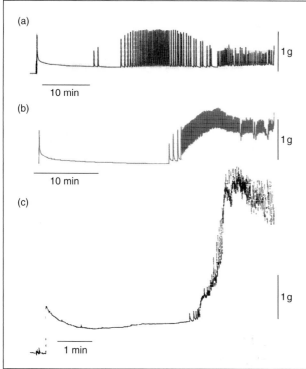

Figure 3.5
Spontaneous contractile activity. Patterns of contractile activity shown by isolated human detrusor muscle strips. (a) Phasic: repetitive contractions of about 30 s duration, each returning to baseline. (b) Tonic: a sustained rise in tension, often with superimposed phasic activity. (c) Fused tetanic contraction: rarely exhibited by muscle strips from normal bladders.

spontaneous mechanical activity. Spontaneous action potentials can be recorded in individual detrusor myocytes.[61] Microelectrode recording from intact smooth muscle strips has been successful predominantly with tissue from small mammals,[48,51,62,86–88] a few studies combining electrical and mechanical recording. In these animals, spontaneous action potentials occur continuously.

Excitatory innervation

The bladder is densely innervated, the ratio of axons to muscle cells in several species approximating to 1:1.[89,90] In the human, detrusor cells are separated from the nearest nerve fiber by a maximum of 200 nm.[56] This arrangement means that there is the potential for near-synchronous activation of the entire detrusor, either by direct nerve stimulation of each cell or by widespread nerve stimulation and limited intercellular propagation.

Acetylcholine is the main neuromuscular transmitter in the parasympathetic nervous system. It is stored in vesicles in the nerve fibers of the detrusor; it is released as a consequence of action potentials and diffuses in the vicinity of the muscle cells. Acetylcholine is active until the molecule undergoes enzymatic degradation by acetylcholinesterase. The choline component diffuses back to the nerve fibers where it is taken up by specific transport mechanisms for recycling. It was formerly thought that neurotransmitter is released from varicosities to diffuse nonspecifically to adjacent muscle cells, but it is now recognized that there are specialized structural relations between nerve fibers and detrusor cells,[91] akin to neuroeffector junctions elsewhere. This observation has experimental significance, as it means the receptors activated pharmacologically during evoked-response experiments in isolated muscle strips are not necessarily those involved physiologically in neuromuscular transmission.[92]

Atropine, a cholinergic antagonist, eliminates virtually all muscular response to nerve stimulation in normal humans,[84,93–96] indicating the predominant role of acetylcholine. Nevertheless, nerves often release cotransmitters simultaneously with the classically recognized transmitters (reviewed in Lundberg[97]). Accordingly, detrusor response to nerve stimulation is partly atropine resistant in most species,[98–101] the atropine-resistant component varying between species and with the stimulus frequency.[102] In fact, variation of the experimental parameters has revealed a 30% atropine-resistant component in humans at low frequencies.[103] ATP has emerged as the most likely non-adrenergic, non-cholinergic (NANC) transmitter mediating atropine-resistant excitation.[104] The release of ATP by intrinsic innervation of the rat bladder has been reported.[105] It causes muscle contraction until enzymatic degradation by an ectoATPase.[106] There is currently little evidence of separate cholinergic and purinergic innervation; the two neurotransmitters are probably co-released.[107] Human detrusor smooth muscle shows a concentration-dependent contraction in response to ATP in the perfusing solution *in vitro*, but the physiological role of ATP in humans has yet to be established.

A wide range of other possible transmitters is present in nerve fibers in the detrusor.[93,108] Adrenergic fibers are few and far between in the body of the bladder, but they are more numerous nearer the bladder outlet.[108,109] Neuropeptide Y-immunoreactive fibers lacking norepinephrine (nonadrenaline) are present in human detrusor[93] and persist after chemical sympathectomy in the rat.[110] Galanin is present in the terminal innervation of the rat and human urinary tract.[111] Vasoactive intestinal polypeptide (VIP) often acts as a cotransmitter with ACh in parasympathetic nerves and is present in the human detrusor innervation.[93] Nitric oxide synthase-like immunoreactivity is also present in detrusor innervation.[112]

The role of these substances *in vivo* is currently uncertain, but it is possible they have a modulatory role. Neuropeptide Y (NPY) has an inhibitory effect on the cholinergic component of electrically induced contractions in the bladder.[113] Prejunctional P_1 receptors are present in the rat bladder,[114] suggesting that the ATP metabolite adenosine may be a neuromodulator. In the human, adenosine reduces responses to electrical stimulation.[115] Several other substances can modulate transmitter release by binding presynaptically, including serotonin,[116,117] the enkephalins,[118] galanin,[119] and histamine.[120] Prejunctional muscarinic receptors influence acetylcholine release: M_1 is facilitatory,[121] whereas M_2[122] and M_4[123] are inhibitory. Modulation might also be mediated by prostanoid substances, either on muscle directly or through effects on innervation,[124] following their release in response to various stimuli such as stretch,[125] nerve stimulation,[126] inflammation,[127] and urothelial injury.[128]

The mechanism by which the efferent innervation achieves muscle contraction is debatable. In small mammals acetylcholine causes little depolarization of the membrane,[51,88,129] although it may cause a delayed increase in action potential frequency. Muscarinic receptor stimulation has been shown to raise intracellular IP_3 levels, implicating release of intracellular stored Ca^{2+} in the initiation of contraction.[130,131] In cultured human detrusor smooth muscle cells, muscarinic receptor activation has been shown to raise intracellular Ca^{2+}, probably via M_3 receptors.[132] After M_3 receptor stimulation, desensitization of the resulting IP_3 response occurs,[133] potentially representing a cellular mechanism for regulation of detrusor contraction. Stimulation of the intrinsic nerves results in depolarizing junction potentials in small mammals[48,51,88,134,135] and in the pig.[51] In the guinea pig, these excitatory junction potentials are caused by release of ATP from the motor nerve supply. Under normal circumstances these junction potentials trigger action potentials, but in the presence of L-type Ca^{2+} channel blockers, the junction potentials can be recorded in isolation. They are unaffected by muscarinic receptor blockade, but abolished by desensitization[51] or blockade[135] of purinergic receptors. Activation of P_{2x} purinoceptors triggers entry of extracellular calcium through voltage-operated Ca^{2+} channels and nonselective cation channels in the cell membrane, leading to depolarization and increased action potential frequency.[51,136]

Myofibroblasts

Myofibroblasts are fibroblastic cells with certain characteristics of smooth muscle,[137] of which the interstitial cell of Cajal (ICC) from the gastrointestinal tract is an example. The myofibroblast group has a role in pacemaker activity and transmission of excitation in the gut[138] and possibly the upper urinary tract.[139] Consequently, the presence of myofibroblasts in the bladder may prove significant physiologically and in the etiology of pathophysiological conditions. Unfortunately, identification of myofibroblasts is hampered by the lack of specific microscopic criteria diagnostic of the group. Accordingly, a panel of features has to be assessed, based on morphology, immunophenotype, and ultrastructural characteristics.[140]

One study has confirmed a myofibroblast population located suburothelially in the human bladder (Figure 3.6), though not in the detrusor.[54] Cells morphologically resembling ICCs have been described in human detrusor[19,141,142] and guinea pig detrusor,[143] but since these studies did not assess ultrastructure, the presence of myofibroblasts in the human detrusor remains unconfirmed. Nevertheless, a widespread network of unidentified cellular processes ramifying throughout the detrusor has been observed in several studies, which may have implications for current understanding of dissemination of excitation through the bladder wall. The potential functional significance of the myofibroblast is underlined by the observation of spontaneous calcium waves in ICC-like cells in the guinea pig detrusor, suggesting that they may act as pacemakers[143] or as intermediaries in neuromuscular transmission.[139]

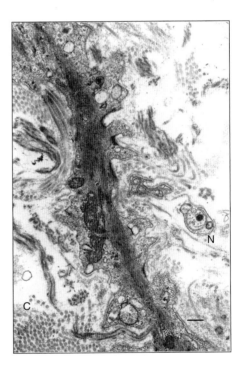

Figure 3.6
A bladder myofibroblast. Electron micrograph of a myofibroblast from the lamina propria of a human bladder, showing several characteristic ultrastructural features, including an incomplete basal lamina, membrane caveolae, and cytoplasmic stress fibers. An unmyelinated nerve fiber with a Schwann cell sheath (N) and several collagen fibers (C) are seen nearby. Scale bar=500 nm. (Picture courtesy of Professor DN Landon, Institute of Neurology, London.)

The micturition cycle

The bladder alternates between phases of filling, in which urine is stored at low pressure, and voiding, where the detrusor contracts and the outlet relaxes. The physiological events during the two phases of the cycle are very different.

Bladder filling

The bladder stores urine for expulsion at an appropriate time. During urine storage, the predominant muscular mechanisms involve adaptation to accommodate rising intravesical volumes, ranging from 0 to 500 ml or more. The range of intravesical volumes necessitates substantial adjustments within the detrusor and urothelium, such that individual smooth muscle cells elongate many times their resting length without increased tension.[144] Several investigators have proposed that the ability of the bladder to stretch with minimal increase in intravesical pressure might be achieved through action of a relaxant factor. Nerve-induced detrusor relaxation involving nitric oxide (NO) has been reported,[145] but other investigators have been unable to find detrusor relaxation in response to nerve stimulation.[146] Detrusor cells express some receptors which can mediate relaxation, including β_3 adrenoceptors[147] and P_{2y} purinoceptors.[148,149] Studies in the rat have suggested the presence of an unidentified relaxant factor released by muscarinic receptor activation[150] and stretch of cultured rat detrusor cells stimulates the release of parathyroid hormone-related protein, which opposes carbachol-induced detrusor contraction.[151] The significance of these observations in normal bladder function has yet to be established.

Because the bladder is able to expel urine regardless of the volume contained, ergonomic considerations require that the ratio of the surface area to the volume is kept to its minimum, optimizing the bladder configuration for voiding if required. The ability to maintain tone without generalized contraction despite considerable stretch may arise in part from spontaneous action potentials unrelated to the innervation,[152] resulting in localized contractile activity. This will tend to maintain tone in the organ as a whole and allow adjustment to the increase in volume, without synchronous mass contraction of the entire bladder.

During bladder filling, several species show transient rises in intravesical pressure unrelated to micturition[153] particularly when the bladder is filled at physiological rates.[154,155] The mechanisms responsible for these non-micturition contractions (NMCs) are not understood but phasic fluctuations in intravesical pressure have been reported in several preparations where pathways of the micturition reflex have been interrupted.[155–158] Intramural contractile activity with minimal pressure rise has also been reported during bladder filling, taking the form of localized shortenings, termed 'micromotions',[159] or propagating waves.[158] These observations indicate that peripheral mechanisms can generate bladder activity independent of the central nervous system (CNS) and that NMCs are based on different mechanisms from micturition. Some understanding of these phenomena may be gained by comparison with the upper urinary tract, where autonomous areas of localized contractility ('pacemakers') synchronize and initiate peristalsis in response to distention.[160] A corresponding arrangement into peripheral autonomous modules has been proposed in the bladder.[161] In this model, modules are proposed as functional contractile units within the detrusor, analogous to the motor unit arrangement of skeletal muscle (Figure 3.7). Each module would be capable of contracting in isolation, perhaps consequent upon pacemaker activity, resulting in a localized contraction. The coordination of activity in neighboring modules would lead to organized contraction of a greater proportion of the bladder wall. Coordination of separate modules might occur through a 'myovesical plexus', comprising a functional interaction between the myofibroblast network and the peripheral innervation, equivalent to the myenteric plexuses of the gut. Alternatively, synchronization of separate areas in guinea pig bladder by myogenic transmission has been reported.[162]

The peripheral autonomous module hypothesis may provide some insight into the basis of NMC and micromotion activity. Preliminary data in support of a modular arrangement of the detrusor are provided by the potential for isolated whole bladders from small mammals to manifest both localized contractions and propagating contraction waves (Figure 3.8).[163]

Voiding

Voiding is initiated by the CNS, which activates the parasympathetic efferents, resulting in widespread synchronous detrusor contraction and consequent increase in intravesical pressure. Simultaneously, a complex series of reflexes ensures appropriate configuration of the bladder outlet and relaxation of the continence mechanisms, resulting in urine flow. In order to ensure complete emptying, force of contraction has to be sustained throughout the voiding phase. A particular feature of the detrusor is the ability to sustain near-maximal force generation in the face of significant length changes.[144] This is influenced both by ergonomic considerations, as alluded to above, and also the maintenance of the stimulus to contract until complete emptying has been achieved. Implicitly, sustained efferent activity will achieve the latter, but conceivably peripheral mechanisms underlying NMC activity could make an important contribution.

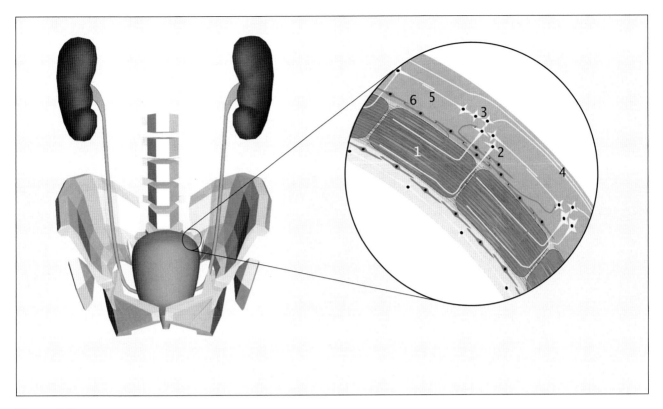

Figure 3.7
The peripheral autonomous module hypothesis of the detrusor. The bladder wall, showing muscle blocks (1) defined by
the region of distribution of axons of dominant motor neurons within intramural ganglia (2). These cells are influenced
by a circuit made up of other neurons in the ganglion (3), which integrate information from diverse inputs, such as collaterals
from suburothelial afferents (4) and axons from neighboring modules (5). Once a dominant motor neuron reaches a
threshold of excitation, it fires action potentials, resulting in autonomous contraction localized to the muscle block supplied.
Communications between modules across a hypothetical 'myovesical plexus', in the form of axons connecting
the integrative circuitry of neighboring modules (5), or myofibroblast processes passing between muscle blocks (6), result in
coordinated activity in a greater proportion of the bladder wall. This physiological proposal has implications in the
comprehension of pathophysiological processes underlying conditions such as detrusor overactivity, since pathologically
enhanced activity within modules or enhanced coordination of neighboring modules could facilitate uninhibited detrusor
contraction outwith volitional control.

Regionalization in the bladder

Functional distinctions can be drawn between various
regions of the bladder musculature. The body of the detrusor
serves to store and expel urine periodically. The bladder
base, particularly the trigone, differs in terms of the
microanatomical arrangement of the muscle, the profile of
receptors expressed,[164] and the predominantly sympathetic
innervation.[165] This region may have a role in sensory
return, and anatomical configuration of the bladder outlet
and vesicoureteric junctions during voiding. The bladder
neck in men provides a sphincter function to ensure
prograde propulsion on ejaculation.

Urothelium and suburothelial region

The urothelium maintains a barrier function, but it also
appears to exhibit sensory and signaling properties that
allow response to the chemical and physical surroundings
and reciprocal communication with subjacent structures.
The urothelium secretes factors that can influence muscle
contractility.[166] Substances released by the urothelium significantly increase the contractile response to carbachol[167]
and electrical field stimulation,[168] whereas a diffusible
inhibitory substance can reduce detrusor contractility.[167]
Urothelium in the trigone releases a relaxant factor in
response to stimulation with carbachol and histamine.[169]

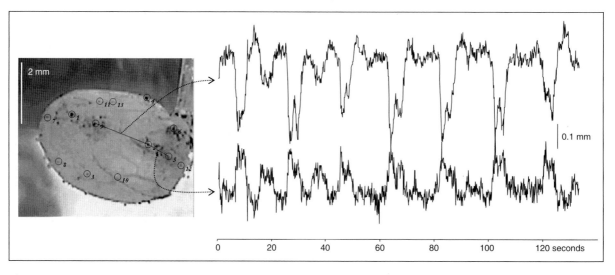

Figure 3.8

Activity in an autonomous module. Localized activity arising spontaneously in an isolated mouse bladder. Separation of multiple markers on the bladder surface was assessed, indicated on the photograph in the left panel. On the right are plotted marker separations in two regions. In one, spontaneous localized shortenings were observed, with concurrent elongations in the neighboring region, indicating autonomous behavior in discrete areas, i.e. functional modularity. Markers outside these regions maintained a constant separation.

The mechanisms involved have yet to be clarified, but the urothelium does release ATP[170] and other substances[171] in response to stretch, proportionate to the degree of intravesical distention.[172] The stretch response could result from the presence of mechanosensitive sodium channels,[173] the density of which varies according to changes in the local conditions.[174] Urothelial cells express a range of receptors and release substances that can regulate the activity of underlying nerves.[175] The suburothelial region is densely innervated and a wide range of putative neurotransmitters is present,[93] which may be released locally ('sensory efferents').[176] In addition, there is an extensive network of myofibroblastic interstitial cells.[54] Clearly, there is much to learn before a full understanding of the complexities can be realized.

The physiology of the urethra

Bladder outlet function is derived from a complex integration of skeletal muscle in the pelvic floor and urethral wall, urethral smooth muscle, lamina propria, and urothelium. There are marked regional variations, even in just the smooth muscle component.[177] The female pig urethra is arranged in three smooth muscle layers – an inner longitudinal, a mid circular, and an outer longitudinal layer – whereas the female human urethra has a smooth muscle bilayer consisting of an inner longitudinal and an outer circular layer.[178] The longitudinal muscle is anatomically continuous with the detrusor,

implying a possible role in bladder neck opening and urethral shortening at the onset of voiding.[178] The circular layer is not continuous with the detrusor and is arranged in a disposition typical of a muscular sphincter, so it may be important for maintaining urethral closure. These anatomical distinctions may contribute to the functional attributes of the urethra in preventing leakage during storage, yet allowing urine flow during voiding. At this stage, however, understanding of the underlying processes is patchy.

Molecular cell biology of the urethra

Receptors

Adrenergic receptors are important in maintenance of urethral closure, the α_{1A} subtype predominating,[179] but with the possible existence of an atypical α_{1L} subtype.[180]

Muscarinic receptors show regional and interspecies variation. Cholinergic contraction of the normal pig urethra appears to be mediated via M_2 and, to a lesser extent, M_3 receptors in circular muscle but only by M_3 receptors in longitudinal muscle.[181] M_1, M_2, and M_3 receptors may be involved in carbachol-induced contraction of the circular muscle of the rabbit urethra.[182,183] The circular muscles have been reported to show a minimum or no response to muscarinic stimulation *in vitro*.[184]

Ion channels

Potassium channels

Urethral smooth muscle seems to be unique in responding to depolarization with high K^+ solutions by relaxation, rather than the contractile response seen with other smooth muscles.[185] Exposure to the potassium channel opener levcromakalim causes relaxation of strips of proximal urethral smooth muscle from the female pig, associated with hyperpolarization and an outward K^+ current, both of which are blocked by glibenclamide.[186] The channel responsible is inhibited by intracellular ATP, reactivated by nucleoside diphosphates, and may be regulated by intracellular magnesium levels.[187] The channel was felt to differ from the ATP-sensitive channel in the guinea pig bladder, because of different conductance and reactivation properties. Another potassium channel opener, nicorandil, appears to induce relaxation in proximal pig urethra through two independent mechanisms.[188] Further components of the outward K^+ current are a Ca^{2+}- and voltage-sensitive BK current and a voltage-activated, Ca^{2+}-insensitive DK current.[28] The resting membrane potential in proximal urethral smooth muscle cells varies according to species and gender between -50.8 mV and -39 mV,[186,189–192] with spontaneous hyperpolarizations and depolarizations apparent in a minority of cells.[189]

Other channels

In urethral smooth muscle of the sheep, guinea pig, and rabbit, L-type Ca^{2+} channels and Ca^{2+}-dependent Cl^- currents have been identified.[190–192] The former seem to be responsible for the upstroke of the action potential.

Cell and tissue physiology of the urethra

Innervation

The bladder outlet receives neuronal inputs from several sources, both somatic and autonomic, mediating voluntary and involuntary mechanisms.[193] Nerve-mediated contractions and relaxations occur in urethral smooth muscle, depending on the stimulation parameters[194,195] and the urethra appears to have both excitatory and inhibitory innervation, differing from the detrusor where direct innervation appears to be solely excitatory.[189] The predominant excitatory innervation is noradrenergic.[72] In addition, a parasympathetic cholinergic excitatory input to the urethra has been identified in male rats, but not in females,[196,197] and there may also be a purinergic component.[193] Nitrergic innervation from nerves with cell bodies in the major pelvic

ganglia is also present[198] and is primarily inhibitory. The constitutive carbon monoxide-producing enzyme heme oxygenase-2 coexists with neuronal nitric oxide synthase in nerve trunks of the human urethra.[199]

Generation of tonic contraction

Smooth muscle tension is one of the factors contributing to the maintenance of intraurethral pressure at a level exceeding the intravesical pressure, thereby ensuring continence. *In-vivo* studies of the effects of cholinergic and adrenergic agonists and antagonists on urethral pressure in humans have had variable results, but suggest that there is a tonic activity in the sympathetic innervation, with minimal contribution from cholinergic stimulation.[200] Overall, sympathetic nervous activity is crucial to maintenance of urethral closure.

Urethral smooth muscle generates spontaneous tone,[194,201] which is greater in strips from the proximal urethra than the distal urethra *in vitro*.[177] This may be dependent on electrical membrane events,[189,190,192,202] the force of contraction depending on the amplitude and duration of the plateau of electrical 'slow waves'.[202] L-type Ca^{2+} current and Ca^{2+}-activated Cl^- current both seem to contribute to the generation of slow waves,[191] whereas BK and DK currents appear to oppose depolarization during the plateau phase of the slow wave and may therefore modulate Ca^{2+} entry.[28] Neither atropine nor guanethidine affect tonic contraction, suggesting, respectively, that it does not depend on cholinergic or adrenergic innervation.[194]

Rabbit urethra appears to contain specialized pacemaking cells that may be responsible for initiating slow waves in smooth muscle cells.[203] Partial tissue dissection with collagenase reveals a small population of branched cells, which may be myofibroblasts. These cells exhibit regular spontaneous depolarizations, which increase in frequency when exposed to norepinephrine (nonadrenaline) and are blocked by perfusion with calcium-free solution. They show Ca^{2+}-activated Cl^- current and spontaneous transient inward currents, which can be blocked by Cl^- channel blockers. Accordingly, generation of tone may result from pacemaker activity of a small group of cells in the urethra, rather than intrinsic properties of the smooth muscle cells themselves.

Urethral relaxation

The urethral pressure drops during micturition, prior to increase in intravesical pressure.[204,205] When cholinergic and adrenergic responses are blocked, intrinsic nerve stimulation relaxes the tone of urethral muscle strips. Nerve-mediated relaxation is at least partly nitrergic,[194,206,207] acting by activating soluble guanylate cyclase.[208] The urothelium in the proximal urethra may enhance nerve-mediated smooth muscle relaxation by releasing nitric oxide.[209] Carbon monoxide may also act as an inhibitory transmitter, although with significantly lower potency than nitric oxide.[210,211] The response to carbon monoxide occurs by a mechanism independent of K^+ channels[212] and is greatly increased by prior sensitization of soluble guanylate cyclase.[213] In contrast, relaxation of detrusor muscle does not occur with carbon monoxide exposure[212] and heme oxygenase enzymes have not been identified in normal detrusor innervation.[93]

Several other mediators may influence urethral tone. Prostaglandins could increase or decrease both longitudinal and circular smooth muscle layer tension.[214] Prostaglandin synthesis inhibitors increase tension and spontaneous activity in pig urethral smooth muscle, whereas E series prostaglandins and VIP have the opposite effect.[215,216] Serotonin produces substantial relaxation, partly inhibited by specific 5-HT receptor antagonists. However, these do not affect nerve-mediated relaxation, suggesting that 5-HT may have no physiological role in urethral smooth muscle relaxation.[217] In proximal urethra from the female dog, capsaicin produces relaxation in strips precontracted with norepinephrine, probably through an effect on primary afferent nerves.[218]

Presynaptic modulation. Activation of α_2 adrenoceptors and muscarinic receptors can inhibit both the release of norepinephrine from adrenergic nerve terminals[219] and the release of acetylcholine from cholinergic nerve terminals.[220] This was interpreted as negative feedback control, indicating that the components of the urethral dual innervation may cross-regulate. The release of NO from nitrergic nerves in the rabbit urethra is reduced and increased by stimulation of prejunctional α_1 and α_2 adrenergic receptors, respectively,[221] whereas nitric oxide inhibits release of norepinephrine from adrenergic nerves.[222] NPY has an inhibitory effect on the adrenergic component of electrically induced contractions in the urethra.[113]

Conclusion

The physiology of smooth muscles of the detrusor and urethra is complex and must be viewed in the context of the integrative function of the entire lower urinary tract and the functional requirements to achieve storage, voiding, and voluntary control. There are several levels of control and integration, including the brainstem, sacral spinal cord, peripheral ganglia, and intramural mechanisms, with a substantial voluntary input. This makes the study of smooth muscle physiology fascinating, but intellectually demanding. We remain far from a complete understanding of how the substantial number of pieces of the jigsaw gathered so far fit together, though substantial progress has been made.

References

1. Turner WH, Brading AF. Smooth muscle of the bladder in the normal and the diseased state: pathophysiology, diagnosis and treatment. Pharmacol Ther 1997; 75:77–110.

2. Turner WH. Physiology of the smooth muscles of the bladder and urethra. In: Corcos J, Schick E, eds. The urinary sphincter. New York: Marcel Dekker, 2001.

3. Kuriyama H, Kitamura K, Itoh T, Inoue R. Physiological features of visceral smooth muscle cells, with special reference to receptors and ion channels. Physiol Rev 1998; 78:811–920.

4. Levin RM, Ruggieri MR, Wein AJ. Identification of receptor subtypes in the rabbit and human urinary bladder by selective radio-ligand binding. J Urol 1988; 139:844–848.

5. Igawa Y, Yamazaki Y, Takeda H, et al. Relaxant effects of isoproterenol and selective beta3-adrenoceptor agonists on normal, low compliant and hyperreflexic human bladders. J Urol 2001; 165:240–244.

6. Malloy B, Price D, Price R, et al. a1-adrenergic receptor subtypes in human detrusor. J Urol 1998; 160:937–943.

7. Eglen RM, Hegde SS, Watson N. Muscarinic receptor subtypes and smooth muscle function. Pharmacol Rev 1996; 48:531–565.

8. Yamaguchi O, Shisda K, Tamura K, et al. Evaluation of mRNAs encoding muscarinic receptor subtypes in human detrusor muscle. J Urol 1996; 156:1208–1213.

9. Kondo S, Morita T, Tahshima Y. Muscarinic cholinergic receptor subtypes in human detrusor muscle studied by labeled and nonlabeled pirenzipine, AFDX-116 and 4DAMP. Urol Int 1995; 54:150–153.

10. Wang P, Luthin GR, Ruggieri MR. Muscarinic acetylcholine receptor subtypes mediating urinary bladder contractility and coupling to GTP binding proteins. J Pharmacol Exp Ther 1995; 273:959–966.

11. Longhurst PA, Leggett RE, Briscoe JAK. Characterization of the functional muscarinic receptors in the rat urinary bladder. Br J Pharmacol 1995; 116:2279–2285.

12. Hegde SS, Choppin A, Bonhaus D, et al. Functional role of M2 and M3 muscarinic receptors in the urinary bladder of rats in vitro and in vivo. Br J Pharmacol 1997; 120:1409–1418.

13. Moore KH, Ray FR, Barden JA. Loss of purinergic P2X(3) and P2X(5) receptor innervation in human detrusor from adults with urge incontinence. J Neurosci 2001; 21 (RC166): 1–6.

14. Lee HY, Bardini M, Burnstock G. Distribution of P2X receptors in the urinary bladder and the ureter of the rat. J Urol 2000; 163:2002–2007.

15. O'Reilly BA, Kosaka AH, Chang TK, et al. A quantitative analysis of purinoceptor expression in human fetal and adult bladders. J Urol 2001; 165:1730–1734.

16. Elneil S, Skepper JN, Kidd EJ, et al. Distribution of P2X(1) and P2X(3) receptors in the rat and human urinary bladder. Pharmacology 2001; 63:120–128.

17. Yunaev MA, Barden JA, Bennett MR. Changes in the distribution of different subtypes of P2X receptor clusters on smooth muscle cells in relation to nerve varicosities in the pregnant rat urinary bladder. J Neurocytol 2000; 29:99–108.

18. Khanna OP, DeGregorio GJ, Sample RC, McMichael RF. Histamine receptors in urethrovesical smooth muscle. Urology 1977; 10:375–381.

19. Ost D, Roskams T, van der Aa F, De ridder D. Topography of the vanilloid receptor in the human bladder: more than just the nerve fibers. J Urol 2002; 168:293–297.

20. Yiangou Y, Facer P, Ford A, et al. Capsaicin receptor VR1 and ATP-gated ion channel P2X3 in human urinary bladder. BJU Int 2001; 87:774–779.

21. Avelino A, Cruz C, Nagy I, Cruz F. Vanilloid receptor 1 expression in the rat urinary tract. Neuroscience 2002; 109:787–798.

22. Quayle JM, Nelson MT, Standen NB. ATP-sensitive and inwardly rectifying potassium channels in smooth muscle. Physiol Rev 1997; 77:1165–1232.

23. Klockner U, Isenberg G. Action potentials and net membrane currents of isolated smooth muscle cells (urinary bladder of the guinea-pig). Pflugers Arch 1985; 405:329–339.

24. Cotton KD, Hollywood MA, Thornbury KD, McHale NG. Effect of purinergic blockers on outward current in isolated smooth muscle cells of the sheep bladder. Am J Physiol 1996; 270:C969–C973.

25. Hirano M, Imaizumi Y, Muraki K, et al. Effects of ruthenium red on membrane ionic currents in urinary bladder smooth muscle cells of the guinea-pig. Pflugers Arch 1998; 435:645–653.

26. Hollywood MA, Cotton KD, McHale NG, Thornbury KD. Enhancement of Ca^{2+}-dependent outward current in sheep bladder myocytes by Evans blue dye. Pflugers Arch 1998; 435:631–636.

27. Trivedi S, Potter-Lee L, Li JH, et al. Calcium dependent K-channels in guinea pig and human urinary bladder. Biochem Biophys Res Commun 1995; 213:404–409.

28. Hollywood MA, McCloskey KD, McHale NG, Thornbury KD. Characterization of outward K(+) currents in isolated smooth muscle cells from sheep urethra. Am J Physiol Cell Physiol 2000; 279:C420–C428.

29. Herrera GM, Nelson MT. Differential regulation of SK and BK channels by Ca(2+) signals from Ca(2+) channels and ryanodine receptors in guinea-pig urinary bladder myocytes. J Physiol (Lond) 2002; 541:483–492.

30. Bonev AD, Nelson MT. ATP-sensitive potassium channels in smooth muscle cells from guinea pig urinary bladder. Am J Physiol 1993; 264:C1190–C1200.

31. Trivedi S, Stetz S, Levin R, et al. Effect of cromakalim and pinacidil on 86Rb efflux from guinea pig urinary bladder smooth muscle. Pharmacology 1994; 49:159–166.

32. Green ME, Edwards G, Kirkup AJ, et al. Pharmacological characterization of the inwardly-rectifying current in the smooth muscle cells of the rat bladder. Br J Pharmacol 1996; 119:1509–1518.

33. Petkov GV, Heppner TJ, Bonev AD, et al. Low levels of K(ATP) channel activation decrease excitability and contractility of urinary bladder. Am J Physiol Regul Integr Comp Physiol 2001; 280:R1427–R1433.

34. Fujii K, Foster CD, Brading AF, Parekh AB. Potassium channel blockers and the effects of cromakalim on the smooth muscle of the guinea-pig bladder. Br J Pharmacol 1990; 99:779–785.

35. Kotlikoff MI, Herrera G, Nelson MT. Calcium permeant ion channels in smooth muscle. Rev Physiol Biochem Pharmacol 1999; 134:147–199.

36. Nakayama S. Effects of excitatory neurotransmitters on Ca^{2+} channel current in smooth muscle cells isolated from guinea-pig urinary bladder. Br J Pharmacol 1993; 110:317–325.

37. Nakayama S, Brading AF. Evidence for multiple open states of the Ca^{2+} channels in smooth muscle cells isolated from the guinea-pig detrusor. J Physiol (Lond) 1993; 471:87–105.

38. Nakayama S, Brading AF. Long Ca^{2+} channel opening induced by large depolarization and Bay K 8644 in smooth muscle cells isolated from guinea-pig detrusor. Br J Pharmacol 1996; 119:716–720.

39. Sui GP, Wu C, Fry CH. Inward Ca^{2+} currents in cultures and freshly isolated human detrusor smooth muscle cells. J Urol 2001; 165:627–631.

40. Inoue R, Brading AF. Human, pig and guinea-pig bladder smooth muscle cells generate similar inward currents in response to purinoceptor activation. Br J Pharmacol 1991; 103:1840–1841.

41. Wellner MC, Isenberg G. Properties of stretch-activated channels in myocytes from the guinea-pig urinary bladder. J Physiol (Lond) 1993; 466:213–227.

42. Wellner MC, Isenberg G. Stretch effects on whole-cell currents of guinea-pig urinary bladder myocytes. J Physiol (Lond) 1994; 480(Pt 3):439–448.

43. Wellner MC, Isenberg G. cAMP accelerates the decay of stretch-activated inward currents in guinea-pig urinary bladder myocytes. J Physiol (Lond) 1995; 482 (Pt 1):141–156.

44. Hamill OP, McBride DW Jr. The pharmacology of mechanogated membrane ion channels. Pharmacol Rev 1996; 48:231–252.

45. Heppner TJ, Bonev AD, Nelson MT. Ca^{2+}-activated K^+ channels regulate action potential repolarization in urinary bladder smooth muscle. Am J Physiol 1997; 273:C110–C117.

46. Mostwin JL, Karim NS, van Koeveringe G. Electrical properties of obstructed guinea pig bladder. Adv Exp Med Biol 1995; 385:21–28.

47. Fry CH, Wu C, Sui GP. Electrophysiological properties of the bladder. Int Urogynecol J Pelvic Floor Dysfunct 1998; 9:291–298.

48. Bramich NJ, Brading AF. Electrical properties of smooth muscle in the guinea-pig urinary bladder. J Physiol (Lond) 1996; 492:185–198.

49. Fry CH, Cooklin M, Birns J, Mundy AR. Measurement of intercellular electrical coupling in guinea-pig detrusor smooth muscle. J Urol 1999; 161:660–664.

50. Parekh AB, Brading AF, Tomita T. Studies of longitudinal tissue impedance in various smooth muscles. Prog Clin Biol Res 1990; 327:375–378.

51. Fujii K. Evidence for adenosine triphosphate as an excitatory transmitter in guinea-pig, rabbit and pig urinary bladder. J Physiol (Lond) 1988; 404:39–52.

52. Foster CD, Speakman MJ, Fujii K, Brading AF. The effects of cromakalim on the detrusor muscle of human and pig urinary bladder. Br J Urol 1989; 63:284–294.

53. Ballaro A, Mundy AR, Fry CH, Craggs MD. A new approach to recording the electromyographic activity of detrusor smooth muscle. J Urol 2001; 166:1957–1961.

54. Sui GP, Rothery S, Dupont E, et al. Gap junctions and connexin expression in human suburothelial interstitial cells. BJU Int 2002; 90:118–129.

55. Gabella G, Uvelius B. Urinary bladder of rat: fine structure of normal and hypertrophic musculature. Cell Tissue Res 1990; 262:67–79.

56. Daniel EE, Cowan W, Daniel VP. Structural bases for neural and myogenic control of human detrusor muscle. Can J Physiol Pharmacol 1983; 61:1247–1273.

57. Neuhaus J, Wolburg H, Hermsdorf T, et al. Detrusor smooth muscle cells of the guinea-pig are functionally coupled via gap junctions in situ and in cell culture. Cell Tissue Res 2002; 309:301–311.

58. Edwards G, Henshaw M, Miller M, Weston AH. Comparison of the effects of several potassium-channel openers on rat bladder and rat portal vein in vitro. Br J Pharmacol 1991; 102:679–680.

59. Gallegos CR, Fry CH. Alterations to the electrophysiology of isolated human detrusor smooth muscle cells in bladder disease. J Urol 1994; 151:754–758.

60. Wammack R, Jahnel U, Nawrath H, Hohenfellner R. Mechanical and electrophysiological effects of cromakalim on the human urinary bladder. Eur Urol 1994; 26:176–181.

61. Montgomery BS, Fry CH. The action potential and net membrane currents in isolated human detrusor smooth muscle cells. J Urol 1992; 147:176–184.

62. Creed KE, Ishikawa S, Ito Y. Electrical and mechanical activity recorded from rabbit urinary bladder in response to nerve stimulation. J Physiol (Lond) 1983; 338:149–164.

63. Nagai R, Kuro-o M, Babij P, Periasamy M. Identification of two types of smooth muscle myosin heavy chain isoforms by cDNA cloning and immunoblot analysis. J Biol Chem 1989; 264:9734–9737.

64. Chacko S, DiSanto M, Menon C, et al. Contractile protein changes in urinary bladder smooth muscle following outlet obstruction. In: Baskin, Hayward, eds. Advances in bladder research. New York: Kluwer Academic/Plenum, 1999.

65. Kelley CA, Takahashi M, Yu JH, Adelstein RS. An insert of seven amino acids confers functional differences between smooth muscle myosins from the intestines and vasculature. J Biol Chem 1993; 268:12848–12854.

66. Malmqvist U, Arner A. Correlation between isoform composition of the 17 kDa myosin light chain and maximal shortening velocity in smooth muscle. Pflugers Arch; Eur J Physiol 1991; 418:523–530.

67. Horowitz A, Menice CB, Laporte R, Morgan KG. Mechanisms of smooth muscle contraction. Physiol Rev 1996; 76:967–1003.

68. Conti MA, Adelstein RS. The relationship between calmodulin binding and phosphorylation of smooth muscle myosin kinase by the catalytic subunit of 3′:5′ cAMP-dependent protein kinase. J Biol Chem 1981; 256:3178–3181.

69. Somlyo AP, Somlyo AV. Signal transduction and regulation in smooth muscle. Nature 1994; 372:231–236.

70. Chambers P, Neal DE, Gillespie JI. Ryanodine receptors in human bladder smooth muscle. Exp-Physiol 1999; 84:41–46.

71. Ganitkevich VY, Isenberg G. Depolarization-mediated intracellular calcium transients in isolated smooth muscle cells of guinea-pig urinary bladder. J Physiol (Lond) 1991; 435:187–205.

72. Andersson K-E. Pharmacology of lower urinary tract smooth muscle and penile erectile tissue. Pharm Rev 1993; 45:253–308.

73. Masters JG, Neal DE, Gillespie JI. The contribution of intracellular Ca^{2+} release to contraction in human bladder smooth muscle. Br J Pharmacol 1999; 127:996–1002.

74. Fry CH, Skennerton D, Wood D, Wu C. The cellular basis of contraction in human detrusor smooth muscle from patients with stable and unstable bladders. Urology 2002; 59:3–12.

75. Mostwin JL. Receptor operated intracellular calcium stores in the smooth muscle of the guinea pig bladder. J Urol 1985; 133:900–905.

76. Yoshikawa A, van Breemen C, Isenberg G. Buffering of plasmalemmal Ca^{2+} current by sarcoplasmic reticulum of guinea pig urinary bladder myocytes. Am J Physiol 1996; 271:C833–C841.

77. Herrera GM, Heppner TJ, Nelson MT. Voltage dependence of the coupling of $Ca(2+)$ sparks to $BK(Ca)$ channels in urinary bladder smooth muscle. Am J Physiol Cell Physiol 2001; 280:C481–C490.

78. Zhao Y, Wein A, Levin RM. Role of calcium in mediating the biphasic reaction of the rabbit urinary bladder. Gen Pharmacol 1993; 24:727–731.

79. Bilgen A, Wein A, Zhao Y, Levin RM. Effects of anoxia on the biphasic response of isolated strips of rabbit bladder to field stimulation, bethanechol, methoxamine and KCl. Pharmacology 1992; 44:283–289.

80. Uvelius B, Arner A. Changed metabolism of detrusor muscle cells from obstructed rat urinary bladder. Scand J Urol Nephrol Suppl 1997; 184:59–65.

81. Haugaard N, Wein AJ, Levin RM. In vitro studies of glucose metabolism of the rabbit urinary bladder. J Urol 1987; 137:782–784.

82. Zhao Y, Wein AJ, Bilgen A, Levin RM. Effect of anoxia on in vitro bladder function. Pharmacology 1991; 43:337–344.

83. Wendt IR, Gibbs CL. Energy expenditure of longitudinal smooth muscle of rabbit urinary bladder. Am J Physiol 1987; 252:C88–C96.

84. Sibley GN. A comparison of spontaneous and nerve-mediated activity in bladder muscle from man, pig and rabbit. J Physiol (Lond) 1984; 354:431–443.

85. Brading AF, Williams JH. Contractile responses of smooth muscle strips from rat and guinea-pig urinary bladder to transmural stimulation: effects of atropine and alpha,beta-methylene ATP. Br J Pharmacol 1990; 99:493–498.

86. Mostwin JL. The action potential of guinea pig bladder smooth muscle. J Urol 1986; 135:1299–1303.

87. Creed KE. Membrane properties of the smooth muscle membrane of the guinea-pig urinary bladder. Pflugers Arch 1971; 326:115–126.

88. Hashitani H, Suzuki H. Electrical and mechanical responses produced by nerve stimulation in detrusor smooth muscle of the guinea-pig. Eur J Pharmacol 1995; 284:177–183.

89. el-Badawi A, Schenk EA. Dual innervation of the mammalian urinary bladder. A histochemical study of the distribution of cholinergic and adrenergic nerves. Am J Anat 1966; 119:405–427.

90. Kluck P. The autonomic innervation of the human urinary bladder, bladder neck and urethra: a histochemical study. Anat Rec 1980; 198:439–447.

91. Gabella G. The structural relations between nerve fibres and muscle cells in the urinary bladder of the rat. J Neurocytol 1995; 24:159–187.

92. Hirst GDS, Chaote JK, Cousins HM, et al. Transmission by postganglionic axons of the autonomic nervous system: the importance of the specialised neuroeffector junction. Neuroscience 1996; 73:7–23.

93. Drake MJ, Hedlund P, Mills IW, et al. Structural and functional denervation of human detrusor after spinal cord injury. Lab Invest 2000; 80:1491–1499.

94. Chen TF, Doyle PT, Ferguson DR. Inhibition in the human urinary bladder by gamma-amino-butyric acid. Br J Urol 1994; 73:250–255.

95. Kinder RB, Mundy AR. Atropine blockade of nerve-mediated stimulation of the human detrusor. Br J Urol 1985; 57:418–421.

96. Sjogren C, Andersson KE, Husted S, et al. Atropine resistance of transmurally stimulated isolated human bladder muscle. J Urol 1982; 128:1368–1371.

97. Lundberg JM. Pharmacology of cotransmission in the autonomic nervous system: integrative aspects on amines, neuropeptides, adenosine triphosphate, amino acids and nitric oxide. Pharmacol Rev 1996; 48:113–178.

98. Dumsday B. Atropine-resistance of the urinary bladder innervation. J Pharm Pharmacol 1971; 23:222–225.

99. Carpenter FG. Atropine resistance and muscarinic receptors in the rat urinary bladder. Br J Pharmacol 1977; 59:43–49.

100. Krell RD, McCoy JL, Ridley PT. Pharmacological characterization of the excitatory innervation to the guinea-pig urinary bladder in vitro: evidence for both cholinergic and non-adrenergic-non-cholinergic neurotransmission. Br J Pharmacol 1981; 74:15–22.

101. Longhurst PA, Belis JA, O'Donnell JP, et al. A study of the atropine-resistant component of the neurogenic response of the rabbit urinary bladder. Eur J Pharmacol 1984; 99:295–302.

102. Brading AF, Inoue R. Ion channels and excitatory transmission in the smooth muscle of the urinary bladder. Z Kardiol 1991; 7:47–53.

103. Luheshi GN, Zar MA. Presence of non-cholinergic motor transmission in human isolated bladder. J Pharm Pharmacol 1990; 42:223–224.

104. Burnstock G, Cocks T, Kasakov L, Wong HK. Direct evidence for ATP release from non-adrenergic, non-cholinergic ('purinergic') nerves in the guinea-pig taenia coli and bladder. Eur J Pharmacol 1978; 49:145–149.

105. Tong YC, Hung YC, Shinozuka K, et al. Evidence of adenosine 5′-triphosphate release from nerve and P2x-purinoceptor mediated contraction during electrical stimulation of rat urinary bladder smooth muscle. J Urol 1997; 158:1973–1977.

106. Westfall TD, Kennedy C, Sneddon P. The ecto-ATPase inhibitor ARL 67156 enhances parasympathetic neurotransmission in the guinea-pig urinary bladder. Eur J Pharmacol 1997; 329:169–173.

107. Hoyes AD, Barber P, Martin BG. Comparative ultrastructure of the nerves innervating the muscle of the body of the bladder. Cell Tissue Res 1975; 164:133–144.

108. Crowe R, Burnstock G. A histochemical and immunohistochemical study of the autonomic innervation of the lower urinary tract of the female pig. Is the pig a good model for the human bladder and urethra? J Urol 1989; 141:414–422.

109. Gosling JA. The distribution of noradrenergic nerves in the human lower urinary tract. Clin Sci 1986; 70 (Suppl. 14):3s–6s.

110. Milner P, Lincoln J, Corr LA, et al. Neuropeptide Y in non-sympathetic nerves of the rat: changes during maturation but not after guanethidine sympathectomy. Neuroscience 1991; 43:661–669.

111. Bauer FE, Christofides ND, Hacker GW, et al. Distribution of galanin immunoreactivity in the genitourinary tract of man and rat. Peptides 1986; 7:5–10.

112. Persson K, Alm P, Johansson K, et al. Nitric oxide synthase in pig lower urinary tract: immunohistochemistry, NADPH diaphorase histochemistry and functional effects. Br J Pharmacol 1993; 110:521–530.

113. Zoubek J, Somogyi GT, De Groat WC. A comparison of inhibitory effects of neuropeptide Y on rat urinary bladder, urethra, and vas deferens. Am J Physiol 1993; 265:R537–R543.

114. Acevedo CG, Contreras E, Escalona J, et al. Pharmacological characterization of adenosine A1 and A2 receptors in the bladder: evidence for a modulatory adenosine tone regulating non-adrenergic non-cholinergic neurotransmission. Br J Pharmacol 1992; 107:120–126.

115. Husted S, Sjogren C, Andersson KE. Direct effects of adenosine and adenine nucleotides on isolated human urinary bladder and their influence on electrically induced contractions. J Urol 1983; 130:392–398.

116. Sellers DJ, Chess-Williams R, Chapple CR. 5-hydroxytryptamine-induced potentiation of cholinergic responses to electrical field stimulation in pig detrusor muscle. BJU Int 2000; 86:714–718.

117. Chen HI. Evidence for the presynaptic action of 5-hydroxytryptamine and the involvement of purinergic innervation in the rabbit lower urinary tract. Br J Pharmacol 1990; 101:212–216.

118. Klarskov P. Enkephalin inhibits presynaptically the contractility of urinary tract smooth muscle. Br J Urol 1987; 59:31–35.

119. Maggi CA, Santicioli P, Patacchini R, et al. Galanin: a potent modulator of excitatory neurotransmission in the human urinary bladder. Eur J Pharmacol 1987; 143:135–137.

120. Fredericks CM. Characterization of the rabbit detrusor response to histamine through pharmacologic antagonism. Pharmacology 1975; 13:5–11.

121. Somogyi GT, Tanowitz M, Zernova G, de Groat WC. M1 muscarinic receptor-induced facilitation of ACh and noradrenaline release in the rat bladder is mediated by protein kinase C. J Physiol (Lond) 1996; 496:245–254.

122. Braverman AS, Kohn IJ, Luthin GR, Ruggieri MR. Prejunctional M1 facilitatory and M2 inhibitory muscarinic receptors mediate rat bladder contractility. Am J Physiol 1998; 274:R517–R523.

123. D'Agostino G, Bolognesi ML, Lucchelli A, et al. Prejunctional muscarinic inhibitory control of acetylcholine release in the human isolated detrusor: involvement of the M4 receptor subtype. Br J Pharmacol 2000; 129:493–500.

124. Maggi CA. Prostanoids as local modulators of reflex micturition. Pharmacol Res 1992; 25:13–20.

125. Poggesi L, Nicita G, Castellani S, et al. The role of prostaglandins in the maintenance of the tone of the rabbit urinary bladder. Invest Urol 1980; 17:454–458.

126. Khalaf IM, Lehoux JG, Elshawarby LA, Elhilali MM. Release of prostaglandins into the pelvic venous blood of dogs in response to vesical distension and pelvic nerve stimulation. Invest Urol 1979; 17:244–247.

127. Nakahata N, Ono T, Nakanishi H. Contribution of prostaglandin E2 to bradykinin-induced contraction in rabbit urinary detrusor. Jpn J Pharmacol 1987; 43:351–359.

128. Downie JW, Karmazyn M. Mechanical trauma to bladder epithelium liberates prostanoids which modulate neurotransmission in rabbit detrusor muscle. J Pharmacol Exp Ther 1984; 230:445–449.

129. Callahan SM, Creed KE. Electrical and mechanical activity of the isolated lower urinary tract of the guinea-pig. Br J Pharmacol 1981; 74:353–358.

130. Noronha-Blob L, Lowe V, Patton A, et al. Muscarinic receptors: relationships among phosphoinositide breakdown, adenylate cyclase inhibition, in vitro detrusor muscle contractions and in vivo cystometrogram studies in guinea pig bladder. J Pharmacol Exp Ther 1989; 249:843–851.

131. Iacovou JW, Hill SJ, Birmingham AT. Agonist-induced contraction and accumulation of inositol phosphates in the guinea-pig detrusor: evidence that muscarinic and purinergic receptors raise intracellular calcium by different mechanisms. J Urol 1990; 144:775–779.

132. Harriss DR, Marsh KA, Birmingham AT, Hill SJ. Expression of muscarinic M3-receptors coupled to inositol phospholipid hydrolysis in human detrusor cultured smooth muscle cells. J Urol 1995; 154:1241–1245.

133. Marsh KA, Harriss DR, Hill SJ. Desensitization of muscarinic receptor-coupled inositol phospholipid hydrolysis in human detrusor cultured smooth cells. J Urol 1996; 155:1439–1443.

134. Brading AF, Mostwin JL. Electrical and mechanical responses of guinea-pig bladder muscle to nerve stimulation. Br J Pharmacol 1989; 98:1083–1090.

135. Creed KE, Callahan SM, Ito Y. Excitatory neurotransmission in the mammalian bladder and the effects of suramin. Br J Urol 1994; 74:736–743.

136. Inoue R, Brading AF. The properties of the ATP-induced depolarization and current in single cells isolated from the guinea-pig urinary bladder. Br J Pharmacol 1990; 100:619–625.

137. Gabbiani G, Ryan GB, Majne G. Presence of modified fibroblasts in granulation tissue and their possible role in wound contraction. Experientia 1971; 27:549–550.

138. Powell DW, Mifflin RC, Valentich JD, et al. Myofibroblasts. I. Paracrine cells important in health and disease. Am J Physiol 1999; 277:C1–9.

139. Klemm MF, Exintaris B, Lang RJ. Identification of the cells underlying pacemaker activity in the guinea-pig upper urinary tract. J Physiol (Lond) 1999; 519 (Pt 3):867–884.

140. Faussone-Pellegrini MS, Thuneberg L. Guide to the identification of interstitial cells of Cajal. Microsc Res Tech 1999; 47:248–266.

141. Drake MJ, Hussain IF, Hedlund P, et al. Characterisation of intramuscular myofibroblasts in human detrusor. BJU Int 2000; 86:367–368.

142. Smet PJ, Jonavicius J, Marshall VR, de Vente J. Distribution of nitric oxide synthase-immunoreactive nerves and identification of the cellular targets of nitric oxide in guinea-pig and human urinary bladder by cGMP immunohistochemistry. Neuroscience 1996; 71:337–348.

143. McCloskey KD, Gurney AM. *kit*-positive cells in the guinea pig bladder. J Urol 2002; 168:832–836.

144. Uvelius B, Gabella G. Relation between cell length and force production in urinary bladder smooth muscle. Acta Physiol Scand 1980; 110:357–365.

145. James MJ, Birmingham AT, Hill SJ. Partial mediation by nitric oxide of the relaxation of human isolated detrusor strips in response to electrical field stimulation. Br J Clin Pharmacol 1993; 35:366–372.

146. Triguero D, Prieto D, Garcia Pascual A. NADPH-diaphorase and NANC relaxations are correlated in the sheep urinary tract. Neurosci Lett 1993; 163:93–96.

147. Takeda M, Obara K, Mizusawa T, et al. Evidence for beta3-adrenoceptor subtypes in relaxation of the human urinary bladder detrusor: analysis by molecular biological and pharmacological methods. J Pharmacol Exp Ther 1999; 288:1367–1373.

148. McMurray G, Dass N, Brading AF. Purinoceptor subtypes mediating contraction and relaxation of marmoset urinary bladder smooth muscle. Br J Pharmacol 1998; 123:1579–1586.

149. Igawa Y, Yamazaki Y, Takeda H, et al. Functional and molecular biological evidence for a possible beta3-adrenoceptor in the human detrusor muscle. Br J Pharmacol 1999; 126:819–825.

150. Fovaeus M, Fujiwara M, Hogestatt ED, et al. A non-nitrergic smooth muscle relaxant factor released from rat urinary bladder by muscarinic receptor stimulation. J Urol 1999; 161:649–653.

151. Steers WD, Broder SR, Persson K, et al. Mechanical stretch increases secretion of parathyroid hormone-related protein by cultured bladder smooth muscle cells. J Urol 1998; 160:908–912.

152. Brading AF. Physiology of the urinary tract smooth muscle. In: Webster GD, Kirby RS, King LR, Goldwasser B, eds. Reconstructive urology. Boston: Blackwell Scientific, 1993.

153. Vaughan CW, Satchell PM. Urine storage mechanisms. Prog Neurobiol 1995; 46:215–237.

154. Igawa Y, Mattiasson A, Andersson KE. Micturition and premicturition contractions in unanesthetized rats with bladder outlet obstruction. J Urol 1994; 151:244–249.

155. Klevmark B. Motility of the urinary bladder in cats during filling at physiological rates. II. Effects of extrinsic bladder denervation on intramural tension and on intravesical pressure patterns. Acta Physiol Scand 1977; 101:176–184.

156. Mills IW, Drake MJ, Noble JG, Brading AF. Are unstable detrusor contractions dependent on efferent excitatory innervation? Neurourol Urodyn 1998; 17:352–354.

157. Sethia KK, Brading AF, Smith JC. An animal model of non-obstructive bladder instability. J Urol 1990; 143:1243–1246.

158. Sugaya K, de Groat WC. Influence of temperature on activity of the isolated whole bladder preparation of neonatal and adult rats. Am J Physiol Regul Integr Comp Physiol 2000; 278:R238–R246.

159. Coolsaet BL, Van Duyl WA, Van Os-Bossagh P, De Bakker HV. New concepts in relation to urge and detrusor activity. Neurourol Urodyn 1993; 12:463–471.

160. Constantinou CE, Yamaguchi O. Multiple-coupled pacemaker system in renal pelvis of the unicalyceal kidney. Am J Physiol 1981; 241:R412–R418.

161. Drake MJ, Mills IW, Gillespie JI. Model of peripheral autonomous modules and a myovesical plexus in normal and overactive bladder function. Lancet 2001; 358:401–403.

162. Hashitani H, Fukuta H, Takano H, et al. Origin and propagation of spontaneous excitation of the guinea-pig urinary bladder. J Physiol (Lond) 2001; 530:273–286.

163. Drake MJ, Chambers P, Neal DE, Gillespie JI. Complexity of contractile activity of the isolated whole guinea pig bladder: evidence for autonomous modules in detrusor muscle. BJU Int 2001; 88:285.

164. Downie JW, Dean DM, Carro-Ciampi G, Awad SA. A difference in sensitivity to alpha-adrenergic agonists exhibited by detrusor and bladder neck of the rabbit. Can J Physiol Pharmacol 1975; 53:525–530.

165. Ek A, Alm P, Andersson KE, Persson CG. Adrenergic and cholinergic nerves of the human urethra and urinary bladder. A histochemical study. Acta Physiol Scand 1977; 99:345–352.

166. Maggi CA, Santicioli P, Parlani M, et al. The presence of mucosa reduces the contractile response of the guinea-pig urinary bladder to substance P. J Pharm Pharmacol 1987; 39:653–655.

167. Hawthorn MH, Chapple CR, Cock M, Chess-Williams R. Urothelium-derived inhibitory factor(s) influences on detrusor muscle contractility in vivo. Br J Pharmacol 2000; 129:416–419.

168. Levin RM, Wein AJ, Krasnopolsky L, et al. Effect of mucosal removal on the response of the feline bladder to pharmacological stimulation. J Urol 1995; 153:1291–1294.

169. Templeman L, Chapple CR, Chess-Williams R. Urothelium derived inhibitory factor and cross-talk among receptors in the trigone of the bladder of the pig. J Urol 2002; 167:742–745.

170. Ferguson DR, Kennedy I, Burton TJ. ATP is released from rabbit urinary bladder epithelial cells by hydrostatic pressure changes – a possible sensory mechanism? J Physiol (Lond) 1997; 505:503–511.

171. Burnstock G. Release of vasoactive substances from endothelial cells by shear stress and mechanosensory transduction. J Anat 1999; 194:335–342.

172. Vlaskovska M, Kasakov L, Rong W, et al. P2X3 knock-out mice reveal a major sensory role for urothelially released ATP. J Neurosci 2001; 21:5670–5677.

173. Tempest H, Turner WH, Ferguson D. Expression of epithelial sodium channels in the epithelium of the human urinary bladder. Neurourol Urodyn 2002; 21:404–405.

174. Burton TJ, Edwardson JM, Ingham J, et al. Regulation of Na(+) channel density at the apical surface of rabbit urinary bladder epithelium. Eur J Pharmacol 2002; 448:215–223.

175. Birder LA, Kanai AJ, de Groat WC, et al. Vanilloid receptor expression suggests a sensory role for urinary bladder epithelial cells. Proc Natl Acad Sci USA 2001; 98:13396–13401.

176. Maggi CA, Meli A. The sensory-efferent function of capsaicin-sensitive sensory neurons. Gen Pharmacol 1988; 19:1–43.

177. Bridgewater M, Davies JR, Brading AF. Regional variations in the neural control of the female pig urethra. Br J Urol 1995; 76:730–740.

178. Dass N, McMurray G, Greenland JE, Brading AF. Morphological aspects of the female pig bladder neck and urethra: quantitative analysis using computer assisted 3-dimensional reconstructions. J Urol 2001; 165:1294–1299.

179. Nasu K, Moriyama N, Fukasawa R, et al. Quantification and distribution of alpha1-adrenoceptor subtype mRNAs in human proximal urethra. Br J Pharmacol 1998; 123:1289–1293.

180. Kava MS, Blue DR, Vimont RL, et al. Alpha1L-adrenoceptor mediation of smooth muscle contraction in rabbit bladder neck: a model for lower urinary tract tissues of man. Br J Pharmacol 1998; 123:1359–1366.

181. Yamanishi T, Chapple CR, Yasuda K, et al. The role of M2 muscarinic receptor subtypes mediating contraction of the circular and longitudinal smooth muscle of the pig proximal urethra. J Urol 2002; 168:308–314.

182. Nagahama K, Tsujii T, Morita T, et al. Differences between proximal and distal portions of the male rabbit posterior urethra in the physiological role of muscarinic cholinergic receptors. Br J Pharmacol 1998; 124:1175–1180.

183. Mutoh S, Latifpour J, Saito M, Weiss RM. Evidence for the presence of regional differences in the subtype specificity of muscarinic receptors in rabbit lower urinary tract. J Urol 1997; 157:717–721.

184. Ek A, Alm P, Andersson KE, Persson CG. Adrenoceptor and cholinoceptor mediated responses of the isolated human urethra. Scand J Urol Nephrol 1977; 11:97–102.

185. Brading AF, Chen HI. High potassium solution induces relaxation in the isolated pig urethra. J Physiol (Lond) 1990; 430:118P.

186. Teramoto N, Brading AF. Activation by levcromakalim and metabolic inhibition of glibenclamide-sensitive K channels in smooth muscle cells of pig proximal urethra. Br J Pharmacol 1996; 118:635–642.

187. Teramoto N, McMurray G, Brading AF. Effects of levcromakalim and nucleoside diphosphates on glibenclamide-sensitive K$^+$ channels in pig urethral myocytes. Br J Pharmacol 1997; 120:1229–1240.

188. Teramoto N, Brading AF. Nicorandil activates glibenclamide-sensitive K$^+$ channels in smooth muscle cells of pig proximal urethra. J Pharmacol Exp Ther 1997; 280:483–491.

189. Creed KE, Oike M, Ito Y. The electrical properties and responses to nerve stimulation of the proximal urethra of the male rabbit. Br J Urol 1997; 79:543–553.

190. Hashitani H, Van Helden DF, Suzuki H. Properties of spontaneous depolarizations in circular smooth muscle cells of rabbit urethra. Br J Pharmacol 1996; 118:1627–1632.

191. Cotton KD, Hollywood MA, McHale NG, Thornbury KD. Ca^{2+} current and Ca(2+)-activated chloride current in isolated smooth muscle cells of the sheep urethra. J Physiol (Lond) 1997; 505 (Pt 1):121–131.

192. Hashitani H, Edwards FR. Spontaneous and neurally activated depolarizations in smooth muscle cells of the guinea-pig urethra. J Physiol (Lond) 1999; 514 (Pt 2):459–470.

193. de Groat WC, Fraser MO, Yoshiyama M, et al. Neural control of the urethra. Scand J Urol Nephrol 2001; Suppl 207:35–43.

194. Bridgewater M, MacNeil HF, Brading AF. Regulation of tone in pig urethral smooth muscle. J Urol 1993; 150:223–228.

195. Klarskov P, Gerstenberg TC, Ramirez D, Hald T. Non-cholinergic, non-adrenergic nerve mediated relaxation of trigone, bladder neck and urethral smooth muscle in vitro. J Urol 1983; 129:848–850.

196. Kakikazi H, Fraser MO, de Groat WC. Reflex pathways controlling urethral striated and smooth muscle function in the rat. Am J Physiol Regul Integr Comp Physiol 1997; 272:R1647–R1656.

197. Flood HD, Liu JL, Fraser MO, de Groat WC. Sex difference in the nitric oxide (NO) mediated smooth muscle component and striated muscle component of urethral relaxation in rats. Neurourol Urodyn 1995; 14:517–519.

198. Vizzard MA, Erdman SL, Forstermann U, de Groat WC. Differential distribution of nitric oxide synthase in neural pathways to the urogenital organs (urethra, penis, urinary bladder) of the rat. Brain Res 1994; 646:279–291.

199. Ho KM, Ny L, McMurray G, et al. Co-localization of carbon monoxide and nitric oxide synthesizing enzymes in the human urethral sphincter. J Urol 1999; 161:1968–1972.

200. Thind P. The significance of smooth and striated muscles in sphincter function of the urethra in healthy women. Neurourol Urodyn 1995; 14:585–618.

201. Greenland JE, Dass N, Brading AF. Intrinsic urethral closure mechanisms in the female pig. Scand J Urol Nephrol Suppl 1996; 179:75–80.

202. Ito Y, Kimoto Y. The neural and non-neural mechanisms involved in urethral activity in rabbits. J Physiol (Lond) 1985; 367:57–72.

203. Sergeant GP, Hollywood MA, McCloskey KD, et al. Specialised pacemaking cells in the rabbit urethra. J Physiol (Lond) 2000; 526 (Pt 2):359–366.

204. Tanagho EA. The anatomy and physiology of micturition. Clin Obstet Gynaecol 1978; 5:3–26.

205. Brading AF. The physiology of the mammalian urinary outflow tract. Exp Physiol 1999; 84:215–221.

206. Ehren I, Iversen H, Jansson O, et al. Localization of nitric oxide synthase activity in the human lower urinary tract and its correlation with neuroeffector responses. Urology 1994; 44:683–687.

207. Persson K, Andersson KE. Nitric oxide and relaxation of pig lower urinary tract. Br J Pharmacol 1992; 106:416–422.

208. Dokita S, Smith SD, Nishimoto T, et al. Involvement of nitric oxide and cyclic GMP in rabbit urethral relaxation. Eur J Pharmacol 1994; 266:269–275.

209. Pinna C, Eberini I, Puglisi L, Burnstock G. Presence of constitutive endothelial nitric oxide synthase immunoreactivity in urothelial cells of hamster proximal urethra. Eur J Pharmacol 1999; 367:85–89.

210. Werkstrom V, Alm P, Persson K, Andersson KE. Inhibitory innervation of the guinea-pig urethra; roles of CO, NO and VIP. J Auton Nerv Syst 1998; 74:33–42.

211. Naseem KM, Mumtaz FH, Thompson CS, et al. Relaxation of rabbit lower urinary tract smooth muscle by nitric oxide and carbon monoxide: modulation by hydrogen peroxide. Eur J Pharmacol 2000; 387:329–335.

212. Werkstrom V, Ny L, Persson K, Andersson KE. Carbon monoxide-induced relaxation and distribution of haem oxygenase isoenzymes in the pig urethra and lower oesophagogastric junction. Br J Pharmacol 1997; 120:312–318.

213. Schroder A, Hedlund P, Andersson KE. Carbon monoxide relaxes the female pig urethra as effectively as nitric oxide in the presence of YC-1. J Urol 2002; 167:1892–1896.

214. Andersson KE, Ek A, Persson CG. Effects of prostaglandins on the isolated human bladder and urethra. Acta Physiol Scand 1977; 100:165–171.

215. Klarskov P, Gerstenberg T, Ramirez D, et al. Prostaglandin type E activity dominates in urinary tract smooth muscle in vitro. J Urol 1983; 129:1071–1074.

216. Klarskov P, Gerstenberg T, Hald T. Vasoactive intestinal polypeptide influence on lower urinary tract smooth muscle from human and pig. J Urol 1984; 131:1000–1004.

217. Klarskov P, Horby-Petersen J. Influence of serotonin on lower urinary tract smooth muscle in vitro. Br J Urol 1986; 58:507–513.

218. Nishizawa S, Igawa Y, Okada N, Ohhashi T. Capsaicin-induced nitric-oxide-dependent relaxation in isolated dog urethra. Eur J Pharmacol 1997; 335:211–219.

219. Mattiasson A, Andersson KE, Sjogren C. Adrenoceptors and cholinoceptors controlling noradrenaline release from adrenergic nerves in the urethra of rabbit and man. J Urol 1984; 131:1190–1195.

220. Mattiasson A, Andersson KE, Sjogren C. Inhibitory muscarinic receptors and alpha-adrenoceptors on cholinergic axon terminals in the urethra of rabbit and man. Neurourol Urodyn 1988; 6:449.

221. Seshita H, Yoshida M, Takahashi W, et al. Prejunctional alpha-adrenoceptors regulate nitrergic neurotransmission in the rabbit urethra. Eur J Pharmacol 2000; 400:271–278.

222. Yoshida M, Akaike T, Inadome A, et al. The possible effect of nitric oxide on relaxation and noradrenaline release in the isolated rabbit urethra. Eur J Pharmacol 1998; 357:213–219.

4

Physiology of the striated muscles

John FB Morrison

INTRODUCTION

This chapter is concerned with the physiological control of the external urethral sphincter, the pelvic floor muscles, and other striated muscles functionally associated with the pelvic diaphragm in the set of conditions described collectively as the 'neurogenic bladder' or 'overactive bladder (OAB)'. Following spinal cord lesions, striated muscles generally develop spasticity – e.g. following a cervical or thoracic spinal cord transection – and a corresponding increase in tone is seen in the striated muscle of the external urethral sphincter and pelvic floor. Alternatively, muscle tone in the pelvis can be flaccid, if there is a lower motoneuron lesion affecting the cauda equina. Partial and mixed lesions also occur and reflex activities can be modified in the remodeling of the neural networks that regulate these muscles, or by the denervation and reinnervation of neurons or skeletal muscle. The muscles themselves also respond to these changes in activity, and, for example, hypoplastic changes and replacement by fibrous tissue can also occur as a result of denervation.

There have been a number of reviews and books on the subject[1–8] during the last couple of decades, and recently there has been a substantial body of genetic and molecular data concerning the mechanisms that operate in muscles of different types, and the mechanisms that operate to maintain the stability of the link between motoneuron and muscle at the nerve–muscle junction. The striated muscles of the lower urinary tract are specialized in function, and are subject to neural coordination that causes them to work together as a functional group. Within this overall concept, there remain areas of muscle that are specialized for different tasks related to the visceral systems with which they are principally associated. Examples include the puborectalis or the fibers of levator ani that loop behind the urethra, and there are also differences between the mechanisms controlling the urethral sphincter, the associated paraurethral muscles, and the muscle fibers that compose the bulk of levator ani. These differences extend to the histological and biochemical properties of the muscle fibers, the pattern and source of innervation, the reflex behavior and the role in voluntary control of the lower urinary tract.

NORMAL STRUCTURE AND FUNCTION

Morphology of the striated muscle of the lower urinary tract

Gross anatomy

Striated muscle occurs in the pelvic floor and within the urethra and both of these contribute to continence mechanisms; smooth muscle as well as skeletal muscle occurs within the urethra, and the roles of these are sometimes difficult to separate. *In-vivo* recordings of intraurethral pressure have been made following blockade of the nicotinic receptors in various mammals,[9–11] and all suggest that the somatic innervation of the striated muscle of this region plays a part in generating the resting urethral pressure.

Striated muscle of the rhabdosphincter

The external urethral sphincter consists of circular striated muscle concentrated over about 40% of the length of the urethra (from 20% to 60% of its length in humans). In the rat, the distribution of striated muscle in the urethra is similar, but there is also a mass of muscle that forms an arch at the perineal membrane that can compress the urethra from above in the lower third.[12]

In the human female the striated muscle is said to form an outer sleeve (the external urethral sphincter or rhabdosphincter), and this surrounds the inner smooth muscle (Figure 4.1). This female rhabdosphincter is separate from the muscle of the anterior pelvic floor. The fibers are

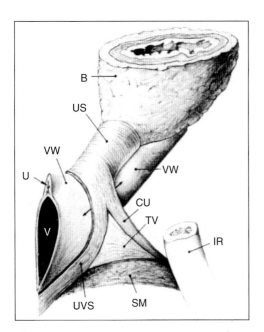

Figure 4.1
Striated urogenital sphincter muscle showing its urethral sphincter (US), compressor urethrae (CU), and urethrovaginal sphincter (UVS). Also shown, B, bladder; IR, ischiopubic ramus; SM, smooth muscle; TV transverse vaginal muscle; U, urethra; V, vagina; VW, vaginal wall. (After Oelrich.)[39]

oriented in a circular direction and are thickest in the middle third of the urethra, but the posterior segment, adjacent to the vaginal wall, is thinner than elsewhere. These striated muscle cells are smaller than in the pelvic floor and exert tone upon the urethral lumen for long periods of time, and this muscle also aids closure. In the human male, the striated muscle also encircles the urethra and, unlike the female, these small fibers merge with larger-diameter fibers of adjacent muscles. One possibility is that these larger fibers are a proximal extension of striated muscle from the bulb of the penis.[7] Other views relate to observations on the striated muscle of the prostatic capsule, where fast and slow fibers are present.[8] In tissues taken from transplant donors it was found that the male rhabdosphincter consists of 35% fast and 65% slow fibers, whereas in the female only 13% of fibers are fast-twitch fibers (see later).

Levator ani

The levator ani is a sling of muscle in the shape of a thin broad sheet attached to the pubis anteriorly and laterally as far as the ischial spine; anteriorly, the muscle is absent in the midline and a fat-filled space lies immediately behind the pubic symphysis. In the human male a few fibers attach to the perineal body behind the prostate to form the levator prostatae. In the female these fibers attach to the lateral vaginal wall to form the pubovaginalis or sphincter

vaginae. Other fibers attach to the anorectal flexure and fuse with the deep part of the external anal sphincter to form puborectalis; other components are called pubococcygeus and iliococcygeus, which tend to merge into one. Levator ani plays an important role in maintaining the position of the pelvic viscera. On contraction of the pelvic floor, the anterior movement of the vagina produces some compressive action on the urethra against the pubis near the location of the urethral sphincter, reinforcing its action, e.g. during coughing.[7]

In the human female, the paraurethral tissues are joined with muscle fibers of the most medial portion of the levator ani in the region of the proximal urethra. At this site, the medial fibers of levator ani insert into the vaginal wall and provide an arching mechanism that can constrict the urethra.[13] It has also been suggested that the medial fibers of the levator ani muscle have a specific role in controlling vesical neck position and in urinary continence mechanisms.[14] The role of the levator ani appears to be to support the proximal urethra and to pull the bladder neck in an anterior direction, such that the lumen is constricted between arching fibers and connective tissue of the levator ani and a connective tissue band (endopelvic fascia) anteriorly. When the levator ani relaxes, the bladder neck can descend, and the lumen can open because the external compression is reduced; at this stage support is provided by the connective tissue of the arcus tendineus fasciae.[13,15] Acute spinal anesthesia has been used to block nerve impulses to the pelvic floor and its effect is to disrupt the active muscular mechanism that supports the bladder neck in healthy continent women.[16] A significant loss of support was demonstrable during spinal anesthesia, indicating that activity originating in the spinal cord and pelvic floor muscles was a major factor responsible for support of the bladder neck.

The distribution and properties of different types of striated muscle fibers

Functional properties of fast and slow muscle

Striated muscle fibers can be divided into different types depending on their speed of contraction and their susceptibility to fatigue. Ranvier's classical observations[17] on slowly contracting 'red' and fast-contracting 'white' muscle indicated that there were at least two types of striated muscle fibers, and studies of the mechanical properties indicated human muscles contain slow-twitch and fast-twitch fibers (Figure 4.2), which take about 100 ms and 30 ms to reach the peak of their contractions, respectively. The fast units often develop much larger forces, and those that upon the temporal pattern of impulses in different pudendal motoneurons. It is only relatively recently that the relationship between function and histochemical properties has been intensively investigated.

Histochemistry

The dominance of oxidative enzymes, such as succinate dehydrogenase, in slow-twitch (type I) fibers and the lack of these in fast fatigable (type II) fibers is an important histochemical correlate. In the human urethral sphincter, the presence of small-diameter fibers containing oxidative enzymes suggests that these are slow fibers, which are adapted to produce a steady tension. There is some evidence that there may also be a few larger fibers that have less ATP-ase reactivity, and these may be involved less with tonic activity and more with squeezing the urethra at times of transient stresses, such as during coughing. The blood supply of the slow (type I) is rich, whereas the capillary supply in fast fibers is less. This correlation may be due to the production and release of angiogenic factors – factors that cause the growth of blood vessels – and this will be discussed briefly below.

The periurethral fibers of the levator ani contain both type I and larger, type II (fast-twitch) fibers, which are more concerned with rapid motor responses such as voluntary squeeze;[20] in contrast, the striated fibers of the external urethral sphincter consist mainly of type I (slow-twitch) fibers, which are associated with the generation of tone. However, as stated previously, there are sex differences, and, in the male rhabdosphincter, approximately one-third of striated muscle fibers are fast fibers, whereas in the female only about one-eighth of fibers are fast-twitch fibers.

Fast and slow muscle fibers differ in their content of oxidative enzymes, creatine kinase, and myoglobin, have different forms of myosin, differences in the expression of transcription factors, and differences in the distribution of nitric oxide synthase in the sarcolemma. The following subsections contain some details on these differences.

Creatine kinase. Fast and slow muscle contractions are both dependent on ATP availability, and the enzyme creatine kinase (CK), which is normally responsible for energy storage and catalyzes the exchange of high-energy phosphate between creatine phosphate and ATP, is present in highest concentration in the fast fibers. Dahlstedt et al[21] used a mutant animal that was deficient in creatine kinase and showed that the fast fibers fatigued more quickly and this may be related to changes in phosphate concentration on crossbridge function and the handling of ionized calcium by the sarcoplasmic reticulum. A reduction in maximum tetanic force production has also been observed in CK-deficient animals.[22]

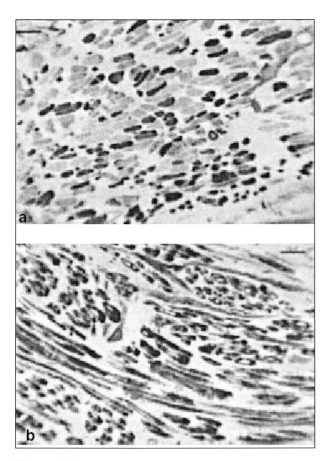

Figure 4.2
Sections from the proximal third of the human male urethra (a) and the female membranous urethra (b) stained for ATPase at pH 4.3, in which the slow-twitch fibers appear darkly stained. Note that most of the female striated muscle is slow twitch, whereas a significant proportion of the male fibers are fast twitch.[8]

produce the greatest force are fatigable (the force generated declines on repetitive stimulation); this is the basis of the subdivision of the fast fibers into two subgroups: fatigable and fatigue resistant. In contrast, the slow units tend to produce smaller forces, and are resistant to fatigue. The proportions of these vary between different muscles.[18]

The fast fibers are innervated by larger alpha motoneurons, whereas the slow fibers are innervated by alpha motoneurons of smaller diameter and lower conduction velocity. The latter are generally tonically active, whereas the former are only activated in a phasic or transient manner; this is known as the 'size principle'.[19] One consequence of the size principle is that the smaller, type I, slow fibers are tonically active and the tonic activity is a result of the regular firing of action potentials along the motoneurons: thus, the tonic activity of the striated muscle of the urethral sphincter is generated within the spinal cord and dependent

Myoglobin. An oxygen storage protein, myoglobin occurs in striated muscle fibers, and is present in higher concentrations in the type I slow muscles of the sort that predominate in the urethral sphincter.[23] Myoglobin is present in oxidative skeletal muscle fibers and facilitates oxygen delivery during periods of high metabolic demand. Its role in muscle performance has been studied in animals that are genetically deficient in myoglobin. Myoglobin-deficient mice have striated muscle fibers that have adapted to the deficiency by converting type I to type II in the soleus muscle as well as other changes, including the expression of angiogenic and endothelial growth factors, which may account for preserved exercise capacity of these models.[24]

Myosin. Biochemical analysis of the myosin chains in different muscles has indicated that the muscle of the rabbit external urethral sphincter has types of myosin more closely associated with fast red muscles than slow white ones.[25,26] Biochemical analysis of the human external urethral sphincter suggested that there is a degree of diversity in the proportions of fast and slow myosin molecules in different specimens, and this was not related to age.[27,28] In rabbits, fast-type myosin exceeded slow type in amount. The ratio of fast to slow myosins in the female was different from that in the male external urethral sphincter (EUS), and there appears to a selective decrease in the volume of type 2 (fast) muscle fibers and/or conversion of type 2 to type 1 (slow) muscle fibers with age and multiparity.[29,30] In male rabbits, the urethral striated muscle appeared to have mainly fast myosin but slow myosin occurred in higher amounts in the proximal region and tended to decrease toward the distal end of the urethra.[31,32] As mentioned earlier, the presence of fast myosin may correlate with the existence of fast muscle extending downwards from the prostatic capsule.

Nitric oxide synthase. The essential enzyme in the formation of nitric oxide, nitric oxide synthase is a mediator in smooth muscle and the nervous system. However, it has been found recently that nitric oxide synthase, which generates the neuromodulator nitric oxide, is present in the sarcolemma of urethral striated muscle fibers.[33] Generally speaking, it is found in fast fibers, but there are reports of it also in the larger slow-twitch fibers in the human membranous urethra. In somatic muscles, the presence of nitric oxide synthase in some sarcolemmal membranes appears to be associated with the syntrophin group of proteins that contain multiple protein interaction motifs, and are associated closely with dystrophin. Alpha-syntrophin also has an important role in synapse formation and in the organization of utrophin, the acetylcholine receptor, and acetylcholinesterase at the neuromuscular synapse.[34]

Transcription factors. The development of slow and fast contractile properties in striated muscle fibers may be related to the levels of certain transcription factors that are involved in myogenesis. One such factor is MyoD, and the mRNA levels of this factor differ between slow and fast muscle; it is associated particularly with the nuclei of the fastest muscle fibers.[35]

Relationship of muscle contractile properties to innervation

Fast fibers are innervated by faster-conducting alpha-motoneurons, and the slow-twitch fibers are innervated by the slower alphamotoneurons. The fast fatigable fibers also have larger diameters than the fast, fatigue-resistant fibers, which, in turn are larger than the slow fibers. The nature of the motor innervation of muscle appears to play an important role in determining the contractile properties of the muscle fibers they innervate. Buller et al[36] transacted the nerves to the fast flexor digitorum longus and the slow soleus, and reconnected them so that the motoneurons that originally innervated one of these now grew back to reinnervate the other. Their findings were that fast muscle becomes slower and slow muscle becomes faster after cross-innervation. These results have been confirmed by others; however, it is suggested that only about 50% of the cross-reinnervated fibers undergo a change in histochemical type.

The results above indicate that there is a gradation in the properties of striated muscles in the pelvic floor and associated structures, and structures that are specialized for production of tone usually contain a majority of slow-twitch fibers. These smaller-diameter muscle fibers are innervated by smaller-diameter alpha motoneurons, which also conduct more slowly than those that innervate the fast striated muscle fibers. However, there is increasing evidence of a spectrum of properties, which is not surprising given that the striated muscle of the lower urinary tract must maintain tone, but also respond to transient needs, such as during coughing.

Development of the striated muscle of the urethral sphincter and of its innervation

In humans, the urethral sphincter first develops as a condensation of mesenchyme around the urethra after the division of the cloaca, and puborectalis appears soon after, following the opening of the anal membrane. Striated muscle fibers can be clearly differentiated at 15 weeks.[37] At this time, the smooth muscle layer also becomes thicker at the level of the bladder neck and forms the inner part of the urethral musculature. The urethral sphincter is a functional unit composed of central smooth muscle fibers and peripheral striated muscle fibers, which develops mainly in the anterior wall of the urethra. It appears to have an omega-shaped configuration that is recognizable after 10 weeks of gestation in both sexes.[38] The rectovesical septum was found to be well developed in neonates, and studies of various markers suggested that this membrane was unlikely to lead to apoptosis of muscle cells in the posterior part of the external sphincter in males after birth. These authors also concluded that the function of the muscle may change during development because of neuronal maturation. Oelrich[39] described the male urethral sphincter as a striated muscle in contact with the urethra from the base of the bladder to the perineal membrane. This muscle develops before the prostate, which develops as a growth from the urethra through the striated muscle sphincter. The muscle fibers of the urethral sphincter are 25–30% smaller than those in adjacent muscles.

Borirakchanyavat et al[40] studied the sequential expression of smooth and striated muscle proteins in the intrinsic urethral sphincter, where smooth and striated muscle are in adjacent positions, in embryos, neonates, and in adult rats of different ages. Sections of the urethra and adjacent levator ani muscles were studied histologically with hematoxylin and eosin, anti-alpha-smooth muscle actin, anti-alpha-sarcomeric actin, and anti-striated muscle myosin heavy chain antibodies. Striated muscle myosin heavy chain protein was absent in the urethral sphincter of the embryo and neonate, and was expressed only in the mature myotubule of adults. Alpha-smooth muscle actin was expressed throughout the urethral sphincter of embryonic and neonatal animals. In adults, alpha-smooth muscle actin was confined to the smooth muscle component of the urethra. Co-expression of alpha-smooth and alpha-sarcomeric muscle actin by the striated sphincter myotubule was noted only in neonates. These authors concluded that the development of the intrinsic urethral sphincter is characterized by sequential expression of well-characterized muscle marker proteins. Given the co-expression of smooth and striated muscle markers by developing sphincter myotubule, the authors were tempted to suggest the possibility that trans-differentiation of smooth to striated muscle occurs in the developing genitourinary tract.

Many of the details of these processes have been worked out on animal models, but there has recently been a paper in which the expression of a protein (p27kip1) has been studied in the muscle fibers of levator ani muscle from aging women and has been related to cell differentiation and degeneration in aging.[41] This protein shows changing expression in differentiating skeletal muscle cells during development, and relatively high levels of p27 RNA were detected in the normal human skeletal muscles. These authors indicated that pelvic floor disorders are associated with an appearance of moderate cytoplasmic p27 expression in perimenopausal patients, and are accompanied by hypertrophy and transition of type II into type I fibers. Elderly patients show shrinking and fragmentation of muscle fibers associated with strong cytoplasmic p27 expression relative to a control group of premenopausal patients.

Innervation of the pelvic floor musculature

During the course of development, each muscle fiber is normally innervated by more than one motoneuron, and these are progressively withdrawn so that in the adult each muscle fiber is innervated by only one alpha motoneuron. The process of synapse elimination in rats appears to be dependent on the removal of factors that tend to favor polyneuronal innervation, including basic fibroblast growth factor and ciliary neurotrophic factor.[42] Some of these factors are considered in more detail in the section on the Cell biology of striated muscle. In the child and the adult human the following details apply.

Peripheral motor nerves

The peripheral innervation of the striated muscle has been described recently in reviews.[5,6] Onuf's nucleus is a group of cell bodies of motoneurons that innervates the striated muscle of the anal, urethral, and vaginal sphincters, the pelvic floor, and bulbocavernosus, and is situated in the ventral horn of the sacral cord.

While the striated muscle of the external urethral sphincter appears to be innervated mainly by the pudendal nerve, there is also evidence of a minor innervation that reaches the muscle via a pathway traversing the pelvis or using the pelvic nerve.[43–47] This appears to be the case in the rat, dog, and human, although some authors believe that the pelvic pathway is absent in the dog.[48] The innervation of the distal urethra by the pudendal nerve appears to be essentially unilateral,[49] as is the innervation of the pelvic floor.[50] Some of the innervation of the urethral sphincter, probably sensory in nature, arises from branches of the dorsal nerve of the penis.[51] The role of the pudendal innervation of the striated muscles in generating resistance has been studied and the conclusion made that the pudendal nerve was of major importance in maintaining urethral resistance in healthy human females.[52] However, there are some recent rat studies that suggest that the pudendal nerve can also play a role in urethral relaxation.[53] It has been generally assumed that the innervation of striated muscle in this region is akin to that found in other parts of the somatic musculature.

Pudendal motoneurons are smaller in diameter than many somatic neurons, in keeping with the size of the muscle fibers they innervate, and they also have a spontaneous repetitive discharge. This tonic activity gives rise to the periurethral skeletal muscle tone and about one-third of the intraurethral pressure at rest is attributable to the tonic activity in the motoneurons that innervate these striated muscles.[54] Not only are these motoneurons smaller in size but also their conduction velocities are less[55] and there are few synaptic contacts on their surface,[56] which possibly reflects the lack of muscle spindle afferents in urethral muscle, and the lack of Ia afferent input to these motoneurons.[57] There were relatively few monosynaptic inputs from primary afferents in sphincteric motoneurons.[56,58] In addition, Renshaw cell inhibition and crossed disynaptic inhibition are absent.[56,59]

In humans the tonic activity of the pudendal nerves has been studied by infiltration of local nerve block,[60] during which the rate of urine flow during voluntary micturition fell to about 50% of the control values. Pudendal nerve degeneration during childbirth has been offered as a reason for denervation of both the anal and the urethral sphincter in women.[61–63] In contrast, electromyographic (EMG) studies on the urethral sphincter have shown that in some women who experience urinary retention there is an altered activity of the EUS, which was described as bizarre repetitive discharges (Figure 4.3).[63–65]

Reflex control

One of the unique features of the pelvic floor muscles is that they react to afferent stimuli originating from the skin and muscle of the lower limbs as well as to the state of distention of the bladder and colon: if the bladder is relaxed and filling slowly, then one particular response may occur; however, if the bladder is full and contracting, the behavior

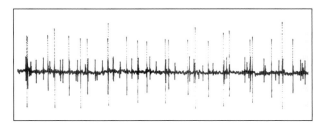

Figure 4.3
Recording of the EMG of the urethral striated muscle in a normal woman during the filling phase of the micturition cycle. The recording was made with a concentric needle electrode. The electrode is picking up signals from at least four different motor units, distinguishable by the amplitude of the spikes. A large increase in the number of units firing is seen during maneuvers that increase intra-abdominal pressure. (From Fowler and Fowler.)

of the pelvic floor may be completely different. Reflex control has been considered previously[5,6] and the following is a short summary of the conclusions.

Somatic reflexes

Cutaneous stimulation of sacral dermatomes is particularly effective in modulating the activity of the pelvic floor and external urinary sphincter. Light touch of the perineal area is known to cause reflex contraction of the pelvic floor muscles and external anal sphincter, and has been used as a clinical test of segmental nerves to this region. Mechanical stimulation of the urethra in both sexes elicits a complex urethrogenital reflex which includes activation of all of the perineal muscles and clonic activity in some. These reflexes show a coordinated pattern of reflex activity involving the somatic, sympathetic, and parasympathetic systems innervating reproductive organs, dependent on a central motor pattern generator within the spinal cord.[66] Painful stimuli in the perineal skin induce a marked increase in EMG activity in periurethral striated muscle;[67] cooling the perineal skin caused a smaller excitation.

Contraction or relaxation of the pelvic floor can also occur in response to proprioceptive stimuli that arise during movement or postural change. Convergence of such afferent inputs from different sources on the activity of pelvic floor and sphincteric muscles is the potential role of afferent impulses from muscles or joints as an adjunct in bladder training and pelvic floor exercises. A variety of maneuvers can cause changes in pelvic floor/sphincteric tone, including attempts to relax and contract the pelvic floor, the Valsalva maneuver, coughing, hip adduction, gluteal contraction, backward tilting of the pelvis, and sit-ups. During hip adduction and gluteal muscle contraction, the urethra contracts concomitantly with the pelvic floor muscles, but not during contraction of the abdominal muscles.

Viscerosomatic reflexes

A guarding reflex that maintains continence by causing urethral sphincter contraction during flow has been described.[68] However, when urethral flow is associated with a bladder contraction, this guarding reflex is overpowered by another reflex that promotes voiding, when relaxation of the sphincter accompanies a rise in bladder pressure or a micturition contraction. Micturition has a major inhibitory influence on the pelvic floor activity in humans. Relaxation of the external anal sphincter occurs at the start of the rise in bladder pressure, and precedes the start of urine flow;[69] it is thought to occur concomitantly with the relaxation of the pelvic floor that allows descent of the bladder.[70] The inhibition extends not only to a depression of tonic activity at rest but also causes a reduction in the excitability of pudendal motoneurons involved in reflex functions.[71] In animal models, colonic distention and stimulation of anal afferents also suppress periurethral muscle EMG activity.[67,72–76]

However, this simple explanation becomes more complicated by studies of the periurethral muscle EMG using fine-wire electrodes directly inserted into the region of the urethral sphincter in anesthetized animals. In some animal models, bladder contractions were accompanied by an alternating oscillatory pattern of on–off bursting in EMG activity during the period when the bladder pressure was rising most rapidly. These periods of oscillatory firing in the periurethral EMG during the rising phase of micturition contraction were never seen in spinal animals, and some authors believe that they are generated by supraspinal mechanisms.[77] A fuller account of the reflex activity of the urethral sphincter can be found in References 5 and 6.

Role of central pathways in the control of the pelvic floor musculature

Anatomy

The central nervous control over the pelvic floor muscles and associated sphincters depends on important descending pathways from regions of the brainstem (particularly the pons and medulla) and the hypothalamus. The dorsolateral pons contains two regions, one of which excites, and the other inhibits tonic activity in the pelvic floor muscles. These regions are close to Barrington's micturition center of the cat and the dorsolateral pontine tegmentum of the rat.[79,80,82] These projections are fairly specific in that they target pudendal motoneurons innervating the urethral sphincter, but not those supplying the anal sphincter. In animals, descending pathways from the pontine micturition center appear to be involved directly in inhibiting the pudendal motoneurons in Onuf's nucleus, whereas those from the L-region facilitate and excite the sphincteric motoneurons (Figure 4.4). Interneurons that utilize γ-aminobutyric acid (GABA)

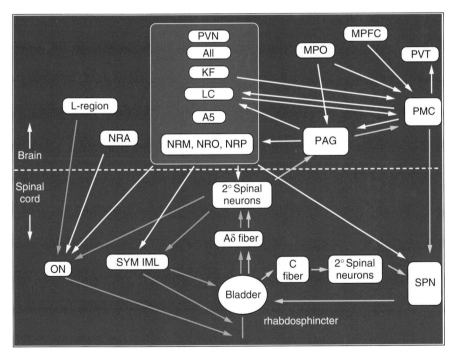

Figure 4.4
Diagram of documented neuroanatomical connections of the primary and secondary components of storage and micturition reflexes. The connections of the primary components of the storage reflexes are shown in red, whereas the connections of the primary components of the micturition reflexes are shown in gold. The connections of the secondary (or modulatory) components of the reflexes are shown in white. Abbreviations: A11, A11 group of dopaminergic neurons; A5, A5 group of noradrenergic neurons; KF, Kollicke–Fuse nucleus; LC, locus coeruleus; MPFC, medial prefrontal cortex; MPO, medial preoptic nucleus of the hypothalamus; NRA, nucleus retroambiguus; NRM, nucleus raphe magnus; NRO, nucleus raphe obscuris; NRP, nucleus raphe pallidus; ON, Onuf's nucleus; PAG, periaqueductal gray; PMC, pontine micturition center; PVN, paraventricular nucleus; PVT, periventricular thalamic nucleus; SPN, sacral parasympathetic nucleus; SYM IML, sympathetic intermediolateral nucleus.

appear to be responsible for the reciprocal inhibition of the sphincteric motoneurons during micturition mediated within the sacral cord (see Figure 4.6).[6,78,83]

The paraventricular nuclei of the hypothalamus (which contain oxytocin), and nuclei in the brainstem, including the ipsilateral caudal pontine lateral reticular formation, and the contralateral caudal nucleus retroambiguus also project to the pudendal motoneurons in Onuf's nucleus[81] via the ipsilateral anterior and contralateral white matter in the spinal cord.

The medullary raphe nuclei and nucleus gigantocellularis reticularis also have a predominantly inhibitory action on bladder motility and sphincteric reflexes.[65,84,85] We now have results from positron emission tomography (PET) studies and transcortical stimulation that indicate that in humans there are mechanisms that correlate well with what was found in previous animals studies.

The nucleus retroambiguus, located in the caudal ventrolateral medulla, contains motoneurons involved in respiration and control of abdominal musculature. In addition, this nucleus has a prominent projection to Onuf's nucleus.[80,86] It has been speculated that this projection activates sphincter motoneurons coincident with activation of the abdominal muscles during forceful expiration such as coughing, laughing, and sneezing. More detailed pharmacological data on these pathways are available.[6]

The CNS control of the striated muscle of the lower urinary tract during micturition in humans

Brainstem

Several PET studies have provided evidence that the brainstem is involved in the control of micturition and the external sphincters: men and women were studied during micturition and showed an increased blood flow in the dorsal part of the pons close to the fourth ventricle, an area analogous to the pontine micturition center in the cat (Figure 4.5).[87,88] A second group of volunteers was asked to micturate during scanning, but were unable to do so. These individuals showed no activation in the dorsal pons, but did have an area of high blood flow in the ventral pons, similar to the location of the 'L-region' – the pontine storage center in cats. It would appear that these subjects contracted their urethral sphincters and withheld their urine, although they had a full bladder and tried to urinate. There is therefore a reasonable correlation between the information in cats and humans concerning the brainstem regulation of voiding and urine storage (Figure 4.6).[88]

Cortex and hypothalamus: the voluntary control of the striated muscle of the lower urinary tract

PET scanning studies in humans have shown that two cortical areas – the cingulate gyrus and the prefrontal cortex, and the hypothalamus, including the preoptic area – are activated during micturition.[87–90] Cerebral blood flow in the cingulate gyrus was significantly decreased during voluntary withholding of urine and during the urge to void. The prefrontal cortex is active when micturition takes place and during involuntary urine withholding. Possibly, activation of the prefrontal cortex and the anterior cingulate gyrus do not reflect specific involvement in micturition, but more in general mechanisms, such as attention and response selection. The prefrontal cortex plays a role in making the decision whether or not micturition should take place at that particular time and place. Forebrain lesions including the anterior cingulate gyrus are known to cause urge incontinence.[91] The cingulate gyrus influences strongly descending pathways involved in the facilitation of motoneurons and interneurons.

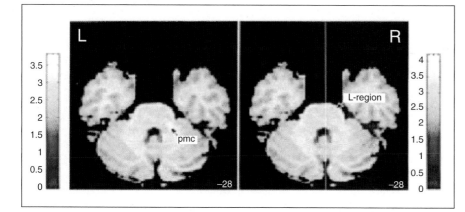

Figure 4.5
PET scan of brainstem with increased activity in vicinity of pontine micturition center (PMC) during voiding. Alternatively, increased activity in L-region association with holding of urine. (After Blok et al [88])

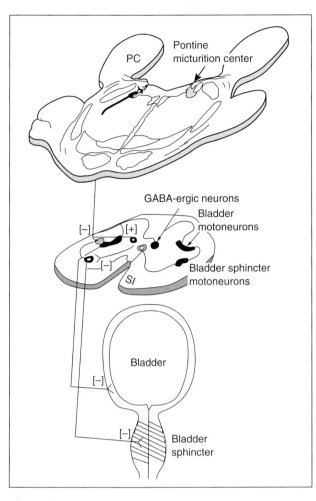

Figure 4.6
Coordination of voiding with external urethral sphincter.
Descending glutamatergic input to sacral spinal cord excites
bladder neurons in sacral parasympathetic neurons (SPN).
Simultaneous activation of GABA neurons inhibits sphincter
neurons in Onuf's nucleus. Conversely, during attempts at urine
storage activation of GABA neurons provide input to bladder
neurons while providing excitatory input to sphincter neurons.

Another PET study on adult female volunteers to
identify brain structures involved in the voluntary motor
control of the pelvic floor focused on four conditions:

- rest
- repetitive pelvic floor straining
- sustained pelvic floor straining
- sustained abdominal straining.

These investigations show that two separate areas of the
motor cortex are activated during pelvic floor contraction
and during contraction of the abdominal musculature.
Concomitant activations of the cerebellum, supplementary

motor cortex, and thalamus were also commonly present,
and the anterior cingulate gyrus was also activated during
sustained pelvic floor straining.

Patients with lesions restricted to the basal ganglia or
thalamus appear to have normal urethral sphincter function. These patients can voluntarily contract the striated
sphincter and abort or considerably lessen the effect of the
abnormal micturition reflex, when an impending involuntary contraction or its onset is sensed. In contrast, patients
with cerebrovascular lesions in the cerebral cortex and/or
internal capsule are unable to forcefully contract the
striated sphincter under these circumstances.

In humans, electrophysiological studies by Hansen[92] also
support the view that cortical centers are involved in the
descending control of pelvic floor muscles. He provided
evidence that the state of the bladder has a significant
influence on sphincteric reflex function. Voluntary influences on the pelvic floor, anal sphincter, urethral sphincter,
and bulbocavernosus muscles of man were studied by
transcranial cortical stimulation using either high voltages
or short-duration magnetic pulses.[92–95] In contrast to the
effects of a small stimulus to the cortex, which causes a
short burst of activity in leg muscles, the responses of the
anal and urethral sphincters were maintained for 1–2 s,
despite the short latency. Voluntary contraction of the
external anal sphincter could cause facilitation of the
response to cortical stimulation in a number of other muscles, such as tibialis anterior. In humans, it had been
believed that pelvic floor muscles increase their activity
during bladder filling. Hansen[92] also showed that the
excitability of pudendal motoneurons could be altered by
bladder filling: initially, when bladder volume is low, there
appears to be some inhibition of pudendal motoneurons,
but when the bladder is full, the motoneurons are facilitated. This facilitation may have been voluntary, as a consequence of sensory information from the bladder.
Changes in the excitability of pudendal motoneurons have
been reported in humans and in cats.[71,85,96]

STRUCTURE AND FUNCTION
FOLLOWING NEUROLOGICAL
LESIONS
Cell biology of striated muscle
and the peripheral nerve and
muscle junction

The amount of specific knowledge on the striated muscle of
the lower urinary tract is relatively sparse compared with that
on other somatic muscles; however, there is a large and
increasing body of information derived from the application

of molecular and gene knockout techniques to somatic muscles that is relevant to the maintenance and regeneration/reinnervation of the muscles of the lower urinary tract. This information, if applied to the muscles of the lower urinary tract, will provide a tremendous impetus to investigate the potential of the new molecules that are being recognized as playing a part in some of the cellular responses associated with stress and strain in pelvic tissues. For example, we are now beginning to understand the molecular basis of the muscle response to stress and the replacement of muscle with fibrous tissue; similarly, we are beginning to understand the factors that operate when stretch of nerves results in partial muscle denervation, and, more importantly, the functional reinnervation of the tissues. The following section aims to highlight some of the mechanisms that operate in the maintenance of the mechanical properties of muscles and the nerves that innervate them, nerve–muscle junction, the factors that are essential for new functional connections following stress and strain injuries, and the factors that operated during development. Some of the molecules and genes that regulate these processes will be considered individually and in greater detail towards the end of this section.

Denervation-induced atrophy

Denervation-induced atrophy is a common clinical observation that is used in diagnosis of disorders of the lower motoneuron, and there should be no surprise that changes in various muscle proteins occur in this condition. For example, Boudriau et al[97] showed that the cytoskeletal lattice in rat fast- and slow-twitch skeletal muscle atrophied following denervation. However, the relative content of dystrophin and desmin were reduced in the slow-twitch muscle (soleus), whereas significant increases were shown in the fast-twitch gastrocnemius muscle. In both muscles, a major increase in alpha-tubulin levels was observed, associated with a distinct rearrangement of the microtubule network toward a predominantly longitudinal alignment. It was concluded that slow-twitch muscles are relatively more susceptible to denervation-induced atrophy.

Concomitant changes occur in the sarcoplasmic reticulum, where the activity of the calcium pump appears to be decreased in both fast- and slow-twitch muscles following denervation, and these changes were associated with prolongation of twitch contraction times and slowed rates of tension development.[98] These results, however, contrast with some of the earlier findings[99] which suggested that denervation resulted in decreases in calcium pump activity in fast- but not slow-twitch muscle. Other calcium-binding proteins, such as calsequestrin and parvalbumin, were present in higher concentrations in fast-twitch muscles following denervation. Neuromuscular activity has a modulatory effect, and the expression of parvalbumin is greatly enhanced by phasic, and drastically decreased by tonic, motor neuron activity.

Effects of axotomy on motoneurons: reinnervation following axotomy

Following axotomy, changes occur in the distal portion of the nerve (fragmentation of the axons and degeneration of the Schwann cells) and changes of dendritic fields and other paraments in the cell bodies within the spinal cord. As the cut neuron terminals begin to grow back toward the peripheral tissues, dramatic changes can be seen, including up-regulation of ciliary neurotrophic factor alpha (CNTF alpha) observed in denervated rat muscle[100] and other neurotrophins as well as their receptors.[101] These neurotrophins are produced endogenously by the lesioned nerve and are capable of significantly accelerating the regeneration of both sensory and motor axons after peripheral nerve damage.

Schwann cells also play a role in guiding growing or regenerating nerve terminals back into paralyzed and partially denervated muscles. Trachtenberg and Thompson[102] found that application of a soluble neuregulin isoform, glial growth factor II (GGF2), to developing rat muscles alters the morphology of the Schwann cells at the motoneuron terminal, the nerve terminals themselves, and postjunctional region of the muscle fibers. The Schwann cells put out processes and migrate away from the synapse, and the nerve terminals retract from acetylcholine receptor-rich synaptic sites, and their axons grow, in association with Schwann cells, to the ends of the muscle. These axons made effective synapses only after withdrawal of the GGF2.

Our understanding of the basic events underlying synapse formation, maintenance, and plasticity has progressed considerably over the last few years, primarily because of the numerous studies that have focused on the nerve–muscle junction and the use of electrophysiological, morphological, pharmacological, and recombinant DNA technology. We will consider two scenarios: first, that occurring during development; and second, that pertinent to reinnervation following injury.

Molecular factors involved in stability of synapses

Neurotrophins and other trophic factors

Neurotrophins, a family of protein growth factors structurally related to the nerve growth factor (NGF), include neurotrophin-1 (nerve growth factor; NGF), brain-derived neurotrophic factor (BDNF), neurotrophin-3 (NT-3), and neurotrophin-4/5 (NT-4/5). Other growth factors include basic fibroblast growth factor (bFGF), glial-derived neurotrophic factor (GDNF), and ciliary neurotrophic factor (CNTF).

A variety of neurotrophins and growth factors are expressed in the skeletal muscle during the critical period of synapse formation.[103] The relationship between neurotrophins and the development of the nerve–muscle junction during development is not completely worked out, but it is known that during fetal life the molecular nature of the nicotinic receptor differs from the adult: the gamma subunit of the acetylcholine receptor (AChR) in the fetus is replaced by the epsilon subunit in the adult. This changeover in postsynaptic molecular organization can be interfered with by genetic manipulation that prevents the normal development of the receptor.[104] The result was that the structural development of the endplate was compromised and there was a severely reduced AChR density and a profound reorganization of AChR-associated components of the postsynaptic membrane and cytoskeleton. The development of the motor endplate appears to depend on the activity of muscle cell nuclei that are located in the vicinity of the postsynaptic membrane. NT-3 appears to be involved in this process.[103] Jasmin et al[105] proposed that transcription processes in these nuclei are functionally different to those of nuclei of the extrasynaptic sarcoplasm. Thus, renewal of proteins concerned with neuromuscular transmission in the postsynaptic membrane appear to occur via a mechanism involving the activation of genes in nuclei adjacent to the nerve–muscle junction using chemical signals originating from motoneurons. Such interaction between presynaptic nerve terminals and the postsynaptic sarcoplasm indicates that the entire signal transduction pathway is compartmentalized at the level of the neuromuscular junction.

Such chemical signals are discussed later and include neuregulin (NRG) and agrin, and there is evidence that these are involved both during development and recovery from injury. NT-4 can be produced by myocytes, and influences the development of presynaptic neuronal terminals, and such regulation is specific to the axonal branch that innervates that myocyte;[106] a consequence of this is that neurotrophin-induced synaptic changes can be spatially restricted to the site of neurotrophin secretion and appears not to spread to neighboring synapses, i.e. the part of the motor unit subjected to NT-4 is targeted individually, and the effects do not spread to other terminals of the motoneuron.

CNTF is a member of the neurotrophin family that, amongst other things, regulates agrin-induced postsynaptic differentiation,[107] induces axons and their nerve terminals to sprout within adult skeletal muscles,[108] has trophic actions on denervated skeletal muscle,[109] and is highly correlated with the reinnervation activity of Schwann cells.[110]

Neuregulin

Nicotinic acetylcholine receptors (nAChRs) are present locally in the sarcolemma at the neuromuscular junction as a result of the expression of genes in the nuclei of the muscle fibers immediately underneath the endplate. The motor nerve terminal seems to influence the induction of these genes within sub-endplate nuclei because of locally released factors, including neuregulin and agrin, that derive from presynaptic endings, and some neurotrophins. Neuregulin activates a Ras/MAP kinase signaling cascade, which ultimately induces nAChR epsilon-subunit gene expression in the sub-endplate nuclei.[111] Neuregulin appears to act on the postsynaptic erbB3 and erbB4 receptors by a tyrosine phosphorylation step, and these receptors are located at synaptic sites.[112,113] Curare, which blocks nicotinic receptors, reduces synaptic neuregulin expression in a dose-dependent manner, yet has little effect on synaptic agrin or a muscle-derived heparan sulfate proteoglycan. This modulation of postsynaptic structures by alterations of synaptic activity and the expression of synaptic regulatory factors is part of the mechanism by which nerves influence the function of muscle. A number of factors change as a result of such blockade of electrical activity, including an increase in the number and a decrease in the size of AChRs, reductions in brain-derived neurotrophic factor and NT-3, and these were thought to indicate the existence of a local, positive feedback loop between synaptic regulatory factors that translates activity into structural changes at neuromuscular synapses.[114] This loop was targeted in some studies in which the neuroregulin-1 gene was disrupted: knockouts showed peripheral neuronal projections defasciculated and displayed aberrant branching patterns within their targets. Motor nerve terminals were transiently associated with broad bands of postsynaptic AChR clusters. Initially, Schwann cell precursors accompanied peripheral projections; but later, Schwann cells were absent from axons in the periphery. Following initial stages of synapse formation, sensory and motor nerves withdrew and degenerated. These studies suggest that NRG-1-mediated signaling is involved in the normal maintenance of synapses; however, the interactions are more complex, involving the motoneuron terminal, muscle, and the Schwann cells at the nerve–muscle junction. It appears that NRG-1 plays a central role in the normal maintenance of peripheral synapses, and ultimately in the survival of CRD-NRG-1-expressing neurons.[115]

Agrins

Neuregulin, however, is not the only signal that influences the expression of the nicotinic receptors: another is a factor, agrin, which causes the aggregation of the nicotinic receptor molecules at synaptic sites.[112] Agrin was originally isolated from the basal lamina of the synaptic cleft, and has been found to be synthesized and secreted by motoneurons. It triggers formation of AChR clusters on cultured myotubes,[116] and, when deficient, the postsynaptic AChR aggregates are markedly reduced in number, size, and density in muscles of agrin-deficient mutant mice. These results support the hypothesis that agrin is a critical organizer of postsynaptic differentiation. Animals deficient in this factor show abnormal intramuscular nerve branching and presynaptic differentiation.

The same group[117] found that differentiation of the postsynaptic membrane at the neuromuscular junction requires (a) agrin (derived from the presynaptic nerve), (b) MuSK, a component of the agrin receptor in muscle, and (c) rapsyn, a protein that interacts with AChRs. From a functional viewpoint, it appears that agrin works through MuSK to determine a synaptogenic region within which synaptic differentiation occurs.[117]

Rapsyn

The role of rapsyn in the organization of the nerve–muscle junction was studied by Bartlett et al,[118] who found that its absence resulted in pre- and postsynaptic defects, including failure to cluster AChRs. The mRNA level for CNTF was decreased in the rapsyn-deficient muscles compared with those of controls, although those for NGF, BDNF, NT-3, and TGF-beta$_2$ were not affected. These authors suggested that failure to form postsynaptic specializations in rapsyn-deficient mice caused an alteration in the CNTF cytokine signaling pathway within skeletal muscle, which may, in turn, account for the increased muscle–nerve branching and motoneuron survival seen in rapsyn-deficient mice. This conclusion is supported by the observations of English and Schwartz[42] who found that the postnatal elimination of polyneuronal innervation can be inhibited by bFGF and CNTF.

These new data indicate the complexity of the dynamic relationships that maintain the nerve–muscle junction and offer some hope that new molecular methods will become available to aid reinnervation after trauma.

Regeneration of striated muscle: interactions with connective tissue

The recovery of muscle function following injury is a challenging problem if techniques are to be developed to improve striated muscle function when it is weakened by injury. Kasemkijwattana et al,[119,120] and Menetrey et al[121] observed a massive muscle regeneration occurring in the first 2 weeks following injury that is subsequently followed by the development of muscle fibrosis. The possibility of enhancement of muscle growth and regeneration, as well as the prevention of fibrotic development, was considered, and three growth factors capable of enhancing myoblast proliferation and differentiation *in vitro* and improving the healing of the injured muscle *in vivo* were identified. The three growth factors capable of improving muscle regeneration and improving muscle force in an injured muscle were bFGF, insulin-like growth factor (IGF), and NGF. The same group considered the use of gene transfer using an adenovirus to deliver an efficient and persistent expression of these growth factors to the injured muscle. These studies may indicate a new strategy to aid efficient muscle healing with complete functional recovery, following muscle contusion and strain injury.

Another helpful molecule in muscle regeneration following crush injury appears to be leukemia inhibitory factor (LIF). Targeted infusion of LIF in both normal and LIF knockout animals stimulated muscle regeneration, but the stimulation observed was much greater in the mutant animals than in controls.[122]

The process of fibrosis may be associated with the activities of another family of membrane proteins, the integrins, which are responsible for the regulation of interactions between the myocytes and the extracellular matrix.[123] Integrin beta-1D provides a strong link between the cytoskeleton and extracellular matrix necessary to support mechanical tension during muscle contraction. It is expressed in the cell membranes of striated muscle tissues, and binds to both cytoskeletal and extracellular matrix proteins.

Angiogenesis and capillary density

Insulin-like growth factor-1 (IGF-1) also appears to be involved in the regulation of size of myocytes and the capillary density.[124] Muscle hypoplasia results from disruption of the IGF-1 gene, and its effects are seen on cell proliferation, differentiation, and apoptosis during development; the concomitant reduction in capillary density may result from both direct and indirect influences on angiogenesis.

Reflex control of the striated muscle of the lower urinary tract following spinal injury

It has been known for over 50 years that somatic events influence the bladder of paraplegic patients,[125] and recently there is increasing evidence for a role of viscero or somatic convergence in the control of the human pelvic floor. Such interactions are particularly true in patients with overactive bladders. Another feature of human paraplegia is that some patients develop automatic bladders and achieve some degree of sphincter inhibition during micturition, whereas others have a hypertonic sphincter and require regular catheterization. In experimental studies for the last 30 years, scientists have reported that the motor pathway to the external sphincters and pelvic floor is subject to control from events in viscera and the segmental innervation of somatic structures. The pathways that control the striated muscle of the external sphincter as well as the detrusor smooth muscle are summarized in Figures 4.4 and 4.6. Figure 4.4 indicates that certain nuclei in the brainstem are of particular importance in the regulation of the external sphincter, including the L-region and the nucleus retroambiguus which have major projections to Onuf's nucleus, and are of particular importance in maintaining continence and facilitating urine storage.[6]

In a study of chronic spinal cats, Sasaki et al[126] found detrusor–sphincter dyssynergia in about 50%, whereas the other 50% achieved some sphincter inhibition during bladder contractions. Sphincteric responses to stimuli were affected by the state of bladder filling, and when the bladder was empty, tactile stimulation of the perineal skin caused an increase in EUS activity and detrusor contractions in spinal animals, the opposite of what occurs in animals with a normal intact neuroaxis. In contrast, when the bladder was full, rhythmic detrusor contractions were present, and tactile stimulation caused EUS activity and bladder contractions, and noxious stimulation of the skin resulted in an immediate contraction of the bladder, followed by some depression of ongoing rhythmic contractions. The effects on the sphincter depended on the state of the sphincter, and when dyssynergia was present, innocuous tactile stimulation was accompanied by a prolonged increase in EUS activity that was not inhibited during micturition contractions. Reflex responses of the sphincter induced by electrical stimulation of afferents in the pudendal nerve were inhibited in spinal animals with a normal synergic relationship between the bladder and urethra, but in dyssynergia, relaxation of the sphincter and inhibition of pudendal nerve reflex responses during bladder contractions were absent.

The clinical literature clearly distinguishes between lesions of the spinal cord in which the peripheral innervation of the striated muscle of the pelvic floor and sphincters is intact, and lesions in which there is peripheral denervation. There may also be a small group where there is a mix of a high lesion and some peripheral denervation. Perlow and Diokno[127] found that a neurogenic bladder developed in spinal patients with lesions at T7 and above, whereas peripheral denervation was common in lesions at vertebral T11 and below. Vesicosphincteric dyssynergia developed in about two-thirds of their patients with neurogenic bladders; the increased excitability of pudendal motoneurons was associated with increased excitability of the bulbocavernosus reflex.[128] During the phase of spinal shock following spinal cord injury in humans, bladder filling was found to be accompanied by an increased urethral resistance in the bladder neck region, not associated with an increased EMG activity of the pelvic floor,[129] presumably associated with smooth muscle activity. Areflexia could also be present. In some patients with spinal cord injuries, bladder contraction and distention of the rectum resulted in inhibition of EMG activity in the external urethral and anal sphincters, whereas in the levator ani there was sometimes an initial excitation of the muscle.[130]

Rossier et at,[131] using pudendal nerve blockade and injections of phentoamine to dissociate the effects of striated and smooth muscle, found that the dyssynergia was due to the passage of impulses along the pudendal nerves, and that about two-thirds of the urethral pressure was due to striated muscle tone developed by this impulse activity – rather more than in normal subjects.[60] Rossier et al[131] commented that there was no evidence of a sympathetic innervation of striated muscle. However, more recent experiments on cats have suggested that the cholinergic preganglionic fibers of the sympathetic system can grow and form functional contacts with denervated striated muscle following the experimental section of spinal roots.[132] Possibly a more detailed study of reinnervation of the striated muscle of the lower urinary tract in humans would support this possibility.

Investigation of the neural connectivity can now be performed using a variety of neurophysiological and radiological techniques. Thiry and Deltenre[133] found that electrical stimulation of the head can be used to assess the volitional as well as segmental and suprasegmental influences on the behavior of the external urethral sphincter; however, subjects were not tolerant of the electrical stimuli. Magnetic stimulation of the brain, spinal cord, and peripheral nerves, however, has been pioneered in the last decade or so and appears to be tolerated better; its use has had considerable impact on the study of the neural control of the striated muscle of the anal sphincter.[95,134–143] It has most recently enabled the study of the control of different parts of the sphincteric apparatus around the anus, and has allowed the effects of birth trauma on different parts of the external anal sphincter to be defined.[144–146] In the lower urinary tract there were early demonstrations of the usefulness of the technique in studying the central and peripheral pathways to the external urethral sphincter,[93,147] perineum,[148] pelvic floor,[149] and bulbocavernosus.[95,139,150] Magnetic stimulation has also been used to confirm the presence of complete or partial lesion of the spinal cord and functional characteristics of the latter.[151] The potential therapeutic use of magnetic stimulation has been pioneered by Craggs in hyperreflexic states.[152,153]

An alternative approach to the hypertonic sphincter has been used by Phelan et al[154] who reported the results following injection of botulinus toxin into the spastic urethral sphincter. Botulinus toxin (Botox) acts presynaptically to prevent the release of acetylcholine at the nerve–muscle junction. It is a very powerful lethal neurotoxin and is delivered in very small doses in these studies, and acts to dissociate the link between high frequencies of impulses in the pudendal motoneurons and the contractile response. These authors claimed that this could be a useful treatment for some patients' sphincter dyssynergia.

In a recent study of the lower urinary tract in patients with neurological disorders, Sakakibara et al[155] studied patients with detrusor–sphincter dyssynergia, and found that one group had uninhibited external sphincter relaxation. In these patients there was an abnormal reduction of external urethral sphincter pressure (by 64 ± 27 cmH$_2$O (mean $\pm$ standard deviation)) and variation in both the sphincteric pressure and EMG. Fluoroscopy showed that bladder neck opening was commonly associated with extreme urge sensation. This appears possibly to be the normal reflex response to bladder contraction involving a major reduction in efferent activity to the striated muscle. However, other patients with detrusor–external sphincter dyssynergia failed to relax their sphincters during attempted voiding, and fluoroscopic imaging showed an incomplete or absent urethral opening at the external sphincter. The mean reduction of urethral pressure during attempted voiding in this group was only 6.4 ± 6.7 cmH$_2$O and 5.0 ± 9.5 cmH$_2$O (females and males, respectively). Possibly this group were unable to inhibit the pudendal motoneuron activity. These results correlate reasonably well with the study on cats by Sasaki et al.[126]

Reflex control of the striated muscle of the lower urinary tract following other neurological lesions

Parkinson's disease

Chemical or surgical lesions of dopamine-containing neurons in the basal ganglia in the rat cause changes in motor activity akin to those seen in Parkinson's disease, and the urodynamic results suggest that the bladder of these animals is overactive. The dopaminergic nerves that are affected in Parkinson's disease projections of dopamine-containing fibers from the substantia nigra have opposing effects on the bladder, depending on whether the D1 or D2 receptors are activated. Activation of D2 receptors are excitatory to micturition, whereas D1 receptors are inhibitory.

In humans, Pavlakis et al[156] described detrusor dyssynergia in the majority of Parkinson's disease patients studied, and the EMG investigations showed that a few patients had a voluntary contraction of the perineal floor in an attempt to prevent leakage, whereas others had sphincter bradykinesia which was associated with the generalized skeletal muscle

hypertonicity found in parkinsonism. This has been reinvestigated recently by Stocchi et al,[157] who found that incomplete pelvic floor relaxation was present in about one-quarter of patients, whereas another quarter had hyperreflexia associated with vesicosphincteric synergy; a further 10% had hyperreflexia with vesicosphincteric synergy associated with incomplete pelvic floor relaxation. Urological manifestations of Parkinson's disease tend to be associated with the severity and duration of the condition.

Stroke

A commonly used experimental model of stroke involves ligation of the middle cerebral artery of the rat, which results in cerebral ischemia and infarction. The urodynamic status of this model is characterized by bladder overactivity consistent with the loss of cerebral inhibition of the lower urinary tract.[86,158] Urodynamic studies on incontinent patients following a stroke showed a disturbance in the function of the striated muscle of the lower urinary tract including detrusor–sphincter dyssynergia.[159] Sakakibara et al[160] reported bladder hyperreflexia, detrusor–sphincter dyssynergia, and uninhibited sphincter relaxation in patients with stroke. More recently the same group[161] demonstrated that frontal lobe disease may cause disorders of storage as well as of voiding; they observed uninhibited sphincter relaxation and unrelaxing sphincter on voiding and disturbances of bladder function in these patients.

Regeneration within the central nervous system

This is not the place for a review of regeneration of neural connections with the CNS, but the topic is worth a mention because such a lot of effort is currently going into this area and producing results. Spinal rats have been able to show some recovery of motor function as a result of these experiments and they provide hope for the future. Examples are the use of neurotrophins to overcome the barrier that exists for muscle sensory nerve regeneration in the dorsal root entry zone, through to the use of stem cells to facilitate the development of new functional connections across a spinal cord lesion.[162–165] The literature is large, and these examples are provided as an indication that spinal transection, previously viewed as a permanent, irrecoverable situation, may yet be conquered.

Conclusions

The control of striated muscle during neurological lesions is an active area of study, and is producing results that are relevant to the problems of the overactive or neurogenic bladder, whether these are caused by peripheral nerve or CNS lesions.

This chapter encompasses the structure and function of the sphincteric muscles and their innervation, looking at the molecular, structural, and physiological factors that are responsible for the generation of skeletal muscle tone, and the changes that can occur following denervation, and during development and aging. The physiological organization of Onuf's nucleus and the reflex control of the tonic activity that is essential for the generation of maintained force in slow-twitch muscle fibers is an important part of the normal function of this system. However, following denervation, say as a result of trauma, the function of the system changes and we are beginning to understand some of the molecular signals necessary for reinnervation, and some of the factors that influence the conversion of denervated muscle into fibrous tissue, and the changes in vascularization that may limit muscular performance. It is in this area that a substantial body of new work can be expected to yield molecules that may be developed as therapeutic agents in manipulating the cellular responses to injuries.

CNS lesions give rise to changes in striated muscle tone in the lower urinary tract and elsewhere, and sections concerned with the changes in striated muscle function following spinal cord injury and other neurological lesions, such as parkinsonism and stroke, are included. Recovery of function following CNS lesions is mentioned briefly because of the importance of the topic and the current excitement in relation to recovery from spinal injuries.

References

1. Torrens M, Morrison JFB. The physiology of the lower urinary tract. London: Springer-Verlag, 1987.

2. Jordan D. The central control of autonomic function. In: Burnstock G, ed. The autonomic nervous system. Amsterdam: Overseas Publishers Association, 1997:304.

3. Morrison JFB. Central nervous control of the bladder. In: Jordan D, ed. Central nervous control of autonomic function, Vol. 11, The Autonomic nervous system. Amsterdam: Overseas Publishers Association, 1997:304.

4. de Groat WC, Downie JW, Levin RM, et al. Basic neurophysiology and neuropharmacology. In: Abrams P, Khoury S, Wein A, eds. Incontinence. UK: Health Publications, 1999:105–154.

5. Morrison JFB. Physiology of the pelvic floor. In: Corcos J, Schick E, eds. The urinary sphincter. New York: Marcel Dekker, 2001:71–87.

6. Morrison JFB, Brading A, Steers WD, et al. Neurophysiology and neuropharmacology: 2nd International Consultation on Incontinence, Paris 2001. In: Abrams P, Khoury S, Wein A, eds. Incontinence, 2nd edn. UK: Health Publications, 2002:83–164.

7. Gosling J, Alm P, Bartsch G, et al. Gross anatomy of the urinary tract. In: Abrams P, Khoury S, Wein A, eds. Incontinence, 1st edn. UK: Health Publications, 1999:21–56.

8. DeLancey J, Gosling J, Creed K, et al. Gross anatomy and cell biology of the urinary tract. In: Abrams P, Cardozo L, Khoury S, Wein A, eds. Incontinence, 2nd edn. UK: Health Publications, 2002:17–82.

9. Greenland JE, Brading AF. Urinary bladder blood flow changes during the micturition cycle in a conscious pig model. J Urol 1996; 156:1858–1861.

10. Xiao CG, de Groat WC, Godec et al. "Skin-CNS-bladder" reflex pathway for micturition after spinal cord injury and its underlying mechanisms. J Urol 1999;162:936–942.

11. Thind P. The significance of smooth and striated muscles in sphincter function of the urethra in healthy women. Neurourol Urodyn 1995; 14:585.

12. Andersson PO, Malmgren A, Uvelius B. Functional responses of different muscle types of the female rat urethra in vitro. Acta Physiolog Scand 1990; 140(3):365–372.

13. DeLancey JO. Functional anatomy of the female lower urinary tract and pelvic floor. Ciba Found Symp 1990; 151:57–69.

14. DeLancey JO, Starr RA. Histology of the connection between the vagina and levator ani muscles. Implications for urinary tract function. J Reprod Med 1990; 35:765–771.

15. DeLancey JO. The pathophysiology of stress urinary incontinence in women and its implications for surgical treatment. World J Urol 1997; 15:268–274.

16. Haeusler G, Sam C, Chiari A, et al. Effect of spinal anaesthesia on the lower urinary tract in continent women. Br J Obst Gynaecol 1998; 105(1):103–106.

17. Ranvier L. De quelques faits relatifs a l'histologie et a la physiologie des muscles stries. Arch Physiol Norm Pathol 1874; 1:5–18.

18. Burke RE. Motor units: anatomy, physiology and functional organisation. In: Brookhart JM, Mountcastle VB, eds. Handbook of physiology, Sect. 1, the nervous system, Vol. II, Part 1. American Physiological Society 1981:345–422.

19. Henneman E, Olson CB. Relations between structure and function in the design of skeletal muscles. J Neurophysiol 1965; 28:581–598.

20. Gosling JA, Dixon JS, Critchley HO, Thompson SA. A comparative study of the human external sphincter and periurethral levator ani muscles. Br J Urol 1981; 53:35–41.

21. Dahlstedt AJ, Katz A, Westerblad H. Role of myoplasmic phosphate in contractile function of skeletal muscle: studies on creatine kinase-deficient mice. J Physiol 2001; 533:379–388.

22. Steeghs K, Oerlemans F, de Haan A, et al. Cytoarchitectural and metabolic adaptations in muscles with mitochondrial and cytosolic creatine kinase deficiencies. Mol Cell Biochem 1998; 184:183–194.

23. Jansson E, Sylven C. Myoglobin concentration in single type I and type II muscle fibres in man. Histochemistry 1983; 78(1):121–124.

24. Grange RW, Meeson A, Chin E, et al. Functional and molecular adaptations in skeletal muscle of myoglobin-mutant mice. Am J Physiol Cell Physiol 2001; 281:C1487–C1494.

25. Tokunaka S, Murakami U, Ohashi K, et al. Electrophoretic and ultrastructural analysis of the rabbit's striated external urethral sphincter. J Urol 1984; 132:1040–1043.

26. Tokunaka S, Murakami U, Okamura K, et al. The fiber type of the rabbits' striated external urethral sphincter: electrophoretic analysis of myosin. J Urol 1986; 135:427–430.

27. Tokunaka S, Okamura K, Fujii H, Yachiku S. The proportions of fiber types in human external urethral sphincter: electrophoretic analysis of myosin. Urol Res 1990; 18:341–344.

28. Okamura K, Tokunaka S, Yachiku S. Histochemical study of human external urethral sphincter. Nippon Hinyokika Gakkai Zasshi (Jpn J Urol) 1991; 82:1487–1493.

29. Tokunaka S, Fujii H, Okamura K, et al. Biochemical analysis of the external urethral sphincter of female rabbits. Nippon Hinyokika Gakkai Zasshi (Jpn J Urol) 1992; 83:493–497.

30. Tokunaka S, Fujii H, Hashimoto H, Yachiku S. Proportions of fiber types in the external urethral sphincter of young nulliparous and old multiparous rabbits. Urol Res 1993; 21:121–124.

31. Fujii H, Tokunaka S, Okamura K, et al. Biochemical analysis of the external striated urethral sphincter of male rabbits. Difference in the proportions of muscle fiber types in the male rabbit external urethral sphincter by axial subdivisional study. Nippon Hinyokika Gakkai Zasshi (Jpn J Urol) 1994; 85:1534–1542.

32. Fujii H, Tokunaka S, Yachiku S. Effects of chronic low-frequency electrical stimulation on the external urethral sphincter of male rabbits – electrophoretic analyses of myosin light and heavy chain isoforms. Nippon Hinyokika Gakkai Zasshi (Jpn J Urol) 1995; 86:1240–1248.

33. Ho KM, McMurray G, Brading AF, et al. Nitric oxide synthase in the heterogeneous population of intramural striated muscle fibres of the human membranous urethral sphincter. J Urol 1998; 159:1091–1096.

34. Adams ME, Kramarcy N, Krall SP, et al. Absence of alpha-syntrophin leads to structurally aberrant neuromuscular synapses deficient in utrophin. J Cell Biol 2000; 150:1385–1398.

35. Hughes SM, Koishi K, Rudnicki M, Maggs AM. MyoD protein is differentially accumulated in fast and slow skeletal muscle fibres and required for normal fibre type balance in rodents. Mech Dev 1997; 61:151–163.

36 Buller AJ, Eccles JC, Eccles RM. Interactions between motoneurones and muscles in respect of the characteristic speeds of their responses. J Physiol 1960; 150:417–439.

37. Bourdelat D, Barbet JP, Butler-Browne GS. Fetal development of the urethral sphincter. Eur J Pediatr Surg 1992; 2:35–38.

38. Ludwikowski B, Oesch HI, Brenner E, Fritsch H. The development of the external urethral sphincter in humans. BJU Int 2001; 87:565–568.

39. Oelrich TM. The urethral sphincter muscle in the male. Am J Anat 1980; 158:229–246.

40. Borirakchanyavat S, Baskin LS, Kogan BA, Cunha GR. Smooth and striated muscle development in the intrinsic urethral sphincter. J Urol 1997; 158:1119–1122.

41. Bukovsky A, Copas P, Caudle MR, et al. Abnormal expression of p27kip1 protein in levator ani muscle of aging women with pelvic floor disorders – a relationship to the cellular differentiation and degeneration. BMC Clin Pathol 2001; 1:4.

42. English AW, Schwartz G. Both basic fibroblast growth factor and ciliary neurotrophic factor promote the retention of polyneuronal innervation of developing skeletal muscle fibers. Dev Biol 1995; 169:57–64.

43. Morita T, Nishizawa O, Noto H, Tsuchida S. Pelvic nerve innervation of the external sphincter of urethra as suggested by urodynamic and horse-radish peroxidase studies. J Urol 1984; 131:591–595.

44. De Leval J, Chantraine A, Penders L. The striated sphincter of the urethra. 1: Recall of knowledge on the striated sphincter of the urethra. J d' Urol 1984; 90:439–454.

45. Zvara P, Carrier S, Kour NW, Tanagho EA. The detailed neuroanatomy of the human striated urethral sphincter. Br J Urol 1994; 74:182–187.

46. Borirakchanyavat S, Aboseif SR, Carroll PR, et al. Continence mechanism of the isolated female urethra: an anatomical study of the intrapelvic somatic nerves. J Urol 1997; 158:822–826.

47. Hollabaugh RS Jr, Dmochowski RR, Steiner MS. Neuroanatomy of the male rhabdosphincter. Urology 1997; 49:426–434.

48. Creed KE, Van Der Werf BA, Kaye KW. Innervation of the striated muscle of the membranous urethra of the male dog. J Urol 1998; 159:1712–1716.

49. Morita T, Kizu N, Kondo S, et al. Ipsilaterality of motor innervation of canine urethral sphincter. Urol Int 1988; 43:149–156.

50. Dubrovsky B, Martinez-Gomez M, Pacheco P. Spinal control of pelvic floor muscles. Exp Neurol 1985; 88(2):277–287.

51. Narayan P, Konety B, Aslam K, et al. Neuroanatomy of the external urethral sphincter: implications for urinary continence preservation during radical prostate surgery. J Urol 1995; 153:337–341.

52. Thind P, Lose G, Colstrup H, Andersson KE. The urethral resistance to rapid dilation: an analysis of the effect of autonomic receptor stimulation and blockade and of pudendal nerve blockade in healthy females. Scand J Urol Nephrol 1995; 29(1):83–91.

53. le Feber J, van Asselt E. Pudendal nerve stimulation induces urethral contraction and relaxation. Am J Physiol 1999; 277:R1368–R1375.

54. Rud T, Andersson KE, Asmussen M, et al. Factors maintaining the intraurethral pressure in women. Inv Urol 1980; 17(4):343–347.

55. Sasaki M. Membrane properties of external urethral and external anal sphincter motoneurones in the cat. J Physiol 1991; 440:345–366.

56. Mackel R. Segmental and descending control of the external urethral and anal sphincters in the cat. J Physiol 1979; 294:105–122.

57. Jankowska E, Riddell JS. A relay for input from group II muscle afferents in sacral segments of the cat spinal cord. J Physiol 1993; 465:561–580.

58. Fedirchuk B, Hochman S, Shefchyk SJ. An intracellular study of perineal and hindlimb afferent inputs onto sphincter motoneurons in the decerebrate cat. Exp Brain Res 1992; 89:511–516.

59. Jankowska E, Padel Y, Zarzecki P. Crossed disynaptic inhibition of sacral motoneurones. J Physiol 1978; 285:425–444.

60. Brindley GS, Rushton DN, Craggs MD. The pressure exerted by the external sphincter of the urethra when its motor nerve fibres are stimulated electrically. Br J Urol 1974; 46:453–462.

61. Womack NR, Morrison JFB, Williams NS. The role of pelvic floor denervation in the aetiology of idiopathic faecal incontinence. Br J Surg 1986; 73:404–407.

62. Deindl FM, Vodusek DB, Hesse U, Schussler B. Pelvic floor activity patterns: comparison of nulliparous continent and parous urinary stress incontinent women. A kinesiological EMG study. Br J Urol 1994; 73(4):413–417.

63. Fowler CJ, Kirby RS, Harrison MJ, et al. Individual motor unit analysis in the diagnosis of disorders of urethral sphincter innervation. J Neurol Neurosurg Psych 1984; 47(6):637–641.

64. Fowler CJ, Kirby RS, Harrison MJ. Decelerating burst and complex repetitive discharges in the striated muscle of the urethral sphincter, associated with urinary retention in women. J Neurol Neurosurg Psych 1985; 48(10):1004–1009.

65. Stein R. Possible significance of the urethral paramyotoni outbursts for micturition reflex activation. Scand J Urol Nephrol Suppl 1995; 175:55–56.

66. McKenna KE, Marson L. Spinal and brainstem control of sexual function. In: Jordan D, ed. Central nervous control of autonomic function, Vol 11. The autonomic nervous system. Amsterdam: Overseas Publishers Association, 1997:151–187.

67. Morrison JFB, Sato A, Sato Y, Yamanishi T. The influence of afferent inputs from skin and viscera on the activity of the bladder and the skeletal muscle surrounding the urethra in the rat. Neurosci Res 1995; 23:195–205.

68. Garry RC, Roberts TDM, Todd JK. Reflexes involving the external urethral sphincter in the cat. J Physiol 1959; 149:653–665.

69. Scott FB, Quesada EM, Cardus D. Studies on the dynamics of micturition: observations on healthy men. J Urol 1964; 92:455–463.

70. Tanagho EA. The anatomy and physiology of micturition. Clin Obstet Gynaecol 1978; 5:3–26.

71. Dyro FM, Yalla SV. Refractoriness of urethral striated sphincter during voiding: studies with afferent pudendal reflex arc stimulation in male subjects. J Urol 1986; 135(4):732–736.

72. de Groat WC. Inhibition and excitation of scarl parasympathetic neurons by visceral and cutaneous stimuli in the cat. Brain Res 1971; 33:399–503.

73. McMahon SB, Morrison JFB. Factors that determine the excitability of parasympathetic reflexes to the bladder. J Physiol 1982; 322:35–44.

74. Floyd K, McMahon SB, Morrison JFB. Inhibitory interactions between colonic and vesical afferents in the micturition reflex of the cat. J Physiol 1982; 322:45–52.

75. Conte B, Maggi CA, Meli A. Vesico-inhibitory responses and capsaicin-sensitive afferents in rats. Naunyn-Schmiedebergs Arch Pharmacol 1989; 339(1–2):178–183.

76. Jiang CH, Lindstrom S. Prolonged increase in micturition threshold volume by anogenital afferent stimulation in the rat. Br J Urol 1998; 82:398–403.

77. Kakizaki H, Fraser MO, de Groat WC. Reflex pathways controlling urethral striated and smooth muscle function in the male rat. Am J Physiol 1997; 272(5 Pt 2):R1647–1656.

78. Fedirchuk B, Shefchyk SJ. Membrane potential changes in sphincter motoneurons during micturition in the decerebrate cat. J Neurosci 1993; 13:3090–3094.

79. Holstege G, Griffiths D, de Wall H, Dalm E. Anatomical and physiological observations on supraspinal control of bladder and urethral sphincter muscles in the cat. J Comp Neurol 1986; 250:449–461.

80. Holstege G, Tan J. Supraspinal control of motoneurons innervating the striated muscles of the pelvic floor including urethral and anal sphincters in the cat. Brain 1987; 110(Pt 5):1323–1344.

81. Kohama T. Neuroanatomical studies on pontine urine storage facilitatory areas in the cat brain. Part II. Output neuronal structures from the nucleus locus subcoeruleus and the nucleus reticularis pontis oralis. Nippon Hinyokika Gakkai Zasshi (Jpn J Urol 1992; 83:1478–1483.

82. Ding YQ, Takada M, Tokuno H, Mizuno N. Direct projections from the dorsolateral pontine tegmentum to pudendal motoneurons innervating the external urethral sphincter muscle in the rat. J Comp Neurol 1995; 357(2):318–330.

83. Kruse MN, Mallory BS, Noto H, et al. Properties of the descending limb of the spinobulbospinal micturition reflex pathway in the cat. Brain Res 1991; 556:6–12.

84. McMahon SB, Spillane K. Brainstem influences on the parasympathetic supply to the urinary bladder of the cat. Brain Res 1982; 234:237–249.

85. McMahon SB, Morrison JFB, Spillane K. An electrophysiological study of somatic and visceral convergence in the reflex control of the external sphincters. J Physiol 1982; 328:379–387.

86. Yokoyama O, Yoshiyama M, Namiki M, de Groat WC. Influence of anesthesia on bladder hyperactivity induced by middle cerebral artery occlusion in the rat. Am J Physiol 1997; 273:R1900.

87. Blok BFM, Sturms LM, Holstege G. Brain activation during micturition in women. Brain 1998; 121:2033–2042.

88. Blok BFM, Willemsen ATM, Holstege G. A PET study on brain control of micturition in humans. Brain 1997; 120:111–121.

89. Athwal BS, Berkley KJ, Hussain I, et al. Brain responses to changes in bladder volume and urge to void in healthy men. Brain 2001; 124:369–377.

90. Ramirez LV, Ulfhake B, Arvidsson U, et al. Serotoninergic, peptidergic and GABAergic innervation of the ventrolateral and dorsolateral motor nuclei in the cat S1/S2 segments: an immunofluorescence study. J Chem Neuroanat 1994; 7:87–103.

91. Andrew J, Nathan PW. Lesions of the anterior frontal lobes and disturbances of micturition and defaecation. Brain 1964; 87:233–262.

92. Hansen M. Spinal influences on the pelvic floor muscles. Scand J Urol Nephrol 1995; 29(Suppl 175):37–39.

93. Eardley I, Nagendran K, Kirby RS, Fowler CJ. A new technique for assessing the efferent innervation of the human striated urethral sphincter. J Urol 1990; 144:948–951.

94. Eardley I, Quinn NP, Fowler CJ, et al. The value of urethral sphincter electromyography in the differential diagnosis of parkinsonism. Br J Urol 1989; 64(4):360–362.

95. Ertekin C, Hansen MV, Larsson LE, Sjodahl R. Examination of the descending pathway to the external anal sphincter and pelvic floor muscles by transcranial cortical stimulation. Electroencephal Clin Neurophysiol 1990; 75:500–510.

96. Fedirchuk B, Downie JW, Shefchyk SJ. Reduction of perineal evoked excitatory postsynaptic potentials in cat lumbar and sacral motoneurons during micturition. J Neurosci 1994; 14:6153–6159.

97. Boudriau S, Cote CH, Vincent M, et al. Remodeling of the cytoskeletal lattice in denervated skeletal muscle. Muscle Nerve 1996; 19:1383–1390.

98. Schulte L, Peters D, Taylor J, et al. Sarcoplasmic reticulum Ca^{2+} pump expression in denervated skeletal muscle. Am J Physiol 1994; 267:C617–C622.

99. Leberer E, Seedorf U, Pette D. Neural control of gene expression in skeletal muscle. Calcium-sequestering proteins in developing and chronically stimulated rabbit skeletal muscles. Biochem J 1986; 239:295–300.

100. Ip FC, Fu AK, Tsim KW, Ip NY. Differential expression of ciliary neurotrophic factor receptor in skeletal muscle of chick and rat after nerve injury. J Neurochem 1996; 67:1607–1612.

101. Funakoshi H, Risling M, Carlstedt T, et al. Targeted expression of a multifunctional chimeric neurotrophin in the lesioned sciatic nerve accelerates regeneration of sensory and motor axons. Proc Natl Acad Sci 1998; 95:5269–5274.

102. Trachtenberg JT, Thompson WJ. Nerve terminal withdrawal from rat neuromuscular junctions induced by neuregulin and Schwann cells. J Neurosci 1997; 17:6243–6255.

103. Fu AK, Ip FC, Lai KO, et al. Muscle-derived neurotrophin-3 increases the aggregation of acetylcholine receptors in neuron–muscle co-cultures. Neuroreport 1997; 8:3895–3900.

104. Missias AC, Mudd J, Cunningham JM, et al. Deficient development and maintenance of postsynaptic specializations in mutant mice lacking an 'adult' acetylcholine receptor subunit. Development 1997; 124:5075–5086.

105. Jasmin BJ, Gramolini AO, Adatia FA, et al. Nerve-derived trophic factors and DNA elements controlling expression of genes encoding synaptic proteins in skeletal muscle fibers. Can J Appl Physiol 1998; 23:366–376.

106. Wang X, Berninger B, Poo M. Localized synaptic actions of neurotrophin-4. J Neurosci 1998; 18:4985–4992.

107. Wells DG, McKechnie BA, Kelkar S, Fallon JR. Neurotrophins regulate agrin-induced postsynaptic differentiation. Proc Natl Acad Sci USA 1999; 96:1112–1117.

108. Jordan CL. Morphological effects of ciliary neurotrophic factor treatment during neuromuscular synapse elimination. J Neurobiol 1996; 31:29–40.

109. Helgren ME, Squinto SP, Davis HL, et al. Trophic effect of ciliary neurotrophic factor on denervated skeletal muscle. Cell 1994; 76:493–504.

110. Hiruma S, Shimizu T, Huruta T, et al. Ciliary neurotrophic factor immunoreactivity in rat intramuscular nerve during reinnervation through a silicone tube after severing of the rat sciatic nerve. Exp Mol Pathol 1997; 64:23–30.

111. Goldman D, Sapru MK. Molecular mechanisms mediating synapse-specific gene expression during development of the neuromuscular junction. Can J Appl Physiol 1998; 23:390–395.

112. Jo SA, Zhu X, Marchionni MA, Burden SJ. Neuregulins are concentrated at nerve–muscle synapses and activate ACh-receptor gene expression. Nature 1995; 373:158–161.

113. Zhu X, Lai C, Thomas S, Burden SJ. Neuregulin receptors, erbB3 and erbB4, are localized at neuromuscular synapses. EMBO J 1995; 14:5842–5848.

114. Loeb JA, Hmadcha A, Fischbach GD, et al. Neuregulin expression at neuromuscular synapses is modulated by synaptic activity and neurotrophic factors. J Neurosci 2002; 22:2206–2214.

115. Wolpowitz D, Mason TB, Dietrich P, et al. Cysteine-rich domain isoforms of the neuregulin-1 gene are required for maintenance of peripheral synapses. Neuron 2000; 25:79–91.

116. Gautam M, Noakes PG, Moscoso L, et al. Defective neuromuscular synaptogenesis in agrin-deficient mutant mice. Cell 1996; 85:525–535.

117. Gautam M, DeChiara TM, Glass DJ, et al. Distinct phenotypes of mutant mice lacking agrin, MuSK, or rapsyn. Brain Res Dev Brain Res 1999; 114:171–178.

118. Bartlett SE, Banks GB, Reynolds AJ, et al. Alterations in ciliary neurotrophic factor signaling in rapsyn deficient mice. J Neurosci Res 2001; 64:575–581.

119. Kasemkijwattana C, Menetrey J, Somogyl G, et al. Development of approaches to improve the healing following muscle contusion. Cell Transplant 1998; 7:585–598.

120. Kasemkijwattana C, Menetrey J, Bosch P, et al. Use of growth factors to improve muscle healing after strain injury. Clin Orthop 2000; (370)272–285.

121. Menetrey J, Kasemkijwattana C, Day CS, et al. Growth factors improve muscle healing in vivo. J Bone Joint Surg Br 2000; 82:131–137.

122. Kurek JB, Bower JJ, Romanella M, et al. The role of leukemia inhibitory factor in skeletal muscle regeneration. Muscle Nerve 1997; 20:815–822.

123. Tarone G, Hirsch E, Brancaccio M, et al. Integrin function and regulation in development. Int J Dev Biol 2000; 44:725–731.

124. Fournier M, Lewis MI. Influences of IGF-I gene disruption on the cellular profile of the diaphragm. Am J Physiol Endocrinol Metab 2000; 278:E707–E715.

125. Guttmann L. Spinal cord injuries. Oxford: Blackwell, 1976:731.

126. Sasaki M, Morrison JFB, Sato Y, Sato A. Effect of mechanical stimulation of the skin on the external urethral sphincter muscles in anaesthetised cats. Jpn J Physiol 1994; 44:575–590.

127. Perlow DL, Diokno AC. Predicting lower urinary tract dysfunctions in patients with spinal cord injury. Urology 1981; 18:531–535.

128. Walter JS, Wheeler JS Jr, Dunn RB. Dynamic bulbocavernosus reflex: dyssynergia evaluation following SCI. J Am Paraplegia Soc 1994; 17:140–145.

129. Rossier AB, Fam BA, DiBenedetto M, Sarkarati M. Urodynamics in spinal shock patients. J Urol 1979; 122(6):783–787.

130. Rodriquez AA, Awad E. Detrusor muscle and sphincteric response to anorectal stimulation in spinal cord injury. Arch Phys Med Rehab 1979; 60(6):269–272.

131. Rossier AB, Fam BA, Lee IY, et al. Role of striated and smooth muscle components in the urethral pressure profile in traumatic neurogenic bladders: a neuropharmacological and urodynamic study. Preliminary report. J Urol 1982; 128:529–535.

132. Kakizaki H, Koyanagi T, Shinno Y, et al. An electromyographic study on the urethral rhabdosphincter in normal and chronically rhizotomized cats: analysis of electrical potentials evoked by sympathetic nerve stimulation. J Urol 1994; 151:238–243.

133. Thiry AJ, Deltenre PF. Neurophysiological assessment of the central motor pathway to the external urethral sphincter in man. Br J Urol 1989; 63:515–519.

134. Hamdy S, Enck P, Aziz Q, et al. Spinal and pudendal nerve modulation of human corticoanal motor pathways. Am J Physiol 1998; 274:G419–G423.

135. Hamdy S, Enck P, Aziz Q, et al. Laterality effects of human pudendal nerve stimulation on corticoanal pathways: evidence for functional asymmetry. Gut 1999; 45:58–63.

136. Jost WH, Schimrigk K. A new method to determine pudendal nerve motor latency and central motor conduction time to the external anal sphincter. Electroencephalogr Clin Neurophysiol 1994; 93:237–239.

137. Loening-Baucke V, Read NW, Yamada T, Barker AT. Evaluation of the motor and sensory components of the pudendal nerve. Electroencephalogr Clin Neurophysiol 1994; 93:35–41.

138. Morren GL, Walter S, Lindehammar H, et al. Evaluation of the sacroanal motor pathway by magnetic and electric stimulation in patients with fecal incontinence. Dis Colon Rectum 2001; 44:167–172.

139. Opsomer RJ, Caramia MD, Zarola F, et al. Neurophysiological evaluation of central-peripheral sensory and motor pudendal fibres. Electroencephalogr Clin Neurophysiol 1989; 74:260–270.

140. Pelliccioni G, Scarpino O, Piloni V. Motor evoked potentials recorded from external anal sphincter by cortical and lumbo-sacral magnetic stimulation: normative data. J Neurol Sci 1997; 149:69–72.

141. Shafik A. Magnetic pudendal neurostimulation: a novel method for measuring pudendal nerve terminal motor latency. Clin Neurophysiol 2001; 112:1049–1052.

142. Turnbull GK, Hamdy S, Aziz Q, et al. The cortical topography of human anorectal musculature. Gastroenterology 1999; 117:32–39.

143. Welter ML, Dechoz S, Leroi AM, Weber J. Evoked mechanical and electrical anal sphincter responses after cortical and lumbar magnetic stimulation. Neurophysiol Clin 2000; 30:246–253.

144. Sato T, Nagai H. Pudendal nerve 'complete' motor latencies at four different levels in the anal sphincter system in young adults. Dis Colon Rectum 2002; 45:923–927.

145. Sato T, Konishi F, Kanazawa K. Variations in motor evoked potential latencies in the anal sphincter system with sacral magnetic stimulation. Dis Colon Rectum 2000; 43:966–970.

146. Sato T, Konishi F, Minakami H, et al. Pelvic floor disturbance after childbirth: vaginal delivery damages the upper levels of sphincter innervation. Dis Colon Rectum 2001; 44:1155–1161.

147. Brodak PP, Bidair M, Joseph A, et al. Magnetic stimulation of the sacral roots. Neurourol Urodyn 1993; 12:533–540.

148. Ghezzi A, Callea L, Zaffaroni M, et al. Perineal motor potentials to magnetic stimulation, pudendal evoked potentials and perineal reflex in women. Neurophysiol Clin 1992; 22:321–326.

149. Bemelmans BL, Van Kerrebroeck PE, Notermans SL, et al. Motor evoked potentials from the bladder on magnetic stimulation of the cauda equina: a new technique for investigation of autonomic bladder innervation. J Urol 1992; 147:658–661.

150. Zhu GY, Shen Y. Application of pudendal evoked potentials in diagnosis of erectile dysfunction. Asian J Androl 1999; 1:145–150.

151. Bondurant CP, Haghighi SS. Experience with transcranial magnetic stimulation in evaluation of spinal cord injury. Neurol Res 1997; 19:497–500.

152. McFarlane JP, Foley SJ, de Winter P, et al. Acute suppression of idiopathic detrusor instability with magnetic stimulation of the sacral nerve roots. Br J Urol 1997; 80:734–741.

153. Kirkham AP, Shah NC, Knight SL, et al. The acute effects of continuous and conditional neuromodulation on the bladder in spinal cord injury. Spinal Cord 2001; 39:420–428.

154. Phelan MW, Franks M, Somogyi GT, et al. Botulinum toxin urethral sphincter injection to restore bladder emptying in men and women with voiding dysfunction. J Urol 2001; 165:1107–1110.

155. Sakakibara R, Hattori T, Uchiyama T, et al. Neurogenic failures of the external urethral sphincter closure and relaxation; a videourodynamic study. Auton Neurosci 2001; 86:208–215.

156. Pavlakis AJ, Siroky MB, Goldstein I, Krane RJ. Neurourologic findings in Parkinson's disease. J Urol 1983; 129:80–83.

157. Stocchi F, Carbone A, Inghilleri M, et al. Urodynamic and neurophysiological evaluation in Parkinson's disease and multiple system atrophy. J Neurol Neurosurg Psychiatry 1997; 62:507–511.

158. Kanie S, Yokoyama O, Komatsu K, et al. GABAergic contribution to rat bladder hyperactivity after middle cerebral artery occlusion. Am J Physiol Regul Integr Comp Physiol 2000; 279(4): R1230–R1238.

159. Gelber DA, Good DC, Laven LJ, Verhulst SJ. Causes of urinary incontinence after acute hemispheric stroke. Stroke 1993; 24:378–382.

160. Sakakibara R, Hattori T, Yasuda K, Yamanishi T. Micturitional disturbance after acute hemispheric stroke: analysis of the lesion site by CT and MRI. J Neurol Sci 1996; 137:47–56.

161. Sakakibara R, Fowler CJ, Hattori T. Voiding and MRI analysis of the brain. Int Urogynecol J Pelvic Floor Dysfunct 1999; 10: 192–199.

162. Raisman G. Repair of corticospinal axons by transplantation of olfactory ensheathing cells. Novartis Found Symp 2002; 231:94–97; discussion 97–109.

163. Raisman G. Olfactory ensheathing cells – another miracle cure for spinal cord injury? Nat Rev Neurosci 2001; 2:369–375.

164. Ramer MS, Duraisingam I, Priestley JV, McMahon SB. Two-tiered inhibition of axon regeneration at the dorsal root entry zone. J Neurosci 2001; 21:2651–2660.

165. Ramer MS, Bishop T, Dockery P, et al. Neurotrophin-3-mediated regeneration and recovery of proprioception following dorsal rhizotomy. Mol Cell Neurosci 2002; 19:239–249.

5

Pharmacology of the lower urinary tract

Karl-Erik Andersson and Annette Schröder

Introduction

The normal bladder functions, storage and elimination of urine, are based on a coordinated interplay of reciprocal contraction and relaxation of the bladder and the outflow region. This interaction is regulated by neural circuits in the brain and spinal cord, which coordinate the activity of the detrusor and that of the smooth and striated muscles of the outflow region. The nervous mechanisms for this control involve a complex pattern of efferent and afferent signaling in parasympathetic, sympathetic, and somatic nerves.

This chapter will briefly review the principles of nervous control of micturition, and then focus on the peripheral mechanisms involved in the contraction and relaxation of the bladder and urethra.

Bladder

Nervous control

The central nervous mechanisms for regulation of micturition are still not completely known. The normal micturition reflex is mediated by a spinobulbospinal pathway, passing through relay centers in the brain. In principle, the central pathways are organized as on-off switching circuits (Figures 5.1 and 5.2).[1] During bladder filling, once threshold tension is achieved, afferent impulses, conveyed mainly by the pelvic nerve, reach centers in the central nervous system (CNS). It has been proposed that the afferent neurons send information to the periaqueductal gray (PAG), which in turn communicates with the pontine tegmentum, where two different regions involved in micturition control have been described in cats.[2] One is a dorsomedially located M region, corresponding to Barrington's nucleus or the pontine micturition center (PMC). A more laterally located L-region may serve as a pontine urine storage center (PSC), which has been suggested to suppress bladder contraction and regulate the external sphincter muscle

activity during urine storage. The M- and L-regions may represent separate functional systems, acting independently.[3]

The peripheral nervous mechanisms for bladder emptying and urine storage involve efferent and afferent signaling in *parasympathetic*, *sympathetic*, and *somatic* nerves.

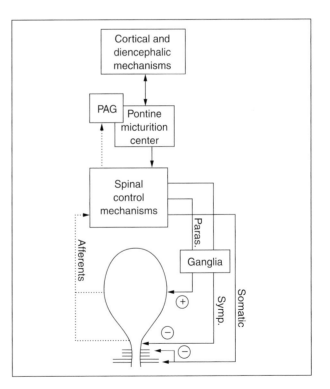

Figure 5.1
Voiding reflexes involve supraspinal pathways, and are under voluntary control. During bladder emptying, the spinal parasympathetic (paras.) outflow is activated, leading to bladder contraction. Simultaneously, the sympathetic (symp.) outflow to urethral smooth muscle and the somatic outflow to urethral and pelvic floor striated muscles are turned off, and the outflow region relaxes. PAG = periaqueductal grey.

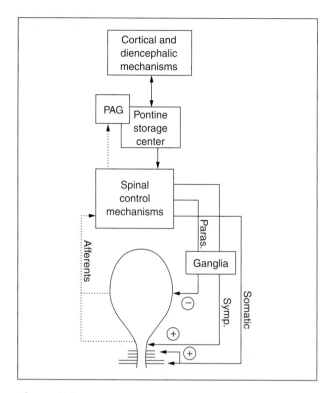

Figure 5.2
During storage, there is continuous and increasing afferent activity from the bladder. There is no spinal parasympathetic (paras.) outflow that can contract the bladder. The sympathetic (symp.) outflow to urethral smooth muscle and the somatic outflow to urethral and pelvic floor striated muscles keep the outflow region closed. Whether or not the sympathetic innervation to the bladder (not indicated) contributes to bladder relaxation during filling in humans has not been established. PAG = periaqueductal grey.

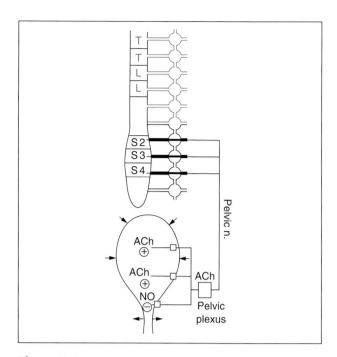

Figure 5.3
The parasympathetic (pelvic nerve) innervation mediates contraction of the bladder (acetylcholine = ACh, muscarinic receptors) and relaxation of the urethra (NO = nitric oxide). T = thoracic, L = lumbar, and S = sacral segments.

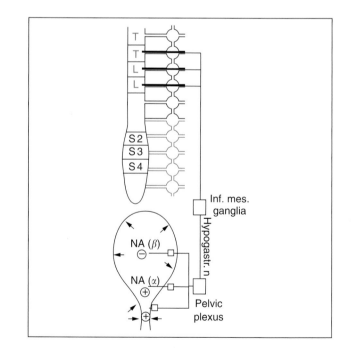

Figure 5.4
Sympathetic innervation (hypogastric nerve) mediates contraction of the bladder outlet and urethral smooth muscle (NA = noradrenaline, α-adrenoceptors) and relaxes the bladder (NA = noradrenaline, β-adrenoceptors). T = thoracic, L = lumbar, and S = sacral segments.

These nerves either maintain the bladder in a relaxed state, while the outflow region is contracted, enabling urine storage at low intravesical pressure, or they initiate micturition by relaxing the outflow region and contracting the bladder smooth muscle. Parasympathetic activation excites the bladder and relaxes the outflow region (Figure 5.3), and sympathetic activation inhibits the bladder body and excites bladder outlet and urethra (Figure 5.4). Somatic nerves activate the striated urethral sphincter (rhabdosphincter; Figure 5.5).

The *sensory* (afferent) innervation, which anatomically can be found in the parasympathetic, sympathetic, and somatic nerves, transmits information about bladder filling and contractile bladder activity to the CNS.

Parasympathetic neurons, mediating contraction of the detrusor smooth muscle and relaxation of the outflow region, are located in the sacral parasympathetic nucleus in the spinal cord at the level of S2–S4.[4] The axons pass through the pelvic nerve and synapse with the postganglionic nerves in either the pelvic plexus, in ganglia on the

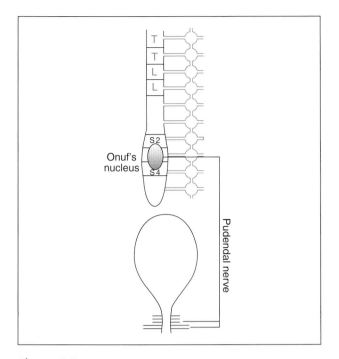

Figure 5.5
During storage, activity in somatic nerves (pudendal nerve) keeps the striated urethral sphincter (rhabdosphincter) closed. During micturition, this activity is suppressed. T = thoracic, L = lumbar, and S = sacral segments.

surface of the bladder (vesical ganglia), or within the walls of the bladder and urethra (intramural ganglia).[5] The preganglionic neurotransmission is mediated by acetylcholine (ACh) acting on nicotinic receptors. This transmission can be modulated by adrenergic, muscarinic, purinergic, and peptidergic presynaptic receptors.[4] The postganglionic neurons in the pelvic nerve mediate the excitatory input to the human detrusor smooth muscle by releasing ACh acting on muscarinic receptors. However, an atropine-resistant component has been demonstrated, particularly in functionally and morphologically altered human bladder tissue (see below). The pelvic nerve also conveys parasympathetic fibers to the outflow region and the urethra. These fibers exert an inhibitory effect and thereby relax the outflow region. This is mediated partly by nitric oxide, although other transmitters might be involved.[6–9]

Most of the *sympathetic* innervation of the bladder and urethra originates from the intermediolateral nuclei in the thoracolumbar region (T10–L2) of the spinal cord. The axons travel either through the inferior mesenteric ganglia and the hypogastric nerve, or pass through the paravertebral chain and enter the pelvic nerve. Thus, sympathetic signals are conveyed in both the hypogastric and pelvic nerves.

The predominant effects of the sympathetic innervation of the lower urinary tract in man are inhibition of the parasympathetic pathways at spinal and ganglion levels, and mediation of contraction of the bladder base and the urethra. However, in several animals, the adrenergic innervation of the detrusor is believed to relax the detrusor directly.[10] Noradrenaline is released in response to electrical stimulation of detrusor tissues *in vitro*, and the normal response of detrusor tissues to released noradrenaline is relaxation.[10]

Somatic motoneurons, activating the external urethral sphincter (EUS), are located in the Onuf's nucleus, a circumscribed region of the sacral ventral horn at the level of S2–S4. EUS motoneurons send axons to the ventral roots and into the pudendal nerves.[1]

The *sensory* (afferent) nerves monitor the urine volume and pressure during urine storage, transmitting the information to the CNS.[11] Most of the sensory innervation of the bladder and urethra reaches the spinal cord via the pelvic nerve and dorsal root ganglia. In addition, some afferents travel in the hypogastric nerve. The afferent nerves of the EUS travel in the pudendal nerve to the sacral region of the spinal cord.[5] There are several populations of afferents in the bladder. The most important for the micturition process are myelinated Aδ fibers and unmyelinated C fibers. The Aδ fibers respond to passive distention and active contraction (low threshold afferents), thus conveying information about bladder filling.[12] The activation threshold for Aδ fibers is 5–15 mmH$_2$O, which is the intravesical pressure at which humans report the first sensation of bladder filling.[4] C fibers have a high mechanical threshold and respond primarily to chemical irritation of the bladder mucosa or cold.[13,14] Following chemical irritation, the C-fiber afferents exhibit spontaneous firing when the bladder is empty, and increased firing during bladder distention.[13] These fibers are normally inactive and are therefore termed 'silent fibers'.

Local control of the bladder

The cholinergic and adrenergic mechanisms involved in bladder storage and emptying functions have been extensively investigated.[1,10,15] Non-adrenergic, non-cholinergic (NANC) bladder mechanisms, on the other hand, have been studied mainly in research animals, and their relevance in humans has not been established.

Cholinergic mechanisms

Cholinergic nerves. Although histochemical methods that stain for ACh esterase (AChE) are not specific for ACh-containing nerves, AChE staining has been used as an indirect marker of cholinergic nerves.[5] The vesicular ACh transporter (VACht) is a marker specific for cholinergic nerve terminals.[16] In rats, for example, bladder smooth muscle bundles were supplied with a very rich number of VAChT-positive terminals also containing neuropeptide Y (NPY), nitric oxide synthase (NOS), and vasoactive intestinal polypeptide (VIP).[17] Similar findings have been made in human bladders of neonates and children.[18] The muscle coat of the bladder showed a rich cholinergic innervation and small VAChT-immunoreactive neurons were found scattered throughout the detrusor muscle. VAChT-immunoreactive nerves were also observed in a suburothelial location in the bladder. The function of these nerves is unclear, but a sensory function or a neurotrophic role with respect to the urothelium cannot be excluded.[18]

Muscarinic receptors. Five distinct genes for muscarinic receptors have been revealed by molecular cloning, and five receptor subtypes (M_1–M_5) correspond to these gene products.[19] The muscarinic receptors are coupled to G proteins. The signal transduction system involved varies, but M_1, M_3, and M_5 preferentially couple to phosphoinositide hydrolysis, leading to mobilization of intracellular calcium, whereas activation of muscarinic M_2 and M_4 receptors inhibits adenylyl cyclase activity.[19] It has been suggested that muscarinic receptor stimulation may also inhibit K_{ATP} channels in smooth muscle cells from urinary bladder through activation of protein kinase C.[20]

Detrusor smooth muscle from various species contains muscarinic receptors of the M_2 and M_3 subtype.[21] In the human bladder, the occurrence of mRNAs encoding M_2 and M_3 subtypes has been demonstrated, whereas no mRNA encoding M_1 receptors was found.[22] The M_3 receptors in the human bladder are believed to cause a direct smooth muscle contraction through phosphoinositide hydrolysis, whereas the role for the M_2 receptors has not been clarified.[23] M_2 receptors may oppose sympathetically initiated smooth muscle relaxation, mediated by β adrenoceptors, since activation of M_2 receptors results in an inhibition of adenylyl cyclase.[24] Contractile mechanisms involving M_2 muscarinic receptors, such as activation of a nonspecific cationic channel and inactivation of potassium channels, may be operative in the bladder.[21]

There is general agreement that M_3 receptors are mainly responsible for the normal micturition contraction. Studies in human tissue where the M_3 receptor has been blocked selectively revealed that M_3 is the predominant, if not exclusive receptor mediating bladder contraction.[21,25] In M_3 receptor knockout mice, the contractile response to muscarinic stimulation of the bladder *in vitro* was virtually abolished.[26,27] Even in the obstructed rat bladder, M_3 receptors were found to play a predominant role in mediating detrusor contraction.[28] On the other hand, in certain disease states, M_2 receptors may contribute to contraction of the bladder. Thus, in the denervated rat bladder, M_2 receptors, or a combination of M_2 and M_3 receptors, mediated contractile responses.[29,30]

Muscarinic receptors are also located on prejunctional nerve terminals and participate in the regulation of transmitter release. The inhibitory prejunctional muscarinic receptors have been classified as muscarinic M_2 in the rabbit and rat, and M_4 in the guinea pig and human urinary bladder.[31–34] Prejunctional facilitatory muscarinic receptors appear to be of the M_1 subtype in the rat and rabbit urinary bladder, and prejunctional muscarinic facilitation has also been detected in human bladders.[33–35]

The muscarinic receptor functions may be changed in different urological disorders, such as outflow obstruction, neurogenic bladders, idiopathic detrusor overactivity, and diabetes.[36]

Adrenergic mechanisms

Adrenergic nerves. Fluorescence histochemical studies have shown that the body of the detrusor receives a relatively sparse innervation by noradrenergic nerves. The density of noradrenergic nerves increases markedly towards the bladder neck, where the smooth muscle receives a dense noradrenergic nerve supply, particularly in the male. The importance of the noradrenergic innervation of the bladder body has been questioned since patients with a deficiency in dopamine β-hydroxylase, the enzyme that converts dopamine to noradrenaline, void normally.[37] Noradrenergic nerves also occur in the submucosa of the bladder, only some of which are related to the vascular supply. Their functional significance remains to be shown.

α Adrenoceptors. In the human detrusor, β adrenoceptors (β ARs) dominate over α adrenoceptors (α ARs) and the normal response to noradrenaline is relaxation.[10] The number of α ARs in the human detrusor was found to be low, the order of abundance being $\beta > \alpha_2 \gg \alpha_1$. Goepel et al found the amount of α_1 ARs was too small for a reliable quantification.[38] However, Malloy et al reported that even if the total α_1-AR expression was low, it was reproducible. Among the high-affinity receptors for prazosin, only α_{1A} and α_{1D} mRNAs were expressed in the human bladder. The relation between the different subtypes was $\alpha_{1D} = 66\%$ and $\alpha_{1A} = 34\%$, with no expression of α_{1B}.[39]

Even if the α ARs have no significant role in normal bladder contraction, there is evidence that there may be changes after, for example, bladder outlet obstruction.[40] However, Nomiya et al concluded that neither an up-regulation of α_1 ARs, nor a down-regulation of β ARs, occurs in human obstructed bladder, and that it was not likely that detrusor α_1 ARs are responsible for the overactivity observed in patients with bladder outflow obstruction.[41]

β Adrenoceptors. The β ARs of the human bladder were shown to have functional characteristics typical of neither β_1 nor β_2 ARs.[42,43] Normal as well as neurogenic human detrusors are able to express β_1, β_2, and β_3 AR mRNA, and selective β_3 AR agonists effectively relaxed both types of detrusor muscle.[44,45] An investigation comparing the subpopulations of β ARs in research animals revealed significant differences amongst species.[46] Studies in human detrusor tissue revealed an expression of β_3 AR mRNA of 97% over β_1 (1.5%) and β_2 (1.4%) AR mRNA, concluding that if the amount of mRNA reflects the population of receptor protein, β_3 AR mediates bladder relaxation.[47] This is in accordance with several *in-vitro* studies, and it seems that atypical β AR-mediated responses reported in early studies of β AR antagonists, are mediated by β_3 ARs.[44,45] It can also partly explain why the clinical effects of selective β_2 AR agonists in bladder overactivity have been controversial and largely inconclusive.[48] It has been speculated that in detrusor overactivity associated with outflow obstruction, there is a lack of an inhibitory β AR-mediated noradrenaline response, but this has never been verified in humans.[41,49,50] Several β_3 AR agonists have shown promising profiles *in vitro* and in animal models, but no proof concept studies seem to have been performed.[44,45,51–53] Whether or not β_3 AR stimulation will be an effective way of treating detrusor overactivity has to await such studies.

Non-adrenergic, non-cholinergic mechanisms

In most animal species, the bladder contraction induced by stimulation of nerves consists of at least two components: one atropine-resistant and one mediated by NANC mechanisms.[10] NANC contractions have been reported to occur in normal human detrusor, even if not representing more than a few percent of the total contraction in response to nerve stimulation.[54–56] However, a significant degree of NANC-mediated contraction may exist in morphologically and/or functionally changed human bladders, and has been reported to occur in hypertrophic bladders, idiopathic detrusor instability, interstitial cystitis bladder, neurogenic bladders, and in the aging bladder.[55,57–63] In such bladders, the NANC component of the nerve-induced response may be responsible for up to 40–50% of the total bladder contraction.

Adenosine triphosphate. There is good evidence that the transmitter responsible for the NANC component is ATP, acting on P2X receptors found in the detrusor smooth muscle membranes of rats and humans.[64–66] The receptor subtype predominating in both species seemed to be the P2X$_1$ subtype. Moore et al reported that detrusor from patients with idiopathic detrusor instability had a selective absence of P2X$_3$ and P2X$_5$ receptors, and suggested that this specific lack might impair control of detrusor contractility and contribute to the pathophysiology of urge incontinence.[67] On the other hand, O'Reilly et al found that in patients with idiopathic detrusor instability, P2X$_2$ receptors were significantly elevated, whereas other P2X receptor subtypes were significantly decreased.[60] They

were unable to detect a purinergic component of nerve-mediated contractions in control (normal) bladder specimens, but there was a significant purinergic component of approximately 50% in unstable bladder specimens. They concluded that this abnormal purinergic transmission in the bladder might explain symptoms in these patients. The same group confirmed that the P2X$_1$ receptor was the predominant purinoceptor subtype also in the human male bladder.[66] They found that the amount of P2X$_1$ receptor per smooth muscle cell was larger in obstructed than in control bladders. This suggests an increase in purinergic function in the overactive bladder arising from bladder outlet obstruction.

Evidence suggesting that ATP may be involved in afferent signaling in the urinary bladder was first presented by Ferguson et al, who showed that ATP was released from the rabbit urothelium in response to stretch.[68] They postulated that the released ATP could activate suburothelial sensory nerves, thus generating a signal that could activate the micturition reflex. That ATP can be produced by and released from the urothelium has been confirmed by other investigators.[69] The postulated target for ATP, the P2X$_3$ receptor, has been shown to be expressed on small-diameter primary sensory neurons.[70,71] In the bladder, P2X$_{2/3}$ receptors have been demonstrated not only on suburothelial nerves but also on the urothelium.[69,72–74] Namasivayam et al, using an *in-vitro* pelvic nerve-afferent rat model, showed that afferent activity induced by bladder distention was reduced by up to 75% after desensitization with $\alpha\beta$-methylene ATP, results consistent with the view that ATP is released from the bladder urothelium by distention, and activates pelvic nerve afferents.[75] Further supporting the role of ATP, cystometry in P2X$_3$-deficient mice revealed decreased voiding frequency, increased bladder capacity and voiding volume, but normal bladder pressures.[72] Based on these findings, the authors suggested that P2X$_3$ receptors are involved in the normal physiological regulation of afferent pathways controlling volume reflexes in the urinary bladder, and thus that P2X$_3$ receptor-containing neurons may serve as volume receptors.

Further supporting a role for ATP in urothelial signaling, Pandita and Andersson found that intravesical instillation of ATP could induce bladder overactivity in unanesthetized, freely moving rats.[76] The ATP-induced effects were effectively counteracted by the P2X$_3$-receptor antagonist, TNP-ATP, which by itself caused an increase in bladder capacity. Interestingly, the effects of ATP could be prevented by pretreatment with L-arginine, and by the NK-2 receptor antagonist SR 48968, suggesting that both nitric oxide (NO) and tachykinins could interfere with the actions of ATP.[76]

Neuropeptides. Various bioactive peptides have been demonstrated to be synthesized, stored, and released in the human lower urinary tract, including atrial natriuretic peptide (ANP), bradykinin, calcitonin gene-related peptide (CGRP), endothelin, enkephalins, galanin, neuropeptide Y, somatostatin, substance P (SP), and vasoactive intestinal polypeptide (VIP).[10] However, their functional roles have not been established.[77–79] In human bladder, Uckert et al found contractant effects of SP and ET-1, a relaxant effect of VIP, and very little effects of ANP and CGRP.[79]

As discussed by Maggi, neuropeptide-containing, capsaicin-sensitive primary afferents in the bladder and urethra may not only have a sensory function ('sensory neuropeptides') but also a local effector or efferent function.[77,78] In addition, they may play a role as neurotransmitters and/or neuromodulators in the bladder ganglia and at the neuromuscular junctions. As a result, the peptides may be involved in the mediation of various effects, including micturition reflex activation, smooth muscle contraction, potentiation of efferent neurotransmission, and changes in vascular tone and permeability. Evidence for this is based mainly on experiments in animals. Studies on isolated human bladder muscle strips have failed to reveal any specific local motor response attributable to a capsaicin-sensitive innervation.[77] However, cystometric evidence that capsaicin-sensitive nerves may modulate the afferent branch of the micturition reflex in humans has been presented.[80] In a small number of patients suffering from bladder hypersensitivity disorders, intravesical capsaicin produced a long-lasting, symptomatic improvement. It has been discussed whether peptides are involved in the pathogenesis of detrusor overactivity. Results from immunohistochemical studies have provided evidence that outflow obstruction, which is commonly associated with detrusor overactivity, causes a reduction in the density of peptide-containing nerves.[81]

Tachykinins. Endogenous tachykinins, SP, neurokinin A (NKA), and neurokinin B (NKB), are widely distributed in the central and peripheral nervous system. They are found in afferent pathways of the bladder and urethra, and there is considerable evidence that they act as transmitters in sensory nerves.[77] In addition, these peptides have been shown to produce diverse biological effects, such as smooth muscle contraction, facilitation of transmitter release from nerves, vasodilatation, and increased plasma permeability. Their actions are mediated by activation of three distinct receptor types, termed NK-1, NK-2, and NK-3. Rat and guinea pig detrusors contain both NK-1 and NK-2 receptors, whereas the NK-2 receptor seems to be the only mediator of contractile responses to tachykinins in human bladder smooth muscle, where the potency of neurokinins was shown to be NKA > NKB ≫ SP.[82] Nociceptive transmission is mainly mediated through NK_1 receptors.

The potential role of tachykinins, particularly SP, in the atropine-resistant component of the contractile response induced by electrical stimulation, has been studied by several investigators.[10,79] With few exceptions, these studies did not favor the view that SP, released from postganglionic nerve-terminals, has an excitatory transmitter role. However, evidence has been presented that SP may play a role in the afferent branch of the micturition reflex.[1,10]

Endothelins. Endothelins (ET-1, ET-2, ET-3) and ET (ET_A, ET_B) receptors have been demonstrated in the bladder. Via their receptors, ETs can initiate both short-term (contraction) and long-term (mitogenesis) events in targets cells in the bladder and urethra. Saenz de Tejada et al demonstrated ET-like immunoreactivity in the transitional epithelium, serosal mesothelium, vascular endothelium, smooth muscles of the detrusor (nonvascular) and vessels, and in fibroblasts of the human bladder.[83] This cellular distribution was confirmed in *in-situ* hybridization experiments. The authors suggested that ETs may act as an autocrine hormone in the regulation of the bladder wall structure and smooth muscle tone, and that it may regulate cholinergic neurotransmission by a paracrine mechanism. In patients with benign prostatic hypertrophy (BPH), the density of ET receptors in the bladder was significantly lower than in men without this disorder.[84] ET-1 is known to induce contraction in animal as well as human detrusor muscle.[10,79] The contractile effect of ETs seems to be mediated mainly by the ET_A receptor, and the ET_B receptor could not be linked to contraction.[85] However, in human bladder smooth muscle, ETs may not only have a contractile action but also could be linked to proliferative effects. Supporting this view, Khan et al found that ET_A- and ET_B-receptor antagonists inhibited rabbit detrusor and bladder neck smooth muscle cell proliferation, and they suggested that ET-1 antagonists may prevent smooth muscle cell hyperplasia associated with partial bladder outflow obstruction.[86]

Many authors have suggested that ET may play a pathophysiological role in bladder outlet obstruction associated with BPH. In the bladder, ETs may be implicated in detrusor hypertrophy and its functional consequences.

Vasoactive intestinal polypeptide. Vasoactive intestinal polypeptide (VIP) was shown to inhibit spontaneous contractile activity in isolated detrusor muscle from several animal species and from humans, but to have little effect on contractions induced by muscarinic receptor stimulation or by electrical stimulation of nerves.[10] Uckert et al found a moderate relaxant effect of VIP on isolated, carbachol-contracted human detrusor, and a less than twofold increase in intracellular cyclic AMP concentration.[79] In isolated rat bladder, VIP had no effect, and in isolated guinea pig bladder, VIP produced contraction. Stimulation of the pelvic nerves in cats increased the VIP output from the bladder, and increased bladder blood flow, although moderately.[87] VIP injected intravenously induced bladder relaxation in dogs.[88] On the other hand, VIP given intravenously to patients in a dose causing increases in heart rate had no effect on cystometric parameters.[89] Plasma concentrations of VIP were obtained, which, in other clinical investigations, had been sufficient to cause relaxation of smooth muscle.[89] Even if a decrease in VIP concentrations has been found in bladders from patients with idiopathic detrusor overactivity, the role of this peptide in bladder function has not been established.[90]

Calcitonin gene-related peptide. Calcitonin gene-related peptide (CGRP) is widely distributed in nerve endings in the bladder, and considered a sensory neuromodulator.[77] However, if CGRP has a role in the control of bladder motility it is controversial. In pig detrusor, CGRP did not alter the response to potassium, carbachol, SP, or electrical field stimulation (EFS).[91] In hamsters, CGRP caused dose-dependent inhibition of the response to EFS, but about 20% of the preparations did not respond.[92] In human detrusor strips the relaxing effect of CGRP on carbachol-induced contraction was negligible, despite a slight increase in cGMP levels.[79] Most probably, the main role of CGRP is that of a sensory neuromodulator.

Neuropeptide Y. Neuropeptide Y (NPY) and noradrenaline are stored in separate vesicles at sympathetic nerve terminals, and NPY is preferentially released at high frequencies of stimulation.[93] In rat bladders, abundant NPY-containing nerves were found, and exogenously added NPY contracted detrusor strips and potentiated the non-cholinergic motor transmission. A possible motor transmitter function of the peptide in the rat bladder was suggested.[10,94] However, other investigators studying rat and guinea pig bladders found no contractile response to exogenous NPY, but inhibitory effects on cholinergic and NANC-induced contractions.[95,96] The human bladder is richly endowed with NPY-containing nerves.[97–100] In neonates and children, small ganglia scattered throughout the detrusor muscle of urinary bladder were found, of which approximately 95% contained NPY.[18] It seems as if NPY can be found in adrenergic as well as cholinergic nerves. However, in the human bladder, only very few if any functional NPY receptors were found.[101] Thus, a role for NPY in bladder function remains to be established.

Prostanoids. Prostanoids are synthesized from a common precursor, arachidonic acid, a process catalyzed by the enzyme cyclooxygenase (COX). This process occurs locally in both bladder muscle and mucosa, and is initiated by various physiological stimuli such as stretch of the detrusor muscle, but also by injuries of the vesical mucosa, nerve stimulation, and by agents such as ATP and mediators of inflammation.[102–105] There seem to be species variations in the spectrum of prostanoids and the relative amounts synthesized and released by the urinary bladder. Biopsies from the human bladder were shown to release

prostanoids in the following quantitative order: $PGI_2 > PGE_2 > PGF_{2\alpha} > TXA_2$.[106]

$PGF_{2\alpha}$, PGE_1, and PGE_2 contract isolated detrusor muscle, whereas PGE_1 and $PGF_{2\alpha}$ relax or have no effect on urethral smooth muscle.[10] Even if prostaglandins have contractile effects on the human bladder, it is still unclear whether they contribute to the pathogenesis of detrusor overactivity. Prostanoids may affect the bladder in two ways: directly by effects on the smooth muscle and/or indirectly via effects on the neurotransmission.[105] Probably, prostanoids do not act as true effector messengers along the efferent arm of the micturition reflex, but rather as a neuromodulator of the efferent and afferent neurotransmission.[105,107] An important physiological role might be sensitization of sensory nerves. Evidence for a sensitizing effect of PGE_2 has also been demonstrated *in vivo*. It was shown in the rat urinary bladder that intravesical instillation of PGE_2 lowered the threshold for reflex micturition, an effect which was blocked by systemic capsaicin desensitization. Indometacin pretreatment and systemic capsaicin increased the micturition threshold without affecting the amplitude of the micturition contraction.[105] Since intravesical PGE_2 did not reduce the residual volume in capsaicin-pretreated animals, it was suggested that endogenous prostanoids enhance the voiding efficiency through an effect, direct or indirect, on sensory nerves.

Prostanoids may also be involved in the pathophysiology of different bladder disorders. As pointed out by Maggi, in cystitis there may be an exaggerated prostanoid production, leading to intense activation of sensory nerves, increasing the afferent input.[105]

Cyclooxygenase is the pivotal enzyme in prostaglandin synthesis. It has been established that this enzyme exists in two isoforms, one constitutive (COX-1) and one inducible (COX-2).[108] The constitutive form is responsible for the normal physiological biosynthesis, whereas the inducible COX-2 is activated during inflammation.[109,110] Park et al demonstrated that the expression of COX-2 was increased as a consequence of bladder outflow obstruction.[111] If prostaglandins generated by COX-2 contribute to bladder overactivity, selective inhibitors of COX-2 would, theoretically, be one possible target for pharmacological therapy. Whether or not available selective COX-2 inhibitors would be useful as treatment for bladder overactivity remains to be established.

Nitric oxide. Evidence has accumulated that L-arginine-derived nitric oxide (NO) is responsible for the main part of the inhibitory NANC responses in the lower urinary tract.[10] However, NO may have different roles in the bladder and the urethra.

Nitrergic nerves: In biopsies taken from the lateral wall and trigone regions of the human bladder, a plexus of NADPH-diaphorase-containing nerve fibers was found.[112] Samples from the lateral bladder wall contained many NADPH-reactive nerve terminals, particularly in the subepithelial region immediately beneath the urothelium; occasionally, they penetrated into the epithelial layer. Immunohistochemical investigations of pig bladder revealed that the density of NO synthase (NOS) immunoreactivity was higher in trigonal and urethral tissue than in the detrusor.[113]

Functional effects of NO: Relaxations to electrical stimulation were found in small biopsy preparations of the human detrusor.[114] The relaxations were sensitive to the NOS-inhibitor L-NOARG, but insensitive to tetrodotoxin, and it was suggested that NO, generated from the detrusor, was important for bladder relaxation during the filling phase. However, Elliott and Castleden were unable to demonstrate a nerve-mediated relaxation in human detrusor.[115] In the pig detrusor, the NO-donor SIN-1, and exogenous NO relaxed muscle preparations, which were pre-contracted by carbachol and endothelin-1, by approximately 60%. However, isoprenaline was about 1000 times more potent than SIN-1 and NO and caused complete relaxation. Nitroprusside, SIN-1, and NO were only moderately effective in relaxing isolated rat, pig, and rabbit detrusor muscle, compared to their effects on the urethral muscle.[113,116,117]

It appears to be unlikely that NO has a major role as a neurotransmitter causing direct relaxation of the detrusor smooth muscle, since the detrusor sensitivity to NO and agents acting via the cyclic GMP system is low.[118] This is also reflected by the finding in rabbits that cyclic GMP is mainly related to urethral relaxation, and cyclic AMP to urinary bladder relaxation.[119] However, this does not exclude that NO may modulate the effects of other transmitters, or that it has a role in afferent neurotransmission.

Summary

There is abundant evidence that cholinergic neurotransmission is predominant in the activation of the human detrusor: this may not be the case in animals, and should be considered when animal models are used for the study of bladder function. Release of ACh, which stimulates M_3 and M_2 receptors on the detrusor smooth muscle cells, will lead to bladder contraction. Other neurotransmitters/modulators (e.g. ATP) have been demonstrated in the bladder of both animals and humans, but their roles in the human bladder remain to be established.

Urethra

Sufficient contraction of the urethral smooth muscle is an important function to provide continence during the storage phase of the micturition cycle. Equally important is

a coordinated and complete relaxation during the voiding phase. The normal pattern of voiding in humans is characterized by an initial drop in urethral pressure followed by an increase in intravesical pressure.[10,120] The mechanism of this relaxant effect has not been definitely established, but several factors may contribute. One possibility is that the drop in intraurethral pressure is caused by stimulation of muscarinic receptors on noradrenergic nerves, diminishing noradrenaline release and thereby tone in the proximal urethra. Another is that contraction of longitudinal urethral smooth muscle in the proximal urethra, produced by released ACh, causes shortening and widening of the urethra, with a concomitant decrease in intraurethral pressure. A third possibility is that an NANC mechanism mediates this response.[10]

Cholinergic mechanisms
Cholinergic nerves

The urethral smooth muscle receives a rich cholinergic innervation, of which the functional role is largely unknown. Most probably, the cholinergic nerves cause relaxation of the outflow region at the start of micturition by releasing NO and other relaxant transmitters, based on the principle of co-transmission, as multiple transmitters were found to be co-localized in cholinergic nerves. In pig urethra co-localization studies revealed that AChE-positive and some NOS-containing nerves had profiles that were similar. These nerves also contained NPY and VIP. NO-containing nerves were present in a density lower than that of the AChE-positive nerves, but higher than the density of any peptidergic nerves.[121] Coexistence of ACh and NOS in the rat major pelvic ganglion was demonstrated by double immunohistochemistry.[122] In the rat urethra, co-localization studies confirmed that NOS and VIP are contained within a population of cholinergic nerves.[16]

Muscarinic receptors

In rabbits, there are fewer muscarinic receptor binding sites in the urethra than in the bladder.[123] Muscarinic receptor agonists contract isolated urethral smooth muscle from several species, including humans, but these responses seem to be mediated mainly by the longitudinal muscle layer.[10] Investigating the whole length of the female human urethra, it was found that ACh contracted only the proximal part and the bladder neck.[124] If this contractile activation is exerted in the longitudinal direction, it should be expected that the urethra is shortened and that the urethral pressure decreases. Experimentally, *in-vitro* resistance to flow in the urethra was only increased by high concentrations of ACh.[125,126] However, in humans, tolerable doses of bethanechol and emeprone had little effect on intra-urethral pressure.[127,128]

Prejunctional muscarinic receptors may influence the release of both noradrenaline and ACh in the bladder neck/urethra. In urethral tissue from both rabbit and humans, carbachol decreased and scopolamine increased concentration-dependently the release of [^{3}H] noradrenaline from adrenergic, and of [^{3}H] choline from cholinergic nerve terminals.[129] This would mean that released ACh could inhibit noradrenaline release, thereby decreasing urethral tone and intraurethral pressure.

Studies in the pig urethra show that M_2 receptors are predominant over M_3. Additionally, contraction of the circular muscle appears to be mediated by M_2 and M_3, while the longitudinal response is mainly mediated by M_3 receptors.[130] This may have clinical interest since subtype-selective antimuscarinic drugs (M_3) are being introduced as a treatment of bladder overactivity.

Adrenergic mechanisms

Adrenergic nerves

The well-known anatomical differences between the male and female urethra are also reflected in the innervation. In the human male, the smooth muscle surrounding the preprostatic part of the urethra is richly innervated by both cholinergic and adrenergic nerves, and considered a 'sexual sphincter', contracting during ejaculation and thus preventing retrograde transport of sperm.[131] The role of this structure in maintaining continence is unclear, but probably not essential.

In the human female, the muscle bundles run obliquely or longitudinally along the length of the urethra, and in the whole human female urethra, as well as in the human male urethra below the preprostatic part, there is only a scarce supply of adrenergic nerves.[5,132] Fine varicose nerve terminals can be seen along the bundles of smooth muscle cells, running both longitudinally and transversely. Adrenergic terminals can also be found around blood vessels. Co-localization studies in animals have revealed that adrenergic nerves, identified by immunohistochemistry using tyrosine hydroxylase (TH), also contain NPY.[133] Chemical sympathectomy in rats resulted in a complete disappearance of the adrenergic nerves, while NOS-containing nerve fibers were not affected by the treatment.[134] This suggests that NOS is not contained within adrenergic nerves.

Both α and β ARs have been found in isolated urethral smooth muscle from animals as well as humans.[125,135–137]

α Adrenoceptors

In humans, up to about 50% of the intraurethral pressure is maintained by stimulation of α ARs, as judged from results obtained with α-AR antagonists and epidural anesthesia in urodynamic studies.[138,139] In human urethral smooth muscle, both functional and receptor binding studies have suggested that the α_1 AR subtype is the predominating postjunctional α AR.[10,140] However, most in-vitro investigations of human urethral α ARs were done in males, and the results support the existence of a sphincter structure in the male proximal urethra, which cannot be found in the female. Other marked differences between sexes in the distribution of α_1 and α_2 ARs (as found in, for example, rabbits), or in the distribution of α_1 AR subtypes, do not seem to occur.[141]

Separating the entire length of the isolated female human urethra into seven parts, from the external meatus to the bladder neck, it was found that noradrenaline (α_1 and α_2), but not clonidine (α_2), produced concentration-dependent contractions in all parts, with a peak in middle to proximal urethra.[124] Also, a similarity in patterns between noradrenaline-induced contraction and the urethral pressure profile in the human urethra was demonstrated.

Among the three high-affinity α_1 AR subtypes (α_{1A}, α_{1B}, α_{1D}) identified in molecular cloning and functional studies, α_{1A} seems to predominate in the human lower urinary tract. However, a receptor with low affinity for prazosin (the α_{1L} AR) was found to be prominent in the human male urethra and may represent a functional phenotype of the α_{1A} AR.[142,143] In the human female urethra, the expression and distribution of α_1 AR subtypes were determined and mRNA for the α_{1A} subtype was predominant. Autoradiography confirmed the predominance of the α_{1A} AR.[141]

The studies cited above suggest that the sympathetic innervation helps to maintain urethral smooth muscle tone through α_1 AR receptor stimulation. If urethral α_1 ARs are contributing to the lower urinary tract symptoms (LUTS), which can occur also in women, an effect of α_1 AR antagonists should be expected in women with these symptoms.[144,145] This was found to be the case in some studies, but was not confirmed in a randomized, placebo-controlled pilot study, which showed that terazosin was not effective for the treatment of 'prostatism-like' symptoms in aging women.[146]

Urethral α_2 ARs are able to control the release of noradrenaline from adrenergic nerves, as shown in in-vitro studies. In the rabbit urethra, incubated with [^{3}H] noradrenaline, electrical stimulation of nerves caused a release of [^{3}H] which was decreased by noradrenaline and clonidine, and increased by the α_2 AR antagonist rauwolscine.[129] Clonidine was shown to reduce intraurethral pressure in humans, an effect that may be attributed partly to a peripheral effect on adrenergic nerve terminals.[147] More probable, however, this effect is exerted on the central nervous system with a resulting decrease in peripheral sympathetic nervous activity. The subtype of prejunctional α_2 AR involved in [^{3}H] noradrenaline secretion in the isolated guinea pig urethra was suggested to be of the α_{2A} subtype.[31]

Prejunctional α_2-AR regulation of transmitter release is not confined to adrenergic nerves.[10] Electrical field stimulation (EFS; frequencies above 12 Hz) of spontaneously contracted smooth muscle strips from the female pig urethra evoked long-lasting, frequency-dependent relaxations in the presence of prazosin, scopolamine, and the NOS inhibitor L-NOARG, suggesting the release of an unknown relaxation-producing mediator. Treatment with a selective α_2 AR agonist markedly reduced the relaxations evoked by EFS at all frequencies tested (16–30 Hz). This inhibitory effect was completely antagonized by the α_2 AR antagonist rauwolscine, and the results suggested that the release of the unknown mediator in the female pig urethra can be modulated via α_2 ARs.[148]

β Adrenoceptors

In humans, the β ARs in the bladder neck were suggested to be of the β_2 subtype, as shown by receptor-binding studies using subtype-selective antagonists.[149] However, β_3 ARs can be found in the striated urethral sphincter.[150]

Although the functional importance of urethral β ARs has not been established, they have been targets for therapeutic intervention. Selective β_2 AR agonists have been shown to reduce intraurethral pressure, while β AR antagonists did not influence intraurethral pressure in acute studies.[151–154] The theoretical basis for the use of β AR antagonists in the treatment of stress incontinence is that blockade of urethral β ARs may enhance the effects of noradrenaline on urethral α ARs. Even if propranolol has been reported to have beneficial effects in the treatment of stress incontinence, this does not seem to be an effective treatment.[10]

After selective β_2 AR antagonists have been used as a treatment of stress incontinence, it seems paradoxical that the selective β_2 AR agonist, clenbuterol, was found to cause significant clinical improvement in women with stress incontinence.[155] The positive effects were suggested to be a result of an action on urethral striated muscle and/or the pelvic floor muscles.[150,156]

Non-adrenergic, non-cholinergic mechanisms

The mechanical responses to autonomic nerve stimulation and to intra-arterial ACh injection on resistance to flow in the proximal urethra, was tested in male cats. It was found that sacral ventral root stimulation produced an atropine-sensitive constriction when basal urethral resistance was low, but dilatation when resistance was high.[157] The latter response was reduced, but not abolished, by atropine. When urethral constriction had been produced by phenylephrine, injection of ACh produced a consistent decrease in urethral resistance, which was then not reduced by atropine. It was suggested that parasympathetic dilatation of the urethra may be mediated by an unknown NANC transmitter released from postganglionic neurons. The predominant transmitter is believed to be NO.

Nitric oxide

NO has shown to be an important inhibitory neurotransmitter in the lower urinary tract.[10,158] NO-mediated responses in smooth muscle preparations are found to be linked to an increase in cyclic GMP (cGMP) formation, which has been demonstrated in several urethra preparations.[117,119,159,160] Subsequent activation of a cGMP-dependent protein kinase (cGK) has been suggested to hyperpolarize the cell membrane, probably by causing a leftward shift of the activation curve for the K^+ channels, thereby increasing their open probability.[161,162] There have also been reports suggesting that NO in some smooth muscles might act directly on the K^+ channels.[163,164] Other mechanisms for NO-induced relaxations, mediated by cGMP, might involve reduced intracellular Ca^{2+} levels by intracellular sequestration, or reduced sensitivity of the contractile machinery to Ca^{2+}, both mechanisms acting without changing the membrane potential.[165] Electrophysiological registrations from urethral smooth muscle are scarce: however, following NANC stimulation in some preparations of urethral smooth muscle from male rabbits, a hyperpolarization was found.[166]

Persson et al investigated the cGMP pathway in mice lacking cGK type I (cGKI). In the wild type controls, EFS elicited frequency-dependent relaxations in urethral preparations. The relaxations were abolished by L-NOARG, and instead a contractile response occurred. In cGKI $-/-$ urethral strips, the response to EFS was practically absent, but a small relaxation generally appeared at high stimulation frequencies (16–32 Hz). This relaxant response was not inhibited by L-NOARG, suggesting the occurrence of additional relaxant transmitter(s).[167]

The abundant occurrence of NOS-immunoreactive (IR) nerve fibers in the rabbit urethra also supports the present view of NO as the main inhibitory NANC mediator.[117] Using cGMP antibodies, target cells for NO were localized in rabbit urethra. Spindle-shaped cGMP-IR cells, distinct from the smooth muscle cells, formed a network around and between the urethral smooth muscle bundles.[168] Similar cGMP IR interstitial cells were found in guinea pig and human bladder/urethra, but in contrast to the findings in rabbits, smooth muscle cells with cGMP immunoreactivity were found in the urethra tissues, following stimulation with sodium nitroprusside.[169] The occurrence of cGMP immunoreactivity in smooth muscle cells seems logical, since NO is believed to stimulate guanylyl cyclase with subsequent cGMP formation in the cells.

The function of the interstitial cells has not been established, but since they have morphological similarities to the interstitial cells of Cajal (ICC) in the gut, which are considered pacemaker cells, it has been speculated that they may also have a similar function in the lower urinary tract. Studies performed in rabbit urethral tissue showed regular spontaneous depolarization of these interstitial cells, suggesting that they indeed may have pacemaker function.[170] The specific marker for ICC, c-kit, was used to demonstrate these cells also in the guinea pig bladder, further suggesting the existence of this mechanism in the lower urinary tract.[171]

Carbon monoxide

The role of CO in urethral function is still controversial. It has been assumed that CO causes relaxation through the cGMP pathway. A weak relaxant effect of exogenous CO, compared to NO, was found in the rabbit urethra, suggesting that CO is not an important mediator of relaxation in this tissue.[168] However, there are known interspecies differences of urethral relaxant responses to CO. In guinea pig urethras the maximal relaxant response to CO did not exceed $15 \pm 3\%$, compared to $40 \pm 7\%$ in pigs.[160,172] The distribution of the CO-producing enzymes heme oxygenases, HO-1 and HO-2, was investigated in urethral smooth muscle of several species. In guinea pigs, HO-2 immunoreactivity was found in all nerve cell bodies of intramural ganglia, localized between smooth muscle bundles in the detrusor, bladder base, and proximal urethra.[172] In the pig urethra, HO-2 immunoreactivity was found in coarse nerve trunks, and HO-1 immunoreactivity in nerve cells, coarse nerve trunks, and varicose nerve fibers within urethral smooth muscle. In strip preparations, exogenously applied CO evoked a small relaxation associated with a small increase in cGMP, but not cAMP, content.[173] However, HO-2 and the NO-producing enzyme neuronal NO synthase (nNOS) were found coexisting in nerve trunks of human male and female urethras, suggesting the possibility of interaction between both systems.[174]

Nassem et al found that in the presence of hydrogen peroxide, the relaxation responses to both CO and NO in the rabbit urethra were significantly increased, and it was suggested that hydrogen peroxide may amplify NO- and CO-mediated responses.[175] In pigs an even more pronounced increase in relaxant response to CO in female pig urethra, using YC-1, a stimulator of sGC, suggested a possible messenger function role for CO in urethral relaxation.[160]

Vasoactive intestinal polypeptide

In various species, VIP-containing urethral ganglion cells have been demonstrated, and numerous VIP-IR nerve fibers have been observed around ganglion cells, in the bladder neck, in the urethral smooth muscle layers, in lamina propria, and in association with blood vessels.[5] However, whether the findings have relevance in man is not proven.

In the pig urethra, VIP and NOS seem to be partly co-localized within nerve fibers.[121] In the rabbit urethra VIP-IR nerve fibers occurred throughout the smooth muscle layer, although the number of nerves was lower than that of NOS-IR structures and a marked relaxation of the isolated rabbit urethral muscle to VIP was reported.[168] Both pelvic and hypogastric nerve stimulation in dogs increased the bladder venous effluent VIP concentration, supporting the view that VIP can be released also from urethral nerves.[88] VIP had a marked inhibitory effect on the isolated female rabbit urethra contracted by noradrenaline or EFS, without affecting noradrenaline release, but in human urethral smooth muscle, relaxant responses were less consistent. However, a modulatory role in neurotransmission could not be excluded.[176] Infusion of VIP in humans in amounts that caused circulatory side-effects, had no effects on urethral resistance, despite the fact that plasma concentrations of VIP were obtained which, in other clinical investigations, had been sufficient to cause relaxation of the lower esophageal sphincter and to depress uterine contractions.[89] Therefore, the physiological importance of VIP for the lower urinary tract function in humans was questioned, and it is still unclear whether or not VIP contributes to NANC-mediated relaxation of the human urethra.[89]

Adenosine triphosphate

ATP has been found to cause smooth muscle relaxation via G-protein coupled P2Y receptors.[177] ATP may also induce relaxation via breakdown to adenosine. In strips of precontracted guinea pig urethra, it was found that ATP caused relaxation and inhibited spontaneous electrical activity.[178] In precontracted preparations, ATP had almost no effect on EFS-induced relaxation in isolated male rabbit circular urethral smooth muscle; however, suramin, a nonselective P2Y-purinoceptor antagonist, and L-NOARG, both concentration-dependently attenuated the relaxation. ATP and related purine compounds (adenosine, AMP, and ADP) each reduced induced tonic contractions in a concentration-dependent manner. The outflow of ATP, measured using the luciferase technique, was markedly increased by EFS.[179] The findings suggested that P2Y purinoceptors exist in the male rabbit urethra, and that ATP and related purine compounds may play a role in NANC neurotransmission. This conclusion was further supported in studies on circular strips of hamster proximal urethra precontracted with arginine vasopressin. EFS caused frequency-dependent relaxations, which were attenuated by suramin and reactive blue. Exogenous ATP produced concentration-related relaxations, which were also attenuated by suramin and reactive blue.[180] The relevance of this system in man remains to be established.

Summary

Available information supports the idea that sympathetic activity, via release of noradrenaline and stimulation of urethral smooth muscle α_1 ARs, is a main factor in the maintenance of intraurethral pressure and, thus, of continence. NO, produced by NOS within cholinergic nerves, seems to be the predominant inhibitory neurotransmitter in the urethra, even if there is good evidence for the existence of other, as yet unidentified, inhibitory transmitters.

References

1. Morrison JF, Steers W, Brading AF, et al. Neurophysiology and neuropharmacology. In: Abrams P, Cardozo L, Khoury S, Wein A, eds. Incontinence, Vol. 1. Plymbridge: Plymbridge Distributors Ltd, UK, 2002:83–163.

2. Griffiths D, Holstege G, Dalm E, de Wall H. Control and coordination of bladder and urethral function in the brainstem of the cat. Neurourol Urodyn 1990; 9:63–82.

3. Blok BF, Holstege G. Two pontine micturition centers in the cat are not interconnected directly: implications for the central organization of micturition. J Comp Neurol 1999; 403:209–218.

4. de Groat WC, Boot AM, Yoshimura N. Neurophysiology of micturition and its modification in animal models of human diseases. In: Maggi CA, ed. Nervous control of the urogenital system, Vol. 3. London: Harwood Academic Publishers, 1993:227–290.

5. Lincoln J, Burnstock G. Autonomic inervation of the urinary bladder and urethra. In: Maggi CA, ed. Nervous control of the urogenital system, Vol. 3. London: Harwood Academic Publishers, 1993:33–68.

6. Andersson KE, Persson K. Nitric oxide synthase and the lower urinary tract: possible implications for physiology and pathophysiology. Scand J Urol Nephrol Suppl 1995; 175:43–53.

7. Bridgewater M, MacNeil HF, Brading AF. Regulation of tone in pig urethral smooth muscle. J Urol 1993; 150:223–228.

8. Hashimoto S, Kigoshi S, Muramatsu I. Nitric oxide-dependent and -independent neurogenic relaxation of isolated dog urethra. Eur J Pharmacol 1993; 231:209–214.

9. Werkstrom V, Persson K, Ny L, et al. Factors involved in the relaxation of female pig urethra evoked by electrical field stimulation. Br J Pharmacol 1995; 116:1599–1604.

10. Andersson KE. Pharmacology of lower urinary tract smooth muscles and penile erectile tissues. Pharmacol Rev 1993; 45:253–308.

11. Yoshimura N, de Groat WC. Neural control of the lower urinary tract. Int J Urol 1997; 4:111–125.

12. Janig W, Morrison JF. Functional properties of spinal visceral afferents supplying abdominal and pelvic organs, with special emphasis on visceral nociception. Prog Brain Res 1986; 67:87–114.

13. Habler HJ, Janig W, Koltzenburg M. Activation of unmyelinated afferent fibres by mechanical stimuli and inflammation of the urinary bladder in the cat. J Physiol 1990; 425:545–562.

14. Fall M, Lindstrom S, Mazieres L. A bladder-to-bladder cooling reflex in the cat. J Physiol 1990; 427:281–300.

15. de Groat WC, Yoshimura N. Pharmacology of the lower urinary tract. Annu Rev Pharmacol Toxicol 2001; 41:691–721.

16. Arvidsson U, Riedl M, Elde R, Meister B. Vesicular acetylcholine transporter (VAChT) protein: a novel and unique marker for cholinergic neurons in the central and peripheral nervous systems. J Comp Neurol 1997; 378:454–467.

17. Persson K, Andersson KE, Alm P. Choline acetyltransferase and vesicular acetylcholine transporter protein in neurons innervating the rat lower urinary tract. Proc Soc Neurosci 1997; 596.

18. Dixon JS, Jen PY, Gosling JA. The distribution of vesicular acetylcholine transporter in the human male genitourinary organs and its co-localization with neuropeptide Y and nitric oxide synthase. Neurourol Urodyn 2000; 19:185–194.

19. Caulfield MP, Birdsall NJ. International Union of Pharmacology. XVII. Classification of muscarinic acetylcholine receptors. Pharmacol Rev 1998; 50:279–290.

20. Bonev AD, Nelson MT. Muscarinic inhibition of ATP-sensitive K+ channels by protein kinase C in urinary bladder smooth muscle. Am J Physiol 1993; 265:C1723–1728.

21. Hegde SS, Eglen RM. Muscarinic receptor subtypes modulating smooth muscle contractility in the urinary bladder. Life Sci 1999; 64:419–428.

22. Yamaguchi O, Shishido K, Tamura K, et al. Evaluation of mRNAs encoding muscarinic receptor subtypes in human detrusor muscle. J Urol 1996; 156:1208–1213.

23. Harriss DR, Marsh KA, Birmingham AT, Hill SJ. Expression of muscarinic M3-receptors coupled to inositol phospholipid hydrolysis in human detrusor cultured smooth muscle cells. J Urol 1995; 154:1241–1245.

24. Hegde SS, Choppin A, Bonhaus D, et al. Functional role of M2 and M3 muscarinic receptors in the urinary bladder of rats in vitro and in vivo. Br J Pharmacol 1997; 120:1409–1418.

25. Fetscher C, Fleichman M, Schmidt M, et al. M(3) muscarinic receptors mediate contraction of human urinary bladder. Br J Pharmacol 2002; 136:641–644.

26. Matsui M, Motomura D, Karasawa H, et al. Multiple functional defects in peripheral autonomic organs in mice lacking muscarinic acetylcholine receptor gene for the M3 subtype. Proc Natl Acad Sci USA 2000; 97:9579–9584.

27. Stengel PW, Yamada M, Wess J, Cohen ML. M(3)-receptor knockout mice: muscarinic receptor function in atria, stomach fundus, urinary bladder, and trachea. Am J Physiol Regul Integr Comp Physiol 2002; 282:R1443–1449.

28. Krichevsky VP, Pagala MK, Vaydovsky I, et al. Function of M3 muscarinic receptors in the rat urinary bladder following partial outlet obstruction. J Urol 1999; 161:1644–1650.

29. Braverman A, Legos J, Young W, et al. M2 receptors in genito-urinary smooth muscle pathology. Life Sci 1999; 64:429–436.

30. Braverman AS, Luthin GR, Ruggieri MR. M2 muscarinic receptor contributes to contraction of the denervated rat urinary bladder. Am J Physiol 1998; 275:R1654–1660.

31. Alberts P. Classification of the presynaptic muscarinic receptor subtype that regulates 3H-acetylcholine secretion in the guinea pig urinary bladder in vitro. J Pharmacol Exp Ther 1995; 274:458–468.

32. D'Agostino G, Bolognesi ML, Lucchelli A, et al. Prejunctional muscarinic inhibitory control of acetylcholine release in the human isolated detrusor: involvement of the M4 receptor subtype. Br J Pharmacol 2000; 129:493–500.

33. Somogyi GT, de Groat WC. Evidence for inhibitory nicotinic and facilitatory muscarinic receptors in cholinergic nerve terminals of the rat urinary bladder. J Auton Nerv Syst 1992; 37:89–97.

34. Tobin G, Sjogren C. In vivo and in vitro effects of muscarinic receptor antagonists on contractions and release of [3H]acetylcholine in the rabbit urinary bladder. Eur J Pharmacol 1995; 281:1–8.

35. Somogyi GT, de Groat WC. Function, signal transduction mechanisms and plasticity of presynaptic muscarinic receptors in the urinary bladder. Life Sci 1999; 64:411–418.

36. Andersson KE. New roles for muscarinic receptors in the pathophysiology of lower urinary tract symptoms. BJU Int 2000; 86: 36–43.

37. Gary T, Robertson D. Lessons learned from dopamine beta-hydroxylase deficiency in humans. News Physiol Sci 1994; 9:35–39.

38. Goepel M, Wittmann A, Rubben H, Michel MC. Comparison of adrenoceptor subtype expression in porcine and human bladder and prostate. Urol Res 1997; 25:199–206.

39. Malloy BJ, Price DT, Price RR, et al. Alpha1-adrenergic receptor subtypes in human detrusor. J Urol 1998; 160:937–943.

40. Hampel C, Dolber PC, Smith MP, et al. Modulation of bladder alpha1-adrenergic receptor subtype expression by bladder outlet obstruction. J Urol 2002; 167:1513–1521.

41. Nomiya M, Shishido K, Uchida H, Yamaguchi O. A quantitative analysis of mRNA expression of α_1- and β-adrenoceptor subtypes and their functional roles in human normal and obstructed bladders. Neurourol Urodyn 2002; 21:299–300.

42. Nergardh A, Boreus LO, Naglo AS. Characterization of the adrenergic beta-receptor in the urinary bladder of man and cat. Acta Pharmacol Toxicol (Copenh) 1977; 40:14–21.

43. Larsen JJ. Alpha and beta-adrenoceptors in the detrusor muscle and bladder base of the pig and beta-adrenoceptors in the detrusor muscle of man. Br J Pharmacol 1979; 65:215–222.

44. Igawa Y, Yamazaki Y, Takeda H, et al. Functional and molecular biological evidence for a possible beta3-adrenoceptor in the human detrusor muscle. Br J Pharmacol 1999; 126:819–825.

45. Takeda M, Obara K, Mizusawa T, et al. Evidence for beta3-adrenoceptor subtypes in relaxation of the human urinary bladder detrusor: analysis by molecular biological and pharmacological methods. J Pharmacol Exp Ther 1999; 288:1367–1373.

46. Yamazaki Y, Takeda H, Akahane M, et al. Species differences in the distribution of beta-adrenoceptor subtypes in bladder smooth muscle. Br J Pharmacol 1998; 124:593–599.

47. Yamaguchi O. Beta3-adrenoceptors in human detrusor muscle. Urology 2002; 59:25–29.

48. Andersson KE, Chapple C, Wein A. The basis for drug treatment of the overactive bladder. World J Urol 2001; 19:294–298.

49. Rohner TJ, Hannigan JD, Sanford EJ. Altered in vitro adrenergic responses of dog detrusor muscle after chronic bladder outlet obstruction. Urology 1978; 11:357–361.

50. Tsujii T, Azuma H, Yamaguchi T, Oshima H. A possible role of decreased relaxation mediated by beta-adrenoceptors in bladder outlet obstruction by benign prostatic hyperplasia. Br J Pharmacol 1992; 107:803–807.

51. Igawa Y, Yamazaki Y, Takeda H, et al. Relaxant effects of isoproterenol and selective beta3-adrenoceptor agonists on normal, low compliant and hyperreflexic human bladders. J Urol 2001; 165: 240–244.

52. Tanaka N, Tamai T, Mukaiyama H, et al. Beta(3)-adrenoceptor agonists for the treatment of frequent urination and urinary incontinence: 2-[4-(2-[[(1S,2R)-2-hydroxy-2-(4-hydroxyphenyl)-1-methylethyl]amino]ethyl)phenoxy]-2-methylpropionic acid. Bioorg Med Chem 2001; 9:3265–3271.

53. Woods M, Carson N, Norton NW, et al. Efficacy of the beta3-adrenergic receptor agonist CL-316243 on experimental bladder hyperreflexia and detrusor instability in the rat. J Urol 2001; 166: 1142–1147.

54. Luheshi GN, Zar MA. Presence of non-cholinergic motor transmission in human isolated bladder. J Pharm Pharmacol 1990; 42: 223–224.

55. Sjogren C, Andersson KE, Husted S, et al. Atropine resistance of transmurally stimulated isolated human bladder muscle. J Urol 1982; 128:1368–1371.

56. Sibley GN. A comparison of spontaneous and nerve-mediated activity in bladder muscle from man, pig and rabbit. J Physiol 1984; 354:431–443.

57. Smith DJ, Chapple C. In vitro response of human bladder smooth muscle in unstable obstructed male bladders: a study of pathophysiological causes. Neurourol Urodyn 1994; 134:14–15.

58. Bayliss M, Wu C, Newgreen D, et al. A quantitative study of atropine-resistant contractile responses in human detrusor smooth muscle, from stable, unstable and obstructed bladders. J Urol 1999; 162:1833–1839.

59. Saito M, Kondo A, Kato T, Miyake K. Response of the human neurogenic bladder induced by intramural nerve stimulation. Nippon Hinyokika Gakkai Zasshi 1993; 84:507–513.

60. O'Reilly BA, Kosaka AH, Knight GF, et al. P2X receptors and their role in female idiopathic detrusor instability. J Urol 2002; 167:157–164.

61. Palea S, Artibani W, Ostardo E, et al. Evidence for purinergic neurotransmission in human urinary bladder affected by interstitial cystitis. J Urol 1993; 150:2007–2012.

62. Wammack R, Weihe E, Dienes HP, Hohenfellner R. Die Neurogene Blase in vitro. Akt Urol 1995; 26:16–18.

63. Yoshida M, Homma Y, Inadome A, et al. Age-related changes in cholinergic and purinergic neurotransmission in human isolated bladder smooth muscles. Exp Gerontol 2001; 36:99–109.

64. Burnstock G. Purine-mediated signalling in pain and visceral perception. Trends Pharmacol Sci 2001; 22:182–188.

65. Lee HY, Bardini M, Burnstock G. Distribution of P2X receptors in the urinary bladder and the ureter of the rat. J Urol 2000; 163:2002–2007.

66. O'Reilly BA, Kosaka AH, Chang TK, et al. A quantitative analysis of purinoceptor expression in the bladders of patients with symptomatic outlet obstruction. BJU Int 2001; 87:617–622.

67. Moore KH, Ray FR, Barden JA. Loss of purinergic P2X(3) and P2X(5) receptor innervation in human detrusor from adults with urge incontinence. J Neurosci 2001; 21:RC166.

68. Ferguson DR, Kennedy I, Burton TJ. ATP is released from rabbit urinary bladder epithelial cells by hydrostatic pressure changes – a possible sensory mechanism? J Physiol 1997; 505:503–511.

69. Vlaskovska M, Kasakov L, Rong W, et al. P2X3 knock-out mice reveal a major sensory role for urothelially released ATP. J Neurosci 2001; 21:5670–5677.

70. Chen CC, Akopian AN, Sivilotti L, et al. A P2X purinoceptor expressed by a subset of sensory neurons. Nature 1995; 377:428–431.

71. Dunn PM, Zhong Y, Burnstock G. P2X receptors in peripheral neurons. Prog Neurobiol 2001; 65:107–134.

72. Cockayne DA, Hamilton SG, Zhu QM, et al. Urinary bladder hyporeflexia and reduced pain-related behaviour in P2X3-deficient mice. Nature 2000; 407:1011–1015.

73. Elneil S, Skepper JN, Kidd EJ, et al. Distribution of P2X(1) and P2X(3) receptors in the rat and human urinary bladder. Pharmacology 2001; 63:120–128.

74. Yiangou Y, Facer P, Ford A, et al. Capsaicin receptor VR1 and ATP-gated ion channel P2X3 in human urinary bladder. BJU Int 2001; 87:774–779.

75. Namasivayam S, Eardley I, Morrison JF. Purinergic sensory neurotransmission in the urinary bladder: an in vitro study in the rat. BJU Int 1999; 84:854–860.

76. Pandita RK, Andersson KE. Intravesical adenosine triphosphate stimulates the micturition reflex in awake, freely moving rats. J Urol 2002; 168:1230–1234.

77. Maggi CA. The dual, sensory and "efferent" function of the capsaicin-sensitive primary sensory neurons in the urinary bladder and urethra. In: Maggi CA, ed. Nervous control of the urogenital system, Vol. 3. London: Harwood Academic Publishers, 1993:383–422.

78. Maggi CA. The mammalian tachykinin receptors. Gen Pharmacol 1995; 26:911–944.

79. Uckert S, Stief CG, Lietz B, et al. Possible role of bioactive peptides in the regulation of human detrusor smooth muscle – functional effects in vitro and immunohistochemical presence. World J Urol 2002; 20:244–249.

80. Maggi CA, Barbanti G, Santicioli P, et al. Cystometric evidence that capsaicin-sensitive nerves modulate the afferent branch of micturition reflex in humans. J Urol 1989; 142:150–154.

81. Chapple CR, Milner P, Moss HE, Burnstock G. Loss of sensory neuropeptides in the obstructed human bladder. Br J Urol 1992; 70:373–381.

82. Giuliani S, Patacchini R, Barbanti G, et al. Characterization of the tachykinin neurokinin-2 receptor in the human urinary bladder by means of selective receptor antagonists and peptidase inhibitors. J Pharmacol Exp Ther 1993; 267:590–595.

83. Saenz de Tejada I, Mueller JD, de Las Morenas A, et al. Endothelin in the urinary bladder. I. Synthesis of endothelin-1 by epithelia, muscle and fibroblasts suggests autocrine and paracrine cellular regulation. J Urol 1992; 148:1290–1298.

84. Kondo S, Morita T, Tashima Y. Benign prostatic hypertrophy affects the endothelin receptor density in the human urinary bladder and prostate. Urol Int 1995; 54:198–203.

85. Okamoto-Koizumi T, Takeda M, Komeyama T, et al. Pharmacological and molecular biological evidence for ETA endothelin receptor subtype mediating mechanical responses in the detrusor smooth muscle of the human urinary bladder. Clin Sci (Lond) 1999; 96:397–402.

86. Khan MA, Shukla N, Auld J, et al. Possible role of endothelin-1 in the rabbit urinary bladder hyperplasia secondary to partial bladder outlet obstruction. Scand J Urol Nephrol 2000; 34: 15–20.

87. Andersson PO, Bloom SR, Mattiasson A, Uvelius B. Bladder vasodilatation and release of vasoactive intestinal polypeptide from the urinary bladder of the cat in response to pelvic nerve stimulation. J Urol 1987; 138:671–673.

88. Andersson PO, Sjogren C, Uvnas B, Uvnas-Moberg K. Urinary bladder and urethral responses to pelvic and hypogastric nerve stimulation and their relation to vasoactive intestinal polypeptide in the anaesthetized dog. Acta Physiol Scand 1990; 138:409–416.

89. Klarskov P, Holm-Bentzen M, Norgaard T, et al. Vasoactive intestinal polypeptide concentration in human bladder neck smooth muscle and its influence on urodynamic parameters. Br J Urol 1987; 60:113–118.

90. Gu J, Restorick JM, Blank MA, et al. Vasoactive intestinal polypeptide in the normal and unstable bladder. Br J Urol 1983; 55:645–647.

91. Persson K, Garcia-Pascual A, Andersson KE. Difference in the actions of calcitonin gene-related peptide on pig detrusor and vesical arterial smooth muscle. Acta Physiol Scand 1991; 143:45–53.

92. Giuliani S, Santicioli P, Lippi A, et al. The role of sensory neuropeptides in motor innervation of the hamster isolated urinary bladder. Naunyn Schmiedebergs Arch Pharmacol 2001; 364:242–248.

93. Lacroix JS, Stjarne P, Anggard A, Lundberg JM. Sympathetic vascular control of the pig nasal mucosa (III): Co-release of noradrenaline and neuropeptide Y. Acta Physiol Scand 1989; 135:17–28.

94. Iravani MM, Zar MA. Neuropeptide Y in rat detrusor and its effect on nerve-mediated and acetylcholine-evoked contractions. Br J Pharmacol 1994; 113:95–102.

95. Zoubek J, Somogyi GT, De Groat WC. A comparison of inhibitory effects of neuropeptide Y on rat urinary bladder, urethra, and vas deferens. Am J Physiol 1993; 265:R537–543.

96. Lundberg JM, Hua XY, Franco-Cereceda A. Effects of neuropeptide Y (NPY) on mechanical activity and neurotransmission in the heart, vas deferens and urinary bladder of the guinea-pig. Acta Physiol Scand 1984; 121:325–332.

97. Crowe R, Noble J, Robson T, et al. An increase of neuropeptide Y but not nitric oxide synthase-immunoreactive nerves in the bladder neck from male patients with bladder neck dyssynergia. J Urol 1995; 154:1231–1236.

98. Dixon JS, Jen PY, Gosling JA. A double-label immunohistochemical study of intramural ganglia from the human male urinary bladder neck. J Anat 1997; 190:125–134.

99. Gu J, Blank MA, Huang WM, et al. Peptide-containing nerves in human urinary bladder. Urology 1984; 24:353–357.

100. Iwasa A. Distribution of neuropeptide Y (NPY) and its binding sites in human lower urinary tract. Histological analysis. Nippon Hinyokika Gakkai Zasshi 1993; 84:1000–1006.

101. Davis B, Goepel M, Bein S, et al. Lack of neuropeptide Y receptor detection in human bladder and prostate. BJU Int 2000; 85:918–924.

102. Brown WW, Zenser TV, Davis BB. Prostaglandin E2 production by rabbit urinary bladder. Am J Physiol 1980; 239:F452–458.

103. Downie JW, Karmazyn M. Mechanical trauma to bladder epithelium liberates prostanoids which modulate neurotransmission in rabbit detrusor muscle. J Pharmacol Exp Ther 1984; 230:445–449.

104. Jeremy JY, Dandona P. Fluoride but not phorbol esters stimulate rat urinary bladder prostanoid synthesis: investigations into the roles of G proteins and protein kinase C. Prostaglandins Leukot Med 1987; 29:129–139.

105. Maggi CA. Prostanoids as local modulators of reflex micturition. Pharmacol Res 1992; 25:13–20.

106. Jeremy JY, Tsang V, Mikhailidis DP, et al. Eicosanoid synthesis by human urinary bladder mucosa: pathological implications. Br J Urol 1987; 59:36–39.

107. Andersson KE, Sjogren C. Aspects on the physiology and pharmacology of the bladder and urethra. Prog Neurobiol 1982; 19:71–89.

108. Feng L, Sun W, Xia Y, et al. Cloning two isoforms of rat cyclooxygenase: differential regulation of their expression. Arch Biochem Biophys 1993; 307:361–368.

109. Pairet M, Engelhardt G. Distinct isoforms (COX-1 and COX-2) of cyclooxygenase: possible physiological and therapeutic implications. Fundam Clin Pharmacol 1996; 10:1–17.

110. Vane JR, Botting RM. Mechanism of action of anti-inflammatory drugs. Scand J Rheumatol Suppl 1996; 102:9–21.

111. Park JM, Yang T, Arend LJ, et al. Cyclooxygenase-2 is expressed in bladder during fetal development and stimulated by outlet obstruction. Am J Physiol 1997; 273:F538–544.

112. Smet PJ, Edyvane KA, Jonavicius J, Marshall VR. Distribution of NADPH-diaphorase-positive nerves supplying the human urinary bladder. J Auton Nerv Syst 1994; 47:109–113.

113. Persson K, Alm P, Johansson K, et al. Nitric oxide synthase in pig lower urinary tract: immunohistochemistry, NADPH diaphorase histochemistry and functional effects. Br J Pharmacol 1993; 110:521–530.

114. James MJ, Birmingham AT, Hill SJ. Partial mediation by nitric oxide of the relaxation of human isolated detrusor strips in response to electrical field stimulation. Br J Clin Pharmacol 1993; 35:366–372.

115. Elliot RA, Castleden CM. Nerve mediated relaxation in human detrusor muscle. Br J Clin Pharmacol 1993; 36:479.

116. Persson K, Igawa Y, Mattiasson A, Andersson KE. Effects of inhibition of the L-arginine/nitric oxide pathway in the rat lower urinary tract in vivo and in vitro. Br J Pharmacol 1992; 107:178–184.

117. Persson K, Andersson KE. Non-adrenergic, non-cholinergic relaxation and levels of cyclic nucleotides in rabbit lower urinary tract. Eur J Pharmacol 1994; 268:159–167.

118. Andersson KE. Pathways for relaxation of detrusor smooth muscle. Adv Exp Med Biol 1999; 462:241–252.

119. Morita T, Tsujii T, Dokita S. Regional difference in functional roles of cAMP and cGMP in lower urinary tract smooth muscle contractility. Urol Int 1992; 49:191–195.

120. Tanagho EA, Miller ER. Initiation of voiding. Br J Urol 1970; 42:175–183.

121. Persson K, Alm P, Johansson K, et al. Co-existence of nitrergic, peptidergic and acetylcholine esterase-positive nerves in the pig lower urinary tract. J Auton Nerv Syst 1995; 52:225–236.

122. Persson K, Alm P, Uvelius B, Andersson KE. Nitrergic and cholinergic innervation of the rat lower urinary tract after pelvic ganglionectomy. Am J Physiol 1998; 274:R389–397.

123. Johns A. Alpha- and beta-adrenergic and muscarinic cholinergic binding sites in the bladder and urethra of the rabbit. Can J Physiol Pharmacol 1983; 61:61–66.

124. Taki N, Taniguchi T, Okada K, et al. Evidence for predominant mediation of alpha1-adrenoceptor in the tonus of entire urethra of women. J Urol 1999; 162:1829–1832.

125. Persson CG, Andersson KE. Adrenoceptor and cholinoceptor mediated effects in the isolated urethra of cat and guinea-pig. Clin Exp Pharmacol Physiol 1976; 3:415–426.

126. Andersson KE, Persson CG, Alm P, et al. Effects of acetylcholine, noradrenaline, and prostaglandins on the isolated, perfused human fetal urethra. Acta Physiol Scand 1978; 104:394–401.

127. Ek A, Andersson KE, Ulmsten U. The effects of norephedrine and bethanechol on the human urethral closure pressure profile. Scand J Urol Nephrol 1978; 12:97–104.

128. Ulmsten U, Andersson KE. The effects of emeprone on intravesical and intra-urethral pressure in women with urgency incontinence. Scand J Urol Nephrol 1977; 11:103–109.

129. Mattiasson A, Andersson KE, Sjogren C. Adrenoceptors and cholinoceptors controlling noradrenaline release from adrenergic nerves in the urethra of rabbit and man. J Urol 1984; 131:1190–1195.

130. Yamanishi T, Chapple CR, Yasuda K, et al. The role of M2 muscarinic receptor subtypes mediating contraction of the circular and longitudinal smooth muscle of the pig proximal urethra. J Urol 2002; 168:308–314.

131. Gosling JA, Dixon JS, Lendon RG. The autonomic innervation of the human male and female bladder neck and proximal urethra. J Urol 1977; 118:302–305.

132. Ek A, Alm P, Andersson KE, Persson CG. Adrenergic and cholinergic nerves of the human urethra and urinary bladder. A histochemical study. Acta Physiol Scand 1977; 99:345–352.

133. Alm P, Zygmunt PK, Iselin C, et al. Nitric oxide synthase-immunoreactive, adrenergic, cholinergic, and peptidergic nerves of the female rat urinary tract: a comparative study. J Auton Nerv Syst 1995; 56:105–114.

134. Persson K, Johansson K, Alm P, et al. Morphological and functional evidence against a sensory and sympathetic origin of nitric oxide synthase-containing nerves in the rat lower urinary tract. Neuroscience 1997; 77:271–281.

135. Levin RM, Wein AJ. Quantitative analysis of alpha and beta adrenergic receptor densities in the lower urinary tract of the dog and the rabbit. Invest Urol 1979; 17:75–77.

136. Latifpour J, Kondo S, O'Hollaren B, et al. Autonomic receptors in urinary tract: sex and age differences. J Pharmacol Exp Ther 1990; 253:661–667.

137. Ek A, Alm P, Andersson KE, Persson CG. Adrenoceptor and cholinoceptor mediated responses of the isolated human urethra. Scand J Urol Nephrol 1977; 11:97–102.

138. Appell RA, England HR, Hussell AR, McGuire EJ. The effects of epidural anesthesia on the urethral closure pressure profile in patients with prostatic enlargement. J Urol 1980; 124:410–411.

139. Furuya S, Kumamoto Y, Yokoyama E, et al. Alpha-adrenergic activity and urethral pressure in prostatic zone in benign prostatic hypertrophy. J Urol 1982; 128:836–839.

140. Brading AF, McCoy R, Dass N. Alpha1-adrenoceptors in urethral function. Eur Urol 1999; 36:74–79.

141. Nasu K, Moriyama N, Fukasawa R, et al. Quantification and distribution of alpha1-adrenoceptor subtype mRNAs in human proximal urethra. Br J Pharmacol 1998; 123:1289–1293.

142. Daniels DV, Gever JR, Jasper JR, et al. Human cloned alpha1A-adrenoceptor isoforms display alpha1L-adrenoceptor pharmacology in functional studies. Eur J Pharmacol 1999; 370:337–343.

143. Fukasawa R, Taniguchi N, Moriyama N, et al. The alpha1L-adrenoceptor subtype in the lower urinary tract: a comparison of human urethra and prostate. Br J Urol 1998; 82:733–737.

144. Chai TC, Belville WD, McGuire EJ, Nyquist L. Specificity of the American Urological Association voiding symptom index: comparison of unselected and selected samples of both sexes. J Urol 1993; 150:1710–1713.

145. Lepor H, Machi G. Comparison of AUA symptom index in unselected males and females between fifty-five and seventy-nine years of age. Urology 1993; 42:36–40; discussion 40–41.

146. Lepor H, Theune C. Randomized double-blind study comparing the efficacy of terazosin versus placebo in women with prostatism-like symptoms. J Urol 1995; 154:116–118.

147. Nordling J, Meyhoff HH, Christensen NJ. Effects of clonidine (Catapresan) on urethral pressure. Invest Urol 1979; 16:289–291.

148. Werkstrom V, Persson K, Andersson KE. NANC transmitters in the female pig urethra – localization and modulation of release via alpha 2-adrenoceptors and potassium channels. Br J Pharmacol 1997; 121:1605–1612.

149. Levin RM, Ruggieri MR, Wein AJ. Identification of receptor subtypes in the rabbit and human urinary bladder by selective radio-ligand binding. J Urol 1988; 139:844–848.

150. Morita T, Iizuka H, Iwata T, Kondo S. Function and distribution of beta3-adrenoceptors in rat, rabbit and human urinary bladder and external urethral sphincter. J Smooth Muscle Res 2000; 36:21–32.

151. Laval KU, Hannappel J, Lutzeyer W. Effects of beta-adrenergic stimulating and blocking agents on the dynamics of the human bladder outlet. Urol Int 1978; 33:366–369.

152. Rao MS, Bapna BC, Sharma PL, et al. Clinical import of beta-adrenergic activity in the proximal urethra. J Urol 1980; 124:254–255.

153. Vaidyanathan S, Rao MS, Bapna BC, et al. Beta-adrenergic activity in human proximal urethra: a study with terbutaline. J Urol 1980; 124:869–871.

154. Thind P, Lose G, Colstrup H, Andersson KE. The influence of beta-adrenoceptor and muscarinic receptor agonists and antagonists on the static urethral closure function in healthy females. Scand J Urol Nephrol 1993; 27:31–38.

155. Ishiko O, Ushiroyama T, Saji F, et al. Beta(2)-Adrenergic agonists and pelvic floor exercises for female stress incontinence. Int J Gynaecol Obstet 2000; 71:39–44.

156. Morita T, Kihara K, Nagamatsu H, et al. Effects of clenbuterol on rabbit vesicourethral muscle contractility. J Smooth Muscle Res 1995; 31:119–127.

157. Slack BE, Downie JW. Pharmacological analysis of the responses of the feline urethra to autonomic nerve stimulation. J Auton Nerv Syst 1983; 8:141–160.

158. Burnett AL. Nitric oxide control of lower genitourinary tract functions: a review. Urology 1995; 45:1071–1083.

159. Dokita S, Smith SD, Nishimoto T, et al. Involvement of nitric oxide and cyclic GMP in rabbit urethral relaxation. Eur J Pharmacol 1994; 266:269–275.

160. Schroder A, Hedlund P, Andersson KE. Carbon monoxide relaxes the female pig urethra as effectively as nitric oxide in the presence of YC-1. J Urol 2002; 167:1892–1896.

161. Peng W, Hoidal JR, Farrukh IS. Regulation of Ca(2+)-activated K+ channels in pulmonary vascular smooth muscle cells: role of nitric oxide. J Appl Physiol 1996; 81:1264–1272.

162. Robertson BE, Schubert R, Hescheler J, Nelson MT. cGMP-dependent protein kinase activates Ca-activated K channels in cerebral artery smooth muscle cells. Am J Physiol 1993; 265:C299–303.

163. Bolotina VM, Najibi S, Palacino JJ, et al. Nitric oxide directly activates calcium-dependent potassium channels in vascular smooth muscle. Nature 1994; 368:850–853.

164. Koh SD, Campbell JD, Carl A, Sanders KM. Nitric oxide activates multiple potassium channels in canine colonic smooth muscle. J Physiol 1995; 489:735–743.

165. Warner TD, Mitchell JA, Sheng H, Murad F. Effects of cyclic GMP on smooth muscle relaxation. Adv Pharmacol 1994; 26:171–194.

166. Ito Y, Kimoto Y. The neural and non-neural mechanisms involved in urethral activity in rabbits. J Physiol 1985; 367:57–72.

167. Persson K, Pandita RK, Aszodi A, et al. Functional characteristics of urinary tract smooth muscles in mice lacking cGMP protein kinase type I. Am J Physiol Regul Integr Comp Physiol 2000; 279:R1112–1120.

168. Waldeck K, Ny L, Persson K, Andersson KE. Mediators and mechanisms of relaxation in rabbit urethral smooth muscle. Br J Pharmacol 1998; 123:617–624.

169. Smet PJ, Jonavicius J, Marshall VR, de Vente J. Distribution of nitric oxide synthase-immunoreactive nerves and identification of the cellular targets of nitric oxide in guinea-pig and human urinary bladder by cGMP immunohistochemistry. Neuroscience 1996; 71:337–348.

170. Sergeant GP, Hollywood MA, McCloskey KD, et al. Role of IP(3) in modulation of spontaneous activity in pacemaker cells of rabbit urethra. Am J Physiol Cell Physiol 2001; 280:C1349–1356.

171. McCloskey KD, Gurney AM. Kit positive cells in the guinea pig bladder. J Urol 2002; 168:832–836.

172. Werkstrom V, Alm P, Persson K, Andersson KE. Inhibitory innervation of the guinea-pig urethra; roles of CO, NO and VIP. J Auton Nerv Syst 1998; 74:33–42.

173. Werkstrom V, Ny L, Persson K, Andersson KE. Carbon monoxide-induced relaxation and distribution of haem oxygenase isoenzymes in the pig urethra and lower oesophagogastric junction. Br J Pharmacol 1997; 120:312–318.

174. Ho KM, Ny L, McMurray G, et al. Co-localization of carbon monoxide and nitric oxide synthesizing enzymes in the human urethral sphincter. J Urol 1999; 161:1968–1972.

175. Naseem KM, Mumtaz FH, Thompson CS, et al. Relaxation of rabbit lower urinary tract smooth muscle by nitric oxide and carbon monoxide: modulation by hydrogen peroxide. Eur J Pharmacol 2000; 387:329–335.

176. Sjogren C, Andersson KE, Mattiasson A. Effects of vasoactive intestinal polypeptide on isolated urethral and urinary bladder smooth muscle from rabbit and man. J Urol 1985; 133:136–140.

177. Dalziel HH, Westfall DP. Receptors for adenine nucleotides and nucleosides: subclassification, distribution, and molecular characterization. Pharmacol Rev 1994; 46:449–466.

178. Callahan SM, Creed KE. Electrical and mechanical activity of the isolated lower urinary tract of the guinea-pig. Br J Pharmacol 1981; 74:353–358.

179. Ohnishi N, Park YC, Kurita T, Kajimoto N. Role of ATP and related purine compounds on urethral relaxation in male rabbits. Int J Urol 1997; 4:191–197.

180. Pinna C, Puglisi L, Burnstock G. ATP and vasoactive intestinal polypeptide relaxant responses in hamster isolated proximal urethra. Br J Pharmacol 1998; 124:1069–1074.

6

Integrated physiology of the lower urinary tract

Naoki Yoshimura, Satoshi Seki, and Michael B Chancellor

Introduction

The urinary bladder and its outlet, the urethra, serve two main functions: (1) storage of urine without leakage and (2) periodic release of urine. These two functions are dependent on central as well as peripheral autonomic and somatic neural pathways.[1–6] Since the lower urinary tract switches in an all-or-none manner between storage and elimination of urine, many of the neural circuits controlling voiding exhibit phasic patterns of activity rather than tonic patterns occurring in autonomic pathways to other viscera. Micturition is also a special visceral mechanism because it is dependent on voluntary control which requires the participation of higher centers in the brain, whereas many other visceral functions are regulated involuntarily. Because of these complex neural regulations, the central and peripheral nervous control of the lower urinary tract is susceptible to a variety of neurological disorders. This chapter will summarize clinical and experimental data to describe the complexity of the peripheral and central nervous systems controlling urine storage and elimination in the lower urinary tract.

Peripheral nervous system

Efferent pathways of the lower urinary tract

During urine storage, the bladder outlet is closed and detrusor (bladder smooth muscle) is quiescent, allowing intravesical pressure to remain low over a wide range of bladder volumes. On the other hand, during voluntary voiding, the initial event is a relaxation of striated urethral muscles, followed by a detrusor muscle contraction. These two different activities are mediated by three sets of peripheral nerves: parasympathetic (pelvic), sympathetic (hypogastric), and somatic (pudendal) nerves (Figure 6.1):[7]

1. Pelvic parasympathetic nerves, which arise at the sacral level of the spinal cord, provide an excitatory input to the bladder and an inhibitory input to the urethral smooth muscle to eliminate urine.

2. Hypogastric sympathetic nerves, which arise at the upper lumbar level of the spinal cord, excite the internal sphincter smooth muscle and inhibit the detrusor to storage urine.

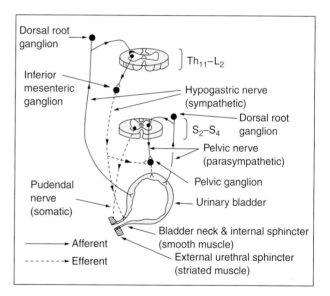

Figure 6.1

Sympathetic, parasympathetic, and somatic innervation of the lower urinary tract. Sympathetic preganglionic pathways emerge from the thoracolumbar cord ($Th_{11}–L_2$) and pass to the inferior mesenteric ganglia. Preganglionic and postganglionic sympathetic axons then travel in the hypogastric nerve to the pelvic ganglia and lower urinary tract. Parasympathetic preganglionic axons which originate in the sacral cord ($S_2–S_4$) pass in the pelvic nerve to ganglion cells in the pelvic ganglia and postganglionic axons innervate the bladder and urethral smooth muscle. Sacral somatic pathways are contained in the pudendal nerve, which provides an innervation to the external urethral sphincter striated muscles. Afferent axons from the lower urinary tract are carried in these three nerves. (Reproduced from Yoshimura and de Groat with permission.)[7]

3. Pudendal somatic nerves, which arise at the sacral level of the spinal cord, elicit excitatory effects to the external sphincter striated muscle to facilitate urine storage in the bladder .

Parasympathetic pathways

Parasympathetic preganglionic neurons (PGN) innervating the lower urinary tract are located in the lateral part of the sacral intermediate gray matter in a region termed the sacral parasympathetic nucleus (SPN).[1,8–11] Parasympathetic PGN send axons through the ventral roots to peripheral ganglia where they release the excitatory transmitter acetylcholine (ACh) which activates postsynaptic ganglionic-type nicotinic receptors.[2,6,7] Parasympathetic postganglionic neurons in humans are located in the detrusor wall layer and not as an independent ganglion, which is known as the major pelvic ganglion in the rodent. Parasympathetic postganglionic nerve terminals release ACh, which can excite various muscarinic receptors in bladder smooth muscles, leading to bladder contractions.[12–15]

The postganglionic parasympathetic input to the urethra elicits inhibitory effects mediated at least in part via the release of nitric oxide (NO), which directly relaxes the urethral smooth muscle.[16–22] Thus, the excitation of sacral parasympathetic efferent pathways induces a bladder contraction and urethral relaxation to promote bladder emptying during voiding (Figure 6.2).

Sympathetic pathways

Sympathetic outflow from the rostral lumbar spinal cord provides a noradrenergic excitatory and inhibitory input to the bladder and urethra[16] to facilitate urine storage. The peripheral sympathetic pathways follow a complex route which passes through the sympathetic chain ganglia to the interior mesenteric ganglia and then via the hypogastric nerves to the pelvic ganglia (see Figure 6.1).[23] Sympathetic PGNs make synaptic connections with postganglionic neurons in the inferior mesenteric ganglion as well as with postganglionic neurons in the paravertebral ganglia and pelvic ganglia.[1,2,24,25] Ganglionic transmission in sympathetic pathways is also mediated by ACh acting on ganglionic-type nicotinic receptors. Sympathetic postganglionic terminals which release norepinephrine elicit contractions of bladder base and urethral smooth muscle and relaxation of the bladder body.[1,2,16,26]

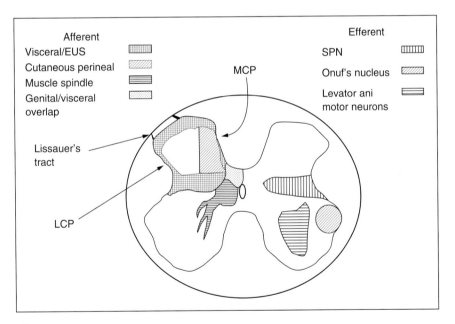

Figure 6.2
Neuroanatomical distribution of primary afferent and efferent components of storage and micturition reflexes within the sacral spinal cord. Afferent components are shown on the left side, whereas efferent components are shown on the right side. Both components are distributed bilaterally and thus overlap extensively. Visceral afferent components represent bladder and urethral afferents contained in the pelvic nerve. External urethral sphincter (EUS) afferents have the same distribution as visceral afferents. Genital (glans penis/clitoris) afferent fibers are contained in the pudendal nerves. Cutaneous perineal afferent components represent afferent fibers that innervate the perineal skin and that are contained in the pudendal nerve. Muscle spindle afferent components represent Iα/β afferent fibers contained in the levator ani nerve that innervate muscle spindles in the levator ani muscle. SPN, sacral parasympathetic nucleus; LCP, lateral collateral afferent projection; MCP, medial collateral afferent projection. (Reproduced from de Groat et al with permission.)[76]

Somatic pathways

Somatic efferent motoneurons which innervate the external striated urethral sphincter muscle and the pelvic floor musculature are located along the lateral border of the ventral horn in the sacral spinal cord, commonly referred to as the Onuf's nucleus (see Figure 6.2).[27] Sphincter motor neurons also exhibit transversely oriented dendritic bundles that project laterally into the lateral funiculus, dorsally into the intermediate gray matter, and dorsomedially toward the central canal. Somatic nerve terminals release ACh, which acts on skeletal muscle type nicotinic receptors to induce a muscle contraction (see Figure 6.1).

Combined activation of sympathetic and somatic pathways elevates bladder outlet resistance and contributes urinary continence.

Afferent pathways of the lower urinary tract

The pelvic, hypogastric, and pudendal nerves also contain afferent axons that transmit information from the lower urinary tract to the lumbosacral spinal cord.[7,28,29] The primary afferent neurons of the pelvic and pudendal nerves are contained in sacral dorsal root ganglia; whereas afferent innervation in the hypogastric nerves arises in the rostral lumbar dorsal root ganglia (see Figure 6.1). The central axons of the dorsal root ganglion neurons carry the sensory information from the lower urinary tract to second-order neurons in the spinal cord.[10,11,27,28] Visceral afferent fibers of the pelvic[11] and pudendal[27] nerves enter the cord and travel rostrocaudally within Lissauer's tract (see Figure 6.2).

Sensory information, including the feeling of bladder fullness or bladder pain, is conveyed to the spinal cord via afferent axons in the pelvic and hypogastric nerves.[29,30] Pelvic nerve afferents, which monitor the volume of the bladder and the amplitude of the bladder contractions consist of small myelinated Aδ and unmyelinated C axons. Electrophysiological studies in cats and rats have revealed that the normal micturition reflex is mediated by myelinated Aδ-fiber afferents, which respond to bladder distention (Figure 6.3).[4,29,31]

While sensing bladder volume is of particular relevance during urine storage, afferent discharges that occur during a bladder contraction have an important reflex function and appear to reinforce the central drive that maintains bladder contractions.[32] Afferent nerves that respond both to distention and contraction, i.e. 'in series tension receptors', have been identified in the pelvic and hypogastric nerves of cats and rats.[33–36] Afferents that respond only to bladder filling have been identified in the rat bladder,[37] and appear to be volume receptors, possibly sensitive to stretch of the mucosa. In the cat bladder, some 'in series tension

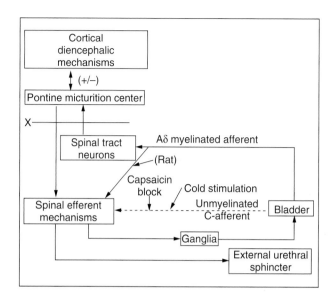

Figure 6.3

The central reflex pathways that regulate micturition in the cat and rat. In animals such as cats and rats with an intact neuraxis, micturition is initiated by a supraspinal reflex pathway passing through the pontine micturition center (PMC) in the brainstem. The pathway is triggered by myelinated afferents (Aδ) connected to tension receptors in the bladder wall (Bladder). Spinal tract neurons carry information to the brain. PMC is controlled by excitatory and inhibitory pathways (+/−) in cortical and diencephalic mechanism. In spinalized animals, connection of the brainstem and the sacral spinal cord are interrupted (X) and micturition is initially blocked. In chronic SCI animals, a spinal reflex mechanism emerges which is triggered by unmyelinated (C-fiber) bladder afferents. The C-fiber reflex pathway is usually weak or undetectable in animals with an intact nervous system. Capsaicin blocks the C-fiber reflex in chronic SCI animals. Cold stimulation also activates the C-fiber-mediated micturition reflex. However, following SCI voiding, reflex in the rat is still triggered by myelinated Aδ afferents connecting to spinal efferent mechanisms (Rat), whereas voiding reflex in the cat is totally abolished by capsaicin treatment.

receptors' may also respond to bladder stretch.[38] In the rat there is now evidence that many C-bladder afferents are volume receptors that do not respond to bladder contractions, a property that distinguishes them from 'in series tension receptors'.[37]

During inflammation and neuropathic conditions there is recruitment of C-fiber bladder afferents, which form a new functional afferent pathway that can cause bladder overactivity and bladder pain (Figure 6.3).[39] In cats, C-fiber afferents have high thresholds and are usually unresponsive to mechanical stimuli such as bladder distention and therefore have been termed 'silent C fibers'. However many of these fibers do respond to chemical, noxious, or cold stimuli.[30,40,41] Previous studies in the rat using patch clamp techniques revealed that C-fiber afferent neurons are relatively inexcitable due to the presence of high-threshold, tetrodotoxin-resistant sodium channels and low-threshold A-type potassium channels.[42] Activation of C-fiber afferents by chemical irritation induces bladder hyperreflexia, which is blocked by administration of capsaicin, a neurotoxin of C-fiber afferents.[1,43,44] However, since capsaicin does not block normal micturition in cats as well as rats, it appears that C-fiber afferents are not essential for normal conscious voiding (Figure 6.3).[1,43,45–47]

Afferent fibers innervating the urethra are also important to modulate lower urinary tract function (Figure 6.4). Talaat[48] has reported in dogs that urethral afferent fibers in the pelvic and pudendal nerves are sensitive to the passage of the urine and that during saline flow through the urethra pudendal nerve afferents were activated at a much lower pressure in comparison to pelvic nerve afferents, discharges of which were induced by high-pressure flow that caused a distention of the urethra. High thresholds (over 60 cmH$_2$O) for activation of urethral afferents in the pelvic nerves were also recently identified in rats.[49] It has also been documented that conduction velocities of cat pudendal nerve afferent fibers responding to electrical stimulation of the urethra are

approximately twice as fast (45 m/s) as pelvic nerve afferent fibers responding to the same stimulation (20 m/s).[50] In addition, urethral afferents in the pudendal and pelvic nerves of the cat seem to have different receptor properties. Pudendal nerve afferents responding to urine flow, some of which may be connected to Pacinian corpuscle-like structures in the muscle layers and the deeper parts of urethral mucosa, exhibited a slowly adapting firing pattern,[51] whereas small myelinated or unmyelinated urethral afferents in the hypogastric nerves and myelinated urethral afferents in the pelvic nerves responding to urine flow or urethral distention are reportedly connected to rapidly adapting receptors.[35,52]

Nociceptive C fibers are also present in pelvic and pudendal nerves innervating the urethra.[53,54] Previous studies have demonstrated that C-fiber afferent fibers identified with positive staining of calcitonin gene-related peptide (CGRP) or substance P were found in the subepithelium, the submucosa, and the muscular layer in all portions of the urethra.[55,56] Moreover, the activation of these urethral C fibers induced by urethral capsaicin application elicited nociceptive behavioral responses, which disappeared after pudendal nerve transection,[57] and increased electromyographic (EMG) activity of pelvic floor striated muscle, including the external urethral sphincter (EUS).[53,54] It is also known that urethral C-fiber activation by capsaicin suppressed reflex bladder contractions.[58]

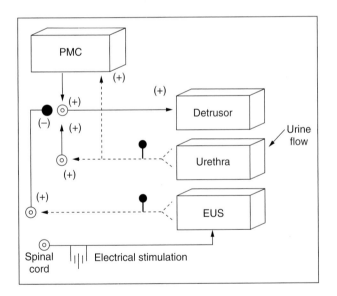

Figure 6.4
Urethra-to-bladder reflexes. Activity in afferent nerves (dashed lines) from the urethra can facilitate parasympathetic efferent outflow to the detrusor via a supraspinal pathway passing through the pontine micturition center (PMC) as well as by a spinal reflex pathway. Afferent input from the external urethral sphincter (EUS) can inhibit parasympathetic outflow to the detrusor via a spinal reflex circuit. Electrical stimulation of motor axons in the S1 ventral root elicits EUS contractions and EUS afferent firing, which in turn inhibits reflex bladder activity; (+) excitatory and (−) inhibitory mechanisms. (Reproduced from de Groat et al with permission.)[76]

Interaction between urothelium and afferent nerves

There is increasing evidence that bladder epithelial cells play an important role in modulation of bladder activity by responding to local chemical and mechanical stimuli and then sending chemical signals to the bladder afferent nerves, which then convey information to the central nervous system (Figure 6.5).[59] It has been shown that urothelial cells express nicotinic, muscarinic, tachykinin, and adrenergic receptors,[1,14] as well as vanilloid receptors,[60] and can respond to mechanical as well as chemical stimuli and in turn release chemicals such as adenosine triphosphate (ATP), prostaglandins, and NO (Figure 6.5).[59,61–63] These agents are known to have excitatory and inhibitory actions on afferent neurons, which are located close to or in the urothelium.[7,64,65] Recent studies using P2X$_3$, an ATP receptor, in knockout mice have revealed that urothelially released ATP during bladder distention can interact with P2X$_3$ receptors in bladder afferent fibers to modulate bladder activity and that a loss of P2X$_3$ receptors resulted in bladder hypoactivity.[61,66] It has also been demonstrated that vanilloid receptor (TRPV1)-knockout mice exhibited reduced NO and ATP release from urothelial cells, as well as alterations in bladder function.[67]

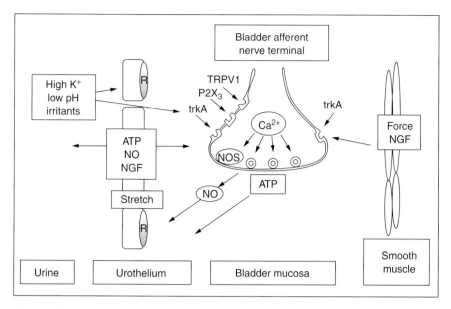

Figure 6.5

Interactions between chemical mediators released from bladder epithelial cells and smooth muscles and afferent nerve endings in the bladder mucosa. ATP and NO can be released from the urothelium and may sensitize the mechanoreceptors via an activation of $P2X_3$ and TRPV1 receptors, respectively, which respond to stretch of the mucosa during bladder distention. This mechanism can be induced by the presence of high urinary potassium concentrations, and possibly by other sensitizing solutions within the bladder lumen, such as those with high osmolality or low pH; the presence in the tissues of inflammatory mediators may also sensitize the endings. The smooth muscle can generate force that may influence some mucosal endings, and the production of nerve growth factor (NGF) is another mechanism that can influence the mechanosensitivity of the sensory ending, via the trkA receptor. NOS, nitric oxide synthase.

The urothelium also appears to modulate contractile responses of the detrusor smooth muscle to muscarinic and other stimulation. Hawthorn and associates[68] recently demonstrated in the pig bladder that there is a greater muscarinic receptor density in the urothelium than in the detrusor smooth muscle. Contractions of urothelium-denuded muscle strip were inhibited in the presence of a second bladder strip with an intact urothelium but not if the second strip was denuded. Thus, the detrusor smooth muscle is sensitive to a diffusible inhibitory factor release from the urothelium.

Overall, it seems likely that urothelial cells exhibit specific signaling properties that allow them to respond to their chemical and physical environments and engage in reciprocal communication with neighboring nerves and smooth muscles in the bladder wall.

Reflex circuitry controlling micturition

Coordinated activities of the peripheral nervous system innervating the bladder and urethra during urine storage and voiding depend upon multiple reflex pathways organized in the brain and spinal cord. The central pathways controlling lower urinary tract function are organized as

on-off switching circuits that maintain a reciprocal relationship between the urinary bladder and urethral outlet.[1,69] The principal reflex components of these switching circuits are listed in Table 6.1 and illustrated in Figure 6.6.

The storage phase of the bladder

The bladder functions as a low-pressure reservoir during urine storage. In both humans and animals, bladder pressures remain low and relatively constant when bladder volume is below the threshold for inducing voiding (Figure 6.7). The accommodation of the bladder to increasing volumes of urine is primarily a passive phenomenon dependent on the intrinsic properties of the vesical smooth muscle and the quiescence of the parasympathetic efferent pathway.[1,4,7] The bladder-to-sympathetic reflex also contributes as a negative feedback or urine storage mechanism that promotes closure of the urethral outlet and inhibits neurally mediated contractions of the bladder during bladder filling[70] (Table 6.1). Reflex activation of the sympathetic outflow to the lower urinary tract can be triggered by afferent activity induced by distention of the urinary bladder.[1,70] This reflex response is organized in the lumbosacral spinal

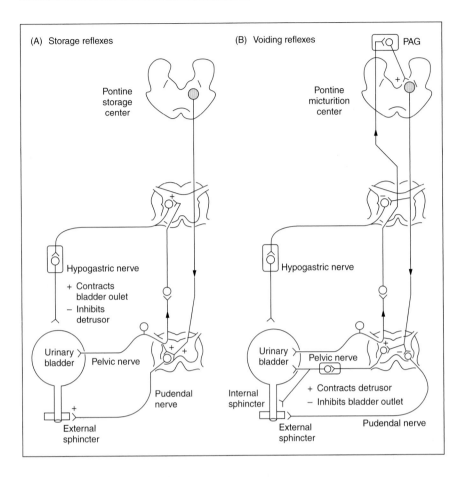

Figure 6.6
Neural circuits controlling continence and micturition. (A) Storage reflexes. During urine storage, bladder distention produces low-level firing in bladder afferent pathways, which in turn stimulates (1) the sympathetic outflow to the bladder outlet (bladder base and urethra) and (2) pudendal outflow to the external sphincter muscle. These responses are elicited by spinal reflex pathways. Sympathetic firing also inhibits detrusor muscle and transmission in bladder ganglia. A region in the rostral pons (the pontine storage center) increases external urethral sphincter activity. (B) Voiding reflexes. During elimination of urine, intense bladder afferent firing activates spinobulbospinal reflex pathways passing through the pontine micturition center, which stimulate the parasympathetic outflow to the bladder and internal sphincter smooth muscle and inhibit the sympathetic and pudendal outflow to the bladder outlet. Ascending afferent input from the spinal cord may pass through relay neurons in the periaqueductal gray (PAG) before reaching the pontine micturition center. (Reproduced from Yoshimura and de Groat with permission.)[7]

Table 6.1 *Reflexes to the lower urinary tract*

Afferent pathways	Efferent pathways	Central pathways
Urine storage Low-level vesical afferent activity (pelvic nerve)	1. External sphincter contraction (somatic nerves) 2. Internal sphincter contraction (sympathetic nerves) 3. Detrusor inhibition (sympathetic nerves) 4. Ganglionic inhibition (sympathetic nerves) 5. Sacral parasympathetic outflow inactive	Spinal reflexes
Micturition High-level vesical afferent activity (pelvic nerve)	1. Inhibition of external sphincter activity 2. Inhibition of sympathetic outflow 3. Activation of parasympathetic outflow to the bladder 4. Activation of parasympathetic outflow to the urethra	Spinobulbospinal reflexes Spinal reflex

cord and persists after transection of the spinal cord at the thoracic levels (Figure 6.7).[71]

During bladder filling the activity of the sphincter electromyogram also increases (see Figure 6.7), reflecting an increase in efferent firing in the pudendal nerve and an increase in outlet resistance that contributes to the maintenance of urinary continence. Pudendal motoneurons are activated by bladder afferent input (the guarding reflex).[72] External urethral sphincter (EUS) motoneurons are also activated by urethral/perineal afferents in the pudendal nerve.[73] This reflex may represent, in part, a continence mechanism that is activated by proprioceptive afferent input from the

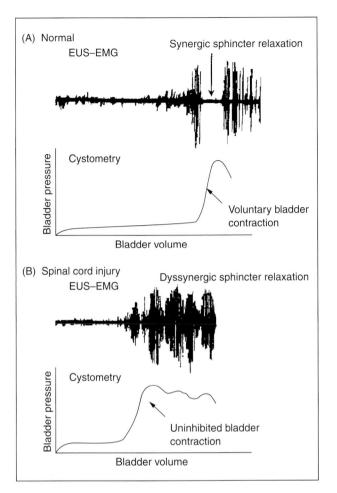

Figure 6.7

Combined cystometry and external urethral sphincter electromyography (EUS–EMG) recordings comparing reflex voiding responses in a normal adult (A, Normal) and in a spinal cord injury (SCI) patient (B, SCI). The abscissas represents bladder volume and the ordinates in cystometrograms represent bladder pressure. In panel A, a slow infusion of fluid into the bladder induces a gradual increase of EMG activity, but no apparent changes in bladder pressure. When a voluntary voiding starts, an increase of bladder pressure (voluntary bladder contraction) is associated with a cessation of EUS–EMG activity (synergic sphincter relaxation). On the other hand, in a SCI patient (B), the reciprocal relationship between bladder and sphincter is abolished. During bladder filling, uninhibited bladder contraction occurs in association with an increase in sphincter activity (detrusor-sphincter dyssynergia). Loss of the reciprocal relationship between bladder and sphincter in SCI patients interferes with bladder emptying. (Reproduced from Yoshimura with permission.)[71]

urethra/pelvic floor and which induces closure of the urethral outlet. These excitatory sphincter reflexes are organized in the spinal cord. It is also reported that a supraspinal urine storage center is located in the dorsolateral pons. Descending inputs from this region activate the pudendal motoneurons to increase urethral resistance (see Figure 6.6).[74,75]

Sphincter-to-bladder reflexes

During the urine storage phase the bladder-to-external urethral sphincter guarding reflex which triggers sphincter contractions during bladder filling could in turn activate sphincter muscle afferents, which initiate an inhibition of the parasympathetic excitatory pathway to the bladder.[76] Previous studies in cats and monkeys have demonstrated that contractions of the EUS stimulate firing in muscle proprioceptive afferents in the pudendal nerve, which then activate central inhibitory mechanisms to suppress the micturition reflex (see Figure 6.4).[76] It is also known that stimulation of somatic afferent pathways projecting in the pudendal nerve to the caudal lumbosacral spinal cord can inhibit voiding function. The inhibition can be induced by activation of afferent input from various sites, including the penis, vagina, rectum, perineum, urethral sphincter, and anal sphincter.[1,77] Electrophysiological studies in cats showed that the inhibition was mediated by suppression of interneuronal pathways in the sacral spinal cord and also by direct inhibitory input to the parasympathetic preganglionic neurons.[78] A similar inhibitory mechanism has been identified in monkeys by directly stimulating the anal sphincter muscle.[79] In monkeys at least part of the inhibitory mechanism is localized in the spinal cord because it persisted after chronic spinal cord injury.

The emptying phase of the bladder

The storage phase of the bladder can be switched to the voiding phase either involuntarily (reflexly) or voluntarily (Figure 6.7). The former is readily demonstrated in the human infant or in patients with neuropathic bladder. When bladder volume reaches the micturition threshold, afferent activity originating in bladder mechanoceptors triggers micturition reflexes. The afferent fibers which trigger micturition in the rat and cat are small myelinated Aδ fibers (see Figure 6.3).[31,80,81] These bladder afferents in the pelvic nerve synapse on neurons in the sacral spinal cord, which then send their axons rostrally to a micturition center (the pontine micturition center) in the dorsolateral pons (see Figure 6.6).[80–85]

Activation of this center reverses the pattern of efferent outflow to the lower urinary tract, producing firing in the sacral parasympathetic pathways and inhibition of sympathetic and somatic pathways (see Figure 6.6). The expulsion phase consists of an initial relaxation of the urethral sphincter followed in a few seconds by a contraction of the bladder, resulting in the flow of urine through the urethra. Relaxation of the urethral smooth muscle during micturition is mediated by activation of a parasympathetic pathway to the urethra that triggers the release of nitric oxide[16,19] and by removal of excitatory inputs to the urethra (see Figure 6.6). Studies in the rat and cat indicate that activity ascending from the spinal cord may pass through a relay center in the periaqueductal gray before reaching the pontine micturition center (see Figure 6.6).[86–90] Thus, voiding reflexes depend on a spinobulbospinal pathway which passes through an integrative center in the brain (see Figure 6.6B). Secondary reflexes elicited by flow of urine through the urethra also facilitate bladder emptying.[1,4,58] Inhibition of EUS reflex activity during micturition is dependent, in part, on supraspinal mechanisms because it is weak or absent in chronic spinal cord injured animals and humans, resulting in simultaneous contractions of bladder and urethral sphincter (i.e. detrusor-sphincter dyssynergia) (see Figure 6.7).[71,91,92]

Urethra-to-bladder reflexes

It has been reported that myelinated afferents innervating the urethra could contribute bladder emptying during the voiding phase. Barrington[93,94] reported that urine flow or mechanical stimulation of the urethra with a catheter could excite afferent nerves that in turn facilitated reflex bladder contractions in the anesthetized cat (see Figure 6.4). He proposed that this facilitatory urethra-to-bladder reflex could promote complete bladder emptying. A recent study[58] in the anesthetized rat has provided additional support for Barrington's findings. Measurements of reflex bladder contractions under isovolumetric conditions during continuous urethral perfusion (0.075 ml/min) revealed that the frequency of micturition reflexes was significantly reduced when urethral perfusion was stopped or following infusion of lidocaine (lignocaine) (1%) into the urethra. Intraurethral infusion of nitric oxide donors (S-nitroso-N-acetylpenicillamine, SNAP, or nitroprusside, 1–2 mmol) markedly decreased urethral perfusion pressure (approximately 30%) and decreased the frequency of reflex bladder contractions (45–75%), but did not change the amplitude of bladder contractions. It was thus concluded that activation of urethral afferents during urethral perfusion could modulate the micturition reflex.

Barrington also identified two components of this facilitatory urethra-to-bladder reflex during voiding. One component was activated by a somatic afferent pathway in the pudendal nerve and produced facilitation by a supraspinal mechanism involving the pontine micturition center.[93] The other component was activated by a visceral afferent pathway in the pelvic nerve and produced facilitation by a spinal reflex mechanism.[94] Afferent fibers which respond to urine flow in the urethra were found in the pelvic, hypogastric, and pudendal nerves although it has been reported that the properties of urethral afferents in pelvic/hypogastric and pudendal nerves are different, as described above.

Spinal and supraspinal pathways involved in the micturition reflex

Spinal cord

In the spinal cord, afferent pathways terminate on second-order interneurons that relay information to the brain or to other regions of the spinal cord. Since spinal reflex pathways controlling bladder and urethral activities are mediated by disynaptic or polysynaptic pathways, interneuronal mechanisms play an essential role in the regulation of lower urinary tract function. Electrophysiological[10,80,95,96] and neuroanatomical techniques[97–100] have identified interneurons in the same regions of the spinal cord that receive afferent input from the bladder. As shown in Figure 6.2, horseradish peroxidase (HRP) labeling techniques in the cat revealed that afferent projections from the EUS and levator ani muscles (i.e. pelvic floor) project into different regions of the sacral spinal cord. The EUS afferent terminals are located in the superficial layers of the dorsal horn and at the base of the dorsal horn, whereas the levator ani afferents project into a region just lateral to the central canal and extending into the medial ventral horn. The EUS afferents overlap very closely with the central projections of visceral afferents in pelvic nerve that innervate the bladder and urethra (Figure 6.2).[11] Intracellular labeling experiments also showed that the dendritic patterns of EUS motoneurons[101] and parasympathetic PGN[9] are similar. Pharmacological experiments revealed that glutamic acid is the excitatory transmitter in these pathways. In addition, approximately 15% of interneurons located medial to the sacral parasympathetic nucleus in laminae V–VII make inhibitory synaptic connections with the PGN.[10,102] These inhibitory neurons release γ-aminobutyric acid (GABA) and glycine. Reflex pathways which control the external sphincter muscles also utilize glutamatergic excitatory and GABAergic/glycinergic inhibitory interneuronal mechanisms.

Central and spinal neural pathways controlling lower urinary tract function have also been identified by transneuronal tracing studies using neurotropic viruses such as pseudorabies virus (PRV) (Figure 6.8). PRV can be injected into a target organ and then move intra-axonally from the periphery to the central nervous system. Because PRV can be transported across many synapses it could sequentially infect all the neurons that connect directly or indirectly to the lower urinary tract.[98–100] Interneurons identified by retrograde transport of PRV injected into the urinary bladder are located in the region of the sacral parasympathetic nucleus (SPN), the dorsal commissure (DCM), and the superficial laminae of the dorsal horn (see Figure 6.8).[10,98,100] A similar distribution of labeled interneurons has been noted after injection of virus into

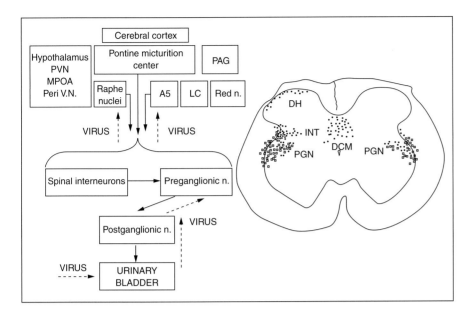

Figure 6.8

Transneuronal virus tracing of the central pathways controlling the urinary bladder of the rat. Injection of pseudorabies virus into the wall of the urinary bladder leads to retrograde transport of virus (dashed arrows) and sequential infection of postganglionic neurons, preganglionic neurons, and then various central neural circuits synaptically linked to the preganglionic neurons. At long survival times, virus can be detected with immunocytochemical techniques in neurons at specific sites throughout the spinal cord and brain, extending to the pontine micturition center in the pons (i.e. Barrington's nucleus or the laterodorsal tegmental nucleus) and to the cerebral cortex. Other sites in the brain labeled by virus are (1) the paraventricular nucleus (PVN), medial preoptic area (MPOA), and periventricular nucleus (Peri V.N.) of the hypothalamus; (2) periaqueductal gray (PAG); (3) locus coeruleus (LC) and subcoeruleus; (4) red nucleus (Red N.); (5) medullary raphe nucleus; and (6) the noradrenergic cell group designated A5. L6 spinal cord section showing the distribution of virus labeled parasympathetic preganglionic neurons (□) and interneurons (●) in the region of the parasympathetic nucleus 72 h after injection of the virus into the bladder. Interneurons (INT) in the dorsal commissure and the superficial laminae of the dorsal horn (DH) are also shown. The left side shows the entire population of preganglionic neurons (PGN) labeled by axonal tracing with fluorogold injected into the pelvic ganglia. The right side shows the distribution of PRV-labeled bladder PGN (□) among the entire population of FG-labeled PGN (□). Bladder PGN were labeled with PRV and FG. Composite diagram of neurons in 12 spinal sections (42 μm). (Reproduced from de Groat et al with permission.)[95]

the urethra[99] or the EUS,[98] indicating a prominent overlap of the interneuronal pathways controlling the various target organs of the lower urinary tract.

The micturition reflex can be modulated at the level of the spinal cord by interneuronal mechanisms activated by afferent input from cutaneous and striated muscle targets. Micturition reflex can also be modulated by inputs from other visceral organs.[1,4,7,69,80,103–106] Stimulation of afferent fibers from various regions (anus, colon/rectum, vagina, uterine cervix, penis, perineum, pudendal nerve) can inhibit the firing of sacral interneurons evoked by bladder distention.[79] This inhibition may occur as a result of presynaptic inhibition at primary afferent terminals or due to direct postsynaptic inhibition of the second-order neurons. Direct postsynaptic inhibition of bladder PGN can also be elicited by stimulation of somatic afferent axons in the pudendal nerve or by visceral afferents from the distal bowel.[104,107]

Pontine micturition center

The dorsal pontine tegmentum has been firmly established as an essential control center for micturition in normal subjects. First described by Barrington,[108] it has subsequently been called 'Barrington's nucleus', the 'pontine micturition center' (PMC),[109] or the 'M region'[74,88,110] due to its medial location.

Studies in animals using brain-lesioning techniques revealed that neurons in the brainstem at the level of the inferior colliculus have an essential role in the control of the parasympathetic component of micturition.[1,4,7] Removal of areas of brain above the colliculus by intercollicular decerebration usually facilitates micturition by elimination of inhibitory inputs from more rostral centers, whereas transections at any point below the colliculi abolish micturition.[111] In addition, bilateral lesions in the region of the locus coeruleus in the cat or the dorsolateral tegmental nucleus in the rat abolish micturition, whereas electrical or chemical stimulation of this region induces a bladder contraction and a reciprocal relaxation of the urethra, leading to bladder emptying.[74,82–85,112]

In addition to providing axonal inputs to the locus coeruleus and the sacral spinal cord,[113–115] neurons in the PMC also send axon collaterals to the paraventricular thalamic nucleus, which is thought to be involved in the limbic system modulation of visceral behavior.[115] Some neurons in the pontine micturition center also project to the periaqueductal gray region[116] which regulates many visceral activities as well as pain pathways.[117] Thus, neurons in the PMC communicate with multiple supraspinal neuronal populations that may coordinate micturition with other functions. Although the circuitry in humans is uncertain, brain imaging studies have revealed increases in blood flow in this region of the pons during micturition.[118] In addition, it has been reported that in a case study of the multiple sclerosis patient, coordinated bladder contraction and urethral relaxation was induced by ectopic activation of a region in the dorsolateral pontine tegmentum.[119] Thus the pontine micturition center appears critical for the normal micturition reflex across species.

Neurons in the PMC provide direct synaptic inputs to sacral PGN,[109] as well as to GABAergic neurons in the sacral DCM.[109] The former neurons carry the excitatory outflow to the bladder, whereas the latter neurons are thought to be important in mediating an inhibitory influence on EUS motoneurons during voiding.[116] As a result of these reciprocal connections, the PMC can promote coordination between the bladder and urethral sphincter.

Central pathways modulating the micturition reflex

Transneuronal tracing studies using PRV injected into the lower urinary tract also identified various areas in the brain (see Figure 6.8).[98,99,100,120] Thus, central control of voiding is likely to be complex. Injection of PRV into the rat bladder labeled many areas of the brainstem, including the laterodorsal tegmental nucleus (the pontine micturition center); the medullary raphe nucleus, which contains serotonergic neurons; the locus coeruleus, which contains noradrenergic neurons; periaqueductal gray; and noradrenergic cell group A5. Several regions in the hypothalamus and the cerebral cortex also exhibited virus-infected cells (see Figure 6.8). Neurons in the cortex were located primarily in the medial frontal cortex. Similar brain areas were labeled after injection of virus into the urethra and urethral sphincter, suggesting that coordination between different parts of the lower urinary tract is mediated by a similar population of neurons in the brain.[98–100,120]

Studies in humans indicate that voluntary control of voiding is dependent on connections between the frontal cortex and the septal/preoptic region of the hypothalamus as well as connections between the paracentral lobule and the brainstem.[1] Lesions to these areas of cortex appear to directly increase bladder activity by removing cortical inhibitory control. Brain imaging studies[109,121] in human volunteers have implicated both the frontal cortex and the anterior cingulate gyrus in control of micturition and have indicated that micturition is controlled predominately by the right side of the brain.

Positron emission tomography (PET) scans were also used to examine which brain areas are involved in human micturition.[122] In their study, when 17 right-handed male volunteers were scanned, 10 volunteers were able to micturate during scanning. Micturition was associated with increased blood flow in the right dorsomedial pontine tegmentum, the periaqueductal gray (PAG), the hypothalamus, and the right inferior frontal gyrus. Decreased blood flow was found in the right anterior cingurate gyrus when urine was withheld. The other seven volunteers were not able to micturate during scanning, although they had a full bladder and tried vigorously to micturate. In this group, during these unsuccessful attempts to micturate, increased blood flow was detected in the right ventral pontine tegmentum. It has been reported that descending inputs from this area can activate the pudendal motoneurons to increase urethral resistance during urine storage in cats.[74,110,123] Another study using PET scans in 11 healthy male subjects also revealed that increased brain activity related to increasing bladder volume was seen in the PAG, in the midline pons, in the mid-cingulate cortex, and bilaterally in the frontal lobe area, suggesting that the PAG receives information about bladder fullness and relays this information to areas involved in the control of bladder storage.[124]

Increased blood flow also occurred in the right inferior frontal gyrus during unsuccessful attempts to micturate, and decreased blood flow occurred in the right anterior cingulate gyrus during the withholding of urine. The results suggest that the human brainstem contains specific nuclei responsible for the control of micturition, and that the cortical and pontine regions for micturition are predominantly on the right side. A PET study[122] was also conducted in adult female volunteers to identify brain structures involved in the voluntary motor control of the pelvic floor. The results revealed that the superomedial precentral gyrus and the most medial portion of the motor cortex are activated during pelvic floor contraction, and the superolateral precentral gyrus is activated during contraction of the abdominal musculature. In these conditions, significant activations were also found in the cerebellum, supplementary motor cortex, and thalamus. The right anterior cingulate gyrus was activated during sustained pelvic floor straining.

Overall, these results in animals and humans indicate that various regions in the central nervous system are necessary for voluntary control of lower urinary tract function.

Developmental changes of bladder reflexes

The neural mechanisms involved in storage and elimination of urine undergo marked changes during postnatal development.[125] In a postnatal period in humans, as well as animals, supraspinal neural pathways controlling lower urinary tract function are immature, and voiding is regulated by primitive reflex pathways organized in the spinal cord (Figure 6.9). In the neonate animals such as rats and cats, voiding is dependent on an exteroceptive somato-bladder reflex mechanism triggered when the mother licks the genital or perineal region of the young animal. This exteroceptive perineal-to-bladder reflex is regulated by primitive reflex pathways organized in the sacral spinal cord (see Figure 6.9). In humans, the neonatal bladder is more of a conduit of urine than a storage organ and, without control from the central nervous system, the bladder will reflexively empty into a diaper when it reaches functional capacity. Primitive reflex activities organized in the spinal cord such as perineal-bladder reflexes are also observed in infants.[95]

Previous studies have also reported that bladder cooling reflexes are positive in neurologically normal infants and children about age 4 years.[126] The bladder ice water cooling test is performed by quickly instilling up to 100 ml of 4°C sterile saline. The normal adult can maintain a stable bladder without uninhibited bladder contractions. The bladder cooling response is triggered by activation of cold receptors within the bladder wall supplied by unmyelinated C-fiber afferents, and organized by segmental spinal reflex pathways.[41,127] Overall, it appears that during a postnatal period, primitive reflex activities organized in the spinal cord such as perineal-bladder reflexes or C-fiber-mediated cooling reflexes are dominant, due to immature control of the central nervous system (Figure 6.9).

However, transneuronal tracing studies using PRV have demonstrated that micturition reflex pathways in the spinal cord and brain are already connected anatomically at birth despite the fact that voiding in neonatal rats does not depend on neural mechanisms in the brain.[100] When PRV was injected into the bladder of 2- and 10-day-old rat pups, the labeled neurons were found in various sites in the brain, such as the pontine micturition center, the nucleus raphe magnus, A5 and A7 regions, parapyramidal reticular formation, the periaqueductal gray, locus coeruleus, the lateral hypothalamus, medial preoptic area, and the frontal cortex (see Figure 6.8).[100] Thus, even in neonatal animals, supraspinal pathways may already be connected, but

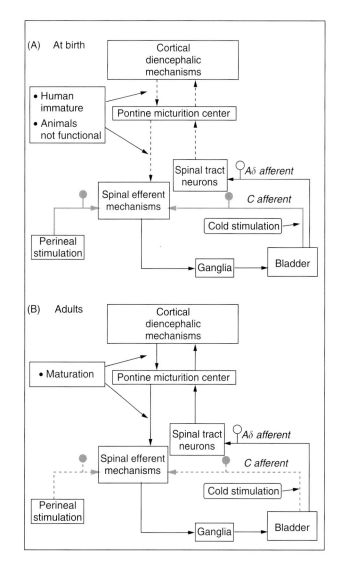

Figure 6.9

Organization of micturition reflex pathways in a postnatal (A) and adult periods (B). A, Since in a postnatal period in humans, as well as animals, supraspinal neural pathways controlling lower urinary tract function are immature, voiding is regulated by primitive reflex pathways organized in the spinal cord. In the neonate animals such as rats and cats, voiding is dependent on an exteroceptive somato-bladder reflex mechanism triggered when the mother licks the genital or perineal region of the young animal (perineal stimulation). Similar reflexes are also observed in infants. Bladder cooling reflexes mediated by C-fiber bladder afferents are positive in neurologically normal infants (Cold stimulation). B, When the central nervous system matures in adults (Maturation), reflex voiding is brought under voluntary control, which originates in the higher center of the brain and, at the same time, primitive spinal reflex activities such as perineal-bladder reflexes or C-fiber-mediated cooling reflexes are masked. However, the primitive neonatal micturition reflexes could be unmasked by pathological processes that disturb the descending neuronal control of normal voiding, such as spinal cord injury (also see Figure 6.3).

either be non-functioning or functioning in an inhibitory manner to suppress the spinobulbospinal micturition reflex, allowing micturition to be induced by primitive spinal reflex mechanisms.[125]

As the central nervous system matures during the postnatal period, reflex voiding is brought under voluntary control, which originates in the higher center of the brain and, at the same time, primitive spinal reflex activities such as perineal-bladder reflexes or C-fiber-mediated cooling reflexes are masked (see Figure 6.9).[125] Electrophysiological studies using patch-clamp recording techniques in rat spinal cord slice preparations indicate that developmental changes in sacral parasympathetic pathways are due in part to alterations in excitatory synaptic transmission between interneurons and preganglionic neurons.[96] However, the primitive neonatal micturition reflexes such as positive bladder cooling responses and/or spinal perineal-to-bladder reflexes could be unmasked by pathological processes that disturb the descending neuronal control of normal voiding, such as spinal cord injury (see Figures 6.3 and 6.9).[95,125]

References

1. de Groat WC, Booth AM, Yoshimura N. Neurophysiology of micturition and its modification in animal models of human disease. In: Maggi CA, ed. The autonomic nervous system, Vol. 3, Nervous control of the urogenital system. London: Harwood Academic Publishers, 1993:227–290.

2. de Groat WC, Booth AM. Synaptic transmission in pelvic ganglia. In: Maggi CA, ed. The autonomic nervous system, Vol. 3, Nervous control of the urogenital system. London: Harwood Academic Publishers, 1993:291–347.

3. Van Arsdalen K, Wein AJ. Physiology of micturition and continence. In: Krane RJ, Siroky M, eds. Clinical neuro-urology. New York: Little Brown & Company, 1991:25–82.

4. Torrens M, Morrison JFB. The physiology of the lower urinary tract. Berlin: Springer-Verlag, 1987.

5. Chai TC, Steers WD. Neurophysiology of micturition and continence. Urol Clin North Am 1996; 23:221–236.

6. Chancellor MB, Yoshimura N. Physiology and pharmacology of the bladder and urethra. In: Walsh PC, Retik AB, Vaughan C, Wein A, eds. Campbell's urology, Vol. 2. Philadelphia: Saunders, 2002:831–886.

7. Yoshimura N, de Groat WC. Neural control of the lower urinary tract. Int J Urol 1997; 4:111–125.

8. Nadelhaft I, de Groat WC, Morgan C. Location and morphology of parasympathetic preganglionic neurons in the sacral spinal cord of the cat revealed by retrograde axonal transport of horseradish peroxidase. J Comp Neurol 1980; 193:265–281.

9. Morgan CW, de Groat WC, Felkins LA, Zhang SJ. Intracellular injection of neurobiotin or horseradish peroxidase reveals separate types of preganglionic neurons in the sacral parasympathetic nucleus of the cat. J Comp Neurol 1993; 331:161–182.

10. de Groat WC, Vizzard MA, Araki I, Roppolo JR. Spinal interneurons and preganglionic neurons in sacral autonomic reflex pathways. In: Holstege G, Bandler R, Saper C, eds. The emotional motor system, Progress in brain research. Amsterdam: Elsevier Science Publishers, 1996:97–111.

11. Morgan C, Nadelhaft I, de Groat WC. The distribution of visceral primary afferents from the pelvic nerve to Lissauer's tract and the spinal gray matter and its relationship to the sacral parasympathetic nucleus. J Comp Neurol 1981; 201:415–440.

12. Eglen RM, Hegde SS, Watson N. Muscarinic receptor subtypes and smooth muscle function. Pharmacol Rev 1996; 48:531–565.

13. Maeda A, Kubo T, Mishina M, Numa S. Tissue distribution of mRNAs encoding muscarinic acetylcholine receptor subtypes. FEBS Lett 1988; 239:339–342.

14. Kondo S, Morita T, Tashima Y. Muscarinic cholinergic receptor subtypes in human detrusor muscle studied by labeled and nonlabeled pirenzepine, AFDX-116 and 4DAMP. Urol Int 1995; 54:150–153.

15. Yamaguchi O, Shishido K, Tamura K, et al. Evaluation of mRNAs encoding muscarinic receptor subtypes in human detrusor muscle. J Urol 1996; 156:1208–1213.

16. Andersson K-E. Pharmacology of lower urinary tract smooth muscles and penile erectile tissues. Pharmacol Rev 1993; 45:253–308.

17. Lundberg JM. Pharmacology of cotransmission in the autonomic nervous system: integrative aspects on amines, neuropeptides, adenosine triphosphate, amino acids and nitric oxide. Pharmacol Rev 1996; 48:113–178.

18. Fraser MO, Flood HD, de Groat WC. Urethral smooth muscle relaxation is mediated by nitric oxide (NO) released from parasympathetic postganglionic neurons. J Urol 1995; 153:461A.

19. Bennett BC, Kruse MN, Roppolo JR, et al. Neural control of urethral outlet activity in vivo: role of nitric oxide. J Urol 1995; 153:2004–2009.

20. Persson K, Igawa Y, Mattiasson A, Andersson K-E. Effects of inhibition of the L-arginine/nitric oxide pathway in the rat lower urinary tract in vivo and in vitro. Br J Pharmacol 1992; 107:178–184.

21. Thornbury KD, Hollywood MA, McHale NG. Mediation by nitric oxide of neurogenic relaxation of the urinary bladder neck muscle in sheep. J Physiol 1992; 451:133–144.

22. Takeda M, Lepor H. Nitric oxide synthase in dog urethra: a histochemical and pharmacological analysis. Br J Pharmacol 1995; 116:2517–2523.

23. Kihara K, de Groat WC. Sympathetic efferent pathways projecting to the bladder neck and proximal urethra in the rat. J Auton Nerv Syst 1997; 62:134–142.

24. Janig W, McLachlan EM. Organization of lumbar spinal outflow to distal colon and pelvic organs. Physiol Rev 1987; 67:1332–1404.

25. Lincoln J, Burnstock G. Autonomic innervation of the urinary bladder and urethra. In: Maggi CA, ed. The autonomic nervous system, Vol. 3, Nervous control of the urogenital system. London: Harwood Academic Publishers, 1993:33–68.

26. Levin RM, Ruggieri MR, Wein AJ. Identification of receptor subtypes in the rabbit and human urinary bladder by selective radioligand binding. J Urol 1988; 139:844–848.

27. Thor KB, Morgan C, Nadelhaft I, et al. Organization of afferent and efferent pathways in the pudendal nerve of the female cat. J Comp Neurol 1989; 288:263–279.

28. de Groat WC. Spinal cord projections and neuropeptides in visceral afferent neurons. Prog Brain Res 1986; 67:165–187.

29. Janig W, Morrison JFB. Functional properties of spinal visceral afferents supplying abdominal and pelvic organs, with special emphasis on visceral nociception. Prog Brain Res 1986; 67:87–114.

30. Habler HJ, Janig W, Koltzenburg M. Activation of unmyelinated afferent fibres by mechanical stimuli and inflammation of the urinary bladder in the cat. J Physiol 1990; 425:545–562.

31. Mallory B, Steers WD, de Groat WC. Electrophysiological study of micturition reflexes in rats. Am J Physiol 1989; 257:R410–R421.

32. Kruse MN, Mallory BS, Noto H, et al. Properties of the descending limb of the spinobulbospinal micturition reflex pathway in the cat. Brain Res 1991; 556:6–12.

33. Iggo A. Tension receptors in the stomach and the urinary bladder. J Physiol 1955; 128:593–607.

34. Floyd K, Hick VE, Morrison JF. Mechanosensitive afferent units in the hypogastric nerve of the cat. J Physiol 1976; 259:457–471.

35. Bahns E, Ernsberger U, Janig W, Nelke A. Functional characteristics of lumbar visceral afferent fibres from the urinary bladder and the urethra in the cat. Pflugers Archiv 1986; 407:510–518.

36. Morrison JF. The physiological mechanisms involved in bladder emptying. Scand J Urol Nephrol Suppl 1997; 184:15–18.

37. Morrison JFB. ATP may be a natural modulator of the sensitivity of bladder mechanoreceptors during slow distensions. First International Consultation on Incontinence, Monaco, 1998.

38. Downie JW, Armour JA. Mechanoreceptor afferent activity compared with receptor field dimensions and pressure changes in feline urinary bladder. Can J Physiol Pharmacol 1992; 70:1457–1467.

39. Yoshimura N, Seki S, Chancellor MB, et al. Targeting afferent hyperexcitability for therapy of the painful bladder syndrome. Urology 2002; 59:61–67.

40. Janig W, Koltzenburg M. Pain arising from the urogenital tract. In: Maggi CA, ed. The autonomic nervous system, Vol. 3, Nervous control of the urogenital system. London: Harwood Academic Publishers, 1993:525–578.

41. Fall M, Lindström S, Mazieres L. A bladder-to-bladder cooling reflex in the cat. J Physiol 1990; 427:281–300.

42. Yoshimura N, White G, Weight FF, de Groat WC. Different types of NA^+ and A-type K^+ currents in dorsal root ganglion neurons innervating the rat urinary bladder. J Physiol 1996; 494:1–16.

43. Maggi CA. The dual, sensory and efferent function of the capsaicin-sensitive primary sensory nerves in the bladder and urethra. In: Maggi CA, ed. The autonomic nervous system, Vol. 3, Nervous control of the urogenital system. London: Harwood Academic Publishers, 1993:383–422.

44. Birder LA, Roppolo JR, Erickson VE, de Groat WC. Increased c-*fos* expression in lumbosacral projection neurons and preganglionic neurons after irritation of the lower urinary tract in the rat. Brain Res 1999; 834:55–65.

45. Cheng C-L, Ma C-P, de Groat WC. Effects of capsaicin on micturition and associated reflexes in the rat. Am J Physiol 1993; 265:R132–R138.

46. de Groat WC, Kawatani M, Hisamitsu T, et al. Mechanisms underlying the recovery of urinary bladder function following spinal cord injury. J Auton Nerv Syst 1990; 30 (Suppl):S71–S77.

47. Cheng C-L, Ma C-P, de Groat WC. Effect of capsaicin on micturition and associated reflexes in chronic spinal rats. Brain Res 1995; 678:40–48.

48. Talaat M. Afferent impulses in the nerves supplying the urinary bladder. J Physiol (London) 1937; 89:1–13.

49. Feber JL, van Asselt E, van Mastrigt R. Neurophysiological modeling of voiding in rats: urethral nerve response to urethral pressure and flow. Am J Physiol 1998; 274:R1473–R1481.

50. Bradley W, Griffin D, Teague C, Timm G. Sensory innervation of the mammalian urethra. Invest Urol 1973; 10:287–289.

51. Todd JK. Afferent impulses in the pudendal nerves of the cat. Q J Exp Physiol 1964; 49:258–267.

52. Bahns E, Halsband U, Janig W. Responses of sacral visceral afferents from the lower urinary tract, colon and anus to mechanical stimulation. Pflugers Arch 1987; 410:296–303.

53. Conte B, Maggi CA, Giachetti A, et al. Intraurethral capsaicin produces reflex activation of the striated urethral sphincter in urethane-anesthetized male rats. J Urol 1993; 150:1271–1277.

54. Thor KB, Muhlhauser MA. Vesicoanal, urethroanal, and urethrovesical reflexes initiated by lower urinary tract irritation in the rat. Am J Physiol 1999; 277:R1002–R1012.

55. Hokfelt T, Schultzberg M, Elde R, et al. Peptide neurons in peripheral tissues including the urinary tract: immunohistochemical studies. Acta Pharmacol Toxicol (Copenh) 1978; 43:79–89.

56. Warburton AL, Santer RM. Sympathetic and sensory innervation of the urinary tract in young adult and aged rats: a semi-quantitative histochemical and immunohistochemical study. Histochem J 1994; 26:127–133.

57. Lecci A, Giuliani S, Lazzeri M, et al. The behavioral response induced by intravesical instillation of capsaicin rats is mediated by pudendal urethral sensory fibers. Life Sci 1994; 55:429–436.

58. Jung SY, Fraser MO, Ozawa H, et al. Urethral afferent nerve activity affects the micturition reflex; implication for the relationship between stress incontinence and detrusor instability. J Urol 1999; 162:204–212.

59. Ferguson DR, Kennedy I, Burton TJ. ATP is released from rabbit urinary bladder epithelial cells by hydrostatic pressure changes – a possible sensory mechanism? J Physiol 1997; 505:503–511.

60. Birder LA, Kanai AJ, de Groat WC, et al. Vanilloid receptor expression suggests a sensory role for urinary bladder epithelial cells. Proc Natl Acad Sci USA 2001; 98:13396–13401.

61. Vlaskovska M, Kasakov L, Rong W, et al. P2X3 knock-out mice reveal a major sensory role for urothelially released ATP. J Neurosci 2001; 21:5670–5677.

62. Birder LA, Apodaca G, De Groat WC, Kanai AJ. Adrenergic- and capsaicin-evoked nitric oxide release from urothelium and afferent nerves in urinary bladder. Am J Physiol 1998; 275:F226–F229.

63. Birder LA, Nealen ML, Kiss S, et al. Beta-adrenoceptor agonists stimulate endothelial nitric oxide synthase in rat urinary bladder urothelial cells. J Neurosci 2002; 22:8063–8070.

64. Bean BP, Williams CA, Ceelen PW. ATP-activated channels in rat and bullfrog sensory neurons: current–voltage relation and single-channel behavior. J Neurosci 1990; 10:11–19.

65. Dmitrieva N, Burnstock G, McMahon SB. ATP and 2-methyl thioATP activate bladder reflexes and induce discharge of bladder sensory neurons. Soc Neurosci Abstr 1998; 24:2088.

66. Cockayne DA, Hamilton SG, Zhu QM, et al. Urinary bladder hyporeflexia and reduced pain-related behaviour in P2X3-deficient mice. Nature 2000; 407:1011–1015.

67. Birder LA, Nakamura Y, Kiss S, et al. Altered urinary bladder function in mice lacking the vanilloid receptor TRPV1. Nat Neurosci 2002; 5:856–860.

68. Hawthorn MH, Chapple CR, Cock M, Chess-Williams R. Urothelium-derived inhibitory factor(s) influences on detrusor muscle contractility in vitro. Br J Pharmacol 2000; 129:416–419.

69. de Groat WC. Nervous control of the urinary bladder of the cat. Brain Res 1975; 87:201–211.

70. de Groat WC, Theobald RJ. Reflex activation of sympathetic pathways to vesical smooth muscle and parasympathetic ganglia by electrical stimulation of vesical afferents. J Physiol 1976; 259:223–237.

71. Yoshimura N. Bladder afferent pathway and spinal cord injury: possible mechanisms inducing hyperreflexia of the urinary bladder. Progress in Neurobiology 1999; 57:583–606.

72. Park JM, Bloom DA, McGuire EJ. The guarding reflex revisited. Br J Urol 1997; 80:940–945.

73. Fedirchuk B, Hochman S, Shefchyk SJ. An intracellular study of perineal and hindlimb afferent inputs onto sphincter motoneurons in the decerebrate cat. Exp Brain Res 1992; 89:511–516.

74. Holstege G, Griffiths D, De Wall H, Dalm E. Anatomical and physiological observations on supraspinal control of bladder and urethral sphincter muscles in the cat. J Comp Neurol 1986; 250:449–461.

75. Kohama T. [Neuroanatomical studies on the urine storage facilitatory areas in the cat brain. Part I. Input neuronal structures to the nucleus locus subcoeruleus and the nucleus radicularis pontis oralis]. Nippon Hinyokika Gakkai Zasshi 1992; 83:1469–1477.

76. de Groat WC, Fraser MO, Yoshiyama M, et al. Neural control of the urethra. Scand J Urol Nephrol Suppl 2001:35–43; discussion 106–125.

77. de Groat WC, Booth AM, Krier J, et al. Neural control of the urinary bladder and large intestine. In: Brooks CM, Koizumi K, Sato A, eds. Integrative functions of the autonomic nervous system. Tokyo: Tokyo Univ. Press, 1979:50–67.

78. de Groat WC, Booth AM, Milne RJ, Roppolo JR. Parasympathetic preganglionic neurons in the sacral spinal cord. J Auton Nerv Syst 1982; 5:23–43.

79. McGuire EJ, Morrissey SG, Schichun Z, Horwinsk E. Control of reflex detrusor activity in normal and spinal injured non-human primates. J Urol 1983; 129:197–199.

80. de Groat WC, Nadelhaft I, Milne RJ, et al. Organization of the sacral parasympathetic reflex pathways to the urinary bladder and large intestine. J Auton Nerv Syst 1981; 3:135–160.

81. Vera PL, Nadelhaft I. Conduction velocity distribution of afferent fibers innervating the rat urinary bladder. Brain Res 1990; 520:83–89.

82. Kuru M. Nervous control of micturition. Physiol Rev 1965; 45:425–494.

83. Nishizawa O, Sugaya K, Noto H, et al. Pontine micturition center in the dog. J Urol 1988; 140:872–874.

84. Mallory BS, Roppolo JR, de Groat WC. Pharmacological modulation of the pontine micturition center. Brain Res 1991; 546:310–320.

85. Noto H, Roppolo JR, Steers WD, de Groat WC. Excitatory and inhibitory influences on bladder activity elicited by electrical stimulation in the pontine micturition center in rat. Brain Res 1989; 492:99–115.

86. Noto H, Roppolo JR, Steers WD, de Groat WC. Electrophysiological analysis of the ascending and descending components of the micturition reflex pathway in the rat. Brain Res 1991; 549:95–105.

87. Blok BF, Holstege G. Direct projections from the periaqueductal gray to the pontine micturition center (M-region). An anterograde and retrograde tracing study in the cat. Neurosci Lett 1994; 166:93–96.

88. Blok BF, De Weerd H, Holstege G. Ultrastructural evidence for a paucity of projections from the lumbosacral cord to the pontine micturition center or M-region in the cat: a new concept for the organization of the micturition reflex with the periaqueductal gray as central relay. J Comp Neurol 1995; 359:300–309.

89. Matsuura S, Allen GV, Downie JW. Volume-evoked micturition reflex is mediated by the ventrolateral periaqueductal gray in anesthetized rats. Am J Physiol 1998; 275:R2049–R2055.

90. Matsuura S, Downie JW, Allen GV. Micturition evoked by glutamate microinjection in the ventrolateral periaqueductal gray is mediated through Barrington's nucleus in the rat. Neuroscience 2000; 101:1053–1061.

91. Blaivas JG. The neurophysiology of micturition: a clinical study of 550 patients. J Urol 1982; 127:958.

92. Rossier AB, Ott R. Bladder and urethral recordings in acute and chronic spinal cord injury patients. Int J Urol 1976; 31:49–59.

93. Barrington FJF. The component reflexes of micturition in the cat. Parts I and II. Brain 1931; 54:177–188.

94. Barrington FJF. The component reflexes of micturition in the cat. Part III. Brain 1941; 64:239–243.

95. de Groat WC, Araki I, Vizzard MA, et al. Developmental and injury induced plasticity in the micturition reflex pathway. Behav Brain Res 1998; 92:127–140.

96. Araki I, de Groat WC. Developmental synaptic depression underlying reorganization of visceral reflex pathways in the spinal cord. J Neurosci 1997; 17:8402–8407.

97. Birder LA, de Groat WC. Induction of c-fos gene expression of spinal neurons in the rat by nociceptive and non-nociceptive stimulation of the lower urinary tract. Am J Physiol 1993; 265:R643–R648.

98. Nadelhaft I, Vera PL. Neurons in the rat brain and spinal cord labeled after pseudorabies virus injected into the external urethral sphincter. J Comp Neurol 1996; 375:502–517.

99. Vizzard MA, Erickson VL, Card JP, et al. Transneuronal labeling of neurons in the adult rat brainstem and spinal cord after injection of pseudorabies virus into the urethra. J Comp Neurol 1995; 355:629–640.

100. Sugaya K, Roppolo JR, Yoshimura N, et al. The central neural pathways involved in micturition in the neonatal rat as revealed by the injection of pseudorabies virus into the urinary bladder. Neurosci Lett 1997; 223:197–200.

101. Sasaki M. Morphological analysis of external urethral and external anal sphincter motoneurones of cat. J Comp Neurol 1994; 349:269–287.

102. Araki I. Inhibitory postsynaptic currents and the effects of GABA on visually identified sacral parasympathetic preganglionic neurons in neonatal rats. J Neurophysiol 1994; 72:2903–2910.

103. de Groat WC. Excitation and inhibition of sacral parasympathetic neurons by visceral and cutaneous stimuli in the cat. Brain Res 1971; 33:499–503.

104. de Groat WC. Inhibitory mechanisms in the sacral reflex pathways to the urinary bladder. In: Ryall RW, Kelly JS, eds. Iontophoresis and transmitter mechanisms in the mammalian central nervous system. Amsterdam: Elsevier, 1978:366–368.

105. Morrison JF, Sato A, Sato Y, Yamanishi T. The influence of afferent inputs from skin and viscera on the activity of the bladder and the skeletal muscle surrounding the urethra in the rat. Neurosci Res 1995; 23:195–205.

106. McGuire EJ. Experimental observations on the integration of bladder and urethral function. Trans Am Assoc Genitourin Surg 1976; 68:38–42.

107. de Groat WC, Ryall RW. Reflexes to sacral parasympathetic neurones concerned with micturition in the cat. J Physiol 1969; 200:87–108.

108. Barrington FJF. The relation of the hind-brain to micturition. Brain 1921; 4:23–53.

109. Blok BFM, DeWeerd H, Holstege G. The pontine micturition center projects to sacral cord GABA immunoreactive neurons in the cat. Neurosci Lett 1997; 233:109–112.

110. Blok BFM, Holstege G. Neuronal control of micturition and its relation to the emotional motor system. Prog Brain Res 1996; 107:113–126.

111. Tang PC, Ruch TC. Localization of brain stem and diencephalic areas controlling the micturition reflex. J Comp Neurol 1956; 106:213–245.

112. Sugaya K, Matsuyama K, Takakusaki K, Mori S. Electrical and chemical stimulations of the pontine micturition center. Neurosci Lett 1987; 80:197–201.

113. Valentino RJ, Chen S, Zhu Y, Aston-Jones G. Evidence for divergent projections to the brain noradrenergic system and the spinal parasympathetic system from Barrington's nucleus. Brain Res 1996; 732:1–15.

114. Ding YQ, Takada M, Tokuno H, Mizuno N. Direct projections from the dorsolateral pontine tegmentum to pudendal motoneurons innervating the external urethral sphincter muscle in the rat. J Comp Neurol 1995; 357:318–330.

115. Otake K, Nakamura Y. Single neurons in Barrington's nucleus projecting to both the paraventricular thalamic nucleus and the spinal cord by way of axon collaterals: a double labeling study in the rat. Neurosci Lett 1996; 209:97–100.

116. Blok BF, van Maarseveen JT, Holstege G. Electrical stimulation of the sacral dorsal gray commissure evokes relaxation of the external urethral sphincter in the cat. Neurosci Lett 1998; 249:68–70.

117. Valentino RJ, Pavcovich LA, Hirata H. Evidence for corticotropin-releasing hormone projections from Barrington's nucleus to the periaqueductal gray and dorsal motor nucleus of the vagus in the rat. J Comp Neurol 1995; 363:402–422.

118. Blok BFM, Willemsen ATM, Holstege G. A PET study on the brain control of micturition in humans. Brain 1997:111–121.

119. Yoshimura N, Nagahama Y, Ueda T, Yoshida O. Paroxysmal urinary incontinence associated with multiple sclerosis. Urol Int 1997; 59:197–199.

120. Marson L. Identification of central nervous system neurons that innervate the bladder body, bladder base, or external urethral sphincter of female rats: a transneuronal tracing study using pseudorabies virus. J Comp Neurol 1997; 389:584–602.

121. Fukuyama H, Matsuzaki S, Ouchi Y, et al. Neural control of micturition in man examined with single photon emission computed tomography using 99mTc-HMPAO. Neuroreport 1996; 7:3009–3012.

122. Blok BF, Sturms LM, Holstege G. A PET study on cortical and subcortical control of pelvic floor musculature in women. J Comp Neurol 1997; 389:535–544.

123. Holstege JC, Van Dijken H, Buijs RM, Goedknegt H, Gosens T, Bongers CM. Distribution of dopamine immunoreactivity in the rat, cat and monkey spinal cord. J Comp Neurol 1996; 376:631–652.

124. Athwal BS, Berkley KJ, Hussain I, et al. Brain responses to changes in bladder volume and urge to void in healthy men. Brain 2001; 124:369–377.

125. de Groat WC, Araki I. Maturation of bladder reflex pathways during postnatal development. Adv Exp Med Biol 1999; 462:253–263.

126. Geirsson G, Lindstrom S, Fall M. The bladder cooling reflex and the use of cooling as stimulus to the lower urinary tract. J Urol 1999; 162:1890–1896.

127. Chancellor MB, de Groat WC. Intravesical capsaicin and resiniferatoxin therapy: spicing up the ways to treat the overactive bladder. J Urol 1999; 162:3–11.

Part II

Functional pathology of the lower urinary tract

7

Epidemiology of the neurogenic bladder

Patrick B Leu and Ananias C Diokno

Introduction

The neurogenic bladder is an entity with many different characteristics. It is not a disease in and of itself, but rather the manifestation of multiple different neurologic processes capable of exerting effects on the bladder by way of its innervation. The outward expression of these effects by the bladder is as varied as the conditions that cause them, ranging from essentially no bladder function at all to extreme overactivity. The long-term consequences cover a spectrum just as broad, ranging from little to no consequence to the patient to severe debility and even death.

This chapter aims to outline for the reader the many neurologic processes which can affect the bladder. While a brief description of some diseases will be given, the main focus is the prevalence and type of neurogenic bladder involvement in many of these conditions. Prevalence of neurogenic bladder is the frequency with which bladder dysfunction is observed among the population of neurologically impaired patients at a given time period. Organization of this chapter is based on location of neurologic injury: above the brainstem, the spinal cord, and the peripheral nervous system.

Cerebrovascular accident

Cerebrovascular accident (CVA) or 'stroke' is a major cause of morbidity and mortality, especially among the elderly. It is defined as the acute onset of a focal neurologic deficit. Causes include cerebral embolus, atherosclerotic thrombus, and hemorrhage. The prevalence is approximately 60/1000 patients older than 65 years and 95/1000 in those older than 75 years.[1] More than 500,000 cerebrovascular accidents occur annually in the United States. One-third are fatal, one-third necessitate long-term nursing care, and another third allow patients to return to home with normal or near-normal ability to function. Risk factors include hypertension, diabetes mellitus, smoking, high serum cholesterol, alcohol consumption, obesity, stress, and a sedentary lifestyle.[2]

Cerebrovascular accidents can have profound effects on the genitourinary system. Voiding dysfunction can range from urinary retention to total incontinence. Evaluation and management can be complicated due to associated comorbidities, which may also contribute to voiding dysfunction in this patient population.

Many studies have demonstrated urologic findings as predictors of prognosis in stroke patients. In an analysis of 532 stroke patients, Wade and Hewer noted that of those with urinary incontinence within the first week after the event, half died within 6 months.[3] They also noted an association between early incontinence and decreased chance of regaining mobility. Taub et al evaluated 639 CVA patients and found that initial incontinence was the best single indicator of future disability.[4]

Acute urinary retention, commonly known as cerebral shock, is often seen immediately after stroke. The neurophysiologic mechanism of this is unknown and it may not necessarily be the result of the stroke. It may be the consequence of inability to communicate the need to void, impaired consciousness, temporary overdistention, restricted mobility, associated comorbidities (i.e. diabetes, benign prostatic hyperplasia (BPH)) or medications. Urodynamic studies soon after unilateral CVA have demonstrated a 21% prevalence of overflow incontinence due to detrusor hyporeflexia; however, several of these patients were either diabetic or receiving anticholinergics.[5]

Urinary incontinence is common after stroke. It may be due to detrusor hyperreflexia secondary to loss of cortical inhibition, cognitive impairment with normal bladder function, or overflow incontinence secondary to detrusor hyporeflexia secondary to neuropathy or medication. Underlying dementia, BPH, or stress urinary incontinence may also contribute.[2]

Incontinence after stroke is frequently transitory. While the incidence of early post-stroke urinary incontinence is 57–83%, many of these patients have been found to recover continence with time, with as many as 80% being continent at 6 months post-CVA.[6]

Irritative voiding symptoms of frequency, urgency, and incontinence are most commonly seen after resolution of the cerebral shock. These are manifestations of detrusor hyperreflexia. In a review of recent literature, Marinkovic and Badlani found that 69% of patients had detrusor hyperreflexia, 10% had detrusor hypocontractility, 31% had uninhibited external sphincter relaxation, and 22% had detrusor-sphincter dyssynergia (DSD). Furthermore, they note that attempts at correlating either the site or mechanism (ischemic vs hemorrhagic) of injury with urodynamic findings have been inconclusive.[2]

Cerebellar ataxia

Ataxia refers to a heterogeneous spectrum of abnormal motor phenomena associated with cerebellar deficiency. Histologically, Purkinje's cells are abnormal and decreased in number. The location of nervous system involvement may extend from the cerebellum to the brainstem, spinal cord, and dorsal nerve roots. The disease is classified based on etiologies. Acute ataxia is secondary to various intoxicants, cerebellar tumors, viral infections, hyperpyrexia, demyelinating diseases, and vascular accidents. Subacute ataxia may be secondary to alcohol abuse, paraneoplastic syndromes, or cerebellar tumors. Chronic childhood ataxias may include Friedreich's ataxia, ataxia telangiectasia, and ataxias associated with inherited metabolic derangements. Adult forms include olivopontocerebellar atrophy and cortical cerebellar degeneration.

On examination, these patients manifest initially with poor leg coordination, with subsequent involvement of the upper extremities. Decreased deep tendon reflexes with decreased vibratory sensation and proprioception can be seen. Dysmetria of the arms, dysarthria, choreiform movements, and horizontal nystagmus may also be present.

Urodynamic evaluation by Leach et al of 15 ataxic patients, ranging in age from 8 to 58 years, found that 8 (53%) had hyperreflexia with bladder-sphincteric coordination, 1 (7%) had hyperreflexia without bladder-sphincteric coordination, 2 (13%) had normal bladder contraction without sphincteric coordination, and 4 (27%) had acontractile bladders.[7]

Tumors of the cerebrum

Incontinence of urine can occur in frontal tumors as part of a frontal lobe syndrome of indifference, disinhibition, and self-neglect. However, it can also present with urinary frequency, urgency, and incontinence without signs of cognitive or intellectual impairment. This was first described by Andrew and Nathan in 1964, who reported this with a variety of frontal lobe lesions and concluded what is known to be true today: there exists a micturition control center in the superomedial part of the frontal lobes.[8] Ten years later, 7 further cases were reported by Maurice-Williams in

a series of 50 consecutive frontal lobe tumors (14%) over a 29-month time span. After evaluation of 100 consecutive intracranial tumors he observed that this constellation of symptoms was seen only with frontal tumors.[9]

Blaivas reported results of urodynamic studies on 550 patients. Twenty-seven (4.9%) of them had pathologic cystometric findings attributable solely to a focal suprapontine lesion. Thirteen of these patients had brain tumors and 14 of them had strokes. Incontinence was their only clinical manifestation, although not all of them were able to void.[10]

Lang et al reported on two cases of urinary retention and space-occupying lesions of the frontal cortex in 1996. The first case involved an 87-year-old woman who regained her ability to void with minimal post-void residual after evacuation of a subdural hematoma. The second patient was a 63-year-old woman who presented with increasing difficulty voiding over $2\frac{1}{2}$ years. She was found to have detrusor hypocontractility and mild bilateral hyperreflexia. She refused surgery for a large left frontal meningioma. During the 4-year follow-up she eventually required suprapubic catheterization before dying of increasing intracranial pressure from the expanding tumor.[11]

Normal pressure hydrocephalus

Normal pressure hydrocephalus (NPH) is a syndrome of progressing dementia and gait disturbance in patients with normal spinal fluid pressure yet distended cerebral ventricles. This was first described in 1965. While some patients can have an identifiable mechanical reason for dilation of cerebral ventricles (obstructing tumor, subarachnoid hemorrhage), the cause of this disease is not identifiable in many patients. Some have suggested failure of cerebrospinal fluid (CSF) to flow into the parasagittal subarachnoid space (where most fluid resorption occurs) as the most likely mechanism.

In 1975, Jonas and Brown evaluated 5 NPH patients with urinary incontinence by performing cystometry. These patients had urinary frequency, urgency, and urge incontinence. Four of the patients exhibited pressure spikes from involuntary bladder contractions. The other patient exhibited low-volume involuntary voiding at 200 ml of fluid. These findings are consistent with the so-called 'uninhibited neurogenic bladder,' as described by Lapides. This is secondary to loss of cortical inhibition of primitive bladder reflex contractions.[12]

Cerebral palsy

Cerebral palsy (CP) is a nonprogressive disorder of the brain, resulting in a variety of motor abnormalities often accompanied by intellectual impairment, convulsive disorders, or other cerebral dysfunction. Strict definitions exclude spinal cord involvement. Approximately one-third of children with CP have lower urinary tract symptoms.

McNeal et al published urodynamic results on 50 patients between the ages of 8 and 29 years. They found enuresis in 28%, stress incontinence in 26%, urgency in 18%, and dribbling in 6%. Overall, 36% had some form of voiding dysfunction and some had multiple symptoms.[13]

Decter et al evaluated 57 children with cerebral palsy and lower urinary tract symptoms. Incontinence occurred in 49/57 (86%) patients. Eleven of the children had wetting limited to day or night, while the remaining 38 experienced wetting during both the day and night. Of the 8 who were totally continent, 3 suffered from severe urgency and frequency, 2 presented with urinary tract infections, 2 complained of difficulty initiating urination, and 1 was in urinary retention.

Although general neurologic examination revealed only minor findings in some patients, urodynamic studies identified definite abnormalities in a majority of patients. On urodynamic evaluation, 70% of the incontinent patients had uninhibited contractions that could not be suppressed, 6% had overflow incontinence with incomplete emptying secondary to detrusor-sphincter dyssynergia (DSD), 4% had hypertonia causing intermittent leaking, and 2% had periodic relaxation of the external sphincter during filling. Overall, 49 of the 57 (86%) patients (continent and incontinent) were found to have purely upper motor neuron lesions.

Urinary tract infection was seen in 11% of the patients. Four of the 6 had bladder outlet obstruction secondary to DSD and 1 had elevated residual volumes owing to poor detrusor contraction. Radiologic abnormalities were seen in all 6 children.[14]

Mental retardation

Mental retardation may result from a heterogeneous group of disorders and is seldom the result of deficient intelligence alone.[15] Etiologies include infection, toxin exposure (maternal overdose), perinatal injury, metabolic disturbances (hypercalcemia, hypoglycemia, phenylketonuria), malformations (hydrocephaly, microcephaly, and others), genetic disorders (Down's syndrome), and cerebral palsy.[16]

In 1981 Mitchell and Woodthorpe published data on prevalence and disability of mentally handicapped people born between 1958 and 1963 in three London boroughs. They reported that nocturnal enuresis occurred in over a quarter of patients and 12% experienced both day and nighttime incontinence.[16] Another British study by Reid et al evaluated behavioral syndromes in a sample of 100 severely (49) and profoundly (51) retarded adults. Sixty-five percent of patients in this study of hospitalized patients were incontinent.[17]

Hellstrom et al studied 21 mentally retarded patients (16 men, 5 women; average age 36 years) referred for long-standing urinary problems. The most common urinary symptoms were incontinence, nocturnal enuresis, and urinary retention/poor bladder emptying. The most common urodynamic findings were detrusor areflexia (7) and detrusor hyperreflexia (5). Four patients had normal urodynamic studies. High micturition pressure was found in 3 patients and large bladder capacity in 1 patient. Poor flow with high residual volume was seen in 2 patients. Some patients had more than one finding.[15]

Parkinson's disease

Parkinson's disease is a leading cause of neurologic disability among the elderly population. The estimated prevalence of the disease in the United States is 100 to 150 per 100,000 population and the incidence per annum is 20 per 100,000. Pathogenesis of the disease involves degeneration of the pigmented dopamine-rich substantia nigra of the brain. The resultant dopamine deficiency results in imbalance between dopamine and acetylcholine concentrations. This manifests clinically as tremor, rigidity and bradykinesia.[18] Urinary symptoms associated with onset of tremor in some Parkinsonian patients were described as early as 1936 and later studies in the 1960s and 1970s demonstrated a 37–71% incidence of bladder dysfunction with Parkinson's disease.[19–21] It is felt that the effect of the normal basal ganglia on micturition is inhibitory in nature.

Pavlakis et al in 1983 reported urodynamic findings on 30 patients (22 men and 8 women) with Parkinson's disease and voiding dysfunction. Fifty-seven percent complained of irritative symptoms, 23% obstructive symptoms and 20% had a combination of the two.

Ninety-three percent of the 30 CO_2 cystometrographs (CMGs) performed demonstrated detrusor hyperreflexia and 7% (women only) detrusor areflexia. No patient had a normal CMG. Of patients with detrusor hyperreflexia, 75% demonstrated appropriate sphincter relaxation, 7% showed pseudo-dyssynergia (voluntary contraction of the perineal floor at the time of detrusor contraction in an attempt to prevent leakage), 11% demonstrated sphincter bradykinesia (involuntary electromyographic (EMG) activity persisting through at least the initial part of the expulsive phase of the CMG), and 7% showed neuropathic sphincter potentials. In the two women with detrusor areflexia there was no evidence of detrusor denervation based on supersensitivity testing, nor was there any evidence of sphincter denervation based on EMG studies. These two patients were on anticholinergics, and this may have been the etiology of their areflexia.

Maximum flow rate was decreased in 10 of the 17 men who underwent uroflow analysis. All 10 had prostatic enlargement and 8 presented with obstructive symptoms. Eight of the 10 demonstrated detrusor hyperreflexia with normal sphincter relaxation and the other 2 had pseudo-dyssynergia.[18]

A more recent study from Araki et al reported urodynamic findings on 70 patients (30 men and 40 women) with Parkinson's disease. No male with evidence of prostatic enlargement based on transrectal ultrasound and retrograde urethrocystography was included.

Detrusor hyperreflexia was present in 67% of patients and hyporeflexia or areflexia was seen in 16%. Other findings were hyperreflexia with impaired contractile function in 9%, hyperreflexia with detrusor-sphincter dyssynergia in 3%, and normal detrusor function in 6%. Detrusor-sphincter dyssynergia and detrusor hyperreflexia with impaired contractile function were observed only at advanced stages, whereas bladder function was normal only at mild or moderate stages. Abnormal urodynamic findings increased with disease severity.[22]

Shy–Drager syndrome

Shy–Drager syndrome is a rare syndrome which manifests as orthostatic hypotension, urinary incontinence and retention, and associated neurologic dysfunction. It was first described in 1960. The complete syndrome may also include rectal incontinence, anhydrosis, iris atrophy, external ocular palsies, rigidity, tremor, impotence, fasciculations, myasthenia, and anterior horn cell neuropathy. Although the disease mostly affects men, it can also affect women; it is a slowly progressive disease. Urinary symptoms occur early and orthostatic hypotension appears later.[23]

Salinas et al studied 9 patients (7 men and 2 women, mean age 71 years) referred for urologic evaluation. Thirty-three percent of patients had difficulty or inability to void, 44% had stress urinary incontinence, 33% had urinary frequency, and 33% had urge incontinence. Two-thirds of patients had lax anal tone and 45% had absent voluntary anal control. Electromyography of the periurethral striated muscle revealed normal response to cough/Valsalva in 56% and weak or absent activity in the remaining patients. Voluntary sphincter control, likewise, was present in 56% and weak or absent in 44%. Two of the three patients who were able to void had synchronous cessation of EMG activity and the other patient exhibited sporadic sphincteric activity. On CMG, 67% failed to demonstrate reflex or voluntary detrusor contractions. Poor bladder compliance was seen in 4 out of the 9 patients. Involuntary contractions were seen in one-third of patients.[24]

Multiple sclerosis

Multiple sclerosis (MS) is a disabling neurologic disease caused by a demyelinating process affecting the central nervous system. It is characterized by exacerbations and remissions, with associated changes in signs and symptoms. It is the most common neurologic disorder in the 20–45-year-old age group and affects women and men in a 2:1 ratio. It affects 1 of 1000 Americans.[25] Eighty to 90% of patients with MS will have urologic manifestations, and as many as 10% will present with urologic dysfunction. Patients may exhibit symptoms of urgency, urge incontinence, frequency and urinary retention. These are secondary to detrusor hyperreflexia, detrusor-sphincter dyssynergia, and hypocontractility.[26] Litwiller et al recently performed a review of the literature on multiple sclerosis and the involvement of the genitourinary system. In evaluating 22 studies involving 1882 patients, they found urodynamic evidence of detrusor hyperreflexia in 62% of patients, detrusor-sphincter dyssynergia in 25%, and detrusor hypocontractility in 20% of patients. Less than 1% of patients had renal deterioration.[27]

The manifestations of the disease can also change during its course. Ciancio et al recently published data on urodynamic pattern changes in multiple sclerosis. They evaluated 22 patients with MS who underwent at least 2 urodynamic evaluations with a mean follow-up interval of 42 ± 45 months between the studies. Overall, 55% of the patients demonstrated a change in their urodynamic patterns and/or compliance. Sixty-four percent of patients had the same or worsening of the same symptoms and 36% had new urologic symptoms. Forty-three percent of patients with no new symptoms and 75% of patients with new symptoms had significant changes found with follow-up urodynamic testing.[28]

Myelodysplasia

Myelodysplasia, also known as spina bifida, is a condition of malformation of the caudal end of the neural tube and vertebral arches. It is the most common cause of neuropathic bladder in children. Spina bifida cystica refers to protrusion of a sac through the vertebral arch defect. This sac may contain parts of nervous tissue, meninges, spinal fluid, and fat. If this sac contains only meninges, the condition is referred to as a meningocele. If there is some element of spinal cord present with the meninges, it is referred to as a myelomeningocele. This is the case in 90% of patients with spina bifida cystica. A lipomyelomeningocele occurs if a fatty growth of tissue is protruding into the sac with spinal cord elements. Myeloschisis occurs when the spinal cord is completely open without any meningeal covering.

Myelodysplasia occurs in approximately 1 in 1000 births in the United States. It can involve all levels of the spinal column, including the lumbar 26%, lumbosacral 47%, sacral 20%, thoracic 5%, and cervical spine 2%. Eighty-five percent of children have an associated Arnold–Chiari malformation.

The neurologic lesion produced can be quite variable and depends on which neural elements have everted with the meningocele sac. The level of the bony defect gives little clue to the clinical manifestation of the patient. The height of the bony level and the highest extent of the neurologic lesion may vary from 1 to 3 vertebral levels in either direction. Furthermore, the differential growth rates between the veterbral bodies and the elongating spinal cord add a factor of dynamism in the developing child. Because of fibrosis surrounding the spinal cord at the site of meningocele closure, the cord can become tethered during growth, leading to changes in bowel, bladder, and lower extremity function. Urodynamic evaluation of these patients is therefore a critical component of their management.[29]

Urodynamic studies in the newborn period have shown that 57% of myelodysplastic infants have bladder contractions. In children with upper lumbar or thoracic lesions where the sacral cord is spared, 50% have bladder contractions.[30] EMG studies of the external sphincter demonstrate 48% of newborns with intact sacral reflex arcs and no lower motor neuron denervation, 23% with partial denervation, and 29% with complete loss of sacral cord function.[31]

In 1981, McGuire et al demonstrated the relation between intravesical pressure at the time of urethral leakage and presence/development of upper tract changes in myelodysplastic patients. No patient with an intravesical pressure less than 40 cmH_2O at the time of urethral leakage developed vesicoureteral reflux and only 10% demonstrated ureteral dilatation on excretory urography. Sixty-eight percent of patients with higher leak point pressures developed vesicoureteral reflux and 81% showed ureteral dilatation on excretory urography.[32]

A major problem and risk factor for developing upper urinary tract deterioration is the presence of dyssynergia between the external sphincter and the bladder. Urodynamic evaluation of 36 infants with myelodysplasia demonstrated 50% with dyssynergia, 25% with synergy, and 25% with no sphincter activity. Seventy-two percent of the group with dyssynergia were found to exhibit hydroureteronephrosis by 2 years of age. This was present in only 22% of those with synergy and 11% with absent activity. Of those patients with synergy who went on to develop upper tract deterioration, it occurred only after development of incoordination between the detrusor and external sphincter. The one patient with absent sphincter activity who developed upper tract changes had an elevated fixed urethral resistance at 1 year of age. This is felt to be secondary to fibrosis of the striated external urethral sphincter. Treatment by catheterization or cutaneous vesicostomy improved drainage of the urinary tract in each patient.[33]

The tethered cord syndrome, resulting from fibrosis around the cord and differential growth rates of vertebral bodies and the spinal cord, can be seen in children and adults after neurosurgical closure of the primary defect. Symptoms of bladder dysfunction may be seen in 56% of patients at presentation.[34] Adamson et al reported on 5 adults with tethered cord syndrome revealing a full spectrum of bladder dysfunction ranging from retention in 2 of the 5 and frequency and or urgency/incontinence in 3 of the 5 patients.[35] Flanigan et al reported urodynamic results of 24 children prior to operative cord release. Seventy-one percent had areflexia and 29% had hyperreflexic bladders.[36] Pang and Wilberger reported preoperative urodynamic study results on 8 patients. Five demonstrated small capacity, spastic unstable bladders while 3 had hypotonic bladders.[34]

Sacral agenesis

Sacral agenesis is defined as the absence of all or part of two or more vertebral bodies at the lower end of the spinal column. Defective development of the second to fourth sacral nerves accompanying the bony abnormalities leads to variable patterns of neuropathic bladder. The incidence of sacral agenesis is about 0.09–0.43% of births. It is seen more frequently in children of diabetic mothers. It is also seen in 12% of children with high imperforate anus. Approximately 20% of children with sacral agenesis are not identified until they are 3–4 years old and present with difficulty in toilet training.[29]

The urodynamic pattern in children with sacral agenesis is varied. Guzman et al reported upper motor lesions at a rate of 35%, including detrusor hyperreflexia, detrusorsphincter dyssynergia, exaggerated sacral reflexes, and no voluntary control over sphincter function. Forty percent demonstrated lower motor lesions, including detrusor areflexia and absent sacral reflexes. The remaining 25% were unaffected.[37]

Another study by Koff and Deridder evaluated 13 patients with sacral agenesis. Urodynamic studies revealed a 31% rate of lower motor lesions (flaccid bladder), 23% had an upper motor lesion, and 31% had a mixed pattern.[38]

Spinal cord injury

Spinal cord injury (SCI) affects over 200,000 persons in the United States, with an estimated 8000–10,000 new cases occurring annually.[39] Bladder dysfunction after SCI can be classified as either lower motor neuron (LMN) dysfunction or upper motor neuron (UMN) dysfunction.[40]

In patients with hyperreflexia following spinal cord injury, it is imperative to know whether the external sphincter is coordinated (synergic) with the detrusor contraction or if the sphincter is uncoordinated (dyssynergic) with the involuntary detrusor contraction. Diokno et al reported a 66% rate of dyssynergia among 47 patients with a reflex neurogenic bladder.[41]

Kaplan et al reported videourodynamic results obtained from 489 patients with spinal cord lesions secondary to a variety of causes: trauma (284), myelomeningocele (75), spinal stenosis (54), tumors (39), sacral agenesis (5), and other conditions (34). Their analysis found that while there was a general correlation between the neurologic level of injury and the expected vesicourethral function, it was neither absolute nor specific. For example, some patients with cervical cord lesions exhibited detrusor areflexia and some with sacral cord lesions exhibited detrusor hyperreflexia or DSD.[42]

In 2000, Weld and Dmochowski reported urodynamic findings of 243 SCI patients. All but 3 patients were male. Of 196 patients with suprasacral injuries, 95% demonstrated hyperreflexia and/or DSD. Forty-two percent had low bladder compliance and 40% had high detrusor leak point pressures. Of 14 patients with sacral injuries, 86% manifested areflexia, 79% had low compliance, and 86% had high leak point pressures. Of 33 patients with combined suprasacral and sacral injuries, 68% demonstrated hyperreflexia and/or DSD, 27% exhibited areflexia, 58% had low compliance, and 61% had high leak point pressures. Hyperreflexia was seen in 42%, 54%, 32%, 14%, and 33% of cervical, thoracic, lumbar, sacral, and multilevel cord injuries, respectively. Detrusor-sphincter dyssynergia was seen in 68%, 50%, 39% 14%, and 45% of these same lesions. Areflexia was seen in 0%, 0%, 21%, 86%, and 27%, respectively. Normal urodynamic findings were found in 1%, 4%, 4%, 0%, and 3% of injuries at the aforementioned levels. These findings further reinforce that while general correlations between level of injury and the clinical manifestation exist, they are not exact or exclusive.[43]

The central cord syndrome is caused by incomplete cervical spinal cord injury and is characterized by incomplete quadriplegia with disproportionately worse impairment of the upper than the lower extremities. Central cord syndrome may involve 9–16% of all spinal cord injuries and is more predominant in the elderly. Smith et al recently reported videourodynamic testing results from 22 men with central cord syndrome. Studies were done an average of 34.5 months after injury and after spinal shock had resolved. Results demonstrated normal evaluations in 14%, detrusor areflexia in 18%, detrusor hyperreflexia with synergy in 5%, DSD in 50%, and detrusor hypocontractility in 5%.[44]

Nath et al reported different findings based on urodynamic studies of 20 men with central cord syndrome and voiding difficulties. Carbon dioxide cystometrography with EMG revealed detrusor hyperreflexia without dyssynergia in 15 (75%) patients and DSD in 5 patients (25%). The differences in these studies may be based on methodology (videourodynamics vs CO_2) or timing of the study with respect to injury. Regardless, urodynamic evaluation is important in evaluating and forming appropriate treatment strategies for these patients.[45]

The status of innervation and function of the external sphincter or periurethral striated muscle is as important as the type of detrusor innervation and function following a spinal cord injury, or for that matter any neurologic condition affecting the lower urinary tract. A paralytic external sphincter due to total or partial injury to the anterior motor neuron will certainly cause reduction to the urethral resistance at the sphincteric level, predisposing the individual to stress incontinence. In patients with areflexic bladder, Diokno et al reported 60% of patients with complete denervation of the external sphincter and the rest had partial denervation.[41]

Diabetes

Diabetes is the most common metabolic disease and affects over 5 million people in the United States. Neuropathy is the most frequent of the many complications associated with the disease. The cause is thought to be due to a combination of ischemic nerve injury secondary to vasculopathy associated with the disease, as well as nerve injury secondary to deranged metabolic function. Neuropathy can occur in either insulin-dependent or non-insulin-dependent diabetes. Tests of autonomic function have shown impairment in roughly 20–40% of diabetic patients.[46]

Diabetic cystopathy is the constellation of clinical and urodynamic findings associated with long-term diabetes mellitus. Classically, it has been described as decreased bladder sensation, increased bladder capacity, and impaired detrusor contractility. It is frequently insidious in onset and progression and many patients may have minimal symptoms. Impaired bladder sensation is the most common initial presentation. Patients may void only once or twice a day. Eventually, they may have difficulty initiating and maintaining voiding. Urodynamic testing of unselected diabetics reveals diabetic cystopathy in 26–87% of patients. The finding of cystopathy correlates directly with the duration of symptoms, which generally occur about 10 years after the onset of diabetes. It frequently coexists with signs of peripheral neuropathy. Many diabetics have coexisting other urologic problems such as benign prostatic hyperplasia, stress incontinence, bladder or prostate cancer or infection, causing voiding symptoms which may be similar to or different from the classically described diabetic bladder.[47]

Kaplan et al reported urodynamic findings of 115 male and 67 female consecutive diabetic patients referred for evaluation of voiding symptoms. Mean duration of diabetes was 58 months, and mean duration of voiding symptoms was 27 months. The most common symptoms were nocturia greater than 2 times in 87%, urinary frequency in 78%, urinary hesitancy in 62%, decreased force of stream in 52%, and sensation of incomplete emptying in 45%. No differences between men or women in the above symptoms were noted.

First sensation of filling was 298 ml. Mean bladder capacity was 485 ml. Fifty-two percent had detrusor instability, 23% had impaired detrusor contractility, 11% had indeterminate findings, 10% had detrusor areflexia, 24% had poor compliance, and 1% was normal. Of the 47 patients with peripheral neuropathy, 70% had detrusor instability, 57% had bladder outlet obstruction, 13% had indeterminate findings, 30% had detrusor areflexia, and 66% had evidence of sacral cord signs.

Bladder outlet obstruction was present in 36% of men. It was an isolated finding in 36% of them and associated with another urodynamic finding in 67%. Nine percent of patients (13) had urinary retention, which in men was secondary to bladder outlet obstruction in 7 and detrusor areflexia in 5. All 4 women with retention had areflexia. Patients with sacral cord signs were more likely to exhibit intermittent detrusor contractions/impaired contractility and detrusor areflexia, while those without sacral cord signs were more likely to demonstrate detrusor instability.[48]

Kitami performed urodynamic studies on 173 diabetics. Patients in this study did have classic findings of increased volume at first desire and decreased maximum vesical pressure (67%), but they also demonstrated overactive bladder (14.5%), low-compliance bladder (11%), and detrusor-external sphincter dyssynergia (32%).[49]

Frimodt-Moller, who coined the term 'diabetic cystopathy', reported on 124 patients with diabetes. Thirty-eight percent had what are now recognized as classic cystopathic findings and 26% had bladder outlet obstruction.[50]

Disc disease

Symptoms from lumbar disc protrusion are most often secondary to posterolateral protrusion, occurring frequently at the L4–L5 and L5–S1 levels. However, more central (posterior) protrusion may disturb nerves leading to the bladder, perineal floor, and cavernous tissue of the penis. The intrathecal sacral nerve roots have been affected in 1–15% of reported cases of lumbar disc prolapse verified at operation, and the most common associated disorder is urinary retention. Fanciullacci et al studied 22 patients with lumbar central disc protrusion and neuropathic bladder. All patients except 2 women with urinary incontinence had urinary retention at presentation. Urodynamic studies performed at the onset of disease revealed areflexia with normal compliance in all patients. Bladder sensation was absent in 16 (73%) and reduced in 6 (27%). EMG showed signs of severe denervation. Postoperative urodynamic evaluation in 17 patients revealed 65% had persistent areflexia, 29% had normoreflexia, 6% had areflexia, and all had normal compliance. Bladder sensation was absent in 35%, reduced in 47%, and normal in 18%. EMG studies of the periurethral muscles showed good recovery of voluntary contraction in 76% of patients.[51]

O'Flynn et al reviewed the records of 30 patients with lumbar disc prolapse and bladder dysfunction who underwent laminectomy and disc removal. Preoperatively, 87% of the patients developed urinary symptoms. Fifty-three percent required catheterization for urinary retention. Postoperative urodynamics revealed 37% of patients had areflexic bladders and voided by straining, 13% exhibited detrusor hyperreflexia with urinary incontinence, and 7% had low compliance with opening of the bladder neck during filling. Thirty-seven percent demonstrated genuine stress incontinence at bladder volumes greater than 300 ml. Only one patient regained normal detrusor activity postoperatively.[52]

Bartolin et al prospectively analyzed 114 patients with lumbar intervertebral disc protrusion requiring surgical treatment. Patients with acute central disc protrusion (cauda equina syndrome) were not included. Urodynamic studies revealed detrusor areflexia in 27.2% of patients. They did not find a significant difference in the rate of areflexia based on the level of disc herniation (L5 vs L4). All patients with detrusor areflexia reported difficult voiding with straining.[53]

The same author evaluated bladder function after surgery. Ninety-eight patients underwent urodynamic evaluation before and after surgery. Twenty-eight percent of patients exhibited detrusor areflexia preoperatively. Only 22% of these patients had a return to normal function after surgery. Of the 71 patients with normal urodynamic findings preoperatively, 4 (6%) developed detrusor hyperreflexia and 3 (4%) developed areflexia postoperatively.[54]

The cauda equina syndrome is a relatively rare constellation of symptoms for herniated lumbar discs. It is characterized by bilateral sciatica, lower extremity weakness, saddle-type hypesthesia, and bowel and bladder dysfunction. Cauda equina syndrome occurs in approximately 1–10% of cases of lumbar disc herniation. Early operative decompression is advocated, but may not always restore normal function. Chang et al evaluated the incidence and long-term outcome of patients with this condition. They identified 4 of 144 (2.8%) consecutive surgical cases of lumbar disc herniation with urinary retention. All patients regained voluntary voiding within 6 months, 1, 3, and 4 years of surgery.[55]

Infectious diseases
Acquired immune deficiency syndrome

Patients with acquired immune deficiency syndrome (AIDS) have not made up a large portion of most urologists' practices. However, due to the large number of people with this disease and increased survival with new medications, urologists can expect to see more patients with AIDS.

Neurologic involvement occurs in 30–40% of patients with AIDS, and involves the central and peripheral nervous systems.[56–58] Neurologic involvement may be the result of infection, immunologic injury to target organs, or neoplasia.

Khan et al performed urodynamic studies on 11 of 677 AIDS patients. Voiding dysfunction secondary to neurogenic bladder was found in 9 of 11 (82%) patients. Urinary retention in 6 of the 11 (55%) patients was the most common presenting symptom. Three patients (27%) presented with urinary incontinence, 1 (9%) with urinary frequency, 1 (9%) with poor urinary flow. Urodynamic study demonstrated areflexia in 4 (36%) patients, hyperreflexia in 3 (27%), hyporeflexia in 2 (18%), and urinary outflow obstruction without evidence of neurologic involvement in 2 (18%).

Electromyographic studies of the urinary sphincter were done in 8 of the patients. Only 2 of them had abnormalities: one with myelopathy exhibited poor recruitment of neuronal activity and the remaining patient with cauda equina syndrome had many fibrillatory potentials.[59]

Menendez et al reported urodynamic evaluations of 3 patients with AIDS and neurogenic bladder. Two of the patients had areflexic bladder secondary to ascending myelitis by herpes simplex virus type II in 1 patient, and cerebral abscess from toxoplasmosis in the other patient. A third patient with AIDS dementia complex exhibited a hyperreflexic detrusor. Voiding symptoms improved in all 3 patients with institution of antiviral, antibiotic, and anticholinergic medications, respectively.[60]

Guillain–Barré syndrome

Guillain–Barré syndrome is an idiopathic polyradiculopathy frequently related to viral illnesses or vaccination. Lesions of the motor neuron in the spinal nerve are seen on pathological examination. Clinically, it is characterized by motor paralysis initially in the lower extremities and progressing cephalad.

Kogan et al first reported urodynamic findings in 2 patients with Guillain–Barré syndrome in 1981. Both patients were found to have motor paralytic bladders on cystometrogram evaluation.[61]

Wheeler et al reported urodynamic findings on 7 patients with Guillain–Barré syndrome. Impaired voiding with large residuals was present in all 7 patients. Urodynamic studies revealed 4 patients with detrusor areflexia and nonrelaxation of the perineal muscles with a positive bethanechol supersensitivity test. Three of these 4 patients had abnormal perineal EMG studies that demonstrated a decreased interference pattern with polyphasic potentials, which is characteristic of motor denervation. Three of the 7 patients had detrusor hyperreflexia with

appropriate sphincter relaxation. Intravesical sensation, although decreased, was present in 6 patients and completely absent in 1 patient.[62]

Another study by Sakakibara et al described urologic findings in 28 patients with Guillain–Barré syndrome. Micturitional symptoms were seen in 25% of patients and included voiding difficulty in 6, transient urinary retention in 3, nocturnal urinary frequency in 3, urinary urgency in 3, diurnal urinary frequency in 2, urge incontinence in 2, and stress incontinence in 1. Urodynamic evaluation in 4 patients revealed disturbed sensation in 1 patient, bladder areflexia in 1, and absence of bulbocavernosus reflex in another. Cystometry showed decreased bladder volume in 2 and bladder overactivity in 2, one of whom had urge urinary incontinence and the other urinary retention.[63]

Herpes

Herpes zoster infection is a viral syndrome characterized by a painful vesicular eruption involving one or more dermatomes and inflammation of the corresponding dorsal root ganglia. Both sensory and motor neurons can be affected.

Cohen et al reviewed the literature of herpes zoster associated with bladder and/or bowel dysfunction since 1970. Thirty-two cases had been reported. Urinary retention was present in 28 (88%), symptoms of cystitis (dysuria, frequency, hesitancy) in 13 (41%), symptoms of both retention and cystitis in 11 (34%), and constipation and/or fecal incontinence in 20 (63%) patients. Sacral dermatomes (S2–S4) were involved in 78% of cases; lumbar and thoracic dermatomes were affected in 16% and 2% of patients, respectively. Men were affected more commonly than women (66% vs 34%). Patients tended to present in the sixth to eighth decades of life, although some women in their twenties have been reported. Cystometrograms typically show absent detrusor spikes or flaccid neurogenic bladders.[64]

In 1993, Brosetta et al published urologic findings on 57 patients diagnosed with and treated for herpes zoster infection. Fifty-four percent of the patients were men and the mean age was 51 years. Thirty-seven percent of patients had some type of immunodeficiency (HIV, hepatic disease, lymphoproliferative disorder). Fifteen of the 57 (26%) had urologic manifestations. Two of the 15 (13%) exhibited urinary retention and were found to have detrusor areflexia on CMG. Three of the 15 (20%) exhibited incontinence and detrusor hyperreflexia on CMG.[65]

Human T-lymphotropic virus

HTLV-I-associated myelopathy (HAM) is a slowly progressive spastic paraparesis caused by infection with human T-lymphotropic virus type I (HTLV-I) and less frequently with HTLV type II. Clinical manifestations result from demyelination and eventual atrophy of the thoracic spinal cord. The myelopathy has a peak incidence in HTLV-infected patients age 40–50 years and women are affected more than men. Co-infection with HIV results in an increased rate of myelopathy among those with HTLV infection. Murphy et al performed a cross-sectional analysis of HTLV-seropositive subjects who were detected from 5 blood donor centers in the United States. Myelopathy was confirmed in 4 of 166 (2.4%) HTLV-I-positive subjects and in 1 of 404 (0.25%) HTLV-II-positive subjects. All 5 patients diagnosed with HAM underwent urodynamic evaluation and all were found to have dyssynergic bladder contractions. In fact, urinary urgency and incontinence were the most common presenting symptoms and 2 of the patients had undergone urodynamic evaluation prior to enrollment in the study.[66]

Lyme disease

Lyme disease is caused by the spirochete *Borrelia burgdorferi*. It is the most common tick-borne disease in the United States and is associated with a variety of neurologic sequelae. Chancellor et al evaluated 7 patients with confirmed Lyme disease and associated lower urinary tract dysfunction. Most of the patients had paraparesis with partial sensory loss and 1 was temporarily in a coma. Two patients had urinary retention, 4 patients had one or more irritative symptoms (frequency, urge incontinence, nocturia), and 1 patient had enuresis. On urodynamic evaluation, 5 of the patients demonstrated detrusor hyperreflexia and 2 had detrusor areflexia. Detrusor-sphincter dyssynergia was not observed in any patient. Of the five patients with detrusor hyper-reflexia, 2 were aware of the involuntary contractions but could not inhibit them and 3 were unaware of the involuntary contractions. With follow-up after intravenous antibiotics ranging from 6 months to 2 years, urologic symptoms resolved completely in 4 patients, while in 3 patients, symptoms improved but with residual urgency and frequency.[67]

Poliomyelitis

Acute poliomyelitis is often associated with urinary retention owing to detrusor areflexia, although bladder function is generally recovered. Uninhibited detrusor contractions with urge incontinence or an atonic bladder with weak, ineffective detrusor contractions may also be seen.[68] Howard et al reported an 11% prevalence of retention in 23 of 203 patients during the acute polio episode, whereas 69/203 (34%) had chronic urinary symptoms persisting after resolution of the acute episode.[69]

Progressive functional deterioration occurring years after an acute episode of poliomyelitis is termed postpolio syndrome (PPS). It manifests as new-onset or progressive motor or visceral dysfunction, or as joint or limb deterioration. It may be present in as many as 78% of patients with a history of polio. Symptoms can be classified into two categories: those associated with orthopedic and joint deterioration and those caused by neurologic deterioration. The symptoms are exacerbated by physical activity or fatigue. The mechanism is not known but may be secondary to premature or accelerated loss of anterior horn cells that innervate large numbers of muscle fibers, loss of neuronal cell terminals that had sprouted to innervate muscle fibers, reactivation of the virus, deterioration of the immune system, and intercurrent neurologic or nonneurologic diseases.[69]

Johnson et al evaluated 330 completed questionnaires mailed randomly to subjects in West Texas with a history of polio. Eighty-seven percent of women and 74% of males reported symptoms of PPS. The mean age of responders was 55 years. The mean age at acute attack was 10 years and the mean interval between the acute episode and the development of PPS was 33 years for females and 36 years for males. Three hundred and six (93%) patients reported urologic symptoms which included change in bladder function, change in sexual function, frequency ≥8 voids/day, nocturia ≥2 voids/night, hesitancy, urgency, intermittency, post-void dribbling, and decreased force of stream. Thirty-five patients (10.6%) reported detrusor instability. Only a few had symptoms compatible with hypocontractile or areflexic bladders, requiring catheterization.

The prevalence of incontinence among females was similar among those with and without PPS (72% vs 77%, respectively); however, the severity of incontinence was worse in those with PPS. Incontinence in men was limited to post-void dribbling or urge incontinence. These symptoms were worse in men with PPS.[70]

Syphilis

Voiding dysfunction related to neurosyphilis had a high prevalence in the pre-penicillin era. Voiding dysfunction caused by decreased vesical sensation resulted in large residual urine and bladder decompensation. Fortunately, improvements in medical care have made neurosyphilis a rare entity.

Neurosyphilis affects males more than females and presents in middle-aged years after a period of latency. Roughly 10% of patients infected with primary syphilis later develop neurosyphilis. Lumbosacral meningomyelitis with involvement of the dorsal cord and/or spinal roots (tabes dorsalis) results in bladder dysfunction. This manifests as decreased bladder sensation, large bladder capacity, and high post-void residuals. In some patients, typically those with general paresis of the insane, incontinence can occur which is usually functional or possibly the result of uninhibited detrusor activity as seen in upper motor neuron lesions.[71]

Brodie reported on 13 patients with neurosyphilis and bladder involvement. Twelve of the 13 had classic detrusor areflexia and decreased bladder sensation, leading to overdistention. One patient had detrusor hyperreflexia.[72]

Garber et al reported on 3 patients with tertiary syphilis. All 3 were found to have hypocompliant bladders with detrusor hyperreflexia, detrusor-sphincter dyssynergia, and elevated residual volumes on videocystometrography. This small group of patients demonstrates how tertiary syphilis can manifest with upper motor neuron bladder dysfunction.[73]

Tuberculosis

Tuberculosis can affect the spine. Spinal tuberculosis is more severe, dangerous, and disabling in children than in adults. Mushkin and Kovalenko studied 32 patients under the age of 16 years with thoracic and lumbar spinal tuberculosis who underwent antibiotic and surgical treatment. Paraplegia occurred in 8 patients and was always associated with bladder and bowel dysfunction. Three other patients without paraplegia also had bladder and bowel dysfunction (34%, overall). Eight of the 11 recovered bladder and bowel function postoperatively. Urodynamic evaluations were not included in this report.[74]

Radical pelvic surgery
Rectal carcinoma/resection

Urinary dysfunction as a consequence of damage to important neuroanatomic structures remains a common complication of radical pelvic surgery, particularly in abdominoperineal resection (APR) for rectal carcinoma. The extent of primary resection and lymphadenectomy are major determinants of degree of postoperative urologic morbidity. The incidence of *de-novo* urinary dysfunction following APR has been reported to be as high as 70%. Urinary retention caused by detrusor denervation is the most common type of voiding dysfunction after APR, and is the result of disruption of detrusor branches of the pelvic nerve. Less commonly, stress urinary incontinence secondary to denervation of the external sphincter or direct injury to the muscle itself can occur.[75]

Voiding dysfunction is more severe after APR than after rectal sphincter-preserving procedures, such as low anterior resection (LAR), and degree of dysfunction is related to the extent of dissection. In a study by Hojo et al, 22 of 25

patients (88%) who underwent preservation of the autonomic nerves were voiding spontaneously by postoperative day 10, whereas 28 of 36 patients (78%) with complete resection of the pelvic autonomic nerves still had urinary retention and were dependent on indwelling catheter drainage by postoperative day 60.[76]

Similar studies by Mitsui et al and Sugihara et al demonstrated that 100% of patients undergoing bilateral nerve sparing with radical resection for rectal carcinoma regained spontaneous voiding postoperativley.[77,78] When unilateral pelvic plexus preservation is performed, over 90% are able to void spontaneously. Thirty percent of patients undergoing complete resection of pelvic autonomic nerves in Sugihara's study required self-catheterization. In Mitsui's series, only 30% of patients in the nonpreserved group voided normally. Interestingly, they noted no significant difference in lower urinary tract function between patients receiving LAR vs APR.

Michelassi and Block reported on 27 patients who underwent either conventional (10) or wide (17) pelvic lymphadenectomy with radical resection for carcinoma of the rectum. They noted that 18% of patients undergoing wide pelvic lymphadenectomy required intermittent self-catheterization postoperatively. All patients in this group were able to stop catheterization within 8 months of the surgery.[79]

Cosimelli et al reported minimal urologic morbidity in 57 male patients undergoing LAR and limited lumboaortic lymphadenectomy. Less than 3% had urinary incontinence and 4.2% experienced urinary retention.[80]

Radical hysterectomy

Voiding dysfunction after radical hysterectomy and pelvic lymphadenectomy for carcinoma of the cervix has typically manifested as bladder atonia. An early report by Ketcham et al revealed an 8% rate of atonia requiring Foley catheter drainage postoperatively.[81]

Seski and Diokno prospectively studied 10 patients before and after radical hysterectomy. Results suggest that a hypertonic phase immediately postoperatively is transient and secondary to myogenic tonicity. By 6–8 weeks postoperatively, bladder capacity and compliance returned to the preoperative level. Only 1/10 (10%) developed significant detrusor denervation, as demonstrated by a positive bethanechol supersensitivity test.[82]

A more recent report by Lin et al reported urodynamic results on patients who underwent either radical hysterectomy, pelvic radiation, or both, and compared them to a control group of patients with cervical cancer before treatment. Detrusor instability or low bladder compliance was found in 57%, 45%, 80%, and 24% of patients, respectively. Each group was found to have decreased bladder capacity.

The frequency of abdominal strain voiding was 100% in all treatment groups, but was 0% in the pretreatment group. Abnormal residual urine was seen in 41%, 27%, 40%, and 24% of patients, respectively.[83]

Spinal stenosis

Lumbar spinal stenosis does not often cause chronic bladder dysfunction. However, when it does, it is considered to be an advanced form and is related to compression of the cauda equina. Kawaguchi et al evaluated 37 patients with lumbar spinal stenosis before and after decompressive laminectomy. Twenty-nine patients had subjective urinary complaints. Preoperative CMG studies revealed 23 patients (62%) with neuropathic bladders (18 underactive, 5 overactive). Thirty-eight percent had normal CMG studies. Postoperative CMG studies in 9 patients with neuropathic bladders demonstrated a normal pattern in 6 patients, with 3 exhibiting a persistent underactive bladder.[84]

Cervical spondylosis is a generalized disease process which can affect all levels of the cervical spine. When the pathology is located laterally, spondylosis causes only radicular symptoms, whereas a central or paracentral location can cause cord compression in addition to root lesions. Lower urinary tract sphincter disturbances and bladder dysfunction (frequency, urgency, urge incontinence) can be seen along with lower extremity signs such as gait disturbance, lower extremity spasticity, and hyperactive tendon reflexes. Tammela et al performed urodynamic studies on 30 consecutive patients with clinically and radiologically verified cervical spondylosis causing radiculopathy and/or myelopathy. Sixty-one percent of patients complained of irritative bladder symptoms, and detrusor hyperactivity was demonstrated urodynamically in 46%. Twenty-five percent had hyperreflexic detrusor contractions with ice water provocation. Sensitivity to cold was lacking in 39%. Eleven percent described difficulty emptying the bladder and all were found to have hypotonic detrusors.[85]

Spine surgery

The incidence of voiding dysfunction after spinal surgery has been shown to be as high as 60%.[86] Boulis et al reported an incidence of 38% of 503 patients undergoing routine cervical or lumbar laminectomy or discectomy. Neither the rate nor the duration of retention between men and women was significantly different. Patients undergoing cervical or lumbar laminectomy were found to have longer duration of retention than those undergoing cervical or lumbar discectomy. Preoperative use of beta-blockers was associated with increased risk of urinary retention postoperatively. Patients who developed urinary retention were

older on average than those who did not develop retention (51.9 years vs 48.4 years). The rate of retention did not differ significantly between groups who did and did not have intraoperative Foley catheters placed.[87]

Brooks et al performed urodynamic evaluations on 74 patients who complained of new onset (69) voiding symptoms or exacerbation of underlying voiding symptoms (5) after undergoing lumbosacral laminectomy, discectomy, or both. Sixty percent were found to have pathologic urodynamic findings. Sixteen percent were found to have a hypoesthetic bladder and 24% demonstrated a hyperesthetic bladder. Fourteen percent had bladder capacities less than 200 ml while another 14% had capacities greater than 500 ml.[86]

Other causes of neurogenic bladder

Non-neurogenic neurogenic bladder

Non-neurogenic neurogenic bladder, also known as Hinman's syndrome is a functional bladder outlet obstruction caused by voluntary contractions of the external urethral sphincter during voiding. It is a learned voiding dysfunction developed early in life by children in response to uncontrolled bladder contractions. Typically, patients present with frequency, urgency, urinary incontinence, recurrent urinary tract infections, or occasionally encopresis. The voiding dysfunction is usually acquired after toilet training and tends to resolve after puberty.[88,89] The syndrome is rare in children. Reports on the prevalence of Hinman's syndrome in adults vary. Jorgensen et al reported a 0.5% prevalence rate among patients referred for urodynamic evaluation.[90]

In scanning a urodynamic database of 1015 consecutive adults referred for evaluation of voiding dysfunction, Groutz et al identified 21 (2%) patients (13 women, 8 men) who met criteria for Hinman's syndrome. Ninety-five percent of the patients exhibited obstructive symptoms and more than half had frequency, nocturia, and urgency. On non-invasive uroflow evaluation, all patients exhibited an intermittent flow pattern. On urodynamic study, first-sensation volume was significantly lower in women than in men (123 vs 272 ml). This trend was also seen in first urge, strong urge, and bladder capacity volumes. Fourteen percent (3) were also found to have detrusor instability. Detrusor pressure at maximum flow and maximum detrusor pressure during voiding were both found to be significantly higher in men than in women. The authors concluded that the prevalence of this condition among the adult population may actually be higher than 2%.[89]

Myasthenia gravis

Myasthenia gravis (MG) is an autoimmune disorder whereby antibodies against the nicotinic cholinergic receptors of neuromuscular transmission result in muscle weakness and easy fatigability. It typically affects striated muscle, although antibodies against smooth muscle muscarinic receptors have been identified as well. Voiding dysfunction in association with the disease is rare.[91]

There are reports in the literature which note an association between MG and incontinence in men with prostatic bladder outlet obstruction. It has been hypothesized that thorough resection led to injury to a sphincter already compromised by the underlying neurologic disorder and the authors recommended incomplete resection to prevent this complication.[92] Another small series of 8 men with MG and prostatic resection found that patients who underwent TURP (transurethral resection of the prostate) with blended current all became incontinent, but men who underwent TURP with either high-frequency unblended current, partial proximal resection, or open prostatectomy remained dry.[93] Khan and Bhola published a report of 1 patient who underwent open prostatectomy and remained dry. EMG studies revealed that although his sphincter functioned normally, it did demonstrate easy fatigability.[94]

There are 4 reports in the literature of voiding dysfunction in patients with no history of TURP. Howard et al reported a 31-year-old female with recurrent incontinence after undergoing bladder neck suspension for stress incontinence. She was found to have an open bladder neck, inability to sustain a pelvic floor contraction, and hyperreflexia which occurred concomitantly with deterioration of her myasthenia gravis.[95] Three other publications reported patients with myasthenia gravis and voiding dysfunction with either detrusor hyporeflexia or areflexia.[96–98]

References

1. Nitti VW, Adler H, Combs AJ. The role of urodynamics in the evaluation of voiding dysfunction in men after cerebrovascular accident. J Urol 1996; 155:263–266.

2. Marinkovic SP, Badlani G. Voiding and sexual dysfunction after cerebrovascular accidents. J Urol 2001; 165:359–370.

3. Wade DT, Hewer RL. Outlook after an acute stroke: urinary incontinence and loss of consciousness compared in 532 patients. Q J Med 1985; 56:601–608.

4. Taub NA, Wolfe CD, Richardson E, Burney PG. Predicting the disability of first-time stroke sufferers at 1 year. 12-month follow-up of a population-based cohort in Southeast England. Stroke 1994; 25:352–357.

5. Gelber DA, Good DC, Laven LJ, Verhulst SJ. Causes of urinary incontinence after acute hemispheric stroke. Stroke 1993; 24:378–382.

6. Brocklehurst JC, Andrews K, Richards B, Laycock PJ. Incidence and correlates of incontinence in stroke patients. J Am Geriatr Soc 1985; 33:540–542.

7. Leach GE, Farsaii A, Kark P, Raz S. Urodynamic manifestations of cerebellar ataxia. J Urol 1982; 128:348–350.

8. Andrew J, Nathan PW. Lesions of the anterior frontal lobes and disturbances of micturition and defaecation. Brain 1964; 87:233–262.

9. Maurice-Williams RS. Micturition symptoms in frontal tumors. J Neurol Neurosurg Psychiatr 1974; 37:431–436.

10. Blaivas JG. The neurophysiology of micturition: a clinical study of 550 patients. J Urol 1982; 127:958–963.

11. Lang EW, Chestnut RM, Hennerici M. Urinary retention and space-occupying lesions of the frontal cortex. Eur Neurol 1996; 36:43–47.

12. Jonas S, Brown J. Neurogenic bladder in normal pressure hydrocephalus. Urology 1975; 5:44–50.

13. McNeal DM, Hawtrey CE, Wolraich ML, Mapel JR. Symptomatic neurogenic bladder in a cerebral-palsied population. Dev Med Child Neurol 1983; 25:612–616.

14. Decter RM, Bauer SB, Khoshbin S, et al. Urodynamic assessment of children with cerebral palsy. J Urol 1987; 138:1110–1112.

15. Hellstrom PA, Jarvelin M, Kontturi MJ, Huttunen NP. Bladder function in the mentally retarded. Br J Urol 1990; 66:475–478.

16. Mitchell SJF, Woodthorpe J. Young mentally handicapped adults in three London boroughs: prevalence and degree of disability. J Epidemiol Comm Health 1981; 35:59–64.

17. Reid AH, Ballinger BR, Heather BB. Behavioural syndromes identified by cluster analysis in a sample of 100 severely and profoundly retarded adults. Psychol Med 1978; 8:399–412.

18. Pavlakis AJ, Siroky MB, Goldstein I, Krane RJ. Neurourologic findings in Parkinson's disease. J Urol 1983; 129:80–83.

19. Langworthy OR, Lewis LG, Dees JE, Hesser FH. Clinical study of control of bladder by central nervous system. Bull Johns Hopkins Hosp 1936; 58:89.

20. Murnaghan GF. Neurogenic disorders of the bladder in parkinsonism. Br J Urol 1961; 33:403–409.

21. Porter RW, Bors E. Neurogenic bladder in parkinsonism: effect of thalamotomy. J Neurosurg 1971; 34:27–32.

22. Araki I, Kitahara M, Oida T, Kuno S. Voiding dysfunction and Parkinson's disease: urodynamic abnormalities and urinary symptoms. J Urol 2000; 164:1640–1643.

23. Shy GM, Drager GA. A neurological syndrome associated with orthostatic hypotension: a clinico-pathologic study. Arch Neurol 1960; 2:511–527.

24. Salinas JM, Berger Y, De La Rocha RE, Blaivas JG. Urological evaluation in the Shy Drager syndrome. J Urol 1986; 135:741–743.

25. Fingerman JS, Finkelstein LH. The overactive bladder in multiple sclerosis. JAOA 2000; 100:S9–S12.

26. Rashid TM, Hollander JB. Multiple sclerosis and the neurogenic bladder. Phys Med Rehabil Clin N Am 1998; 9:615–629.

27. Litwiller SE, Frohman EM, Zimmern PE. Multiple sclerosis and the urologist. J Urol 1999; 161:743–757.

28. Ciancio SJ, Mutchnik SE, Rivera VM, Boone TB. Urodynamic pattern changes in multiple sclerosis. Urology 2001; 57:239–245.

29. Selzman AA, Elder JS, Mapstone TB. Urologic consequences of myelodysplasia and other congenital abnormalities of the spinal cord. Urol Clin N Am 1993; 20:485–504.

30. Pontari MA, Keating M, Kelly M, et al. Retained sacral function in children with high level myelodysplasia. J Urol 1995; 154:775–777.

31. Spindel MR, Bauer SB, Dyro FM, et al. The changing neurourologic lesion in myelodysplasia. JAMA 1987; 258:1630–1633.

32. McGuire EJ, Woodside JR, Borden TA, Weiss RM. Prognostic value of urodynamic testing in myelodysplastic patients. J Urol 1981; 126:205–209.

33. Bauer SB, Hallett M, Khoshbin S, et al. Predictive value of urodynamic evaluation in newborns with myelodysplasia. JAMA 1984; 252:650–652.

34. Pang D, Wilberger JE. Tethered cord syndrome in adults. J Neurosurg 1982; 57:32–47.

35. Adamson AS, Gelister J, Hayward R, Snell ME. Tethered cord syndrome: an unusual cause of adult bladder dysfunction. Br J Urol 1993; 71:417–421.

36. Flanigan RC, Russell DP, Walsh JW. Urological aspects of tethered cord. Urology 1989; 33:80–82.

37. Guzman L, Bauer SB, Hallet M, et al. Evaluation and management of children with sacral agenesis. Urology 1983; 22:506–510.

38. Koff SA, Deridder PA. Patterns of neurogenic dysfunction in sacral agenesis. J Urol 1977; 118:87–89.

39. Waites KB, Canupp KC, DeVivo MJ, et al. Compliance with annual urologic evaluations and preservation of renal function in persons with spinal cord injury. J Spinal Cord Med 1995; 18:251–254.

40. Burns AS, Rivas DA, Ditunno JF. The management of neurogenic bladder and sexual dysfunction after spinal cord injury. Spine 2001; 26:S129–S136.

41. Diokno AC, Koff SA, Anderson W. Combined cystometry and perineal electromyography in the diagnosis and treatment of neurogenic urinary incontinence. J Urol 1976; 115:161–163.

42. Kaplan SA, Chancellor MB, Blaivas JG. Bladder and sphincter behavior in patients with spinal cord lesions. J Urol 1991; 146:113–117.

43. Weld KJ, Dmochowski RR. Association of level of injury and bladder behavior in patients with post-traumatic spinal cord injury. Urology 2000; 55:490–494.

44. Smith CP, Kraus SR, Nickell KG, Boone TM. Video urodynamic findings in men with the central cord syndrome. J Urol 2000; 164:2014–2017.

45. Nath M, Wheeler JS, Walter JS. Urologic aspects of traumatic central cord syndrome. J Am Paraplegia Soc 1993; 16:160–164.

46. Ross MA. Neuropathies associated with diabetes. Med Clin N Am 1993; 77:111–124.

47. Kaplan SA, Blaivas JG. Diabetic cystopathy. J Diabet Complications 1988; 2:133–139.

48. Kaplan SA, Te AE, Blaivas JG. Urodynamic findings in patients with diabetic cystopathy. J Urol 1995; 153:342–344.

49. Kitami K. Vesicourethral dysfunction of diabetic patients. Nippon Hinyokika Gakkai Zasshi 1991; 82:1074–1083.

50. Moller CF. Diabetic cystopathy. I: A clinical study of the frequency of bladder dysfunction in diabetics. Dan Med Bull 1976; 23:267–278.

51. Fanciullacci F, Sandri S, Politi P, Zanollo A. Clinical, urodynamic and neurophysiological findings in patients with neuropathic bladder due to a lumbar intervertebral disc protrusion. Parapelgia 1989; 27:354–358.

52. O'Flynn KJ, Murphy R, Thomas DG. Neurogenic bladder dysfunction in lumbar intervertebral disc prolapse. Br J Urol 1992; 69:38–40.

53. Bartolin Z, Gilja I, Bedalov G, Savic I. Bladder function in patients with lumbar intervertebral disk protrusion. J Urol 1998; 159:969–971.

54. Bartolin Z, Vilendecic M, Derezic D. Bladder function after surgery for lumbar intervertebral disk protrusion. J Urol 1999; 161:1885–1887.

55. Chang HS, Nakagawa H, Mizuno J. Lumbar herniated disc presenting with cauda equina syndrome: long-term follow-up of four cases. Surg Neurol 2000; 53:100–105.

56. Britton CB, Miller JR. Neurologic complications in acquired immunodeficiency syndrome (AIDS). Neurol Clin 1984; 2:315–339.

57. Levy RM, Bredesen DE, Rosenblum ML. Neurological manifestations of acquired immunodeficiency syndrome: experiences at UCSF and review of the literature. J Neurosurg 1985; 62:475–495.

58. Snider WD, Simpson DM, Nielsen S, et al. Neurological complications of acquired immune deficiency syndrome: analysis of 50 patients. Ann Neurol 1983; 14:403–418.

59. Khan Z, Singh VK, Yang WC. Neurogenic bladder in acquired immune deficiency syndrome (AIDS). Urology 1992; 40:289–291.

60. Menendez V, Valls J, Espuna M, et al. Neurogenic bladder in patients with acquired immunodeficiency syndrome. Neurourol Urodyn 1995; 14:253–257.

61. Kogan BA, Solomon MH, Diokno AC. Urinary retention secondary to Landry–Guillain–Barré syndrome. J Urol 1981; 126:643–644.

62. Wheeler JS, Siroky MB, Pavlakis A, Krane RJ. The urodynamic aspects of the Guillain–Barré syndrome. J Urol 1984; 131:917–919.

63. Sakakibara R, Hattori T, Kuwabara S, et al. Micturitional disturbance in patients with Guillain–Barré syndrome. J Neurol Neurosurg Psychiatr 1997; 63:649–653.

64. Cohen LM, Fowler JF, Owen LG, Callen JP. Urinary retention associated with herpes zoster infection. Int J Dermatol 1993; 32:24–26.

65. Broseta E, Osca JM, Morera J, et al. Urological manifestations of herpes zoster. Eur Urol 1993; 24:244–247.

66. Murphy EL, Fridey J, Smith JW, et al. HTLV-associated myelopathy in a cohort of HTLV-I and HTLV-II-infected blood donors. Neurology 1997; 48:315–320.

67. Chancellor MB, McGinnis DE, Shenot PJ, et al. Urinary dysfunction in Lyme disease. J Urol 1993; 149:26–30.

68. Timmermans L, Bonnet F, Maquinay C. Urological complications of poliomyelitis and their treatment. Acta Urol Belg 1965; 33:409–426.

69. Howard RS, Wiles CM, Spencer GT. The late sequelae of poliomyelitis. Q J Med 1988; 66:219–232.

70. Johnson VY, Hubbard D, Vordermark JS. Urologic manifestations of postpolio syndrome. JWOCN 1996; 23:218–223.

71. Wheeler JS, Culkin DJ, O'Hara RJ, Canning JR. Bladder dysfunction and neurosyphilis. J Urol 1986; 136:903–905.

72. Brodie EL, Helfert I, Phifer IA. Cystometric observations in asymptomatic neurosyphilis. J Urol 1940; 43:496–510.

73. Garber SJ, Christmas TJ, Rickards D. Voiding dysfunction due to neurosyphilis. Br J Urol 1990; 66:19–21.

74. Mushkin AY, Kovalenko KN. Neurological complications of spinal tuberculosis in children. Int Orthop 1999; 23:210–212.

75. Hollabaugh RS, Steiner MS, Sellers KD, et al. Neuroanatomy of the pelvis: implications for colonic and rectal resection. Dis Colon Rectum 2000; 43:1390–1397.

76. Hojo K, Vernava AM, Sugihara K, Katumata K. Preservation of urine voiding and sexual function after rectal cancer surgery. Dis Colon Rectum 1991; 34:532–539.

77. Mitsui T, Kobayashi S, Matsuura S, et al. Vesicourethral dysfunction following radical surgery for rectal carcinoma: change in voiding pattern on sequential urodynamic studies and impact of nerve-sparing surgery. Int J Urol 1998; 5:35–38.

78. Sugihara K, Moriya Y, Akasu T, Fujita S. Pelvic autonomic nerve preservation for patients with rectal carcinoma: oncologic and functional outcome. Cancer 1996; 78:1871–1880.

79. Michelassi F, Block GE. Morbidity and mortality of wide pelvic lymphadenectomy for rectal adenocarcinoma. Dis Colon Rectum 1992; 35:1143–1147.

80. Cosimelli M, Mannella E, Giannarelli D, et al. Nerve-sparing surgery in 302 resectable rectosigmoid cancer patients: genitourinary morbidity and 10-year survival. Dis Colon Rectum 1994; 37:S42–46.

81. Ketcham AS, Hoye RC, Taylor PT, et al. Radical hysterectomy and pelvic lymphadenectomy for carcinoma of the uterine cervix. Cancer 1971; 28:1272–1277.

82. Seski JC, Diokno AC. Bladder dysfunction after radical abdominal hysterectomy. Am J Obstet Gynecol 1977; 128:643–651.

83. Lin HH, Sheu BC, Lo MC, Huang SC. Abnormal urodynamic findings after radical hysterectomy or pelvic irradiation for cervical cancer. Int J Gynaecol Obstet 1998; 63:169–174.

84. Kawaguchi Y, Kanamori M, Ishihara H, et al. Clinical symptoms and surgical outcome in lumbar spinal stenosis patients with neuropathic bladder. J Spinal Disord 2001; 14:404–410.

85. Tammela TLJ, Heiskari MJ, Lukkarinen OA. Voiding dysfunction and urodynamic findings in patients with cervical spondylotic spinal stenosis compared with severity of the disease. Br J Urol 1992; 70:144–148.

86. Brooks ME, Moreno M, Sidi A, Braf ZF. Urologic complications after surgery on lumbosacral spine. Urology 1985; 26:202–204.

87. Boulis NM, Mian FS, Rodriguez D, et al. Urinary retention following routine neurosurgical procedures. Surg Neurol 2001; 55:23–28.

88. Hinman F. Nonneurogenic neurogenic bladder (the Hinman syndrome): 15 years later. J Urol 1986; 136:769–777.

89. Groutz A, Blaivas JG, Pies C, Sassone AM. Learned voiding dysfunction (non-neurogenic, neurogenic bladder) among adults. Neurourol Urodynam 2001; 20:259–268.

90. Jorgensen TM, Djurhuus JC, Schroder HD. Idiopathic detrusor sphincter dyssynergia in neurologically normal patients with voiding abnormalities. Eur Urol 1982; 8:107–110.

91. Sandler PM, Avillo C, Kaplan SA. Detrusor areflexia in a patient with myasthenia gravis. Int J Urol 1998; 5:188–190.

92. Greene LF, Ghosh MK, Howard FM. Transurethral prostatic resection in patients with myasthenia gravis. J Urol 1974; 12:226–227.

93. Wise GJ, Gerstenfeld JN, Brunner N, Grob D. Urinary incontinence following prostatectomy in patients with myasthenia gravis. Br J Urol 1982; 54:369–371.

94. Khan Z, Bhola A. Urinary incontinence after transurethral resection of prostate in myasthenia gravis patients. Urology 1989; 34:168–169.

95. Howard JF, Donovan MK, Tucker MS. Urinary incontinence in myasthenia gravis: a single-fiber electromyographic study. Ann Neurol 1992; 32:254(abstr).

96. Matsui M, Enoki M, Matsui Y, et al. Seronegative myasthenia gravis associated with atonic urinary bladder and accommodative insufficiency. J Neurol Sci 1995; 133:197–199.

97. Berger AR, Swerdlow M, Herskovitz S. Myasthenia gravis presenting as uncontrollable flatus and urinary/fecal incontinence. Muscle Nerve 1996; 19:113–114.

98. Sandler PM, Avillo C, Kaplan SA. Detrusor areflexia in a patient with myasthenia gravis. Int J Urol 1998; 5:188–190.

8

Ultrastructural pathology of neurogenic bladder

Ahmad Elbadawi

Two broad neuroanatomic categories of neurogenic bladder (NB), occasionally combined, have traditionally been recognized.[1,2] Upper motoneuron neurogenic bladder (UMNB) results from neuraxial deficits or disorders higher than the parasympathetic vesicomotor nuclei in the sacral spinal cord. Lower motoneuron neurogenic bladder (LMNB) results from lesions involving the vesicomotor nuclei, infraspinal (peripheral) neural pathways – including vesicourethral ganglia, and/or intrinsic vesicourethral innervation. In the decentralization form of LMNB, following spinal cord and/or spinal root lesions, the neural deficit involves preganglionic parasympathetic pathways through sacral nerve roots, the pelvic nerves, or a combination. In the other less common 'denervation' form, e.g. following extensive pelvic surgery[3–8] or therapeutic destruction of the pelvic plexus,[9–11] both parasympathetic and sympathetic postganglionic neurons are involved: within vesicourethral ganglia, their branches forming the pelvic plexus, intrinsic ramifications of the plexus within lower urinary tract organs, or a combination. A population of postganglionic neurons resides within the bladder wall and supplies it with much of its intrinsic innervation,[12] so that the bladder cannot truly be denervated no matter how extensive an infraspinal deficit is responsible or how anatomically close to the bladder it is located.[13]

Detailed microstructural study of NB had been hindered by the tenacious idea that its dysfunction results from and merely reflects compromise of its neuraxial control mechanisms, and by its tacit corollary that there is no reason for the dysfunction to be associated with altered structure of the bladder. Histologic and histochemical studies, however, revealed qualitative changes in intrinsic vesical innervation in the LMNB in several experimental models and in humans.[14–26] Marked increase in intrinsic adrenergic nerves was described in the decentralized detrusor.[17,24,25] Cholinergic nerves were described as absent or markedly reduced in the 'denervated' bladder 4 months to 30 years following radical extirpative pelvic surgery.[19,23] In a histochemical/ultrastructural study of similar material, obtained 5–7 weeks or 7–13 months postoperatively, cholinergic nerves were found to be reduced in short-term and restituted – presumably by regeneration – in long-term samples, but there was no change in adrenergic nerves in either.[20]

Ultrastructural pathology of neurogenic bladder

The pathology of neurogenic bladder (NB) has been studied ultrastructurally in much more detail in several experimental feline lower motoneuron (LM) models,[27–34] and various chronic upper motoneuron (UM) settings in the human[35–37] (Tables 8.1 and 8.2). Changes in intrinsic nerves and smooth

Table 8.1 *Neurogenic bladder studied ultrastructurally*			
Neurogenic bladder	Duration	Neurologic lesion	Structure studied
Lower motoneuron, experimental[a] Unilateral Bilateral	 2–10 weeks 1 day to 12 weeks	 Three feline models Two feline models	 Detrusor Rhabdosphincter; detrusor
Lower + upper motoneuron, clinical	14–28 years	Meningomyelocele	Detrusor
Upper motoneuron, clinical Spinal Supraspinal	 3 months to 33 years 10 months to 43 years	 Spinal cord injury Brainstem/brain disorders	 Detrusor Detrusor

[a]Details given in Table 8.2.

Table 8.2 *Experimental models of lower motoneuron neurogenic bladder (LMNB)*[27–34,44,117]

Model[a]	Postoperative specimen collection[f]		Parasympathetic innervation[g]			Sympathetic innvervation[g]			Somatomotor innervation[h]
	Early (short-term)	Established (long-term)	Pregang	Postgang	Afferent	Pregang	Postgang	Afferent	
Bladder decentralization models:									
Sacral ventral rhizotomy, unilateral (SVR)[b]	2–4 wk	8,10 wk	×	✔	✔	✔	✔	✔	×
* Sacral ventral rhizotomy, bilateral (BSVR)[b]	1,2 wk	4,6,10 wk	×	✔	✔	✔	✔	✔	×
* BSVR + bilateral hypogastric neurectomy (HN)[c]	1–4 wk	6–10 wk	×	✔	✔	×	✔	×	×
Pelvic neurectomy, unilateral (PN)[d]	2,3 wk	10 wk	×	×	×	×	×	✔	✔
Infraspinal bladder 'denervation' model:									
Pelvic plexus neurectomy, unilateral (PPN)[e]	1–4 d, 3 wk	7–12 wk	×	×	×	×	×	×	✔

[a]Neuraxial pathway (parasympathetic and sympathetic spinal cord nuclei, cerebrospinal pathways, brainstem and cerebral centers and pathways) remain intact; * = models used for study of rhabdosphincter.

[b]7th lumbar through 1st coccygeal roots sectioned; achieves pure parasympathetic decentralization of the bladder plus somatic denervation of rhabdosphincter.

[c]Hypogastric nerves excised between origin from inferior mesenteric ganglion and entry into pelvis plexus; combined SVR and HN achieves combined sympathetic/parasympathetic decentralization of the bladder (and interrupts sympathetic conveyed vesical afferent pathway).

[d]Nerve excised between its points of origin and branching; achieves parasympathetic decentralization of the bladder and interrupts parasympathetic conveyed vesical afferent pathway; intact somatomotor innervation of rhabdosphincter.

[e]Plexus excised (together with contained ganglia) flush with the lateral wall of bladder and urethra; achieves combined sympathetic/parasympathetic postganglionic efferent, and afferent 'denervation' of the bladder.

[f]Duration of animal survival with induced neurogenic bladder: d = days, wk = weeks.

[g]Efferent pathways to bladder and urethra: Pregang = preganglionic component, Postgang = postganglionic neuroeffector component;
  × = interrupted, ✔ = anatomically intact.

[h]Nerves originating in sacral spinal cord to directly innervate rhabdosphincter via pudendal nerve.

muscle of the detrusor have been described in both categories (Table 8.3); changes described in the experimental LMNB remain to be confirmed – or modified if necessary – in human settings by detailed ultrastructural study. The changes observed in experimental models were the outcome of the neural deficits. Unilateral LM models hardly disturb voiding,[27,33] and do not result in vesical distention or smooth muscle hypertrophy that follow bilateral dorsoventral sacral rhizotomy,[16] and per se may lead to structural changes in muscular and neural elements.[38–40] Vesical overdistention and detrusor hypertrophy are avoided in the models of bilateral sacral ventral rhizotomy (BSVR) by twice daily evacuation of the bladder content by Credé expression.[30,34]

Neuromuscular ultrastructure of the detrusor, including topographic arrangement of its smooth muscle as bundles and smaller fascicles,[41] and the components of its intrinsic innervation are generally recognizable microscopically in NB. Intrinsic neural elements include perineurium-bound nerve trunks with mixed Schwann cell enwrapped unmyelinated and myelinated nonvaricose axon segments, Schwann cell ensheathed unmyelinated cholinergic and adrenergic

axon bundles (preterminal axons with varicosities and intervaricose segments), and bare unmyelinated axon terminals (cholinergic and adrenergic) at neuroeffector junctions (cholinergic, adrenergic, diautonomic) with muscle cells.[42] Adrenergic axonal elements are not easy to discern in the human detrusor due to release of their neurotransmitter norepinephrine (noradrenaline) during procurement of material for microscopic study, but their visualization can be enhanced considerably (by intensifying their dense-cored vesicles) in experimental material by preloading the animal *in vivo* with 5-hydroxydopamine as a false adrenergic transmitter that intensifies core densities of intra-axonal vesicles.[27,43]

In the NB, intrinsic nerves of the detrusor display a combination of degenerative, reactive/regenerative, and ultrastructurally normal axon profiles in various proportions depending on the type and duration of NB (Table 8.3). Neurohistochemistry for acetylcholinesterase in cholinergic and norepinephrine in adrenergic nerves has limited value in revealing either early (short-term) or established (long-term) changes in cholinergic innervation in the decentralized bladder (sacral ventral rhizotomy, SVR;

Table 8.3 *Differential ultrastructural features in detrusor*

Neurogenic bladder (NB)	Early (short-term) NB							Established (long-term) NB						
	Unmyelinated efferent axon profiles[a]			Degenerative myelinated axon profiles[d]	Smooth muscle cells			Unmyelinated efferent axon profiles[a]				Smooth muscle cells		
	Normal	Degen	Reactive[c]		Normal	Degen	Regen	Normal[e]	Degen	Regen[f]	Adrenergic hyperinnerv	Normal	Degen	Regen
Experimental lower motoneuron neurogenic bladder models – qualitative data[27–34]														
Decentralized LM (SVR)	⊕ cholin;	+++ cholin;	++ adren;	⊕	++	+	+	+++	∅	+++	+++	++	∅	++
Decentralized LM (PN)	most adren[b]	⊕ adren	+ cholin	+++				cholin						
Decentralized LM (SVR + HN)	⊕ cholin; ⊕ adren	+++ cholin; +++ adren	∅	⊕	++	+	+	⊕	+++	⊖	∅	+++	+	⊖
'Denervated' LM	⊖	early; +++ cholin; +++ adren; ASC	∅	early; +++, ASC	+	early, ++	⊕	⊖	+++; ASC	⊖	∅	most	⊕	∅
Clinical, long-standing, upper motoneuron neurogenic bladder settings – quantitative data[35–37]														
Spinal UM + LM								6%	82%	18%			mostly +	
Spinal UM								8%	72%	20%	∅	generally	to ⊖; rarely	indefinite
Supraspinal UM								33%	57%	14%		++/+++	++/+++	

[a] Include neuroeffector junctions.

[b] Includes cholinergic ⇌ adrenergic axoaxonal synapses (interstitial axon bundles; at neuroeffector junctions).

[c] Presumably represent early regeneration.

[d] Includes afferent and preganglionic efferent nerves.

[e] Includes restituted neuroeffector junctions.

[f] Axon sprouts and/or copeptidergic axons.

degen = degeneration, regen = regeneration, hyperinnerv = hyperinnervation.

cholin = cholinergic, adren = adrenergic, ASC = axonless Schwann cells (interstitial axon bundles; perineurium-bound nerve trunks).

Extent of distribution of ultrastructural feature: +++ = widespread, ++ = abundant, + = focal, ⊕ = sporadic, ⊖ = rare, ∅ = absent.

% = median percent of observed profiles with tabulated feature; details in text.

pelvic neurectomy, PN models), but is useful in detecting both short- and long-term cholinergic and adrenergic hypoinnervation in the 'denervated' bladder (pelvic plexus neurectomy: PPN model) as well as long-term adrenergic hyperinnervation in the established decentralized bladder.[44] Ultrastructural observations on intrinsic detrusor innervation point out crucial differences between the decentralized and 'denervated' forms of LMNB[33] (Table 8.3). Corresponding differences in functional behavior and pharmacologic responses (including detrusor supersensitivity) need to be investigated.

The neural changes are associated with: (a) muscle cell degeneration and regeneration, also in different proportions in various NB settings; (b) changes characteristic of additional vesical dysfunction (neurogenic or non-neurogenic) when present: complete dysjunction, full degeneration and myohypertrophy patterns, respectively associated with detrusor overactivity, impaired detrusor contractility, and bladder outlet obstruction.[13,36,37,45–48] Detrusor-sphincter dyssynergia, however, was not associated with any particular pattern of detrusor ultrastructure.[36]

Intrinsic innervation in experimental lower motoneuron neurogenic bladder

Axonal degeneration

Widespread axonal degeneration of cholinergic axons is observed within 3–4 weeks in all experimental LMNB models. It is observed in 1–4 days in more peripheral neurectomy models (PN and PPN), in which degeneration of *all* myelinated axons is evident. Degeneration of both cholinergic and adrenergic axons is observed in the PPN model as well as the model of decentralization by SVR combined with hypogastric neurectomy (HN).

The ultrastructural features of degenerated unmyelinated and myelinated axon profiles resemble those described in various models of experimentally induced or pathologic axonal degeneration.[49–72] Segregated intra-axonal clustering, and reduction to depletion of small vesicles are the hallmark of unmyelinated axonal degeneration (Figure 8.1).

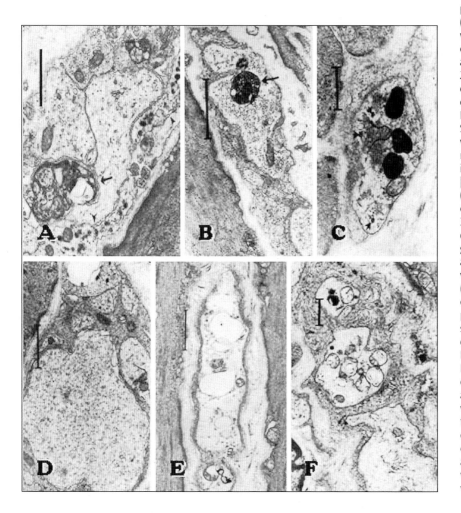

Figure 8.1
LMNB, axonal degeneration – preterminal unmyelinated axon profiles. (A) Electron-dense form. Axon bundle with one profile occupied by confluent electron-dense bodies (*arrow*), 2 intact adrenergic profiles (*arrowheads*), and 2 cholinergic profiles (*left*) with reduced content and central clustering of small clear vesicles [SVR, 2 weeks; Neg # 18855]. (B) Electron-dense form. Schwann cell ensheathed axon varicosity with membrane-bound electron-dense multivesicular body (*arrow*) and adjacent irregular dense patch of uneven density [SVR, 3 weeks; Neg # 19277]. (C) Electron-dense form. Schwann cell ensheathed axon varicosity contains 3 intensely dense myelin figures, uneven dense patches, deformed mitochondria, glycogen aggregates (*arrowheads*), and small clusters of small clear vesicles [SVR, 4 weeks; Neg # 24167]. (D) Floccular form. Schwann cell-ensheathed cholinergic axon varicosity packed with small dense granules; rare small clear vesicles and no recognizable other organelles [SVR, 3 weeks; Neg # 18320]. (E) Hydropic form. Ensheathed cholinergic axon profile with clear vacuoles distorted mitochondria, and rare small clear vesicles [SVR, 3 weeks; Neg # 16143]. (F) Filamentous form. 3 Schwann cell ensheathed cholinergic axon profiles with rare small clear vesicles, disrupted mitochondria, and a few dense patches, and contain wavy bundles of neurofilaments [SVR, 3 weeks; Neg # 18148]. [Scale bar = 1 μm.]

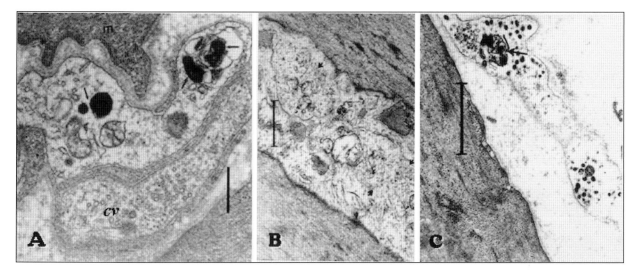

Figure 8.2

LMNB, axonal degeneration – unmyelinated terminals at neuroeffector junctions. (A) Cholinergic neuroeffector junction at muscle cell (m); partially bare cholinergic axon terminal with features of electron-dense degeneration: multiple irregular intensely dense bodies (*arrows*), uneven less dense patches, distorted mitochondria, and marked reduction of small clear vesicles; adjacent cholinergic axon varicosity (*cv*) with reduced and focally clustered small vesicles [SVR + HN, 3 weeks; Neg # 34500]. (B) Cholinergic neuroeffector junction with features of degeneration: widened junctional cleft containing collagen fibers, and bare axon terminal profile with disrupted mitochondria, markedly reduced small clear vesicles, and fuzzy or breached axolemma (*arrowheads*) [SVR, 3 weeks; Neg # 18151]. (C) Adrenergic neuroeffector junction with irregularly widened junctional cleft, and bare terminal axon profile with irregularly lamellated dense body (*arrow*), central zonal depletion of dense-cored small vesicles, and focally fuzzy axolemma; large dense-cored vesicles apparently increased [SVR, 2 weeks; Neg # 18801]. [Scale bar = 1 μm.]

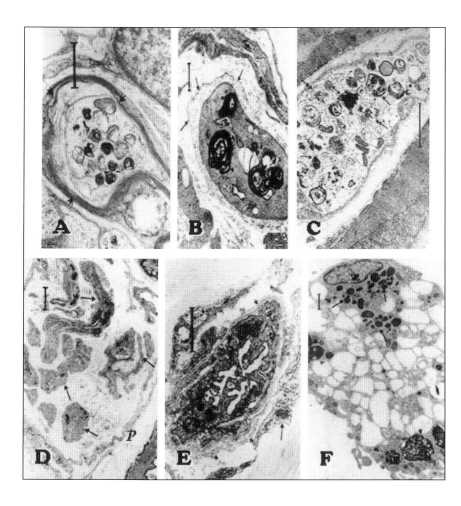

Figure 8.3

LMNB, axonal degeneration – Schwann cell ensheathed axon and nerve bundles. (A) Myelinated axon profile with numerous polymorphous intensely dense bodies, disrupted organelles, and focally split myelin sheath (*arrowheads*) [SVR, 3 weeks; Neg # 19451]. (B) Collapsed myelinated axon profiles with distorted myelin sheaths (*arrowheads*); redundant basal lamina of ensheathing Schwann cell (*arrows*) [PPN, 4 days; Neg # 22448]. (C) Interstitial Schwann cell ensheathed axon profile with extensive degenerative features: dense intra-axonal bodies and patches (*arrows*), disrupted mitochondria (*arrowheads*), depleted vesicles, and multivesicular dense body (*double-headed arrow*) [PPN, 4 days; Neg # 22443]. (D) Nerve bundle with collapsed axonless Schwann cell elements (*arrows*), retracted from perineurium (*p*) and widely separated by collagen; ensheathed axons presumably disintegrated and eliminated [PPN, 3 weeks; Neg # 22445]. (E) Collapsed axonless Schwann cell elements with redundant and replicated basal lamina (*arrowheads*); adjacent fibroblast (*arrow*) that normally lacks basal lamina [PPN, 10 weeks; Neg # 22501]. (F) Active phagocytic Schwann cell: cytoplasm with abundant empty spaces, numerous lysosomes (*arrows*) and multiple dense bodies of myelin debris, [PPN, 4 days; Neg # 22438]. [Scale bar = 1 μm.]

Most degenerative profiles have electron dense bodies, occasionally myelin figures, and some display a floccular, filamentous or empty-appearing hydropic (vacuolated) axoplasm[64,65] (Figures 8.1 and 8.2); the axolemma of some profiles may appear fuzzy or retracted from enclosing Schwann cells or adjacent muscle cells (Figure 8.2B,C). Neuroeffector junctions with degenerative axon terminal profiles may be preserved or have widened (up to ± 500 nm) junctional clefts (Figure 8.2). Degenerative myelinated axon profiles in nerve trunks, and Schwann cells devoid of ensheathed axon profiles, in smooth muscle interstitium or within nerve trunks, may be observed[27,33] (Figure 8.3). These features are sporadic in the SVR but widespread and evident in the PN model, which eliminates afferent (myelinated) innervation supplied by peripheral (infraspinal) vesical projections of sacral dorsal root ganglia, as well as the PPN model which – in addition – interrupts the preganglionic component (also myelinated) of efferent autonomic vesical innervation.[33] Axonless Schwann cell elements (Figure 8.3C,D), often with replicated basal lamina, appear collapsed, retracted (from perineurium), and widely separated by collagen fibers.[33] Early widespread axonal degeneration following PPN, however, is associated with structurally active Schwann cells that become engaged in phagocytosis of axonal debris (Figure 8.3E), as described in previous studies on axotomized somatic and autonomic neural systems.[73–75] These Schwann cells may become extinct or persist as interstitial macrophages.

Axonal change in the LM model of infraspinal (postganglionic) neurectomy (PPN)[23] conforms with the known *primary degeneration* of the distal stump of a peripheral nerve following axotomy, or chemical or pathologic injury of intrinsic visceral postganglionic nerves.[39,40,49,53,54,57,59,62,63,66,70–72] The degeneration in other LM models (and in UMNB) involves axons of *intact (nonaxotomized) postganglionic nerves*, occurring across one synaptic relay (in peripheral ganglia) in the LM model (or multiple interneuronal synapses at successive neuraxial levels in UMNB). Such *transsynaptic (transneuronal) degeneration*, which can occur across 2–4+ synaptic relays, had been known in central neural pathways (optic, cochlear, vestibular, olfactory, trigeminal, cervical chain sympathetic),[76] and in somatomotor neurons caudal to spinal cord lesions.[77] The rapidity of onset of axonal degeneration is proportional to the length of axonal stump in primary degeneration, and of the multisynaptic pathway involved in transsynaptic degeneration.[49,60,76] Ultrastructural changes of degeneration thus become established in 1–4 days after PPN (in essence a postganglionic neurectomy), but are relatively delayed (2–3 weeks) after decentralization (a preganglionic neurectomy) by PN and SVR.[33]

Widespread degeneration of adrenergic axons with loss of their neuroeffector junctions following parasympathetic decentralization by SVR combined with HN results from: (a) primary degeneration of postganglionic sympathetic fibers conveyed by the hypogastric nerves,[24] and more importantly (b) interruption of the preganglionic efferent sympathetic component of the nerve with subsequent transsynaptic degeneration of the postganglionic adrenergic axon component of intrinsic detrusor innervation,[34] which in the cat originates caudal to the site of neurectomy, in vesicourethral ganglia of the pelvic plexus and intramural ganglia within the bladder wall.[12]

Axonal regeneration

Axonal regeneration is represented by reactive and/or regenerative profiles. Reactive axon profiles are packed with mitochondria, small vesicles, and lamellar membranous bodies, and regenerative profiles – representing early axonal sprouting – display less mitochondria and vesicles but abound in axoplasmic reticulum and neurofilaments[27,64] (Figures 8.4A and 8.5A). The regeneration is widespread and prominent in SVR and PN models of LMNB, but is very limited and sporadic in the SVR + HN model, and is virtually absent (with resultant cholinergic and adrenergic hypoinnervation) in the PPN model.[28,33,34] Intact efferent sympathetic innervation therefore has a key role in regenerative reinnervation of the LMNB.[34] It would be interesting to find out whether an intact efferent parasympathetic innervation has a similar (or a different) role – if any – in regard to adrenergic detrusor innervation. In other words, whether sympathetic decentralization alone (by thoracolumbar ventral rhizotomy or HN) results in a pattern of innervation that is the reverse of that following parasympathetic decentralization (by SVR or PN), i.e. early transsynatic degeneration of intrinsic adrenergic axons with eventual long-term cholinergic hyperinnervation.

Axonal regeneration is manifested by:[28,78,79] (a) restitution of cholinergic neural elements and neuroeffector junctions (Figure 8.4); (b) increased adrenergic axon terminals, varicosities, and intervaricose segments (Figures 8.4 and 8.5) with overall adrenergic hyperinnervation; (c) cholinergic and adrenergic axonal sprouts, some forming neuroeffector junctions with detrusor muscle cells (Figure 8.5); (d) abundant copeptidergic axons replete with large densecored vesicles (Figure 8.5), also some forming neuroeffector junctions. Differences in axonal regeneration between models of LMNB[28,33,34] suggest that:[80] (a) restitution of cholinergic axons is established by sprouting as a reaction to degeneration of effector (tissue-innervating) axons, as demonstrated in central cephalic or spinal and peripheral somatic or autonomic neural systems; (b) adrenergic hyperinnervation, demonstrated histochemically and pharmacologically in other experimental models,[15,17,24,25] is achieved by sprouting of structurally normal preserved intrinsic adrenergic axons (derived from hypogastric nerve conveyed efferent pathways remaining anatomically intact)

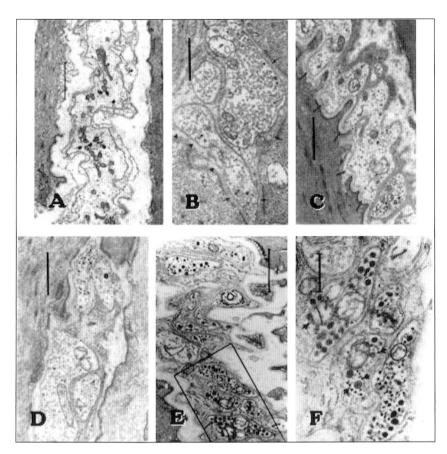

Figure 8.4

LMNB, axonal regeneration. (A) Schwann cell ensheathed intervaricose unmyelinated axon segment with abundant mitochondria, neurofilaments, neurotubules, and stellar clusters of highly electron-dense glycogen particles (*thick arrows*) [SVR, 10 weeks; Neg # 23100]. (B) Ultrastructurally normal cholinergic neuroeffector junctions; basal lamina like material (*arrows*) and elastin (*arrowheads*) in junctional clefts [SVR + HN, 10 weeks; Neg # 35070]. (C) Cholinergic neuroeffector junction with ultrastructurally normal axon terminals (*arrows*) and normally wide clefts; adjacent Schwann cell ensheathed, normal adrenergic axon profile [PN, 10 weeks; Neg # 22884]. (D) Ultrastructurally normal cholinergic (*c*) and adrenergic (*a*) axon varicosity profiles at diautonomic close neuroeffector junctions with normally wide cleft [SVR, 2 weeks; Neg # 18573]. (E) Schwann cell process between muscle cells enclosing ultrastructurally normal cholinergic (*midleft*) and adrenergic axon profiles containing abundant large dense-cored vesicles (about 120 nm diameter), deposits of glycogen, and some enlarged mitochondria with partially clear matrix (boxed profiles enlarged in Figure 8.4F) [SVR, 10 weeks; Neg # 20693]. (F) Small clear vesicles in 2 cholinergic axon profiles (*left*), and small dense-cored vesicles in an adrenergic profile (*top right*); abundant large dense-cored vesicles in 4 profiles, some of which contain enlarged partially clear mitochondria and clusters of glycogen particles (*arrowheads*). [Enlargement of boxed field in Figure 8.4E, Scale bar = 1 μm.]

in the SVR and PN models, and possibly those participating in cholinergic ⇌ adrenergic axoaxonal synapses within the detrusor (see below) – possibly as an expression of mutual cholinergic/adrenergic neurotrophism.[28]

Morphologically normal axons

Axon profiles of normal ultrastructure are virtually absent in early and established NB following PPN, in which peripheral postganglionic cholinergic parasympathetic and adrenergic sympathetic nerves are interrupted.[33] In the other models, sparse normal cholinergic and variable proportions of normal adrenergic axonal elements may be observed in early, and more adrenergic plus cholinergic elements of normal ultrastructure (including regenerated axons) in established NB.[27,28,33,34] Many of the morphologically normal axonal profiles in the early LMNB are observed at preserved diautonomic (dual cholinergic and adrenergic) neuroeffector junctions[81] and/or cholinergic ⇌ adrenergic axoaxonal synapses[82] (Figure 8.4D, Figure 8.6). It is possible that the diautonomic neuroeffector junctions and axoaxonal synapses subserve a mutual cholinergic/adrenergic neurotrophic function, in addition – respectively – to their presumptive dual autonomic control of the same muscle cells, and reciprocal prejunctional interaxonal modulation of neuroeffector transmission.[33]

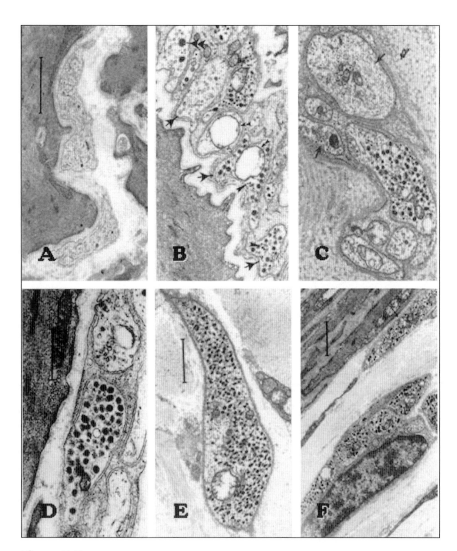

Figure 8.5

LMNB, axonal regeneration. (A) Neuroeffector junction with terminals of cholinergic axon sprout replete with tubulovesicular elements [SVR, 10 weeks; Neg # 22639]. (B) Intercellular Schwann cell process ensheathing regenerative cholinergic (*short arrows*) and adrenergic sprout profiles containing abundant pleomorphic large dense-cored vesicles of variable size and electron density (generally lighter in cholinergic profiles), stellar glycogen deposits (*arrowheads*), and few enlarged mitochondria with largely clear matrix (*double arrowheads*) [SVR, 10 weeks; Neg # 20186]. (C) Interstitial Schwann cell process with enclosed cholinergic axon sprout profiles (*arrows*), and copeptidergic profile containing few mitochondria and abundant polymorphic large vesicles with intensely dark cores [SVR + HN, 10 weeks; Neg # 35037]. (D) Neuroeffector junction with copeptidergic axon varicosity containing abundant pleomorphic large dense-cored and few small clear vesicles [SVR, 10 weeks; Neg # 21504]. (E) Adrenergic axon sprout profile containing few small and abundant pleomorphic large dense-cored vesicles, and tubulovesicular elements (*arrowheads*) [SVR, 10 weeks; Neg # 23770]. (F) Adrenergic axon sprout profiles ensheathed by Schwann cell, and at neuroeffector junction (*arrow*), with abundant pleomorphic large dense-cored vesicles and mitochondria [SVR, 10 weeks; Neg # 23768]. [Scale bar = 1 μm.]

Detrusor smooth muscle in experimental lower motoneuron neurogenic bladder

Muscle cell changes tend to be focal in experimental LMNB.[29] The detrusor displays a combination of cells of normal ultrastructure, cells with features of degeneration, and cells with features of regeneration (Figure 8.7A), with recognizable intermediate cell junctions (Figure 8.7B,C). Muscle cell changes have no constant relationship to changes in spatially close axon bundles. Most degenerative profiles, however, are next to degenerative profiles of cholinergic axon terminals or varicosities with lost neuroeffector junctions. Muscle cells of intact ultrastructure may have intact adrenergic or diautonomic junctions (see above).

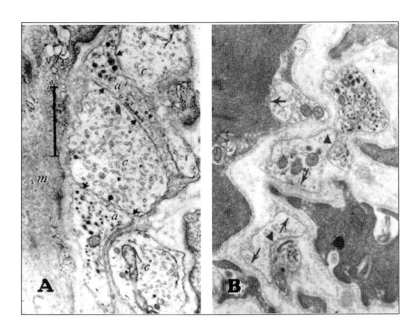

Figure 8.6

LMNB, normal axon profiles. (A) Ultrastructurally normal cholinergic (*c*) and adrenergic (*a*) axon terminal profiles with multiple axoaxonal synapses (*short arrows*) at diautonomic neuroeffector junction with muscle cell (*m*). [SVR, 2 weeks; Neg # 19140]. (B) Cholinergic neuroeffector junctions (*arrows*) and adjacent cholinergic ↔ adrenergic axoaxonal synapses (*arrowheads*) [SVR, 10 weeks; Neg # 22339]. [Scale bar = 1 μm.]

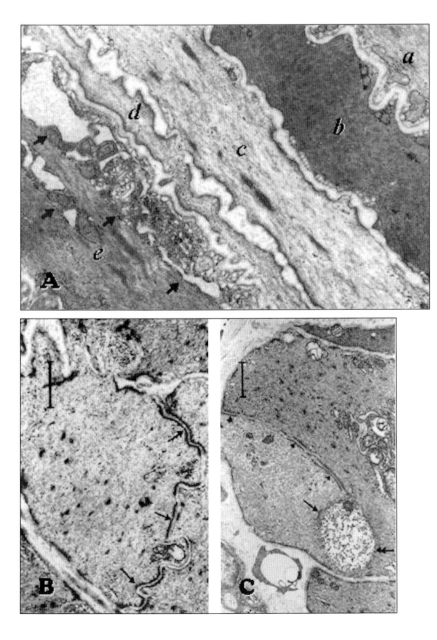

Figure 8.7

LMNB, muscle cell degeneration. (A) Five contiguous muscle cell profiles with variable electron density: (*a*), normal density and ultrastructure; (*b*), degenerative with increased density and clumped myofilaments; (*c,d*), degenerative with rarefied light sarcoplasm and irregularly distributed dense ('cigar') bodies; (*e*), regenerative with very prominent and microcystic subsarcolemmal endoplasmic reticulum (*arrows*) [SVR, 10 weeks; Neg # 23090]. (B) Sarcoplasm with reduced density, focally crowded dense bodies and glycogen clusters; lengthy intermediate cell junctions (*arrows*, about 25 nm junctional cleft) and interspersed intimate junctions with very close (≤12 nm) contact [SVR, 2 weeks; Neg # 18926]. (C) Granular sarcoplasmic disintegration in globular cell protrusion (*arrow*) with intimate cell junction (*double arrow*), and lengthy intermediate junction (*arrowheads*) with adjacent muscle cell [SVR, 2 weeks; Neg # 18448]. [Scale bar = 1 μm.]

Muscle cell degeneration predominates in early (a few days to 4 weeks), and regeneration in established (10 weeks) LMNB, coinciding with dominant axonal degeneration and regeneration, respectively, in the same models. Degeneration persists, however, in the SVR + HN model, with very limited or no regeneration in the established resultant NB.[34] Degenerative profiles have altered sarcoplasmic structure, sarcolemma, organelles, and cell–cell relationship (Figure 8.8). Regenerative profiles may be recognized by normal ultrastructure, active nuclei with nucleoli, and proliferation of certain organelles – particularly sarcoplasmic reticulum (Figure 8.9).

Pathophysiologic considerations

The above-described ultrastructural neuromuscular detrusor changes in the experimental LMNB introduced a potential pathologic basis for its motor dysfunction. These changes allow its decentralization and 'denervation' forms

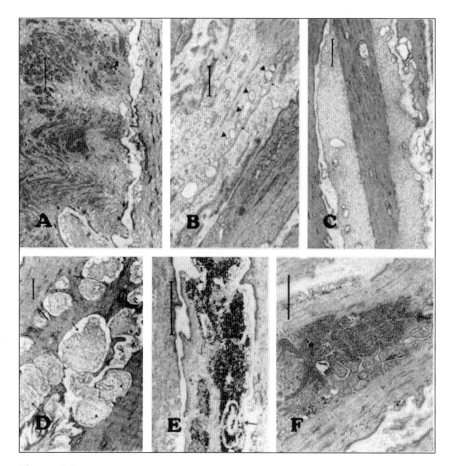

Figure 8.8
LMNB, muscle cell degeneration. (A) Myofilaments irregularly clumped as crowded wavy bundles and dense patches; unevenly thick sarcolemma with indistinct basal lamina [SVR, 10 weeks; Neg # 22958]. (B) Upper cell profile with condensed myofilaments and streaming dense bodies; lower profile with rarefied sarcoplasm – disrupted myofilaments and early hydropic/vacuolar degeneration, disrupted mitochondria (*arrowheads*), dense glycogen clusters, and sarcolemma with long stretches of thin cell membrane (*arrows*) [SVR, 2 weeks; Neg # 18793]. (C) Myofilaments of peripheral sarcoplasm replaced by amorphous particulate matter (floccular degeneration), with multiple hydropic vacuoles; preserved sarcoplasm of cell core, and cells above and below [SVR, 3 weeks; Neg # 19446]. (D) Multiple irregularly shaped sarcoplasmic bodies with floccular degeneration; some may represent blebbing (*arrows*), others degenerated axons engulfed by muscle cells (*arrowheads*) [SVR, 3 weeks; Neg # 16001]. (E) Sarcoplasmic hypergranulation by glycogen deposits; unevenly thick and focally indistinct (*arrow*) sarcolemma [SVR, 10 weeks; Neg # 23096]. (F) Paranuclear hypergranulation by free ribosomes of disrupted sarcoplasmic reticulum; scattered glycogen clusters in peripheral sarcoplasm. [SVR, 3 weeks; Neg # 16154]. [Scale bar = 1 μm.]

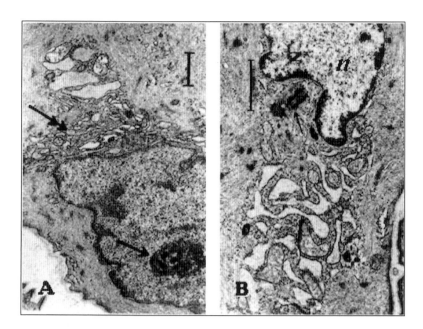

Figure 8.9
LMNB, muscle cell regeneration.
(A) Sarcoplasm with normal density and myofilament organization, nucleus with nucleolus (*arrow*), prominent endoplasmic reticulum with dilated cisternae, and prominent Golgi apparatus (*double arrow*) [SVR, 10 weeks; Neg # 20702]. (B) Paranuclear (*n* = nucleus) proliferated endoplasmic reticulum with moderately dilated cisternae and abundant associated ribosomes; *arrow* marks centrosome [SVR, 2 weeks; Neg # 18982]. [Scale bar = 1 μm.]

to be distinguished ultrastructurally, and may explain in part their different functional behavior.

Concurrence of degenerative and regenerative muscle cell and axonal changes may be the expression of nerve/muscle trophism, well documented in somatomotor but only sketchily in autonomic neuroeffector systems.[83–88] The more restricted distribution of muscular than axonal changes in the decentralization models probably reflects the largely normal adrenergic axonal population as well as intact cholinergic axons remaining at diautonomic neuroeffector junctions and axoaxonal synapses.[29] Degenerating muscle cells often have increased junctions with adjacent muscle cells, with intimate cell junctions resembling gap-junction,[36] possibly to replace hampered or deficient neuroeffector transmission (as the result of axonal degeneration) by enhanced myogenic muscle cell coupling – as indicated in the denervated vas deferens.[89]

Persistent hypoinnervation of the 'denervation' form, with virtual absence of a copeptidergic axon population, indicates profound impedance of neuroeffector transmission in the detrusor, leading to marked alteration of its functional behavior, with enlarged bladder capacity and absence of detrusor overactivity. Whether or not this behavior becomes dependent on myogenic effector transmission requires further study, specially pathophysiologic and pharmacologic aspects of the 'denervated' detrusor. Differences in supersensitivity between the 'denervated' and decentralized detrusor (see below) need to be defined; such differences had been described in relation to adrenergic innervation of the vas deferens.[89]

It appears that the decentralization form initially loses its cholinergic effector excitomotor function as a result of transsynaptic degeneration of intrinsic cholinergic axons

innervating the detrusor. Eventually, however, it acquires a tripartite neoinnervation pattern that comprises restituted cholinergic neuroeffector junctions, adrenergic hyperinnervation, and an emergent population of copeptidergic axons.[28]

In addition to impairment of cholinergic neuroeffector function, cholinergic axonal degeneration is probably accompanied by excessive extraneural leakage of cholinergic neurotransmitter from its stores in axonal vesicles. This may lead to 'denervation' supersensitivity of the detrusor, with (a) exaggerated cholinergic muscular responses, as known clinically,[90] and demonstrated in cholinergic innervation of the rat bladder,[91–93] adrenergic innervation of the cat nictitating membrane,[72] and both cholinergic and adrenergic innervation of salivary glands,[94] and (b) increased sensitivity of muscular responses to the antimuscarinic action of atropine, as demonstrated in a rat denervation model.[95,96] The supersensitivity was considered to be a factor in development of vesical hypertonicity of the decentralizion form of LMNB.[97] Such a bladder, however, acquires a functional state of adrenergic dominance (demonstrated in the cat, rat, and the human[21,24,25,92]), because of preservation of adrenergic axons with early sprouting of many. This dominance, and its eventual reinforcement by adrenergic detrusor hyperinnervation with exaggerated α-adrenergic responses, are additional probable factors in the development of hypertonicity.[21,24,25,98] Concomitant changes in muscle cells that have an impact on their excitation–contraction coupling mechanism may also contribute to supersensitivity, particularly prominent changes in the sarcoplasmic reticulum (major site of Ca^{2+} turnover), and apparently increased cell–cell junctions promoting myogenic cell coupling.[29]

Neodevelopment of prominent peptide content has been documented experimentally in regenerating peripheral somatic axons.[99] The emergence of abundant copeptidergic axons in the detrusor of LMNB has considerable functional significance. The copeptidergic axon population involves many regenerated cholinergic and many reactively sprouted adrenergic axon terminals and varicosities. It is likely that the axons become replenished with one or more neuropeptides, in addition to or instead of their innate classical neurotransmitters (acetylcholine and norepinephrine). Thereby, these axons become a mechanism for adjusting, supplementing, or supplanting altered or deficient cholinergic, as well as altered – possibly exaggerated – adrenergic neuroeffector function in the established decentralized LMNB.[28] It has been shown that autonomic axons can 'switch' functionally from a classical to a putative (specially peptide) neurotransmitter during neurigenesis and in association with reactive/regenerative sprouting.[100–102] Marked increase of VIP-containing nerves was reported in the rat bladder decentralized by pelvic neurectomy.[18] A recent study has described neuropeptide immunoreactivity in the detrusor of UMNB resulting from spinal cord injury.[103] For proper understanding of NB dysfunction, however, it is crucial that peptide cotransmitters in both LMNB and UMNB, short as well as long term (if possible), are identified in detail by immunohistochemistry. The identified peptides need to be catalogued in relation to accurately characterized aspects of detrusor function, as well as various causative entities, to sort out and define the nature, functional impact, and possible therapeutic implications of corresponding peptidergic vesical responses.

Pathology of detrusor in long-standing clinical upper motoneuron neurogenic bladder

Ultrastructural changes in muscle cells and intrinsic axons are qualitatively similar to their respective changes in experimental LMNB. In general, muscle cell degeneration is neither pronounced nor widespread, irrespective of measured detrusor contractility, and muscle cell regeneration is not clearly demonstrable.[36]

Regarding intrinsic innervation, the detrusor has axon profiles with features of degeneration, profiles with features of regeneration, and morphologically normal profiles, varying in proportion with anatomic level of the causative neural deficit[37] (Table 8.3). The changes involve both unmyelinated and myelinated axons, with activation of related Schwann cells in preterminal axon bundles and main nerve trunks.[104–108] Unmyelinated axon profiles discernible ultrastructurally in human UMNB are mostly cholinergic; enhanced visualization of adrenergic axon profiles by 5-hydroxydopamine preloading (as in experimental LMNB models:[31] see above) is inapplicable to the human.

Morphologically normal profiles (Figure 8.10A) in supraspinal UMNB are 4–5.5 times as common as spinal UMNB with or without the LM component (Table 8.3). Accordingly, degenerative profiles are less than twice the normal profiles in supraspinal vs 9–13.5 times more in spinal UMNB. The degenerative profiles, however, are 3.5–4.5 times more than regenerative profiles in both spinal and supraspinal UMNB.

Unmyelinated degenerative axon profiles display reduced to depleted small vesicles (Figure 8.10B), and those with regeneration appear as axon sprouts or copeptidergic axons (Figure 8.10C,D). Copeptidergic axon profiles are identical to sprout profiles, except that they display less (≤3) mitochondria.[35] Myelinated degenerative axon profiles have features similar to Wallerian degeneration[104–108] (Figure 8.10E,F). As in the central models of LMNB (SVR, PN), the observed axonal degeneration/regeneration must be transsynaptic in nature (see above). In long-standing UMNB, these changes appear to represent a dynamic process (Figure 8.11) that is independent of the duration of neurogenic dysfunction.[37] Whether or not a comparable process takes place in long-standing LMNB of months or years duration awaits further investigation. Nonetheless, repression of adrenergic axon sprouts (with degeneration) by reforming cholinergic axons was mentioned in the decentralization form of experimental LMNB.[28] Both persistence, and regression (repression) of 'foreign' axonal sprouts before establishment of functioning synaptic/junctional contacts, have been demonstrated in conjunction with and following regeneration of initially degenerating 'native' axons.[109–114]

In UMNB, muscle cell degeneration tends to be sporadic, regardless of detrusor contractility, and some muscle cell profiles may suggest regeneration.[36] When hyperreflexic, the detrusor displays the ultrastructural complete dysjunction pattern[36] with reduced or lost intermediate (adherence) muscle cell junctions of normal detrusor, dominant intimate cell junctions (including protrusion junctions and ultraclose abutments of non-neurogenic detrusor overactivity[13,41,45–48]) in a >2 : 1 (up to 40+ : 1) ratio of intimate to intermediate junctions, and chain-like linkage of ≥5 cells by the intimate junctions (Figure 8.12).[36,41]

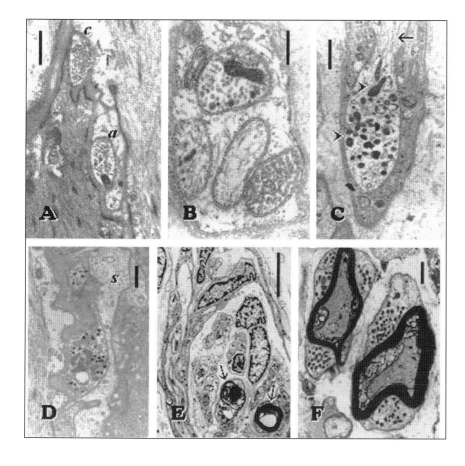

Figure 8.10

Long-standing UMNB, axonal changes.
(A) Diautonomic neuroeffector junction
with cholinergic (*c*) and adrenergic
(*a*) axon terminal profiles of rather
normal ultrastructure [SCI, 2 years;
Neg # 70025]. (B) Interstitial axon
bundle: Schwann cell ensheathed axon
preterminals – one (*bottom right*)
ultrastructurally normal, packed with
cholinergic small clear vesicles, 3
(*top left, bottom left*) with reduced and
fragmented small vesicles, and the
5th (*middle*) depleted of vesicles [SCI,
4 years; Neg # 67491]. (C) Schwann cell
ensheathed axon sprout with abundant
mitochondria (*arrowheads*), large dense-
cored vesicles, and neurotubules
(*arrow*) [SCI, 3 years; Neg # 67051].
(D) Neuroeffector junction with partially
bare sprout axon terminal: abundant
mitochondria, large dense-cored vesicles
and small vesicles (*s* = Schwann cell)
[SCI, 6 months; Neg # 70929]. (E) Mixed
nerve trunk with degenerative profiles of
myelinated (*arrows*) and unmyelinated
axons, some with prominent large
dense-cored vesicles apparently the
result of regressed regeneration (see
Figure 8.11) [SCI, 31 years; Neg # 67790].
(F) Degenerative myelinated axon
profiles: split and irregular myelin
sheaths, with collapse of axon (*right*);
activated ensheathing Schwann cell with
abundant mitochondria [SCI, 10 years;
Neg # j57578]. [All figures: scale
bar = 0.5 μm; Figures 8.10A and C
reproduced (modified) from Elbadawi[35]
with permission from *Journal of Urology*.
Figures 8.10D and F from Haferkamp[37]
with permission from *Journal of
Urology*.]

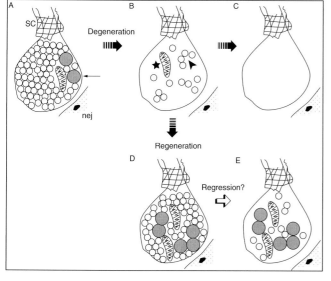

Figure 8.11

Diagram of proposed dynamic axonal changes in longstanding UMNB. (A) Ultrastructurally normal cholinergic axon terminal
profile: abundant small clear vesicles (*empty circles*), 2 large dense-cored vesicles (*arrow*), and almost close neuroeffector junction
(*nej*)[81] with about 40 nm junctional cleft. (B) Degenerative profile: markedly reduced small vesicles (*arrowhead*); no large vesicles,
widened nej; *star* = mitochondrion. (C) Degenerative profile depleted of organelles with empty appearance and widened nej.
(D) 'Stable' regenerative profile, copeptidergic of normal ultrastructure: abundant small clear vesicles, 2 mitochondria, 5 large
dense-cored vesicles; cleft of nej similar to A; profiles (axon terminals or preterminals) with abundant small and large (≥3)
vesicles, mitochondria (≥4) and neurotubules and neurofilaments designated as sprout profiles;[35] (E) 'Regressed' regenerative
profile (presumably axonal degeneration following regeneration):[37] reduced small vesicles but preserved mitochondria and large
vesicles (see Figure 8.10E). [Scale bar = 1 μm.] [Reproduced (modified) from Haferkamp et al [37] with permission from *Journal of
Urology*.]

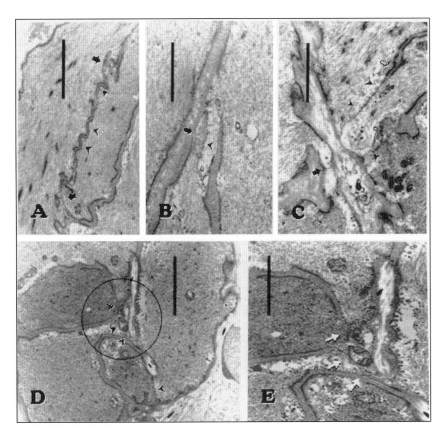

Figure 8.12
Hyperreflexic UMNB, complete dysjunction pattern. (A) Broad digitate intimate cell appositions (ICA, *arrows*) contrast with intermediate junction (IJ, *arrowheads*) [SCI, 2 years; Neg # 70010]. (B) Slender digitate form (protrusion junction) of side-to-side ICA (*arrow*) with quasisyncytial appearance (*arrowhead*) because of focally indiscernible junctional gap – different sarcoplasmic appearance indicates 2 separate cell processes in contact [MMC, 15 years; Neg # 69200]. (C) Barely discernible gap of ICA (marked by sarcolemmal caveolae of the 2 cells) at protrusion junction (*arrow*) and planar ultraclose abutment (*arrowheads*) contrast with about 60 nm gap of adjacent short IJ (*open arrow*) [SCI, 2 years; Neg # 70012]. (D) Chain of 5 muscle cells linked by ICA (*arrowheads*); middle area of 3 adjoined cells (*in circle*) enlarged in Figure 8.12E [SCI, 3 years; Neg # 67040]. (E) Complex ICA of 3 muscle cells (*white arrows*) [Neg # 67041]. [Figures 8.12B,C,D,E: scale bar = 0.5μm; Figure reproduced (modified) from Haferkamp et al,[36] with permission from the *Journal of Urology*.]

Pathologic features of rhabdosphincter in experimental lower motoneuron neurogenic bladder

The feline rhabdosphincter is composed of slow- and fast-twitch myofibers (Figure 8.13),[20] which have somatomotor innervation through classical motor-end-plates, as well as autonomic innervation via nonspecialized surface contacts with myofibers lacking sole-plate (end-plate) differentiation (Figure 8.14).[115] The human rhabdosphincter is similarly composed of slow- and fast-twitch myofibers.[116] It has pudendal nerve derived somatomotor innervation, and its adrenergic innervation has been documented, but its autonomic cholinergic innervation remains to be demonstrated.[12]

Experimental LMNB following BSVR is associated with ultrastructural changes in myofibers of the male feline urethral rhabdosphincter and their innervation[30–32] (Figure 8.14), but neuromuscular pathology of the denervated human rhabdosphincter awaits investigation. SVR deprives the rhabdosphincter of its pudendal nerve conveyed somatic innervation through classical neuromuscular junctions, whereas its nonspecialized autonomic neuromuscular surface contacts are preserved but

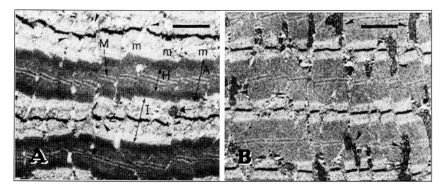

Figure 8.13

Normal feline rhabdosphincter, myofibers – longitudinally sectioned. (A) Fast-twitch myofiber. Sarcomeric band structure marked on myofibrils (*m*): Z disc, M line, A band, I band, H zone. Thin straight Z disc ($\overline{\times}$45 nm), narrow M line (50 nm), sparse mitochondria (*arrow*), well-developed sarcoplasmic reticulum, and T tubules (*arrowheads*), conspicuous glycogen [Neg # 27350]. (B) Slow twitch myofiber: thick jagged Z-disc ($\overline{\times}$95 nm), wide M line (95 nm), abundant mitochondria aligned along myofibrils (*arrowheads*), poorly developed sarcoplasmic reticulum and T tubules, little glycogen [Neg # 27342]. [Scale bar = 1 μm.]

*Normal human rhabdosphincter is similarly composed of fast- and slow-twitch myofibers[116] (figures depicting myofiber ultrastructure in Elbadawi A, Matthews R, Light JK, Wheeler T[116], *Journal of Urology* were inadvertently switched in print).

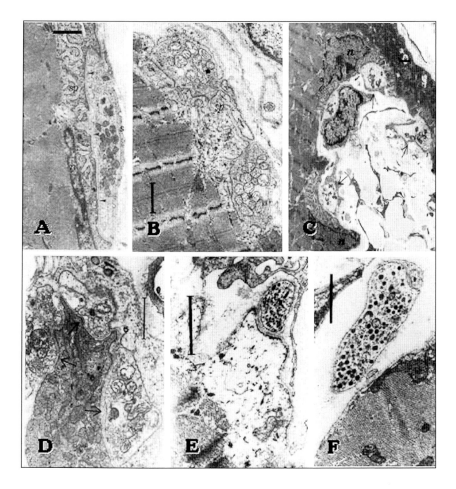

Figure 8.14

Normal feline rhabdosphincter, innervation. (A) Somatomotor neuromuscular junction (nmj), en plaque form: bare aspect of large cholinergic axon terminal profile (abundant small clear vesicles and mitochondria), and underlying sole-plate (*sp*) opposite nucleus (*n*) of myofiber, with 70 nm wide separation gap (primary synaptic cleft) containing central dense line (*arrowheads*); plate has complex sarcoplasmic junctional folds separated by secondary junctional clefts; *s* = Schwann cell covers side of terminal away from myofiber [Neg # 25845]. (B) Nmj, en plaque form: sole-plate (*sp*) in contact with 2 cholinergic axon terminal profiles (appear separate by sectioning artifact); *arrowheads* mark M line [Neg # 26024]. (C) Nmj, en grappe form: cluster of 4 separate and independent nmjs (*arrows*), 3 opposite nucleus (*n*) [Neg # 25935]. (D) Three cholinergic axon terminal profiles in close surface contact (no sole-plate differentiation) with myofiber (*arrows*, 55–100 nm clefts) (see Figure 8.14A) [Neg # 24719]. (E) Adrenergic axon terminal profile in surface contact (66 nm cleft) with protuberance of myofiber [Neg # 26018]. (F) Copeptidergic axon profile (abundant large dense-cored vesicles, few mitochondria) approaches nonspecialized surface of myofiber (about 120 nm gap) [Neg # 24701]. [Scale bar = 1 μm.]

become subject to changes similar to those in intrinsic nerves of detrusor. Neurohistochemistry can detect established but not early changes in innervation of the rhabdosphincter denervated by BSVR, but has no value in revealing any changes in the unilaterally rhizotomized feline model.[117] It seems that the denervated side of the rhabdosphincter rapidly becomes completely reinnervated by sprouts from nerves of the intact side because of small size of the rhabdosphincter, bilateral (crossed) somatomotor innervation, and direct anatomical continuity of its two sides.[117]

Innervation

Early after somatic denervation (1–2 weeks), there is virtual loss of myelinated axons within nerve trunks and interstitial Schwann cell ensheathed axon bundles, with degeneration and loss of cholinergic axon terminals at sole-plates of the neuromuscular junctions[30,118] (Figure 8.15A–C). Nonspecialized autonomic surface contacts with myofibers are preserved (Figure 8.15D–F).

With established denervation (4–10 weeks), axonless sole-plates acquire a simplified structure or partially retain their junctional complexity (Figure 8.16A,B). Many plates become reinnervated by cholinergic and/or adrenergic – occasionally copeptidergic – axon terminals, and nonspecialized autonomic axon/myofiber surface contacts appear to be increased.[31] Cholinergic ⇌ adrenergic axoaxonal synapses of surface-innervating terminals at residual simplified sole-plates may be observed (Figure 8.16E). Axons of intact ultrastructure in myofiber contact (Figure 8.16F) or within interstitial axon bundles (Figure 8.17) may display features of sprouting or copeptidergic axons. Some interstitial axon bundles may still enclose degenerating axons (Figure 8.15B).

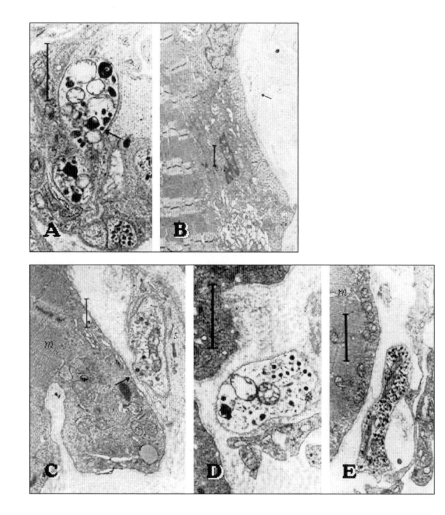

Figure 8.15

Somatic denervated rhabdosphincter, myofiber innervation. (A) Degenerative profile of unmyelinated axon (*arrow*; depleted small vesicles, dense bodies, disrupted mitochondria) within interstitial Schwann cell [SVR, 10 weeks; Neg # 23692]. (B) Preserved sole-plate and degenerative profile of related axon terminal (*arrow*, no vesicles or mitochondria, floccular granular material) [SVR, 2 weeks; Neg # 24199]. (C) Partially Schwann cell ensheathed *(s)* cholinergic axon terminal profile in nonspecialized (no sole-plate) surface contact (*arrow*) with myofiber *m* [SVR, 2 weeks; Neg # 24715]. (D) Profile of cholinergic axon terminal (small clear vesicles) with numerous large dense-cored vesicles in nonspecialized surface contact with myofiber [SVR, 1 week; Neg # 24721]. (E) Profile of adrenergic axon terminal (small dense-cored vesicles) with abundant pleomorphic large dense-cored vesicles in nonspecialized surface contact with myofiber *m* [SVR, 2 weeks; Neg # 24169]. [Scale bar = 1 μm.]

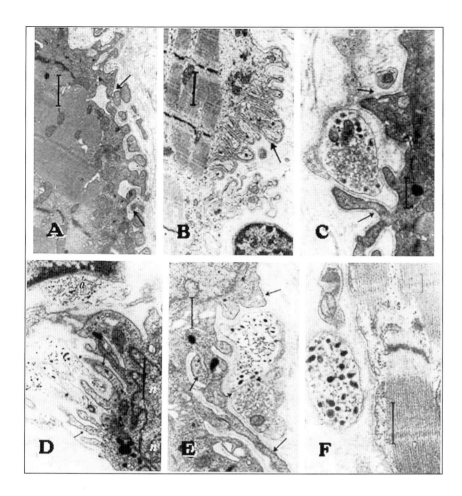

Figure 8.16

Somatic denervated rhabdosphincter, myofiber innervation. (A) Axonless sole-plate (*between arrows*) with simplified structure: junctional folds shallower, less complex, more widely separated than normal (see Figure 8.14A) [SVR, 4 weeks; Neg # 25303]. (B) Axonless sole-plate (*arrow*) with preserved structure and complexity of junctional folds [SVR, 10 weeks; Neg # 24380]. (C) Sole-plate of simplified structure (*between arrows*) reinnervated by cholinergic axon terminal [SVR, 4 weeks; Neg # 25311]. (D) Sole-plate of preserved complexity (*between arrows*), next to myofiber nucleus (*n*), reinnervated by adrenergic axon terminal extending as processes (*arrowheads*) into secondary junctional clefts; terminal continuous (in serial section) with outlying adrenergic axon (*a*) [SVR, 4 weeks; Neg # 24967]. (E) Sole-plate of simplified structure (*between arrows*), reinnervated by cholinergic (*right*) and adrenergic (*left*) axon terminals in axoaxonal synapse (*arrowheads*) [SVR, 4 weeks; Neg # 25317]. (F) Bare copeptidergic/cholinergic axon terminal (small clear vesicles, abundant pleomorphic large dense-cored vesicles, few mitochondria) in nonspecialized surface contact with myofiber [SVR, 10 weeks; Neg # 24080]. [Scale bar = 1 μm.]

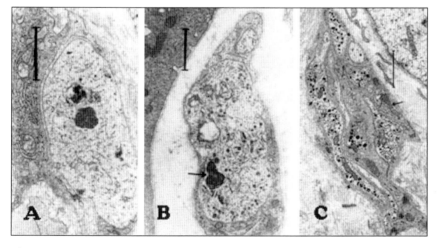

Figure 8.17

Somatic denervated rhabdosphincter, regenerative innervation. (A) Early regeneration. Interstitial partially Schwann cell ensheathed axon sprout profile containing 3 dense bodies and packed with neurotubules and tubulovesicular elements of axoplasmic reticulum [SVR, 2 weeks; Neg # 24206]. (B) Established regeneration. Schwann cell ensheathed axon sprout profile containing mitochondria and laminated dense body (*arrow*), packed with neurotubules, tubulovesicular reticulum, and large dense-cored vesicles, next to nonspecialized surface of myofiber (no sole plate) [SVR, 4 weeks; Neg # 25309]. (C) Established regeneration. Interstitial Schwann cell ensheathing 1 cholinergic (*arrow*) and 6 adrenergic axon profiles, some of which (*short arrows*) appear copeptidergic (abundant pleomorphic large dense-cored vesicles) [SVR, 10 weeks; Neg # 24441]. [Scale bar = 1 μm.]

Myofibers

The somatically denervated rhabdosphincter displays a combination of ultrastructurally normal, degenerative, and regenerative profiles of its myofibers (see Figure 8.20A).[32] Degenerative profiles are most prominent early (1–2 weeks) after denervation and display changes in myofibrils, sarcoplasm and sarcoplasmic organelles, without myofiber atrophy or interstitial fibrosis. The degenerative changes include[119–130] disorganization of myofibrils and sarcomeric

band structure, altered sarcoplasmic organelles, sarcoplasmic inclusion bodies, proliferation of T tubules of triad system, and protuberant sarcoplasmic bulgings of variable ultrastructure (Figures 8.18 and 8.19). Regenerative profiles are observed focally in early and are most prominent with established (4–6 weeks) denervation. They are manifested by central active nuclei, active myosatellite cells and formation of myoblasts and myotubes[119,131–135] (Figures 8.20 and 8.21).

None of the degenerative changes described in the denervated rhabdosphincter is specific for denervated

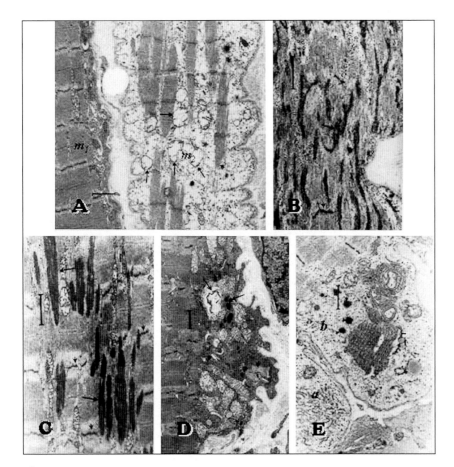

Figure 8.18

Somatic denervated rhabdosphincter, myofiber degeneration. (A) Two myofibers: m_1 with preserved ultrastructure (thick jagged Z disc, wide well-defined M line, few mitochondria); m_2 with features of degeneration: bloated mitochondria (*arrows*), disorganized and frayed myofibrils (*arrowhead*), clarified granular sarcoplasm [SVR, 4 weeks; Neg # 24918]. (B) Largely lost sarcomeric band structure, electron-dense Z discs irregularly streamed in rows (*arrow*) perpendicular to residual Z discs (*arrowhead*); compared to 'nemaline' rods (see Figure 8.18C), streams are less dense and thinner, irregular in configuration and associated with loss of mitochondria [SVR, 10 weeks; Neg # 24478]. (C) Highly electron-dense Z line 'nemaline' rods (*arrows*) perpendicular to residual Z discs (*arrowheads*) [SVR, 4 weeks; Neg # 24942]. (D) Afibrillary protuberant sarcoplasmic mass with myelin figure (*arrow*), lysosomes (*double arrow*), lipid droplets (*arrowheads*), enlarged mitochondria with complex cristae; nonaligned Z discs of contiguous myofibrils [SVR, 4 weeks; Neg # 25117]. (E) Two protruberant afibrillary sarcoplasmic masses: (*a*), dominated by dilated tubulovesicular elements of sarcoplasmic reticulum; (*b*), bilamellar cytomembranous inclusions, lysosomes (*arrowheads*) and lipid bodies (*arrows*) [SVR, 2 weeks; Neg # 24297]. [Scale = 1 μm.].

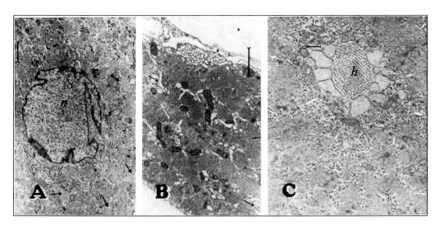

Figure 8.19
Somatic denervated rhabdosphincter – proliferation of triad system. (A) Centrally located nucleus (*n*) and marked proliferation of T tubules appearing as cross-sectioned honeycomb structures (*arrows*) [SVR, 6 weeks; Neg # 25124]. (B) Abundant mitochondria and dilated T tubules (*arrows*); subsarcolemmal honeycomb structure communicating with extracellular space (*arrowhead*) [SVR, 4 weeks; Neg # 25300]. (C) Roughly hexagonal honeycomb structure (*h*) of T-tubule origin; outlying dilated sacs of sarcoplasmic reticulum, abundant mitochondria, and dense clusters of free ribosomes [SVR, 6 weeks; Neg # 25126]. [Scale = 1 μm.]

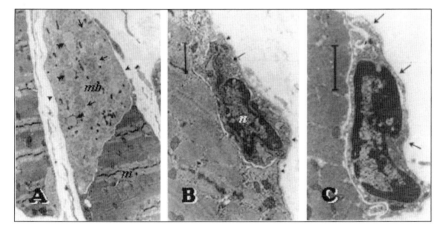

Figure 8.20
Somatic denervated rhabdosphincter, myofiber regeneration. (A) Early myoblast probably (*mb*) derived from myosatellite cell of myofiber *m* (enclosed by its basal lamina: *arrowheads*); sarcoplasm contains abundant mitochondria, tubulovesicular elements of sarcoplasmic reticulum, clusters of unorganized myofibrils (*arrows*), and lipid droplets (*double arrowheads*) [SVR, 6 weeks; Neg # 24953]. (B) Active myosatellite cell (see Figure 8.20C) enclosed by basal lamina of myofiber (*arrowheads*); expanded cytoplasm (*arrow*) with many mitochondria and dilated cisterns of rough endoplasmic reticulum; *n* = nucleus [SVR, 6 weeks; Neg # 25134]. (C) Normal myosatellite cell apposed to myofiber and enclosed by its basal lamina (*arrows*); large nucleus and sparse organelle-free cytoplasm [Neg # 27938]. [Scale = 1 μm.]

striated muscle. Many have been described in neurogenic as well as non-neurogenic diseases such as muscle dystrophy, pathologic, toxic or drug-induced myopathy, polymyositis, Parkinson's disease, and various neuropathies[119,122,123,125,126] Furthermore, myoblasts and myotubes, the hallmark of regenerating striated muscle, have been described in developing and growing striated muscle.[127,130–134]

Pathophysiologic considerations

The neuromuscular changes described above need to be investigated, and confirmed – or modified if necessary – in the somatically denervated human rhabdosphincter. It appears that the denervated male feline rhabdosphincter acquires *exclusive* autonomic neural control, initially

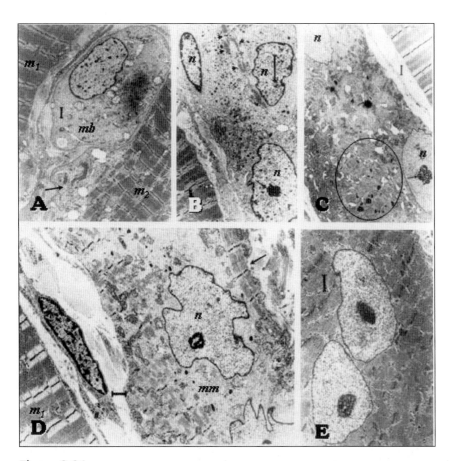

Figure 8.21

Somatic denervated rhabdosphincter, myofiber regeneration – myoblast/myotube formation. (A) Early myoblast (*mb*) with granular sarcoplasm, mitochondria, and unorganized myofibrils (*dark zone*); myofiber m_1 has normal and m_2 degenerative features (*arrow*) [SVR, 6 weeks; Neg # 24298]. (B) Early myotube: 3 nuclei (*n*), one with nucleolus (*arrow*), densely granular sarcoplasm containing abundant mitochondria, free ribosomes, lysosomes, and myofibrils in early organization – parallel sarcomeric alignment and appearance of band structure (*arrowheads*); adjacent myofiber of normal ultrastructure [SVR, 6 weeks; Neg # 24207]. (C) Late myotube formation: 2 central nuclei (*n*), one with nucleolus (*arrow*), organelle-rich sarcoplasm (abundant mitochondria, dilated sarcoplasmic reticulum), organizing myofibrils (*in ellipse*) [SVR, 6 weeks; Neg # 24815]. (D) Maturing myofiber (*mm*): central nucleus (*n*) with nucleolus, paranuclear zone of myofibril-free sarcoplasm, intermediate zone of disorganized sarcomeres, peripheral zone of largely normal ultrastructure (*arrow*); m_1 = adjacent myofiber of normal ultrastructure [SVR, 2 weeks; Neg # 24304]. (E) Well-developed myofibrils with banded sarcomeres; 2 central nuclei with nucleoli [SVR, 6 weeks; Neg # 25123]. [Scale = 1 μm.]

by its nonspecialized axon/myofiber surface contacts, and eventually by these contacts as well as autonomically reinnervated residual sole-plates rendered axonless initially. The persistent surface nerve/myofiber contacts and reinnervated sole-plates are ultrastructurally sound as vehicles for neurotransmission, and thus potentially provide the denervated rhabdosphincter with excitatory neural influence.[31] The presumed excitatory influence remains to be characterized, however, according to physiopharmacologic responses of the normal as well as denervated feline rhabdosphincter – which also need to be studied. In particular, the functional significance of autonomic innervation of the normal rhabdosphincter, and of sole-plate reinnervation by adrenergic axons – including those with axoaxonal synapse as well as the copeptidergic axon population – require full investigation. Information on denervated striated muscle, in general, suggests that the excitatory influence, exercised by autonomic fibers with much slower conduction velocity than the myelinated nerves of normal neuromuscular junctions,[136] may have delayed onset,[137–139] and may not generate normal or effective responses of myofibers,[140,141] including their functioning as fast- or slow-twitch myofibers.[142–145]

Rhabdosphincter myofibers undergoing early degeneration after denervation are neither eliminated nor persistent, but are induced to regenerate, probably by the trophic influence of sustained autonomic innervation, as experimentally demonstrated in relation to sympathetic and parasympathetic ganglia both *in vivo* and *in vitro*.[146–149] The somatically denervated feline rhabdosphincter lacks atrophy and fibrosis, both of which have been described in the human urethral striated sphincter in the LM neurogenic dysfunction associated with myelodysplasia.[150] This, however, differs in its developmental immaturity, and perhaps maldevelopment, from the denervation model in fully mature cats.[32] The lack of atrophy and fibrosis allows the rhabdosphincter to remain functional after somatic denervation, albeit not necessarily normally or fully – in view of its eventual exclusively autonomic innervation (see above). The observed postdenervation structural changes include prominent alteration of myofiber content and orientation of mitochondria, which tend to obfuscate the structural identity of myofibers as functionally fast- or slow-twitch.[32] The reported subsarcolemmal aggregates of ribosomes probably are the source of neogenesis of autonomic neurotransmitter receptors, assumed to result in postdenervation supersensitivity (to acetylcholine and catecholamines) of striated muscle, until reinnervated.[142,151–161]

Concluding remarks

Ultrastructural studies revealed that both lower and upper motoneuron neurogenic bladder are associated with neuromuscular structural changes in the detrusor that may cause or contribute to resultant voiding dysfunction. These changes are readily recognizable, and may help in the diagnosis of the neurogenic nature of a voiding dysfunction, and possibly also in disclosing an occult neurogenic factor in a dysfunction that clinically appears to be nonneurogenic. Observed variable proportions of the changes in different types of NB may allow distinction of the anatomic level of the responsible neural factor, i.e. upper vs lower motoneuron, and infraspinal 'denervation' vs decentralization form of the latter (Table 8.3). *First*, widespread degeneration of intrinsic axons combined with axonal regeneration (axon sprout and/or copeptidergic axon profiles) is probably sufficient to distinguish a neurogenic from a non-neurogenic dysfunction. Whereas the full ultrastructural degeneration pattern of non-neurogenic impaired detrusor contractility has widespread nerve degeneration as a constant component, it lacks neural elements with features of regeneration.[45] Further investigation is needed to identify and possibly catalogue the various neuropeptide cotransmitters in regenerative neural populations, as a possible guide to both the

pathophysiology and future management of neurogenic dysfunctions. *Secondly*, presence of the regeneration as a minor component of intrinsic neural change might suggest infraspinal lower motoneuron NB. *Thirdly*, prominent adrenergic innervation in combination with nerve regeneration in the decentralization form of LMNB distinguishes it from both its infraspinal 'denervation' form and from UMNB. *Fourthly*, coexistence of abundant ultrastructurally normal with both degenerative and regenerative intrinsic axon profiles appears to be an important feature of supraspinal vs spinal UMNB.[37] It might be helpful to study the detrusor of various etiologic types of NB, both early and long-standing if possible, including various brain disorders – individually, in search for possible specific ultrastructural 'markers' of different causative entities. One important aspect of such a study would be detailed characterization of any identified copeptidergic neurotransmitter component(s).

It seems inevitable to conclude that the rhabdosphincter plays an important role in NB dysfunction, although the exact nature and scope of that role still need to be determined. The neuromuscular changes described in the feline rhabdosphincter following bilateral sacral ventral rhizotomy need to be studied, and confirmed or modified, in a unilateral rhizotomy model and in the human with LMNB or UMNB. Both the feline and the human rhabdosphincter also need to be fully studied physiologically, urodynamically, and pharmacologically to determine the functional impact and correlates of the postdenervation changes that have been and may yet be described.

Acknowledgment

Studies that led to the presented material were supported over two decades by grants AM-28000, NS-17144, AG-4390, and AG-08812 from the National Institutes of Health, USA, and the Pathology Medical Group Research Fund, Upstate Medical Center, State University of New York, Syracuse, NY. The author remains very grateful to the urologists who successively contributed with great skill, dedication, and effort to the various studies: Professors Doctors Mohamed Adel Atta and Ahmed Gamal ElDeen Hanno, University of Alexandria, Egypt, and Axel Haferkamp, University of Bonn, Germany. The suggestions, scientific input, and encouragement over many years of Professors Drs John W. Downie, Dalhousie University, Nova Scotia, Canada, Neil M. Resnick, University of Pittsburgh, Pennsylvania, USA, and Subbarao V. Yalla, Harvard University, Boston, Massachusetts, USA, have been inspirational and deeply appreciated. The author owes a great debt of gratitude to the numerous specialists who contributed to the immense technical aspects of the various studies.

References

1. Bors E, Comarr AE. Neurological urology. New York: Karger, 1971.

2. Gibbon NOK. Nomenclature of neurogenic bladder. Urology 1976; 8:423–431.

3. Forney JP. The effect of radical hysterectomy on bladder physiology. Am J Obstet Gynecol 1980; 138:374–382.

4. Gerstenberg TC, Nielsen ML, Clausen S, et al. Bladder function after abdominoperineal resection of the rectum for anorectal cancer. Urodynamic investigation before and after operation in consecutive series. Ann Surg 1980; 191:81–86.

5. McGuire EJ, Yalla SV, Elbadawi A. Abnormalities of vesicourethral function following radical pelvic extirpative surgery. In: Yalla SV, McGuire EJ, Elbadawi A, Blaivas JG, eds. Neurourology and urodynamics: principles and practice. New York: McMillan, 1988: 331–337.

6. Seski JC, Diokno A. Bladder dysfunction after radical abdominal hysterectomy. Am J Obstet Gynecol 1977; 128:643–651.

7. Smith PH, Ballantyne B. The neuroanatomical basis for denervation of the urinary bladder following major pelvic surgery. Br J Surg 1968; 55:929–932.

8. Yalla SV, Andriole GL. Vesicourethral dysfunction following pelvic visceral ablative surgery. J Urol 1984; 132:503–509.

9. Blackford HN, Murray K, Stephenson TP, Mundy AR. Results of transvesical infiltration of the pelvic plexus with phenol in 116 patients. Br J Urol 1984; 56:647–649.

10. Ewing R, Bultitude MI, Shuttleworth KED. Subtrigonal phenol injection for urge incontinence secondary to detrusor instability in females. Br J Urol 1982; 54:689–692.

11. Mundy AR, Stephenson TP. Transvesical injection of the pelvic plexus with phenol for treatment of detrusor hyperreflexia/instability and bladder hypersensitivity. Proc 14th Ann Mtg Int Cont Soc 1984: 55–56.

12. Elbadawi A. Functional anatomy of the organs of micturition. Urol Clin N Am 1996; 23:177–210.

13. Elbadawi A. Functional pathology of urinary bladder muscularis: the new frontier in diagnostic uropathology. Sem Diagn Pathol 1993; 10:314–354.

14. Alm P, Elmér M. Adrenergic and cholinergic innervation of the rat urinary bladder. Acta Physiol Scand 1975; 94:36–45.

15. Alm P, Elmér M. Adrenergic reinnervation of the denervated rat urinary bladder. Experientia 1979; 35:1387–1388.

16. Carpenter FG. Histological changes in parasympathetically denervated feline bladder. Am J Physiol 1951; 166: 692–698.

17. Dahlström A. The adrenergic innervation of the urinary bladder of the cat and man in the normal state and after parasympathetic denervation. Acta Pharmacol Toxicol 1978; 43:19–25.

18. Gu J, Blank M, Morrison J, et al. Origin of vasoactive intestinal polypeptide containing nerves in the urinary bladder of rat. Presented at 1st Symposium on VIP and Related Peptides, 1983.

19. Kirby RS, Fowler CJ, Gilpin SA, et al. Bladder muscle biopsy and urethral sphincter EMG in patients with bladder dysfunction after pelvic surgery. J Roy Soc Med 1986; 79:270–273.

20. Neal DE, Bogue PR, Williams RE. The histology of the innervation of the bladder in patients with denervation after excision of the rectum for carcinoma. Br J Urol 1982; 54:658–666.

21. Norlén L. The autonomous bladder: a clinical and experimental study. Scand J Urol Nephrol 1976; (Suppl 36):1–28.

22. Norlén L, Dahlström A, Sundin T, Svedmyr N. The adrenergic innervation and adrenergic receptor activity of the feline urinary bladder and urethra in the normal state and after hypogastric and/or parasympathetic denervation. Scand J Urol Nephrol 1976; 10:177–184.

23. Parsons KF, Scott AG, Traer S. Endoscopic biopsy in the diagnosis of peripheral denervation of the bladder. Br J Urol 1980; 52:455–459.

24. Sundin T, Dahlström A. The sympathetic innervation of the urinary bladder and urethra in the normal state and after parasympathetic denervation at the spinal root level. An experimental study in cats. Scand J Urol Nephrol 1973; 7:131–149.

25. Sundin T, Dahlström A, Norlén L, Svedmyr N. The sympathetic innervation and adrenoreceptor function of the human lower urinary tract in the normal state and after parasympathetic denervation. Invest Urol 1977; 14:322–328.

26. van Poppel H, Stessens R, Baert L et al. Vasoactive intestinal polypeptidergic innervation of the human urinary bladder in normal and pathological conditions. Urol Int 1988; 43: 205–210.

27. Elbadawi A, Atta MA, Franck JI. Intrinsic neuromuscular defects in the neurogenic bladder. I. Short-term ultrastructural changes in muscular innervation of the decentralized feline bladder base following unilateral sacral ventral rhizotomy. Neurourol Urodyn 1984; 3:93–113.

28. Atta MA, Franck JI, Elbadawi A. Intrinsic neuromuscular defects in the neurogenic bladder. II. Long-term innervation of the unilaterally decentralized feline bladder base by regenerated cholinergic, increased adrenergic and emergent probable "peptidergic" nerves. Neurourol Urodyn 1984; 3:185–200.

29. Elbadawi A, Atta MA. Intrinsic neuromuscular defects in the neurogenic bladder. III. Transjunctional, short- and long-term changes in muscle cells of the decentralized feline bladder base following unilateral sacral ventral rhizotomy. Neurourol Urodyn 1984; 3:245–270.

30. Atta MA. Elbadawi A. Intrinsic neuromuscular defects in the neurogenic bladder. IV. Loss of somatomotor and preservation of autonomic innervation of the male feline rhabdosphincter following bilateral sacral ventral rhizotomy. Neurourol Urodyn 1985; 4:219–229.

31. Elbadawi A, Atta MA. Intrinsic neuromuscular defects in the neurogenic bladder. V. Autonomic reinnervation of the male feline rhabdosphincter following somatic denervation by bilateral sacral ventral rhizotomy. Neurourol Urodyn 1986; 5:65–85.

32. Elbadawi A, Atta MA. Intrinsic neuromuscular defects in the neurogenic bladder. VI. Myofiber ultrastructure in the somatically denervated male feline rhabdosphincter. Neurourol Urodyn 1986; 5:453–473.

33. Elbadawi A, Atta MA. Hanno AG-E. Intrinsic neuromuscular defects in the neurogenic bladder. VIII. Effects of unilateral pelvic and pelvic plexus neurectomy on ultrastructure of the feline bladder base. Neurourol Urodyn 1988; 7:77–92.

34. Hanno AG-E, Atta MA, Elbadawi A. Intrinsic neuromuscular defects in the neurogenic bladder. IX. Effects of combined parasympathetic decentralization and hypogastric neurectomy on neuromuscular ultrastructure of the feline bladder base. Neurourol Urodyn 1988; 7:93–111.

35. Elbadawi A, Resnick NM, Dörsam J, et al. Structural basis of neurogenic bladder dysfunction. I. Methods of prospective ultrastructural study and overview of the findings. J Urol 2003; 169:540–546.

36. Haferkamp A, Dörsam J, Resnick NM, et al. Structural basis of neurogenic bladder dysfunction. II. Myogenic basis of detrusor hyperreflexia. J Urol 2003; 169:547–554.

37. Haferkamp A, Dörsam J, Resnick NM, et al. Structural basis of neurogenic bladder dysfunction. III. Intrinsic detrusor innervation. J Urol 2003; 169:555–562.

38. Gabella G. Hypertrophy of intestinal smooth muscle. Cell Tis Res 1975; 163:199–214.

39. Sehn JT. Anatomic effect of distension therapy in unstable bladder. New Approach. Urology 1978; 11:581–587.

40. Sehn JT. The ultrastructural effect of distension on the neuromuscular apparatus of the urinary bladder. Invest Urol 1979; 16:369–375.

41. Hailemariam S, Elbadawi A, Yalla SV, Resnick NM. Structural basis of geriatric voiding dysfunction. V. Standardized protocols for routine ultrastructural study and diagnosis of endoscopic detrusor biopsies. J Urol 1997; 157:1783–1801.

42. Elbadawi A. Neuromorphologic basis of vesicourethral function. I. Histochemistry, ultrastructure, and function of intrinsic nerves of the bladder and urethra. Neurourol Urodyn 1982; 1:3–50.

43. Tranzer JP, Thoenen H. Electron microscopic localization of 5-hydroxydopamine (3,4,5-trihydroxyphenyl-ethylamine), a new "false" sympathetic transmitter. Experientia 1967; 23:743–744.

44. Elbadawi A, Atta MA. Intrinsic neuromuscular defects in the neurogenic bladder. X. Value and limitations of neurohistochemistry. Neurourol Urodyn 1989; 8:263–276.

45. Elbadawi A, Yalla SV, Resnick NM. Structural basis of geriatric voiding dysfunction. II. Aging detrusor: normal versus impaired contractility. J Urol 1993; 150:1657–1667.

46. Elbadawi A, Yalla SV, Resnick NM. Structural basis of geriatric voiding dysfunction. III. Detrusor overactivity. J Urol 1993; 150:1668–1680.

47. Elbadawi A, Yalla SV, Resnick NM. Structural basis of geriatric voiding dysfunction. IV. Bladder outlet obstruction. J Urol 1993; 150:1681–1695.

48. Elbadawi A, Hailemariam S, Yalla SV, Resnick NM. Structural basis of geriatric voiding dysfunction. VI. Validation and update of diagnostic criteria in 71 detrusor biopsies. J Urol 1997; 157:1802–1813.

49. Bareggi S, Dahlström A, Häggendal J. Intra-axonal transport and degeneration of adrenergic nerve terminals after axotomy with long and short nerve stump. Med Biol 1974; 52:327–335.

50. Bennett T, Burnstock G, Cobb JLS, Malmfors T. An ultrastructural and histochemical study of the short-term effects of 6-hydroxydopamine on adrenergic nerves in the domestic fowl. Br J Pharmacol 1970; 38:802–809.

51. Blümcke S, Dengler HJ. Noradrenalin content and ultrastructure of adrenergic nerves of rabbit iris after sympathectomy and hypoxia. Virch Arch 1970; 6:281–293.

52. Bray GM, Peyronnard JM, Aguayo AJ. Reaction of unmyelinated nerve fibers to injury – an ultrastructural study. Brain Res 1972; 42:297–309.

53. Dail WG Jr, Evan AP, Gerristen GC, Dublin WE. Abnormalities in pelvic visceral nerves. A basis for neurogenic bladder in the diabetic Chinese hamster. Invest Urol 1977; 15:161–166.

54. Dvorak AM, Osage JE, Monahan RA, Dickersin GR. Crohn's disease: transmission electron microscopic studies. III. Target tissues, Proliferation of and injury to smooth muscle and the autonomic nervous system. Human Pathol 1980; 11:620–634.

55. Fehér E, Csányi K, Vajda J. Degeneration analysis of the efferent nerves to the urinary bladder in the cat. Acta Anat 1980; 107:80–90.

56. Garrett JR. Changes in autonomic nerves of salivary glands on degeneration and regeneration. Prog Brain Res 1971; 34:475–488.

57. Gordon-Weeks P, Gabella G. Degeneration of varicose axons and their phagocytosis by smooth muscle cells. J Neurocytol 1977; 6:711–721.

58. Hámori J, Lánge E, Simon L. Experimental degeneration of the preganglionic fibers in the superior cervical ganglion of the cat. An electron microscopic study. Z Zellforsch 1968; 90:37–52.

59. Heath JW, Evans BK, Burnstock G. Axon retraction following guanethidine treatment. Studies of sympathetic neurons in vivo. Z Zellforsch 1973; 146:439–451.

60. Iwayama T. Ultrastructural changes in the nerves innervating the cerebral artery after sympathectomy. Z Zellforsch 1970; 109:465–480.

61. Joó F, Lever JD, Ivens C, et al. A fine structural and electron histochemical study of the axon terminals in the rat superior cervical ganglion after acute and chronic preganglionic denervation. J Anat 1971; 110:181–189.

62. Kapeller K, Mayor D. An electron microscopic study of the early changes distal to a constriction in sympathetic nerves. Proc Roy Soc London [Biol Sci] 1969; 172:53–63.

63. Knoche H, Terwort H. Elektronenmikroskopischer Beitrag zur Kenntnis von Degenerationsformen der vegetativen Endstrecke nach Durchschneidung postganglionärer Fasern. Z Zellforsch 1973; 141:181–202.

64. Lampert PW. A comparative electron microscopic study of reactive, degenerative, regenerating, and dystrophic axons. J Neuropathol Exp Neurol 1967; 26:345–368.

65. Mugnaini E, Friedrich VL Jr. Electron microscopy: identification and study of normal and degenerating neural elements by electron microscopy. In: Hiemer L, Robards MJ, eds., Neuroanatomical tract – tracing methods. New York: Plenum Press, 1980:377–406.

66. Révész E, van der Zypen E. Ultrastructural changes in adrenergic neurons following chemical sympathectomy. Acta Anat 1979; 105:198–208.

67. Roth CD, Richardson KC. Electron microscopical studies on axonal degeneration in the rat iris following ganglionectomy. Am J Anat 1969; 123:341–360.

68. Sporrong B, Alm P, Owman C, et al. Ultrastructural evidence of adrenergic nerve degeneration in the guinea pig uterus during pregnancy. Cell Tis Res 1978; 195:189–193.

69. Thomas PK, King RHM. The degeneration of unmyelinated axons following nerve section: an ultrastructural study. J Neurocytol 1974; 3:497–512.

70. Tranzer JP, Thoenen H. An electron microscopic study of selective, acute degeneration of sympathetic nerve terminals after administration of 6-hydroxydopamine. Experientia 1967; 24:155–156.

71. Uemura E, Fletcher TP, Dirks VA, Bradley WE. Distribution of sacral afferent axons in cat urinary bladder. Am J Anat 1973; 136:305–314.

72. van Orden LS III, Bensch KG, Langer SZ, Trendelenburg U. Histochemical and fine structural aspects of the onset of denervation supersensitivity in the nictitating membrane of the spinal cat. J Pharmacol Exp Ther 1967; 157:274–283.

73. Holtzman E, Novikoff AB. Lysosomes in the rat sciatic nerve following crushing. J Cell Biol 1965; 27:651–669.

74. Nageotte J. Sheaths of the peripheral nerves, nerve degeneration and regeneration. In: Penfield W, ed. Cytology and cellular pathology of the nervous system. New York: Hafner, 1965; 1:189–239.

75. Weiss P, Wang H. Transformation of adult Schwann cells into macrophages. Proc Soc Exp Biol Med 1945; 58:273–275.

76. Cowan WM. Antegrade and retrograde transneuronal degeneration in the central and peripheral nervous system. In: Nauta WJH, Ebbesson SOL, eds. Contemporary research methods in neuroanatomy. New York: Springer-Verlag, 1970:217–251.

77. Eidelberg E, Nguyen LH, Polich R, Walden JG. Transsynaptic degeneration of motoneurones caudal to spinal cord lesions. Brain Res Bull 1989; 22:39–45.

78. Blümcke S, Niedorf HR. Fluoreszenzmikroskopische und Elektronenmikroskopische untersuchungen an regenerierenden adrenergischen Nervenfasern. Z Zellforsch 1965; 68:724–732.

79. Blümcke S, Niedorf HR. Elektronenoptische Untersuchungen an Wachstumsendkolben regenerierenden peripherer Nervenfasern. Virch Arch Pathol Anat 1965; 340:93–104.

80. Diamond J, Cooper E, Turner C, Macintyre L. Trophic regulation of nerve sprouting. Science 1976; 193:371–377.

81. Elbadawi A. Autonomic innervation of the vesical outlet and its role in micturition. In: Hinman F Jr, ed. Benign prostatic hypertrophy. New York: Springer-Verlag, 1983:330–348.

82. Elbadawi A. Ultrastructure of vesicourethral innervation. II. Postganglionic axoaxonal synapses in intrinsic innervation of the vesicourethral lissosphincter. J Urol 1984;131:781–790.

83. Bevan RD, Tsuru H. Long-term denervation of vascular smooth muscle causes not only functional but structural changes. Blood Vess 1979; 16:109–112.

84. Campbell GR, Gibbins I, Allan I, Gannon B. Effects of long term denervation on smooth muscle of the chicken expansor secundarorium. Cell Tiss Res 1977; 176:143–156.

85. Drachman DB. Trophic interactions between nerves and muscles: the role of cholinergic transmission (including usage) and other factors. In: Goldberg AM, Hanin I, eds. Biology of cholinergic function. New York: Raven Press, 1976:161–186.

86. Gutmann E. Neurotrophic relations. Ann Rev Physiol 1976; 38:177–216.

87. Tweedle CD. The development and maintenance of smooth muscle in control and aneurogenic amphibians (Ambystoma). Cell Tiss Res 1976; 166:275–283.

88. Varon SS, Bunge RP. Trophic mechanisms in the peripheral nervous system. Ann Rev Neurosci 1978; 1:327–361.

89. Westfall DP, Lee TJ-F, Stitzel RE. Morphological and biochemical changes in supersensitive smooth muscle. Fed Proc 1975; 34:1985–1989.

90. Lapides J, Friend CR, Ajemian EP, Reus WS. Denervation supersensitivity as a test for neurogenic bladder. Surg Gynecol Obstet 1962: 114:241–244.

91. Elmér M. Degeneration activity in the rat urinary bladder. Acta Physiol Scand 1973; 87:223–227.

92. Elmér M. Action of drugs on the innervated and denervated urinary bladder of the rat. Acta Physiol Scand 1974; 91:289–297.

93. Ekström J, Elmér M, Banns H. Transient supersensitivity in the partially denervated rat urinary bladder. Acta Pharmacol Toxicol 1978; 43:318–322.

94. Emmelin N, Trendelenburg U. Denervation activity after parasympathetic or sympathetic denervation. Ergeb Physiol 1968; 66:147–211.

95. Elmér M. Atropine sensitivity of the rat urinary bladder during nerve degeneration. Acta Physiol Scand 1975; 93:202–205.

96. Ekström J, Elmér P. Compensatory increase of responses to nerve stimulation of the partially denervated rat urinary bladder. Acta Physiol Scand 1980; 110:21–29.

97. El-Salmy S, Downie JW, Awad SA. Bladder and urethral function and supersensitivity to subcutaneously administered bethanechol in cats with chronic cauda equina lesions. J Urol 1985; 134:1011–1018.

98. Norlén L, Sundin T. Alpha-adrenolytic treatment in patients with autonomous bladders. Acta Pharmacol Toxicol 1978; 43:31–34.

99. Müller HW, Ignatius MJ, Shooter EM. Degeneration and regeneration-associated polypeptides in rat peripheral nerve. Soc Neurosci Abst 1983; 9:45.

100. Ceccarelli B, Clementi F, Mantegazza P. Adrenergic reinnervation of smooth muscle of nictitating membrane by preganglionic sympathetic fibers. Arch Int Pharmacodyn Thér 1972; 196:293–295.

101. Jan YN, Jan LY. Coexistence and corelease of cholinergic and peptidergic transmitters in frog sympathetic ganglia. Fed Proc 1983; 42:2929–2933.

102. Landis SC. Development of cholinergic sympathetic neurons: evidence for transmitter plasticity in vivo. Fed Proc 1983; 42:1633–1638.

103. Drake MJ, Hedland P, Mills IW, et al. Structural and functional denervation of human detrusor after spinal core injury. Lab Invest 2000; 80:1491–1499.

104. Fries RP, Martinez TJ. Analysis of axon-sheath relations during early Wallerian degeneration. Brain Res 1970; 19:199–212.

105. Blümcke S, Niedorf HR. Electron microscope studies of Schwann cells during the Wallerian degeneration with special reference to the cytoplasmic filaments. Acta Neuropathol 1966; 6:46–60.

106. Nathaniel EJH, Pease DC. Collagen and basement membrane formation by Schwann cells during nerve regeneration. J Ultrastruc Res 1963; 9:550–560.

107. Payer AF. An ultrastructural study of Schwann cell response to axonal degeneration. J Comp Neurol 1979; 183:365–384.

108. Vial JD. The early changes in the axoplasm during Wallerian degeneration. J Biophys Biochem Cytol 1958; 4:551–567.

109. Bennett MR, Raftos J. The formation and regression of synapses during the re-innervation of axolotl striated muscles. J Physiol 1977; 265:264–295.

110. Fangboner RF, Vanable JW Jr. Formation and regression of inappropriate nerve sprouts during trochlear nerve regeneration in Xenopus laevis. J Comp Neurol 1974; 157:391–406.

111. Frank E, Jansen JKS, Lømo T, Westgaard RH. The interaction between foreign and original motor nerves innervating the soleus muscle of rats. J Physiol 1975; 247:725–743.

112. Kemplay S. Inhibition of parasympathetic axonal sprouting in the cat submandibular gland by sympathetic axons. A histochemical study. Cell Tiss Res 1980; 207:155–163.

113. Purves D. Persistent innervation of mammalian sympathetic neurones by native and foreign fibers. Nature 1975; 256:589–590.

114. Shimahara T, Tauc L. Multiple interneuronal afferents to the giant cells in Aplysia. J Physiol 1975; 247:299–319.

115. Elbadawi A, Atta MA. Ultrastructure of vesicourethral innervation. IV. Evidence for somatomotor plus autonomic innervation of the male feline rhabdosphincter. Neurourol Urodyn 1985; 4:23–36.

116. Elbadawi A, Matthews R, Light JK, Wheeler T. Immunohistochemical and ultrastructural study of rhabdosphincter component of prostatic capsule. J Urol 1997; 158:1819–1828.

117. Atta MA, Elbadawi A. Intrinsic neuromuscular defects in the neurogenic bladder. VII. Neurohistochemistry of the somatically denervated male feline rhabdosphincter. Neurourol Urodyn 1987; 6:47–56.

118. Manolov S. Initial changes in the neuromuscular synapses of denervated rat diaphragm. Brain Res 1974; 63:303–316.

119. Cullen MJ, Johnson MA, Mastaglia FL. Pathological reactions of skeletal muscle. In: Mastaglia FL, Walton JN, eds. Skeletal muscle pathology. Edinburgh: Churchill Livingstone, 1992:123–184.

120. Engel WK. Muscle target fibers, a newly recognized sign of denervation. Nature 1961; 191:389–390.

121. Gori A. Proliferation of the sarcoplasmic reticulum and the T system in denervated muscle fibers. Virch Arch (Abt B) Zell Pathol 1972; 11:147–160.

122. Jennekens FGI. Neurogenic disorders of muscle. In: Mastaglia FL, Walton JN, eds. Skeletal muscle pathology. Edinburgh: Churchill Livingstone, 1992:563–597.

123. Kovarsky J, Schochet SS, McCormick WF. The significance of target fibers: a clinicopathologic review of 100 patients with neurogenic atrophy. Am J Clin Pathol 1973; 59:790–797.

124. Mair WGP, Tomé FMS. Atlas of the ultrastructure of diseased human muscle. Edinburgh: Churchill Livingstone, 1972.

125. Pellegrino C, Franzini C. An electron microscopic study of denervation atrophy in red and white skeletal muscle. fibers. J Cell Biol 1963; 17:327–349.

126. Price HM. Ultrastructural pathologic characteristics of the skeletal muscle fiber: an introductory survey. In: Pearson CM, Mostofi FK, eds. The striated muscle. Baltimore: Williams & Wilkins, 1973:144–184.

127. Schochet SS Jr, Lampert PW. Diagnostic electron microscopy of skeletal muscle. In: Trump BF, Jones RT, eds. Diagnostic electron microscopy. New York: Wiley, 1978:209–251.

128. Shafiq SA, Milhorat AT, Gorycki MA. Fine structure of human muscle in neurogenic atrophy. Neurology 1967; 17:934–948.

129. Stennington HH, Engel AG. Normal and denervated muscle: a morphometric study of fine structure. Neurology 1973; 23:714–724.

130. Tomanek RJ, Lund DD. Degeneration of different types of skeletal muscle fibers. I. Denervation. J Anat 1973; 116:395–407.

131. Carlson BM. The regeneration of skeletal muscle. A review. Am J Anat 1973; 137:119–150.

132. Dubowitz V. Pathology of experimentally reinnervated skeletal muscle. J Neurol Neurosurg Psychiat 1967; 30:99–110.

133. Reznik M. Origin of myoblast during skeletal muscle regeneration. Electron microscopic observations. Lab Invest 1969; 20:353–363.

134. Reznik M. Current concepts of skeletal muscle regeneration. In: Pearson CM, Mostofi FK, eds. The striated muscle. Baltimore: Williams & Wilkins, 1973:185–225.

135. Shafiq SA, Gorycki MA. Regeneration in skeletal muscle of mouse: some electron microscopic observations. J Pathol Bacteriol 1965; 90:123–127.

136. Dudel J. Excitation of nerve and muscle. In: Schmidt RF, ed. Fundamentals of neurophysiology. New York: Springer-Verlag, 1978:19–71.

137. Dennis MJ, Miledi R. Non-transmitting neuromuscular junctions during an early stage of end-plate reinnervation. J Physiol (London) 1974; 239:553–570.

138. Dennis MJ, Miledi R. Characteristics of transmitter release in regenerating frog neuromuscular junctions. J Physiol (London) 1974; 239:571–594.

139. Miledi R. Properties of regenerating neuromuscular synapses in the frog. J Physiol (London) 1960; 154:190–205.

140. Beranék R, Vyskočil F. The action of tubocurarine and atropine on the normal and denervated rat diaphragm. J Physiol (London) 1967; 188:53–66.

141. Feltz A, Mallart A. Ionic permeability changes induced by some cholinergic agonists in normal and denervated frog muscles. J Physiol (London) 1971; 218:101–116.

142. Guth L. "Trophic" influences of nerve on muscle. Physiol Rev 1968; 48:645–687.

143. Gutman E. Neurotrophic relations. Ann Rev Physiol 1976; 38:177–216.

144. Margreth A, Salviati G, Di Mauro S, Turati G. Early biochemical consequences of denervation in fast and slow skeletal muscles and their relationship to neural control over muscle differentiation. Biochem J 1972; 126:1099–1110.

145. Miledi R, Stefani E. Nonselective re-innervation of slow and fast muscle fibers in the rat. Nature 1969; 222:569–571.

146. Crain SM, Peterson ER. The regeneration of skeletal muscle, a review. Ann NY Acad Sci 1974; 228:6–34.

147. Kobayachi T, Tsukagoshi H, Shimizu Y. Trophic effects of sympathetic ganglia on normal and dystrophic chicken skeletal muscle in tissue culture. Exp Neurol 1982; 77:241–253.

148. Landmesser L. Pharmacological properties, cholinesterase activity, and anatomy of nerve–muscle junctions in vagus-innervated frog sartorius. J Physiol (London) 1972; 220:243–256.

149. Mendez J, Aranda LC, Luco JV. Antifibrillary effect of adrenergic fibers on denervated striated muscles. J Neurophysiol 1970; 33:882–890.

150. Bauer SB, Labib KB, Dieppa RA, Retik AB. Urodynamic evaluation of boy with myelodysplasia and incontinence. Urology 1977; 10:354–362.

151. Axelsson J, Thesleff S. A study of supersensitivity in denervated mammalian skeletal muscle. J Physiol (London) 1959; 178:193.

152. Harris TJ. Inductive functions of the nervous system. Ann Rev Physiol 1974; 36:251–305.

153. McArdle JJ, Albuquerque EX. A study on the reinnervation of the fast and slow mammalian muscles. J Gen Physiol 1973; 61:1–23.

154. Miledi R. The acetylcholine sensitivity of frog muscle fibres after complete or partial denervation. J Physiol 1960; 151:1–23.

155. Banerjee SP, Sharma VK, Kung LS. β-adrenergic receptors in innervated and denervated skeletal muscle. Biochim Biophys Acta 1977; 470:123–127.

156. Bowman WC, Raper C. The effects of sympathomimetic amines on chronically denervated skeletal muscles. Br J Pharmacol 1965; 24:98–109.

157. Bowman WC, Raper C. Adrenotropic receptors in skeletal muscle. Ann NY Acad Sci 1967; 139:741–753.

158. Eakins KE, Katz RP. The effects of sympathetic stimulation and epinephrine on the superior rectus muscle of the cat. J Pharmacol Exp Ther 1967; 157:524–531.

159. Paterson G. The dual action of adrenaline on denervated skeletal muscle. Biochem Pharmacol 1963; 12(Suppl):85.

160. Rodger IW, Bowman WC. Adrenoreceptors in skeletal muscle. In: Kunos G, ed. Adrenoreceptors and catecholamine action, Part B. New York: Wiley and Sons, 1983:123–125.

161. Yamada K, Harigaya S. Contractile response to sympathomimetic amines in isolated rat muscle after chronic denervation. Jpn J Pharmacol 1974; 24:2187–2190.

9

Pathophysiology of the overactive bladder

Alison F Brading

Introduction

In the proceedings of the Second International Consultation on Incontinence, the overactive bladder is described as one which fails to remain relaxed until an appropriate time for urination.[1] The resulting symptom syndrome includes the symptoms of urgency, with or without urge incontinence, usually with frequency and nocturia. International Continence Society (ICS) terminology in 2002[2] classifies the overactive bladder as one in which the symptoms are suggestive of urodynamically demonstrable detrusor overactivity (involuntary detrusor contraction) during the filling phase, which may be spontaneously provoked. Detrusor overactivity is thus a urodynamic observation, and the term replaces detrusor instability. It can be subdivided into neurogenic (when there is a relevant neurological condition) or non-neurogenic (including idiopathic overactivity, and overactivity related to outflow obstruction and aging).

The very fact that the symptom syndrome is found in patients with all the different associations of detrusor overactivity suggests that there may well be common underlying pathological changes in the bladder wall, and indeed examination of the physiological properties and ultrastructure of bladder wall obtained from human overactive bladders or bladder from animal models of overactivity supports this assertion. In this chapter the common pathophysiological features of the overactive bladder will be discussed and their significance examined. The possible causes of the changes will then be explored, and the chapter will end with a consideration of the origin of probably the most 'bothersome' of the symptoms, that is urgency.

The following changes in the detrusor are routinely seen:

- increased spontaneous myogenic activity
- fused tetanic contractions
- altered responsiveness to stimuli
- characteristic changes in smooth muscle ultrastructure.

Examination of the peripheral innervation and the micturition reflex in animals and humans with overactive bladders also shows common changes:

- patchy denervation of the bladder wall
- enlarged sensory neurons
- enlarged parasympathetic ganglion cells
- increased effectiveness of a spinal micturition pathway.

All these common features make it very likely that whatever the etiology of the condition, the underlying causative mechanisms are the same or very similar. I will first discuss the normal properties of the detrusor and then consider the changes seen in more detail.

Smooth muscle of the bladder wall

Normal properties of the detrusor

Smooth muscle strips dissected from normal animal or human detrusor have characteristic properties. A proportion of them will develop spontaneous contractile behavior, featuring small transient rises in pressure from a low or zero baseline tone, the size of which is considerably smaller than that of evoked contractions (Figure 9.1). These spontaneous contractions are myogenic, and are not abolished either by tetrodotoxin which blocks conducted action potentials in nerves, or by receptor antagonists.[3] The strips can be activated by transmural stimulation of the intrinsic nerves with short electrical current pulses in a frequency-dependent manner, or directly activated by longer current pulses. Contraction mediated by intrinsic nerves can be totally abolished in normal human bladder by the muscarinic receptor antagonist atropine[4] (Figure 9.2), although in animal bladders there is usually an atropine-resistant component which predominates at low frequencies and is

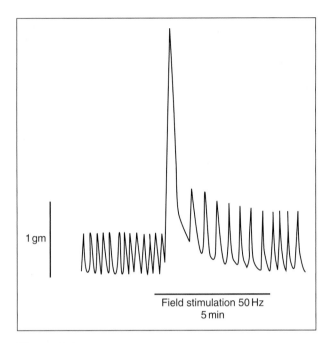

Figure 9.1
Spontaneous contractile activity in a strip of smooth muscle dissected from the detrusor of a pig bladder. At the arrow the intramural nerves were stimulated for 5 s at 50 Hz.

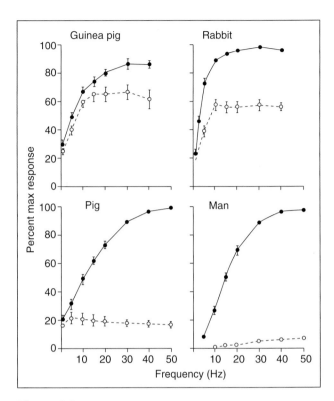

Figure 9.3
Frequency–response curves of detrusor strips from various animals under control conditions (filled symbols) and in the presence of atropine (open symbols). Note the species dependency of the size of the atropine-resistant responses. These curves were further suppressed in the presence of tetrodotoxin with the exception of the human bladder, where the atropine-resistant contractions were also TTX resistant, and presumably due to direct smooth muscle stimulation (not shown).

mediated by neuronal release of ATP (Figure 9.3; for references see Brading[3]).

This purinergic innervation may be used to produce small spurts of urine without bladder emptying for territorial marking. Strips from animal and human bladders will also respond by contracting in a dose-dependent manner to depolarization with high potassium solutions and application of muscarinic and P2x purinoceptor agonists, although activation of purinoceptors cannot initiate the full contractile response available to the strip.

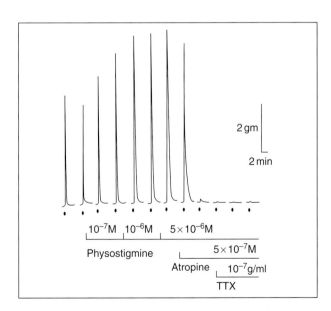

Figure 9.2
Contractile responses in a strip of human detrusor to transmural field stimulation (20 Hz, 5 s) of the intrinsic nerves. Note that the size of the response is enhanced by the cholinesterase inhibitor physostigmine, and almost completely blocked by the muscarinic antagonist atropine. (Reproduced from Sibley with permission.)[5]

Changes to the smooth muscle of the bladder wall

Spontaneous activity

Smooth muscle strips dissected from overactive bladders often show increases in spontaneous contractile activity.

This has been seen in human bladder strips from obstructed overactive bladders[5] and from neuropathic overactive bladders.[6] A change in the pattern of the spontaneous activity is also seen which is very characteristic of bladder overactivity. Strips from overactive bladders show fused tetanic contractions[7–10] (Figure 9.4), reminiscent of the activity typically shown by well-coupled smooth muscles such as in the gut. Similar fused tetanic contractions are seen in bladders from pigs with instability secondary to outflow obstruction; indeed in those with well-developed instability, bizarre patterns are often observed[11] (Figure 9.5).

Altered responsiveness to stimuli

Alterations are also seen in the responses of overactive detrusor to stimulation with agonists and to transmural electrical stimulation (either direct or via activation of intrinsic nerves). In this case, there are differences in the patterns seen in tissues from overactive bladders of different etiology. In obstructed bladders there is a supersensitivity to muscarinic agonists and KCl with a reduced contraction to intrinsic nerve stimulation.[5,12–14] Similar changes are seen in animal models of bladder overactivity (pig[15,16] and rabbit[17]) (Figure 9.6). In neuropathic bladders from patients with spina bifida (Figures 9.7 and 9.8), supersensitivity is again seen to cholinergic agonists and KCl, but there is no change in the sensitivity of the contractile response to intrinsic nerve stimulation, although the size of the response is smaller.[6] In idiopathic overactivity, bladder strips show supersensitivity to KCl, but not to muscarinic agonists (Figure 9.9) and there is a reduced contractile response to intrinsic nerve stimulation.[10] We have also found evidence that overactive strips are more easily activated by direct electrical stimulation of the smooth muscle (showing contractions elicited by transmural nerve stimulation that are resistant to the nerve blocking action of tetrodotoxin (TTX) (Figure 9.10).[18]

Ultrastructural changes

At an ultrastructural level, a common feature seen in overactive detrusor is the presence of protrusion junctions and ultra-close abutments between the smooth muscle cells, features occurring only rarely in normal tissue.[19] Again, development of these junctions has been seen in animal models.[20]

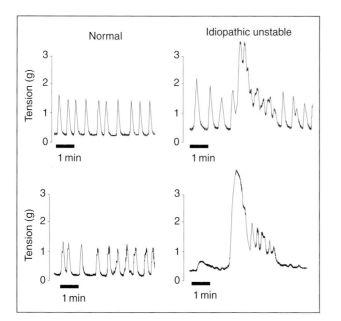

Figure 9.4
Spontaneous contractile activity in detrusor strips dissected from normal (left) and idiopathically overactive (right) human bladders. Note the typical small phasic contractions of the normal detrusor strips, and the larger fused contractions in strips from overactive bladders. (Reproduced from Mills with permission.)[42]

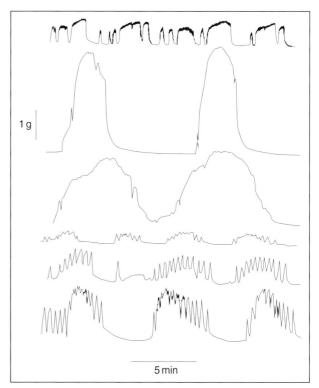

Figure 9.5
Bizarre spontaneous contractile activity in strips of smooth muscle dissected from the bladders of pigs with an overactive bladder due to partial bladder outlet obstruction. Note the spontaneous large fused tetanic contraction, which can reach an amplitude larger than the response to transmural stimulation (not shown). (Reproduced from Turner with permission.)[11]

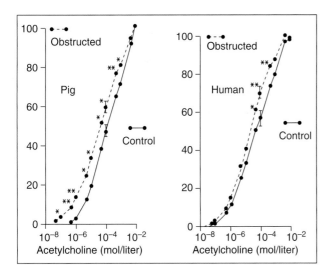

Figure 9.6
Concentration–contractile response curve to 10 s applications of carbachol to strips from normal human (right) and pig (left) bladders (straight line curve) and bladders from patients and pigs with overactive bladders secondary to bladder outflow obstruction (dotted line curve). Note the increased sensitivity of the smooth muscle to the muscarinic agonist. (Stars indicate significant difference from control.) (Reproduced from Sibley.[5])

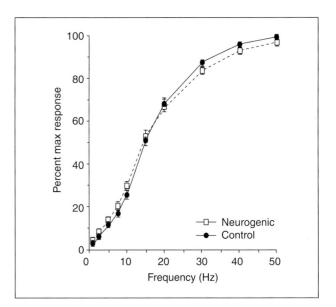

Figure 9.8
Frequency–response curve to transmural nerve stimulation of strips from normal human bladders (circles) and bladders from patients with overactive bladders secondary to spina bifida (squares). Expressed as a percentage of the maximal response of each strip, there is no significant difference between the two curves, indicating that the sensitivity to stimulation is unchanged, although the absolute size of the response is smaller in strips from the overactive bladders. (Reproduced from German et al with permission.)[6]

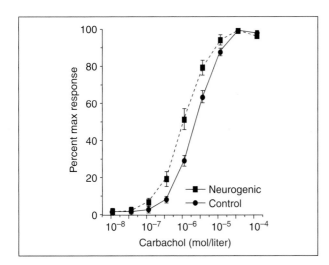

Figure 9.7
Concentration–contractile response curve to 10 s applications of carbachol to strips from normal human bladders (circles) and bladders from spina bifida patients with neurogenic overactive bladders (squares). Expressed as a percentage of the maximal response of each strip, strips from the overactive bladders are significantly more sensitive to muscarinic agonists. (Reproduced from German et al with permission.)[6]

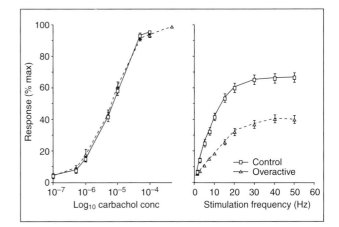

Figure 9.9
Log concentration–response curves (to 10 s carbachol) and frequency response curves of human bladder strips from normal (straight line curve) bladders and bladders from patients with idiopathic detrusor overactivity (dotted line curve).

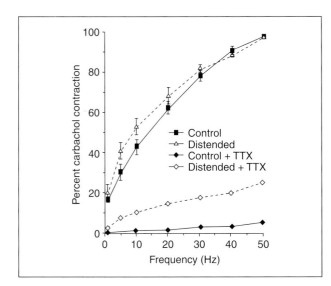

Figure 9.10
Frequency–response curves of strips from pig bladders to electrical field stimulation and the effects of tetrodotoxin (TTX) in normal pigs (black curves), and those with overactive bladders secondary to previous overdistention (red curves). Note the TTX resistant contractions in the strips from overactive bladders. (Reproduced from Sethia with permission.)[18]

Significance of these changes

The properties of the normal detrusor suggest that the smooth muscle bundles are not as well coupled electrically as are most visceral smooth muscles. This suggestion is supported by the fact that spontaneous myogenic contractions only produce a fraction of the tension available on synchronous activation of the whole strip and by the lack of clearly defined gap junctions between the smooth muscle cells (e.g. see Daniel et al[21]). Immunohistochemical studies do, however, demonstrate the presence of connexins (the gap-junction proteins) in the detrusor,[22] and electrophysiological measurements in the guinea pig[23–25] show that individual cells within a bundle are electrically coupled to their neighbors, but that spread of current between cells in the axial direction is poor, with current spread rarely occurring between pairs of cells separated by more than 40 μm in the axial direction. This poorly developed electrical coupling prevents synchronous activation of all the smooth muscles in the strip from spontaneous action potentials, and is likely to account for the small size of the spontaneous contractions. In the whole bladder, the great compliance of the bladder wall means that intravesical pressure will only rise when there is synchronous contraction of the majority of smooth muscle cells in the wall. The lack of good coupling means that *in-vivo* electrical activity will be able to control the length of individual cells without the risk of generating a rise in intravesical pressure. Synchronous activation of the muscle and a rise in intravesical pressure during micturition

requires coordinated activation of the smooth muscle, and is achieved through the dense parasympathetic innervation in which varicosities form close junctions with the great majority of the smooth muscle cells.[21,26]

The changes that occur in the smooth muscle of the overactive bladders strongly suggest that the cells are better coupled by some means, so that spontaneous activity will spread and initiate synchronous contractions in many more smooth muscle cells. This would account for the fused tetanic contractions seen in the overactive bladder strips; the close abutments and protrusion junctions seen ultrastructurally may be the morphological correlates of this connectivity. In the whole bladder, the increased excitability of the smooth muscle combined with the greater connectivity results in the situation where a focus of electrical activity can spread to activate the whole detrusor and produce an overactive contraction. Such a focus of activity could arise myogenically or could be evoked by activation of a few motor nerves, which in the normal bladder would not elevate intravesical pressure. A myogenic origin of the spontaneous pressure rises seen in pigs with overactive bladders is certainly suggested since they persist after section of the sacral roots[18] (Figure 9.11), and can still occur in the presence of TTX[11] (Figure 9.12).

Why should such changes occur in the smooth muscle of overactive bladders? Smooth muscle, along with most innervated tissues, is capable of altering its responses to changes in its pattern of activation. The types of change that are seen in the detrusor smooth muscle are reminiscent of the changes due to experimental denervation.[27] It seems very likely that the changes in detrusor properties are caused by altered patterns of activation. This will be explored below.

Changes in peripheral innervation and the micturition reflex

Changes in the bladder wall

Another common feature of overactive detrusor is a change in the macroscopic structure of the bladder wall. Regardless of the etiology of the condition, sections of the bladder wall from overactive human bladder frequently show patchy denervation of the muscle bundles. Some muscle bundles may be completely denervated, whereas neighboring ones appear normal (Figures 9.13 and 9.14) and in other areas sparser innervation is also seen.[6,10,20,28,29] A similar pattern is seen in animal models (pigs,[30] guinea pigs,[31] and rabbit[17]), although interestingly not in the rat,[26] where the postganglionic neurons are all in the pelvic ganglia and not in the bladder wall. The denervated and sparsely innervated areas of the bladder wall become infiltrated with connective tissue elements such as collagen and elastin

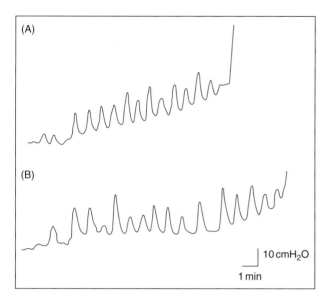

Figure 9.11
Overactive pressure rises in a pig during artificial filling. This animal had been made overactive by a partial bladder outflow obstruction several months earlier. (A) The situation when the spinal roots are intact and (B) after section of the dorsal and ventral spinal roots L7–S3. (Reproduced from Sethia with permission.)[18]

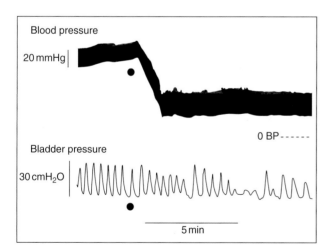

Figure 9.12
Urodynamic experiment in an anesthetized mini-pig. Upper trace, blood pressure; lower trace, intravesical pressure. The animal had an overactive bladder secondary to bladder outflow obstruction. At the dot, tetrodotoxin (TTX) was infused in an amount sufficient to prevent action potentials in the autonomic and somatic nerves. Note the rapid fall in blood pressure (removal of sympathetic tone), but persistence of bladder overactivity. Artificial ventilation was applied after TTX infusion, since respiration stopped. (Reproduced from Turner with permission.)[11]

(Figure 9.15),[6,20,28] and in the completely denervated areas in tissue from idiopathic and neuropathic overactive bladders, hypertrophy of the smooth muscle cells is seen.[28]

Changes in neuronal structure

Animal experiments (carried out mainly in the rat) have demonstrated that procedures such as spinal section or urethral obstruction, as well as leading to the development of bladder instability, also lead to an increase in size of both the afferent neurons in the dorsal root ganglia (L6–S1[32]) and the efferent neurons in the pelvic plexus (after obstruction[33,34] and after spinal section[35]). We have seen a similar increase in the size of the neurons in bladder wall ganglia in the obstructed guinea pig (unpublished work).

Changes in the micturition reflex

Changes have also been seen in the micturition reflex in animals after recovery from spinal shock following spinal

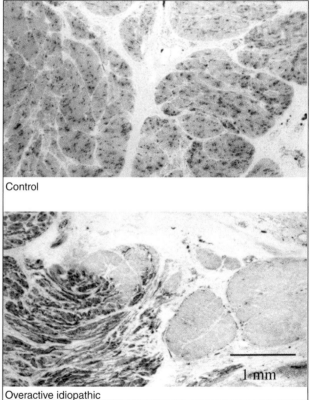

Figure 9.13
Sections of human detrusor stained to show the presence of acetylcholinesterase on the axons of intramural nerves. Upper trace from a normal bladder: note uniform dense staining of the smooth muscle bundles. Lower trace from a patient with idiopathic instability (note the patchy denervation of the smooth muscle bundles). (Reproduced from Mills et al with permission.)[10]

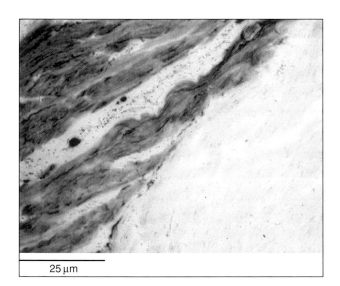

25 µm

Figure 9.14
Section of a human detrusor from a patient with an unstable bladder secondary to spina bifida. Note the exceptionally dense brown innervation of one muscle bundle adjacent to another completely denervated bundle.

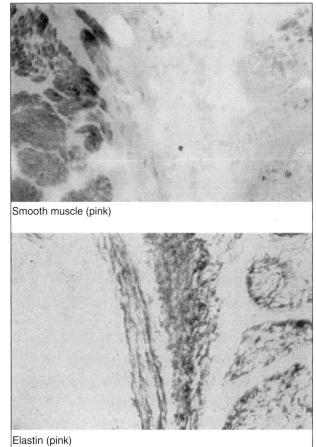

Smooth muscle (pink)

Elastin (pink)

Figure 9.15
Two adjacent sections of human detrusor from a spina bifida patient with an overactive bladder. Top panel stained with Masson's trichrome (smooth muscle seen in pink); bottom panel stained for the presence of elastin. In these sections normal muscle bundles are present on the left, and on the right damaged bundles with less smooth muscle, and also denervation (not shown). Note the increased elastin distribution in the damaged bundles.

injury. Electrophysiological measurements of the central delay in the micturition reflex show a shorter delay in animals with spinal injury (for references see de Groat[36]) than in intact animals, suggesting that there has been reorganization of the micturition pathway from a spino-bulbo-spinal pathway to a purely spinal pathway. Also, activation of specific C-fiber afferents can trigger micturition in overactive bladders but not in normal bladders. This latter observation is thought to be true in humans, since in normal humans the ice water test (instillation of the bladder with cold water), which is thought to activate specific C fibers, does not trigger micturition, but does so in many patients with overactive bladders.[37,38] In fact, intravesical administration of selective C-fiber neurotoxins such as capsaicin and resiniferatoxin is an effective treatment in many patients with neuropathic instability.[39]

Possible causes of these changes

It seems inherently likely that the changes associated with the overactive bladder are the result of alterations in the activity in the neuronal pathways controlling the detrusor. The sensory neurons are likely to encounter increased stimulation after outflow obstruction or inflammation of the urothelium, which could result in the hypertrophy of

the dorsal root ganglion neurons and also of the autonomic ganglia, since presumably increased parasympathetic activation will result. The patchy denervation suggests that there has been death of some of the intrinsic neurons in the bladder wall. The most likely cause of this is bladder wall ischemia. The bladder has been shown to be susceptible to ischemia,[40–42] since anything that raises intravesical pressure to more than 30–40 cmH_2O seriously compromises blood flow in the wall. Enhanced intravesical pressure and bladder wall ischemia could result from prostatic obstruction or, in cases of spinal injury, from detrusor sphincter dyssynergia. In outflow obstruction where there is a significant hypertrophy of the wall, increased metabolic demands[43] and reduced blood flow[41] can lead to

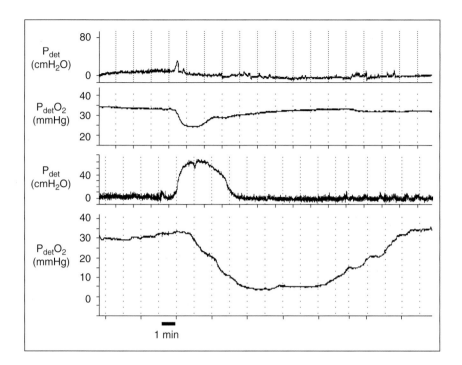

1 min

Figure 9.16
Urodynamic tracings from pigs. The top of each pair of tracings is the intravesical pressure, and the bottom trace is oxygen tension in the bladder wall, recorded with an oxygen electrode. The traces show bladder filling and a micturition. The top traces are from a normal pig, and show a small rise in intravesical pressure during voiding, and an associated more prolonged reduction in oxygen tension. The bottom traces are from a pig with a bladder outflow obstruction. Note the increased and prolonged pressure rise during the void, and the drastic extended fall in oxygen tension, which does not return to baseline for about 14 min. (Reproduced from Greenland and Brading with permission.)[53]

significant periods of anoxia, which might result eventually in neuronal death (Figure 9.16). We have recently shown that 1 hour of bladder ischemia produced in anesthetized guinea pigs by occlusion of the terminal aorta, followed by 1 hour reperfusion, resulted in expression of apoptotic-associated markers in the ganglia in the bladder wall[44] (Figure 9.17).

The changes in the reflex pathway that occur after spinal injury probably result from the loss of descending pathways. This may trigger the production of growth factors and the resultant sprouting of axon terminals in surviving pathways to make new and abnormal connections; for instance, the C fibers may increase their connections to the interneurons or motor neurons in the segmental spinal parasympathetic pathways. The enhanced size of the efferent postganglionic neurons in obstructed bladders appears to be the result of the liberation of nerve growth factor (NGF) by the detrusor, since autoimmunization of rats against NGF reduces the neuronal hypertrophy.[45] Presumably, the stimulus for the production of NGF may be the increased work load of the obstructed bladder.[46]

The problem of urgency

Everyday experience would suggest that urgency is a separate sensation from that of bladder fullness. Animal experiments recording from afferent nerves during bladder filling and contraction[47–50] have shown increased activity in a unimodal population of small myelinated and unmyelinated (Aδ and C) fibers in response to intravesical pressure and detrusor contraction, suggesting that there are in-series stretch receptors in the bladder wall whose activity correlates with the sensations of bladder filling and fullness. However, it seems unlikely that fibers with such properties mediate the sensation of urgency. Again, from everyday experience, urgent desire to void disappears as soon as micturition starts – at a time when intravesical pressure and detrusor activity will both be high. Unfortunately, the relationship between urgency and detrusor activity cannot be investigated in animals, since we cannot know what sensations they perceive. In humans, however, it is clear from both normal and ambulatory cystometry that overactive pressure rises may occur without eliciting any apparent sensations. A sensible theory about urgency has been proposed by Coolsaet et al.[51] They suggest that urgency is triggered by local distortions in the bladder wall, caused by activity in some muscle bundles but not others. Such a condition would arise in normal bladders if a small population of low-threshold postganglionic parasympathetic neurons were activated, e.g. towards the end of bladder filling. Because of relatively poor coupling between bundles, such diffuse activity would not cause a rise in intravesical pressure, but could activate a population of sensory nerve fibers that might specifically mediate the sensation of urgency and play a useful role in encouraging the initiation of normal micturition. In overactive bladders, however, such diffuse activation of some muscle bundles might spread because of the increased connectivity to give rise to the overactive

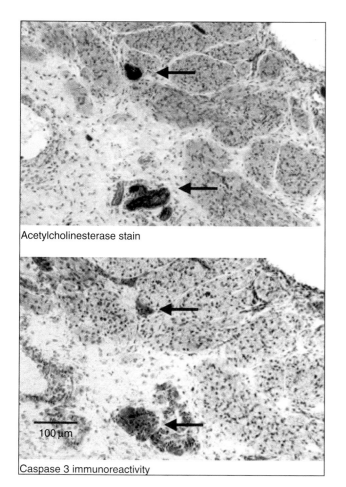

Acetylcholinesterase stain

100 μm

Caspase 3 immunoreactivity

Figure 9.17
Two adjacent sections from a guinea pig bladder that had been subjected to ischemic conditions. The top section localizes intramural ganglia which show acetylcholinesterase activity. In the bottom section the ganglia can be seen to react with antibodies to caspase 3, a pro-apoptotic marker. (Reproduced from Symes[44] with permission; sections prepared by Lucia Esposito.)

pressure rises. An increase in the sensitivity of fibers mediating urgency may be responsible for the enhanced urgency seen in inflammatory conditions, interstitial cystitis, and other examples of sensory urgency.

Conclusions

It is clear that we are still some way from really understanding what causes bladder overactivity. However, there are sufficient clues from the observations and experimental results described above to suggest that we are dealing with the consequences of altered patterns of activation of the nerves in the micturition pathways and the resultant effects

of this on the smooth muscle in the detrusor. In cases of severe overactivity and urge incontinence, the process has probably been ongoing for years. Some factors such as detrusor-sphincter dyssynergia, outflow obstruction, or abnormal rises in intra-abdominal pressure have caused periodic bladder wall ischemia and this has reached a stage in which neurons in the bladder wall have actually died; the smooth muscle in the detrusor has then become able to generate synchronous contractions and these result in the overactive pressure rises seen. What precise mechanism triggers these overactive contractions is not yet clear, although it is likely that premature activation through some local or supraspinal pathway of the remaining parasympathetic ganglia is usually involved.

It may be that the most likely scenario for urge incontinence which is associated with overactive contractions is as follows: activity in some muscle bundles generated either by stretch or by diffuse activity in parasympathetic fibers causes local distortions of the bladder wall; this both activates the sensation of urgency and spreads to cause synchronous activation of the bladder wall, resulting in an overactive pressure rise. The sequence of events recorded should be urgency occurring first, followed almost immediately by an overactive contraction. What happens after this may vary. If the contraction is large enough to overcome the outflow resistance, leakage will occur. This could, in its turn, activate receptors in the urethra and trigger secondary changes (transient opening of the bladder neck, etc.), but often the pressure and sensation of urgency will subside. Synchronous detrusor contraction will itself reduce the sensation of urgency and the bladder pressure may return to normal. Activation of the detrusor smooth muscle, unless supported by continuous neural input, is self-limiting, since the muscles possess calcium-activated potassium channels which ensure that the membrane hyperpolarizes and spontaneous action potentials will be switched off transiently.[52] Normally, urge incontinence does not result in complete bladder emptying, but if there is a well-developed segmental spinal micturition reflex and loss of any descending control, activation of the pressure/stretch receptors may reinforce the activity and produce bladder emptying.

References

1. Koelbl H, Mostwin JL, Boiteux JP, et al. Pathophysiology. In: Abrams P, Cardozo L, Khoury S, Wein A, eds. Incontinence. Plymouth, UK: Health Publications, 2002:205–241.

2. Abrams P, Cardozo L, Fall M, et al. The standardisation of terminology of lower urinary tract function: report from the Standardisation Sub-committee of the International Continence Society. Neurourol Urodyn 2002; 21(2):167–178.

3. Brading AF. Physiology of bladder smooth muscle. In: Torrens MJ, Morrison JFB, eds. The physiology of the lower urinary tract. New York: Springer Verlag, 1987:161–191.

4. Sibley GNA. A comparison of spontaneous and nerve-mediated activity in bladder muscle from man, pig and rabbit. J Physiol (Lond) 1984; 354:431–443.

5. Sibley GNA. The response of the bladder to lower urinary tract obstruction [D.M.]. Oxford, 1984.

6. German K, Bedwani J, Davies J, et al. Physiological and morphometric studies into the pathophysiology of detrusor hyperreflexia in neuropathic patients. J Urol 1995; 153(5):1678–1683.

7. Kinder RB, Mundy AR. Atropine blockade of nerve-mediated stimulation of the human detrusor. Br J Urol 1985; 57(4):418–421.

8. Turner WH, Brading AF. Smooth muscle of the bladder in the normal and the diseased state: pathophysiology, diagnosis and treatment. Pharmacol Ther 1997; 75(2):77–110.

9. Mills IW, Greenland JE, McCoy R, et al. Spontaneous myogenic contractile activity of isolated human detrusor smooth muscle in idiopathic instability. JU 1999; 161 (AUA Suppl 4):253.

10. Mills IW, Greenland JE, McMurray G, et al. Studies of the pathophysiology of idiopathic detrusor instability: the physiological properties of the detrusor smooth muscle and its pattern of innervation. J Urol 2000; 163(2):646–651.

11. Turner WH. An experimental urodynamic model of lower urinary tract function and dysfunction [D.M.]. Cambridge, 1997.

12. Brading AF. Alterations in the physiological properties of urinary bladder smooth muscle caused by bladder emptying against an obstruction. Scand J Urol Nephrol Suppl 1997; 184:51–58.

13. Sibley GNA. Developments in our understanding of detrusor instability. Br J Urol 1997; 80(Suppl 1):54–61.

14. Brading AF, Turner WH. The unstable bladder: towards a common mechanism. Br J Urol 1994; 73(1):3–8.

15. Sibley GNA. An experimental model of detrusor instability in the obstructed pig. Br J Urol 1985; 57(3):292–298.

16. Speakman MJ, Brading AF, Gilpin CJ, et al. Bladder outflow obstruction – a cause of denervation supersensitivity. J Urol 1987; 138(6):1461–1466.

17. Harrison SC, Ferguson DR, Doyle PT. Effect of bladder outflow obstruction on the innervation of the rabbit urinary bladder. Br J Urol 1990; 66(4):372–379.

18. Sethia KK. The pathophysiology of detrusor instability [D.M.]. Oxford, 1988.

19. Elbadawi A, Yalla SV, Resnick NM. Structural basis of geriatric voiding dysfunction. III. Detrusor overactivity. J Urol 1993; 150 (5 Part 2):1668–1680.

20. Brading AF, Speakman MJ. Pathophysiology of bladder outflow obstruction. In: Whitfield H, Kirby R, Hendry WF, Duckett J, eds. Textbook of genitourinary surgery, 2nd edn. Oxford: Blackwell Science, 1998:465–479.

21. Daniel EE, Cowan W, Daniel VP. Structural bases for neural and myogenic control of human detrusor muscle. Can J Physiol Pharmacol 1983; 61(11):1247–1273.

22. Sui GP, Rothery S, Dupont E, Fry CH, Severs NJ. Gap junctions and connexin expression in human suburothelial interstitial cells. BJU Int 2002; 90(1):118–129.

23. Bramich NJ, Brading AF. Electrical properties of smooth muscle in the guinea-pig urinary bladder. J Physiol 1996; 492(1):185–198.

24. Fry CH, Cooklin M, Birns J, Mundy AR. Measurement of intercellular electrical coupling in guinea-pig detrusor smooth muscle. J Urol 1999; 161(2):660–664.

25. Hashitani H, Fukuta H, Tkano H, et al. Origin and propagation of spontaneous excitation in smooth muscle of the guinea-pig urinary bladder. J Physiol 2001; 530(2):273–286.

26. Gabella G. The structural relations between nerve fibres and muscle cells in the urinary bladder of the rat. J Neurocytol 1995; 24:159–187.

27. Westfall DP. Supersensitivity of smooth muscle. In: Bülbring E, Brading AF, Jones AW, Tomita T, eds. Smooth muscle: an assessment of current knowledge. London: Arnold, 1981:285–309.

28. Charlton RG, Morley AR, Chambers P, Gillespie JI. Focal changes in nerve, muscle and connective tissue in normal and unstable human bladder. BJU Int 1999; 84(9):953–960.

29. Drake MJ, Hedlund P, Mills IW, et al. Structural and functional denervation of human detrusor after spinal cord injury. Lab Invest 2000; 80(10):1491–1499.

30. Speakman MJ. Studies on the physiology of the normal and obstructed bladder [M.S.]. London, 1988.

31. Williams JH, Turner WH, Sainsbury GM, Brading AF. Experimental model of bladder outflow tract obstruction in the guinea-pig. Br J Urol 1993; 71(5):543–554.

32. Steers WD, Ciambotti J, Etzel B, et al. Alterations in afferent pathways from the urinary bladder of the rat in response to partial urethral obstruction. J Comp Neurol 1991; 310(3):401–410.

33. Steers WD, Ciambotti J, Erdman S, de Groat WC. Morphological plasticity in efferent pathways to the urinary bladder of the rat following urethral obstruction. J Neurosci 1990; 10:1943–1951.

34. Gabella G, Berggren T, Uvelius B. Hypertrophy and reversal of hypertrophy in rat pelvic ganglion neurons. J Neurocytol 1992; 21(9):649–662.

35. Kruse MN, Belton AL, de Groat WC. Changes in bladder and external sphincter function after spinal injury in the rat. Am J Physiol 1993; 264(R):1157–1163.

36. de Groat WC. A neurological basis for the overactive bladder. Urology 1997; 50(Suppl 6A):36–52.

37. Geirsson G, Lindstrom S, Fall M. The bladder cooling reflex in man – characteristics and sensitivity to temperature. Br J Urol 1993; 71(6):675–680.

38. Geirsson G, Fall M, Lindstrom S. The ice-water test – a simple and valuable supplement to routine cystometry. Br J Urol 1993; 71(6):681–685.

39. de Ridder D, Baert L. Vanilloids and the overactive bladder. BJUI Int 2000; 86(2):172–180.

40. Greenland JE, Brading AF. Urinary bladder blood flow changes during the micturition cycle in a conscious pig model. J Urol 1996; 156(5):1858–1861.

41. Brading AF, Greenland JE, Mills IW, et al. Blood supply to the bladder during filling. Scand J Urol Nephrol Suppl 1999; 201:25–31.

42. Mills IW. The pathophysiology of detrusor instability and the role of bladder ischaemia in its aetiology [D.M.]. Oxford, 1999.

43. Levin RM, Haugaard N, Hypolite JA, et al. Metabolic factors influencing lower urinary tract function. Exptl Physiol 1999; 84(1):171–194.

44. Symes SE. Effects of ischaemic-like conditions on guinea-pig urinary bladder. [D. Phil.]. Oxford, 2002.

45. Steers WD, Creedon DJ, Tuttle JB. Immunity to nerve growth factor prevents plasticity following urinary bladder hypertrophy. J Urol 1996; 155(1):379–385.

46. Levin RM, Haugaard N, Levin SS, et al. Bladder function in experimental outlet obstruction: pharmacologic responses to alterations in innervation, energetics, calcium mobilization, and genetics. In: Zderic S, ed. Muscle, matrix, and bladder function. New York: Plenum Press; 1995:7–19.

47. Iggo A. Tension receptors in the stomach and the urinary bladder. J Physiol 1955; 128(3):593–607.

48. Jänig W, Morrison JFB. Functional properties of spinal visceral afferents supplying abdominal and pelvic organs, with special emphasis on visceral nociception. Progress Brain Res 1986; 67:87–114.

49. Morrison JFB. Sensations arising from the lower urinary tract. In: Torrens M, Morrison JFB, eds. The physiology of the lower urinary tract. Berlin: Springer-Verlag, 1987:89–131.

50. Namasivayam S, Eardley I, Morrison JFB. A novel in vitro bladder pelvic nerve afferent model in the rat. Br J Urol 1998; 82(6):902–905.

51. Coolsaet BL, Van Duyl WA, Van Os-Bossagh P, De Bakker HV. New concepts in relation to urge and detrusor activity. Neurourol Urodyn 1993; 12(5):463–471.

52. Wellner MC, Isenberg G. Stretch effects on whole-cell currents of guinea-pig urinary bladder myocytes. J Physiol (Lond) 1994; 480(Pt 3):439–448.

53. Greenland JE, Brading AF. The effect of bladder outflow obstruction on detrusor blood flow changes during the voiding cycle in conscious pigs. J Urol 2001; 165(1):245–248.

10

Pathophysiology of areflexic bladder

Katsumi Sasaki, Jun Nishiguchi, and Michael B Chancellor

Introduction

Detrusor areflexia (DA) is defined as acontractility due to an abnormality of nervous control.[1] In DA, detrusor cannot be demonstrated to contract during urodynamic studies. Impaired contractility of the detrusor (ICD) can be told from DA by weak and faint contractions of the detrusor during urodynamic studies. DA can be developed from various kinds of conditions, when neurologic pathways innervating bladder are mainly damaged. However, it is difficult to ignore myogenic factors.[2]

In this chapter, the authors first review the mechanisms of micturition reflexes and mention several conditions that develop DA. Future treatment strategies for DA are also presented.

The mechanism of micturition reflexes

Pelvic afferent pathways

Efferent outflow to the lower urinary tract can be activated reflexively by spinal afferent pathways as well as input from the brain. Afferent input from the pelvic visceral organs and also somatic afferent pathways from the perineal muscle and skin are very important.[3] Somatic afferent pathways in the pudendal nerves that transmit noxious and non-noxious information from the genital organs, urethra, prostate, vagina, anal canal, and skin can modulate voiding function.[4-6]

Bladder afferent nerves are critical for sending signals of bladder fullness and discomfort to the brain and for initiating the micturition reflex. The bladder afferent pathways are composed of two types of axons: large/medium diameter myelinated $A\delta$-fibers and unmyelinated C-fibers.[7] $A\delta$-fibers transmit signals mainly from mechanoreceptors that detect bladder fullness or wall tension. The C-fibers, on the other hand, mainly detect noxious signals and initiate painful sensations. The bladder C-fiber nociceptors perform a similar function and signal the central nervous system when we have an infection or irritative condition in the bladder.

C-fiber bladder afferents also have reflex functions to facilitate or trigger voiding.[8-10] This can be viewed as a defense mechanism to eliminate irritants or bacteria. The C-fiber bladder afferents have been implicated in the triggering of reflex bladder hyperactivity associated with neurologic disorders such as spinal cord injury and multiple sclerosis. Capsaicin and its ultrapotent analogue resiniferatoxin are specific C-fiber afferent neurotoxins and are undergoing clinical trials for the treatment of lower urinary tract dysfunction relating to C-fiber alterations.[5]

Micturition reflexes

Normal micturition is completely dependent on neural pathways in the central nervous system. These pathways perform three major functions: *amplification, coordination,* and *timing*.[4] The nervous control of the lower urinary tract must be able to *amplify* weak smooth muscle activity to provide sustained increases in intravesical pressures sufficient to empty the bladder. The bladder and urethral sphincter function must be *coordinated* to allow the sphincter to open during micturition but to be closed at all other times. *Timing* represents the voluntary control of voiding in the normal adult and the ability to initiate voiding over a wide range of bladder volumes (Figure 10.1). In this regard, the bladder is a unique visceral organ which exhibits predominantly voluntary rather than involuntary (autonomic) neural regulation. A number of important reflex mechanisms contribute to the storage and elimination of urine and modulate the voluntary control of micturition.[6]

Guarding reflexes (guarding against stress urinary incontinence)

There is an important bladder to urethral reflex that is mediated by sympathetic efferent pathways to the urethra. This is an excitatory reflex that contracts the urethral

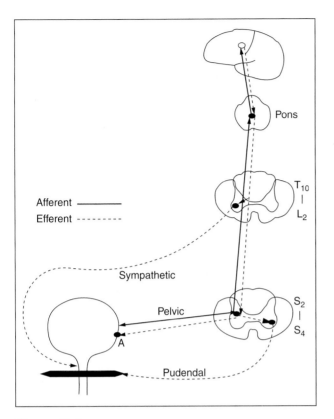

Figure 10.1
Micturition requires positive feedback to ensure complete bladder emptying. As the bladder fills, myelinated Aδ-tension receptors are activated. This afferent signal must reach the pontine micturition center with subsequent activation of parasympathetic efferent outflow.

smooth muscle and thus is called a guarding reflex.[11,12] The positive reflex is not activated during micturition but when bladder pressure is increased such as during a cough or exercise. A second guarding reflex is triggered by the bladder afferents which synapse with sacral interneurons that in turn activate urethral external sphincter efferent neurons that send axons into the pudendal nerves.[13] The activation of pudendal urethral efferents pathways contracts the external urinary sphincter, and prevents stress urinary incontinence (Figure 10.2). The brain inhibits the guarding reflexes during micturition.

Conditions or diseases developing detrusor areflexia or impaired contractility of the detrusor

Detrusor areflexia (DA) or impaired contractility of the detrusor (ICD) is usually observed when the following

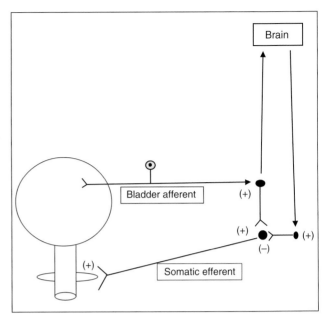

Figure 10.2
The guarding reflex prevents urinary incontinence. When there is a sudden increase in intravesical pressure, such as cough, the urinary sphincter contracts via the spinal guarding reflex to prevent urinary incontinence. The spinal guarding reflex can be turned off by the brain to urinate.

mechanisms are damaged:[14]

- bladder peripheral afferent pathways
- bladder peripheral efferent pathways
- lumbosacral spinal cord (micturition center)
- myogenic failure

These four factors are often mixed in the condition of DA or ICD. In this section, we discuss several kinds of diseases that develop DA or ICD, including the pathogenesis, urodynamic findings, and treatments.

Diabetes mellitus (diabetic cystopathy)

It is widely accepted that diabetes results in sensory and autonomic polyneuropathy. When sensory and/or autonomic neurons innervating the bladder are damaged, bladder dysfunction – which is characterized by impaired sensation of bladder fullness, increased bladder capacity, reduced bladder contractility and increased residual urine – can be observed.[15–17] The sex and age of patients are not the factors related to prevalence, whereas the duration of diabetes is bound up with the prevalence rate of diabetic cystopathy.[18]

It has also been reported that diabetic cystopathy can occur silently and early in the course of diabetes.[17] In those cases, it is not rare that bladder dysfunction induced by diabetes could not be found without careful questions and/or urodynamic testing. Thus, urodynamic testing on diabetic patients is sometimes necessary for early diagnosis of bladder dysfunction induced by diabetes.

Pathogenesis of diabetic cystopathy

Pathological and physiological studies in humans as well as in animals have revealed that diabetic cystopathy is induced by polyneuropathy that predominantly affects sensory and autonomic nerve fibers.[19,20] Historically, it has been accepted that the etiology of diabetic neuropathy is multifocal. Some of the proposed pathogenesis includes altered metabolism of glucose, ischemia, superoxide-induced free-radical formation and impaired axonal transport.[21] However, the absolute pathogenesis of diabetic neuropathy has not been fully clarified.

Recently, the changes of tissue neurotrophic factors such as nerve growth factor (NGF) have been focused on as a convincing pathogenesis of diabetic neuropathy. Some investigators have reported the increase or decrease of tissue NGF levels in diabetic animals and humans.[22–27] The increase or decrease of another neurotrophic factor, neurotrophin-3 (NT-3), has also been reported.[28–30] We have also found that in streptozotocin (STZ)-induced diabetic rats, the decrease of tissue NGF levels in the bladder and bladder afferent pathways was associated with diabetic cystopathy that was induced by dysfunctions of both $A\delta$- and C-fiber bladder afferent pathways.[31] Thus, it is promising that the changes of tissue neurotrophic factor could play a critical role in inducing diabetic cystopathy.

Urodynamic testing on diabetic cystopathy

In most typical cases with diabetic cystopathy, cystometry shows a long curve with lack of sensation, often until bladder capacity is reached, with a low detrusor pressure.[17,32,33] However, it has been reported that this classical type of hypoactive diabetic cystopathy is sometimes modified by concomitant lesions such as bladder outlet obstruction (BOO) or a history of cerebrovascular disease. For example, previous reports have reported a high incidence of detrusor hyperreflexia up to 50–60% when bladder function was examined in a selected population of diabetic patients presenting with positive lower urinary tract symptoms[34] or those with a history of stroke.[35] BOO should also be considered as a differential diagnosis for detrusor hyperreflexia in diabetic patients.[33] BOO is documented by measuring a high or normal pressure in the presence of an impaired urinary flow rate. Some patients with both diabetic cystopathy and BOO exhibit detrusor hyperreflexia and elevated detrusor pressure during low-flow voiding.

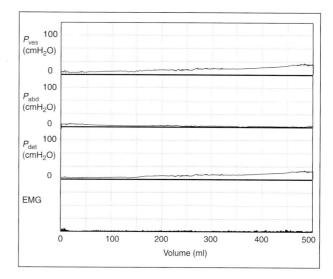

Figure 10.3

Detrusor areflexia in a 62-year-old insulin-depended diabetic woman. The patient is on intermittent catheterization approximately 4 times per 24 hours. P_{ves}, intravesical pressure; P_{abd}, abdominal pressure; P_{det}, detrusor pressure.

However, despite recent reports of a relatively high incidence of detrusor hyperreflexia in symptomatic diabetic patients,[34] one should be aware that autonomic and sensory neuropathy with diminished bladder sensation and bladder contractility is the predominant urological manifestation of diabetic cystopathy when unselected diabetic patients are examined[15–17] (Figure 10.3).

Electromyography (EMG) is usually normal but sometimes exhibits sphincter denervation and uninhibited sphincter relaxation. Uroflowmetry shows low peak flow and prolonged duration of flow associated with increased residual urine. Urethral pressure profiles have not been well studied or validated in diabetic cystopathy.[17,36]

Treatment of diabetic cystopathy

The first step in the management of diabetes is to control the blood glucose level. However, the control of blood glucose level does not mean the prevention of diabetic cystopathy.[18] The treatment for diabetic cystopathy is basically concluded to avoid or eliminate residual urine. For patients with asymptomatic or moderate signs of cystopathy the treatment choices include scheduled time voiding and possibly drug treatment with cholinergic receptor agonists. For severe cases with much residual urine and pyuria, intermittent catheterization may be added.[18,32] However, deficient bladder sensation is irreversible in diabetes and long-term follow-up is necessary. In addition, many patients with diabetic cystopathy may delay seeking urological evaluation because of insidious development of diabetic cystopathy that induces diminished sensation and increased bladder capacity. Thus, careful surveillance for voiding symptoms and screening for elevated residual urine, including urodynamic study, may be useful to prevent long-term complications secondary to diabetic cystopathy.

Future treatment strategies

Conservative treatments for diabetic cystopathy are limited and cannot restore bladder function, as mentioned previously. Recently, new treatment approaches for diabetic polyneuropathy, including diabetic cystopathy, have been reported in both the basic and clinical fields. Most common treatments are the ones using neurotrophic factors. Following the efficacy of nerve growth factor (NGF) treatment in basic studies,[37–39] the efficacy of NGF treatment in the clinical field has been reported.[40–42] We have also studied the feasibility of gene therapy using replication deficient herpes simplex virus (HSV) encoding *rhNGF* genes injected into the bladder wall in diabetic rats.[43] Other reports using neurotrophic factors other than NGF, such as glial cell line-derived neurotrophic factor (GDNF) or neurotrophin-3 (NT-3), have also demonstrated significant efficacies in restorations of nerve functions in diabetic animals.[44,45]

Thus, in the future, neurotrophic factors or other growth factors combined with targeted gene therapy techniques may be beneficial for the therapy of patients with diabetic cystopathy.

Conclusions

Diabetic cystopathy, which is characterized bladder hypoactivity, is common and can develop insidiously. Tests, including urodynamic study in the early stage of the diabetes, are needed. Exciting new approaches to treat diabetic cystopathy are being investigated.

Injury to the spinal cord, cauda equina, and pelvic plexus

Any injury to the spinal cord such as blunt, degenerative, developmental, vascular, infectious, traumatic, and idiopathic injury can cause voiding dysfunction. In this section we will discuss the urodynamic manifestations of some common spinal and cauda equina neurologic processes not previously discussed.

Injury to the cauda equina and peripheral sacral nerves can have a devastating effect on bladder and urethral

sphincter function. The true incidence of lower urinary tract dysfunction as a result of cauda equina and pelvic plexus injury is still unknown, mainly because of the lack of prospective studies with pre- and postoperative neuro-urological evaluation of the patients.

The resulting urinary dysfunction can be a major cause of morbidity in these cases. Lumbosacral spinal cord injury and herniated intervertebral disc are the two most common etiologic factors.[46,47] Other etiologic causes include lumbar spinal stenosis, myelodysplasia, spinal arachnoiditis, arteriovenous malformations, and primary or metastatic tumors of the lumbar spine. It could be also a rare complication of regional anesthesia.

Injury to the pelvic plexus is not common. It is usually iatrogenic, most often occurring after major abdominal and pelvic surgery such as abdominoperineal resection or radical hysterectomy for malignancy. Sometimes the problem may result from a fractured pelvis, or the trauma may be intentional (e.g. transvesical phenol injection) with the intent being to abolish detrusor hyperreflexia in patients who have failed standard treatment regimens.

The true incidence of lower urinary tract dysfunction as a result of pelvic plexus injury is still unknown, mainly because of the lack of prospective studies with pre- and postoperative neuro-urological evaluation of the patients. The issue is made more complex because of three additional factors:

1. Most patients in the age group requiring treatment for pelvic malignancy may have preexisting bladder outlet obstruction or another pathology responsible for the functional derangement of the lower urinary tract.
2. In a significant percentage of patients, recovery of bladder function may occur as time goes on. Up to 80% of the patients with bladder dysfunction following major pelvic surgery will resume normal voiding within 6 months of the procedure.
3. In most early series, the technical means for a comprehensive urodynamic evaluation were not available.

In view of the complexity of neural injury in these cases, which can involve parasympathetic, sympathetic, as well as somatic nerve fibers, it is evident that only modern urodynamic techniques[48,49] can provide exact information on the nature and the extent of the disorder.

Neuroanatomy and pathophysiology

Although it is well established that the pelvic plexus is derived from the ventral rami of S2–4 nerves,[50] there is contradictory information on sacral nerve connections and collateralization.[51] The precise branching and interconnects among the sacral plexus is important because of increasing interest in dorsal rhizotomy and functional electrical stimulation for bladder control.

The pelvic plexus lies deep in the pelvis, oriented in a parasagittal plane alongside the rectum. On most occasions injury to this structure is iatrogenically induced following major pelvic ablative surgery. Involvement of the pelvis with a malignant process or invasive rectal neoplasms in the lateral and posterior or rectal wall may infiltrate the adjacent pararectal autonomic nerves, thus causing pelvic plexus injury.[48,52,53]

Marani et al[51] reported the surgical dissection of the cauda equina and pelvic plexus of 10 human cadavers (5 males and 5 females). In 9 (4 males and 5 females) a branch connecting the ventral rami of the second and third sacral spinal nerves was found. Electron microscopy demonstrated the presence of thick myelinated fibers in this branch. This may contribute to the interaction between detrusor and sphincter contractions. The branches contributing to the pelvic plexus differ greatly individually and intersexually. It is important to be aware of the wide range of branches when decisions have to be made concerning the strategy of neurostimulation and dorsal rhizotomy.

Voiding dysfunction after major pelvic surgery is usually caused by intraoperative injury to pelvic, hypogastric, and pudendal nerves.[49,53] The neuroanatomic basis for the denervation of the bladder has been described on the basis of detailed anatomic dissections.[54] Direct damage to the parasympathetic nerves and the posterior part of the pelvic plexus may occur during dissection on the anterolateral aspect of the lower rectum. In addition, traction injury may occur during mobilization of the lower rectum because of the relationship of the pelvic nerves to the fascial capsule investing the rectum.[55]

During hysterectomy, the main factor producing bladder denervation appears to be extensive dissection inferolateral to the cervix.[52] Damage to the sympathetics in the hypogastric plexus may occur at the pelvic brim medial to the ureters and also in the region lateral to the rectum. Extensive dissection in the vicinity of the cardinal ligaments at the time of radical hysterectomy may also produce sympathetic denervation.[53]

During the perineal portion of an abdominoperineal resection at the time of mobilization of the anus, injury to the pudendal nerve may occur. It is therefore apparent that varying degrees of damage to parasympathetic, sympathetic, and somatic nerves may occur, which can range from neural traction injury, to incomplete or complete nerve ablation.

Pelvic surgery

Many patients in the age group requiring surgical treatment for pelvic malignancy may have preexisting bladder outlet obstruction or pathology responsible for the functional derangement of the lower urinary tract. Also, in a significant percentage of patients undergoing major pelvic surgery, recovery of bladder function may occur as time goes on. Moreover, in many early series, the technical means for a comprehensive urodynamic evaluation were not available.

The incidence of vesicourethral dysfunction has been reported to be 20–68% of patients after abdominal perineal resection, 16–80% after radical hysterectomy, 10–20% after proctocolectomy, and 20–25% after anterior resection.[49,53,55–58] The true incidence of neurogenital bladder dysfunction following pelvic surgery will never be known without prospective pre- and postoperative evaluations.

Pelvic and sacral fractures

Pelvic trauma can result in cauda equina and pelvic plexus injury. The frequency of neurologic injury after pelvic fractures is estimated at between 0.75 and 11%.[59–61] Autopsy findings and clinical studies have showed that neurologic injury accompanying sacral fractures occurs either intradurally or extradurally within the sacral canal. Sacral fractures are associated with pelvic fractures in 90% of the cases,[59,60] and approximately 25% of sacral fractures will result in permanent neurologic deficit.[62,63] The injury most closely correlated with neurologic injury is a transverse sacral fracture. Approximately two-thirds of these patients will have neurogenic bladder.[64]

Because most of the injuries are incomplete, the majority of patients with neuro-urologic injury after pelvic and sacral fractures will notice improvement with time. Delayed neurologic deficit occurring after sacral fracture is a recognized complication.[65,66] The delayed deficits were attributed to scarring, hematoma formation at the fracture site, and untreated spinal instability.

Herniated disc

Some reports indicate that the incidence of voiding dysfunction as a result of disc prolapse may approach 20% of patients.[67,68] Since the data demonstrated that detrusor recovery was rare after treatments once patients showed bladder dysfunctions following lumbar disc prolapse, cauda equina syndrome from lumbar disc herniation might be a diagnostic and surgical emergency.[69,70]

Clinical findings

Patients with known or suspected neurologic injury due to pelvic or sacral injury should have a careful physical examination. The integrity of the sacral dermatomes is tested by assessing perianal sensation, anal sphincter tone, and control of the bulbocavernosus reflex.

The type of the resulting functional disturbance will depend on the nature and extent of nerve injury. Parasympathetic denervation causes detrusor areflexia, whereas sympathetic damage will produce loss of proximal urethral pressure[71] as a result of the compromised alpha-mediated innervation to the smooth muscle fibers of the bladder neck and urethra.[72]

Many patients complain of straining to urinate, incontinence, and sensation of incomplete emptying. The urinary stream may be diminished and interrupted, as many of these patients rely on abdominal straining to urinate. On occasions, symptoms of voiding dysfunction can be the only initial clinical manifestation of a cauda equina lesion.[73] The varied and mixed symptomatologies emphasize the need for a complete neuro-urologic evaluation.

The physical examination may reveal a distended bladder, but the most characteristic features are elicited on a careful neurologic examination. Sensory loss in the perineum or perianal area is associated with S2–4 dermatomes. The extent of perineal anesthesia can be a useful predictive clinical index in patients with lumbar disc prolapse. If 'saddle' anesthesia of the S2–4 dermatomes continues after surgical laminectomy and decompression, the urinary bladder rarely recovers.[74] On the contrary, a unilateral or mild sensory disturbance indicates a better prognosis. Deep tendon reflexes in the lower extremities, clonus, and plantar responses, as well as the bulbocavernosus reflex, should be routinely evaluated.

In a series of patients with cauda equina injury of various etiologies, the bulbocavernosus reflex was absent or significantly diminished in 84% of the cases, whereas the perineal sensation and muscle stretch reflexes were compromised in 77% of the patients.[64] In addition, it was noted that absence of the reflex correlated well with perineal floor denervation.[75]

It is of interest that parasympathetic denervation itself may actually increase adrenergic activity by unmasking already existing alpha receptors or by inducing alpha receptors. It has been demonstrated by histochemical fluorescence studies that the adrenergic nerve terminals of denervated human detrusors were thicker and denser than in neurologically normal detrusors. A complete injury of both pelvic plexuses disrupts the nerve supply to the bladder and the urethra, but most injuries are incomplete. Since most ganglia lie close to or within the bladder wall and large numbers of postganglionic neurons remain intact, any denervation is followed by reinnervation,[76] so that some residual lower tract activity remains. Sensation may be preserved, but, if it is lost, the resultant symptoms are those of retention and overflow incontinence.

Peripheral sympathetic injury results in an open, nonfunctional bladder neck and proximal urethra. Although this could occur as an isolated injury, it typically occurs in association with partial detrusor denervation, but with preservation of sphincter function.[72] The combination of decreased compliance, open bladder neck, and fixed external sphincter resistance results in the paradoxical symptomatology of both leaking across the distal sphincter and the inability to empty the bladder. Under these circumstances, anticholinergics given to make bladder storage pressure lower with bladder evacuation by intermittent catheterization result in the optimal management.

Urodynamic findings

The typical cystometrogram (CMG) finding of cauda equina injury is detrusor areflexia (Figure 10.3).[48,64] On the uroflowmetry, an abdominal straining saw-tooth pattern is generally seen when the patients claim they can urinate (Figure 10.4). Urodynamic abnormalities may be the only aberration documented without other overt neurologic manifestations in some patients with cauda equina injury. On herniated disc, which is not induced by trauma or acute conditions, the protrusion is usually slow and progressive. In these cases, it may result in nerve irritation and consequently detrusor hyperreflexia.[77]

Sphincter denervation – as documented on EMG by a decreased interference pattern, fibrillation, positive sharp waves, and polyphasic potentials – has also been reported.[64] This observation can be attributed to the different location of the detrusor and pudendal motor nuclei within the sacral cord,[78] as well as to the fact that the dominant segment of the pelvic nerve usually arises one segment higher than that of the pudendal nerve.[79]

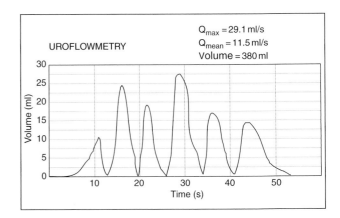

Figure 10.4
Straining uroflowmetry of diabetic woman in Figure 10.2. The patient complained of a sensation of incomplete emptying post-micturition, occasional incontinence, and straining to urinate. Although her maximum flow rate (Q_{max}) is normal (29.1 ml/s), the voiding pattern is classic for Valsalva voiding without true detrusor contractility.

The predominant CMG/EMG pattern is detrusor areflexia associated with sphincter neuropathy. Bladder sensation, however, is preserved in a significant number of patients because of the presence of numerous exteroceptive sensory nerves in the bladder trigone and vesical neck that enter the thoracolumbar spinal segments, thus bypassing the sacral cord.[80]

Peripheral sympathetic injury results in an open, nonfunctional bladder neck and proximal urethra. Although this could occur as an isolated injury, it typically occurs in association with partial detrusor denervation, but with preservation of sphincter function. The combination of decreased compliance, open bladder neck, and fixed external sphincter resistance results in the paradoxical symptomatology of both leaking across the distal sphincter and inability to empty the bladder.

The integrity of the sacral reflex may be further studied with the evaluation of the latency time of the sacral evoked potentials by stimulating the penile skin and recording the response with a needle electrode in the bulbocavernosus muscle.[54,81] In patients with complete cauda equina lesions, the sacral evoked response is either absent or significantly prolonged[82] and this represents a more sensitive indicator of neuropathy than the classic EMG changes.

Rockswold and Bradley[83] reported the use of evoked EMG responses in diagnosing lesions of the cauda equina in 110 patients and correlated the results with clinical myelographic and operative findings. Absent evoked EMG responses were consistently correlated with urinary retention. Delayed evoked EMG responses were less consistently associated with urinary retention and lesions along this reflex pathway. However, normal responses do not exclude significant pathology of the cauda equina. Four patients with normal preoperative evoked EMG responses had arachnoiditis, a congenital lipoma, or a myelomeningocele at the time of the operation. Therefore, the technique cannot be considered in isolation. The technique does provide information regarding lesions involving the sacral nerves distal to the dural sac that were not accessible to myelography. Routine magnetic resonance imaging (MRI) was not available at that study. In conclusion, the major urodynamic features in patients with cauda equina injury are an absent or diminished bulbocavernosus reflex, detrusor areflexia, neuropathic changes on perineal floor EMG, and absent evoked EMG responses.

Lesions of the pudendal nerve

The pudendal nerve arises for anterior primary rami of S2–4 and leaves the pelvis through the greater sciatic foramen below the piriformis muscle and passes forward into the ischiorectal fossa. The nerve is occasionally injured in fractures of the pelvis. Damage produces sensory loss in the perineum and scrotum on the side of the lesion. Bilateral lesions produce bladder disturbances with urinary incontinence and overflow.

Treatment

Individualization of treatment is necessary according to the underlying abnormality. Indwelling or intermittent catheterization should be instituted in the postoperative period. Urodynamic evaluation should be performed after a few weeks. It is better to study the patients after they have had a chance to recover from the major pelvic insult. If the bladder is acontractile, clean intermittent self-catheterization is our recommendation. If bladder compliance diminishes (Figure 10.5) or detrusor hyperreflexia develops, anticholinergics should be started in order to prevent upper tract damage.[48,72]

If the detrusor hyperreflexia or poor filling compliance is unresponsive to aggressive anticholinergic trials, bladder augmentation using a detubularized bowel segment may be used. Prostatectomy in a man who develops urinary retention immediately after a major pelvic operation must be avoided. Not only does resection of the prostate not help

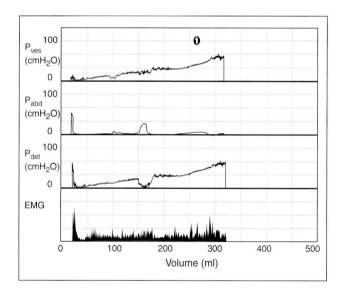

Figure 10.5
Detrusor areflexia and poor bladder compliance 2 years after abdominal perineal resection of patient described in Figure 10.2. The patient has been on intermittent self-catheterization but began to develop urine leakage between catheterization and decreased catheterization volumes. The bladder remains areflexive but detrusor compliance has diminished and she leaked urine at a bladder leak point pressure of 45 cmH₂O at 320 ml.[1] P$_{ves}$, intravesical pressure; P$_{abd}$, abdominal pressure; P$_{det}$, detrusor pressure.

a man to urinate but, it also may result in stress urinary incontinence when there is underlying denervation of the external sphincter.[53] Even when there is clearly documented benign prostatic hyperplasia (BPH) prior to cauda equina surgery or injury, resection of the internal sphincter, the bladder neck, in light of a denervated external sphincter, can render the unhappy patient who has a bladder that does not work worse, because now not only can he not void but he is also completely incontinent and wearing an adult diaper. It is medically unsound to perform an prostatectomy without careful urodynamic testing in this scenario.

The most commonly used pharmacologic agent in the treatment of detrusor areflexia is the cholinergic agent bethanechol chloride. Although the drug increases intravesical pressure, it has not been shown beneficial in promoting adequate bladder emptying.[84,85] In fact, there are no single prospective randomized studies that demonstrate any clinical efficacy of bethanechol chloride in detrusor areflexia. Bethanechol chloride is especially contraindicated in patients with detrusor areflexia and bladder outlet obstruction such as BPH, urethral stricture, or sphincter dyssynergia. In this scenario, increasing intravesical pressure with the existing increased outlet resistance may hasten vesicoureteral reflux, urinary sepsis, and renal damage. Similarly, the performance of Credé's maneuver for detrusor areflexia may trigger a reflex contraction of the perineal floor, thus increasing bladder outlet resistance, a phenomenon that can also impede renal function. An adequate Credé's maneuver or abdominal straining voiding is only effective when both smooth and skeletal muscle resistance are significantly reduced. This is feasible in some women but rarely effective or safe in men. Finally, external stimulation with implantable electrodes has met with many problems, making its routine use impractical.

Stress urinary incontinence secondary to pelvic floor denervation may be difficult to manage. In men, the application of an external condom-type collecting device is the most common solution. In women, however, no external urinary collection device has ever proven effective. Many women choose an indwelling Foley catheter but this is associated with bladder irritation, chronic bacterial colonization, destruction of the sphincter mechanism, and even squamous cell carcinoma of the bladder with prolonged indwelling bladder catheterization.

Treatment options for the destroyed urethral sphincter require major reconstructive urological surgery such as the artificial urinary sphincter implantation, pubovaginal sling procedures, or supravesical urinary diversion such as the ileocystostomy, bladder chimney procedure. Finally, in patients with detrusor and perineal floor denervation but preservation of urethral smooth muscle function, the combination of bladder augmentation with a continent stoma and intermittent catheterization provides a reasonable therapeutic alternative.

Conclusions

Neuro-urologic dysfunction secondary to injury to the cauda equina and pelvic plexus can result in devastating urologic dysfunction, the loss of volitional micturition. Fortunately, most of the initial bladder and urethral dysfunction will recover within 6–12 months unless the injury is severe and bilateral. Conservative bladder management such as clean intermittent self-catheterization guided by urodynamic evaluation is the preferred management. Permanent solutions should be deferred after 1 year.

Infectious neurologic problems
Acquired immune deficiency syndrome

The acquired immune deficiency syndrome (AIDS) is commonly associated with neurologic dysfunction. Neurological involvement occurs in as many as 40% of patients with AIDS. It involves both the central and peripheral nervous systems.

Kahn and associates[86] reported on 11 patients with neurogenic bladder during a 1-year period where 677 cases of AIDS were reported at their institution. Urinary retention was the most common presenting symptom, and was seen in 6 of the 11 patients (55%). Urodynamic evaluation revealed detrusor areflexia in 36%, detrusor hyperreflexia in 27%, and bladder outlet obstruction in 18%. The remaining 19% had normal urodynamic evaluation.

Neurosyphilis (tabes dorsalis)

Neurosyphilis has long been recognized as a cause of central and peripheral nerve abnormalities. Voiding dysfunction related to neurosyphilis was common in the era before penicillin use. Hattori and associates[87] reported decreased bladder sensation in tabes dorsalis. Six of 8 patients had increased bladder capacity at first desire to void and 3 also had an increased maximum cystometric capacity. The most common urodynamic finding in neurosyphilis is detrusor areflexia. Sphincteric EMG activity is generally normal, as the corticospinal tracts are not involved in the disorder.[88]

Herpes zoster and herpes simplex

Herpes zoster is an acute, painful mononeuropathy associated with a vesicular eruption in the distribution of the affected nerve. The viral activity is predominantly located in the dorsal root ganglia or sensory ganglia of the cranial nerves. However, sacral nerve involvement may be associated with loss of bladder and anal sphincter control.[89]

When viral invasion of the lumbosacral dorsal roots occurs there may be visible skin vesicles along the corresponding dermatome, and cystoscopy may reveal a similar grouping of vesicles in the urethral and bladder mucosa. The early stages of lower urinary tract involvement with herpes are manifested as symptomatic detrusor instability with urinary frequency and urgency, but the latter stages include decreased sensation of filling and elevated residual urine or urinary retention.[90] On the positive side, the problem is only temporary and generally spontaneous over several months.

Guillain–Barré syndrome

Guillain–Barré syndrome, also known as postinfectious polyneuritis, is an acute symmetric ascending polyneuropathy occurring 1–4 weeks after an acute infection. The syndrome is characterized by rapidly progressive signs of motor weakness and paresthesias progressing from lower to upper extremities. Paralysis may progress for about 10 days and then remains relatively unchanged for about 2 weeks. The recovery is gradual and may take from 6 months to 2 years for completion. Autonomic disorders are not unusual.

The inflammatory process may involve the afferent sensory neurons as well and produce loss of position and vibration sense. This may explain the urodynamic findings of detrusor motor and sensory deficits with Guillain–Barré syndrome.[91] Retention of urine may occur in the early stages and require bladder catheterization.[92] Long-term urological dysfunction is uncommon.

Lyme disease

Lyme disease, caused by the spirochete *Borrelia burgdorferi*, is associated with a variety of neurologic sequelae. The urological manifestation of Lyme disease can be the primary or late manifestation of the disease affecting both sexes and all ages. Urinary urgency, nocturia, and urge incontinence are the most common urological symptoms.[93,94]

Urodynamic evaluation in a series of 7 patients revealed detrusor hyperreflexia in 5 patients and detrusor areflexia in 2 patients. Detrusor-external sphincter dyssynergia was not noted on EMG in any patient. The urinary tract may be involved in two different ways in the course of Lyme disease. There may be neurogenic voiding dysfunction as a part of neuroborreliosis and there may also be direct invasion of the urinary tract by the spirochete. This is analogous to voiding dysfunction secondary to other neurologic diseases such as multiple sclerosis. Only one patient had direct bladder invasion by the spirochete and he was an unusual case of Lyme disease with a fulminate presentation and multisystem involvement.

Sacral nerve stimulation
Sacral afferent input-modifying micturition reflexes

The guarding and voiding reflexes discussed in the first section (The mechanism of micturition reflexes) are activated at different times under completely different clinical scenarios. However, anatomically they are located in close proximity in the S2–4 levels of the human spinal cord.[95] Both sets of reflexes are modulated by a number of centers in the brain. Thus, these reflexes can be altered by a variety of neurologic diseases, some of which can unmask involuntary bladder activity mediated by C-fibers. It is possible to modulate these reflexes via sacral nerve stimulation (SNS) and restore voluntary micturition (Figure 10.5).

Experimental data from animals indicate that somatic afferent input to the sacral spinal cord can modulate the guarding and bladder–bladder reflexes. de Groat[13] has shown that sacral preganglionic outflow to the urinary bladder receives inhibitory inputs from various somatic and visceral afferents, as well as a recurrent inhibitory pathway.[96,97] The experiments have also provided information about the organization of these inhibitory mechanisms.[98,99] Electrical stimulation of somatic afferents in the pudendal nerve elicits inhibitory mechanisms.[100] This is supported by the finding that interneurons in the sacral autonomic nucleus exhibiting firing correlated with bladder activity and were inhibited by activation of somatic afferent pathways. This electrical stimulation of somatic efferent nerves in the sacral spinal roots could inhibit reflex of bladder hyperactivity mediated by spinal or supraspinal pathways. In neonatal kittens and rats, micturition as well as defecation are elicited when their mother licks the perineal region.[100] This reflex appears to be the primary stimulus for micturition, since urinary retention occurs when the young kittens and rat pups are separated from their mother.

To induce micturition the perineal afferents must activate the parasympathetic excitatory inputs to the bladder but also suppress the urethral sympathetic and sphincter somatic guarding reflexes. A suppression of guarding reflexes by SNS contributes to enhancement of voiding in patients with urinary retention.

The perineal-to-bladder reflex is very prominent during the first four postnatal weeks and then becomes less effective and usually disappears in kittens by the age of 7–8 weeks, which is the approximate age of weaning. In adult animals and humans, perineal stimulation or mechanical stimulation of the sex organs (vagina or penis) inhibits the micturition reflex.[6,11,12,101]

Besides the strong animal research that identified somatic afferent modulation of bladder and urethral reflexes, there are also data from clinical physiological studies supporting the view that stimulation of sacral afferents can modify bladder and urethral sphincter reflexes. Functional electrical stimulation appears to be a favorable non-surgical treatment for many patients with detrusor instability. Stimulation techniques have utilized surface electrodes, anal and vaginal plug electrodes,[102–104] and dorsal penile nerve electrodes.[105,106]

Hypotheses of sacral nerve stimulation mechanisms

How do sacral somatic afferents alter lower urinary tract reflexes to promote voiding? To understand this mechanism, it should be recognized that, in adults, brain pathways are necessary to turn off sphincter and urethral guarding reflexes to allow efficient bladder emptying. Thus, spinal cord injury produces bladder sphincter dyssynergia and inefficient bladder emptying by eliminating the brain mechanisms (Figure 10.6). This may also occur after more subtle neurologic lesions in patients with idiopathic urinary retention such as after a bout of prostatitis or urinary tract infection. Before the development of brain control of micturition, at least in animals, that stimulation of somatic afferent pathways passing through the pudendal nerve to the perineum can initiate efficient voiding by activating bladder efferent pathways and turning off the excitatory pathways to the urethral outlet.[4,5,9] Tactile stimulation of the perineum in the cat also inhibits the bladder-sympathetic reflex component of the guarding reflex mechanism. With the hypothesis that SNS can elicit similar responses in patients with urinary retention and turn off excitatory

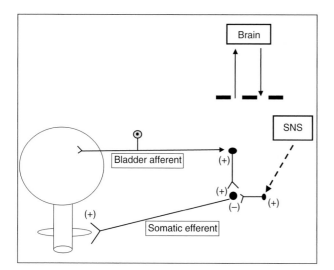

Figure 10.6
In cases of neurologic diseases, the brain cannot turn off the guarding reflex and retention can occur. Sacral nerve stimulation (SNS) restores voluntary micturition in cases of voiding dysfunction and urinary retention but inhibiting the guarding reflex.

outflow to the urethral outlet and promote bladder emptying, Tanagho et al[107] demonstrated the efficacy of sacral nerve stimulation for DA not only in the animal studies but also in clinical studies. The methods for the nerve stimulation also vary – including intraspinal transplantation, nerve root implantation, and transcutaneous stimulation.[107–109] Because sphincter activity can generate afferent input to the spinal cord that can in turn inhibit reflex bladder activity, an indirect benefit of suppressing sphincter reflexes would be a facilitation of bladder activity. This may also be useful in this patient population.

Myogenic sections

Degeneration of or damage to bladder smooth muscle is also an important factor that induces detrusor hyporeflexia or areflexia. Diabetes is the most common disease that shows these conditions. Chronic overdistention can result in detrusor myogenic failure even if the neurologic disease is treated or reversed. Bladder management to avoid overdistention, such as institution of intermittent catheterization after spinal cord injury, may protect the bladder from permanent myogenic damage.

At the present time, detrusor myogenic failure has been impossible to treat or reverse. This is why catheterization, either intermittent or indwelling, has been the most commonly used management. There is potential hope for the future, however, of transplanting muscle stem cells to repair the damaged bladder with or without *ex-vivo* gene therapy.

The aim of *ex-vivo* cell therapy is to replace, repair, or enhance the biological function of damaged tissue or organs. An *ex-vivo* process involves harvesting cells from patients or donors, *in-vitro* manipulation to enhance the therapeutic potential of the harvested cells (*ex-vivo* gene therapy), and subsequent injection or implantation of the cells into the patient. One particular advantage of cellular-based *ex-vivo* gene therapy is that the manufactured cells act like bioreactors. At any stage of the process, cells can be cryopreserved so that therapy can be scheduled according to the patient's requirements.[110] A safety feature of the *ex-vivo* approach is that all genetic manipulation involving viral vectors is performed *in vitro* in a controlled fashion. Therefore, the patients are not directly exposed to the viral vectors. In addition, the amount of gene product expression can be quantitated, leading to controlled protein production at specific sites with decreased system side-effects.[111]

Cell transplantation is not a new concept; however, the field of urologic tissue engineering has just recently grown to new and exciting levels. Because there is a general lack of regenerative ability in the bladder and urethral smooth muscle, research has centered on tissue repair by using pluripotent stem cells derived from other lineages. Our laboratory has focused on the isolation and characterization of a small population of these pluripotent stem cells that were derived from skeletal muscle. Through purifying techniques, we are capable of isolating cells that are highly capable of surviving post-transplantation and differentiating into other lineages.

The rationale for using skeletal muscle for cellular-based gene therapy for the urinary tract is two-fold. In contrast to smooth muscle, skeletal muscle is constantly undergoing repair of its damaged tissue due to the presence of satellite cells.[112] These cells are fusion-competent skeletal muscle precursors and, when differentiated, fuse to form myofibers capable of muscle contraction. Secondly, a small percentage of muscle satellite cells behave like pluripotent stem cells that have the ability to differentiate into another lineage.

We and other investigators have previously demonstrated the ability to harvest muscle-derived cells (MDC) which contain satellite cells and stem cells from a skeletal muscle biopsy.[113,114] MDC have been used for the delivery of secretory nonmuscle protein products such as human growth hormone and coagulation factor IX to the circulation.[115,116] In addition, when MDC differentiate, they form myofibers that become postmitotic and consequently exhibit long-term transgene persistence.[117] Thus, MDC from skeletal muscle might be used as a treatment for detrusor areflexia or impaired bladder contractility.[118,119]

Summary

Detrusor areflexia (DA) or impaired contractility of the detrusor can be observed in many neurologic conditions. Careful examinations not only urodynamically but also neurologically are necessary for the diagnosis of DA. Cholinergic agents, α_1 blockers, and self-intermittent catheterization are the typical conservative treatment options. Sacral nerve stimulation may be an effective treatment option for detrusor areflexia. New concepts such as stem cell therapy[120] and neurotrophic gene therapy[121] are being explored.

References

1. Ostergard DR, Bent AE. Appendices. In: Ostergard DR, eds. Urogynecology and urodynamics. Theory and practice. Baltimore: Williams and Wilkins, 1996:643–660.

2. Chancellor MB, Yoshimura N. Physiology and pharmacology of the bladder and urethra. In: Walsh PC, Retik AB, Vaughan Jr ED, Wein AJ, eds. Campbell urology, 8th edn. Philadelphia: WB Saunders, 2002; 2 (Pt 4):831–886.

3. de Groat WC, Theobald RJ. Reflex activation of sympathetic pathways to vesical smooth muscle and parasympathetic ganglia by electrical stimulation of vesical afferents. J Physiol 1976; 259: 223–237.

4. de Groat WC. Central nervous system control of micturition. In: O'Donnell PD, ed. Urinary incontinence. St. Louis: Mosby, 1997:33–47.

5. Yoshimura N, de Groat WC. Neural control of the lower urinary tract. Int J Urol 1997; 4:111–125.

6. de Groat WC, Araki I, Vizzard MA, et al. Developmental and injury induced plasticity in the micturition reflex pathway. Behav Brain Res 1998; 92:127–140.

7. Yoshimura N, Chancellor MB. Current and future pharmacological therapy for overactive bladder. J Urol 2002; 168:1897–1913.

8. Cheng CL, Ma CP, de Groat WC. Effect of capsaicin on micturition and associated reflexes in rats. Am J Physiol 1993; 265:R132–138.

9. Kruse MN, de Groat WC. Spinal pathways mediate coordinated bladder/urethral sphincter activity during reflex micturition in normal and spinal cord injured neonatal rats. Neurosci Lett 1993; 152:141–144.

10. Cheng CL, Ma CP, de Groat WC. Effect of capsaicin on micturition and associated reflexes in chronic spinal rats. Brain Res 1995; 678:40–48.

11. de Groat WC, Nadelhaft I, Milne RJ, et al. Organization of the sacral parasympathetic reflex pathways to the urinary bladder and large intestine. J Auton Nerv Syst 1981; 3:135–160.

12. de Groat WC, Vizzard MA, Araki I, Roppolo JR. Spinal interneurons and preganglionic neurons in sacral autonomic reflex pathways. In: Holstege G, Bandler R, Saper C, eds. The emotional motor system. Progress in Brain Research. New York: Elsevier Science Publishers, 1996; 107:97.

13. de Groat WC. Inhibitory mechanisms in the sacral reflex pathways to the urinary bladder. In: Ryall RW, Kelly JS, eds. Iontophoresis and transmitter mechanisms in the mammalian central nervous system, Holland: Elsevier, 1978:366–368.

14. Chancellor MB, Blaivas JG. Classification of neurogenic bladder disease. In: Chancellor MB, eds. Practical neuro-urology. Boston: Butterworth-Heinemann, 1995:25–32.

15. Frimodt-Moller C. Diabetic cystopathy: I. A clinical study of the frequency of bladder dysfunction in diabetics. Dan Med Bull 1976; 23:267–278.

16. Ellenburg M. Development of urinary bladder dysfunction in diabetes mellitus. Ann Intern Med 1980; 92:321–323.

17. Ueda T, Yoshimura N, Yoshida O. Diabetic cystopathy: relationship to autonomic neuropathy detected by sympathetic skin response. J Urol 1997; 157:580–584.

18. Frimodt-Moller C. Diabetic cystopathy: epidemiology and related disorders. Ann Intern Med 1980; 92:318–321.

19. Mastri AR. Neuropathology of diabetic neurogenic bladder. Ann Intern Med 1980; 92:316–318.

20. Van Poppel H, Stessens R, Van Damme B, et al. Diabetic cystopathy: neuropathological examination of urinary bladder biopsy. Eur Urol 1988; 15:128–131.

21. Apfel SC. Neurotrophic factors and diabetic peripheral neuropathy. Eur Neurol 1999; 41(Suppl):27–34.

22. Kasayama S, Oka T. Impaired production of nerve growth factor in the submandibular gland of diabetic mice. Am J Physiol 1989; 257:E400–E404.

23. Hellweg R, Hartung HD. Endogenous levels of nerve growth factor (NGF) are altered in experimental diabetes mellitus: a possible role of NGF in the pathogenesis of diabetic neuropathy. J Neurosci Res 1990; 26:258–267.

24. Fernyhough P, Diemel LT, Brewster WJ, Tomlinson DR. Deficits in sciatic nerve neuropeptide content coincide with a reduction in target tissue nerve growth factor messenger RNA in streptozotocin-diabetic rats: effects of insulin treatment. Neuroscience 1994; 62:337–344.

25. Steinbacher BC, Nadelhaft I. Increased level of nerve growth factor in the urinary bladder and hypertrophy of dorsal root ganglion neurons in the diabetic rat. Brain Res 1998; 782:255–260.

26. Diemel LT, Cai F, Anand P, et al. Increased nerve growth factor mRNA in lateral calf skin biopsies from diabetic patients. Diabet Med 1999; 16:113–118.

27. Schmid H, Forman LA, Cao X, et al. Heterogenous cardiac sympathetic denervation and decreased myocardial nerve growth factor in streptozotocin-induced diabetic rats: implications for cardiac sympathetic dysinnervation complicating diabetes. Diabetes 1999; 48:603–608.

28. Ihara C, Shimatsu A, Mizuta H. Decreased neurotrophin-3 expression in skeletal muscles of streptozotocin-induced diabetic rats. Neuropeptides 1996; 30:309–312.

29. Fernyhough P, Diemel LT, Tomlinson DR. Target tissue production and axonal transport of neurotrophin-3 are reduced in streptozotocin-diabetic rats. Diabetologia 1998; 41:300–306.

30. Cai F, Tomlinson DR, Fernyhough P. Elevated expression of neurotorophin-3 mRNA in sensory nerve of streptozotocin-diabetic rats. Neurosci Lett 1999; 263:81–84.

31. Sasaki K, Chancellor MB, Phelan MW, et al. The correlation between bladder dysfunction and decreased nerve growth factor (NGF) levels in the bladder and lumbosacral dorsal root ganglia in diabetic rats. J Urol 2002; 167(Suppl):277A.

32. Frimodt-Moller C. Diabetic cystopathy: a review of the urodynamic and clinical features of neurogenic bladder dysfunction in diabetes mellitus. Dan Med Bull 1978; 25:49–60.

33. Blaivas JG. Neurogenic dysfunction. In: Yalla SU, McGuire EJ, Elbadawi A, Blaivas JG, eds. Neurourology and urodynamics: principles and practice. New York: Macmillan, 1988:347–350.

34. Kaplan SA, Te AE, Blaivas JG. Urodynamic findings in patients with diabetic cystopathy. J Urol 1995; 153:342–344.

35. Starer P, Libow L. Cystometric evaluation of bladder dysfunction in elderly diabetic patients. Arch Intern Med 1990; 150:810–813.

36. Bradley WE. Diagnosis of urinary bladder dysfunction in diabetes mellitus. Ann Intern Med 1980; 92:323–326.

37. Apfel SC, Arezzo JC, Brownlee M, et al. Nerve growth factor administration protects against experimental diabetic sensory neuropathy. Brain Res 1994; 634:7–12.

38. Delcroix JD, Michael GJ, Priestley JV, et al. Effect of nerve growth factor treatment on p75^{NTR} gene expression in lumbar dorsal root ganglia of streptozotocin-induced diabetic rats. Diabetes 1998; 47:1779–1785.

39. Unger JW, Klitzsch T, Pera S, Reiter R. Nerve growth factor (NGF) and diabetic neuropathy in the rat: morphological investigation of the sural nerve, dorsal root ganglion, and spinal cord. Exp Neurol 1998; 153:23–34.

40. Petty BG, Comblath DR, Adornato BT, et al. The effect of systemically administered recombinant human nerve growth factor in healthy human projects. Ann Neurol 1994; 36:244–246.

41. Apfel SC, Kessler JA, Adomato BT, et al. The NGF study group: recombinant human nerve growth factor in the treatment of diabetic polyneuropathy. Neurology 1998; 51:695–702.

42. Apfel SC, Schwartz S, Adomato BT, et al. The rhNGF clinical investigator group: efficacy and safety of recombinant human nerve growth factor in patients with diabetic polyneuropathy. A randomized control trial. JAMA 2000; 284:2215–2221.

43. Sasaki K, Yoshimura N, Phelan MW, et al. Nerve growth factor (NGF) gene therapy mediated by herpes simplex virus (HSV) vectors reverses bladder dysfunction and the decline in NGF expression in L6–S1 afferent neurons in diabetic rats. J Urol 2001; 165(Suppl):274A.

44. Akkina SK, Patterson CL, Wright DE. GDNF rescues nonpeptidergic unmyelinated primary afferents in streptozotocin-treated diabetic mice. Exp Neurol 2001; 167:173–182.

45. Pradat PF, Kennel P, Naimi-Sadaoui S, et al. Continuous delivery of neurotrophin 3 by gene therapy has a neuroprotective effect in experimental models of diabetic and acrylamide neuropathies. Hum Gene Ther 2001; 12:2237–2249.

46. Bradley WE, Andersen JT. Neuromuscular dysfunction of the lower urinary tract in patients with lesions of the cauda equina and conus medullaris. J Urol 1976; 116:620–621.

47. Hellstrom P, Kortelainen P, Kontturi M. Late urodynamic findings after surgery for cauda equina syndrome caused by a prolapsed lumbar intervertebral disk. J Urol 1986; 135:308–312.

48. Woodside JR, Crawford ED. Urodynamic features pelvic plexus injury. J Urol 1980; 124:657–658.

49. Blaivas JG, Barbalias GA. Characteristics of neural injury after abdominoperineal resection of the rectum. J Urol 1983; 129:84–87.

50. Gray H. In: Williams PL, Warwick R, eds. Gray's anatomy, 36th edn. Edinburgh: Churchill Livingstone, 1984:1110–1123.

51. Marani E, Pijl ME, Kraan MC, et al. Interconnections of the upper ventral rami of the human sacral plexus: a reappraisal for dorsal rhizotomy in neurostimulation operations. Neurourol Urodyn 1993; 12:585–598.

52. Forney JP. The effect of radical hysterectomy on bladder physiology. Am J Obstet Gynecol 1980; 138:374–382.

53. Yalla SV, Andriole GL. Vesicourethral dysfunction following pelvic visceral ablative surgery. J Urol 1984; 132:503–509.

54. Siroky MB, Sax DS, Krane RJ. Sacral signal tracing: the electrophysiology of the bulbocavernosus reflex. J Urol 1979; 122:661–664.

55. Smith PH, Ballantyne B. The neuroanatomical basis for denervation of the urinary bladder following major pelvic surgery. Br J Surg 1968; 55:929–933.

56. McGuire EJ. Urodynamic evaluation after abdominal-perineal resection and lumbar intervertebral disc herniation. Urology 1975; 6:63–70.

57. Seski JC, Diokno AC. Bladder dysfunction after radical abdominal hysterectomy. Am J Obstet Gynecol 1977; 128:643–651.

58. Mundy AR. An anatomical explanation for bladder dysfunction following rectal and uterine surgery. Br J Urol 1982; 54:501–504.

59. Patterson FP, Morton KS. Neurologic complications of fractures and dislocations of the pelvis. Surg Gynecol Obstet 1961; 112:702.

60. Brynes DP, Russo GL, Dunker TB, Cowley RA. Sacrum fractures and neurological damage. J Neuorsurg 1977; 47:459–462.

61. Heckman JD, Keats PK. Fracture of the sacrum in children. J Bone Joint Surg Am 1978; 60:404–405.

62. Goodell CL. Neurological deficit associated to pelvic fractures. J Neurosurg 1966; 24:837–842.

63. Fountain SS, Hamilton RD, Jameson RM. Transverse fractures of the sacrum: a report of six cases. J Bone Joint Surg Am 1977; 59:486–489.

64. Pavlakis AJ. Cauda equina and pelvic plexus injury. In: Krane RJ, Siroky MB, eds. Clinical neuro-urology. Boston: Little Brown, 1991:333–334.

65. Dewey P, Browne PSH. Fractures and dislocation of the lumbosacral spine with cauda equina lesion. J Bone Joint Surg Br 1968; 50:635–638.

66. Fardon DF. Displaced fractures of the lumbosacral spine with delayed cauda equina deficit. Clin Orthop 1976; 120:155–158.

67. Scott PJ. Bladder paralysis in cauda equina lesions from disc prolapse. J Bone Joint Surg 1965; 47:244.

68. Bartolin Z, Vilendecic M, Derezic D. Bladder function after surgery for lumber intervertebral disk protrusion. J Urol 1999; 161:1885–1887.

69. O'Flynn KJ, Murphy R, Thomas DG. Neurogenic bladder dysfunction in lumbar intervertebral disc prolapse. Br J Urol 1992; 69:38–40.

70. Shapiro S. Medical realities of cauda equina syndromes secondary to lumbar disc herniation. Spine 2000; 25:348–352.

71. Albert NE, Sparks FC, McGuire EJ. Effect of pelvic and retroperitoneal surgery on the urethral pressure profile and perineal floor electromyogram in dogs. Invest Urol 1977; 15:140–142.

72. McGuire EJ, Wagner FC. The effects of sacral denervation on bladder and urethral function. Surg Gynecol Obstet 1977; 144:343–346.

73. Blaivas JG, Scott MR, Labib KB. Urodynamic evaluation as neurologic test for sacral cord function. Urology 1979; 8:682–687.

74. Scott M. Surgery of the spinal column. Prog Neurol Psychiatry 1965; 20:509–523.

75. Lapides J, Babbitt JM. Diagnostic value of bulbocavernosus reflex. JAMA 1956; 162:971.

76. Neal DE, Boguc PRI, Williams RE. Histological appearances of the nerves of the bladder in patients with denervation of the bladder after excision of the rectum. Br J Urol 1982; 54:658–666.

77. Jones DL, Moore T. The types of neuropathic bladder dysfunction associated with prolapsed lumbar intervertebral discs. Br J Urol 1973; 45:39–43.

78. Kuru M. Nervous control of micturition. Physiol Rev 1965; 45:425.

79. Bradley WE, Teague C. Spinal cord representation of the peripheral neural pathways of the micturition reflex. J Urol 1969; 101:220–223.

80. Bradley WE, Timm GM, Scott FB. Cystometry: V. Bladder sensation. Urology 1975; 6:654–658.

81. Blaivas JG, Zaved AAH, Labib KB. The bulbocavernosus reflex in urology: a prospective study of 299 patients. J Urol 1981; 126:197–199.

82. Krane RJ, Siroky MB. Studies on sacral evoked potentials. J Urol 1980; 124:872–876.

83. Rockswold GL, Bradley WE. The use of evoked electromyographic responses in diagnosing lesions of the cauda equina. J Urol 1977; 118:629–631.

84. Blaivas JG, Labib KB, Michalik SJ, Zayed AA. Failure of bethanechol denervation supersensitivity as a diagnostic aid. J Urol 1980; 123:199–201.

85. Wein A, Raezer D, Malloy T. Failure of the bethanechol supersensitivity test to predict improved voiding after subcutaneous bethanechol administration. J Urol 1980; 123:302–303.

86. Kahn Z, Singh VK, Yang WE. Neurogenic bladder in acquired immune deficiency syndrome (AIDS). Urology 1992; 40:289–291.

87. Hattori T, Yasuda K, Kita K, Hirayama K. Disorders of micturition in tabes dorsalis. Br J Urol 1990; 65:497–499.

88. Wheeler JS Jr, Culkin DJ, O'Hara RJ, Canning JR. Bladder dysfunction and neurosyphilis. J Urol 1986; 136:903–905.

89. Cohen LM, Fowler JF, Owen LG, Callen JP. Urinary retention associated with herpes zoster infection. Int J Dermatol 1993; 32:24–26.

90. Yamanishi T, Yasuda K, Sakakibara R, et al. Urinary retention due to herpes virus infections. Neurol Urodyn 1998; 17:613–619.

91. Wheeler JS Jr, Siroky MB, Pavlakis A, Krane RJ. The urodynamic aspects of the Guillain–Barré syndrome. J Urol 1984; 137:917–919.

92. Kogan BA, Solomon MH, Diokno AC. Urinary retention secondary to Landry Guillain–Barré syndrome. J Urol 1981; 126:643–644.

93. Chancellor MB, McGinnis DE, Shenot PJ, et al. Lyme cystitis and neurogenic bladder dysfunction. Lancet 1992; 339:1237–1238.

94. Chancellor MB, McGinnis DE, Shenot PJ, et al. Urinary dysfunction in Lyme disease. J Urol 1992; 149:26–30.

95. Chancellor MB, Chartier-Kastler EJ. Principles of sacral nerve stimulation (SNS) for the treatment of bladder and urethral sphincter dysfunctions. J Neuromodulation 2000; 3:15–26.

96. de Groat WC, Ryall RW. The identification and antidromic responses of sacral preganglionic parasympathetic neurons. J Physiol 1968; 196:563–577.

97. de Groat WC. Nervous control of the urinary bladder of the cat. Brain Res 1975; 87:201–211.

98. de Groat WC. Inhibition and excitation of sacral parasympathetic neurons by visceral and cutaneous stimuli in the cat. Brain Res 1971; 33:499–503.

99. de Groat WC. Mechanisms underlying recurrent inhibition in the sacral parasympathetic outflow to the urinary bladder. J Physiol 1976; 257:503–513.

100. de Groat WC. Changes in the organization of the micturition reflex pathway of the cat after transection of the spinal cord. In: Veraa RP, Grafstein B, eds. Cellular mechanisms for recovery from nervous systems injury: a conference report. Exp Neurol 1981; 71:22.

101. de Groat WC, Ryall RW. Recurrent inhibition in sacral parasympathetic pathways to the bladder. J Physiol 1968; 196:579–591.

102. Janez J, Plevnik S, Suhet P. Urethral and bladder responses to anal electrical stimulation. J Urol 1979; 122:192–194.

103. Fall M. Electrical pelvic floor stimulation for the control of detrusor instability. Neurourol Urodyn 1985; 4:329.

104. Ohlsson BL, Fall M, Frankenbers-Sommar S. Effects of external and direct pudendal nerve maximal electrical stimulation in the treatment of the uninhibited overactive bladder. Br J Urol 1989; 64:374–380.

105. Wheeler JS Jr, Walter JS, Zaszczurynski PJ. Bladder inhibition by penile nerve stimulation in spinal cord injury patients. J Urol 1992; 147:100–103.

106. Walter JS, Wheeler JS, Robinson CJ, Wurster RD. Inhibiting the hyperreflexic bladder with electrical stimulation in a spinal animal model. Neurourol Urodyn 1993; 12:241–252.

107. Tanagho EA, Schmidt RA. Electrical stimulation in the clinical management of the neurogenic bladder. J Urol 1988; 140:1331–1339.

108. Heine JP, Schmidt RA, Tanagho EA. Intraspinal sacral root stimulation for controlled micturition. Invest Urol 1977; 15:78–82.

109. Crocker M, Doleys DM, Dolce JJ. Transcutaneous electrical nerve stimulation in urinary retention. South Med J 1985; 78: 1515–1516.

110. Huard J, Acsadi G, Jani A, et al. Gene transfer into skeletal muscles by isogenic myoblasts. Hum Gene Ther 1994; 5:949–958.

111. Schindhelm K, Nordon R. Ex vivo cell therapy. San Diego: Academic Press, 1999:1–4.

112. Campion DR. The muscle satellite cell: a review. Int Rev Cytol 1984; 87:225.

113. Rando TO, Blau HM. Primary mouse myoblast purification, characterization, and transplantation for cell-mediated gene therapy. J Cell Biol 1994; 125:1275–1287.

114. Qu Z, Balkir L, van Deutekom JC, Robbins PD, et al. Development of approaches to improve cell survival in myoblast transfer therapy. J Cell Biol 1998; 142:1257.

115. Dhawan J, Pan LC, Pavlath GK, et al. Systemic delivery of human growth hormone by injection of genetically engineered myoblasts. Science 1991; 254:1509.

116. Dai Y, Schwarz EM, Gu D, et al. Cellular and humoral immune responses to adenoviral vectors containing factor IX gene: tolerization of factor IX and vector antigens allow for long-term expression. Proc Natl Acad Sci USA 1995; 92:1401.

117. Jiao S, Guerich V, Wolffe JA. Long-term correction of rat model of Parkinson's disease by gene therapy. Nature 1993; 362:450.

118. Chancellor MB, Yokoyama T, Tirney S, et al. Preliminary results of myoblast injection into the urethra and bladder wall: a possible method for the treatment of stress urinary incontinence and impaired detrusor contractility. Neurourol Urodyn 2000; 19:279–287.

119. Yokoyama T, Dhir R, Qu Z, et al. Persistence and survival of autologous muscle derived cells versus bovine collagen as possible treatment of stress urinary incontinence. J Urol 2001; 165:271–276.

120. Yokoyama T, Huard J, Yoshimura N, et al. Muscle derived cells transplantation and differentiation into the lower urinary tract smooth muscle. Urology 2001; 57:826–831.

121. Sasaki K, Yoshimura N, Chancellor MB. Implications of diabetes mellitus, impotence; neurogenic bladder and renal diseases. Urol Cl N Am 2003; 30:1–2.

11

Pathophysiology of the low compliant bladder

Emmanuel Chartier-Kastler, Jean-Marc Soler, and Pierre Denys

Introduction and physiology

Bladder compliance is defined by the ratio of the increase in intravesical pressure over the increase in bladder volume ($\Delta V / \Delta P$). It reflects the capacity of the detrusor to allow bladder filling at low pressure in order to maintain the functional properties of the urinary system and to avoid deterioration of these properties (vesicorenal reflux, deterioration of the bladder wall, incontinence). It is dependent on both the physical reservoir qualities and the qualitative and quantitative innervation of the bladder (autonomic nervous system).

The urodynamic definition of bladder compliance was proposed by the International Continence Society (ICS) and its various clinical study reports. The individual definition of compliance has been shown to vary as a function of bladder volume at the time of measurement, the filling rate,[1,2] the technique used to measure compliance,[3] repetition of urodynamic investigations,[4] and filling conditions (physiological versus artificial).[5]

The detrusor is normally composed of 70% elastic tissue, consisting of smooth muscle cells, and 30% viscous tissues, consisting of collagen fibers. Smooth muscle fibers behave like elastic elements, i.e. they are able to return to their initial state as soon as the stretching force is removed. Smooth muscle fiber lengthening is proportional to the tension applied. By Hooke's law:

$$T \text{ (tension)} = f \text{ (elastic module)} \times L \text{ (lengthening)}$$

Collagen fibers present the property of being able to delay deformation in response to stretch. Linear viscosity is governed by Newton's law, which states that the deformity of a fiber is directly proportional to the rate of tension. For more than 25 years, there has been an ongoing debate concerning whether bladder tone is determined by the passive properties of the bladder wall or by the autonomic nervous system. In this chapter, we will see that arguments derived from clinical experience of neurogenic bladder and its natural history, as well as our knowledge of detrusor innervation, now explain the important role of the nervous system in disorders of compliance.

In 1994, in an editorial devoted to this subject, McGuire[6] summarized the history of these concepts. The interaction between reflex detrusor contraction and failure of sphincter opening mechanisms inevitably leads to the appearance of disorders of compliance. Introduction of self-catheterization into the management of neurogenic bladder, in which there is no longer any detrusor-sphincter synergy, has demonstrated the positive effect on improvement of bladder compliance. An increase in intravesical pressure, for whatever reason, is universally accepted to be a major factor in disorders of compliance. Various diseases can be responsible for increased intravesical pressure, including myelomeningocele, spinal cord injury, multiple sclerosis, obstructive uropathy, including benign prostatic hyperplasia, and radiotherapy-induced lesions. All of the treatments proposed below are designed to decrease intravesical pressures, as clinical experience has demonstrated the major role of raised intravesical pressure in deterioration of the upper tract and the appearance of voiding disorders with severe repercussions on quality of life.

Natural history of compliance in neurogenic bladder: prognostic factors related to the mode of drainage

Clinical experience provides pathophysiological information about disorders of compliance in neurogenic bladder. A review of large cohorts analyzed according to the level of the spinal cord lesion and the treatment used demonstrates a correlation between high intravesical pressure and disorders of compliance. In a series of 316 patients, Weld et al[7] showed that patients treated by self-catheterization had a significantly higher incidence of normal bladder compliance than those with indwelling catheter, regardless of the level of the lesion. With a follow-up ranging between 16 and 20 years, 75% of patients treated by self-catheterization had normal compliance (>12.5 ml/cm) vs 20% of patients with an indwelling catheter and 60% of patients with reflex voiding. The rate of clinical complications was also proportional to the state of compliance. The level of the lesion also influences the incidence of **low compliant** bladder, which are less frequent in the case of a suprasacral vs sacral lesion, or an incomplete vs complete lesion.

These data were confirmed by other cohort studies.[8–11] Particular attention must be paid to cauda equina lesions, which may be associated with **low** compliance in up to 55% of cases,[12] representing a major threat for the upper urinary tract, requiring strict surveillance and screening. More recently, Beric and Light[13] emphasized the need to clearly distinguish between cauda equina lesions and conus lesions, especially by neurological or electrophysiological examinations. Pure conus lesions without detrusor areflexia may present various abnormalities of compliance on urodynamic studies (5 patients), including decreased compliance with a high risk of functional impairment. This finding has also been reported even more recently by Shin et al.[14]

Myelomeningocele must also be considered separately. Although the extent of the neurological lesions can vary considerably, 40–48%[15] of patients develop upper urinary tract lesions over a period of 7 years. A correlation has been demonstrated between the level of the malformation, as 57% of patients present with upper urinary tract dilatation in the case of thoracolumbar lesion and 90% in the case of thoracic lesion. This is particularly true during early childhood, whereas puberty and the growth period constitute the second high-risk period for the appearance of a major compliance disorder, even despite well-conducted treatment, especially self-catheterization. Boys are more particularly concerned (65%) and the presence of a tethered spinal cord, destabilized by growth, must be detected and treated if necessary, but this does not always prevent the risk of deterioration of probably 'acquired' bladder compliance. This problem must be carefully assessed before treatment of sphincter incompetence, especially by artificial urinary sphincter. De Badiola et al[16] demonstrated the importance of precise preoperative assessment of compliance, which, when abnormal (<2 ml/cm), must be treated by bladder enlargement associated with artificial urinary sphincter in a population predominantly composed of patients with myelomeningocele (18/23). This demonstrates the major role of raised intravesical pressure on deterioration of bladder compliance in the case of artificial increase of sphincter resistance on a reservoir with limited properties. Kaufman et al,[17] in a cohort of 214 children with myelomeningocele, confirmed the often irreversible nature of the disorder of compliance in this population (only 42% improvement after treatment based on a radiologically documented urological indication). Upper tract deterioration, reflecting increased resistance to bladder emptying, should not be detected by radiological surveillance alone, but especially by urodynamic studies.

Clinical experience has confirmed the higher incidence of compliance disorders according to the level (topography) and complete or incomplete nature of the neurological lesion. The available treatments for hyperreflexia and low compliance were limited to bladder enlargement surgery in the case of failure of self-catheterization and parasympatholytics, which have been shown to improve intravesical pressure and compliance.[7,18]

New conservative treatments for hyperreflexia more clearly illustrate the role of neurological tone in the pathogenesis of disorders of compliance.

Data on disorders of compliance derived from conservative treatments of neurogenic bladder

Old data concerning improvement of compliance by urethral dilatation in children with myelomeningocele support the important role of high intravesical pressure as a factor predisposing to disorders of compliance. A short series of 18 children out of 350[19] treated by dilatation (12F to 38F dilators) showed improvement of compliance by 11.66–27.41 ml/cmH$_2$O. The urodynamic results of open or endoscopic sphincterotomy do not specifically concern compliance, but may nevertheless indicate similar changes.

Disafferentation induced by section of the posterior nerve roots performed in the context of implantation of a Brindley stimulator[20] induced a marked improvement of compliance. Brindley,[20] Koldewijn et al,[21] and Madersbacher have reported their experience with this technique. In a publication specifically devoted to this aspect of neurogenic bladder, Koldewijn et al[21] reported a dramatic improvement of compliance at 6 months in 27 patients, which remained less than 20 ml/cmH$_2$O in only 2 patients. This result was not constantly observed at the 5th postoperative day, while hyperreflexia was abolished in the great majority of patients and an increase of compliance was even observed in some cases during the very first postoperative days. Detrusor denervation interrupts the reflex arc and consequently reduces or even abolishes detrusor hyperreflexia and high pressures. Previous denervation techniques failed, probably due to incomplete rhizotomy.

Few papers have reported the use of α-blockers in neurogenic bladder, particularly concerning their effects on bladder compliance. Swierzweski et al[22] prospectively studied the effect of terazosin on compliance in 12 spinal cord injury patients after failure of self-catheterization and maximal pharmacological blockade. Terazosin, at a dosage of 5 mg/day (by month) for 4 weeks, significantly improved bladder compliance during treatment, suggesting an α-blocking effect on detrusor receptors. The bladder compliance of 22 patients was improved by an average of 73% with return to baseline after stopping treatment, reflecting an 'on-off' effect. The feedback effect induced on the urethra could not be analyzed, but cannot be excluded, as indicated by the authors. The authors also reported a significant reduction of episodes of incontinence and dysreflexia. More recently, Schulte-Baukhloh et al[23] reported a study concerning alfuzosin. Seventeen children, mostly with myelomeningocele, with a mean age of 6.3 years, obtained an increase in bladder compliance from 9.3 to 19.6 ml/cmH$_2$O (111%).

The use of adrenergic blocking agents appears to clinically confirm the neurogenic interference on disorders of compliance, which may be due to a cholinergic activity, myogenic activity, or fibrosis, but it can also be mediated by activation of α-adrenergic receptors.[22] The reduction of bladder outlet obstruction has been shown to improve compliance of neurogenic bladders, but these clinical data on alpha blockers tend to suggest a direct effect on detrusor α-adrenergic receptors. None of the patients in this study developed incontinence as a result of terazosin. A more precise pathophysiological explantation cannot be proposed in the absence of a study of bladder leak point. Sundin et al,[24] in 1977, demonstrated the presence of adrenergic nerve endings in the detrusor, specifically in the case of parasympathetic denervation.

The use of vanilloids (resiniferatoxin and capsaicin) is still under evaluation. The treatment strategy consists of inducing pharmacological bladder disafferentation of silent type C afferent fibers. Resiniferatoxin has been demonstrated to be effective on detrusor hyperreflexia,[25] and was able to improve the disorder of compliance of a patient with myelomeningocele not presenting hyperreflexia.[26] According to the authors, this result appears to suggest that type C fibers are partially responsible for signals participating in deterioration of bladder compliance in some patients with myelomeningocele. This result needs to be confirmed on larger cohorts, especially including spinal cord injury patients.

The use of intravesical botulinum toxin is much more interesting in terms of pathophysiology and treatment. Schurch et al reported the effects of intravesical botulinum toxin on continence in spinal cord injury patients,[27] as blockade of the release of acetylcholine into the neuromuscular junction (efferent) induces a variable duration of bladder paralysis, with an estimated mean duration of 6–8 months. The results obtained on bladder compliance in adults and, more recently, in children with myelomeningocele are particularly demonstrative. Bladder compliance was improved from 20.39 to 45.18 ml/cmH$_2$O, i.e. by 121%. Botulinum toxin induces a marked reduction of intravesical pressure by inhibiting reflex contractions, but by acting on the efferent pathway of the reflex arc, thereby transforming the disorder of compliance, provided there is no pre-existing disorder of the bladder wall.

The effect of continuous intrathecal baclofen on compliance has been studied in neurogenic bladder. Steers et al[28] in 1992 and Bushman et al[29] in 1993, respectively, demonstrated the marked effects on bladder compliance in a population of patients with spastic spinal cord injury or hereditary spastic paraplegia. The effect of baclofen may be related to relaxation of the striated sphincter, leading to decreased resistance and/or a central neurological effect.

Data derived from experimental studies

Morphometric studies on human bladder strips and animal models now provide a better understanding of the cellular and intercellular mechanisms of neurological disorders of compliance.

The study very recently published by Backhaus et al[30] is particularly important. Although an increased intravesical pressure participates in the disorder of compliance, and although it is not always easy to distinguish the respective roles of bladder wall disorders and purely neurological disorders, these authors developed, for the first time, an experimental model designed to correlate pressure and the expression of proteolytic enzymes and their endogenous inhibitors (tissue metalloproteinase MMP-1 inhibitors). On human bladder cells, they demonstrated that pressures of 20 or 40 cmH$_2$O interfered with MMP-1 production. The molecular mechanisms responsible for the turnover of intercellular matrix have not been clearly elucidated, but this study showed the link between the pressure applied and the rate of release into the medium of these enzymes responsible for destruction of types I and III collagen. Earlier studies[31] demonstrating that the urothelium could be involved in the production of type I collagen suggest the role of these cells in the synthesis of extracellular matrix also needs to be studied.

The direct participation of type III collagen was demonstrated on human bladder chips by the elevated levels of mRNA observed in the case of non-compliant bladder.[32] Older morphometric studies[33] demonstrated a significant increase of connective tissue with no loss of muscle tissue on neurogenic non-compliant bladder, already suggesting participation of the bladder wall in the disorder of compliance with very probable functional alterations. The chronology of the disorders and their reversible or irreversible nature has not been studied *in vitro*.

Several studies have tried to elucidate the role of blood flow and possible slowing of blood flow on these disorders of the bladder wall. In general and independently of any neurogenic cause for detrusor dysfunction, Kershen et al[34] studied the effect of bladder filling on the blood supply of the wall in 17 conscious patients (Doppler transducer introduced by endoscopy). Blood flow tended to increase with increasing bladder volume and pressure and was mediated by local control mechanisms. In contrast, when the bladder reached its full capacity, blood flow decreased followed by a rebound increase after bladder emptying. The authors found a strong correlation between reduction of detrusor blood flow and bladder wall compliance, suggesting that ischemia participates in structural modifications of the bladder wall. This study provides different, but complementary data, concerning the role of ischemia due to high intravesical pressure in neurogenic bladder. Ohnishi et al[35] had already studied this hypothesis on neurogenic bladders presenting disorders of compliance vs a control group using laser Doppler measurement of blood flow, confirming that blood flow was highly significantly decreased in full non-compliant bladders.

The role of innervation has been studied on models of bilateral hypogastric nerve transection in spinal cord injury rats,[36] as these nerves provide the major sympathetic input to the bladder neck and urethra. Transection of these nerves reduces detrusor dysfunction in paraplegic patients, but did not alter the effects of dopaminergic receptor antagonists on the micturition reflex in spinal cord injury rats. Ten years earlier, the same mechanism was studied in anesthetized, non-spinal cord injury cats. Nerve section induced a reduction of bladder compliance at the end of filling, reflecting the inhibitory effect of sympathetic innervation during the second phase of filling, which probably helps to explain the mechanism of action of α-blockers[22,23] in this type of dysfunction.

Gloeckner et al[37] confirmed that bladder wall disorders induced a loss of viscoelastic properties of the bladder. They used biaxial mechanical testing to study the bladders of spinal cord injury rats vs a control group and demonstrated marked differences, with muscle hypertrophy, in rats with central neurogenic bladder. Human morphometric studies also provide similar findings, showing a significant increase of connective tissue with no loss of muscle tissue in neurogenic bladders. Landau et al[38] studied bladder biopsies in a population of 29 consecutive patients with neurogenic bladder requiring bladder enlargement and demonstrated an increase in the percentage of connective tissue and the connective tissue/muscle tissue ratio.

Hormonal factors also probably play a role. Experiments conducted on pregnant and virgin female rabbits demonstrated loss of compliance in response to hormonal impregnation. Electrical or pharmacological stimulation of bladder strips also considerably altered compliance.[39]

Conclusion

The pathophysiology of disorders of bladder compliance is still poorly understood. Although the presence of high intravesical pressure, facilitated by uncontrolled detrusor

Table 11.1 *Clinical factors influencing low compliant neurogenic bladder*
Type of drainage of the bladder

Type of neurogenic lesion
    Location
    Completeness

Type of treatment of hyperreflexia (bladder pressure)

hyperreflexia or high sphincter resistance, is certainly involved in the pathogenesis of disorders of compliance, the course, deterioration, differentiation between bladder wall factors (irreversible?), and 'neurological' factors are still poorly elucidated (Table 11.1). All of the treatments used in routine clinical practice demonstrate that the main factor ensuring improvement of the disorder of compliance is an action on high intravesical pressure. Studies on bladder biopsies in patients with neuro-urological disease could provide greater insight, especially concerning collagen deposits. New treatments, particularly botulinum toxin, may be useful in the context of a test of reversibility of the disorder of compliance. In the future, molecular biology and the study of cellular interactions should provide a better understanding of the mechanism linking raised intravesical pressure and loss of compliance. A number of aspects remain to be elucidated,[40] especially cellular interactions in wall changes, the reversible or irreversible nature of the various changes observed, the role of local neurotrophic factors, and changes induced on bladder afferent pathways. Similar questions have yet to be resolved concerning bladder aging or abnormalities induced by non-neurological obstruction.

Further studies need to be conducted to develop a preventive treatment for disorders of compliance in neurogenic bladder, other than specific treatment of the underlying disease or bladder drainage, and to determine the adjuvant role of α-blocking drugs in this setting.

References

1. Coolsaet B. Bladder compliance and detrusor activity during the collection phase. Neurourol Urodyn 1985; 4:263–273.

2. Coolsaet B, Elhilali M. Detrusor overactivity. Neurourol Urodyn 1988; 7:541–561.

3. Nordling J, Walter S. Repeated, rapid fill CO_2-cystometry. Urol Res 1977; 5:117–122.

4. Sorensen S, Nielsen J, Norgaard J, et al. Changes in bladder volumes with repetition of water cystometry. Urol Res 1984; 12:205–208.

5. Webb R, Griffiths C, Ramsden P, Neal D. Ambulatory monitoring of bladder pressure in low compliance neurogenic bladder dysfunction. J Urol 1992; 148(5)1477–1481.

6. McGuire E. Editorial: bladder compliance. J Urol 1994; 151:955–956.

7. Weld KJ, Graney MJ, Dmochowski RR. Differences in bladder compliance with time and associations of bladder management with compliance in spinal cord injured patients. J Urol 2000; 163(4):1228–1233.

8. Soler J-M, Amarenco G, Lemaitre D, et al. Corrélations entre données cystométriques et sphinctérométriques et lésions médullaires. Ann Readap Med Phys 1988; 31:465–471.

9. Hackler R, Hall M, Zampieri T. Bladder hypocompliance in the spinal cord injury population. J Urol 1989; 141:1390–1393.

10. Light J, Beric A. Detrusor function in suprasacral spinal cord injuries. J Urol 1992; 148:355–358.

11. Cardenas D, Mayo M, Turner L. Lower urinary changes over time in suprasacral spinal cord injury. Paraplegia 1995; 33:326–329.

12. Rhein F, Audic B, Bor Y, Perrigot M. Etude clinique de la récupération des syndromes de la queue de cheval par hernie discale. A propos de 65 cas. Ann Readapt Med Phys 1985; 28:153–168.

13. Beric A, Light J. Detrusor function with lesions of the conus medullaris. J Urol 1992; 148(1):104–106.

14. Shin J, Parc C, Kim H, Lee I. Significance of low compliance bladder in cauda equina injury. Spinal Cord 2002; 40(12):650–655.

15. Anderson P, Travers A. Development of hydronephrosis in spina bifida patients: predictive factors and management. Br J Urol 1993; 72:958–961.

16. de Badiola F, Castro-Diaz D, Hart-Austin C, Gonzalez R. Influence of preoperative bladder capacity and compliance on the outcome of artificial urinary sphincter implantation in patients with neurogenic sphincter incompetence. J Urol 1992; 148(5):1493–1495.

17. Kaufman A, Ritchey M, Roberts A, et al. Decreased bladder compliance in patients with myelomeningocele treated with radiological observation. J Urol 1996; 156(6):2031–2033.

18. Weld KJ, Dmochowski RR. Effect of bladder management on urological complications in spinal cord injured patients. J Urol 2000; 163(3):768–772.

19. Bloom D, Knechtel J, McGuire E. Urethral dilation improves bladder compliance in children with myelomeningocele and high leak point pressures. J Urol 1990; 144:430–433.

20. Brindley G. The first 500 patients with sacral anterior root stimulator implants: general description. Paraplegia 1994; 32(12):795–805.

21. Koldewijn E, van Kerrebroeck P, Rosier P, et al. Bladder compliance after posterior sacral root rhizotomies and anterior sacral root stimulation. J Urol 1994; 151:955–960.

22. Swierzewski S, Gormely E, Belville W, et al. The effect of terazosin on bladder function in the spinal cord injured patient. J Urol 1994; 151(4):951–954.

23. Schulte-Baukloh H, Michael T, Miller K, Knispel H. Alfuzosin in the treatment of high leak-point pressure in children with neurogenic bladder. BJU Int 2002; 90(7):716–720.

24. Sundin T, Dahlstrom A, Norlin L, Svedmyr N. The sympathetic innervation and adrenoreceptor function of the human lower urinary tract in the normal state and after parasympathetic denervation. Invest Urol 1977; 14:322–325.

25. Chancellor M, de Groat W. Intravesical capsaicin and resiniferatoxin therapy: spicing up the ways to treat the overactive bladder. J Urol 1999; 162:3.

26. Seki N, Ikawa S, Takano N, Naito S. Intravesical instillation of resiniferatoxin for neurogenic dysfunction in a patient with myelodysplasia. J Urol 2001; 166:2368–2369.

27. Schurch B, Hauri D, Rodic B, et al. Botulinum-A toxin as a treatment of detrusor-sphincter dyssynergia: a prospective study in 24 spinal cord injury patients. J Urol 1996; 155:1023–1029.

28. Steers W, Meythalter J, Haworth C, et al. Effects of acute and chronic continuous intrathecal baclofen on genitourinary dysfunction due to spinal cord pathology. J Urol 1992; 148(6):1849–1855.

29. Bushman W, Steers W, Meythalter J. Voiding dysfunction in patients with spastic paraplegia: urodynamic evaluation and response to continuous intrathecal baclofen. Neurourol Urodyn 1993; 12(2): 163–170.

30. Backhaus B, Kaefer M, Haberstroh K, et al. Alterations in the molecular determinants of bladder compliance at hydrostatic pressures less than 40 cm H_2O. J Urol 2002; 168:2600–2604.

31. Baskin L, Howard P, Macarak E. Effect of physical forces on bladder smooth muscle and urothelium. J Urol 1993; 150:601–605.

32. Kaplan E, Richier J, Howard P, et al. Type III collagen messenger RNA is modulated in non-compliant human bladder tissue. J Urol 1997; 157(6):2366–2369.

33. Ohnishi N, Kishima Y, Hashimoto K, et al. Morphometric study of low compliant bladder [in Japanese]. Hinyokika Kiyo 1994; 40(8):657–661.

34. Kershen R, Azadzoi K, Siroky M. Blood flow, pressure and compliance in the male human bladder. J Urol 2002; 168:121–125.

35. Ohnishi N, Kishima Y, Hashimoto K, et al. A new method of measurement of the urinary bladder blood flow in patients with low compliant bladder [in Japanese]. Hinyokika Kiyo 1994; 40(8):663–667.

36. Yoshiyama M, de Groat W. Effect of bilateral hypogastric nerve transection on voiding dysfunction in rats with spinal cord injury. Exp Neurol 2002; 175(1):191–197.

37. Gloeckner D, Sacks M, Fraser M, et al. Passive biaxial mechanical properties of the rat bladder wall after spinal cord injury. J Urol 2002; 167(5):2247–2252.

38. Landau E, Jayanthi V, Churchill B, et al. Loss of elasticity in dysfunctional bladders: urodynamic and histochemical correlation. J Urol 1994; 152:702–705.

39. Lee J, Wein A, Levin R. Effects of pregnancy on urethral and bladder neck function. Urology 1993; 42(6):747–752.

40. Koebl H, Mostwin J, Boiteux J-P, et al. Pathophysiology. In: Abrams P, Cardozo L, Khoury S, Wein A, eds. Incontinence. Plymouth: Health Publications, 2002:203–241.

12

Pathophysiology of detrusor-sphincter dyssynergia

Bertil FM Blok

Introduction

Disorders of the lower urinary tract musculature are common, often causing urinary incontinence or retention. In order to understand the pathophysiology of various neurogenic urological disorders, including bladder sphincter dyssynergia, it is important to be aware of the organization of the central control systems of the urinary bladder and sphincter. Normal micturition consists of a synergic action between the detrusor muscle of the bladder and the external urethral sphincter: five to eight times per day the external urethral sphincter relaxes, followed by a contraction of the detrusor muscle and expulsion of stored urine from the bladder. This synergy between the detrusor and the external urethral sphincter is controlled by a specific area in the caudal brainstem, i.e. the pontine micturition center. Disruption of the pathways between this area and the caudal part of the spinal cord often results in detrusor-sphincter dyssynergia. This means that an involuntary contraction of the detrusor is accompanied by an involuntary contraction of the external urethral sphincter and, consequently, urine is not expelled without force from the bladder. Finally, this results in a low-compliant and thick-walled bladder, elevated retrograde pressures in the ureter and pyelum, hydronephrosis, and even renal scarring and terminal kidney failure. Most treatments of detrusor-sphincter dyssynergia are aimed at circumventing the contracted external urethral sphincter and increasing bladder volume, e.g. by using intermittent self-catheterization, botulinum toxin, baclofen, bladder augmentation, or sphincterotomy.

Damage to higher central regions in the cortex or forebrain do not result in detrusor-sphincter dyssynergia, but in a loss of control over the start of micturition, which causes urge incontinence. This chapter gives an overview of the neural pathways involved in the control of micturition and continence and the pathophysiology of detrusor-sphincter dyssynergia.

Neural control of the bladder and external urethral sphincter

Specific areas of the mammalian nervous system are important for the control of micturition and continence: the peripheral nervous system with autonomic ganglion cells in the bladder wall and sympathetic chain and sensory ganglion cells in the dorsal root chain; the central nervous system, including motoneurons and sensory interneurons in the caudal spinal cord; the caudal brainstem, including the pontine micturition center; and forebrain areas, including the emotional cortex and the hypothalamus. Peripheral nerves, spinal and brainstem neurons comprise the basic components of the micturition reflex and are interconnected via peripheral nerves and central fiber tracts, whereas specific cortical and subcortical structures determine the appropriate moment micturition starts. Normally, we are continent for urine continuously, except for the necessary micturition. Specific lesions of the neural pathways can result in urological dysfunction, which comprises hypoactivity or hyperactivity of the detrusor muscle, hyperactivity of the continence pathways, and a loss of control of the beginning of micturition.

Ganglion cells and sacral neurons

The detrusor muscle of the bladder is innervated by parasympathetic ganglion cells in the bladder wall. These ganglion cells are innervated via the pelvic nerve by preganglionic parasympathetic bladder motoneurons, which are located in the intermediolateral cell column of the sacral cord.[1,2] The parasympathetic outflow controls the bladder contraction during micturition. The bladder neck and the internal urethral sphincter are innervated by sympathetic ganglion cells in the thoracolumbar chain. Preganglionic sympathetic motoneurons of the urinary bladder are located in the intermediolateral cell column of the caudal thoracic and the upper lumbar spinal cord and control sympathetic ganglion cells via hypogastric nerves. The sympathetic outflow plays a role during the end of the urine storage phase[3,4] and provides closure of the bladder neck during orgasm.[5] The striated muscles of the pelvic floor, including the external urethral sphincter, are innervated by motoneurons located in a region known as the nucleus of Onuf of the sacral ventral horn. Onuf's nucleus is located in most species just medial to the motoneurons of the hindlimb and lateral to those of the trunk and axial musculature,[6–8] but there exists a considerable variation among species.[9–11]

Micturition and continence pathways

Since Barrington,[12] it is known that an essential structure of the micturition reflex is located in the dorsal pontine tegmentum, because bilateral lesions in this area result in urinary retention. This Barrington's area projects to bladder motoneurons (Figure 12.1) and is known as the pontine micturition center[13] or M (medial) region.[14] Electrical or chemical stimulation of the pontine micturition center produces a sharp decrease in the urethral pressure, a pelvic floor relaxation, and an increased intravesical pressure,[14,15] mimicking normal micturition. The increased intravesical pressure is caused by the bilateral monosynaptic excitatory pathway from the pontine micturition center to sacral bladder motoneurons,[16] which probably utilizes glutamate as the main transmitter.[17] The relaxation of the urethral sphincter during micturition is caused by a monosynaptic pontine micturition center projection to sacral inhibitory interneurons in the dorsal gray commissure, also known as the intermediomedial cell column.[18,19] These inhibitory dorsal gray commissure interneurons, in turn, inhibit directly sphincter motoneurons in Onuf's nucleus during micturition.[20] The inhibitory transmitters involved in this pathway are γ-aminobutyric acid (GABA)[18] and glycine.[19] Bilateral lesions in the pontine micturition center result in total urinary retention, leading to depressed detrusor activity and increased bladder capacity. Another pontine area located in the ventral pons is known as the pontine continence center or L (lateral) region (Figure 12.2), which projects to sphincter motoneurons in Onuf's nucleus.[14]

Stimulation of the pontine continence center results in contraction of the pelvic floor musculature and an increased urethral pressure. Bilateral lesions in the pontine continence center give rise to an extreme form of urge incontinence: bladder capacity is strongly reduced and

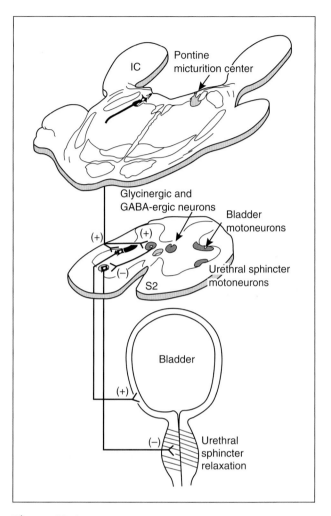

Figure 12.1
Pathways involved in micturition control are present at both sides. IC, inferior colliculus.

urine is expelled prematurely by excessive detrusor activity accompanied by urethral relaxation.[14] The urethral pressure is usually not depressed below normal values, except during micturition. These observations suggest that during the filling phase the pontine continence center produces a continuous excitatory effect on external urethral sphincter motoneurons in the nucleus of Onuf. The drive of this tonic excitatory effect is unknown, but probably originates from areas important for the flight–fight reaction, such as the central nucleus of the amygdala and lateral hypothalamus. Several positron emission tomography (PET) studies have provided evidence that brainstem areas involved in micturition control are comparable in cats and humans. Healthy men and women were able to micturate during scanning and showed an increased regional blood flow during micturition in the dorsal part of the pons close to the fourth ventricle.[21,22] The location of this area was similar to that of the pontine micturition center described in the cat. A second group of volunteers was not able to

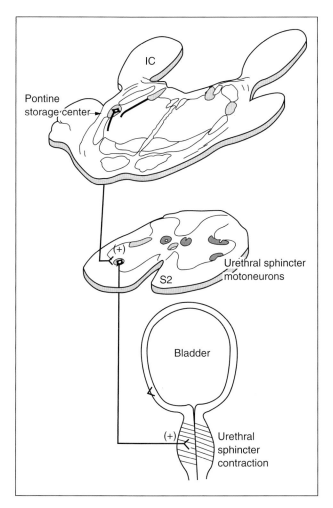

Figure 12.2
Pathways involved in urinary continence control are present at both sides. IC, inferior colliculus.

micturate during scanning. They showed no activation in the dorsal, but in the ventral pons, similar to the location of the pontine continence center in cats. Apparently, the volunteers in this not successful micturition group, probably because they did not feel themselves in a safe environment, contracted their urethral sphincter and withheld their urine, although they had a full bladder and tried to urinate.

Sensory pathways

Afferent fibers from the urinary bladder enter the lumbosacral cord via the pelvic nerve. The peripheral fibers of the dorsal root ganglia neurons of the pelvic nerve contact mechanoreceptors in the bladder wall. The central fibers enter Lissauer's tract and terminate on interneurons in laminae I, V, VII, and the DGC.[2] Bladder-filling information

from these sensory interneurons in the sacral cord must finally reach the pontine micturition center in order to empty the bladder at an appropriate time. Neurons in the lumbosacral cord do not project to pontine micturition center descending projecting neurons in the cat[23] and only to a limited extent in the rat.[24] The micturition reflex is not abolished by precollicular decerebration, which means that lumbosacral projections to forebrain areas, such as the thalamus and hypothalamus, are not essential for this reflex.[25] Several publications have suggested that the mesencephalic periaqueductal gray (PAG) is a critical component of the micturition reflex. Interneurons in the lumbosacral cord project strongly to the lateral and dorsal parts of the PAG.[23] Stimulation of the pelvic nerve results in short latency potentials in the caudal PAG.[26] The PAG is the only caudal brainstem structure known to project specifically to the pontine micturition center.[27] Micturition evoked by glutamate injection in the ventrolateral PAG is mediated by this PAG–pontine micturition center pathway.[28] PET scanning during bladder filling resulted in increased activation in the PAG.[29] These results support the hypothesis that the PAG receives information concerning the sense of bladder fullness and is critically involved in the sensorimotor loop of the micturition reflex.

Forebrain micturition control

Although the forebrain is not essential for the micturition reflex, clinical observations suggest that it is important for the beginning of micturition. In the cat, stimulation of forebrain structures such as the anterior cingulate gyrus, hypothalamus, amygdala, bed nucleus of the stria terminalis, and septal nuclei can elicit bladder contractions.[30] Although most of these regions send fibers to the brainstem, only the hypothalamic preoptic area projects specifically to the pontine micturition center.[31,32] PET scanning studies suggest that this might also be true in humans, because the hypothalamus, including the preoptic area, was activated during micturition.[21] The direct projection from the hypothalamic preoptic area to the pontine micturition center possibly conveys the 'safe signal' to the pontine micturition center to start micturition.

Most of the PET scanning studies on micturition[21,22,29,33] point to two cortical areas: the cingulate gyrus and the prefrontal cortex. Cerebral blood flow in the cingulate gyrus was significantly decreased during voluntary withholding of urine and during urge to void. The prefrontal cortex is active when micturition takes place and during involuntary urine withholding. Possibly, activation of the prefrontal cortex and the anterior cingulate gyrus do not reflect specific involvement in micturition, but more in general mechanisms, such as attention and response selection. The prefrontal cortex plays a role in making the decision whether or not micturition should take place at a particular time and place. Forebrain lesions including the anterior cingulate gyrus are known to cause urge incontinence.[34] The cingulate gyrus strongly influences descending pathways involved in the facilitation or defacilitation of all motoneurons and interneurons. Important examples of these modulatory pathways are the serotonergic raphe and noradrenergic coerulear spinal tracts.

Micturition and urinary continence are controlled by involuntary mechanisms, which have to be distinguished from the voluntary control of the pelvic floor musculature. Both mechanisms are exerting influence on the same motoneurons, but via completely separate pathways. The involuntary descending pathways from the pontine micturition center and pontine continence center have already been discussed previously. PET scanning suggested that voluntary motor pathways involved in pelvic floor control originate in the most medial part of the primary motor cortex.[35] Additional structures involved in voluntary pelvic contraction are the medial cerebellum and the motor thalamus.

Pathophysiology of detrusor-sphincter dyssynergia

The pontine micturition center is connected with the sacral cord via ascending and descending pathways. Following spinal cord transection and disconnection of the pontine–sacral cord pathways, the synergic action between the detrusor and sphincter is lost and, after a few weeks, the external urethral sphincter remains contracted, when the detrusor muscle of the bladder contracts, a condition known as detrusor-sphincter dyssynergia.

To understand the pathophysiology of dyssynergia, knowledge about the neonatal control of micturition is essential. Newborn rats and cats micturate via a somatic–sacral–vesical pathway (Figure 12.3). Licking by the mother of the perineum of the neonate evokes micturition.[36] Skin receptors and their C fibers send, via pudendal somatic sensory afferents, direct or indirect excitatory signals to the parasympathetic preganglionic motoneurons in the sacral cord, resulting in a contraction of the bladder. The contraction of the bladder stops immediately when the skin stimulus, i.e. the licking, discontinues. The descending projections from the pontine micturition center are present in the neonate, but do not have a functional role in the control of micturition at this stage.[37] During weaning neonatal rats or kittens, after about 4–6 weeks the growing connections from the pontine micturition center to the sacral cord compete with the declining connections of the perineal receptors with the sacral cord. Ultimately the strength of pontine–sacral projections overrides that of the segmental perineal–sacral

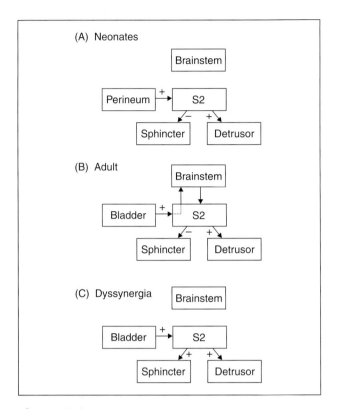

Figure 12.3
Diagram of the control of micturition: in neonates (A), licking of the perineum results in relaxation of the sphincter and contraction of the detrusor; in adults (B), the filled bladder is emptied via the brainstem at the right time and place; and in spinal transection with dyssynergia (C), the sphincter contracts when the detrusor contracts (see text).

connections. This results in the adult control state, with predominance of the sacral–brainstem–sacral switch mechanism: the pontine micturition center is switched on with imminent relaxation of the external urethral sphincter followed by contraction of the detrusor muscle (Figure 12.3). Directly after complete or incomplete spinal cord transection there is a phase of spinal shock with an acontractile bladder and urinary retention, followed in a few weeks by low-volume reflex contractions of the detrusor with hyperactive voiding. It has been suggested that during this period terminals of capsaicin-sensitive C fibers of the segmental 'neonatal' circuits on the sacral bladder motoneurons are increasing, while the terminals of the sacral–brainstem–sacral pathways disappear.[38] Activation of these afferent unmyelinated C fibers can trigger reflex micturition in overactive bladders in spinal injury, but not in normal micturition, which is associated with thin myelinated Aδ afferents. The reorganization of the micturition-related pathways after spinal cord transection is triggered by the release of neural growth factors.

Damage to pelvic and pudendal nerves, cauda equina, or the sacral spinal cord can result in an hypoactive bladder (with urinary retention and overflow incontinence) and external urethral sphincter (with stress incontinence). Patients with suprapontine brain lesions, with the exception of motor cortex damage, do not have detrusor-sphincter dyssynergia. These patients may have urge incontinence (i.e. the micturition pathway is switched on prematurely).

References

1. Nadelhaft I, De Groat WC, Morgan C. Location and morphology of parasympathetic preganglionic neurons in the sacral spinal cord of the cat revealed by retrograde axonal transport of horseradish peroxidase. J Comp Neurol 1980; 193:265–281.

2. Morgan C, Nadelhaft I, De Groat WC. The distribution of visceral primary afferents from the pelvic nerve to Lissauer's Tract and the spinal gray matter and its relationship to the sacral parasympathetic nucleus. J Comp Neurol 1981; 201:415–440.

3. Sato M, Mizuno N, Konishi A. Localization of motoneurons innervating perineal muscles: a HRP study in cat. Brain Res 1978; 140:149–154.

4. Roppolo JR, Nadelhaft I, De Groat WC. The organization of pudendal motoneurons and primary afferent projections in the spinal cord of the rhesus monkey revealed by horseradish peroxidase. J Comp Neurol 1985; 234:475–488.

5. Kuzuhara S, Kanazawa I, Nakanishi T. Topographical localization of the Onuf's nuclear neurons innervating the rectal and vesical striated sphincter muscles: a retrograde fluorescent double labeling in the cat and dog. Neurosci Lett 1980; 16:125–130.

6. Schroder HD. Organization of motoneurons innervating the pelvic muscles of the male rat. J Comp Neurol 1980; 192:567–587.

7. Ulibarri C, Popper P, Micevych PE. Motoneurons dorsolateral to the central canal innervate perineal muscles in the Mongolian gerbil. J Comp Neurol 1995; 356:225–237.

8. Blok BFM, Roukema G, Geerdes B, Holstege G. Location of anal sphincter motoneurons of the female domestic pig. Neurosci Lett 1996; 216:203–206.

9. De Groat WC, Saum WR. Sympathetic inhibition of the urinary bladder and of pelvic ganglionic transmission in the cat. J Physiol 1972; 220:297–314.

10. Vaughan CW, Satchell PM. Role of sympathetic innervation in the feline continence process under natural filling conditions. J Neurophysiol 1992; 68:1842–1849.

11. Kimura Y, Adachi K, Kisaki N, Ise K. Role of alpha-adrenergic receptor mechanism in closure of the internal urethral orifice during ejaculation. Urol Int 1975; 30:341–349.

12. Barrington FJF. The effect of lesions of the hind- and mid-brain on micturition in the cat. Quart J Exp Physiol Cogn Med 1925; 15:81–102.

13. Loewy AD, Saper CB, Baker RP. Descending projections from the pontine micturition center. Brain Res 1979; 172:533–539.

14. Holstege G, Griffiths D, De Wall H, Dalm E. Anatomical and physiological observations on supraspinal control of bladder and urethral sphincter muscles in the cat. J Comp Neurol 1986; 250:449–461.

15. Mallory BS, Roppolo JR, De Groat WC. Pharmacological modulation of the pontine micturition center. Brain Res 1991; 546:310–320.

16. Blok BFM, Holstege G. Ultrastructural evidence for a direct pathway from the pontine micturition center to the parasympathetic preganglionic motoneurons of the bladder of the cat. Neurosci Lett 1997; 222:195–198.

17. Matsumoto G, Hisamitsu T, De Groat WC. Role of glutamate and NMDA receptors in the descending limb of the spinobulbospinal micturition reflex pathway of the rat. Neurosci Lett 1995; 183:58–62.

18. Blok BFM, De Weerd H, Holstege G. The pontine micturition center projects to sacral cord GABA immunoreactive neurons in the cat. Neurosci Lett 1997; 233:109–112.

19. Sie JA, Blok BFM, De Weerd H, Holstege G. Ultrastructural evidence for direct projections from the pontine micturition center to glycine-immunoreactive neurons in the sacral dorsal gray commissure in the cat. J Comp Neurol 2001; 429:631–637.

20. Blok BFM, Van Maarseveen JT, Holstege G. Electrical stimulation of the sacral dorsal gray commissure evokes relaxation of the external urethral sphincter in the cat. Neurosci Lett 1998; 249:68–70.

21. Blok BFM, Willemsen ATM, Holstege G. A PET study on brain control of micturition in humans. Brain 1997; 120:111–121.

22. Blok BFM, Sturms LM, Holstege G. Brain activation during micturition in women. Brain 1998; 121:2033–2042.

23. Blok BFM, De Weerd H, Holstege G. Ultrastructural evidence for the paucity of projections from the lumbosacral cord to the M-region in the cat. A new concept for the organization of the micturition reflex with the periaqueductal gray as central relay. J Comp Neurol 1995; 359:300–309.

24. Blok BFM, Holstege G. The pontine micturition center in rat receives direct lumbosacral input. An ultrastructural study. Neurosci Lett 2000; 282:29–32.

25. Tang PC, Ruch TC. Localization of brain stem and diencephalic areas controlling the micturition reflex. J Comp Neurol 1956; 106:213–245.

26. Noto H, Roppolo JR, Steers WD, De Groat WC. Electrophysiological analysis of the ascending and descending components of the micturition reflex pathway in the rat. Brain Res 1991; 549:95–105.

27. Blok BFM, Holstege G. Direct projections from the periaqueductal gray to the pontine micturition center (M-region). An anterograde and retrograde tracing study in the cat. Neurosci Lett 1994; 166:93–96.

28. Matsuura S, Downie JW, Allen GV. Micturition evoked by glutamate microinjection in the ventrolateral periaqueductal gray is mediated through Barrington's nucleus in the rat. Neuroscience 101; 1053–1061.

29. Athwal BS, Berkley KJ, Hussain I, et al. Brain responses to changes in bladder volume and urge to void in healthy men. Brain 2001; 124: 369–377.

30. Gjone R. Excitatory and inhibitory bladder responses to stimulation of 'limbic', diencephalic and mesencephalic structures in the cat. Acta Physiol Scand 1966; 66:91–102.

31. Holstege G. Some anatomical observations on the projections from the hypothalamus to brainstem and spinal cord: an HRP and autoradiographic tracing study in the cat. J Comp Neurol 1987; 260:98–126.

32. Ding YQ, Wang D, Xu JQ, Ju G. Direct projections from the medial preoptic area to spinally-projecting neurons in Barrington's nucleus: an electron microscope study in the rat. Neurosci Lett 1999; 271:175–178.

33. Nour S, Svarer C, Kristensen JK, et al. Cerebral activation during micturition in normal men. Brain 2000; 123:781–789.

34. Andrew J, Nathan PW. Lesions of the anterior frontal lobes and disturbances of micturition and defaecation. Brain 1964; 87:233–262.

35. Blok BFM, Sturms LM, Holstege G. A PET study on cortical and sub-cortical control of pelvic floor musculature in women. J Comp Neurol 1997; 389:535–544.

36. Thor KB, Blais DP, de Groat WC. Behavioral analysis of the postnatal development of micturition in kittens. Brain Res Dev Brain Res 1989; 46:137–144.

37. Sugaya K, Roppolo JR, Yoshimura N, et al. The central neural pathways involved in micturition in the neonatal rat as revealed by the injection of pseudorabies virus into the urinary bladder. Neurosci Lett 1997; 223:197–200.

38. de Groat WC, Araki I. Maturation of bladder reflex pathways during postnatal development. Adv Exp Med Biol 1999; 462:253–263.

13

Pathophysiology of autonomic dysreflexia

Waleed Altaweel and Jacques Corcos

The role of urology in the management of spinal cord injury (SCI) patients has become increasingly important in the last century, and a better understanding of the pathophysiology of changes occurring in the urinary tract (UT) has led to new ways of evaluation and treatment. Among the changes occurring in the UT of SCI patients, autonomic dysreflexia (AD) has to be considered as a serious condition that might expose the patients to significant complications.

Urologists should be cognizant of manifestations, precipitating factors, and management. Patients with SCI above T5 are generally at risk of developing AD. However, it has also been reported in patients with lesions as low as T8.[1] The two most common names for this syndrome are AD and autonomic hyperreflexia. It is sometimes referred to as paroxysmal hypertension,[2] paroxysmal neurogenic hypertension,[3] autonomic spasticity,[4] sympathetic hyperreflexia,[5] mass reflex,[6] and neurovegetative syndrome.[7]

As a true medical emergency, AD is associated with morbidity and sometimes mortality. Its prevention is the key for successful management.

Historical overview

In 1860, Hilton[8] was the first to report a case consistent with AD. He described recurrent chills and hot flushes in a C5 injured patient. In 1890, Bowlby[9] quoted hot flushes and sweating in C7 injured patients after catheter passage.

In 1917, Head and Riddoch[6] observed episodes of intense sweating associated with slowing pulse in association with bladder filling, blockage catheter, or administration of an enema in SCI patients.

In 1938, Talaat[10] found distention of the bladder with increased blood pressure. Four years later, Guttmann et al[8] described, in a series of SCI patients, how distention viscera led to an autonomic response which induced profound effects on cardiovascular activity in parts of the body above the level of the spinal cord lesion. In 1951 Pollock and his group[11] reported defective regulatory

mechanisms of autonomic nervous system function after SCI. Subsequently, many publications have described AD, its pathophysiology and treatment, including reviews by Trop and Bennett,[12] Vaidyanathan et al,[13] and Karlsson.[14]

Neurophysiology of autonomic dysreflexia after spinal cord injury

The symptomatic triad of AD comprises high blood pressure, bradycardia, and sweating and hot flushes with occasional headaches. All these symptoms are related to a dysfunctional autonomic nervous system, which plays an important role in blood pressure and heart rate control. Major splanchnic outflow from the sympathetic system emanates from T5 to L2 under the inhibitory action of the supraspinal center. After SCI, inhibition of the sympathetic system is absent or decreased, evoking exaggerated reactions to any stimuli below the level of the injury (Figures 13.1 and 13.2). These mechanisms lead to:

1. **High blood pressure**: Sympathetic stimulation increases the blood pressure by augmenting the heart rate and peripheral vascular resistance to flow.
2. **Bradycardia**: The parasympathetic system decreases the blood pressure by reducing the heart rate. High blood pressure stimulates baroreceptors in the wall of the carotid sinus. These receptors give signals that travel via the glossopharyngeal nerve to the tractus solitarius in the medulla where the vasoconstrictor center is inhibited and the vagal center is stimulated. Vagal stimulation leads to decreased heart rate and cardiac contractility that allow for a drop in blood pressure in SCI patients with a lesion above the splanchnic outflow. Dysreflexia occurs because inhibitory impulses from the brainstem cannot reach the effectors organs. The sudden increase in blood pressure caused by arterial spasms stimulates receptors in the carotid sinus and

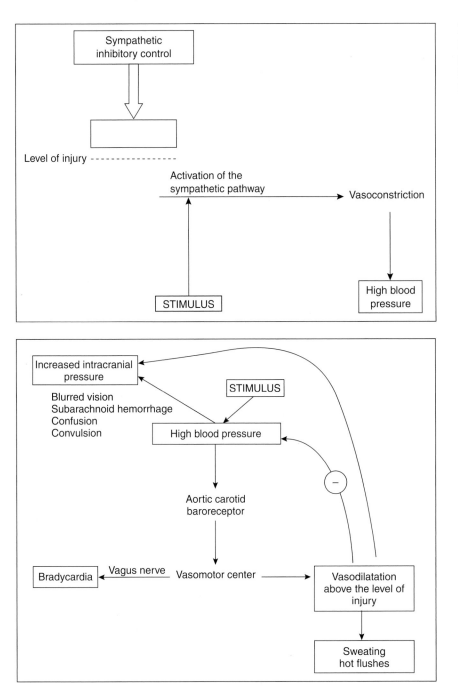

Figure 13.1
Pathophysiology of hypertension in.
(Adapted from J Corcos and E Schick,
Les vessies neurogènes de l'adulte.
Editions Masson, 1996: 205.)

Figure 13.2
Pathophysiology of AD. (Adapted from
J Corcos and E Schik, Les vessies
neurogènes de l'adulte. Editions
Masson, 1996: 205.)

aortic arch. This, in turn, affects the vagus nerve, resulting in marked bradycardia. However, the correction of hypertension is minimal.

3. ***Hot flushes, sweating, and headaches***: Afferent outflow from receptors in the aortic arch and carotid sinus to the vasomotor center in the brainstem results in vasodilatation in the head and neck. These changes explain the hot flushes, profuse sweating, and pounding headaches above the level of the lesion.

Vaidyanathan et al[13] have summarized current concepts of neurophysiological AD in experimental animals and SCI patients. These can be divided into changes in sympathetic preganglionic neurons (SPN), neurobiochemical alterations in the spinal cord caudal to the injury, remodeling of spinal cord circuits after SCI, and hypersensitivity of vascular α-adrenoreceptors.

Changes in sympathetic preganglionic neurons

After spinal cord transection, disruption of descending bulbospinal input to the SPN elicits partial deafferentation that culminates in initial, transient SPN atrophy within

7 days of cord transection or hemisection.[15] The loss of dendritic processes of preganglionic neurons renders the SPN less receptive to excitatory input.

Within 30 days of SCI, the preganglionic neurons re-establish a normal dendritic arbor. This morphologic recovery heralds the advent of AD, which signals the development of abnormal synaptic connection within the spinal cord. The SPN may express new receptors, or up-regulate normally expressed receptors in response to their initial deafferentation.[16]

Neurobiochemical changes in the spinal cord caudal to spinal cord injury

Increased expression of synaptophysin, a phosphopron found in synaptic vesicles of axon terminals, caudal to the cord transection, is consistent with its elevation in synaptic terminals of the gray matter, indicating possible sprouting of local axons of interneurons and signaling new inputs to the SPN that mediate the sympathetic hyperresponsiveness of established AD.[15,17] In chronic spinal rats, expression of the catecholamine-synthesizing enzyme dopamine β-hydroxylase is up-regulated in somata within the intermediate gray matter of spinal segments caudal to the transection. The number of somata immunoreactive to this enzyme increases six-fold by 14 days after cord transection, compared to the few stomata found in control rats.[18]

It has been shown that the expression of substance P is heightened, with its wider distribution in immunoreactive fibers caudal to cord transection.[18] As the effects of substance P on spinal preganglionic neurons can be excitatory, a spinal source could contribute to the development of AD.

An increased central arbor of calcitonin-generated peptide containing primary afferent fibers suggests sprouting of unmyelinated afferent fibers and up-regulation of their excitatory neuropeptide expression.[19]

Remodeling of spinal cord circuits after spinal cord injury

Regrowth occurs after initial retraction of the dendritic tree of SPN.

Partial deafferentation of the sympathetic preganglionic neurons after spinal cord transection stimulates the sprouting of myelinated and unmyelinated primary afferent fibers, and possibly interneurons. Afferent fiber sprouting does not directly reach the autonomic or motor

neurons but may cause hyperreflexia by increasing inputs to the interneurons.[19]

The combination of lost descending pathways to the SPN and formation of new synaptic inputs, which are inappropriate because of their source, leads to the development of exaggerated reflex responses, and abnormal cardiovascular control.

Hypersensitivity of vascular α adrenoreceptors

In tetraplegic patients with a history of AD, venous α adrenoreceptors showed an increased responsiveness to norepinephrine (noradrenaline) in the foot vein, as illustrated by a significant leftward shift of the dose–response curve. The results were similar in all patients and were in marked contrast to those obtained in age-similar normal subjects who required a 6–7-fold increase in norepinephrine concentration to produce a comparable 50% venoconstriction.[20] These data indicated that the hyperresponsiveness of α adrenoreceptors, which was observed in veins, might also be present in the arteries, and the hypersensitivity of vascular α adrenoreceptors may be important in the manifestation of AD in patients with tetraplegia.

Peripheral afferent (bladder) stimulation below the level of the lesion in SCI patients gives rise to a 15-fold increase in leg norepinephrine spillover from basal values of 0.06 to 0.91 pmol/min/100 g. Such pronounced norepinephrine spillover suggests that the amount of transmitter released per nerve impulse may be augmented caudal to the level of SCI.[21]

Incidence and prevalence

AD is seen in patients with SCI at the level of T6 or above. One study of 213 SCI patients reported a 48% incidence of AD.[22] Another study[23] revealed that during urodynamic evaluation of 48 patients with SCI above T6, all patients showed significantly elevated systolic and diastolic blood pressure, although only 20 had blood pressure above 150/100 mmHg, and this was more frequent in subjects with cervical cord injury. In 1991, in a survey of current AD treatment options, 86 physicians estimated a 19% incidence of symptomatic AD. A majority of physicians felt that the incidence was lower than what it was 10 years previously.[24] However, this lower incidence could be due to fewer patients showing symptoms and AD might also be mild or silent in some patients. Another study found that 78% of SCI patients manifested AD during urodynamic evaluation, with 48% disclosing silent AD.[25]

Symptoms

SCI patients may present with one or more of the following signs or symptoms when experiencing an AD episode. However, the symptoms may be minimal or absent, despite the significantly increased blood pressure. Usually, the symptoms start after the spinal shock period. However, AD can be seen at an early stage and it should be considered in the differential diagnosis of patients immediately after SCI.[26]

AD symptoms are diverse and include:

- profuse sweating above the level of the injury, mainly the face, neck, and shoulders, but it could also occur below the level of injury
- pounding headaches
- hot flushes above the injury, especially the face and neck
- piloerection or goose bumps above or below the lesion
- blurred vision and the appearance of spots in the visual field
- nasal congestion and anxiety
- severe headaches, usually occipital, bitemporal, and bifrontal in location, in more than 50% of patients.[27]

Signs

Systolic and diastolic blood pressure increases are mainly severe and sudden, frequently association with bradycardia. Usually, patients with SCI above T6 have normal blood pressure in the range of 90–110 mmHg. Therefore, blood pressure of 20–40 mmHg above baseline may be a sign of AD.[28] However, systolic blood pressure above 300 mmHg and diastolic blood pressure above 220 mmHg have been reported.[27,29,30]

Other objective signs that might be associated with AD include:

- tachycardia
- atrial fibrillation, premature ventricular contraction, atrioventricular conduction abnormalities
- cutaneous vasodilatation or vasoconstriction
- erection
- changes in skin and rectal temperature
- changes in the level of consciousness
- visual field defects
- cardiac enlargement.

Differential diagnosis

The differential diagnosis of AD includes essential hypertension, pheochromocytoma, migraine, cluster headaches, toxemia of pregnancy, and posterior fossa neoplasm.[27]

Pheochromocytoma signs and symptoms involve most of the body, whereas AD diaphoresis and flushing are seen above the level of injury. Tachycardia is a characteristic of pheochromocytoma, whereas bradycardia is more common in AD.[31]

Posterior fossa neoplasm may mimic pheochromocytoma or AD, but neurological deficits and papilledema occur with posterior fossa tumors.[27,32]

Migraine and cluster headaches are associated with increased blood pressure. However, the cluster headaches are usually unilateral, brief, intense, periorbital, or frontal. A positive family history is consistent with cluster headache or migraine.

Pregnancy-induced hypertension occurs in women with SCI. In AD the blood pressure elevation is transient and returns to normal after removal of the triggering factor, whereas pregnancy-induced hypertension persists until delivery.

Causes

Afferent peripheral stimulation below the lesion in SCI patients provokes AD. If more than one stimulus presents at the same time the reaction tends to be more severe (Table 13.1).

Distention of the bladder and then of the rectum is the most common cause. Catheterization, urinary tract infection, cystoscopy, bladder or kidney stones, blocked catheter, abnormal urodynamics, and bladder percussion are all well-known precipitating factors.[23,33] However, it has been shown that flexible cystoscopes reduce the risk of AD, and are safer than rigid scopes.[34] Gastrointestinal diseases such as acute abdomen,[35] gastric ulcers, gastroesophageal reflux,[36] colorectal disease, and hemorrhoids[37] can cause AD. Sexual activity and vaginal manipulation or sexually transmitted diseases also can elicit AD.

Pregnant women with SCI and a history of AD have an increased frequency of AD.[38,39] It is more serious during labor and has been reported in two-thirds of women with SCI above T6. Blood pressure may be very high and two cases of intraventricular hemorrhage during labor have been recorded.[40]

Pathological conditions, such as skeletal fractures[41,42] or hip dislocation,[43] deep vein thrombosis or pulmonary embolism can cause AD.

Electroejaculation and vibrators have been reported to be associated with increased blood pressure in SCI patients.

Morbidity

Autonomic dysreflexia is a life-threatening condition that can lead to serious events. The increase in blood pressure might cause neurological symptoms such as blurred vision.

Table 13.1 *Causes of autonomic dysreflexia in spinal cord injury patients*

Urinary system	*Reproductive system*
Bladder distention	Sexual intercourse
Blocked catheter	Sexually transmitted disease
Catheterization	Male:
Bladder or renal stones	Ejaculation
Cystoscopy	Epididymitis
Urodynamics	Scrotal compression
Detrusor-sphincter dyssynergia	Electroejaculation and vibratory stimulation
Urinary tract infection	Female:
Extra corporal shock wave lithotripsy	Menstruation
	Pregnancy
	Delivery
Gastrointestinal system	Vaginitis
Fecal impaction	
Acute abdomen	
GI instrumentation	
Hemorrhoids	*Other systems*
Gastric ulcers	Deep vein thrombosis
Abdominal distention	Excessive caffeine or other diuretics
Gallstone	Excessive alcohol
	Fractures or trauma
	Pulmonary emboli
Integument system	Substance abuse
Constrictive clothing, shoes, appliances	Surgical or invasive diagnostic procedures
Blisters	
Burns, sunburn	
Ingrown toe nail	
Pressure ulcer	

However, it might also lead to very serious events like seizures,[44] and intracerebral and subarachnoid hemorrhage, which might result in death.[45,46] Autonomic dysreflexia can alter heart rate and cause arrhythmias such as premature ventricular contractions and second-degree heart block, which have been reported during labor.[28] Episodes of atrial fibrillation following AD have been observed in SCI patients.[47,48] Pulmonary edema has been found in one case of prolonged AD.[49] It is important to recognize the signs and symptoms of AD in order to treat it, and to eliminate the triggering factors to avoid serious morbidity.

Pregnancy and autonomic dysreflexia

Pregnancy is associated with cardiovascular changes such as increased cardiac output and heart rate, decreased blood pressure in the first and second trimesters, as well as systemic resistance. Hypertension can occur during pregnancy secondary to preeclampsia, gestational hypertension, and essential hypertension.

Obstetricians and midwives should be aware of the symptoms and emergency management of AD. It has been reported that AD causes intracranial hemorrhage and death in pregnant women.[40,50] Autonomic dysreflexia in

pregnancy presents with the same signs, symptoms, and pathophysiology as AD in nonpregnant women. Vaginal examinations, labor, and delivery can trigger its onset.

Children

The pathophysiology, signs, symptoms, and management of AD in children are similar to those in adults with SCI. In children, however, the variations in blood pressure according to age should be known along with the use of appropriately sized pressure cuffs. As children may be unable to communicate their symptoms, the family should receive instruction on the signs and symptoms of AD as well as its precipitating causes, and should understand the measures needed to prevent it.[51]

Conclusion

The prevention of AD must be a constant concern to health care professionals in charge of SCI patients. This life-threatening event occurs mainly during medical care and simple measures can avoid irreversible consequences. A good understanding of the pathophysiology of this syndrome is the key to accurate management and prevention.

References

1. Erickson, RP. Autonomic hyperreflexia, pathophysiology and medical management. Arch Phys Med Rehabil 1980; 61:431.

2. Thompson CE, Witham AC. Paroxysmal hypertension in spinal cord injuries. Engl J Med 1948; 239:291.

3. Mathias CJ, Christensen NJ, Corbett JL, et al. Plasma catecholamines during paroxysmal neurogenic hypertension in quadriplegic men. Circ Res 1976; 39:204.

4. McGuire TJ, Kumar VN. Autonomic dysreflexia in spinal cord injury: what physicians should know about this medical emergency. Postgrad Med 1986; 80:81.

5. Young JS. Use of guanethidine in the control of sympathetic hyperreflexia in persons with cervical cord lesions. Arch Phys Med Rehabil 1963; 44:204.

6. Head H, Riddoch G. The autonomic bladder, excessive sweating, and some other reflex conditions in gross injuries of the spinal cord. Brain 1917; 40:188.

7. Ascoli R. The new vegetative syndrome of vesicle distension in paraplegics. Prevention therapy. Paraplegia 1971; 9:82.

8. Hilton J. Pain and therapeutic influence of mechanical physiological rest in accident and surgical disease. Lancet 1860; 2:401.

9. Bowlby AA. The reflexes in cases of injury to the spinal cord. Lancet 1890; 1:1071.

10. Talaat M. Afferent impulses in nerves supplying the bladder. J Physiol 1938; 32:121.

11. Pollock LJ, Boshes B, Chor H. Defects in the regulatory mechanism of autonomic function in injuries to the spinal cord. Neurophysiol 1951; 14:85.

12. Trop CS, Bennett CJ. Autonomic dysreflexia and urological implications. A review. J Urol 1991; 146:1461.

13. Vaidyanathan S, Soni BM, Sett P, et al. Pathophysiology of autonomic dysreflexia: long term treatment with terazosin in adult and pediatric spinal cord injury patients manifesting recurrent dysreflexic episodes. Spinal Cord 1998; 36:761.

14. Karlssan AK. Autonomic dysreflexia. Spinal Cord 1999; 37:363.

15. Krassioukov AV, Weaver LC. Morphological changes in sympathetic preganglionic neurons after spinal cord injury in rats. Neuroscience 1996; 70:211.

16. Krassioukov AV, Weaver LC. Episodic hypertension due to autonomic dysreflexia in acute and chronic spinal cord injured rats. Am J Physiol 1995; 37:268.

17. Krassioukov AV, Weaver LC. Reflex and morphological changes in spinal preganglionic neurons after cord injury in rats. Clin Exp Hypertens 1995; 17:361.

18. Cassam AK, Lewellyn-Smith IJ, Weaver LC. Catecholamine enzymes and neuropeptides are expressed in fibers and stomata in the intermediate gray matter in chronic spinal rats. Neuroscience 1997; 78:89.

19. Krenz NR, Weaver LC. Sprouting of primary afferent fibers after spinal cord transection in rats. Neuroscience 2001; 18:1119.

20. Arnold J, Feng QP, Delaney GA, Teasll RW. Autonomic dysreflexia in tetraplegic patients; evidence for alpha-adrenoceptor hyperresponsivness. Clin Autonom Res 1995; 5:267.

21. Karlsson AK, Friberg P, Lonnroth P, et al. Regional sympathetic function in high spinal cord injury during mental stress and autonomic dysreflexia. Brain 1998; 121:1711.

22. Lindian R. Incidence and clinical features of autonomic dysreflexia in patients with spinal cord injury. Paraplegia 1980; 18:285.

23. Giannantoni A, Distasi SM, Scirolletto G, et al. Autonomic dysreflexia during urodynamics. Spinal Cord 1999; 37:308.

24. Braddom RL, Rocco JF. Autonomic dysreflexia survey of current treatment. Am J Phys Med Rehabil 1991; 70:234.

25. Linsenmeyer TA, Campagnolo DI, Chou IH. Silent autonomic dysreflexia during voiding in man with spinal cord injuries. J Urol 1996; 155(2):519.

26. Silver JL. Early autonomic dysreflexia. Spinal Cord 2000; 38:229.

27. Kewalramani LS. Autonomic dysreflexia in traumatic myelopathy. Am J Phys Med 1980; 59:1.

28. Gutman L, Frakle H, Paeslack V. Cardiac irregularities in paraplegic women. Paraplegia 1965; 3:144.

29. Arieff AJ, Tigay EL, Pyzik SW. Acute hypertension induced by urinary bladder distension. Arch Neurol 1962; 6:248.

30. Lindan R, Joiner E, Frahafer A, Hazel C. Incidence and clinical features of autonomic dysreflexia in patient with spinal cord injury. Paraplegia 1980; 18:285.

31. Manger WM, Davis SW, Chu DS. Autonomic hyperreflexia and its differentiation from pheochromocytoma. Arch Phys Med Rehab 1979; 60:159.

32. Evans CH, Westfall V, Atuk NO. Astrocytoma mimicking the features of pheochromocytoma. N Engl J Med 1972; 286:1397.

33. Perkash I. Autonomic dysreflexia and detrusor sphincter dysenergia in spinal cord injury patients. J Spinal Cord Med 1997; 20:365.

34. Rivasda, Chancellor MB, et al. Flexible cystoscopy during in spinal cord injured patients. Paraplegia 1994; 32(7):454–462.

35. Baron Z, Ohry A. The acute abdomen in spinal cord injury individuals. Paraplegia 1995; 33:704.

36. Donald IP, Gear MW, Wilkinson SP. A life threatening respiratory complication of gastroesophageal reflux in patient with tetraplegia. Postgrad Med J 1987; 63:397.

37. Hawkins RL, Bailey HR, Donnovan WH. Autonomic dysreflexia resulting from prolapsed hemorrhoids. Report of a case. Dis Colon Rect 1917; 40:188.

38. Craig DI. The adaptation to pregnancy of spinal cord injured women. Rehabil Nurse 1990; 15:6.

39. Craig DI. Spinal cord injury and pregnancy: the stories of two women. S C I Nurse 1994; 11:100.

40. McGregor JA, Meeuwesen J. Autonomic hyperreflexia: a mortal danger for spinal cord damaged women in labor. Am J Obstet Gynecol 1985; 151:330.

41. Beard JP, Wade WH, Barber DB. Sacral insufficiency stress fractures as etiology of positional autonomic dysreflexia. Case report. Paraplegia 1996; 34:173.

42. Givre S, Freed HA. Autonomic dysreflexia a potential fatal complication of somatic stress in quadriplegics. J Emer Med 1989; 7:461.

43. Graham GP. Recurrent dislocation of the hip in adult paraplegics. Paraplegia 1992; 30:587.

44. Yarkony GM, Katz RT, Wu YC. Seizures secondary to autonomic dysreflexia. Arch Phys Med Rehabil 1986; 67:834.

45. Kursh ED, Freehafer A, Persky L. Complications of autonomic dysreflexia. J Urol 1977; 118:70.

46. Eltorai I, Kim R, Vulpe M, Kasravi H, Ho W. Fatal cerebral hemorrhage due to autonomic dysreflexia in a tetraplegic patient: case report and review. Paraplegia 1992; 30(5):355–360.

47. Pine ZM, Miller SD, Alonso JA. Atrial fibrillation associated with autonomic dysreflexia. Am J Phys Med Rehabil 1991; 70(5):271–273.

48. Forrest GP. Atrial fibrillation associated with autonomic dysreflexia in patients with tetraplegia. Arch Phys Med Rehabil 1991; 72(8):592–594.

49. Kiker JD, Woodside JR, Jelinek GE. Neurogenic pulmonary edema associated with autonomic dysreflexia. J Urol 1982; 128:1038.

50. Abouleish EL, Hanley ES, Palmer SM. Can epidural fentanyl control autonomic dysreflexia in quadriplegic patients? Anasth Analg 1989; 68:523.

51. Bray GP. Rehabilitation of spinal cord injury: family approach. J Appl Rehabil Counseling 1978; 9:70.

14

Pathophysiology of spinal cord injury

Magdy Hassouna, Nader Elmayergi, and Mazen Abdelhady

Introduction

The functions of the lower urinary tract are to store and periodically eliminate urine. This function implies a reciprocal relationship between the reservoir (bladder) and outlet (urethra and sphincter) component of the lower urinary tract. The functions of the bladder and urethral sphincter are regulated by a complex neural control system located in the brain and spinal cord.[1,2] Spinal cord injury (SCI) initially induces an areflexic bladder and urinary retention due to loss of supraspinal excitatory stimulation.

Recognition of the problem of SCI and the associated lower urinary tract dysfunction dates back to at least 1700 BC with the description in the *Edwin Smith surgical papyrus*: 'One having a dislocation in a vertebra of his neck while he is unconscious of his two legs and his two arms, and his urine dribbles. An ailment not to be treated'.[3]

Innervation of the lower urinary tract

The bladder is innervated by three sets of peripheral nerves: parasympathetic (pelvic), sympathetic (hypogastric), and somatic (pudendal) nerves[4] (Figure 14.1). Afferent sensory fibers from the bladder can exit along either the sympathetic or parasympathetic pathway. Also, these nerves contain afferent axons innervating the lower urinary tract; the most important afferents for initiating micturition are those carried in the pelvic nerve[1,5] (see Figure 14.1).

Parasympathetic preganglionic axons originate in the intermediolateral column of the S2–S4 spinal cord and terminate on postganglionic neurons in the bladder wall and in the pelvic plexus, which is a rectangular network located on the lateral surface of the rectum in humans (see Figure 14.1). The portion of the pelvic plexus that specifically supplies the bladder is sometimes called the vesical plexus. The plexus receives input from the S2–S4 spinal cord segments by means of the presacral nerve. The

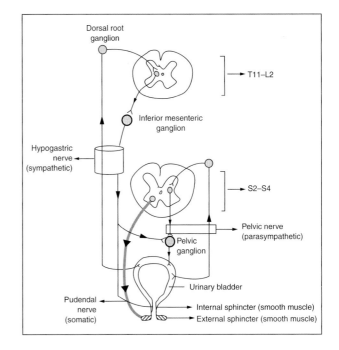

Figure 14.1
Innervation of bladder by parasympathetic, sympathetic and somatic nerves.

primary supply to the detrusor is by parasympathetic nerves, which are uniformly and diffusely distributed throughout the detrusor.[6]

A rich plexus of sympathetic nerve terminals supplies the bladder neck smooth muscle in males. In contrast, in the female numerous parasympathetic nerves, which are identical to that innervating the detrusor, supply the bladder neck and urethral muscle. In the female the bladder muscle and the urethra receive a poor supply of sympathetic innervation.[7]

The sympathetic preganglionic nuclei are located in the 1st and 2nd lumbar segments, and possibly the 12th thoracic segment.

The superior hypogastric plexus is a fenestrated network of fibers anterior to the lower abdominal aorta. The hypogastric nerves exit bilaterally at the inferior poles of the superior hypogastric plexus, which lie at the level of the sacral promontory. The network of nerve structures is located between the endopelvic fascia and the peritoneum. The hypogastric nerves unite the superior hypogastric plexus and the inferior hypogastric plexus or pelvic plexus bilaterally.[8] The superior hypogastric plexus and hypogastric nerves are mainly sympathetic, the pelvic splanchnic nerves are mainly parasympathetic, and the inferior hypogastric plexus has both types of nerves.

Bladder afferent fibers convey mechanoreceptive input essential for voiding. These visceral afferent fibers also transmit sensations of bladder fullness, urgency, and pain.

The pudendal nerve is a mixed nerve carrying motor and sensory fibers. It is a part of the pelvic plexus, and its fibers are derived from the somatic components of the 2nd, 3rd, and 4th sacral nerves. Nerve branches combine to form one major trunk of the pudendal nerve.[9]

The parasympathetic preganglionic axons release acetylcholine (ACh), which activates postsynaptic nicotinic receptors.[10,11] Nicotinic transmission at ganglionic synapses can be regulated by various modulatory synaptic mechanisms which involve muscarinic, adrenergic, and enkephalinergic receptors[1] (Table 14.1). Parasympathetic postganglionic neurons in turn provide an excitatory input to the bladder smooth muscle. Parasympathetic postganglionic nerve terminals release ACh, which can excite different types of muscarinic receptors (M_2 and M_3) that are present in the detrusor muscle,[12–14] (see Table 14.1). Muscarinic receptors are also involved in a presynaptic inhibition (M_2) and facilitation (M_1) of ACh release from postganglionic nerve terminals in the bladder[15,16] (see Table 14.1). Adenosine triphosphate

(ATP), which is a co-transmitter also released from parasympathetic postganglionic terminals, induces a rapid onset, transient contraction of the bladder[17,18] (see Table 14.1). On the other hand, the parasympathetic input to the urethra elicits inhibitory effects mediated at least in part via the release of nitric oxide (NO), which directly relaxes the urethral smooth muscle.[11,19,20] In contrast to other transmitters which are stored and released from synaptic vesicles by exocytosis, NO is not stored but is synthesized immediately prior to release by the enzyme nitric oxide synthase (NOS). NOS-containing nerve terminals are found more densely in the bladder base and urethra than in the detrusor.[21] Thus, it seems reasonable to assume that the excitation of sacral parasympathetic efferent pathways induces a bladder contraction via ACh/ATP release and urethral relaxation via NO release (see Table 14.1). Sympathetic preganglionic neurons located within the intermediolateral cell column of the T11–L2 spinal cord make synaptic connections with postganglionic neurons in the inferior mesenteric ganglion as well as with postganglionic neurons in the paravertebral ganglia and pelvic ganglia[1,10,22] (see Figure 14.1). Ganglionic transmission in sympathetic pathways is also mediated by ACh acting on nicotinic receptors. Sympathetic postganglionic terminals, which release norepinephrine, elicit contractions of the bladder base and urethral smooth muscle and relaxation of the bladder body mediated through adrenoceptors[19,22] (see Table 14.1). In addition, postganglionic sympathetic input to bladder parasympathetic ganglia can facilitate and inhibit parasympathetic ganglionic transmission.[22] Somatic efferent pathways which originate from the motoneurons in Onuf's nucleus of the anterior horn of the S2–S4 spinal cord

Table 14.1 *Receptors in peripheral nervous pathways regulating lower urinary tract function. Facilitatory and inhibitory responses are indicated by plus and minus in parentheses, respectively*

		Efferent			Afferent
		Parasympathetic	Sympathetic	Somatic	
Ganglia	(+)	N, M, VIP	N, M, α_1,[b] β[b]		
	(−)	ENK, δ[a]	α_2[b]		
Bladder	(+)	M_2, M_3, P_{2X}, M_1[a]			NK_1, NK2, CGRP, H_1, B_2, vanilloid
	(−)	M_1,[a] NPY[a]	β_1, β_2, NPY[a]		VIP
Bladder neck and urethra	(+)	M_2, M_3	α_1, α_2		
	(−)	NO			
Striated urethral sphincter	(+)			N	
	(−)				

[a]Presynaptic receptors.

[b]Heterosynaptic inputs onto parasympathetic ganglion cells.

ENK, enkephalin; VIP, vasoactive intestinal peptide; NO, nitric oxide; NPY, neuropeptide Y; N, nicotinic receptor; M_1, M_2, and M_3, muscarinic receptors; α_1, α_2, β_1, and β_2, adrenergic receptors; P_{2X}, purinergic receptor; CGRP, calcitonin gene-relating peptide receptors; NK_1 and NK_2, tachykinin receptors; δ, opioid receptors; H_1, histamine receptor; B_2, bradykinin receptor.

innervate the external striated urethral sphincter muscle and the pelvic floor musculature (see Figure 14.1). Somatic nerve terminals release ACh, which acts on nicotinic receptors to induce a muscle contraction (see Table 14.1). Combined activation of sympathetic and somatic pathways elevates bladder outlet resistance and contributes to urinary continence. Several other non-adrenergic–non-cholinergic transmitters such as leucine enkephalin (ENK), vasoactive intestinal polypeptide (VIP), and neuropeptide Y have been identified as modulators of efferent inputs to the lower urinary tract[22,23] (Table 14.1).

Physiology of urine storage and micturition

The bladder functions as a low-pressure reservoir during urine storage. The bladder pressures remain low and relatively constant when bladder volume is below the threshold for inducing voiding. This is mainly due to the combined effect of the viscoelastic properties of the bladder wall and quiescence of the parasympathetic pathway to the bladder.[1,4] During urine storage, the bladder outlet is closed and the bladder smooth muscle is quiescent, allowing intravesical pressure to remain low over a wide range of bladder volumes. Sensory information, including the feeling of bladder fullness or bladder pain, is conveyed to the

spinal cord via afferent axons in the pelvic and hypogastric nerves.[5,24] Neuronal bodies of these afferent nerves are located in the dorsal root ganglia (DRG) at S2–S4 and T11–L2 spinal segmental levels (see Figure 14.1). The afferent fibers carry impulses from tension receptors and nociceptors in the bladder wall to neurons in the dorsal horn of the spinal cord. Afferent fibers passing in the pelvic nerve to the sacral cord are responsible for initiating the micturition reflex. These bladder afferents have myelinated (Aδ-fiber) or unmyelinated (C-fiber) axons.[25–27]

In addition, during bladder filling, afferent activity derived from the bladder activates a sacral–thoracolumbar intersegmental spinal reflex pathway, which triggers firing in sympathetic pathways to the bladder.[28] Activation of sympathetic efferents then mediates an inhibition of bladder activity and contraction of the bladder neck and proximal urethra.[29] Pudendal motoneurons are also activated by vesical afferent input as the bladder fills, thereby inducing a contraction of the striated sphincter muscle, which contributes to urinary continence.[30,31] Thus, urine storage is mainly controlled by reflexes integrated in the spinal cord (Figure 14.2). However, it is also reported that a supraspinal urine storage center is located in the dorsolateral pons. Descending inputs from this region activate the pudendal motoneurons to increase urethral resistance[32] (see Figure 14.2).

When bladder volume reaches the micturition threshold, afferent activity originating in bladder mechanoceptors triggers micturition reflexes, which consist of firing in

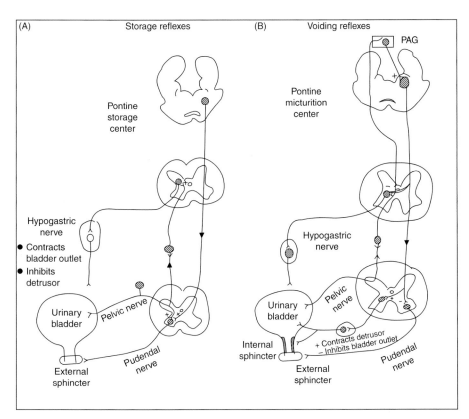

Figure 14.2 Storage and voiding reflexes of the bladder.

the sacral parasympathetic pathways and inhibition of symptathetic and somatic pathways. This leads to a contraction of the bladder and a concomitant relaxation of the urethra. The afferent fibers which trigger micturition in the rat and cat are myelinated Aδ fibers.[25,26] These bladder afferents in the pelvic nerve synapse on neurons in the sacral spinal cord, which then send their axons rostrally to a micturition center in the dorsolateral pons. This center contains neurons that are essential for inducing voiding reflexes.[33–35] It has been demonstrated that activity ascending from the spinal cord may pass through a relay center in the periaqueductal gray before reaching the pontine micturition center.[30,31]

Thus, voiding reflexes depend on a spino-bulbospinal pathway which passes through an integrative center in the brain (see Figure 14.2). This center functions as an 'on-off' switch, activated by afferent activity derived from bladder mechanoceptors, and also receives inhibitory and excitatory inputs from the brain regions rostral to the pons. Reflex voiding is also facilitated by afferent inputs from the urethra. This urethrovesical reflex triggered by urine flow into the urethra enhances bladder contractions.[2] During voiding reflexes, activity in the pudendal efferent pathway to the striated urethral sphincter is suppressed to reduce outlet resistance.[1,35] This mechanism is mainly due to an inhibition of the pudendal motoneurons by the descending inputs from the dorsolateral pons.[25,36,37] An excitation of the sacral parasympathetic pathway also directly induces a relaxation of urethral smooth muscle mediated by the release of NO.

During voluntary voiding, relaxation of the pelvic floor and striated urethral sphincter muscles occurs, followed by a detrusor muscle contraction and opening of the bladder neck. Reflex inhibition of the smooth and striated urethral sphincter muscles also occurs during micturition.

In the human bladder smooth muscle, only two muscarinic receptor subtypes (M_2 and M_3) have been identified. Although the M_2 receptor subtype is the predominant subtype in the bladder (approximately 80%), the contractions of the bladder are mediated by M_3 receptors.[38] Muscarinic receptors (M_1 subtype) are also located prejunctionally on cholinergic nerve terminals in the bladder.[39] Voiding reflexes are mediated by myelinated (Aδ-fiber) bladder afferents, which activate a supraspinal micturition reflex that passes through neural circuits in the rostral brainstem.[40] Also, unmyelinated (C-fiber) bladder afferents are present and they are found to be silent in normal cats and do not respond to bladder distention.

roots. On each side, the anterior and dorsal nerve roots combine to form the spinal nerve as it exits from the vertebral column through the neuroforamina. The spinal cord extends from the base of the skull and terminates near the lower margin of the LI vertebral body. Thereafter, the spinal canal contains the lumbar, sacral, and coccygeal spinal nerves that comprise the cauda equina. Therefore, injuries below L1 are not considered SCIs because they involve the segmental spinal nerves and/or cauda equina. Spinal injuries proximal to L1, above the termination of the spinal cord, often involve a combination of spinal cord lesions and segmental root or spinal nerve injuries.

The primary watershed area of the spinal cord is the midthoracic region. Vascular injury may cause a cord lesion at a level several segments higher than the level of spinal injury. For example, a lower cervical spine fracture may result in disruption of the vertebral artery that ascends through the affected vertebra. The resulting vascular injury may cause an ischemic high cervical cord injury. At any given level of the spinal cord, the central part is a watershed area. Cervical hyperextension injuries may cause ischemic injury to the central part of the cord, causing a central cord syndrome.

The effect of SCI on the lower urinary tract depends on the level, duration, and completeness of the cord lesion. According to the level, it may give the picture of an upper motor neuron lesion, which corresponds with damage to the spinal cord rostral to the sacral cord, and lower motor neuron diseases in which damage occurs to the sacral cord and/or cauda equina that give rise to the parasympathetic and somatic pathway to the bladder and urethral sphincter.[41,42] Among patients with SCI, upper motoneuron disease such as cervical and thoracic vertebral injuries forms the major group.[41] Upper motoneuron type of SCI initially leads to a phase of spinal shock that is followed by a recovery phase during which neurologic changes emerge. During the period of spinal shock immediately after SCI, there is a flaccid paralysis and absence of reflex activity below the level of the lesion; thus, the urinary bladder becomes areflexic. However, activity of the internal and external sphincter persists or rapidly recovers after suprasacral injuries. Therefore, because sphincter tone is present, urinary retention develops and patients have to be treated with intermittent or continuous catheterization to eliminate urine from the urinary bladder. Following the spinal shock phase, reflex detrusor activity reappears after 2–12 weeks in most cases.[41,42]

Effects of spinal cord injury on micturition

The spinal cord is divided into 31 segments, each with a pair of anterior (motor) and dorsal (sensory) spinal nerve

The pathophysiology of spinal cord injury

It is now generally accepted that acute SCI is a two-step process involving primary and secondary mechanisms.[43,44]

The primary mechanism involves the initial mechanical injury due to local deformation and energy transformation, whereas the secondary mechanism encompasses a cascade of biochemical and cellular processes that are initiated by the primary process and may cause ongoing cellular damage and even cell death.[45]

Throughout the recent medical literature the whole process of spinal cord injury has been explained in detail, with the term spinal shock used sparingly. It is at best intertwined within SCI, at worst disregarded completely.

In common use 'spinal shock' is a misnomer.[46] The concept of 'spinal shock' has recently been criticized for a number of reasons. Importantly, there is no universal agreement on the time at which the phase of spinal shock ends. Furthermore, the state of spinal shock has no prognostic significance. The concept of 'spinal shock' as it relates to neurologic dysfunction should therefore be reconsidered.[46]

From the pathophysiological perspective, the same mechanisms of SCI are the cause of the simultaneous 'shock,' whether neurologic or from hypotensive causes. To properly discuss spinal shock, and all the mechanisms leading to it, would be incomplete without explaining in detail the bigger picture of SCI.

Primary mechanism

The primary mechanism (see Table 14.2) of SCI is a combination of both the initial impact and the subsequent persisting compression. This is common in injuries like fracture dislocation, missile injuries, ruptured discs, and burst fractures. Clinical scenarios where impact alone occurs without ongoing compression may include severe ligamentous injuries in which the spinal column dislocates and then spontaneously reduces.[45] Similarly, spinal cord laceration from sharp bone fragments or missile injuries can produce a mixture of spinal cord laceration, contusion, and compression or concussion.[47]

Secondary mechanisms

The primary mechanical injury initiates a cascade of secondary injury mechanisms (Table 14.3), including the following:

1. vascular changes[44,48,49]
2. free radical production[50–52]
3. ionic derangements[53,54]
4. programmed cell death or apoptosis[55,56]
5. neurotransmitter accumulation (excitotoxic cell injury)[57,58]
6. inflammation

7. loss of adenosine triphosphate-dependent cellular processes[59]
8. edema[60]
9. endogenous opioids.[61,62]

Table 14.2 *Primary mechanism of acute spinal cord injury*

- Acute compression
- Impact
- Missile
- Distraction
- Laceration
- Shear

Table 14.3 *Secondary mechanisms of spinal cord injury*

Systemic vascular effects:
- Heart rate: brief tachycardia, then prolonged bradycardia
- Blood pressure: brief hypertension, then prolonged hypotension
- Peripheral resistance: decreased
- Cardiac output: decreased
- Hypoxia
- Hyperthermia
- Injudicious movement of the unstable spine, leading to worsening compression

Local vascular changes:
- Loss of autoregulation
- Systemic hypotension (neurogenic shock)
- Hemorrhage
- Loss of microcirculation
- Reduction in blood flow
  - Vasospasm
  - Thrombosis

Free radical production:
- Lipid peroxidation

Ionic derangements:
- Increased intracellular calcium
- Increased intracellular potassium
- Increased intracellular sodium and sodium permeability

Apoptosis

Neurotransmitter accumulation:
- Excitotoxic amino acids

Inflammation

Loss of energy metabolism:
- Decreased ATP production

Edema

Endogenous opioids:
- Endorphins

Vascular changes

One of the most critical elements in the evolution of bio-chemical and morphologic alterations following spinal cord trauma is the condition of vascular flow to the tissue. Blood flow, which is present or lacking in the spinal cord tissue after trauma, is a reflection of the damage provoked.[56]

Blood supply of the spinal cord. Blood is supplied to the vertebral column by way of segmental arteries that arise near it from the aorta, or from adjacent arteries in the areas beyond the extent of the aorta. These include the costocervical and intercostal arteries in the thorax, the lumbar and iliolumbar arteries in the lumbar region, and the lateral sacral arteries in the pelvis.

The anterior spinal artery (ASA) is supplied by a series of 5–10 unpaired radicular arteries (that originate from the vertebral arteries, and aorta and its branches). This single artery runs in the ventral midline from the foramen magnum to the filum terminale. The posterior spinal arteries are fed by smaller radicular arteries at nearly every spinal level.

The centripetal blood supply is derived from the posterior spinal and pial arteries. The pial arteries are lateral branches from the ASA and they communicate extensively with lateral branches originating from the posterior spinal arteries. The centrifugal supply is by the sulcal arteries. These arteries number approximately 4–5 per centimeter of spinal cord, and often bifurcate in the anterior median sulcus. The centrifugal sulcal arterial system supplies the anterior gray matter, the anterior half of the posterior gray matter, the inner half of the anterior and lateral white columns, and the anterior half of the posterior white columns.[49] The intervening watershed zones are supplied by both the centripetal and centrifugal systems.

After an acute SCI, both local and systemic changes occur to affect the spinal cord blood flow (SCBF) (see Table 14.4).

Systemic effects. Acute SCI can cause numerous cardiovascular and hemodynamic effects, the magnitude of which is related directly to the level and severity of the SCI, with the largest changes occurring in complete cervical injuries.[48] It is also one of the causes of neurogenic shock,[63] typically being related to the magnitude and severity of the cord injury. Neurogenic shock is characterized by severe autonomic dysfunction, resulting in hypotension, relative bradycardia, peripheral vasodilation, and hypothermia. It usually does not occur with SCI below the level of T6. Decreased sympathetic tone, unopposed cardiac vagal tone, and other cardiac changes are all contributory.[64] At its extreme, systemic effects including hypotension and bradycardia may be profound. These changes may persist for an extended period of time, sometimes months. In concert with these changes, total peripheral resistance and cardiac output may also remain depressed for a prolonged period of time.

The main cause for most of these effects is impairment of autoregulation following an acute SCI.[65–67] The systemic hypotension (preceded by a transient hypertension) that occurs as a result of this can cause further decreases in SCBF with induced hypertension (see Endogenous opioids section) not necessarily reversing the ischemia, but rather causing marked hyperemia at adjacent sites.[44,68] The reason for this transient hypertension is unknown but may be mediated by both the thoracic sympathetic ganglions and the adrenal glands.[69] Experimentally, it has been shown in animal studies that autoregulation is intact during the initial 60–90 min after SCI but is then lost coincident with the onset of ischemia. It has been suggested that the ischemic response to SCI is mediated both by the loss of autoregulation and by relative constriction of the resistance vessels.[66]

Disturbances of venous drainage may play a role in the secondary damage that occurs after acute SCI, particularly in terms of exacerbating ischemia of the posterior columns.[70–72] This hypothesis gains weight by studies that

Table 14.4 *Systemic and local vascular effects with acute SCI*	
Systemic effects (neurogenic shock)	Local effects (cord microcirculation)
Heart rate (increased then decreased)	Mechanical disruption of spinal cord vessels
Blood pressure (brief increase then prolonged decrease)	Hemorrhage
Peripheral resistance (decreased)	Loss of microcirculation
Cardiac output (decreased)	Loss of autoregulation
Catecholamines (increased, then decreased)	Reduction of spinal cord blood flow (SCBF)
	Vasospasm
	Thrombosis

show that venous occlusion in various pathologic conditions causes white matter lesions.[73–75] It may be that peculiarities of the venous drainage of the spinal cord make it more susceptible to damage.[71]

Local effects

Microcirculation: There is a major reduction in the microcirculation of the traumatized spinal cord and lack of perfusion. Also, major areas lack filling of the arterioles, capillaries, and venules. This occurs both at the injury site, and for a considerable distance cephalad and caudad in the cord. The ischemic zones encompass a large portion of the gray matter and the surrounding white matter, and are especially severe in white matter adjacent to hemorrhages in the gray matter.[49] This may be due to obstruction of the anterior sulcal arteries that leads to the hemorrhagic necrosis and subsequent central myelomalacia seen at the site of injury.

There also seems to be a secondary injury to the microcirculation such as thrombosis or vasospasm of arterioles traversing the gray matter to supply the white matter. The large vessels of the cord such as the anterior spinal artery and the anterior sulcal arteries, however, almost always remain patent even after severe cord injury.

Axonal conduction: The relationships among the severity of acute SCI, motor and somatosensory evoked potentials (MEPs and SSEPs), and SCBF were studied. A linear relationship was found between the severity of acute SCI and the reduction in SCBF at the injury site. Also the reduction in amplitude of the MEP and SSEP was significantly correlated with the reduction of post-traumatic SCBF. Both the severity of cord injury and the degree of post-traumatic ischemia were significantly related to post-traumatic axonal dysfunction. Thus, these studies provide quantitative evidence linking post-traumatic ischemia to axonal dysfunction following acute SCI.[48]

Histology: Histologically, there are many changes that occur after an SCI. Though there are petechial and more confluent hemorrhages in the gray matter, there is an initial absence of cellular and tissue necrosis. A progressive necrotizing process and an inflammatory cell infiltration that affects the gray matter and extends into the white matter follows this early period. Throughout these changes the main arteries remain patent, and this has led to the conclusion that much of the vascular damage occurs primarily in the intramedullary vascular system.

Also, the principal site of vascular damage is the endothelial cells, either by direct physical trauma or secondary to the resultant ischemia. These alterations in endothelial cell function cause an increase in vascular permeability and edema formation.[76–78] Endothelial damage occurs early, with the formation of craters, adherence of noncellular debris, overriding of endothelial cell junctions, and microglobular formations occurring 1–2 hours after acute SCI.[79]

Free radical pathology and lipid peroxidation

Molecules are composed of atoms bonded together. This bonding process is accomplished by the sharing of electrons. When two atoms come together and their electrons pair up, a bond is created. Paired electrons are quite stable; nearly 100% of all electrons in the human body exist in a paired state, and a general principle of quantum chemistry is that only 2 electrons can exist in one bond.

If the bond between atoms is broken, the electrons either stay together (i.e. one atom gets both electrons and the other atom gets none) or they split up (each atom gets one electron). If the electrons split up, the atoms are called *free radicals* (molecules with an unpaired electron). This electron split is what makes free radicals both useful and dangerous.

It is important to mention that there are several essential biochemical pathways and cell biologic phenomena that depend on free radicals. Examples include (but are not limited to) mitochondrial electron transport, phagocytosis by macrophages and polymorphonuclear leukocytes, and hydroxylation reactions in the endoplasmic reticulum.

However, among biomolecules, the unsaturated acyl chains in cell membrane phospholipids and cholesterol in membranes are highly susceptible to pathologic free radical damage. This is due to:

1. Their inherent structure (polyunsaturated acyl chains are normally unconjugated and the α-methylenic carbons between carbons with double bonds have allylic hydrogen that can readily enter into free radical reactions).
2. The 700% greater solubility of molecular oxygen within nonpolar compared to aqueous environments (the most nonpolar regions of a cell are generally the hydrophobic portion of the membranes; the phospholipid acyl chains and the cholesterol comprise the hydrophobic portion of cell membranes, with the exception that organelle membranes are usually devoid of cholesterol, which is usually found in close association with phospholipids only in the plasma membrane and myelin).
3. Molecular oxygen has outer orbitals that have unpaired electrons, thereby conferring upon oxygen certain properties of free radicals, such as magnetic susceptibility (due to the magnetic moment of an unpaired electron in orbit) and the ability to initiate free radical chain reactions among susceptible molecules that lack sufficient antioxidant neighboring molecules.[50]

The consumption of a major CNS antioxidant, ascorbic acid, in the ischemic or traumatized tissues occurs before the loss of the lipids, and is an important factor in establishing the free radical nature of some of the pathologic changes.

Free radicals most commonly form from molecular oxygen. Superoxide (O_2) is formed by incomplete electron transport in mitochondria. Superoxide is converted to H_2O_2 by superoxide dismutase and this in turn to H_2O and O_2 by catalase. In the presence of free iron, released from hemoglobin, transferrin, or ferritin by either lowered pH or oxygen radicals, H_2O_2 forms highly reactive hydroxyl radicals (HO). These, if unchecked, can cause geometrically progressive lipid peroxidation, spreading over the cellular surface and causing impairment of phospholipid-dependent enzymes, disruption of ionic gradients, and if severe enough, membrane lysis. This process also forms more lipid peroxides and consequently more free radicals.[50]

Though still not completely established, in SCI the initiation of the free radical reactions following impact is probably mediated by the initial extravasation of blood in the central gray matter and perhaps by coenzyme Q autoxidation when spinal cord ischemia (hypoxia) occurs. The hemorrhages are minute and petechial, but they provide inorganic iron and copper from the plasma, as well as iron and copper from red blood cells (RBCs) that extravasate and lyse. Iron compounds such as hematin can accelerate the autoxidation of unsaturated lipids by five orders of magnitude. Further, the concentration of highly polyunsaturated fatty acyl (PUFA) chains in membrane phospholipids is greatest in the central gray matter; PUFAs are very susceptible to free radical reactions, particularly in the presence of iron, or copper.[50]

Ionic derangements

Potassium and calcium. Potassium ions (K^+) and calcium ions (Ca^{2+}) play important roles in the central nervous system (CNS). Intracellular K^+ activity ($[K^+]i$) is normally at least 20 times greater than extracellular K^+ activity ($[K^+]e$). The resultant transmembrane K^+ gradient controls membrane potentials, action potential conduction, and active transport of sodium ions (Na^+). Increases in cell membrane permeability to K^+ produce rises in $[K^+]e$. Because normal $[K^+]e$ is 3–4 mmol/liter (mM), small changes in (K^+)e profoundly alter neuronal activity. Cells typically maintain very low intracellular Ca^{2+} activity ($[Ca^{2+}]i$), <100 nmol/liter (nM) in contrast to extracellular Ca^{2+} activity ($[Ca^{2+}]e$) of >1.0 mM. Owing to this very large gradient, Ca^{2+} ions readily enter cells when membrane permeability increases. Ca^{2+} entry into cells links membrane activity with cellular functions. Large Ca^{2+} influxes into cells have been postulated to kill hepatocytes, myocytes, peripheral nerves, myelin, and spinal axons.[54]

Potassium changes: Contusion that occurs causes a disruption of a large proportion of cells at the impact site.

This disruption leads to a large increase in extracellular K, with a rise from 4 mM to 54 mM. One hour after impact, approximately 50% of K is lost from the impact site. By 3 hours, only 35% of pre-injury tissue K remains at the impact site.

Consequences of potassium depletion: Cells do not repossess K^+ ions released into the extracellular space at the impact site. Potassium is gone from the impact site, not merely equilibrated between the intra- and extracellular compartments. The cells not initially disrupted by the contusion also lose intracellular K^+, due to increased permeability of cell membranes depolarized by elevated $[K^+]e$.

The surviving cells tend to distribute in the outer rim of the spinal cord, the part least susceptible to ischemia. Note that the effects of $[K^+]i$ depletion are likely to outlast the $[K^+]e$ changes. Potassium ions released into extracellular space should be rapidly cleared by diffusion and glial transport.[80–84] Restoration of $[K^+]i$ depends on active ionic transport.

Ironically, rapid recovery of $[K^+]e$ to normal levels will force ionic restitution mechanisms to work against steeper transmembrane ionic gradients. One consequence of low $[K^+]i$ will be depolarization of cells in the presence of normal $[K^+]e$. This may explain the paradoxical loss of spontaneous activity or conduction block occasionally observed in ischemia and spinal cord injury even when $[K^+]e$ appears to be normalized.[54]

Potassium diffusion: The K^+ spilled from the damaged cells is absorbed either into the spinal cord itself, into the cerebrospinal fluid (CSF), or into the blood. The far majority (70%) of K^+ is absorbed into the cord surrounding the impact site. Three hours after the injury (the time it takes for the blood–brain barrier to break down) increased amounts of K^+ are lost into the CSF. However, diffusion into the CSF and blood is negligible during the periods of ischemia[85–87] and spreading depression.[81,83,88] Spreading depression is a transient, slowly propagating wave of tissue depolarization that can be evoked by mechanical stimulation, and has been associated with ischemia or traumatic brain injury. Each wave lasts for 1–2 min; waves of spreading depression have been observed to occur for several days after injury. In a model of ischemia, these waves have been shown by magnetic resonance imaging (MRI) to precede neural damage, with infarct volume increasing by up to 23% after each wave. Spreading depression is of non-neuronal origin, being mediated by astrocytes, and neurons are only secondarily affected. Two different, interacting mechanisms help to propagate spreading depression from cell to cell: a gap junction-mediated pathway and an ATP-purinergic pathway. While most of the work on spreading depression has been done in the brain, recent studies have shown that spinal cord astrocytes can mediate spreading depression via the ATP-purinergic pathway after edema.

Calcium changes: Extracellular calcium $[Ca^{2+}]e$ recorded with ion-selective microelectrodes is typically greater than 1.2 mM in uninjured spinal cords and brain. $[Ca^{2+}]i$ in the spinal cord is not known with certainty, but some estimates suggest <100 nM^3, negligible compared to $[Ca^{2+}]e$. The amounts of Ca changes at the impact site appear small when compared with the K changes. On an ion-by-ion basis, the Ca shifts constitute a minor fraction of the ionic changes at the impact site. But the Ca changes must be considered in light of the lower pre-injury $[Ca^{2+}]e$ levels and the higher proportion of bound Ca vs free Ca^{2+} in the spinal cord. $[Ca^{2+}]e$ remains at <0.1 mM for hours after the injury at the impact site.

Calcium diffusion. Uptake of Ca by intact cells plays only a small role in the persistent low $[Ca^{2+}]e$ levels found after injury at the impact site. Active uptake into the CSF is very difficult, due to the large concentration gradient and rapid drop of $[Ca^{2+}]e$. Inorganic phosphate plays a major role.

Phosphate binds strongly with Ca^{2+} to form phosphate complexes, most notably hydroxyapatite or $Ca_5(PO_4)_3(OH)$. The association constant of Ca^{2+} with the phosphate ion (H_2PO_4) is pK -7.2.[89,90] Tissue concentrations of inorganic phosphates often exceed 5 mM. Calcium phosphate is quite insoluble. Hydroxyapatite has a solubility product of pK 58.6 and is less sensitive to pH than other Ca complexes.[91] At pH <6.5, other Ca complexes transform to hydroxyapatite when phosphates are available.[92–94] Ca^{2+} ions diffusing to the impact site sequester inorganic phosphates and precipitate as hydroxyapatites or other complexes, i.e. 'amorphous calcium deposits'.

There are sufficient phosphates in the tissue to buffer large quantities of Ca^{2+}. ATP turnover, for example, can provide 1–2 mM of phosphate. Extreme depletion of cellular phosphates due to sequestration by Ca^{2+} explains the rapid losses of ATP and other metabolic derangements in injured spinal cords.[95,96]

Pathological consequences of calcium influx: The finding of early Ca accumulation at the impact site preceding onset of gross tissue necroses argues for a causative role of Ca^{2+} in cell damage. The intracellular volume of axons at the impact site is likely to be a tiny fraction of the total axoplasm available to buffer Ca^{2+} ions entering the axon. Furthermore, the critical metabolic apparatus of cells giving rise to the axons is situated far from the lesion site and therefore is not as accessible to the entering Ca^+ ions. In contrast, cell bodies situated at the lesion site are more vulnerable to the damaging effects of Ca^{2+} influx.[54]

Apoptosis (programmed cell death)

Cell death that occurs after SCI occurs either through necrosis or apoptosis. Necrotic cell death occurs passively, resulting from the actual tissue mechanical damage and resultant release of destructive lysozymes, ion fluxes, and disturbed cell membranes producing an inflammatory response that has long been understood to be the sole component of neuronal tissue death and the ultimate clinical neurologic ramifications of acute spinal cord injury.

In contradistinction to necrotic cell injury, apoptosis is associated with physiologic or programmed cell death.[97,98] It is an actively regulated response and there is a variety of morphologic criteria that distinguish apoptotic from necrotic cell death.

Apoptotic cell death occurs a single cell at a time, whereas necrotic cells normally die in groups. Although cell membranes may undergo blebbing during apoptotic cell death, they do not lose their structural integrity as do cells undergoing necrotic cell death. Cells undergoing apoptotic death actually shrink, forming apoptotic cell bodies which contain cleaved DNA. In contrast, necrotic cells swell and lyse, which incites a significant inflammatory response. Thus, although both apoptotic cell bodies and necrotic cells may be phagocytosed by tissue macrophages, apoptotic cell bodies do not incite any type of inflammatory response and thus undergo a 'silent' cell death.

At the molecular level, there are many distinct morphologic and biochemical changes occurring during apoptosis, including chromatin condensation, DNA fragmentation into oligonucleosome-sized fragments, and the compaction of chromatin into uniformly dense masses. The constant biochemical event which occurs in apoptosis is the activation of an endonuclease which cleaves DNA at internucleosomal linker sites.

The biochemical criteria for distinguishing apoptotic from necrotic cell death are also quite well established. Apoptotic cell death is induced by physiologic stimuli, either external or internal, whereas necrotic cell death arises from nonphysiologic disturbances. Apoptotic cell death is a tightly regulated process with a sequence of activation steps that requires energy and specific macromolecular synthesis as well as *de-novo* gene transcription.[99] This precedes the nonrandom oligonucleosomal length DNA fragmentation which is the common final pathway of eventual apoptotic cell death. In contrast, during necrotic cell death there are no energy requirements because there is no *de-novo* gene transcription, and thus no new protein or nucleic acid synthesis occurring.[98,100] The cellular DNA is randomly digested following cell lysis by macrophages that are solicited following the inflammatory response.

There are several features of SCI that suggest apoptosis plays a key role in the pathophysiology.

Increases in intracellular Ca^{2+} occur after SCI and are important in post-traumatic cell death. Ca^{2+}-dependent breakdown of DNA and protein also occurs in apoptosis. Hypoxia and free radical formation follow SCI, and are processes known to trigger p53-mediated DNA repair and apoptosis. Glutamate excitotoxicity has been established as a key event following neural trauma and has also been linked to apoptosis[55] (see Excitotoxins section).

It is thought that oligodendrocytes are the major cell type in compressive SCI that undergoes apoptosis[101,102] seen in areas of wallerian degeneration and detectable between 24 hours and 3 weeks post injury.[103] The mechanism behind this is unclear, but it may occur as a result of adverse changes in the cellular environment resulting in axonal demyelination or as a result of wallerian degeneration, or by a combination of both of these processes.[104,105] Apoptosis occurs around the lesion epicenter as well as within areas of wallerian degeneration in both ascending and descending white matter tracts.[106]

Some forms of experimental treatment of SCI are aimed at limiting the histological injury, such as the oncogene Bcl-2, which regulates the antioxidant pathway, thus limiting free radical generation. Similarly, cycloheximide treatment can improve outcome after contusion trauma in the spinal cords of rats.[107]

Excitotoxins

Endogenously released excitatory amino acids may contribute to injury in the CNS in several different disorders, including epilepsy, neurodegenerative diseases, and cerebral ischemia.[108] The acidic amino acids glutamate and aspartate are widely distributed within the CNS and serve as excitatory neurotransmitters. It has long been recognized that these substances may be neurotoxic.[58]

N-methyl-D-aspartate (NMDA), quisqualate, and kainite are receptors of excitatory amino acids. Selective NMDA receptor antagonists, injected directly into the brain, protect hippocampal neurons from cell death following cerebral ischemia[109] and hypoglycemia.[110] NMDA receptors also play a role in neurotransmission in the spinal cord.[111,112]

Most selective NMDA antagonists do not readily cross the blood–brain barrier, and hence their effects only appear after direct CNS administration. MK-801 [(+)-5-methyl-10,11-dihydro-5H-dibenzol [a,d]cyclo-hepten-5,10-imine maleate] is centrally active following systemic administration. It is a selective, noncompetitive antagonist that is use-dependent, requiring activation of receptors for its effect to be demonstrated.[113]

MK-801 significantly improves neurologic outcome after traumatic spinal cord injury. Moreover, NMDA, but not its levo isomer, significantly exacerbates the consequences of traumatic injury. From these data it is suggested that excitotoxins, released in response to injury and acting in part through the NMDA receptor, contribute to the secondary pathophysiologic effects after trauma that lead to irreversible tissue damage.[58] These findings extend the excitotoxin hypothesis of CNS injury to trauma, in addition to their proposed role in neurodegenerative diseases, epilepsy, and ischemia.[108]

The exact mechanism of how these excitatory amino acids produce their neurotoxic actions is still not clear. One hypothesis suggests that such a toxicity is a result of neuronal depolarization and sustained excitation, leading to accumulation of intracellular Na and Cl and loss of energy reserves, then to cellular edema and lysis.[114] A second hypothesis proposes that neurotoxicity of excitatory amino acids is mediated by an influx of extracellular calcium. A third hypothesis is a mixture of the previous two, with an early response, associated with neuronal swelling, which is dependent upon extracellular sodium and chlorine and can be demonstrated in the absence of extracellular calcium; a more delayed response, leading to cell death, is dependent upon the presence of extracellular calcium.[115]

Inflammation

The CNS is relatively 'immune privileged,' meaning that under normal conditions there is minimal immune surveillance. This is partly due to the blood–brain barrier, a specialized structure made up of endothelia and astrocytic end-feet that separates the circulatory and the central nervous systems, and tightly regulates passage of molecules and cells between them. Thus, few immune cells are found in the healthy CNS. Upon injury, however, the blood–brain barrier is physically and functionally altered, blood vessels become leaky, and cells of the immune system invade the CNS, triggering an inflammatory response. The immediate, but transient, appearance of neutrophils characterizes the early immune response. The next phase of the immediate early inflammatory response that follows SCI is mediated mainly by two groups of leukocytes – T lymphocytes (or T cells) and macrophages. T cells are antigen-specific; each is activated by a specific stimulus (or antigen) that is frequently just a part of a molecule. They reside in the major immune organs, circulate through the body in the lymphatic system, and can home in on sites of injury, where they migrate into the surrounding tissue. If activated by binding to their respective antigen, they increase their release of cytokines and are cytotoxic to target cells. Macrophages, on the other hand, are not antigen-specific. They circulate, but also reside in various tissues. Best known for their phagocytic properties, macrophages also have important functions in antigen presentation, cytokine secretion, and cytotoxicity. Quiescent macrophages residing within the CNS are known as microglia.

The molecular basis of spinal cord inflammation draws from a vast arsenal of known immunologic molecules, including cytokines and chemokines, as well as growth factors, trophic factors, and other agents. Cytokines, of which there are about 60, regulate cell–cell communication between immune cells. They are small proteins that produce local and transient effects. Chemokines are chemotactic molecules that attract immune cells, helping them to 'home' to sites of inflammation. Frequently, the cells producing these regulatory molecules also bear receptors for them, participating in a complex network of self-regulating and local interactions that orchestrate the proliferation of immune cells and then the subsequent decline of immune activity.

The inflammatory response in SCI is both beneficiary and deleterious. If the inflammatory response is deleterious to recovery, one approach might be to eliminate the immune cells that mediate this response. This is still under research.

Loss of ATP-dependent cellular processes

The ATP-dependent cellular processes are affected in SCI in two successive stages: one in the first 4 hours and the second between 4 and 24 hours. Throughout the 24-hour period, the total adenylates and concentrations of ATP, P-Creatine, and lactic acid are relatively constant. However, the difference between the two stages is in the sequence of changes in the lactate/pyruvate ratio, the energy change, and the tissue levels of pyruvate and glucose.

After the first 15 min glucose concentration in the spinal cord declines, due to both the utilization of glucose stores and the impediment of proper glucose transport to the impact site. However, after the initial 15 min until 4 hours there is a rise in glucose, as replenishment occurs.

The tissue levels of both the glucose and pyruvate become supranormal between 4 and 24 hours. Also, there is a slight rise in energy changes and the lactate/pyruvate ratio falls to normal levels.

The increase in tissue glucose and pyruvate levels suggested a stimulation or release of the glycolytic rate from its previously depressed state. Decline in the lactate/pyruvate ratio implies that oxidative pathways are operative. The mechanism(s) responsible for the increased metabolic rate are not known.[59] In those areas where edema was minimal or diminishing, some recovery of metabolic rate would be expected.[116] The rise in tissue glucose levels between 4 and 24 hours may be due to increased perfusion to microregions within the injured segment, perhaps coupled with an augmented glucose transport from blood.[117]

Two theories have previously been advanced to explain the prolonged depression of the adenylate pool and tissue ATP levels in the oligemic cerebrum. First, during ischemia, ATP is dephosphorylated to ADP and AMP, and the size of the adenine nucleotide pool is diminished secondary to the degradation of AMP to inosine monophosphate (IMP) and adenosine.[118] Since many of the AMP metabolites are diffusible and resynthesis of adenine nucleotides is slow, the size of the adenylate pool may be subnormal for extended periods.[119] Consequently, insufficient levels of ADP and AMP may prevent adequate resynthesis of ATP.[120] Secondly, it has been suggested that

lack of ATP resynthesis and persistent depression of total adenylates reflect irreversible tissue damage.[116,120,121] Histological studies after compression injury of the spinal cord showed hemorrhagic necrosis of gray and white matter and prominent ischemic nerve cell change.[122,123] Thus, the injured segment may present a spectrum of tissue injury ranging from normal to necrotic. Consequently, the sequence of metabolic changes may reflect an averaging of these necrotic, anaerobic, and aerobic areas. For the initial 4 hours, anaerobic metabolism likely predominates. However, between 4 and 24 hours there appears to be an increasing percentage of oxidative metabolism in the remaining metabolically viable tissue.[59]

Edema

Edema in the spinal cord is defined as a significant increase in the water content of the tissue. Impact trauma to the spinal cord causes vascular damage at the site of injury, which results in extravasation of serum proteins and an increase in tissue water. There is a direct relationship between the formation and spread of edema and the magnitude of trauma leading to the SCI.

The spread of edema longitudinally, rostrally, and caudally in the white matter after trauma is likely to be associated with the development of tissue pressure gradients between the area adjacent to the injury site and areas more rostral and caudal.

Endogenous opioids

Following SCI, significant vascular changes occur (see Vascular changes section). There is a reduction in SCBF, which begins in the central gray region shortly after trauma and progresses in a centripetal fashion to involve the long white matter tracts in the early hours after injury.[124–126] Since autoregulation of SCBF is often impaired following spinal injury,[127,128] blood flow depends more directly upon blood pressure; thus, the hypotension that often accompanies injuries to the cervical and upper thoracic spinal cord[129] may potentiate the progressive ischemia initiated by spinal trauma. Under these conditions, restoration of blood pressure should augment SCBF and reduce subsequent ischemia, thereby improving neurologic outcome. Unfortunately, pressor agents have not been helpful in improving blood pressure after spinal injury,[130,131] probably due to the rapid development of tachyphylaxis.[132]

It is suggested that endogenous opioid peptides (endorphins) contribute to the hypotension in spinal injury. Naloxone (an opiate antagonist) treatment improves blood pressure and SCBF and is associated with less prominent spinal cord changes and significantly improved neurologic recovery.

References

1. de Groat WC, Booth AM, Yoshimura N. Neurophysiology of micturition and its modification in animal models of human disease. In: Maggi CA, ed. The autonomic nervous system, Vol. 3, Nervous control of the urogenital system. London: Harwood Academic Publishers, 1993:227–290.

2. Chai TC, Steers WC. Neurophysiology of micturition and continence. Urol Clin North Am 1996; 23:221–236.

3. Breasted JH. The Edwin Smith surgical papyrus. Chicago, IL: University of Chicago Press, 1930.

4. Yoshimura N, de Groat WC. Neural control of the lower urinary tract. Int J Urol 1997; 4:111–125.

5. Jänig W, Morrison JFB. Functional properties of spinal visceral afferents supplying abdominal and pelvic organs, with special emphasis on visceral nociception. Prog Brain Res 1986; 67:87–114.

6. Gosling J. The structure of the bladder and urethra in relation to function. Urol Clin North Am 1979; 6:31–38.

7. ACOG Technical Bulletin. Chronic pelvic pain, No. 223. Int J Gynecol Obstet 1996; 54:59–68.

8. Havenga K, DeRuiter MC, Enker WE, Welvaart K. Anatomical basis of autonomic nerve-preserving total mesorectal excision for rectal cancer. Br J Surg 1996; 83:384–388.

9. Juenemann KP, Lue TF, Schmidt RA, Tanagho EA. Clinical significance of sacral and pudendal nerve anatomy. J Urol 1988; 139:74–80.

10. Jänig W, McLachlan EM. Organization of lumber spinal outflow to distal colon and pelvic organs. Physiol Rev 1987; 67:1332–1440.

11. Morris JL, Gibbins IL, Kadowitz PJ, et al. Roles of peptides and other substances in cotransmission from vascular autonomic and sensory neurons. Can J Physiol 1995; 73(5):521–532.

12. Yamaguchi O, Shishido K, Tamura K, et al. Evaluation of mRNAs encoding muscarinic receptor subtypes in human detrusor muscle. J Urol 1996; 156:1208–1213.

13. Kondo S, Morita T, Tashima Y. Muscarinic cholinergic receptor subtypes in human detrusor muscle studies by labelled and non-labelled pirenzepine, AF-DX116 and 4DAMP. Urol Int 1995; 54:150–153.

14. Wang P, Luthin GR, Ruggieri MR. Muscarinic acetylcholine receptor subtypes mediating urinary bladder contractility and coupling to GTP proteins. J Pharmacol Exp Ther 1995; 273:959–966.

15. Somogyi GT, de Groat WC. Evidence for inhibitory nicotinic and facilitatory muscarinic receptors in cholinergic nerve terminals of the rat urinary bladder. J Auton Nerv Syst 1992; 37:89–97.

16. Somogyi GT, Tanowitz M, de Groat WC. M-1 muscarinic receptor mediated facilitation of acetylcholine release in the rat urinary bladder but not in the heart. J Physiol 1994; 80:81–89.

17. Hoyle CHV, Burnstock GP. Postganglionic efferent transmission in the bladder and urethra. In: Maggi CA, ed. The autonomic nervous system, Vol. 3, Nervous control of the urogenital system. London: Harwood Academic Publishers, 1993:349–382.

18. Lundberg JM. Pharmacology of cotransmission in the autonomic nervous system: integrative aspects on amines, neuropeptides, adenosine triphosphate, amine acids and nitric oxide. Pharmacol Rev 1996; 48:113–178.

19. Andersson KE. Pharmacology of lower urinary tract smooth muscles and penile erectile tissues. Pharmacol Rev 1993; 45:253–308.

20. Bennett BC, Roppolo JR, Kruse MN, de Groat WC. Neural control of urethral smooth and striated muscle activity in vivo: role of nitric oxide. J Urol 1995; 153:2004–2009.

21. Persson K, Alm P, Johansson K, et al. Nitric oxide synthase in pig lower urinary tract: immunohistochemistry, NADPH diaphorase histochemistry, and functional effects. Br J Pharmacol 1993; 110:521–530.

22. de Groat WC, Booth AM. Synaptic transmission in pelvic ganglia. In: Maggi CA, ed. The autonomic nervous system, Vol. 3, Nervous control of the urogenital system. London: Harwood Academic Publishers 1993:291–347

23. Tran LV, Somogyi GT, de Groat WC. Inhibitory effects of neuropeptide Y on cholinergic and adrenergic transmission in the rat urinary bladder and urethra. Am J Physiol 1994; 266:R1411–R1417.

24. Häbler HJ, Jänig W, Koltzenburg M. Activation of unmyelinated afferent fibres by mechanical stimuli and inflammation of the urinary bladder in the cat. J Physiol 1990; 425:545–562.

25. Mallory B, Steers WD, de Groat WC. Electrophysiological study of micturition reflexes in rats. Am J Physiol 1989; 257:R410–R421.

26. de Groat WC, Nadelhaft I, Milne RJ, et al. Organization of the sacral parasympathetic reflex pathways to the urinary bladder and large intestine. J Auton Nerv Syst 1981; 3:135–160.

27. Vera PL, Nadelhaft I. Conduction velocity distribution of afferent fibers innervating the rat urinary bladder. Brain Res 1990; 520:83–89.

28. de Groat WC, Lalley PM. Reflex firing in the lumbar sympathetic outflow to activation of vesical afferent fibers. J Physiol 1972; 226:289–309.

29. de Groat WC, Theobald RJ. Reflex activation of sympathetic pathways to vesical smooth muscle and parasympathetic ganglia by electrical stimulation of vesical afferents. J Physiol 1976; 259:223–237.

30. Shimoda N, Takakusaki K, Nishizawa O, et al. The changes in the activity of pudendal motoneurons in relation to reflex micturition evoked in decerebrated cats. Neurosci Lett 1992; 135:175–178.

31. Fedirchuk B, Shefchyk SJ. Membrane potential changes in sphincter motoneurons during micturition in the decerebrate cat. J Neurosci 1993; 13:3090–3094.

32. Holstege G, Griffiths D, de Wall H, Dalm E. Anatomical and physiological observations on supraspinal control of bladder and urethral sphincter muscles in cat. J Comp Neurol 1986; 250:449–461.

33. Nishizawa O, Sugaya K, Noto H, et al. Pontine micturition center in the dog. J Urol 1988; 140:872–874.

34. Noto H, Roppolo JR, Steers WD, de Groat WC. Electrophysiological analysis of ascending and descending components of the micturition reflex pathway in the rat. Brain Res 1991; 549:95–105.

35. Kruse MN, Noto H, Roppolo JR, de Groat WC. Pontine control of the urinary bladder and external urethral sphincter in the rat. Brain Res 1990; 532:182–190.

36. Shimoda N, Takakusaki K, Nishizawa O, et al. The changes in the activity of pudendal motoneurons in relation to reflex micturition evoked in decerebrated cats. Neurosci Lett 1992; 135:175–178.

37. Fedirchuk B, Shefchyk SJ. Membrane potential changes in sphincter motoneurons during micturition in the decerebrate cat. J Neurosci 1993; 13:3090–3094.

38. Hedge SS, Eglen RM. Muscarinic receptor subtypes modulating smooth muscle contractility in the urinary bladder. Life Sci 1999; 64:419–428.

39. Somogyi GT, de Groat WC. Function, signal transduction mechanisms and plasticity of presynaptic muscarinic receptors in the urinary bladder. Life Sci 1999; 64:411–418.

40. Yoshimora N. Bladder afferent pathway and spinal cord injury: possible mechanisms including hyperreflexia of the urinary bladder. Prog Neurobiol 1999; 57:583–606.

41. Fam BA, Sarkarati M, Yalla SV. Spinal cord injury. In: Yalla SV, McGuire EJ, Elbadawi A, Blaivas JG, eds. Neurourology and urodynamics. New York: Macmillan, 1988:291–302.

42. Chancellor MB, Blaivas JG. Spinal cord injury. In: Chancellor MB, Blaivas JG, eds. Practical neuro-urology: genitourinary complications of neurologic disease. Newton: Butterworth-Heinemann, 1996:99–118.

43. Fried LC, Goodkin R. Microangiopathic observations of the experimentally traumatized spinal cord. J Neurosurg 1971; 35:709–714.

44. Tator CH, Fehlings MG. Review of the secondary injury theory of acute spinal cord trauma with emphasis on vascular mechanisms. J Neurosurg 1991; 75:15–26.

45. Sekhon L, Fehling M. Epidemiology, demographics, and pathophysiology of acute spinal cord injury. Spine 2001; 26:S2–S12.

46. Nockels RP. Nonoperative management of acute spinal cord injury. Spine 2001; 26:S31–S37.

47. Tator CH. Update on the pathophysiology and pathology of acute spinal cord injury. Brain Pathol 1995; 5:407–413.

48. Tator CH. Review of experimental spinal cord injury with emphasis on the local and systemic circulatory effects. Neurochirurgie 1991; 37:291–302.

49. Tator CH, Koyanagi I. Vascular mechanisms in the pathophysiology of human spinal cord injury. J Neurosurg 1997; 86:483–492.

50. Demopoulos HB, Flamm ES, Pietronigro DD, et al. The free radical pathology and the microcirculation in the major central nervous system disorders. Acta Physiol Scand Suppl 1980; 492:91–119.

51. Hall ED, Yonkers PA, Horan KL, et al. Correlation between attenuation of posttraumatic spinal cord ischemia and preservation of tissue vitamin E by the 21-aminosteroid U74006F: evidence for an in vivo antioxidant mechanism. J Neurotrauma 1989; 6:169–176.

52. Hung TK, Albin MS, Brown TD, et al. Biomechanical responses to open experimental spinal cord injury. Surg Neurol 1975; 4:271–276.

53. Agrawal SK, Fehlings MG. Mechanisms of secondary injury to spinal cord axons in vitro: role of Na$^+$, Na$^{(+)}$-K$^{(+)}$-ATPase, the Na$^{(+)}$-H$^+$ exchanger, and the Na$^{(+)}$-Ca^{2+} exchanger. J Neurosci 1996; 16:545–552.

54. Young W, Kerch I. Potassium and calcium changes in injured spinal cords. Brain Res 1986; 365:42–53.

55. Casha S, Yu WR, Fehlings MG. Oligodendroglial apoptosis occurs along degenerating axons and is associated with FAS and P75 expression following spinal cord injury. Neuroscience 2001; 103:203–218.

56. De La Torre JC. Spinal cord injury: review of basic and applied research. Spine 1981; 6:315–335.

57. Agrawal SK, Fehlings MG. The role of NMDA and non-NMDA inotropic glutamate receptors in traumatic spinal cord axonal injury. J Neurosci 1997; 17:1055–1063.

58. Faden AI, Simon RP. A potential role for excitotoxins in the pathophysiology of spinal cord injury. Ann Neurol 1988; 23:623–626.

59. Anderson DK, Means ED, Waters TR, et al. Spinal cord energy metabolism following compression trauma to the feline spinal cord. J Neurosurg 1980; 53:375–380.

60. Wagner FC Jr, Stewart WB. Effect of trauma dose on spinal cord edema. J Neurosurg 1981; 54:802–806.

61. Faden AI, Jacobs TP, Holaday JW. Comparison of early and late naloxone treatment in experimental spinal injury. Neurology 1982; 32:677–681.

62. Faden AI, Jacobs TP, Smith MT. Evaluation of calcium channel antagonist nimodipine in experimental spinal cord ischemia. J Neurosurg 1984; 60:796–799.

63. Atkinson PP, Atkinson JL. Spinal shock. Mayo Clin Proc 1996; 71:384–389.

64. Guha A, Tator CH. Acute cardiovascular effects of experimental spinal cord injury. J Trauma 1988; 28:481–490.

65. Kobrine AL, Doyle TF, Rizzoli HV. Altered spinal cord blood flow as affected by changes in systemic arterial blood pressure. J Neurosurg 1975; 42:144–149.

66. Senter HJ, Venes JL. Loss of autoregulation and posttraumatic ischemia following experimental spinal cord trauma. J Neurosurg 1979; 50:198–206.

67. Young W, Decrescito V, Tomasula JJ. Effect of sympathectomy on spinal blood flow autoregulation and posttraumatic ischemia. J Neurosurg 1982; 56:706–710.

68. Guha A, Tator CH, Rochon J. Spinal cord blood flow and systemic blood pressure after experimental spinal cord injury in rats. Stroke 1989; 20:372–377.

69. Young W, Decrescito V, Tomasula JJ, et al. The role of the sympathetic nervous system in pressor responses induced by spinal injury. J Neurosurg 1980; 52:473–481.

70. Koyanagi I, Tator CH, Lea PJ. Three-dimensional analysis of the vascular system in the rat spinal cord with scanning electron microscopy of vascular corrosion casts: 2. Acute spinal cord injury. Neurosurgery 1993; 33:285–292.

71. Koyanagi I, Tator CH, Theriault E. Silicone rubber microangiography of acute spinal cord injury in the rat. Neurosurgery 1993; 32:260–268.

72. Shingu H, Kimura I, Nasu Y, et al. Microangiographic study of spinal cord injury and myelopathy. Paraplegia 1989; 27:182–189.

73. Kim RC, Smith HR, Henbest ML, et al. Nonhemorrhagic venous infarction of the spinal cord. Ann Neurol 1984; 15:379–385.

74. Ohshio I, Hatayama A, Kaneda K, et al. Correlation between histopathologic features and magnetic resonance images of spinal cord lesions. Spine 1993; 18:1140–1149.

75. Rao KR, Donnenfeld H, Chusid JG, et al. Acute myelopathy secondary to spinal venous thrombosis. J Neurol 1982; 56:107–113.

76. Griffiths IR, Miller R. Vascular permeability to protein and vasogenic edema in experimental concussive injuries to the canine spinal cord. J Neurol Sci 1974; 22:291–304.

77. Hsu CY, Hogan EL, Gadsden RHS, et al. Vascular permeability in experimental spinal cord injury. J Neurol Sci 1985; 70:275–282.

78. Stewart WB, Wagner FC. Vascular permeability changes in the contused feline spinal cord. Brain Res 1979; 169:163–167.

79. Demopoulos HB, Yoder M, Gutman EG, et al. The fine structure of endothelial surfaces in the microcirculation of experimentally injured feline spinal cords. In: Becker RP, Johari O, eds. Scanning

electron microscopy II. IL: AMF O'Hare, Scanning Electron Microscopy 1978:677–682.

80. Cordingley GE, Somjen GG. The clearing of excess potassium from extracellular space in spinal cord and cerebral cortex. Brain Res 1978; 151:291–306.

81. Gardner-Medwin AR, Gibson JL, Willshaw DJ. The mechanism of potassium dispersal in brain tissue [proceedings]. J Physiol (London) 1979; 293:37–38.

82. Gardner-Medwin AR. Analysis of potassium dynamics in mammalian brain tissue. J Physiol (London) 1983; 335:393–426.

83. Nicholson C. Dynamics of the brain cell microenvironment. Neurosci Res Bull 1980; 18:177–322.

84. Nicholson C, Philips JM, Gardner-Medin A. Diffusion from an iontophoretic point source in the brain: a role of tortuosity and volume fraction. Brain Res 1979; 164:580–584.

85. Hansen AJ, Gjedde A, Siemkowicz E. Extracellular potassium and blood flow in the post-ischemic rat brain. Pflager's Arch 1980; 389:1–7.

86. Hansen AJ, Lund-Andersen H, Crone C. K$^+$ permeability of the blood brain barrier investigated by aid of a K$^+$-sensitive microelectrode. Acta Physiol Scand 1977; 101:438–445.

87. Hansen AJ. The potassium concentration in cerebrospinal fluid in young and adult rats following complete brain ischemia – effects of pre-treatment with hypoxia. Acta Physiol Scand 1976; 97:519–522.

88. Nicholson C. Modulation of extracellular calcium and functional implications. Fed Proc Fed Am Soc EP Biol 1980; 39:1519–1523.

89. Betts F, Blumenthal NC, Posner AS et al. Atomic structure of intracellular amorphous calcium phosphate deposits. Proc Natl Acad Sci USA 1975; 72:2088–2090.

90. Riley GP, Harrall RL, Constant CR, et al. Prevalance and possible pathological significance of calcium phosphate salt accumulation in tendon matrix degeneration. Ann Rheum Dis 1996; 55(2):109–115.

91. Balentine JD, Spector M. Calcifications of axons in experimental spinal cord trauma. Ann Neurol 1977; 2:520–523.

92. Brown WE. Solubility of phosphates and other sparingly soluble compounds. In: Griffin EJ, Beeton A, Spencer JM, Mitchell DT, eds. Environmental phosphorus handbook. New York: John Wiley, 1973:203.

93. Kretsinger RH. Calcium in neurobiology: a general theory of its function and evolution. In: Schmitt FO, Worden FG, eds. The neurosciences – fourth study program. Cambridge: MIT Press, 1979:617–622.

94. Sillen SG. The physical chemistry of sea water. In: Sears M, ed. Oceanography. Am Assoc for the Advancement of Science, Pub. No. 67, 1961:549–581.

95. Astrup J. Energy-requiring cell functions in the ischemic brain: their critical supply and possible inhibition in protective therapy. J Neurosurg 1982; 56:482–497.

96. Braughler JM, Hall ED. Lactate and pyruvate metabolism in the injured cat spinal cord before and after a single large intravenous dose of methylprednisolone. J Neurosurg 1983; 59:256–261.

97. Abrams JM, White K, Fessler LI, Steller H. Programmed cell death during Drosophila embryogenesis. Development 1993; 117:29–43.

98. Bargmann CL. Death from natural and unnatural causes. Elegant studies of the nematode are providing answers to the question of how programmed cell death and neurodegeneration are regulated. Curr Biol 1991; 1:388–390.

99. Kerr JFR, Wyllie AH, Currie AR. Apoptosis. A basic biological phenomenon with wide-ranging implications in tissue kinetics. Br J Cancer 1972; 26:239–257.

100. Collins WF, Piepmeir J, Ogle E. The spinal cord injury problem. A review. Central Nerv Syst Trauma 1986; 3:317–331.

101. Collins WF. A review and update of experimental and clinical studies of spinal cord injury. Paraplegia 1983; 21:204–219.

102. Li GL, Brodin G, Farooque M, et al. Apoptosis and expression of Bcl-2 after compression trauma to rat spinal cord. J Neuropathol Exp Neurol 1996; 55:280–289.

103. Crowe MJ, Bresnahan JC, Shuman SL, et al. Apoptosis and delayed degeneration after spinal cord injury in rats and monkeys. Nat Med 1997; 3:73–76.

104. Barres BA, Jacobson MD, Schmid R. Does oligodendrocytes survival depend on axons? Curr Biol 1993; 3:489–497.

105. Dusart I, Schwab ME. Secondary cell death and the inflammatory reaction after dorsal hemisection of the rat spinal cord. Eur J Neurosci 1994; 6:712–724.

106. Emery E, Aldana P, Bunge MB, et al. Apoptosis after traumatic human spinal cord injury. J Neurosurg 1998; 89:911–920.

107. Liu XZ, Xu XM, Hu R, et al. Neuronal and glial apoptosis after traumatic spinal cord injury. J Neurosci 1997; 17:5395–5406.

108. Meldrum B. Possible therapeutic applications of antagonists of excitatory amino acid neurotransmitters. Clin Sci 1985; 68:113–122.

109. Feden AI. Pharmacotherapy in spinal cord injury: a critical review of recent developments. Clin Neuropharmacol 1987; 10:193–204.

110. Wieloch T. Hypoglycemia-induced neuronal damage prevented by so N-methyl-D-aspartate antagonist. Science 1985; 230:681–683.

111. Davies J, Watkins JC. Role of excitatory amino acid receptors in mono- and polysynaptic excitation in the cat spinal cord. Exp Brain Res 1983; 49:280–290.

112. Ganoug AH, Lanthorn TH, Cotman CW. Kynurenic acid inhibits synaptic and acidic amino acid-induced responses in the rat. Brain Res 1983; 273:170–174.

113. Wong EHF, Kemp JA, Priestley T. The novel anticonvulsant MK-801 is a potent N-methyl-aspartate antagonist. Proc Natl Acad Sci USA 1986; 83:7104.

114. Olney JW, Ho OL, Rhee V. Cytotoxic effects of acidic and sulphur containing amino acids on the infant mouse central nervous system. Exp Brain Res 1971; 14:61–76.

115. Rivlin AS, Tator CH. Objective clinical assessment of motor function after experimental spinal cord injury in the rat. J Neurosurg 1977; 47:577–581.

116. Welsh FA, Ginsberg MD, Rieder W, et al. Diffuse cerebral ischemia in the cat. II. Regional metabolites during severe ischemia and recirculation. Ann Neurol 1978; 3:493–501.

117. Gatfield PD, Lowry OH, Schulz DW, et al. Regional energy reserves in mouse brain and changes with ischemia and anaesthesia. J Neurochem 1966; 13:185–195.

118. Smith AL, Wollman H. Cerebral blood flow and metabolism. Anesthesiology 1972; 36:378–400.

119. Siesjo BK. Brain energy metabolism. New York: John Wiley and Sons, 1978: 607.

120. Nordstrom CH, Rehncrona S, Siesjo BK. Effects of penobarbital in cerebral ischemia. Part II: restitution of cerebral energy state, as well as glycolytic metabolites, citric acid cycle intermediates and associated amino acids after pronounced incomplete ischemia. Stroke 1978; 9(4):335–343.

121. Atkinson DE. Cellular energy metabolism and its regulation. New York: Academic Press, 1977:293.

122. Means ED, Anderson DK. Histopathology of experimental spinal cord compression injury. Fifth Annual Meeting of the Society for Neuroscience Vol. 1, 1975:698. [Abstract]

123. Means ED, Anderson DK, Gutierrez C. Light and electron microscopy of gray matter following experimental spinal cord compression injury. J Neuropathol Exp Neurol 1976; 35:348. [Abstract]

124. Dohrmann GJ, Wick KM, Bucy PC. Spinal cord blood flow patterns in experimental traumatic paraplegia. J Neurosurg 1973; 38:52–58.

125. Ducker TB, Salcman M, Lucas JT, et al. Experimental spinal cord trauma. II: Blood flow, tissue oxygen, evoked potentials in both paretic and plegic monkeys. Surg Neurol 1978; 10:64–70.

126. Sandler AN, Tator CH. Effect of acute spinal cord compression injury on regional spinal cord blood flow in primates. J Neurosurg 1976; 45:660–676.

127. Ducker TB, Perot PL. Spinal cord blood flow compartments. Trans Am Neurol Assoc 1971; 96:229–231.

128. Osterholm JL. The pathophysiological response to spinal cord injury. J Neurosurg 1974; 40:5–33.

129. Yashon D. Spinal injury. New York: Appleton-Century-Crofts, 1978:248–254.

130. Ducker TB, Salcapan M, Daniell HB. Experimental spinal cord trauma. III: Therapeutic effect of immobilization and pharmacologic agents. Surg Neurol 1978; 10:71–76.

131. Faden AI, Jacobs TP, Woods M. Cardioacceleratory sites in the zona intermedia of the cat spinal cord. Exp Neurol 1978; 61:301–310.

132. Faden AI, Jacobs TP, Mougey MS, Holaday JW. Endorphins in experimental spinal injury: therapeutic effect of naloxone. Ann Neurol 1981; 10:326–332.

Part III

Neurological pathologies responsible for the development of the neurogenic bladder

15

Spina bifida in infancy and childhood

Atsuo Kondo, Momokazu Gotoh, and Osamu Kamihira

Introduction

In 1932, Penfield and Cone[1] successfully operated on 19 of 33 children suffering from spina bifida, cranium bifidum, or rachischisis without mortality. However, up to the 1950s, most children with spinal dysraphism had not been well treated or were simply left to die. In 1960s, many children started to survive as a result of advances in shunting technology (ventriculoperitoneal shunt, ventriculoatrial shunt, or lumboperitoneal shunt), the use of antibiotics, and improvements in surgical techniques. The ileal loop conduit developed by Bricker in 1950[2] was applied extensively to wet children to let them dry for the next two decades. In the 1970s, ethical dilemmas and medical concerns were expressed over whether a myelodysplastic infant should be actively treated or left untreated.[3,4] Lorber[5] suggested criteria for selecting patients based on the degree of paralysis, head circumference, kyphosis, and associated gross congenital anomalies. Continuous reassessment was vital, even after a positive treatment strategy was chosen.

In 1972 Lapides et al[6] established clean intermittent catheterization (CIC) that subsequently altered treatment concepts and surgical strategies dramatically and drastically. For instance, the ileal loop conduit, which once provided continence but created new complications such as urolithiasis, skin ulceration, and psychosomatic problems when the child got older,[7] was not attempted any more and urinary undiversion[8,9] was recommended in combination with intermittent catheterization. In the 1980s and 1990s, bladder augmentation procedures, using either the ileum, colon, or sigma, became the gold standard for urologists in association with antireflux surgery, anti-incontinence sling operation, or implantation of an artificial urinary sphincter[10] when necessary. Most patients with augmented bladder definitely require CIC postoperatively. Mitrofanoff[11] reported usage of the appendix as a catheterizable stoma in 1980 that would not have been invented without the work of Lapides. Ten years later, Malone et al[12] took advantage of the Mitrofanoff procedure to wash out hard stools with antegrade continence enema (ACE).

In the last century, as we saw above, the attitude to and treatment strategies for children with myelodysplasia have swung like a pendulum. Nowadays, in most developed countries, multidisciplinary centers have been established, which provide significant safeguards to counsel parents and children and to present multifaceted as well as comprehensive treatment programs to minimize disability and handicap.

Folic acid and neural tube defects

Folic acid reduces the risk of fetuses being afflicted by neural tube defects (NTDs). During the last two decades, we have seen two major modalities that reduce the number of fetuses with NTDs. One is maternal periconceptional folic acid supplementation. The other is the antenatal diagnosis of NTDs through the serum marker of alpha-fetoprotein values and subsequent termination of the affected fetus. It is obvious that the primary prevention of NTDs by the former modality is more humanistic and valuable than the latter. Herewith, we present the relationship of folic acid and NTDs, and demonstrate our observations on how dietary folate is taken and the targetted serum concentration of folic acid in five groups of women.

What is folic acid?

Dietary folate or pteryolpolyglutamic acid, sometimes called vitamin M, is rich in green-yellow vegetables, fruits, beans, and liver. Because dietary folate is relatively heat labile, considerable amounts of folate are destroyed by cooking, processing, and storage. Consequently, it has to be supplied every day. When folate is digested, it is converted into pteryolmonoglutamic acid by conjugation in the small intestine. Pteryolmonoglutamic acid is the same as folic acid contained in supplements such as multivitamin or folic acid tablets. Bioavailability is approximately 50% in dietary folate, and 85% in folic acid supplements. Folic acid is water-soluble, not known to be toxic, and not only important in the synthesis of DNA and RNA but also necessary for the growth and differentiation of cells. It is now confirmed that maternal periconceptional folic acid supplementation in the critical periods of organ formation is associated with reduced occurrence and recurrence of NTDs, congenital heart defects, obstructive urinary tract anomalies, limb deficiencies, orofacial clefts, and congenital hypertrophic pyloric stenosis. Insufficient maternal intake of folic acid results in preterm deliveries, intrauterine growth retardation, placental abruption, and infarction.[13,14]

Incidence of myelodysplasia

Marked geographic, ethnic, and racial variations exist in the prevalence of spina bifida and anencephaly. They are highest in people of Celtic extraction and the western part of the British Isles, in Newfoundland, Canada, and in the eastern parts of the USA.[15] NTDs occurred in 4.5 in 1000 births in England and Wales in 1970, but significantly declined to 0.18 in 1000 births in 1991. In the State of South Carolina, USA, NTDs and fetal death occurred in 1.89 per 1000 live births in 1992, which decreased to 0.95 in 1998 probably because of the increased periconceptional use of folic acid supplements among women of childbearing age.[16] In the Northern part of China, this ratio was extremely high, 4.4 per 1000 births.[17] The incidence in Japan was estimated to be 0.3–0.4 per 1000 births in 1998.[18] Over the last two decades, there has been an enormous decline in the number of NTD births on a worldwide basis, because of antenatal diagnosis and maternal periconceptional intake of folic acid among young women capable of becoming pregnant or wishing to be pregnant.[19]

NTDs are a spectrum of common and serious malformations of the cranium, spine, and nervous system, including anencephaly, spina bifida, encephalocele, craniorachischisis, and iniencephaly. Development and closure of the neural tube are normally completed within 28 days after conception, i.e. 2 weeks after the first missed menstruation. Since approximately 60% of women are diagnosed as being pregnant in the 5th week after conception, young females are recommended to start folic acid supplementation 4 weeks before conception. Epidemiological studies suggest that environmental and genetic factors play a joint role in causing NTDs. Genetic controls of the cellular mechanisms of closure have yet to be determined, although several possibly associated genes have been identified in animal models.[14] Exposure to specific materials is known to elicit NTDs, e.g. maternal diabetes,[20] maternal use of antiepileptic drugs, valproic acid, phenobarbital,[21] and trimethoprim,[22] maternal development of high fever or hyperthermia in early pregnancy,[23] and maternal obesity.[24]

Randomized controlled trials

In 1964, Hibbard[25] observed that defective folic acid metabolism was responsible for anemia during pregnancy, placental abruption, and a number of abortions and fetal malformations. In 1980, Smithhells et al[26] recruited 449 women who had had NTD infants. Multivitamin tablets containing 360 μg/day of folic acid were given to 185 women starting 4 weeks before conception until well after the time of neural tube closure, while the control group comprised 264 women who received no vitamin tablets. The recurrence rate of NTDs was significantly different: only 0.6% (1/178 infants or fetuses) in the supplemented group vs 5.0% (13/260 infants or fetuses) in the control group.

In 1991, the Medical Research Council Vitamin Research Study[27] made a memorable contribution to humankind. It clearly demonstrated that periconceptional folic acid supplementation was clinically useful to reduce the risk of recurrence of fetuses affected by NTDs in a total number of 1817 women who had had infants or pregnancies with NTDs. This randomized, prospective, double-blind, multicenter prevention trial was performed in seven countries: the UK, France, Canada, Australia, Hungary, Israel, and the USSR. Women in the study group took folic acid tablets of 4000 μg/day from the date of randomization until 12 weeks of pregnancy. The control group received either other vitamins or no vitamins for the same time period. It was found that the study group had 5 NTDs in 514 women (1.0%) vs 18 in the control group of 517 women (3.5%) and that folic acid supplementation reduced the risk of NTD recurrence by 72%.

In 1982, a Hungarian group[28] reported results similar to those of the Medical Research Council. This group studied the efficacy of 800 μg of folic acid in more than 4000 women who had not had any infants/pregnancies affected by NTDs. Six cases of NTDs occurred in 2046 women of the control group (0.3%) compared to no NTDs in 2104 women of the vitamin-supplemented group. In 1999, a Chinese study[29] confirmed that periconceptional intake of 400 μg of folic acid, one-tenth of the dose level used in the Medical Research Council protocol in 1991, is effective in reducing the risk of fetuses with NTDs, proving for the first time that this hypothesis is also applicable to the Mongolian race, which includes Japanese. The rates of NTDs in the control group were 4.8 per 1000 pregnancies in the northern region, and 1.0 per 1000 pregnancies in the folic acid group. Periconceptional use of folic acid reduced the risk of having NTDs by 79% in the north and by 41% in the south.

Case-control studies

When well-prepared, prospective, randomized trials of folic acid assessment are somehow difficult to perform, case-control studies are undertaken. As early as 1989, 2 years prior to the Medical Research Council report from the UK researchers in the USA and Australia supported the hypothesis that folic acid supplementation[30] or dietary folate intake[31] in early pregnancy is associated with reduced risks of NTDs in infants.

In 1993, Werler et al[13] studied 436 mothers who had had pregnancies or infants affected by NTDs and 2615 controls with other major malformations except oral clefts. These subjects were interviewed within 6 months after delivery in regard to vitamin supplements during 6 months before the last menstrual period through the end of pregnancy, a semiquantitative food frequency questionnaire, occupation, family history of birth defects, and so on. Their observation was that daily use of multivitamins containing folic acid in the periconceptional period resulted in a relative risk of 0.4 (95% confidence interval, 0.2–0.7); i.e. 60% of NTDs were successfully prevented by folic acid supplementation. For dietary folate, there was a dose-related decline in risk according to the quintiles of intake. Shaw et al[32] reported a similar case-control study. Women taking vitamins containing folic acid in the 3 months before conception had a lower risk (odds ratio [OR] = 0.65). The OR was also similar for women who took the vitamins 3 months after conception (OR = 0.60).

On the other hand, Mills et al[33] tested the validity of the hypothesis and arrived at the opposite conclusion in 1989. They reviewed three groups of mothers – i.e. 565 mothers with an NTD, 538 mothers with a stillbirth or malformation, and 567 mothers with a normal infant – within 5 months after delivery regarding periconceptional use of folic acid or multivitamins. They found that the mothers of infants or fetuses with NTDs were no less likely to have taken multivitamins or folate around the time of conception than women in the two control groups. Some factors could explain these discordant results: recall bias, differences in questionnaire's design, interviewers' backgrounds, and so on.

Dietary folate and plasma folate concentration

When we explain to young women why folic acid is vital for their pregnancies, it is important to tell them that insufficient intake is one of many, complicated etiologies and that NTDs cannot be completely prevented by folate-rich food or folic acid supplementation. We investigated the dietary intake of folate and plasma folate concentrations.[34] A total of 222 women comprising five groups participated in our study:

- 61 adult women (mean age 37 and body mass index (BMI) of 21.0)
- 66 mothers of myelodysplastic patients (age 42 years and BMI 21.6)
- 18 pregnant women (age 33 years and BMI 21.7)
- 32 myelodysplastic patients (age 24 years and BMI 22.8)
- 45 nursing students (age 20 years and BMI 20.1).

Food frequency questionnaires kept 3 days were analyzed by a dietitian based on the 5th Standard Food Composition Table of Japan. Plasma folate concentrations were measured by chemiluminescent immunoassay. Changes in plasma folate concentrations and possible adverse effects following the folic acid supplementation for 16 weeks were also investigated.

Dietary folate intake, plasma folate concentration, and energy intake averaged 293 μg/day, 8.1 ng/ml, and 1857 kcal, respectively, among the subjects (Table 15.1). Pregnant women consumed the largest amount of dietary folate (350 μg/day) and demonstrated the highest plasma folate concentration (11.9 ng/ml) among the groups. Folate status in the mothers of myelodysplastic patients was not significantly different from that of adult women. Figure 15.1 reports on the amount of dietary folate taken, for a median of 269 μg/day in 218 women. Four women ingested more than 650 μg/day. Figure 15.2 represents data on serum concentration, showing a median of 7.1 ng/ml among 190 women with the exclusion of four subjects who had taken folic acid supplements.

The recommended dietary allowance of folate in Japan is 200 μg/day for adult women and 400 μg/day for pregnant women. Overall, 22% of adult women and 72% of pregnant women failed to meet this amount. Dietary folate was mainly derived (57%) from the 3rd food group (vegetables, potatoes, and fruits), but the 4th food group (cereals, sugar, and fat) was consumed the most, 799 g (Table 15.2). Mean dietary folate was significantly correlated with serum folate concentrations ($p = 0.012$, $r = 0.186$). Consecutive administration of 400 μg supplements increased the baseline plasma value of 8.7 to 32.6 ng/ml 4 months later without any adverse effects, but fell rapidly to 17.3 ng/ml 24 hours later.

In summary, women who are capable of becoming pregnant are recommended to consume much of the 3rd food group, and those who are planning to become pregnant are advised to take 400 μg of folic acid supplements from 4 weeks before to 12 weeks after conception.

Table 15.1 *The daily dietary folate intake, plasma folate concentration, and energy intake were investigated in 222 women. Statistical difference was assessed between adult women and another 4 groups in respect of the 3 parameters (CI = confidence interval)*

Subjects	Dietary folate intake (μg)	Plasma folate concentration (ng/ml)	Energy intake (k/cal)
Adult women (*n* = 61) Mean (95% CI)	338 (305–370)	8.2 (7.6–8.9)	2003 (1900–2107)
Mothers of myelodysplastic patients (*n* = 66) Mean (95% CI)	301 (273–330)	8.2 (7.1–9.4)[a]	1828 (1733–1923)*
Pregnant women (*n* = 18) Mean (95% CI)	350 (299–401)	11.9 (7.1–16.6)[b]	1959 (1772–2145)
Myelodysplastic patients (*n* = 32) Mean (95% CI)	273 (237–308)*	7.3(6.3–8.3)	1747 (1600–1892)**
Nurse students (*n* = 45) Mean (95% CI)	217 (196–238)**	6.8 (6.1–7.4)**	1753 (1622–1885)**
Total (95% CI)	293 (278–309)	8.1 (7.5–8.7)[c]	1857 (1802–1912)

[a]Exclusion of 1 mother of myelodysplastic patients who had had supplementation decreases the value to 7.9 (7.0–8.9) ng/ml.
[b]Exclusion of 3 pregnant women who had had supplementation decreases the value to 8.6 (6.8–10.5).
[c]Exclusion of the above 4 women decreases the value to 7.7 (7.5–8.6).
*$p < 0.05$; **$p < 0.01$.

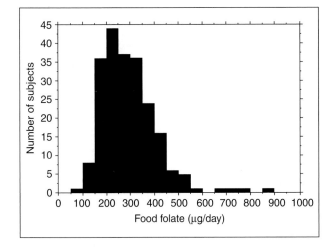

Figure 15.1
Distribution of dietary folate among 218 women. Four women took more than 650 μg/day.

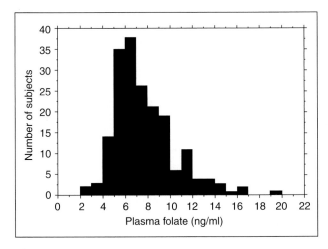

Figure 15.2
Distribution of plasma folate among 190 women. Those who took folic acid supplements were excluded here.

National policies on and awareness of reducing risks with folic acid

As early as 1992, the US Centers for Disease Control was sensitive enough to publicly announce a recommendation of folic acid supplementation to reduce the number of spina bifida cases:[35]

All women of childbearing age in the United States who are capable of becoming pregnant should consume 0.4 mg of folic acid per day for the purpose of reducing their risk of having a pregnancy affected with spina bifida or other NTDs. Because the effects of high intakes are not well known but include complicating the diagnosis of vitamin B12 deficiency, care should be taken to keep total folate consumption at < 1 mg per day, except under the supervision of a physician. Women who have had

Table 15.2 *Mean values of the daily dietary folate intake, dietary folate percent, and food weight consumed in each of 4 food groups where means and 95 percent confidence intervals (CI) were calculated*

Food groups[a]	Dietary folate intake (μg)	Dietary folate percent (%)	Food weight (g/day)	
Group 1 Mean (95% CI)	25 (23–26)	8	166 (150–182)	
Group 2 Mean (95% CI)	42 (34–50)	14	189 (179–199)	
Group 3 Mean (95% CI)	169 (156–181)	57	369 (347–391)	
Group 4 Mean (95% CI)	61 (57–64)	21	799 (759–839)	
Total (95% CI)	293 (278–309)	100	1525 (1470–1579)	

[a]Group 1 comprises milk, milk products, and eggs; group 2 comprises fish, meats, beans, and bean products; group 3 comprises vegetables, potatoes, and fruits; and group 4 comprises cereals, sugar, and fat.

a prior NTD-affected pregnancy are at high risk of having a subsequent affected pregnancy. When these women are planning to become pregnant, they should consult their physicians for advice.

Dutch teams stressed the importance of increasing awareness among the public through newspapers and a mass media campaign that started in 1995.[19] De Walle et al[36] reported that the general goals of the mass media campaign were that 70% of women planning a pregnancy should know of the recommendation and that 65% of women who knew of the advice before pregnancy should follow it during the entire recommended period. They found that after the campaign 78% of women knew in 1998 that folic acid should be taken before conception and 51% in 1998 used folic acid during the recommended period.

Cornel and Erickson[37] collected published information from 13 countries that issued official policies on periconceptional intake of folic acid/folate-rich food to the public. These countries comprised Australia, Canada, China, Denmark, Hungary, Ireland, New Zealand, Norway, South Africa, Spain, the Netherlands, the UK, and the USA. The majority of health agencies recommended a high daily consumption of 4–5 mg of folic acid to prevent recurrence and a low dose of 0.4–0.5 mg to prevent the first occurrence of NTDs. In 2000, the Japanese Government issued public recommendations. First, women of childbearing age should have well-balanced food. Second, women planning a pregnancy should take folic acid supplements of 400 μg/day from 1 month before to 4 months after conception. Third, women who had had a prior conception affected with NTDs should consult their physicians. Fourth, smoking and drinking alcohol should be stopped to allow the fetus to grow normally during pregnancy.[38]

In 1996, the US Food and Drug Administration issued a regulation requiring the addition of 140 μg of folic acid to the cereal grain products of 100 g.[39] Since the fortification process was essentially completed by mid-1997, Jacques et al[40] studied the effect of folic acid fortification on serum folate status in the Framingham Offspring Study cohort. The study group comprising 350 persons who did not use vitamin supplements was examined before and after fortification, and the control group of 756 persons was seen twice before the fortification in a period of 3 years. Mean folate concentrations increased from 4.6 to 10.0 ng/ml, and the prevalence of low folate concentrations (<3 ng/ml) decreased from 22% to 2% in the study group. On the other hand, mean folate concentrations in the control group increased slightly from 4.6 to 4.8 μg/day, and the prevalence of low folate concentrations decreased from 25% to 21% without statistical significance. The results indicated that folate status in a population of middle-aged and older adults substantially improved after fortification of enriched grain products and that the objective of the US Government was accomplished.

Guidelines for clinical management

Our guidelines stem from over 30 years of clinical experience with over 330 myelodysplastic children treated in both Nagoya University Hospital and Komaki Shimin Hospital. They are based on the recommendations prepared by seven urologists for the Ministry of Health and Welfare, Japan, and on 401 articles identified by computer search. The original guidelines were published in 2001 for urologists and other health care providers to properly manage the lower urinary tract of patients. A Medline search from 1966 to

2001 was undertaken according to several combinations of the following seven key words: myelodysplasia, spina bifida, urinary tract, urodynamics, catheterization, vesicoureteral reflux (VUR), and surgery. Eventually, 401 articles were found to be important and are discussed here. Infants and children were divided into two groups: less than 5 years of age and 6–15 years. The following five findings served as the basis of the present guideline formulation:

1. Myelodysplastic patients often suffer lower urinary tract dysfunction, which, in turn, results in renal damage, urinary tract infection, and urinary incontinence.[41]
2. Risk factors of the upper urinary tract comprise leak point pressure (LPP) of more than 40 cmH$_2$O,[42–44] detrusor-sphincter dyssynergia,[45,46] urinary bladder with low compliance,[47] detrusor hyperreflexia,[48] significant residual volume,[49] and recurrent urinary tract infection (UTI).[50]
3. Damage to the upper urinary tract is not always reversible. The risk of bladder augmentation for those with bladder storage disorders is two times as high as for those who are instructed to perform CIC.[51]
4. Early detection of the upper urinary tract deterioration is essential to maintain normal renal and bladder function.[51–53]
5. A combination of CIC and anticholinergics eradicates 60–70% of VUR and improves 70–75% of hydronephrosis and 55–84% of urinary incontinence.[54–58]

The guidelines for neonates and infants 1–5 years of age

Objectives

The fundamental objective is to maintain the bladder as a low-pressure reservoir and to prevent UTI. In other words, the majority of infants could be managed by CIC with or without anticholinergics and microbials, instead of evacuating urine by Credé expression or the Valsalva maneuver. Keeping infants dry at this stage is not as important as in children who socially communicate with others in school. Parents will accept the use of diapers for their infants. Authors witnessed that the majority of patients could be conservatively treated except a few who required surgical intervention in the early stages because renal function had been severely compromised.

Clinical management

Early detection of any upper urinary tract abnormalities and risk factors is extremely important for prompt urological management and intervention, which are illustrated in Figure 15.3. Urinalysis, urinary culture, and abdominal ultrasonography are essential first-line tests. If they suggest the presence of UTI, further invasive studies will be required:

- cystourethrography (CUG) will reveal detrusor-sphincter dyssynergia, VUR, bladder wall trabeculations, bladder neck competence
- urodynamic study (UDS) will disclose the presence of detrusor overactivity, filling bladder pressure, bladder capacity, bladder compliance, bladder sensation, LPP[43]
- intravenous urography (IVU) will demonstrate the presence of hydronephrosis, dilated ureter, urinary bladder shape and size.
- renoscintigraphy will reveal how the renal parenchyma has been compromised.

The presence of any risk factors of elevated LPP (>40 cmH$_2$O), detrusor hyperreflexia, low bladder compliance, or detrusor-sphincter dyssynergia will require CIC institution together with anticholinergics. Catheter size should be 5–8 F, and infants should be catheterized every 2–3 h in the daytime. Aseptic catheterization procedures or

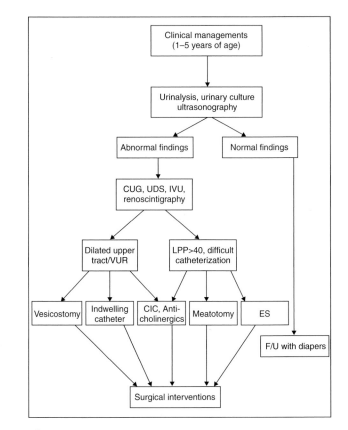

Figure 15.3
Guidelines for clinical management of infants aged from 1 to 5 years. CIC, clean intermittent catheterization; CUG, cystourethrography; UDS, urodynamic study; IVU, intravenous urography; VUR, vesicoureteric reflux; LPP, leak point pressure; ES, electrostimulation; F/U, follow-up.

prophylactic administration of antimicrobials are hardly necessary. Teichman et al[59] observed that patients who were put on CIC for medical reasons sustained renal deterioration more frequently than those in whom it was started for continence and that 21% of patients on CIC ultimately suffered renal deterioration. Intravesical electrostimulation (ES) reported by Katona[60] in 1975 may be beneficial for some patients with incomplete pelvic nerve damage.

A contracted and narrow external urethral meatus will be encountered in a few cases that require prompt meatotomy. Reflux occurs in 16–35% of myelodysplastic children,[61,62] but early institution of CIC and anticholinergics will resolve the reflux or downgrade it. Advanced hydronephrosis and/or VUR may require an indwelling catheter or vesicostomy for a period of 6–12 months. In our experience, a limited number of patients in this age group will need surgical interventions, such as bladder augmentation, antireflux surgery, and strengthening of the urinary sphincter. Any surgical interventions at the bladder level without augmentation procedures are not recommended because surgery itself will later compromise bladder compliance.[63]

Guidelines for children 6–15 years of age

Clinical assessment consists of urinalysis, urinary culture, abdominal ultrasonography, frequency volume chart (FVC), CUG, and UDS. Invasive tests requiring urethral catheterization can be easily performed because the majority of children are already on the CIC regimen. FVCs, CUG, and UDS will reveal the etiologies of urinary incontinence, if present, and will suggest appropriate medical and/or surgical management that will improve the patient's quality of life. If risk factors are not detected, patients are allowed to evacuate urine by abdominal strain or by CIC. Follow-up assessments are repeated every 6 months. An algorithm of clinical management is presented in Figure 15.4. Abnormalities observed in these examinations further require IVU, bowel movement charts (BMCs), and renoscintigraphy.

Conservative treatments primarily comprise CIC with anticholinergics and microbials, enema, laxatives, and diapers. Catheterization with an 8–12 F catheter is necessary 3–6 times a day, depending on tidal urinary volume. CIC is encouraged for all patients. Prophylactic antimicrobials and sterile procedures are not always necessary. Most children feel secure if they wear diapers or pads all the time. In some cases, meatotomy of the external orifice is mandatory. If any one or a combination of urinary incontinence, fecal soiling, reflux, detrusor overactivity, and low bladder compliance are intractable and resistant to nonsurgical treatment strategies, surgery should be considered after

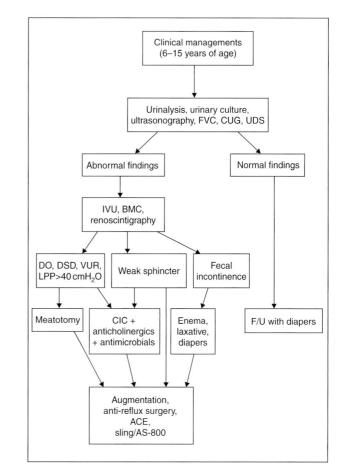

Figure 15.4
Guidelines for clinical management of children aged from 6 to 15 years. ACE, antegrade continence enema; FVC, frequency volume chart; BMC, bowel movement chart; DO, detrusor overactivity; DSD, detrusor-sphincter dyssynergia. Other abbreviations are the same as for Figure 15.3.

the merits and demerits of these interventions have been conveyed to the patient and parents.

Surgical options include enterocystoplasty, antireflux surgery, ACE,[12] sling operation, or implantation of an artificial sphincter.[64,65] Though autoaugmentation[66,67] does not require a segment of the bowel and excludes possible development of bladder malignancy and electrolyte imbalance, there is one uncertainty: that no one can predict the final outcome of surgery in terms of bladder capacity and compliance. We routinely perform antireflux surgery by Orikasa's method,[68] which manipulates the ureteral orifice intravesically and has a significant advantage that it will not compromise blood circulation at the distal end of the ureter. Though it has been reported[69] that antireflux surgery is not necessary provided the bladder is sufficiently augmented, we believe reflux prevention is warranted at the time of surgical intervention.

We previously studied the incidence of fecal incontinence in 94 patients afflicted by myelodysplasia[70] and found that their bowel movements were characterized by repetition of constipation lasting 4–6 days and diarrhea for 1–2 days. It is not surprising that 78% of them mentioned that fecal incontinence or fecal soiling was more troublesome than urinary incontinence and that 65% wore diapers for fecal incontinence. Though the use of suppositories, enemas, or dietary management is said to let these children be socially acceptable, this is not the case for most of the children.[71]

If BMCs are recorded for at least 1 month, it is fairly easy to judge the necessity of ACE in a specific child.

Case reports

Case 1. K.K., a 5-year-old girl, afflicted with lipomeningocele, complained of urinary incontinence in 1997. She underwent lipoma resection 6 months after birth. Her lower extremities functioned normally and she had already been on CIC taught elsewhere. Cystograms showed a moderate degree of trabeculation and a dilated bladder neck, suggesting the presence of detrusor overactivity, but did not reveal any reflux (Figure 15.5, left). Renoscintigraphy did not detect any scar formation (Figure 15.6, left). UDS demonstrated that the LPP was >80 cmH$_2$O and that severe detrusor overactivity was responsible for her urinary incontinence (Figure 15.7, left). Anticholinergics (10 mg of propiverine/day) were prescribed and followed up regularly. Since June 2002 she suffered several times from UTI, which could not be controlled by increased doses of anticholinergics and antimicrobials. Recent studies revealed grade 4 left reflux (see Figure 15.5, right), scar formation in the left kidney, and space-occupying lesions in both kidneys (see Figure 15.6, right). Urodynamically proven detrusor overactivity (see Figure 15.7, right) was responsible for the development of VUR and UTI. She underwent clam cystoplasty and antireflux surgery by Orikasa's method[68] in December 2002. She did not require a sling operation or ACE.

Comments: We could say that we should have increased the dose of anticholinergics to alleviate violent detrusor contractility, but in reality K.K. could not take it because of adverse effects (severe dry mouth and blurred vision).

Case 2. A 10-year-old boy suffered from urinary incontinence and occasional febrile episodes in 1987. Though he was immediately put on CIC, reflux persisted. Transurethral Teflon injection for bilateral reflux was unsuccessful in 1988. He had been operated on in 1989 (Figure 15.8) for reflux, low compliance, and small bladder

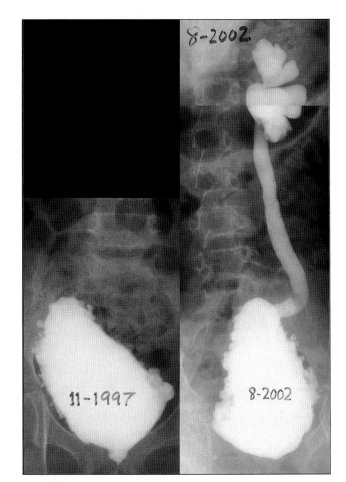

Figure 15.5
Cystograms of case 1.

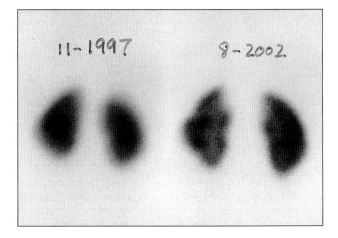

Figure 15.6
Renoscintigrams of case 1.

capacity. He has been on CIC 5–6 times a day and has worked as an occupational therapist in a regional hospital. Although he needs 2–3 pads a day, he is happy to be socially accepted.

Comments: The fact that his bladder neck is open suggests the presence of intrinsic sphincter deficiency (see Figure 15.8, left). It is regretted that sling surgery had not been attempted. Injection of Teflon paste was reported by O'Donnell and Puri[72] in 1984, but the long-term results were disappointing in our hands: i.e. we obtained a 71% success rate in 38 primary reflux ureters and 53% in 17 secondary reflux ureters.[73]

Case 3. A 4-year-old boy, referred by a neurosurgeon in 1991, complained of urinary incontinence. He had undergone lipoma resection in his back at age 3 years. Initial tests revealed grade 4 reflux in the left kidney and low bladder compliance. He underwent antireflux surgery, sling operation, and clam enterocystoplasty in 1993. Figure 15.9 shows his atonic bladder neck (bottom arrow) and left reflux (top arrow) prior to surgery (left: March 1992). His patulons bladder neck was successfully treated by fascia sling (right: August 1993). He has been completely free from urinary incontinence and UTI.

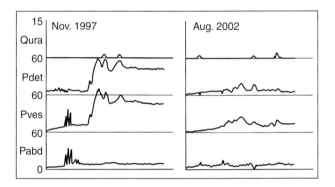

Figure 15.7
Urodynamic tracings of case 1. Qura, urinary flowmetry; Pdet, detrusor pressure; Pves, intravesical pressure; Pabd, abdominal pressure.

Comments: He now plays baseball in a club and does not leak as long as urine is regularly evacuated by CIC.

Case 4. A 9-year-old boy complained of urinary incontinence in 1989. He had worn a urinal to cover his entire external genitalia (Figure 15.10, left), under which severe chronic dermatitis was caused by constant contact with urine (Figure 15.10, right). His renal function was normal, and his bladder was atonic without any uninhibited contractions. He was circumcized and preferred voiding with abdominal strain to CIC.

Comments: Nowadays, this sort of urinal is hardly ever encountered. We assume that he does need surgical intervention for urinary incontinence, but he was lost to follow-up.

Case 5. A 4-year-old boy complained of urinary incontinence and fecal soiling in 1982. He was put on CIC 5 times a day that successfully eradicated his grade 2 bilateral reflux 8 months later. Fourteen years subsequently, he underwent clam enterocystoplasty, sling operation, and ACE. Figure 15.11 illustrates how ACE works. Contrast medium (150 ml) infused through the appendicial stoma demonstrates the ascending colon and sigma. Mark 1 represents the navel, and mark 2 is an orifice of the appendicial stoma. He washes his colon once a week with a tidal volume of 150 ml of saline several times.

Comments: Although 7 patients had been operated on with ACE in our hands, 2 of them abandoned it later. One of these 2 patients found that ACE through the appendicial stoma did not help him much, and the other was reluctant to catheterize the stoma every night.

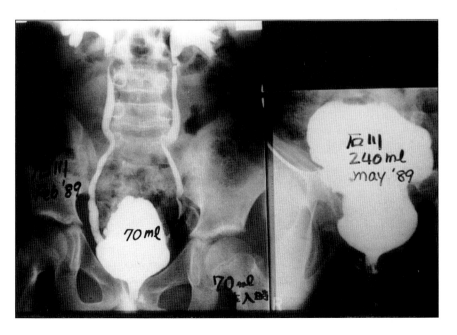

Figure 15.8
Cystograms of case 2 before (left) and after (right) surgery. Intrinsic sphincter deficiency is present.

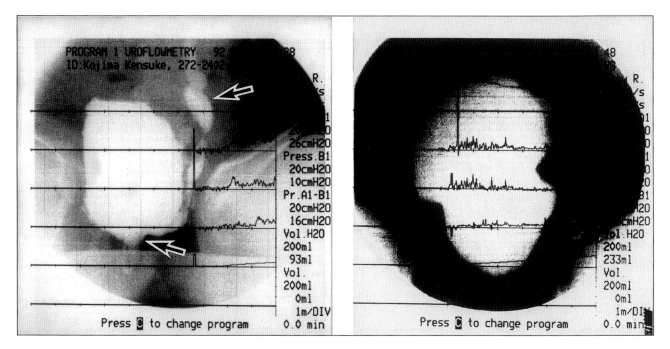

Figure 15.9
Cystograms of case 3 before (left) and after (right) surgery. Left reflux (arrow above) and the incompetent bladder neck (arrow below) are illustrated.

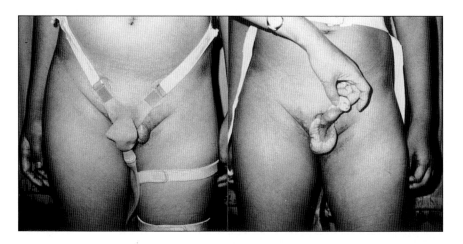

Figure 15.10
A urinal observed in case 4 (left). The prepuce and the scrotum suffered from chronic dermatitis (right).

Case 6. A 3-year-old girl complained of febrile episodes in 1995. Her bladder was not compliant (60 cmH$_2$O per 100 ml), LPP was >80 cmH$_2$O, and grade 5 left reflux was demonstrated. Although she was placed on CIC, we judged that surgical intervention was imminent. She submitted to clam cystoplasty and antireflux surgery 6 months later. In 1998 she complained of hematuria, and plain film (Figure 15.12) showed a bladder stone measuring 33 × 25 mm. The stone was removed transurethrally.

Comments: We recently assessed the incidence of urolithiasis in patients who underwent bladder augmentation.[74] Urolithiasis occurred in 20% of patients undergoing bladder augmentation (10/50 patients) and in 2% of patients

who had not had this operation (5/253 patients). In other words, urolithiasis was 10 times more prevalent in patients subjected to enterocystoplasty than in those without bladder augmentation.

Summary

The primary objective of treating infants and children afflicted by myelodysplasia is to maintain the bladder as a low-pressure reservoir, to prevent UTI, and to keep them dry. Urinalysis is the key to the detection of any changes in the urinary tract. For neonates and infants, conservative

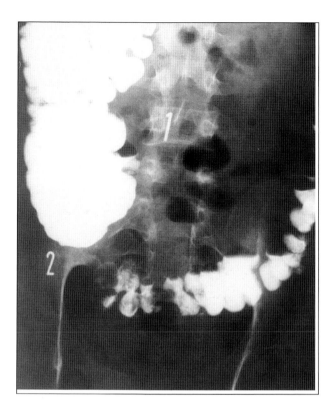

Figure 15.11
Photograph of case 5 illustrates the colon and the sigma where 150 ml of contrast medium was infused through the appendicial stoma of an antegrade continence enema (ACE).

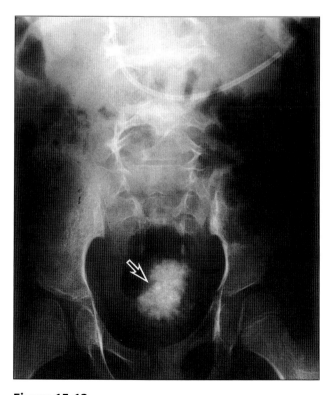

Figure 15.12
A bladder stone shown by an arrow was formed 3 years after clam enterocystoplasty.

treatments comprising CIC with anticholinergics are indicated unless they lose all urine due to weak urinary sphincter function. Although the majority of infants can be treated conservatively, surgical intervention may be necessary in some cases when the upper urinary tract has already been severely compromised.

When children start to go to school, urinary and/or fecal incontinence are the biggest problems for them. Fascia sling surgery and/or ACE will solve these problems, together with bladder augmentation and antireflux surgery. If complete continence fails in a boy, an artificial sphincter (AS-800) can be implanted at the bulbous urethra with a fairly easy technique. Antireflux surgery can be readily undertaken if one chooses Orikasa's method, which does not compromise blood circulation postoperatively at the distal end of the ureter.

Acknowledgments

The senior author sincerely appreciates the hard work and friendship of his longtime colleagues and co-authors. We thank the Guidelines Committee (Y. Igawa, H. Kakizaki, H. Momose, O. Yokoyama, N. Seki, M. Gotoh, and A. Kondo) for allowing us to modify part of their guidelines and to use them.

References

1. Penfield W, Cone W. Spina bifida and cranium bifidum. JAMA 1932; 98:454–461.

2. Bricker EM. Bladder substitution after pelvic evisceration. Surg Clin North Am 1950; 30:1511–1521.

3. Freeman JM. To treat or not to treat: ethical dilemmas of treating the infant with a myelomeningocele. Clin Neurosurg 1997; 20:134–146.

4. Shurtleff DB, Hayden PW, Loeser JD, Kronmal RA. Myelodysplasia: decision for death or disability. N Engl J Med 1974; 291:1005–1011.

5. Lorber J. Results of treatment of myelomeningocele. Develop Med Child Neurol 1971; 13:279–303.

6. Lapides J, Diokno AC, Silber SJ, Lowe BS. Clean intermittent self-catheterization in the treatment of urinary tract disease. J Urol 1972; 107:458–461.

7. Middleton AW Jr, Hendren WH. Ileal conduits in children at the Massachusetts General Hospital from 1955 to 1970. J Urol 1976; 115:591–595.

8. Sundar B, Mackie GG. Urinary undiversion. Montreal Children's Hospital Experience. Urology 1980; 16:172–175.

9. Ahmed A, Carney A. Urinary undiversion in myelomeningocele patients with an ileal conduit diversion. J Urol 1981; 125:847–852.

10. Goldwasser B, Webster GD. Augmentation and substitution enterocystoplasty. J Urol 1986; 135:215–224.

11. Mitrofanoff P. Cystostomie continente trans-appendiculaire dans le traitement des vessies neurologiques. Chir Pediatr 1980; 21:297–305.

12. Malone PS, Ransley PG, Kiely EM. Preliminary report: the antegrade continence enema. Lancet 1990; 336:1217–1218.

13. Werler MM, Shapiro S, Mitchell AA. Periconceptional folic acid exposure and risk of occurrent neural tube defects. JAMA 1993; 269:1257–1261.

14. Botto LD, Moore CA, Khoury MJ, Erickson JD. Neural-tube defects. N Engl J Med 1999; 341:1509–1519.

15. Hall J, Solehdin F. Folic acid for the prevention of congenital anomalies. Eur J Pediatr 1998; 157:445–450.

16. Stevenson RE, Allen WP, Pai GS, et al. Decline in prevalence of neural tube defects in a high-risk region of the United States. Pediatr 2000; 106:677–683.

17. Lian Z-H, Yang H-Y, Li Z. Neural tube defects in Beijing-Tianjin area of China. J Epidemiol Comm Health 1987; 41:259–262.

18. Sumiyosi Y. Study on congenital anomaly monitoring in Japan [in Japanese]. Integrated study on children and family. Ministry of Health and Welfare, Japan, 2000: 3–13.

19. Bekkers RLM, Eskes TKAB. Periconceptional folic acid intake in Nijmegen, Netherlands. Lancet 1999; 353(9149):242

20. Becerra JE, Khoury MJ, Cordero JF, Erickson JD. Diabetes mellitus during pregnancy and the risks for specific birth defects: a population-based case-control study. Pediatrics 1990; 85:1–9.

21. Hernandez-Diaz S, Werler MM, Walker AM, Mitchell AA. Folic acid antagonists during pregnancy and the risk of birth defects. N Engl J Med 2000; 343:1608–1614.

22. Hernandez-Diaz S, Werler MM, Walker AM, Mitchell AA. Neural tube defects in relation to use of folic acid antagonists during pregnancy. Am J Epidemiol 2001; 153:961–968.

23. Graham JM Jr, Edwards MJ, Edwards MJ. Teratogen update: gestational effects of maternal hyperthermia due to febrile illnesses and resultant patterns of defects in humans. Teratology 1998; 58:209–221.

24. Watkins ML, Scanlon KS, Mulinare J, Khoury MJ. Is maternal obesity a risk factor for anencephaly and spina bifida? Epidemiology 1996; 7:507–512.

25. Hibbard BR. The role of folic acid in pregnancy. With particular reference to anaemia, abruption and abortion. J Obstet Gynaecol Br Commonw 1964; 71:529–542.

26. Smithells RW, Sheppard S, Schorah CJ, et al. Possible prevention of neural-tube defects by periconceptional vitamin supplementation. Lancet 1980; i:339–340.

27. MRC Vitamin Study Research Group. Prevention of neural tube defects: results of the medical research council vitamin study. Lancet 1991; 338:131–137.

28. Czeizel AE, Dudas I. Prevention of the first occurrence of neural-tube defects by periconceptional vitamin supplementation. N Engl J Med 1992; 327:1832–1835.

29. Berry RJ, Li Z, Erickson JD, et al. Prevention of neural-tube defects with folic acid in China. N Engl J Med 1999; 341:1485–1490.

30. Milunsky A, Jick H, Jick SS, et al. Multivitamin/folic acid supplementation in early pregnancy reduces the prevalence of neural tube defects. JAMA 1989; 262:2847–2852.

31. Bower C, Stanley FJ. Dietary folate as a risk factor for neural-tube defects: evidence from a case-control study in Western Australia. Med J Aust 1989; 150:613–619.

32. Shaw GM, Schaffer D, Velie EM, et al. Periconceptional vitamin use, dietary folate, and the occurrence of neural tube defects. Epidemiol 1995; 6:219–226.

33. Mills JL, Rhoads GG, Simpson JL, et al. The absence of a relation between the periconceptional use of vitamins and neural-tube defects. N Engl J Med 1989; 321:430–435.

34. Kondo A, Kimura K, Isobe Y, et al. Folic acid reduces risks of having fetus affected with neural tube defects: dietary food folate and plasma folate concentration. Jpn J Urol 2003; 94:551–559.

35. CDC. Recommendations for the use of folic acid to reduce the number of cases of spina bifida and other neural tube defects. MMWR 1992; 41:1–7.

36. De Walle HEK, De Jong-van den Berg LYW, Cornel MC. Periconceptional folic acid intake in the northern Netherlands. Lancet 1999; 353:1187.

37. Cornel MC, Erickson JD. Comparison of national policies on periconceptional use of folic acid to prevent spina bifida and anencephaly (SBA). Teratology 1997; 55:134–137.

38. The Ministry of Health and Welfare of Japan. Periconceptional intake of folic acid reduces the risk of having fetus afflicted with neural tube defects. Official letter, December 2000.

39. Food and Drug Administration. Food standards: amendment of standards of identity for enriched grain products to require addition of folic acid. Fed Regist 1996; 61:8781–8807.

40. Jacques PF, Selhub J, Bostom AG, et al. The effect of folic acid fortification on plasma folate and total homocysteine concentrations. N Engl J Med 1999; 340:1449–1454.

41. Fernandes ET, Reinberg Y, Vernier R, Gonzalez R. Neurogenic bladder dysfunction in children: review of pathophysiology and current management. J Pediatr 1994; 124:1–7.

42. McGuire EJ, Woodside JR, Borden TA, Weiss RM. Prognostic value of urodynamic testing in myelodysplastic patients. J Urol 1981; 126:205–209.

43. McGuire EJ, Cespedes RD, O'Connell HE. Leak-point pressures. Urol Clin North Am 1996; 23:253–262.

44. Ghoniem GM, Roach MB, Lewis VH, Harmon EP. The value of leak pressure and bladder compliance in the urodynamic evaluation of meningocele patients. J Urol 1990; 144:1140–1142.

45. Bauer SB, Hallett M, Khoshbin S, et al. Predictive value of urodynamic evaluation in newborns with myelodysplasia. JAMA 1984; 252: 650–652.

46. Van Gool JD, Dik P, De Jong TPVM. Bladder-sphincter dysfunction in myelomeningocele. Eur J Pediatr 2001; 160:414–420.

47. Kaufman AM, Ritchey ML, Roberts AC, et al. Decreased bladder compliance in patients with myelomeningocele treated with radiological observation. J Urol 1996; 156:2031–2033.

48. Perez LM, Khoury J, Webster GD. The value of urodynamic studies in infants less than 1 year old with congenital spinal dysraphism. J Urol 1992; 148:584–587.

49. Brinkman J, Enrile B, Koff SA. Prophylactic use of intermittent catheterization in children with spina bifida. Br J Urol 1991; 68:643A.

50. Mohler JL, Cowen DL, Flanigan RC. Suppression and treatment of urinary tract infection in patients with an intermittent catheterized neurogenic bladder. J Urol 1987; 138:336–340.

51. Kaefer M, Pabby A, Kelly M, et al. Improved bladder function after prophylactic treatment of the high risk neurogenic bladder in newborns with myelomeningocele. J Urol 1999; 162:1068–1071.

52. Geraniotis E, Koff SA, Enrile B. The prophylactic use of clean intermittent catheterization in the treatment of infants and young children with myelomeningocele and neurogenic bladder dysfunction. J Urol 1988; 139:85–86.

53. Kasabian NG, Bauer SB, Dyro FM, et al. The prophylactic value of clean intermittent catheterization and anticholinergic medication in newborns and infants with myelodysplastic at risk of developing urinary tract deterioration. AJDC 1992; 146:840–843.

54. Cohen RA, Rushton HG, Belman AB, et al. Renal scarring and vesicoureteral reflux in children with myelodysplasia. J Urol 1990; 144:541–544.

55. Anderson PAM, Travers AH. Development of hydronephrosis in spina bifida patients: predictive factors and management. Br J Urol 1993; 72:958–961.

56. Hernadez RD, Hurwitz RS, Foote JE, et al. Nonsurgical management of threatened upper urinary tract and incontinence in children with myelomeningocele. J Urol 1994; 152:1582–1585.

57. Knoll M, Madersbacher H. The chances of a spina bifida patient becoming continent/socially dry by conservative therapy. Paraplegia 1993; 31:22–27.

58. Webster GD, El-Mahrouky A, Stone AR, Zakrzewski C. The urological evaluation and management of patients with myelodysplasia. Br J Urol 1986; 58:261–265.

59. Teichman JMH, Scherz HC, Kim KD, et al. An alternative approach to myelodysplasia management: aggressive observation and prompt intervention. J Urol 1994; 152:807–811.

60. Katona F. Stages of vegetative afferentation in reorganization of bladder control during intravesical electrotherapy. Urol Int 1975; 30:192–203.

61. Gaum LD, Wese FX, Alton DJ, et al. Radiological investigation of the urinary tract in the neonate with myelomeningocele. J Urol 1982; 127:510–512.

62. Kaplan WE, Firlit CF. Management of reflux in the myelodysplastic child. J Urol 1983; 129:1195–1197.

63. Kondo A, Saito M, Gotoh M, et al. Bladder compliance in myelodysplastic children: effect of anti-reflux surgery and conservative treatment. Br J Urol 1991; 67:647–651.

64. Barrett DW, Furlow WL. The management of severe urinary incontinence in patients with myelodysplasia by implantation of the AS 791/792 urinary sphincter device. J Urol 1982; 128:484–486.

65. Venn SN, Greenwell TJ, Mundy AR. The long-term outcome of artificial urinary sphincters. J Urol 2000; 164:702–707.

66. Cartright PC, Snow BW. Bladder autoaugmentation: early clinical experience. J Urol 1989; 142:505–508.

67. Stroehrer M, Kramer A, Goepel M, et al. Bladder autoaugmentation. An alternative for enterocystoplasty: preliminary results. Neurourol Urodyn 1995; 14:11–23.

68. Orikasa S. A new antireflux operation. Eur Urol 1990; 17:330–332.

69. Nasrallah PF, Aliabadi HA. Bladder augmentation in patients with neurogenic bladder and vesico-ureteral reflux. J Urol 1991; 146:563–566.

70. Saito M, Kondo A. Management of bowel problems in the patient with spina bifida. J Neurogenic Bladder Soc 1997; 8:12–18.

71. Leonard CO, Freeman JM. Spina bifida: a new disease. Pediatr 1981; 68:136–137.

72. O'Donnell B, Puri P. Treatment of vesicoureteric reflux by endoscopic injection of Teflon. Br Med J 1984; 289:7–9.

73. Kondo A, Yoshikawa Y, Nagai T, Saito M. Anti-reflux surgery by injection of Teflon paste. Br J Urol 1992; 69:507–509.

74. Kondo A, Gotoh M, Isobe Y, et al. Urolithiasis in those patients with myelodysplasia. Jpn J Urol 2003; 94:15–19.

16

Spina bifida in adults

JLH Ruud Bosch

Introduction

Myelomeningocele (MMC) and spina bifida occulta are the commonest causes of neurogenic bladder dysfunction in childhood, and can also cause significant problems in adults with complications such as incontinence, obstructive uropathy, vesicoureteric reflux, pyelonephritis, and subsequent renal failure. In the majority of the spina bifida cases, the lumbosacral region is involved, leading to neurogenic disturbance of urogenital, colorectal, and pelvic floor function.

The mortality of MMC patients was high before the 1940s. A change in prognosis has developed in a stepwise fashion in the second half of the 20th century. Initially, improved obstetric and neonatal care resulted in an increase of surviving MMC children by the end of the first half of the 20th century. More aggressive neurosurgical management, including early closure of the neural tube defect and shunting techniques for the accompanying hydrocephalus, followed this. Thereafter, many of these children received comprehensive health care. In many developed countries management and follow-up protocols were developed and delivered by multidisciplinary teams. These teams usually involved a pediatric nephrologist, neurosurgeon, orthopedic surgeon, and urologist. A much higher number of severely affected children now reach adulthood and 97% of these have urogenital problems.[1]

A new phase may have been entered since the recognition of the role of folic acid supplementation for all women of childbearing age as an important measure in the prevention of neural tube defects. In the United States and in Australia a statistically significant decrease in the prevalence of neural tube defects has been noticed after enrichment of certain foods with folic acid.[2,3] Therefore, it is recommended that all women of childbearing age consume 0.4 mg of folic acid daily.

An abnormality such as a meningocele that is an extension of the dural sac outside the spinal canal (usually through a posterior defect) may be seen on fetal ultrasound scanning. Although a diagnosis *in utero* by ultrasound and alpha-fetoprotein is now routinely possible, there may be very difficult management decisions to take, including the possibility of terminating the pregnancy. A more widespread use of preventive measures and the diagnosis of neural tube defects in early pregnancy will probably lead to a decrease in the number of adult patients with spina bifida within a few decades.

Urodynamic types of lower urinary tract dysfunction

Four basic types of lower urinary tract dysfunction have been identified in MMC patients. In a series of 111 children the following patterns were found:[4] an 'inactive detrusor plus inactive pelvic floor' in 32%; an 'overactive detrusor and overactive pelvic floor' were seen in 38%. A combination of 'overactive pelvic floor plus inactive detrusor' and 'inactive pelvic floor plus overactive detrusor' was found in 9% and 12%, respectively. In 10%, normal lower urinary tract function was seen. So, more than 50% of the patients either had a normal or a low-pressure detrusor. The 'classic' urodynamic pattern of the lower urinary tract in young adults with MMC was formerly described as the 'inactive detrusor plus inactive pelvic floor' or areflexive bladder with open vesical outlet.[5] This, however was mainly a reflection of the selection and survival of the 'fittest', because these patients are at low risk for upper tract deterioration and only rarely develop vesicoureteral reflux and pyelonephritis.[4] More recently, adult patients with other urodynamic patterns are seen more frequently as well as adult patients who have undergone lower urinary tract reconstruction and those who are candidates for a kidney transplantation and need a low-pressure lower urinary tract to accept the transplant.

Poor bladder compliance is one of the main problems in patients with abnormal detrusor function. Particularly detrimental to the function of the upper tracts and kidneys is the combination of poor compliance and a non-relaxing or uncoordinated outlet. If the pressures in the bladder are almost permanently above 40 cmH$_2$O, ureteral delivery of urine boluses to the bladder stops. Patients with an abdominal leak point pressure above 40 cmH$_2$O are at risk for upper tract damage.[6]

Patients with a normal bladder function all had defects limited to the sacral area that had been surgically closed.[4] A normal lower urinary tract function in the early years of life is no guarantee for the absence of future problems. In fact, these patients should be followed closely into adult age because they are at risk for development of a so-called tethered cord syndrome. The pathogenesis of the tethered cord syndrome is explained by traction on the lumbar spinal cord between two fixation points. The upper fixation point is at the exit site of the posterior and anterior spinal nerve roots and the lower fixation point is at the site of the tethering or the site of scar fixation from the previous neurosurgical closure. The repetitive injury to the small blood vessels due to stretching and kinking leads to a reduction of the blood supply to this section of the cord and consequent neuronal hypoxemia.[7] The alternative explanation based on the concept of 'abnormal ascent' of the spinal cord during growth of the child is wrong: during the 8th week of fetal development the spinal cord has already attained the level of L1–2.[8] The decision to neurosurgically untether the cord in patients with a normal bladder function is a difficult one since there is no solid evidence that the function will deteriorate if the cord is not untethered; alternatively, about 11% of children with a normal bladder develop neurogenic bladder dysfunction after untethering.[9]

Principles of management of lower urinary tract dysfunction

The primary goal in the management of MMC patients is preservation of kidney function. To achieve this goal, the bladder should function as a low-pressure reservoir. Obstructive uropathy and high bladder pressures during a significant part of the filling phase are the most important causes of kidney failure in these patients. If on urodynamic testing the detrusor pressure begins to rise only above a filling volume of 300–400 ml, it is feasible for most patients to limit the high-pressure time by clean intermittent self-catheterization (CISC). If the compliance of the bladder is lower or if the detrusor is hyperreflexive even at relatively small volumes, the combination of anticholinergic drugs and CISC may achieve the goal of reasonable dryness and preservation of the upper tracts. However, if these measures fail, an augmentation cystoplasty should be performed. In patients who have a very thick bladder wall, substitution cystoplasty may be more appropriate.[10] Continuation of CISC in these cases is the rule. Conversion of the lower urinary tract into a low-pressure reservoir by CISC with or without medication, augmentation, or

diversion may not be able to prevent late renal failure if some kidney damage has already occurred.[11] In most adult patients the issue of high pressures will have been taken care of at an earlier age.

An unsolved problem of urinary incontinence may have a serious impact on quality of life. However, most of these patients have lived with their handicaps for their whole life and have often adapted to it in a remarkable way. Contrary to patients who have an acquired neurogenic bladder problem, they have no previous personal experience with normal function of the urinary tract. This is important to keep in mind because this notion may help to understand that those who have a comparable but congenital problem perceive the margin for improvement, which is present in patients with acquired disease, quite differently. Most of the remaining problems cannot be solved without creating new ones! Incontinence is multifactorial: hyperreflexia, decreased compliance, and sphincteric or pelvic floor incompetence all play a role. Hyperreflexia can be addressed by medical treatment and both hyperreflexia and low compliance can be treated by an augmentation cystoplasty, usually in combination with CISC. A weak outlet can be treated by the creation of a fixed outlet resistance. To achieve this, techniques such as injection of bulking agents, colposuspension, or a pubovaginal sling can be employed; again, CISC is usually needed as an adjunctive measure in these situations. The artificial sphincter holds the theoretical promise of near-normal voiding; however, in most patients with MMC this cannot be achieved.

The neural tube defect mainly involves the dorsal part of the spinal cord. The neurological deficit therefore is mainly determined by a sensory defect. In fact, about 90% of the anteriorly located motor neurons are intact in MMC patients.[12] Therefore, despite the fact that the afferent part of the sacral reflex arcs is absent or severely deficient, the efferent nerves to the sphincter and pelvic floor muscles may be responsive to electrical stimulation. Electrical stimulation of the pudendal nerve at the site of the ischial spine may improve urethral and anal sphincteric function in these patients.[13]

The reputation of the artificial urinary sphincter (AUS) in MMC patients is somewhat poor, because placement of an AUS can lead to secondary changes in bladder function that may be detrimental to the upper urinary tract. Bladder overactivity or a decrease in bladder compliance may occur *de novo* after increasing the outflow resistance of the lower urinary tract by the implantation of an artificial sphincter.[14,15] In one series, 32 of 47 implanted patients who were implanted as children could be followed up for a minimum of 10 years (mean 15.4 years). There were 13 removals (due to erosion or infection) and 19 sphincters were still intact (59.4%). Of these patients, 18 were dry and 7 of 19 voided spontaneously. There were 0.03 revisions per patient-year and it was noted that 9 of 13 with placement after 1987 had not needed revisions. This series therefore shows that a long-term successful outcome of the AUS is possible in well-selected patients, even if the device is implanted at a young age.[14]

The main advantage of the AUS is the potential preservation of spontaneous voiding. However, in a population of patients with MMC, only 27% were able to void spontaneously and were continent after the implantation of an AUS.[15] One could therefore reason that other methods to increase the outflow resistance, such as a fascia sling procedure, would be preferable in these patients because the main advantage of the AUS, i.e. preservation of spontaneous voiding, cannot be achieved in these patients anyway.

Concerning the combination of enterocystoplasty and AUS placement, Furness et al have reviewed the literature and their own experience in 17 MMC patients.[16] Of these, 3 had the AUS placed before the augmentation and 4 had the sphincter placed after the bladder augmentation. In 10 patients the procedures were performed simultaneously. Based on the compiled literature data and their own results, they summarized that the infection rates were 14.5% and 6.8% for simultaneous and staged procedures, respectively. However, these rates were not statistically different. Only three of the reviewed papers reported rates for both the staged and the simultaneous procedures. In these papers the differences in infection rates were 40.5%, 18.2%, and 3.7%, with the simultaneous procedures always showing the higher rates. In their own series the difference was 4.3%. Many factors can mitigate the infection rate, but this review did not control for any of the possible factors, such as other simultaneous reconstructive procedures, duration of the procedure, positive preoperative urine cultures, type of bowel used, or antibiotic prophylaxis. Miller et al did not find an influence of these factors, except for type of bowel used.[17] Gastrocystoplasty was associated with a 0% infection rate. The overall AUS infection rate in their series was 6.9%. However, it was 20% excluding the gastrocystoplasties.

Other important questions in relation to the bladder augmentation are: Who needs a bladder augmentation in combination with an AUS? Are there urodynamic parameters that can predict the necessity for enterocystoplasty? In their retrospective review Miller et al[17] found that the average bladder compliance of those in whom an augmentation was performed was 7.8 ml/cmH$_2$O; in two patients the compliance was more than 10 ml/cmH$_2$O and in none of the patients was it less than 2 ml/cmH$_2$O.

Kronner et al[18] found that 15 of 38 MMC patients (39.5%) who were younger than 18 years at the time of the implant, subsequently required augmentation after a mean follow-up of 101 months. The mean time to augmentation was 49 (range 10–118) months. An augmentation was performed if urodynamics had worsened. Repeat urodynamic tests were performed when intractable incontinence and/or upper tract changes occurred. Before the implant of the

AUS, the bladder capacity and the compliance were not significantly different between the patients who were (8.0 ± 4.8 ml/cmH$_2$O) and those who were not (7.0 ± 3.3 ml/cmH$_2$O) treated by bladder augmentation ($p = 0.45$). The authors contended that cut-off values of bladder compliance below which others have recommended simultaneous augmentation, such as bladder compliance below 2 and below 6.7 ml/cmH$_2$O, are inaccurate. In fact, many of their patients had a compliance below one of these cut-off values but did not need an augmentation. It should be noted, however, that the original group consisted of 80 patients; of these, 35 underwent a primary augmentation because of severely decreased compliance or capacity. So it seems that the jury is still out on this subject.

Undiversion and conversion

Today urinary diversion is rarely performed in children with MMC. Those who have reached adulthood and were diverted in the past might wish to become candidates for orthotopic undiversion or conversion to a continent urinary diversion such as an Indiana pouch or one of its alternatives. Although cosmetic reasons do play a role, undiversion is more indicated in those with upper tract problems in order to create a nonrefluxing low-pressure continent reservoir.

Before undiversion, patients should be evaluated with urine cultures, creatinine clearance, a renogram, an intravenous urogram (IVU), and a loop-o-gram to adequately describe function and anatomy. If orthotopic undiversion is contemplated, this should be complemented by videourodynamic studies or a cystogram and retrograde ureterograms if there is no reflux.

Contraindications to undiversion include inability to perform clean intermittent catheterisation (CIC) and poor kidney function. As a general rule, patients with a serum creatinine greater than 2 mg/dl (175 μmol/ml) will have difficulty in coping with the metabolic challenges posed by the use of small or large bowel for a continent reservoir.[19] In MMC patients the lean body mass is decreased and therefore the creatinine clearance is a more reliable parameter than serum creatinine: in MMC patients a creatinine clearance cut off of 50 ml/min would be roughly equivalent to the above-mentioned values. MMC patients with an impaired anal sphincteric function will be at increased risk for fecal incontinence when intestinal function becomes (slightly) impaired due to the use of bowel segments to reconstruct the urinary tract.

In those with a well-working cutaneous diversion and no upper tract complications, the risks of an undiversion should be taken into account. A new anastomosis between the ureters and the bowel segment is more prone to stenosis even if the caliber appears to be large at the time of the undiversion. Probably, the changed tissue quality and vascularity of the ureteral wall is the explanation for this observation. In one series a 22% stenosis rate was reported in a group of 48 neurogenic patients as opposed to only 6.4% in the total group of 374 patients.[20]

Those MMC patients who are wheelchair-bound are not good candidates for an orthotopic undiversion because of the difficulty in performing CISC. For women it is particularly troublesome to have to catheterize through the urethra. In MMC women we often find large labia that complicate CISC via the urethra. Since most of these patients also have an increased body mass index (BMI) with increased diameters of the thighs and limited ranges of movement in the hips, it is much easier for them to be able to catheterize without having to transfer out of the wheelchair. This can be accomplished by a catheterizable stoma at an easily accessible spot on the (upper) abdomen or via the umbilicus. In wheelchair-bound male MMC patients the penis is often concealed due to the abnormal body habitus, making CISC more difficult as well as fitting of a condom catheter.

Adult MMC patients who have previously undergone an enterocystoplasty and those who opt for an undiversion or conversion of a cutaneous stoma into a catheterizable orthotopic or heterotopic reservoir can be confronted with several complications. Urologists following adult MMC patients should be aware of these complications, which include stomal stenosis, stenosis of the ureteroenteric anastomoses, reservoir perforation, mucus production in the reservoir, struvite stone formation, clinically significant urinary tract infections,[21] and metabolic problems such as acid–base disturbances, osteopenia, osmotic diarrhea, fatty diarrhea, calcium oxalate urolithiasis, and vitamin B12 deficiency.[19] Treatment of these complications is according to generally accepted guidelines, not specific for MMC patients. One measure should, however, be highlighted and that is daily irrigation with normal saline, which frees the reservoir of mucus and helps prevent the formation of calculi.

Pretransplant surgical preparation of the lower urinary tract is a special situation in which reconstruction, diversion, or even undiversion may be indicated. When the bladder is not reparable or usable with acceptable results, ileal conduit, continent urinary diversions, and/or bladder augmentation may be required.[22–24] Each method has its specific set of possible complications and these should be thoroughly discussed with individual patients prior to use. A native dilated ureter can be used to augment the bladder and may be the procedure of choice in neurogenic bladder associated with grossly dilated ureters.[25]

Sexual dysfunction

Sexual dysfunction, with both genders having loss of genital sensation, is a common problem. As patients with spina bifida now have increased life expectancy, this is recognized as an important quality-of-life issue. Theoretically, the effects on penile erection, vaginal lubrication, and orgasm are related to the level and completeness of the lesion. In reality, there is a paucity of literature about sexual function in MMC patients. Erections are claimed by about 70% of adolescent males, although most of the erections are probably reflex in nature and not in response to sexual stimuli. The occurrence of erections is positively correlated with a lower sensory level and the presence of an anocutaneous reflex.[26] Theoretically, those with normal bladder function and intact sacral reflexes are likely to have normal sexual function. There are no studies on the use of oral medication, intracorporeal injections, or penile prosthesis specifically on these patients.

In women, pregnancy and vaginal delivery is possible, although complications related to urinary tract dysfunction and deformation of the pelvis occur frequently.[27]

References

1. Durham Smith E. Urinary prognosis in spina bifida. J Urol 1972; 108:815–817.

2. Stevenson RE, Allen WP, Pai GS, et al. Decline in prevalence of neural tube defects in a high risk region of the United States. Pediatrics 2000; 106:677–683.

3. Halliday JL, Riley M. Fortification of foods with folic acid (letter). N Engl J Med 2000; 343:970–971.

4. Van Gool JD. Spina bifida and neurogenic bladder dysfunction: a urodynamic study. Utrecht: Impress, 1986: 219.

5. McGuire EJ, Denil J. Adult myelodysplasia. AUA Update Series 1991; 10:298–303.

6. McGuire EJ, Woodside JR, Borden TA. Upper tract deterioration in patients with myelodysplasia and detrusor hypertonia with a follow up study. J Urol 1983; 129:873.

7. Fujita J, Yamamoto H. An experimental study on spinal cord traction effect. Spine 1989; 14:698–705.

8. Wilson DA, Prince JR. Imaging determination of the location of the normal conus medullaris throughout childhood. AJR 1989; 152:1029–1032.

9. Keating MA, Rink RC, Bauer SB, et al. Neurourological implications of the changing approach in management of occult spinal lesions. J Urol 1988; 140:1299–1301.

10. Stephenson TP, Mundy AR. Treatment of the neuropathic bladder by enterocystoplasty and selective sphincterotomy or sphincter ablation and replacement. Br J Urol 1985; 57:27–31.

11. Brem AS, Martin D, Callaghan J, Maynard J. Long term renal risk factors in children with meningomyelocele. J Pediatr 1987; 110:51–54.

12. Stark GD. The nature and cause of paraplegia in myelomeningocele. Paraplegia 1972; 9:219.

13. Schmidt RA, Kogan BA, Tanagho EA. Neuroprosthesis in the management of incontinence in myelomeningocele patients. J Urol 1990; 143:779–782.

14. Kryger JV, Spencer Barthold J, Fleming P, Gonzales R. The outcome of artificial sphincter placement after a mean 15-year follow-up in a paediatric population. BJU Int 1999; 83:1026–1031.

15. Roth DR, Vyas PR, Kroovand RL, Perlmutter AD. Urinary tract deterioration associated with the artificial urinary sphincter. J Urol 1986; 135:528–530.

16. Furness III PD, Franzoni DF, Decter RM. Bladder augmentation: does it predispose to prosthetic infection of simultaneously placed artificial genitourinary sphincters or in situ ventriculoperitoneal shunts? BJU International 1999; 84:25–29.

17. Miller EA, Mayo M, Kwan D, Mitchell M. Simultaneous augmentation cystoplasty and artificial urinary sphincter placement: infection rates and voiding mechanisms. J Urol 1998; 160:750–753.

18. Kronner KM, Rink RC, Simmons G, et al. Artificial urinary sphincter in the treatment of urinary incontinence: preoperative urodynamics do not predict the need for future bladder augmentation. J Urol 1998; 160:1093–1095.

19. Stamper DS, McDougal WS, McGovern FJ. Metabolic and nutritional complications. Urol Clin N Am 1997; 24:715–722.

20. Stein R, Matani Y, Doi Y, et al. Continent urinary diversion using the Mainz pouch I technique – ten years later. J Urol 1995; 153 (4, Suppl.):241A.

21. Rink RC. Bladder augmentation: options, outcomes, future. Urol Clin N Am 1999; 26:111–123.

22. MacGregor P, Novick AC, Cunningham R, et al. Renal transplantation in end stage renal disease patients with existing urinary diversion. J Urol 1986; 135:686–688.

23. Hatch DA, Belitsky P, Barry JM, et al. Fate of renal allografts transplanted in patients with urinary diversion. Transplantation 1993; 56:838–842.

24. Dawahra M, Martin X, Tajra LC, et al. Renal transplantation using continent urinary diversion: long-term follow-up. Transplant Proc 1997; 29:159–160.

25. Koyle MA, Pfister RR, Kam I, et al. Bladder reconstruction with the dilated ureter for renal transplantation. Transplant Proc 1994; 26:35–36.

26. Diamond DA, Rickwood AMK, Thomas DG. Penile erections in myelomeningocele patients. Br J Urol 1986; 58:434–435.

27. Richmond D, Zaharievski I, Bond A. Management of pregnancy in mothers with spina bifida. Eur J Obstet Reprod Biol 1987; 25:341–345.

17

Syringomyelia and lower urinary tract dysfunction

Marc Le Fort and Jean-Jacques Labat

Introduction

Syringomyelia manifests as a liquid cavity in the spinal cord. It may be accompanied by neurological signs. This type of spinal cord cavity has been known for a long time through autopsies and dissections. The name 'syringomyelia' was coined by Olivier d'Angers in 1824 (*syrinx* = flute used by the Greek god Pan), described in 1867 by Bastian and only accepted as a real entity since the years 1950–1960 after Freeman's studies (1953) and the first report by Barnett and Jousse in 1966. Its evolution is classically slow and can become functionally disabling if untreated. Most syringomyelias occur in a congenital malformative context (primary syringomyelia), with a late clinical expression. A secondary syringomyelia can occur after spinal cord injury (SCI). The diagnosis is made by magnetic resonance imaging (MRI), but the mechanisms of syringomyelia occurrence are not perfectly understood.

Primary syringomyelia

Etiopathogeny

Dysraphic theory[1]

According to this ancient theory, syringomyelia would be due to a closing defect of the neural tube, which normally occurs between the 21st and 28th days of embryonal life. This embryopathy would arise from abnormal constitution of the posterior raphe. Bony anomalies associated with cervico-occipital transition and Chiari malformation would have no physiopathological link.

Hydrodynamic theories

Gardner's theory.[2] In the 1950s, Gardner revolutionized the physiopathological concepts of syringomyelia, introducing the notion of a pathogenic role of cerebrospinal fluid (CSF) dynamics. This primitive embryological disorder comprises a lack or late opening of the roof orifices of the 4th ventricle that links the great cistern with the perimedullary and pericerebral subarachnoid spaces. Thus, a CSF hyperpressure is responsible for downward dilation of the spinal central canal. At birth, this hydromyelia bursts into a zone of lower resistance, the gray posterior commissure. It generates the syringomyelic cavity, which will have a permanent tendency to extend. Prolapse of the cerebellar tonsils, which by itself can hamper CSF circulation, and the cervico-occipital bony abnormalities would be consequences of the hydroencephalomyelia (Arnold–Chiari malformation).

Aboulker's theory.[3] This theory insists on the transition effect. Any effort generating veinous hyperpressure creates growth of CSF pressure in the perimedullary spaces. This hyperpressure is normally transmitted upwards to the cranious spaces. In the case of cervico-occipital bony abnormalities, CSF passage to the great cistern is held up, and the consequent hyperpressure furthers CSF entry into the medullary spaces, about the level of the posterior rootlets. Coalescence of the liquidian lakes forms the syringomyelic cavity.

Clinical signs

Physical examination may provide the diagnosis of medullary cavity and specify its extension that could even involve the high spinal cord (syringobulbomyelia). Its classical description is:

- An upper syndrome combining a lower motoneuron deficiency with dissociative sensory loss: abolished reflexes, amyotrophy, peripheral motor weakness, thermic and pain anesthesia but with relative sparing of light touch and perception.
- A lower syndrome under the lesion level: upper motoneuron weakness and vibratory sensory deficiency.

The actual clinical signs are rarely well caricatured. One symptom can raise suspicions of a spinal cord pathology and should lead to an MRI. However, CSF accumulation within the spinal cord does not necessarily result in clinical neurological deterioration, and the time period between the first sign and the diagnosis is still 6–8 years.[1] Xenos et al[4] mention, in cases of spinal lipomas, a possible role for syringomyelia in accelerating clinical deterioration. The most frequent early functional signs are subjective sensitivity of an upper limb (paresthesiae, pain), walking incapacity, cervical or cephalic pain, vertigo, motor deficiency of a limb, trophic signs (painless burn), and rapidly progressing thoracic scoliosis of adolescence. Electrophysiological exploration may contribute to the early diagnosis, not so much to affirm a syringomyelia as to suspect a pathology of the spinal cord.[5]

Radiological signs

Standard radiographies

There could be indirect signs of an expansive intraspinal process: interpedicle enlargement, pedicle thinning, and spinal scalloping. A cervico-occipital abnormality, an associated bony dysraphism (spina bifida occulta) or kyphoscoliosis should be investigated.

Neuroradiology

MRI supplants myelography. Myeloscans can be useful to study lower dysraphisms.

MRI[6,7] has close to 100% sensitivity and specificity. The signal of a syringomyelic cavity is the same as a CSF signal, and is better seen with T2 exploration. A syrinx is tube-shaped and extends beyond the SCI site to at least two vertebral levels. The signal is homogeneous and clearly delimits the upper and lower limits of the syringomyelia. The extension is always much more significant than the clinics suppose. The syringomyelic cavity may be multiloculated, and neuroradiology also gives information on tension inside the syrinx. MRI can show the associated abnormalities, neuromeningeal or cerebellar.

There seems to be a significant correlation between the location of a segmental cavity in the spinal cord and the type of presenting symptomatology, but in case of a holocord cavity, the different type of signs may be distributed evently.[8]

Urinary signs

Neuro-urological disorders rarely reveal the development of a syringomyelia but are, on the contrary, regarded as a late symptomatology.[9] Nevertheless, they may be present at the time of the diagnosis and should be explored systematically, clinically, or through urodynamic studies. These urinary symptoms appeared after 5.3 years (ranging from 2 months to 13 years) from the occurrence of neurological symptoms in a Japanese study.[9] Neuro-urological signs readily coexist with bowel function and lower extremity abnormalities. Lower urinary tract dysfunction and spinal cord lesions may be suspected in patients with anorectal abnormalities: among 30 patients presenting with anorectal abnormalities, Taskinen et al[10] found 4 syringomyelias on systematic MRIs, with 2 normal on urodynamic evaluation and 2 overactive bladders.

The urinary signs are not specific most of the time, as they constitute a part of the lower syndrome syringomyelia, with an upper motor neuron bladder due to a suprasacral lesion. Their presentation is close to that of incomplete spinal cord lesions: urgency and eventually urge incontinence, pollakiuria, hesitancy, polyphasic micturition, occasional temporary urination impossibility, and even acute urine retention. Dysuria should provoke the search for other apparent causes such as prostate hypertrophy. Urodynamic studies argue in favor of such a spinal cord lesion, showing a poorly inhibited and/or dyssynergic bladder: lasting and ondulatory high contractions are evocative.

Extension of the cavity into the sacral gray matter can give rise to signs of lower motor neuron bladder. Blunted micturition need, impaired perception of urine flow, or a progressively growing functional capacity of the bladder with a lower micturitional frequency can correspond to decreased bladder sensitivity or reflexivity on urodynamic assessment. Acute urinary retention has been described as the first manifestation of syringomyelia and can possibly be triggered by a well-defined factor – the Valsalva maneuver – which would acutely create increased pressure within the intraspinal space and the syrinx,[11] or a pharmacological side-effect of cyproheptadine.[12]

These neurourological disorders will progress in the same way as the disease. Serious disease forms will then combine with other functional incapacities and loss of autonomy. Sakakibara et al,[9] studying 11 primary and 3 secondary syringomyelias, tried to find a relationship between micturitional disturbance and neurological signs. Besides detrusor hyperreflexia, common in patients with Babinski's sign (suprasacral lesion with pyramidal tract involvement), urinary disturbances (detrusor hyperreflexia or voiding difficulty) seem to be linked with other neurological deficiencies, especially disturbed sleep sensation.

Patients are determined to be candidates for treatment on the basis of their clinical status and MRI findings. Surgery of a primary syringomyelia may be complex because of associated malformations. It is difficult to separate symptoms attributed to the syrinx alone, and, when associated with syringomyelia, lipoma excision and cord untethering can, for instance, lead to a reduction in syrinx size: it is controversial whether syrinx cavities should be allowed to drain by themselves.[4] The main goal of surgery is, however, to at least stabilize progression of the symptoms.[8] According to Oakes (editorial comment to La Marca et al[8]) the smaller a symptomatic syrinx is at the time of initial treatment, the more likely a successful therapeutic intervention will be.

Secondary syringomyelia

Syringomyelia can occur without any malformations due to spinal cord pathologies: arachnoiditis, tumors, or overall post-traumatic condition (Figure 17.1). The neuro-urological status of SCI patients may change and raise suspicions of cavity occurrence.

Post-traumatic syringomyelia is defined as an intramedullary cavity that occurs secondarily to SCI. This etiology represents one-quarter of all syringomyelia cases. The incidence of post-traumatic syringomyelias is estimated to be 1.3–5%. Any spinal level can be affected by complete or incomplete lesions. The first clinical signs can occur between 2 months and 36 years.[13]

Etiopathogeny

Pathogenesis theories are still being discussed, but two phases (initial formation and cavity extension) have to be taken into account.

Initial formation of the cavity

The mechanisms that lead to syrinx occurrence are not unequivocal. One is a vascular mechanism, especially secondary necrosis of a myelomalacic zone and a direct action of lysosomal enzymes on the injured parenchyma. The other mechanism is arachnoiditis, which is responsible not only for ischemia but also for permanent stretching of the injured zone during spinal movements.

Cavity extension

This mechanism is a more mechanical one. Williams et al[14] proposed the most compelling theory with a main role for variations in venous pressures. Any rise in pressure of the abdominal or thoracic cavity is transmitted to the epidural veins, squeezing the spinal cord and pushing the eventual intracystic fluid upwards. It is called the 'slosh' effect, an energetic and upward pulsatile movement of fluid, with energy so significant that blockage occurs at the lesion site. These phenomena dissect the spinal cord at the extremities of the cavity where the spinal cord parenchyma is more fragile. The downward extension can be explained by another mechanism – slush – a negative pressure gradient in relation to the upward movement, making liquid enter the cavity.[15,16] The extensions are favored by arachnoiditis, a tethered spinal cord, or persistent compression (Figure 17.2).

Treatment of post-traumatic syringomyelia is essential in cases of intractable pain and progression of a motor deficit, but it may also include the management of canal stenosis and arachnoiditis.[17]

Clinical signs

Pain, the main sign, is often associated with paresthesiae and numbness; it is noted in more than one-half of patients: Rossier et al[18] reported pain in 17 out of 30 cases,

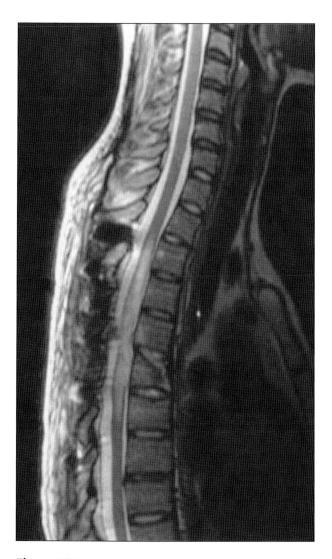

Figure 17.1
Post-traumatic syringomyelia.

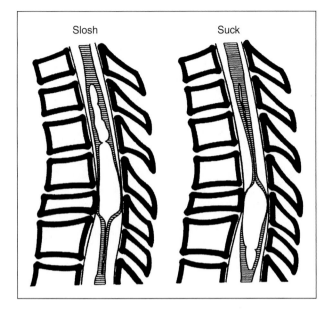

Figure 17.2
According to Williams' theory, secondary extension from the initial necrosis zone is a consequence of increased epidural venous pressure at the origin of intrachordal fluid movements. 'Slush' leads to rostral extension and breaks down the zones of structural weakness; 'slush' is the consequence of a pressure gradient at the origin of the caudal extension and filling of the cavity. These two phenomena are increased in the case of blockage in the subarachnoid space.[14] (Reproduced with permission from Macmillan Publishers Ltd.)

dysesthesia in 8, and motor deficiency in 7. This pain may be impulsive. The other signs are rarely inaugural and isolated. Most of the time, sensitive signs consist of thermoalgesic dissociation with preservation of tactile sensitivity and proprioception. Preservation of normal sensitivity between the injury level and the upper sensory signs is often found.[19] Rossier et al[18] described an ascending sensory level in 28/30 patients; this ascending sensory level is generally unilateral. Increased motor weakness above the level of the lesion and loss of reflexes are early signs that can also be found.[17]

Radiological signs

The diagnosis is also made by MRI, which can disclose the upper and lower levels, a multiloculated cavity, and intracystic turbulences. The signal criteria of syringomyelia are the same. Cross sections transversely localize the cavity in the spinal cord. Perrouin-Verbe et al[20] reported a mean extension of 3.5 segments in asymptomatic patients and 10 segments in symptomatic cases. The persistent bony compression has also been assessed in the genesis of post-traumatic syringomyelia.[17,21]

Urinary signs

The urinary signs are not specific for post-traumatic syringomyelia, but their occurrence in an SCI patient must make them suspect. Dysuria may worsen, due to increased detrusor-sphincter dyssynergia or decreased bladder reflectivity; reflex voiding may disappear. Fading of reflex erections, difficult ejaculation, or deterioration of autonomic dysreflexia can also constitute an alert. These signs of lower motoneuron bladder lead to MRI, in a way investigating the downward extension of the syringomyelic cavity.

Possible lesion evolution imposes neuro-urological follow-up in SCI patients. Clinical analysis must include determination of the level and flaccid or spastic character of the lesion, particularly in the sacral area. The mode of voiding and its eventual changes have to be assessed. Follow-up must be regular during the first 2 years; then, it should become annual, with clinical, urodynamic, and morphological studies. Less frequent follow-up can be discussed in case there is no significant risk factor.[17]

Conclusion

Primary or secondary syringomyelia consists of an evolutive spinal cord syndrome that can lead to lower urinary tract dysfunction. MRI can easily confirm the diagnosis if it has previously been suspected by systematic clinical examination, or directed by functional symptoms. Most of the urinary signs are not specific. Primary syringomyelias correspond to an upper motor neuron bladder (suprasacral lesion), and in the secondary forms, modification of the voiding mode may be due to extension of the cavity into the sacral level. Treatment indications have not yet been perfectly determined, but surgery is decided on the basis of the patient's clinical status and MRI findings.

References

1. Sichez JP, Capelle L. Syringomyélie. Editions techniques, EMC Neurologie, 17077A10, 4-1990.

2. Gardner WJ, Angel J. The mechanism of syringomyelia and its surgical correction. Clin Neurosurg 1959; 6:131–140.

3. Aboulker J. La syringomyélie et les liquides intra-rachidiens. Neurochirurgie (Paris) 1979; 25(S1):9–22.

4. Xenos C, Sgouros S, Walsh R, Hockley A. Spinal lipomas in children. Pediatr Neurosurg 2000; 32:295–307.

5. Anderson NE, Frith RW, Synek VM. Somatosensory evoked potentials in syringomyelia. J Neurol Neurosurg Psychiatry 1986; 49:1407–1410.

6. Wilberger JE, Maroon JC, Prostko ER, et al. Magnetic resonance imaging and intraoperative neurosonography in syringomyelia. Neurosurg 1987; 20:599–606.

7. Aubin ML, Baleriaux D, Cosnard G, et al. IRM dans les syringomyélies d'origine congénitale, infectieuse, traumatique ou idiopathique. A propos de 142 cas. J Neuroradiol (Paris) 1987; 14:313–336.

8. La Marca F, Herman M, Grant JA, MacLone DG. Presentation and management of hydromyelia in children with Chiari type II malformation. Pediatr Neurosurg 1997; 26:57–67.

9. Sakakibara R, Hattori T, Yasuda K, Yamanishi T. Micturitional disturbance in syringomyelia. J Neurol Sci 1996; 143:100–106.

10. Taskinen S, Valanne L, Rintala R. The effect of spinal cord abnormalities on the function of the lower urinary tract in patients with anorectal abnormalities. J Urol 2002; 168:1147–1149.

11. Amoiridis G, Meves S, Schöls L, Przuntek H. Reversible urinary retention as the main symptom in the first manifestation of a syringomyelia. J Neurol Neurosurg Psychiatry 1996; 61: 407–408.

12. Houang M, Leroy B, Forin V, et al. Rétention aiguë d'urines: un mode de révélation rare d'une syringomyélie cervicodorsale à l'occasion de la prise de cyproheptadine. Arch Pédiatrie (Paris) 1994; 1:260–263.

13. Umbach I, Heilporn A. Post spinal-cord injury syringomyelia. Review. Paraplegia 1991; 29:219–221.

14. Williams B, Terry AF, Jones HWF, McSweeney T. Syringomyelia as a sequel to traumatic paraplegia. Paraplegia 1981; 19:67–80.

15. MacLean DR, Miller JDR, Allen PBR, Ezzedin SA. Post traumatic syringomyelia. J Neurosurg 1973; 39:485–492.

16. Ball MJ, Dayan AD. Pathogenesis of syringomyelia. Lancet 1972; 2:799–800.

17. Perrouin-Verbe B, Lenne-Aurier K, Robert R, et al. Post-traumatic syringomyelia and post-traumatic spinal canal stenosis: a direct relationship: review of 75 patients with a spinal cord injury. Spinal Cord 1998; 36:137–143.

18. Rossier AB, Foo D, Shillito J, Dyro FM. Post traumatic cervical syringomyelia: incidence, clinical presentation, electrological studies, syrinx protein and results of conservative and operative treatment. Brain 1985; 108:439–461.

19. Vernon JD, Silver JR, Ohry A. Post traumatic syringomyelia. Paraplegia 1982; 20:339–364.

20. Perrouin-Verbe B, Robert R, Le Fort M, et al. Syringomyélie post-traumatique. Neurochirurgie (Paris) 1999; 45(S1):58–66.

21. Schurch B, Wichmann W, Rossier AB. Post-traumatic syringomyelia (cystic myelopathy): a prospective study of 449 patients with spinal cord injury. J Neurol Neurosurg Psychiatry 1996; 60:61–67.

18

Systemic illnesses: (diabetes mellitus, sarcoidosis, alcoholism and porphyrias)

Ditlev Jensen and Bjørn Klevmark

This chapter on peripheral neuropathies comprises four systemic illnesses. Among these diseases, diabetes mellitus is the only one where neurogenic bladder is a well-known complication. Hence, there is a summary after the diabetes mellitus section, and a short conclusion at the end of the chapter.

Diabetes mellitus

There are two types of idiopathic or primary diabetes mellitus (diabetes). Type I requires treatment with insulin. Type II usually occurs at an older age and can be treated without insulin. The two types seem to be equally susceptible to complications, which are similar for both.[1]

The prevalence of diabetes among adults is difficult to ascertain, but is probably around 1%. The prevalence of both types is increasing worldwide. However, a more rapid increase in type II is expected in the future.[2–5] Among school-age children in the USA the prevalence of type I is 1.9 per 1000. It is increasing with age, from 1 in 1430 children at age 5 to 1 in 360 at age 16; both sexes are almost equally affected. In western Europe the prevalence among children is markedly highest in Denmark and Finland.[6]

Complications

The main complications are the vascular and the neurogenic ones; the latter are probably the most common.[3] Diabetic neuropathy occurs throughout the world, and is equally distributed among men and women. Available information indicates a prevalence of about 50% for patients with diabetes of 25 years' duration. Neuropathy is present in less than 10% when diabetes is discovered.[7] In children the most common complication is peripheral neuropathy, which was found in 11% of diabetic patients from 8 to 15 years of age.[8]

Table 18.1 *Clinical syndromes of diabetic peripheral neuropathy*

Mononeuropathy of cranial, trunk, or limb nerves
Mononeuropathia multiplex
Painful lumbosacral radiculoplexus neuropathy
Atrophic lumbosacral radiculoplexus neuropathy (diabetic amyotrophy)
Symmetrical lower limb proximal neuropathy
Symmetrical upper and lower limb distal polyneuropathy (most common)
Autonomic neuropathy
Mixed forms

Diabetic peripheral neuropathy can be separated into eight clinical syndromes (Table 18.1).[9–11] Autonomic neuropathy is the cause of the neurogenic bladder. It is often combined with one of the other syndromes, most often with the symmetrical upper and lower limb distal polyneuropathy. In that case the clinical manifestations of autonomic neuropathy usually appear at a later stage than those of the other syndromes.

Peripheral innervation

The lower urinary tract has autonomic innervation of the bladder and urethra, and somatic innervation of the striated part of the urethral wall and of the striated periurethral sphincter (m. pubococcygeus). In peripheral neuropathies only lesions of the parasympathetic nerves to the bladder (nn. pelvici) will result in a neurogenic bladder. Both the afferent and efferent arms of the micturition reflex are located in the pelvic nerves. Lesions of somatic nerves (n. pudendalis) can influence voiding by changing the striated sphincter function. Lesions of the sympathetic nerves (nn. hypogastrici) can alter tension in the bladder neck and urethra. Sympathectomy in humans does not change the clinical pattern of voiding. Peripheral local reflexes and feedback mechanisms can be disturbed by peripheral neuropathies.

Pathological anatomy and pathogenesis

In the diabetic autonomic neuropathy, neuron degeneration as well as neurons with vacuoles and granular deposits is found. There is a loss of myelinated nerve fibers in the vagus and splanchnic nerves, and a neuronal loss in the spinal cord intermediolateral columns.[10] Alterations such as beading, thickening, and fragmentation of postganglionic sympathetic axons adjacent to the bladder have been demonstrated.[12] Also shown is a reduced density of acetylcholinesterase-positive-staining nerves in the bladder wall.[13]

The pathogenesis of the neuropathological changes is related to the functional state of the vasa nervorum. If these are blocked by atherosclerosis, ischemia is the cause of the degenerative changes. If the vessels are open, another pathological nerve metabolism will take place. Three hypotheses have been put forward to explain how hyperglycemia may lead to chronic complications in diabetes.[14] The first hypothesis suggests that increased intracellular glucose gives rise to an advanced glycosylation end product that crosslinks proteins, accelerates atherosclerosis, promotes glomerular dysfunction and, induces endothelial dysfunction. The second hypothesis assumes that in the state of increased intracellular glucose, some of the glucose is converted to sorbitol. This substance acts as a tissue toxin, and may be a factor in the pathogenesis of retinopathy, neuropathy, cataracts, nephropathy, and aortic disease.[2,14] The third hypothesis proposes that hyperglycemia increases the formation of diacylglycerol, leading to activation of isoforms of protein kinase C, which in turn alters, among others, extracellular matrix proteins in endothelial cells and neurons. Whether the same pathophysiological processes are responsible for all complications, or whether certain processes predominate in certain organs is not fully understood.[14]

No exact prevalence of the diabetic neurogenic bladder (diabetic cystopathy) is available.[15] In different studies, the figures vary between 20 and 80%,[16] and are by other authors even quoted as between 2 and 83%.[17] Most patients with a diabetic neurogenic bladder show prominent signs of other long-term diabetic complications.[15]

Little information has been obtained on the diabetic neurogenic bladder among children. The few cases found are anecdotal.[18,19]

Examinations

To diagnose dysfunction of the lower urinary tract, some or all of the investigations shown in Table 18.2 may be necessary. The bladder symptoms have an insidious onset, characterized by a progressive failure of bladder emptying. Sensory nerve function is usually impaired at an early stage. Patients are not adequately warned to empty the bladder, and a situation occurs which leads to increased voiding intervals and difficult initiation. This can sometimes result in large volumes of residual urine with chronic retention (overflow incontinence). Males may already have noticed an impairment of erection before the occurrence of bladder symptoms.[17,20–24]

In diabetes, isolated autonomic neuropathy is rare. Most common is the mixed form. At the clinical neurourological investigation of this condition, a diminished superficial and deep sensation may be found in the lower limbs and in the perianal region. Knee and ankle jerks are depressed or wholly absent, and a similar lack of reaction is found in the anal skin reflex and the bulbocavernosus reflex. The digital exploration of the rectum may show a reduced external anal sphincter tonus, with no response to cough and voluntary contraction.

In cases of reduced sensory function the frequency volume chart will show either infrequent voiding of large volumes or frequent voiding of small volumes (chronic retention of urine). Residual urine is measured with ultrasonography. If spontaneous uroflowmetry is not normal

Table 18.2 *Neurogenic bladder: examinations*
History
Clinical examination
Frequency volume chart
Residual urine
Uroflowmetry
Uroflowmetry with rectal pressure recording
Pressure flow study
Cystometry
Ambulatory monitoring
Urethral pressure profile
Electromyography
Evoked responses
Urethrocystoscopy
Ultrasonography
Radiology (urography, micturition urethrocystography)

a flowmetry with rectal pressure recording should be done. This can demonstrate the use of abdominal straining during voiding (Figures 18.1 and 18.2). To evaluate the

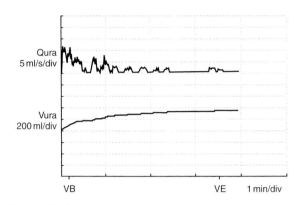

Figure 18.1 Uroflowmetry. Emptying with interrupted flow (Q ura) causing a prolonged voiding time of 216 sec. The voided volume (V ura) is 341 ml, maximum flow rate 12.5 ml/sec, average flow rate 3.0 ml/sec and residual urine 118 ml. VB: void begins, VE: void ends. Prolonged interrupted voiding in a patient with sensory hypoactive neurogenic bladder. Same patient as in Figures 18.3 and 18.4.

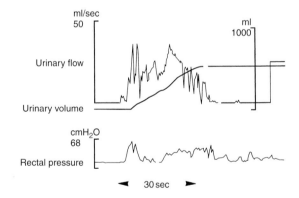

Figure 18.2 Uroflowmetry with rectal pressure measurement. Voiding starts with abdominal straining and continues with a combinaition of detrusor contraction and abdominal straining. Most probably motor hypoactive neurogenic bladder.

strength of detrusor and a bladder outlet obstruction, a pressure flow study is necessary. Cystometry has been performed as conventional cystometry, usually with a filling rate of 50 ml/min.[25,26] However, conventional cystometry is a less-sensitive method than filling at physiological rates.[25] Therefore, the Standardisation Sub-Committee of the International Continence Society recommends that filling rates are divided into physiological and non-physiological rates.[26] The usual finding in a patient with a diabetic neurogenic bladder is a sensory hypoactive bladder with

desire to void at a much larger volume than normal, and often reduced detrusor activity (Figure 18.3).

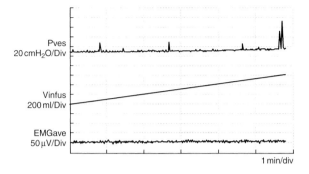

Figure 18.3 Cystometrogram with electromyography. Cystometry with filling rate 100 ml per minute. Moderate intravesical pressure rise (P ves) of 10 cm H_2O at 600 ml of filling (V infus). Filling stopped. No feeling of filling and no detrusor contraction. Small artifacts due to coughing. The electromyographic activity from the periurethral sphincter (female patient) is minimal and does not show the normal increase during filling (concentric needle recording, integrated signal, EMG ave). Sensory hypoactive neurogenic bladder with peripheral neurogenic striated muscle affection.

However, some elderly diabetic patients have suffered vascular complications affecting the brain or the spinal cord above the conus medullaris. In such cases the central nervous lesion may cause increased tendon reflexes and neurogenic detrusor overactivity.[27]

The urethral pressure profile is usually normal. When the striated muscles of the external anal sphincter, the male bulbocavernosus muscle, and the female periurethral muscle, are investigated with needle electrode electromyography, denervation potentials can be demonstrated (Figure 18.4).

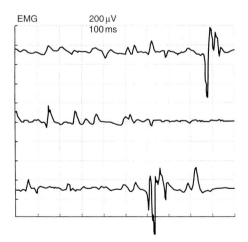

Figure 18.4 Denervation potentials. Concentric needle electromyographic (EMG) recording from the female periurethral sphincter. Two bursts of polyphasic denervation potentials are consistent with peripheral neurogenic striated muscle affection.

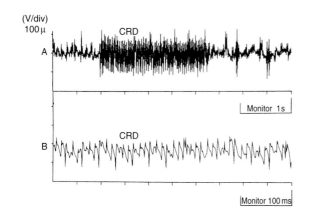

Figure 18.5 Pseudomyotonic electromyographic activity. Concentric needle electromyography from the periurethral female sphincter. A: The normal resting activity is interrupted by bursts of complex repetitive discharges (CRD) of almost regular amplitude and rate. B: The CRD potentials depicted at high speed monitoring. The finding is consistent with peripheral neurogenic striated muscle affection.

Pseudomyotonic activity may also be a sign of peripheral nerve affection of the pelvic floor muscles (Figures 18 and 18.5).[28] The latency of the first component of the evoked bulbocavernosus reflex is delayed only in patients with an advanced peripheral neuropathy. This reflex investigation only assesses conduction velocity in somatic nerves, not in autonomic fibers.[29,30] In men, during urethrocystoscopy, at a level just below the pelvic floor, the voluntary and reflex contraction of the periurethral striated sphincter can be visually evaluated. The bladder wall is usually smooth without trabeculation. The bladder neck may be open or closed. Ultrasonography gives information about the caliber of the upper urinary tract, and the size, form, and consistency (cysts) of the kidney. Urography may often be a necessary screening investigation of the kidneys and the upper urinary tract. Vesicoureteral reflux can, however, only be demonstrated by micturition urethrocystography (MUCG).

Autonomic neuropathy in a patient with diabetes can have many other etiologies. The main groups of such conditions are metabolic, infectious, spinal, and degenerative. Examples are vitamin B12 deficiencies, herpes infections, lumbar disc prolapse, and multiple system atrophy.[31] Therefore, a detailed case history and thorough clinical examination is mandatory.

Summary

Diabetic peripheral neuropathy has eight clinical syndromes. Autonomic neuropathy is the cause of the diabetic neurogenic bladder, and results from pathological metabolic processes in the parasympathetic pelvic nerves. The bladder is usually sensory hypoactive and, to a lesser degree, motor hypoactive. Clinical neuro-urological and urodynamic investigations show characteristic findings. However, many other etiologies than diabetes are possible.

Sarcoidosis

Sarcoidosis, known as Mb. Boeck or Besnier–Boeck–Schaumann disease [Boeck, Caesar, 1808–1875, Professor of Dermatology, Christiania (Oslo)],[32] is a relatively common disease that affects individuals of both sexes, and most all ages, races, and geographical locations. Females seem to be slightly more susceptible than males.[33] Among adults, the prevalence is from 10 to 40 per 100,000 in both the USA and Europe. A high prevalence is found in the Netherlands, Great Britain, and the Scandinavian countries.[34] The peak incidence in both sexes is around the age of 25–30 years. The disease is infrequent below the age of 15, and especially below 9 years of age. It is estimated that about 6% of all affected by the disease are children.[35]

Sarcoidosis is a chronic, multisystem disorder of unknown etiology. Characteristics are an accumulation of lymphocytes and mononuclear phagocytes, noncaseating epithelioid granulomas, as well as derangements of the normal tissue architecture. All the body organs can be affected; the lungs, however, are most frequently affected.[33] In adults, the prevalence of neurogenic involvement is 5%.[10] The proportion of peripheral nervous involvement is 25–50%.[34,36] In some rare cases, multiple sarcoidosis lesions can clinically mimic multiple sclerosis or spinal cord abnormalities.[33] Neurosarcoidosis is unusual in children,[37] but the precise prevalence is not known.[38]

The pathological findings in peripheral nerves are scattered perineural changes and sarcoid granuloma infiltration between nerve fibers,[34,36] giving rise to practically all types of nerve involvement. This includes isolated mononeuritis, mononeuritis multiplex, progressive lesion of the cauda equina, and polyneuropathy. This type of neuropathy is most consistent with axonal degeneration with a multifocal pattern.[39]

If the autonomic nerves innervating the lower urinary tract are affected, a neurogenic bladder, as described in the section on diabetes mellitus, can occur. Likewise, if the central nervous system is affected, a detrusor overactivity can be found. Only few cases of neurogenic bladder due to neurosarcoidosis have been reported: two patients suffered from neurogenic detrusor overactivity with detrusor-sphincter dyssynergia caused by thoracic intramedullary lesions; one patient had neurogenic detrusor overactivity without dyssynergia due to a cervical lesion, and an autonomic dysreflexia as well.[40–42]

Alcoholism

The drinking of ethanol (alcohol) is a universal behavior, and is performed by 90% of all people. One definition of alcoholism (the primary type) is when there is physical evidence that alcohol has harmed a person's health, including signs of an alcoholic withdrawal syndrome.[43] Alcoholism is seen in all races, ethnic, and socioeconomic groups. The exact prevalence of alcoholism is, however, difficult to determine. An estimate is that 10 million men and women in the USA, or approximately 10% of the nation's labor force, has a drinking problem.[44] In addition to the ethanol, the congeners found in alcoholic beverages which may contribute to body injuries with heavy drinking are methanol, butanol, aldehydes, esters, histamine, phenols, tannins, iron, lead, and cobalt.[43]

Alcohol-related neurological disorders affect the brain, brainstem, cerebellum, and the peripheral nerves. Polyneuropathy is the most common chronic disease,[45] affecting 5–15% of alcoholics.[43] The precise prevalence is unknown. In some reports men and women seem to be nearly equally affected, even though three-quarters of alcoholics are men, which suggests that women may be more susceptible to alcoholic polyneuropathy than men.[46] Polyneuropathy is a result of thiamine deficiency and/or a direct toxic effect of ethanol and acetaldehyde.[43]

Alcoholic polyneuropathy usually presents as a gradual development of a distal, symmetrical, sensoric, and motoric disease. Axonal degeneration, as well as segmental demyelination, are main factors in this pathological process.[3,45] The degenerative process is most intense in the distal direction; the nerve roots are spared, except in advanced cases. Unmyelinated fibers are also involved.[9] A loss of sympathetic and parasympathetic nerve fibers as well as ganglion neurons have also been observed.[47]

Clinical manifestations of autonomic dysfunction are unusual in uncomplicated alcoholic peripheral neuropathy.[48] References to affection of the lower urinary tract are sparse.[22,23] If neurogenic bladder occurs, a clinical neuro-urological and urodynamic investigation will show the same findings as for diabetic neurogenic bladder.

Porphyrias

Porphyrias comprise a group of eight hereditary disorders – five hepatic and three erythropoietic – with porphyrin accumulation in either the hepatic or erythropoietic tissues. This disease is due to inherent or acquired disturbances in heme biosynthesis. Each of the eight types is characterized by a specific pattern of overproduction, accumulation, and excretion of metabolic products of heme biosynthesis. In the acute hepatic porphyrias, an overproduction of porphyrin precursors occurs, whereas the substance is porphyrin in the cutaneous types.[7,49–51] Neurological symptoms are present in four of the hepatic porphyrias: delta-aminolevulinic acid dehydratase deficient porphyria (ADP), intermittent acute porphyria (IAP), variegate porphyria (VP), and hereditary coproporphyria

(HCP). The two latter types also have cutaneous manifestations. ADP is an autosomal recessive disorder described in only a few patients. The three other hepatic types in question are transmitted as autosomal dominant disorders. The acute attacks of symptoms are similar, often precipitated by intake of a number of different drugs, including barbiturates, estrogens, contraceptives, sulfonamides, griseofulvin, meprobamate, phenytoin, valproic acid, steroids, and succinamides. Alcohol, starvation, infections, and fever may also give rise to the attacks.[49,52]

IAP (Swedish porphyria) is the most common of the three relevant hepatic types with neurogenic affection, occurring worldwide with a prevalence estimated to be between 1 in 5000 and 1 in 50,000. This type of disorder becomes clinically manifest after puberty, with an onset usually between 20 and 50 years of age. It is far more frequent in females (65%) than in males (35%). The highest prevalence occurs in Scandinavia and the United Kingdom.[49,50,53] VP (South African genetic porphyria) has a higher prevalence of 3 in 1000 in South Africa than elsewhere. Affected individuals in South Africa have been identified as descendants of a Dutch female settler who immigrated in 1688. The disease is, however, distributed worldwide. It is probably less common than IAP, and has no racial or geographic predilection.[49,50] HCP seems to occur less frequently than IAP, but since the disease is more gentle and more likely to express itself only in a latent form, the true frequency is difficult to ascertain. Racial predilections are unknown.[50,54]

In rapidly fatal cases the central and peripheral nervous systems may be without traceable pathological lesions. Otherwise, patchy areas of demyelination with or without destruction of the axis cylinders can be observed throughout the nervous system. Chromolysis may appear in the neurons of the anterior horns, in the cranial nerve nuclei, the spinal ganglia, and the cerebral cortex. The most dramatic changes will, however, be seen in the peripheral nerves and supporting cells. Here, a degeneration of the axons with secondary demyelination is found, whereas inflammatory or vascular lesions are lacking.[10,53,54] Autonomic function studies have demonstrated abnormalities of both sympathetic and parasympathetic nerves.[55]

Clinical symptoms are similarly distributed in the three types of porphyrias in question. Recurrent attacks are reported to last from days to months, varying in frequency and severity. The main features are initial abdominal pain, psychotic symptoms, peripheral acute or subacute proximal or distal polyneuropathy or mononeuritis multiplex, trunkal sensory loss, and the excretion of colorless porphyrinogens in urine, turning red or purple when exposed to light and air.[7,10,49,54] The most common manifestations, including abdominal pain, however, are a result of autonomic neuropathy. Other symptoms, due to autonomic failure include tachycardia, postural hypotension,

Table 18.3 *Autonomic neuropathies which may cause neurogenic bladder*

Disorders without associated somatic peripheral neuropathy: primary disorders
- Acute and subacute autonomic neuropathy
  - Pure pandysautonomia
  - Pure cholinergic dysautonomia
- Chronic
  - Pure autonomic failure

Disorders associated with somatic peripheral neuropathy: secondary disorders
- Hereditary
  - Amyloid disease (also secondary amyloidosis)
  - Porphyrias
- Metabolic
  - Diabetes mellitus
  - Chronic renal failure
  - Chronic hepatic failure
  - Vitamin B12 deficiency
- Alcoholism and nutritional disorders
- Sarcoidosis
- Connective tissue disorders: immune-complex diseases?
  - Systemic lupus erythematosus
  - Rheumatoid arthritis
  - Mixed connective tissue disease
  - The vasculitis syndromes
- Malignancy: paraneoplastic remote effect of cancer
- Toxins
  - Antineoplastic agents, certain other drugs, heavy metals, organic solvents

hypertension, fever, sweating, retinal artery spasm, and urinary retention.[53] In two female patients with porphyria and acute urinary retention cystoscopy was normal, whereas the cystometrogram shifted to the right.[56] The same diagnostic considerations as described for diabetic neurogenic bladder apply for the porphyrias.

Conclusion

Autonomic neuropathy with neurogenic bladder has only rarely been shown in sarcoidosis, alcoholism, and porphyrias. Different classifications of autonomic neuropathy are accounted for in tabular versions.[10,23,48,57,58] A selection relevant for this chapter is given in Table 18.3.

Acknowledgment

The preparation of the sections on diabetes mellitus, sarcoidosis, alcoholism and porphyrias has included a database search in Ovid Medline for the period 1966 to May 2002. Few findings concerning items of interest for our purpose were found. Various other sources gave the information used herein.

References

1. Windebank AJ, McEvoy KM. Diabetes and the nervous system. In: Aminoff MJ, ed. Neurology and general medicine. New York: Churchill Livingstone, 1989:273–304.

2. Foster DW. Diabetes mellitus. In: Braunwald E, Isselbacher KJ, Petersdorf RG, et al, eds. Harrison's principles of internal medicine, 11th edn. New York: McGraw-Hill, 1987:1778–1797.

3. Bosch EP, Mitsumoto H. Disorders of peripheral nerves, plexuses, and nerve roots. In: Bradley WG, Daroff RB, Fenichel GM, Marsden CD, eds. Neurology in clinical practice. Boston: Butterworth-Heinemann, 1991:1719–1818.

4. Herman WH, Sinnock P, Brenner E, et al. An epidemiologic model for diabetes mellitus: incidence, prevalence, and mortality. Diabetes Care 1984; 7:367–371.

5. Powers AC. Diabetes mellitus. In: Braunwald E, Fauci AS, Kasper DL, et al, eds. Harrison's principles of internal medicine, 15th edn. New York: McGraw-Hill, 2001:2109–2137.

6. Sperling MA. Diabetes mellitus. In: Behrman RE, Kliegman RM, Jenson HB, eds. Nelson textbook of pediatrics, 16th edn. Philadelphia: WB Saunders, 2000:1767–1791.

7. Schaumburg HH, Berger AR, Thomas PK, eds. Disorders of peripheral nerves, 2nd edn. Philadelphia: FA Davis, 1992.

8. Eeg-Olofsson O, Petersen I. Childhood diabetic neuropathy. Acta Ped Scand 1966; 53:163–167.

9. Dyck PJ, Low PA, Stevens JC. Diseases of peripheral nerves. In: Joynt RJ, ed. Clinical neurology. Philadelphia: JB Lippincott, 1990:1–126.

10. Adams RD, Victor M, Ropper AH. Principles of neurology, 6th edn. New York: McGraw-Hill, 1997.

11. Thomas PK, Tomlinson DR. Diabetic and hypoglycemic neuropathy. In: Dyck PJ, Thomas PK, Griffin JW, et al, eds. Peripheral neuropathy, 3rd edn. Philadelphia: WB Saunders, 1993:1219–1250.

12. Low PA, Dyck PJ. Pathologic studies and the nerve biopsy in autonomic neuropathies. In: Low PA, ed. Clinical autonomic disorders. Boston: Little, Brown, 1993:331–344.

13. Faerman I, Glocer L, Celener D, et al. Autonomic nervous system and diabetes. Histological and histochemical study of the autonomic nerve fibers of the urinary bladder in diabetic patients. Diabetes 1973; 22:225–237.

14. Powers AC. Diabetes mellitus. In: Braunwald E, Fauci AS, Kasper DL, et al, eds. Harrison's principles of internal medicine, 15th edn. New York: McGraw-Hill, 2001:2109–2137.

15. Frimodt-Møller C. Diabetic cystopathy I: A clinical study of the frequency of bladder dysfunction in diabetics. Dan Med Bul 1976; 23:267–278.

16. Hilsted J, Low PA. Diabetic autonomic neuropathy. In: Low PA, ed. Clinical autonomic disorders. Boston: Little, Brown, 1993:423–443.

17. Bors E, Comarr AE. Neurological urology. Basel: S. Karger, 1971.

18. Ouvrier RA. Peripheral neuropathy. In: Berg BO, ed. Principles of child neurology. New York: McGraw-Hill, 1996:1607–1655.

19. Garg BP. Disorders of micturition and defecation. In: Swaiman KF, ed. Pediatric neurology, principles and practice, 2nd edn. St Louis: Mosby, 1994:271–284.

20. Hopkins WF, Pierce JM. The neurogenic bladder in diabetes mellitus. In: Boyarsky S, ed. The neurogenic bladder. Baltimore: Williams and Wilkins, 1967:155–157.

21. Kendall AR, Karafin L. Classification of neurogenic bladder disease. In: Lapides J, ed. Symposium on neurogenic bladder. The urologic clinics of North America. Philadelphia: WB Saunders, 1974:37–44.

22. Bradley WE. Neurologic disorders affecting the urinary bladder. In: Krane RJ, Siroky MB, eds. Clinical neuro-urology. Boston: Little, Brown, 1979:245–255.

23. Hald T, Bradley WE. The urinary bladder, neurology and dynamics. Baltimore: Williams and Wilkins, 1982.

24. Dasgupta P, Thomas PK. Peripheral neuropathy. In: Fowler CJ, ed. Neurology of bladder, bowel, and sexual dysfunction. Boston: Butterworth-Heinemann, 1999:339–352.

25. Klevmark B. Natural pressure–volume curves and conventional cystometry. Scand J Urol Nephrol 1999; Suppl 201:1–4.

26. Abrams P, Cardozo L, Fall M, et al. The standardisation of terminology of lower urinary tract function: Report from the Standardisation Sub-Committee of the International Continence Society. Neurourol Urodyn 2002; 21:167–178.

27. Starer P, Libow L. Cystometric evaluation of bladder dysfunction in elderly diabetic patients. Arch Intern Med 1990; 150:810–813.

28. Jensen D, Stien R. The importance of complex repetitive discharges in the striated female urethral sphincter and the male bulbocavernosus muscle. Scand J Urol Nephrol 1996; 30(Suppl 179):69–73.

29. Vodusek DB, Fowler CJ. Clinical neurophysiology. In: Fowler CJ, ed. Neurology of bladder, bowel, and sexual dysfunction. Boston: Butterworth-Heinemann, 1999:109–143.

30. Beck RO. Investigation of male erectile dysfunction. In: Fowler CJ, ed. Neurology of bladder, bowel, and sexual dysfunction. Boston: Butterworth-Heinemann, 1999:145–160.

31. Appel RA, Whiteside HV. Diabetes and other peripheral neuropathies affecting lower urinary tract function. In: Krane RJ, Siroky MB, eds. Clinical neuro-urology, 2nd edn. Boston: Little, Brown, 1991: 365–373.

32. Boeck C. Multiple benign sarcoid of the skin. J Cutan Genitourin Dis 1899; 17:543.

33. Crystal RG. Sarcoidosis. In: Braunwald E, Isselbacher KJ, Petersdorf RG, et al, eds. Harrison's principles of internal medicine, 11th edn. New York: McGraw-Hill, 1987:1445–1450.

34. Silberberg DH. Sarcoidosis of the nervous system. In: Aminoff MJ, ed. Neurology and general medicine. New York: Churchill Livingstone, 1989:701–712.

35. Dyken PR. Neurosarcoidosis. In: Berg BO, ed. Principles of child neurology. New York: McGraw-Hill, 1996:889–899.

36. Matthews WB. Sarcoid neuropathy. In: Dyck PJ, Thomas PK, Griffin JW, et al, eds. Peripheral neuropathy, 3rd edn. Philadelphia: WB Saunders, 1993:1418–1423.

37. Weil ML, Levin M. Infections of the nervous system. In: Menkes JH, ed. Textbook of child neurology, 5th edn. Baltimore: Williams and Wilkins, 1995:379–509.

38. Ashwal S, Schneider S. Neurologic complications of vasculitic disorders of childhood. In: Swaiman KF, ed. Pediatric neurology, principles and practice, 2nd edn. St Louis: Mosby, 1994:841–863.

39. Scott TS, Brillman J, Gross JA. Sarcoidosis of the peripheral nervous system. Neurol Res 1993; 15:389–390.

40. Fitzpatrick KJ, Chancellor MB, Rivas DA, et al. Urologic manifestation of spinal cord sarcoidosis. J Spinal Cord Med 1996; 19:201–203.

41. Kim IY, Elliott DS, Husmann DA, Boone TB. An unusual presenting symptom of sarcoidosis: neurogenic bladder dysfunction. J Urol 2001; 165:903–904.

42. Sakakibara R, Uchiyama T, Kuwabara S, et al. Autonomic dysreflexia due to neurogenic bladder dysfunction; an unusual presentation of spinal cord sarcoidosis. [Letter] J Neurol Neurosurg Psychiatry 2001; 71:819–820.

43. Schuckit MA. Alcohol and alcoholism. In: Braunwald E, Isselbacher KJ, Petersdorf RG, et al, eds. Harrison's principles of internal medicine, 11th edn. New York: McGraw-Hill, 1987:2106–2111.

44. Victor M. Neurologic disorders due to alcoholism and malnutrition. In: Joynt RJ, ed. Clinical neurology. Philadelphia: JB Lippincott, 1990:1–94.

45. Messing RO, Greenberg DA. Alcohol and the nervous system. In: Aminoff MJ, ed. Neurology and general medicine. New York: Churchill Livingstone, 1989:533–547.

46. Layzer RB. Neuromuscular manifestations of systemic disease. Philadelphia: FA Davis, 1985.

47. Windebank AJ. Polyneuropathy due to nutritional deficiency and alcoholism. In: Dyck PJ, Thomas PK, Griffin JW, et al, eds. Peripheral neuropathy, 3rd edn. Philadelphia: WB Saunders, 1993:1310–1321.

48. McLeod JG. Autonomic dysfunction in peripheral nerve disease. In: Bannister R (Sir Roger), Mathias CJ, eds. Autonomic failure, 3rd edn. Oxford: Oxford University Press, 1993:659–681.

49. Meyer UA. Porphyrias. In: Braunwald E, Isselbacher KJ, Petersdorf RG, et al, eds. Harrison's principles of internal medicine, 11th edn. New York: McGraw-Hill, 1987:1638–1643.

50. Sassa S. The porphyrias. In: Behrman RE, Kliegman RM, Jenson HB, eds. Nelson textbook of pediatrics, 16th edn. Philadelphia: WB Saunders, 2000:430–439.

51. Desnick RJ. The porphyrias. In: Braunwald E, Fauci AS, Kasper DL, et al, eds. Harrison's principles of internal medicine, 15th edn. New York: McGraw-Hill, 2001:2261–2267.

52. Evans OB, Bock H-GO, Parker C, Hanson RR. Inborn errors of metabolism of the nervous system. In: Bradley WG, Daroff RB, Fenichel GM, Marsden CD, eds. Neurology in clinical practice. Boston: Butterworth-Heinemann, 1991:1269–1322.

53. Glaser GH, Pincus JH. Neurologic complications of internal disease. In: Joynt RJ, ed. Clinical neurology. Philadelphia: JB Lippincott, 1990:1–57.

54. Windebank AJ, Bonkovsky HL. Porphyric neuropathy. In: Dyck PJ, Thomas PK, Griffin JW, et al, eds. Peripheral neuropathy, 3rd edn. Philadelphia: WB Saunders, 1993:1161–1168.

55. Yeung Laiwah AC, Macphee GJA, Boye P, et al. Autonomic neuropathy in acute intermittent porhyria. J Neurol Neurosurg Psychiat 1985; 48:1025–1030.

56. Redeker AG. Atonic neurogenic bladder in porphyria. J Urol 1956; 75:465–469.

57. Low PA, McLeod JG. The autonomic neuropathies. In: Low PA, ed. Clinical autonomic disorders. Boston: Little, Brown, 1993:395–421.

58. Mathias CJ. Autonomic neuropathy: aspects of diagnosis and management. In: Asbury AK, Thomas PK, eds. Peripheral nerve disorders 2. Oxford: Butterworth-Heinemann, 1998:95–117.

19

Other peripheral neuropathies (lumbosacral zoster, genitourinary herpes, tabes dorsalis, Guillain–Barré syndrome)

Vincent WM Tse and Anthony R Stone

Introduction

Peripheral neuropathy is a rare but significant cause of storage and voiding dysfunction. An adequate working knowledge of the underlying pathophysiology, clinical presentation, diagnosis, and management of such a dysfunction are essential in any urologist's armamentarium. The neuropathy affecting the bladder often takes the form of an autonomic neuropathy, which may involve both the sympathetic and parasympathetic, as well as afferent and efferent, innervation of the bladder and urethra, leading to alteration of bladder sensation, the sacral reflex arc, detrusor-sphincter synergy, and detrusor contractility. The cause of the neuropathy can be metabolic, iatrogenic, traumatic, infective, or immunological. The focus of this chapter is on the infective and immunological disorders which may lead to peripheral neuropathy: namely, lumbosacral herpes zoster, genitourinary herpes simplex, tabes dorsalis, and Guillain–Barré syndrome.

Neuropathic bladder associated with infection by the herpes virus family

The herpes virus family consists of DNA viruses which are relatively large and made up of 162 cylindrical capsomeres. Four members of this family affect humans: namely, herpesvirus hominis (herpes simplex virus type 1 and 2), herpes varicellae (varicella-zoster virus), cytomegalovirus, and infectious mononucleosis virus. The first two types are more commonly encountered clinically. However, with respect to neuropathic bladder dysfunction, varicella-zoster infection is a more common cause than anogenital herpes simplex (type 2), although the latter can present with acute urinary retention as a result of micturitional pain rather than a direct viral neurogenic inflammation.[1] Cytomegalovirus and infectious mononucleosis have not been reported to cause neuropathic bladder dysfunction.

Lumbosacral herpes zoster

Pathophysiology

Herpes zoster is a varicella-zoster virus infection manifested by circumscribed painful vesicular eruption of the skin and mucous membrane. Urinary retention afflicts 3.5% of patients with active herpes zoster infection, and is most commonly seen in infection of the sacral dorsal root ganglia (78%), followed by thoracolumbar (11%), and higher thoracic levels (11%).[2] The urinary retention typically presents concurrently with or within a few days following the onset of the rash,[3] and is thought to be due to a sensory neuropathy from inflammatory reaction in the dorsal nerve roots and ganglia, which spreads proximally and distally to the sacral segments of the cord, with interruption of the micturition reflex.[4] If the sacral micturition center is involved, a parasympathetic motor neuropathy may also contribute to the urinary retention.[5] In herpes zoster affecting the thoracic and lumbar segments, urinary retention has been explained by activation of the lumbar sympathetic outflow, resulting in increased tone of the bladder neck and internal urethral sphincter.[6] Virus particles and neurotropic factors have been identified in neurons and supporting satellite cells in the sensory ganglia and within peripheral sensory nerves of the corresponding dermatome, thus explaining the origin of the dermatomal distribution of the rash and associated pain.[7] The virus may also cause inflammation of the spinal cord,[8] which may manifest as a myelitic disorder of the long tracts.[9]

Clinical features

Herpes zoster infections can occur sporadically in healthy subjects with previous exposure to varicella (chickenpox), or in the immunocompromised, most notably the elderly, diabetics, transplant patients, and patients with the acquired immunodeficiency syndrome (AIDS). A distinctive feature is the localization of the rash, which may involve one or two, and sometimes more, adjacent dermatomes. Those with bladder involvement usually have a classical zoster skin eruption in a sacral dermatomal distribution, typically affecting one or more of adjacent S2, S3, or S4 areas. The lesions can be either unilateral or bilateral, though the former predominates. In unilateral skin or bladder mucosal involvement, bilateral depression of the reflex arc, resulting in urinary retention, may still occur. This is because the virus affects not only the ipsilateral dorsal root ganglion and nerve but may also involve the meninges and the contralateral nerve roots.[1] Both sexes are affected equally but bladder involvement is more common in males.[1] There is no age predilection for bladder dysfunction, which may even occur in the pediatric population as young as the neonate or infant.[10]

Focused neurological examination may reveal reduced or absent sensation to light touch and pinprick in the perineal or perianal areas. The anal and bulbocavernosus reflexes are often depressed or absent. The patellar (L2, 3, 4) and Achilles tendon (S1) reflexes may also be impaired, depending on the level of the neuritic inflammation. The Babinski sign is usually negative. Motor function is rarely affected.[1] Digital rectal examination may reveal a loaded rectum consistent with neurogenic rectal involvement.[3,11] Cystoscopy may reveal mucosal eruptions ipsilateral to the side of skin involvement.[12]

Clinical and urodynamic diagnosis

The diagnosis should be suspected in any young, healthy, sexually active individual as well as in those who are immunocompromised and present with acute urinary retention. Attention should be directed at examination of the perineal and perianal skin areas for the typical skin eruptions, which, together with antibodies against the virus (in cerebrospinal fluid and serum), would be diagnostic. Midstream urine should be collected to exclude bacterial infection. Urodynamic study in the acute phase typically reveals detrusor areflexia or hyporeflexia with decreased sensation of bladder filling.[13] Electromyography (EMG) is often difficult to perform in the acute phase due to painful blistering perineal skin. It has been reported that external anal sphincter EMG and bulbocavernosus reflex latency were often normal.[14] All urodynamic changes are reversible and usually resolve within 4–8 weeks. A urinary tract ultrasound, or intravenous pyelography (IVP) if evidence of hematuria, should be performed to exclude

upper tract or pelvic pathology such as hydronephrosis or pelvic mass. A cystoscopy is recommended if there is associated hematuria to exclude bladder involvement or the presence of other intravesical pathology.

Treatment and prognosis

Management of zoster-induced urinary retention consists of simple analgesics, antiviral medications, and clean intermittent catheterization (CIC) for a period of 4–8 weeks during which the detrusor slowly returns to normal. Patients should be reassured that the voiding dysfunction is transient and full return to normal detrusor behavior is expected. Repeat urodynamics should be performed on follow-up to confirm this. Dermatological opinion should be sought at the outset so that appropriate topical management for the blistering rash can be instituted to prevent development of superimposed bacterial cellulitis. Postherpetic neuralgia is rare but may occur.

Genitourinary herpes simplex

Pathophysiology

Infections with the herpes simplex virus (HSV) are common in humans. Like varicella-zoster, the virus may afflict the young and healthy as well as the immunocompromised. There are two types: type 1 is associated with orofacial infections and rarely involves the genitals, whereas type 2 is anogenital and often occurs after the onset of sexual activity.[15] The rash of herpes simplex is very similar to varicella-zoster but the distribution of the former is different, being limited to the face for type 1 and to the genitalia for type 2. Both HSV and the varicella-zoster virus may become dormant in the dorsal root ganglia after the initial infection, a feature called neurotropism. Within the cutaneous nerves that are afferent to the infected ganglia, viral proteins as well as perineural and intraneural inflammation have been demonstrated,[16] giving evidence that neurotropic factors may be transported between cutaneous nerve endings and the corresponding dorsal root ganglia, thus explaining the dermatomal distribution of post-herpetic neuralgia and the development of the characteristic eruption in varicella-zoster.

Clinical features

Urinary retention in patients with anogenital herpes is not uncommon. Most cases are due to severe dysuria caused by direct contact of urine with the blistering urethral mucosa.[17] It is often seen in sexually active young adults, with no sexual predilection; though in men, it is often in the homosexual population. True neurogenic urinary retention in anogenital HSV infection is rare and occurs in less than 1% of cases.[18] In these cases, the onset of bladder dysfunction occurs typically 1–2 weeks after the onset of a vesicular and painful rash in the anogenital region. The pathogenesis of the neurogenic retention with HSV is localized lumbosacral meningomyelitis, with involvement of mainly sacral nerve roots, or infectious neuritis that affects the pelvic nerves,[1] thus resembling varicella-zoster. Aseptic meningoencephalitis and myelitis may occur. Neurogenic bowel may supervene, leading to constipation.

The neurological findings are similar to those of its varicella-zoster counterpart. There may be blunting of sensation to light touch and pinprick over the sacral dermatomes. The bulbocavernous and anal reflexes are often intact, but may be reduced or absent, which suggests sacral involvement. Motor function is not affected.

Clinical and urodynamic diagnosis

The diagnosis can be clinched from the history, characteristic rash, and raised level of anti-HSV immunoglobulin M (IgM) titers. Depending on the patient's sexual habits, a full oropharyngeal, rectal, genital, and vaginal speculum examination should be performed to assess disease extent and to exclude other sexually transmitted diseases. Midstream urine should be collected to exclude bacterial infection, and appropriate investigations should be performed if other sexually transmitted diseases are suspected. Counseling is advised for contact tracing and treatment.

Urodynamically, there is often detrusor areflexia with impaired or absent sensation of bladder fullness. The detrusor is also acontractile. These changes are fully reversible, often within 4–8 weeks, but recovery taking up to months has been reported.[17,19]

Treatment and prognosis

Treatment is directed towards effective bladder drainage during the areflexic and acontractile phase by CIC for about 4–8 weeks. Treat any superimposed urine infection but prophylactic antibiotics are not necessary. Follow-up should include repeat urodynamics to document full recovery of both storage and voiding phases of the micturition cycle. Patient should be reassured that the bladder dysfunction is temporary and reversible. Systemic antiviral therapy may be indicated in some patients to shorten the course of skin lesions. Post-herpetic neuralgia is a rare but significant complication.

Caveat

Although the pathology and management of HSV and HZV are similar, it is important to point out that bladder dysfunction is an uncommon complication of herpes virus infection. Any patients, especially in the younger age group, who present with unexplained bladder dysfunction without the typical skin lesions, should be investigated for neurological pathology, some of which include multiple sclerosis, lumbosacral disc prolapse, lumbar canal stenosis, spinal cord or brain tumors, other forms of viral sacral radiculomyelitis, spina bifida occulta, primary bladder neck obstruction, or Fowler's syndrome.

Neuropathic bladder dysfunction from tabes dorsalis

Pathophysiology

Syphilis is a sexually transmitted disease caused by the spirochete *Treponema pallidum*. Voiding dysfunction secondary to neurosyphilis is nowadays a very rare finding in the developed world but may still be endemic in some underdeveloped countries. Approximately 10% of patients with primary syphilis will develop neurosyphilis. More males are affected than females. There are different types of neurosyphilis: asymptomatic, meningovascular, and parenchymatous.[20] The asymptomatic form only has positive cerebrospinal fluid. The meningovascular form involves the vasculature and meninges. If it affects the lumbosacral spinal cord, bladder dysfunction may result. As the posterior spinal cord mediates sensation, lumbosacral meningomyelitis may cause decreased bladder sensation and increased bladder capacity. Parenchymatous neurosyphilis includes syndromes known as tabes dorsalis and general paresis of the insane. Tabes dorsalis is a demyelinating atrophy of the dorsal spinal cord that affects the posterior column, resulting in impaired bladder sensation, detrusor areflexia, and hence overdistention and eventual detrusor decompensation if left untreated. Out of the three forms of neurosyphilis, parenchymatous neurosyphilis presents the latest, occasionally up to 20 years after the primary infection.

Clinical and urodynamic diagnosis

Definitive diagnosis of syphilis is done by darkfield examination or direct immunofluorescent antibody tests of lesion exudates. Serological diagnosis is complementary. The rapid plasma reagin (RPR) and Venereal Disease Research Laboratory (VDRL) tests are not antibody-based and can be used to gauge disease activity as results are reported quantitatively, whereas the fluorescent treponemal antibody absorption test (FTA-ABS) is antibody-based and its level correlates poorly with disease activity.[21]

False-negatives may occur with the FTA-ABS during the window period of initial infection and in immunocompromised patients. Hence a combination of both antibody and non-antibody-based tests are often necessary in patient management.

Urodynamics often demonstrate detrusor areflexia with reduced or absent bladder sensation and increased bladder capacity. Suprasacral as well as sacral cord involvement may occur, leading to reduced bladder compliance, detrusor hyperreflexia with detrusor-sphincter dyssynergia, or detrusor hypocontractility with large post-void residual urine.[22,23]

Treatment and prognosis

Detrusor areflexia, bladder sensation, and bladder capacity often improve with time after treatment with penicillin, but may not return entirely to normal.[20] Timed voiding can be used to promote bladder drainage in those where contractility is not affected. Intermittent catheterization is necessary if hypocontractility with large post-void residuals is present. A case of hyperreflexia requiring urinary diversion was reported.[23] Appropriate bladder management will facilitate bladder drainage, prevent urinary tract infection, and avoid renal damage.

Neuropathic bladder due to Guillain–Barré syndrome

Pathophysiology

Guillain–Barré syndrome (GBS) is an immune-mediated neurological disorder affecting both small and large myelinated axons, causing acute progressive weakness, usually an ascending paralysis, with 30% of the affected having respiratory paralysis necessitating mechanical ventilation.[24,25] Complete or substantial recovery is the rule. It may manifest either as a demyelinating form or an axonal form. The pathophysiological mechanism is an autoimmune destruction of myelin by antiganglioside antibodies. Activated T cells, macrophages, and increased matrix metalloproteinases may also play a role.[26] Autonomic neuropathy may be present in up to 50% of patients.[27] The lumbosacral spinal roots and thoracolumbar sympathetic chain may be involved, leading to lower urinary tract dysfunction.[28] It is likely that the condition of acute distal autonomic neuropathy is a form of GBS and may affect the pelvic plexus and its associated nerves (sympathetic and parasympathetic), which may result in lower urinary tract dysfunction.[29]

Clinical and urodynamic features

Guillain–Barré syndrome is not directly genetically inherited, but presumed to be an individual's idiosyncratic response to a preceding infection, which may have a genetic basis. It affects both the pediatric and adult populations.[30] Typical presenting signs and symptoms include paresthesia of hands and feet, acute symmetric ascending weakness of limbs with areflexia, and reduced proprioception. Gait disorder is common in all age groups. Autonomic neuropathy may manifest as labile blood pressure, cardiac arrhythmias, paralytic ileus, or bladder dysfunction. Approximately 25% of patients with GBS showed micturition symptoms.[31] These may include hesitancy, poor and prolonged flow, urinary retention, urgency, nocturnal frequency, and urge incontinence, reflecting that both storage and emptying function can be affected. These symptoms are more common in patients with severe weakness (especially those requiring ventilatory assistance) than in those with a mild form of neuropathy, typically present after onset of muscular weakness, and improve gradually with the neurological signs over time.[32] Constipation as well as erectile dysfunction may also occur.

The diagnosis is made with nerve conduction studies, which are the most sensitive test. Lumbar puncture may show elevated protein, with normal white cell count.[33]

Urodynamics commonly reveal detrusor areflexia and impaired bladder sensation with large post-void residuals.[34] Detrusor hyperreflexia, both with and without sphincter dyssynergia, has been reported.[35,36] Decreased bladder capacity may occur with hyperreflexia without radiological evidence of spinal cord involvement, indicating that the overactivity may occur at the peripheral nerve level with probable pelvic nerve irritation.[31]

Treatment and prognosis

From a neurological aspect, the principle of management is hospitalization with monitoring of respiratory function and elective endotracheal intubation for impending respiratory failure. Intravenous immunoglobulin with plasmapheresis is indicated for patients with severe weakness and rapid progression.[37] With respect to autonomic neuropathy, cardiac monitoring is required for arrhythmias, strict bowel regime for constipation and ileus, and CIC or indwelling urethral catheter for detrusor areflexia or detrusor hyperreflexia with sphincter dyssynergia. Urodynamic parameters improve during the course of the disease approximately 6–8 weeks after the onset of weakness. All patients should be educated that full or significant recovery is expected.

References

1. Yamanishi T, Yasuda K, Sakakibara R, et al. Urinary retention due to herpes virus infections. Neurourol Urodyn 1998; 17:613–619.

2. Broseta E, Osca JM, Martinez-Agullo J, Jimenez-Cruz JF. Urological manifestations of herpes zoster. Eur Urol 1993; 24:244–247.

3. Cohen LM, Fowler JF, Owen LG, Callen JP. Urinary retention associated with herpes zoster infection. Int J Dermatol 1993; 32(1):24–26.

4. Gibbon N. A case of herpes zoster with involvement of urinary bladder. Br J Urol 1956; 28:417–421.

5. Kendall AR, Karafin L. Classification of neurogenic bladder disease. Urol Clin N Am 1974; 1:45.

6. Rankin JT, Sutton RA. Herpes zoster causing retention of urine. Br J Urol 1969; 41:238–241.

7. Bastian FO, Rabson AS, Yee CL, Tralka TS. Herpesvirus varicellae: isolated from human dorsal root ganglia. Arch Pathol 1974; 97:331–333.

8. Jellinek EH, Tulloch WS. Herpes zoster with dysfunction of bladder and anus. Lancet 1976; 2:1219–1222.

9. Richmond W. The genitourinary manifestations of herpes zoster. Three case reports and a review of the literature. Br J Urol 1974; 46:193–200.

10. Gold I, Azizi E, Eshel G. Neurogenic bladder due to herpes zoster infection in an infant. Eur J Pediatr 1989; 148(5):468–469.

11. Ginsberg PC, Harkaway RC, Elisco AJ III, Rosenthal BD. Rare presentation of acute urinary retention secondary to herpes zoster. J Am Osteopath Assoc 1998; 98(9):508–509.

12. Ray B, Wise G. Urinary retention associated with herpes zoster. J Urol 1970; 104:422–425.

13. Tsai HN, Wu WJ, Huang SP, et al. Herpes zoster induced neuropathic bladder – a case report. Kaohsiung J Med Sci 2002; 18(1):39–44.

14. Herbaut AG, Nogueira MC, Wespes E. Urinary retention due to sacral myeloradiculitis: a clinical and neurophysiological study. J Urol 1990; 144:1206–1208.

15. Oates JK, Greenhouse PR. Retention of urine in anogenital herpetic infection. Lancet 1978; 1:691–692.

16. Worrell JT, Cockerell CJ. Histopathology of peripheral nerves in cutaneous herpes virus infection. Am J Dermatopathol 1997; 19:133–137.

17. Clason AE, McGeorge A, Garland C, Abel BJ. Urinary retention and granulomatous prostatitis following sacral herpes zoster infection. Br J Urol 1982; 54:166–169.

18. Greenstein A, Matzkin H, Kaver I, Braf Z. Acute urinary retention in herpes genitalis infection. Urology 1988; 31(5):453–456.

19. Riehle RA Jr, Williams JJ. Transient neuropathic bladder following herpes simplex genitalis. J Urol 1979; 122(2): 263–264.

20. Wheeler JS Jr, Culkin DJ, O'Hara RJ, Canning JR. Bladder dysfunction and neurosyphilis. J Urol 1986; 136:903–905.

21. Krieger JN. Sexually transmitted diseases. In: Tanagho E, McAninch J, eds, Smith's general urology, 15th edn. Columbus: McGraw-Hill, 2000:287–299.

22. Garber SJ, Christmas TJ, Rickards D. Voiding dysfunction due to neurosyphilis. Br J Urol 1990; 66(1):19–21.

23. Hattori T, Yasuda K, Kita K, Hirayama K. Disorders of micturition in tabes dorsalis. Br J Urol 1990; 65(5):497–499.

24. Fowler CJ. Neurological disorders of micturition and their treatment. Brain 1999; 122(7):1213–1231.

25. Arnason BGW, Soliven B. Acute inflammatory demyelinating polyradiculoneuropathy. In: Dyck PJ, Thomas PK, eds, Peripheral neuropathy, 3rd edn. Philadelphia: WB Saunders, 1993:1437–1497.

26. Pascuzzi R, Fleck J. Acute peripheral neuropathy in adults. Neurol Clin 1997; 15(3):529–548.

27. Tuck RR, McLeod JG. Autonomic dysfunction in Guillain–Barré syndrome. J Neurol Neurosurg Psychiatry 1981; 52:857–864.

28. Honavar M, Tharakan JKJ, Hughes RAC, et al. A clinicopathological study of the Guillain–Barré syndrome; nine cases and literature review. Brain 1991; 114:1245–1269.

29. Kirby RS, Fowler CJ, Gosling JA, Bannister R. Bladder dysfunction in distal autonomic neuropathy of acute onset. J Neurol Neurosurg Psychiatry 1985; 48:762–767.

30. Evans O, Vedanarayanan V. Guillain–Barré syndrome. Pediatr Rev 1997; 18(1):10–17.

31. Zochodne D. Autonomic involvement in Guillain–Barré syndrome: a review. [Review] Muscle Nerve 1994; 17:1145–1155.

32. Sakakibara R, Hattori T, Kuwabara S, et al. Micturitional disturbance in patients with Guillain–Barré syndrome. J Neurol Neurosurg Psychiatry 1997; 63:649–653.

33. Wexler I. Serial Sensory and motor conduction measurement in Guillain–Barré syndrome. Clin Neurophysiol 1980; 20(2):87–103.

34. Wheeler JS Jr, Siroky MB, Pavlakis A, Krane RJ. The urodynamic aspects of Guillain–Barré syndrome. J Urol 1984; 131(5):917–919.

35. Grbavac Z, Gilja I, Gubarev N, Bozicevic D. Neurologic and urodynamic characteristics of patients with Guillain–Barré syndrome. Lijec Vjesn 1989; 111(1–2):17–20.

36. Kogan BA, Soloman MH, Diokno AC. Urinary retention secondary to Landry–Guillain–Barré syndrome. J Urol 1981; 126:643–644.

37. Bella I, Chad D. Neuromuscular disorders and acute respiratory failure. Neurol Clin 1998; 6(2):391–417.

20

Peripheral neuropathies of the lower urinary tract, following pelvic surgery and radiation therapy

Richard T Kershen and Timothy B Boone

Introduction

Though control and coordination of micturition is relegated to higher centers in the brain and spinal cord, the lower urinary tract (LUT) is ultimately innervated by the 'hard wiring' of peripheral nerves, conveying essential neurotransmission of the autonomic and somatic nervous systems. Iatrogenic damage to peripheral nerves of the bladder, urethra, and pelvic floor during the course of surgical endeavors or radiotherapy may result in significant patient morbidity in terms of resultant vesicourethral dysfunction. Voiding dysfunction resulting from extirpative or ablative therapies aimed at the treatment of cancer may be physically and socially devastating for a patient. It is important for the pelvic surgeon and radiotherapist alike to be familiar with the complex innervation of the bladder and urethra in order to reduce the likelihood of injury to peripheral nerves during the course of therapy. In addition, the urologist must be familiar with the signs, symptoms, and typical urodynamic manifestations of peripheral nerve injury in order to facilitate precise physiologic diagnosis and optimize treatment strategies. It is appropriate to begin our discussion with a review of the anatomy of the peripheral nervous system as it pertains to innervation and neural control of the LUT.

Anatomic considerations in lower urinary tract innervation

Both the autonomic and somatic nervous systems are integrally responsible for innervation of the LUT. In essence, the LUT is innervated by three sets of peripheral nerves, representing the parasympathetic, sympathetic, and somatic nervous systems (Figure 20.1).[1] Each nerve conveys both sensory and motor fibers to and from the central nervous system. The parasympathetic input originates from the sacral spinal cord (S2–4) in the sacral parasympathetic nucleus located in the intermediolateral cell column.[2] Long, preganglionic parasympathetic nerve fibers travel within the pelvic nerve to synapse with their short, postganglionic counterparts in the pelvic plexus or detrusor muscle itself. Stimulation of the parasympathetic system results in detrusor contraction and urethral relaxation. Consequently, damage to the parasympathetic input will result in detrusor hyporeflexia or areflexia.[3] The sympathetic input arises in the intermediolateral cell columns of the thoracolumbar spinal cord (T11–12, L1–3). Preganglionic sympathetic nerve fibers arise from lumbosacral sympathetic chain ganglia traveling in lumbar spanchnic nerves composing the superior hypogastric plexus which then bifurcates below the great vessels, forming paired hypogastric nerves which ultimately synapse with postganglionic sympathetic neurons in the pelvic plexus. Short postganglionic sympathetic nerves then go on to innervate the bladder body, neck, and proximal urethra.[4]

Of note, this arrangement is somewhat atypical for sympathetic nerves, which usually have short preganglionic nerves that synapse far from their target organs. In addition, multiple regions of crossover exist between opposing sides via branches coursing through the inferior mesenteric ganglion. Stimulation of the sympathetic system results in inhibition of bladder contractility as well as an increase in bladder outlet resistance.

Damage to the sympathetic input will result in impaired compliance, bladder outlet incompetence, and retrograde ejaculation. Somatic input arises from motor neurons in Onuf's nucleus at the lateral border of the ventral horn of the sacral spinal cord (S2–4). Sacral nerve roots coalesce, forming the pudendal nerve, which travels through the pelvis and perineum, innervating the striated muscle of the external urethral sphincter.

Afferent information from the LUT is transmitted via pelvic, hypogastric, and pudendal nerves to the

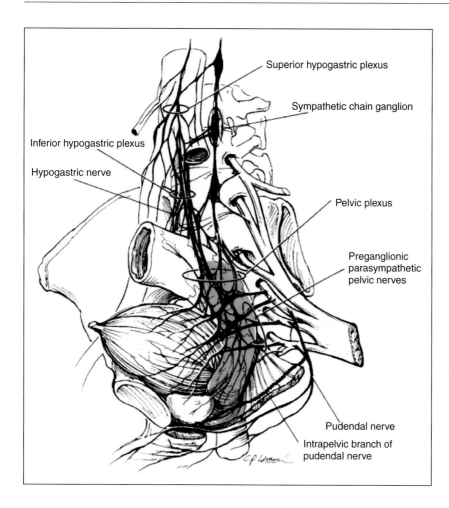

Superior hypogastric plexus

Sympathetic chain ganglion

Inferior hypogastric plexus

Hypogastric nerve

Pelvic plexus

Preganglionic parasympathetic pelvic nerves

Pudendal nerve

Intrapelvic branch of pudendal nerve

Figure 20.1
Peripheral innervation of the lower urinary tract.

lumbosacral spinal cord. Bladder receptors sensing bladder volume and contractility travel in the pelvic nerve to the spinal cord via myelinated Aδ fibers and unmyelinated C fibers. C fibers are also recruited after neurologic insult (spinal cord injury), during times of obstruction or bladder inflammation to convey nociceptive responses.[1]

In the last several years, great strides have been made in our understanding of gross pelvic neuroanatomy due to the work of surgeons who understand the potential for iatrogenic injury during radical pelvic surgery. Hollabaugh and colleagues performed meticulous intrapelvic and perineal dissections under magnification on male and female cadavers hemisected at the level of the sacral promontory.[5] They traced the course of what they called the 'pelvic nerve,' which by description appears to be the confluence of nerves arising from the pelvic plexus, going on to innervate the pelvic viscera. This nerve, originating over the hypogastric artery, represents a confluence of postganglionic sympathetic and parasympathetic fibers running together from the pelvic plexus. This dense intermingling of sympathetic and parasympathetic nerve fibers arising from the pelvic plexus has been described by other authors.[6] As the nerve enters the pelvis, it gives off multiple web-like branches, which travel within the endopelvic

fascial sleeve, innervating the detrusor muscle, and other pelvic viscera (colon, rectum, prostate, vagina, and uterus).

The main branch of the nerve was found to travel inferiolateral to the rectum, deep to the levator ani fascia, coursing through the pelvis towards the external sphincter, where it gives off its terminal innervating branches, anterior to the rectum. The pudendal nerve was also traced from its point of origin in the pelvis through its path in Alcock's canal.

It was noted that the pudendal nerve gives off an intrapelvic branch, which courses beneath the levator ani fascia and joins the distal aspect of the pelvic nerve at the level of the prostatic apex to innervate the external urinary sphincter. The main trunk of the pudendal nerve then enters Alcock's canal and gives off numerous variable branches within the canal and in the perineum, ultimately terminating in the perineal nerve, providing somatic innervation to the urinary rhabdosphincter. Thus, the external urinary sphincter appears to have a dual innervation, both autonomic from the pelvic nerve and somatic from the intrapelvic and perineal branches of the pudendal nerve.

Strasser and colleagues sought to clarify the neuromuscular function and physiology of the urethra and external urinary sphincter.[7] Performing human cadaveric dissections as well as functional studies in sheep, they found, similarly to Hollabaugh's group, that the autonomic fibers which supply the pelvic viscera course as a confluence of nerves lateral to the rectum within the envelope of the levator fascia. In the male, the smooth muscle within the membranous urethra was found to be innervated by autonomic fibers arising from this 'pelvic nerve' via branches derived from a prostatic plexus as well as the periprostatic cavernous nerves which pass through the urogenital hiatus. In the female, the autonomic nerves to the proximal urethral smooth muscle arose from the pelvic nerve and traveled along the lateral aspects of the uterus and vagina to their point of insertion dorsolaterally.

Functionally, Strasser and colleagues found that stimulation of the pelvic plexus generated strong responses in the proximal urethra, but little in the distal urethra or external rhabdosphincter. Pudendal nerve stimulation, however, resulted in distal urethral smooth muscular contraction as well as the expected rhabdosphincter response. These findings suggest autonomic control over proximal urethral function, with the somatic nervous system controlling distal urethral function. It is obvious that the peripheral nerves serving the LUT are diverse, representing multiple targets for injury.

Peripheral neuropathies of the lower urinary tract as a consequence of pelvic surgery

Although peripheral neuropathies affecting bladder and urethral function may result from a variety of causes, including metabolic or infectious disease, degenerative disorders, systemic illnesses, or disc disease, for the purposes of this discussion we will focus on those that arise subsequent to surgical endeavors in the pelvis or ablative radiotherapy.

We will discuss specific mechanisms for injury as well as reported clinical and urodynamic findings correlating with the site of injury. In addition, we will elaborate on methods to prevent and reduce potential injury. Peripheral neuropathy will commonly distort normal motor, sensory, and/or autonomic functions. As the LUT is limited in its ability to express functional pathology, the presence of neurologic injury will manifest in a finite number of ways, including voiding dysfunction, incontinence, and/or pain. Predicting urodynamic findings for individual cases on the basis of symptomatology and neurologic examination alone is often impossible, and therefore therapy should be directed on the basis of clinical history and thorough urodynamic testing.

Extirpative pelvic surgery has long been associated with LUT dysfunction. The incidence of vesicourethral dysfunction has been reported to be 8–70% post-abdominoperineal resection (APR),[5, 8–13] 16–80% post-hysterectomy,[14–16] and 20–25% after low anterior resection.[17] The manifestations of, and mechanisms for dysfunction are broad and may vary with the specific type of surgery performed and the initial indication for surgery (as pelvic malignancies themselves have been implicated in vesicourethral dysfunction).[18]

In general – notwithstanding iatrogenic injury resulting in gross anatomic derangements of the bladder, urethra, or sphincter themselves – neurologic injury is usually implicated as the causative factor. The exact nature of the neurologic lesion may be difficult to predict by history alone however, due to the potential for partial or complete autonomic and/or somatic denervation. Transient neuropraxic injuries may occur due to neural traction during surgery. Urodynamic evaluation has proven invaluable for proper assessment of these patients, aiding in precise characterization of the neurologic lesion. As detailed earlier, our expanding knowledge of pelvic neuroanatomy and the neurophysiology of normal voiding has, in recent years, allowed modifications of extirpative surgical procedures that may reduce or eliminate negative iatrogenic sequelae on the LUT.

For the purposes of this chapter we will discuss specific surgical procedures, elucidating the mechanisms for injury and the clinical spectra of the subsequent neuropathies which develop. Neurologically induced voiding dysfunction from peripheral neuropathy may either resolve during the early postoperative period (weeks to months) or stabilize and persist for years postoperatively. The most typical clinical manifestations of enduring peripheral nerve injury affecting the LUT after pelvic extirpative surgery will include large urinary residuals, incomplete emptying, and Valsalva voiding.[19] The classic functional pathology will include a noncontractile bladder (areflexic or underactive detrusor) with or without a relaxed urinary sphincter (denervated or underactive).[20] Generally, a parasympathetic injury will result in detrusor hypoactivity with varying degrees of bladder paralysis. Sympathetic injury may manifest as alpha- or beta-adrenergic denervation. Beta-adrenergic denervation may result in poor bladder compliance and occasionally detrusor hyperactivity.[19] Alpha-adrenergic denervation typically manifests as bladder neck incompetence. Of note, male patients with autonomic injury related to pelvic neuropathy often complain of coexistent erectile dysfunction.

Neuro-urologic examination

Iatrogenic peripheral nerve injury resulting in LUT dysfunction may have a variable presentation, including sensory and/or motor neuropathy of the bladder with or without urethral sphincteric dysfunction. A focused neuro-urologic exam may provide clues to the underlying nature of the pathology, but may not necessarily be diagnostic. Unlike patients with spinal cord injuries, patients with peripheral nerve injury, with intact central nervous systems, will not exhibit abnormalities in lower extremity tone or reflex response. Competency of the sacral reflex arc may be assessed, however, via elicitation of the bulbocavernosus reflex. The glans penis or clitoris is manually stimulated and the anal sphincteric response is assessed. Absence or prolongation of this reflex suggests peripheral nerve injury in this subset of patients. Decreased or absent anal sphincteric tone may suggest pudendal motor nerve injury. Sensory examination of the perineum to assess vibratory and tactile sense should be performed to determine the likelihood of pudendal sensory neuropathy.

Urodynamic evaluation

The utility of preoperative urodynamics in any patient undergoing extirpative pelvic surgery cannot be adequately emphasized. Such studies may prove invaluable when faced with a patient complaining about postoperative voiding dysfunction. Preoperative voiding dysfunction due to pre-existing bladder outlet obstruction or, potentially, a preoperative peripheral nerve lesion from the primary pelvic pathologic process may be present, and complicate the interpretation of postoperative symptoms if previously undiagnosed. In addition, a pre-existing neuropathy related to tumor infiltration may indicate the potential risk for intraoperative injury during resection.

We typically perform initial postoperative urodynamic evaluations by the 3rd or 4th week after surgery. It is apparent that a variety of sympathetic, parasympathetic, and/or somatic injuries may occur and will require complete urodynamic evaluation to correctly identify the nature of the pathology. Videourodynamics with abdominal and vesical pressure monitoring as well as electromyography (EMG) of the pelvic floor/striated sphincter complex allows precise diagnosis. Abdominal pressure monitoring is essential for the determination of the true detrusor pressure, as many patients will suffer from areflexia.[21]

The absence of a detrusor contraction during urodynamics does not prove areflexia and the presence of abdominal straining will assist in the diagnosis. Pressure–flow evaluation will allow a precise diagnosis of obstruction if present. Indeed, Blaivas and Barbalias found significant obstruction from benign prostatic hyperplasia (BPH) in 4 of 5 males with urinary retention after APR.[13] Pelvic floor needle EMG will assist in determining the presence or absence of denervation potentials within the external sphincter. Sacral evoked potentials may also be performed to more accurately assess integrity of the sacral reflex arc.[22]

Abdominoperineal resection

It has long been recognized that radical rectal excision via APR has been closely associated with postoperative voiding dysfunction.[23] McGuire performed the first urodynamic characterization of voiding dysfunction in these patients in 1975.[24] He described detrusor areflexia in all patients with variable degrees of internal and external sphincteric weakness. Blaivas and Barbalias subsequently performed videourodynamics on 13 men who had undergone APR.[13] Patients presented with a variety of symptoms, including isolated storage problems (incontinence), isolated emptying problems (retention), or combined difficulties with storage and emptying. Interestingly, all patients demonstrated incompetence of the bladder neck (proximal sphincter) on videourodynamic testing, suggesting universal sympathetic denervation. Whether or not a patient was incontinent, however, was dependent upon the degree of concomitant parasympathetic and pudendal denervation. In fact, patients afflicted with the most troublesome sequelae of combined difficulties with storage and emptying (4/13 patients) had evidence of extensive neurologic injury, manifesting detrusor areflexia and an open bladder neck at rest, along with EMG and clinical evidence of a lower motor neuron lesion to the external sphincter (combined parasympathetic, sympathetic, and somatic/pudendal denervation). Overall, clinical and urodynamic evidence of parasympathetic denervation (impaired emptying/areflexia) was present in 38%, and somatic/pudendal denervation was present in 54%.

Yalla and Andriole were interested in the natural history of neurogenically induced vesicourethral dysfunction in patients who had undergone radical pelvic surgery.[19] They performed both early (2 weeks to 4 months) and delayed (18 months to 3 years) postoperative urodynamic evaluations in patients with voiding dysfunction after APR. Early evaluation revealed the presence of an incompetent bladder neck, detrusor hypertonia (impaired compliance), diminished proprioception, and detrusor hypoactivity or inactivity, suggesting combined parasympathethic and sympathetic denervation. Additionally, patients who demonstrated total incontinence manifested diminished urethral closure pressures with absent reflex activity of the external striated sphincter. Interestingly, a recovery phase was noted, with 75% of incontinent patients regaining passive continence within 4 months. This corresponded with the finding of restored urethral closure pressure in the membranous urethra with return of peirurethral striated muscle reflex activity. The bladder neck and prostatic urethra remained incompetent, suggesting recovery of somatic innervation without return of sympathetic urethral innervation. Delayed evaluations revealed persistence of parasympathetic denervation, manifested in a large cystometric capacity with detrusor hypoactivity or inactivity. The presence of bladder neck incompetence, indicative of persistent sympathetic innervation, was variable. Ultimately, 21 of 22 patients had persistent vesicourethral dysfunction with large residuals, and Valsalva voiding after pelvic extirpative surgery.

In summary, the most common urodynamic findings after APR include detrusor hyporeflexia with impaired sensation, increased capacity, and compliance with concomitant incompetence of the bladder neck, suggesting a combined injury to both parasympathetic and sympathetic innervation. Most patients will be continent and have difficulties related to impaired emptying. Incontinent patients after APR will have commonly suffered additional injury to the pudendal nerve, resulting in external sphincteric dysfunction. The more severely incontinent patients may have a higher degree of sympathetic denervation, with a resultant loss of bladder compliance occurring concurrently with decreased or absent proximal and distal sphincteric function. Fortunately, most patients with somatic nerve injury will have recovery of function over time with the return of active and/or passive continence. This may be heralded by the reappearance of the bulbocavernosus reflex. Because slow recovery is the rule, at least 1 year should lapse after APR before consideration of surgical intervention.

Mechanism for, and means for prevention of neurologic injury during abdominoperineal resection

It is clear that the extent of pelvic dissection during APR relates directly to the degree of subsequent vesicourethral dysfunction.[25] Urologic morbidity may be avoided by a detailed understanding of pelvic neuroanatomy. Indeed, Hojo and colleagues demonstrated that complete preservation of autonomic innervation allowed 88% of patients undergoing APR to void spontaneously within 10 days of surgery. Conversely, 78% of patients who underwent complete resection of the pelvic autonomic nerves remained in urinary retention by 2 months postoperatively. Damage along the course of the pelvic nerve may result in isolated bladder dysfunction, proximal urethral dysfunction, and/or external sphincteric dysfunction. It appears that avoidance of dissection beneath the presacral fascia will protect the proximal portions of continence-preserving nerves during rectal resection and mesorectal lymphadenectomy. This may avoid damage to the sympathetic fibers of the hypogastric plexus at the level of the pelvic brim, where they course medial to the ureters. The pelvic nerve is susceptible to injury as it courses inferolateral to the rectum towards the prostatic apex. It may be injured during the course of circumferential rectal dissection and

during levator ani muscular division, resulting in proximal urethral denervation. Levator ani muscle division will also result in damage to the intrapelvic branch of the pudendal nerve, abolishing its ability to provide innervation to the smooth muscular component of the distal urethral sphincter. Injury to these continence-preserving nerves may be averted by respecting the integrity of Denonvilliers' fascia near the prostatic apex, and carefully dividing the levator ani away from the intrapelvic branch of the pudendal nerve traveling close to the ischium.[5] In females, preservation of the vagina will also protect these nerves as they travel to the urethra. During perineal dissection, care should be taken to dissect cautiously near the ischial tuberosity where the terminal branches of the pudendal nerve may be injured as they exit Alcock's canal.

Hysterectomy

Similar to previously outlined experience with APR, the performance of radical hysterectomy has long been associated with the development of postoperative bladder dysfunction.[16,26,27] This relationship owes much to the close anatomic associations between the pelvic plexus and uterosacral and cardinal ligaments.[28] The uterosacral and cardinal ligaments, historically resected in radical hysterectomy, carry autonomic nerve fibers which go on to innervate the bladder and urethra. The uterosacral ligaments themselves contain important pelvic parasympathetic and hypogastric nerve rami. The cardinal ligaments, located at the base of the broad ligaments, surround the cervix and extend laterally to the pelvic sidewalls. Each ligament lies in close proximity to the cervix, at whose inferomedial margin, fibers from the pelvic plexus – predominantly sympathetic in nature – advance in a palpable nerve bundle to eventually innervate the bladder and urethra. As with any radical pelvic operation, damage to the pelvic plexus itself can also occur with aggressive posterior dissection.

Yalla and Andriole noted that after radical hysterectomy nearly all patients have vesicourethral dysfunction related predominantly to parasympathetic denervation.[19] Up to 50% of patients may also have additional sympathetic denervation with the resultant manifestation of vesical hypertonia and incompetency of the bladder neck.[6,14,15,29] Indeed, Iio and colleagues noted urodynamically evident decreases in detrusor compliance and maximal urethral closure pressures in 24 patients who underwent radical hysterectomy.[30] The frequency of sympathetic denervation may correspond to the extent of dissection of the cardinal ligaments and the amount these ligaments are resected.[15]

To avoid this injury and spare the sympathetic innervation of the bladder and its base, maintaining proximal urethral function and continence, more conservative surgical approaches (if allowable by the stage of the cervical cancer involved) that preserve the inferior portions of the cardinal ligaments are warranted. In cases of extensive cervical cancer, vaginal cuff excision may be mandatory and resultant bladder neck incompetence probable. A less-destructive surgical approach, as implemented with simple, supracervical hysterectomy has been felt to reduce the risk of post-hysterectomy bladder dysfunction.[31]

This, however, is not absolute, as evident in the work of Parys and colleagues, who analyzed the clinical spectra of bladder dysfunction after simple hysterectomy.[16] They performed urodynamic studies and sacral reflex latency studies on 126 women with LUT symptoms after hysterectomy. They found that 86% of patients had a demonstrable urodynamic abnormality, with 47% of patients having detrusor instability, 37% having evidence of urethral obstruction, and 25% having evidence of stress incontinence. Sacral reflex latencies were prolonged or absent in 80% of 25 patients studied, suggesting autonomic peripheral neuropathy due to pelvic plexus injury. Recently, Kuwabara and colleagues have proposed using intraoperative electrical stimulation of the cardinal ligaments to identify the location of the vesical branches of the pelvic nerve and they have demonstrated some benefit to this approach.[32]

Radical prostatectomy

It's clear that incontinence after radical prostatectomy is related to intrinsic sphincter deficiency in the majority of patients. Urodynamic studies in postprostatectomy patients have revealed, however, a high prevalence of concomitant detrusor dysfunction – namely, instability and impaired compliance.[33,34] Hubert and colleagues, performed pre- and postoperative bladder biopsies comparing nerve fiber density in the superficial trigone in men undergoing radical prostatectomy.[35] They found that nerve fiber density decreased postoperatively and regenerated over time. Patients with persistent incontinence had less than half the amount of nerve fiber regeneration than continent patients at 6 months postoperatively. Urinary incontinence was associated with trigonal denervation, a high sensory threshold, and a low maximal urethral closure pressure. The authors hypothesized that wide dissection around the prostate, bladder base, and seminal vesicles leads to disruption of bladder and proximal urethral innervation. They suggested that preservation of trigonal innervation may be important for maintenance of continence. When this technique was applied to nerve and seminal vesicle sparing cystectomy, high degrees of urinary continence were achieved, supporting the theory that preservation of the pelvic plexus and trigonal innervation improves urinary continence.[36] Although the etiology may be multifactorial, detrusor dysfunction

after radical prostatectomy may indeed be related to peripheral nervous denervation. More detailed anatomic studies may further elucidate this mechanism in the future.

Ureteral reimplantation

Voiding dysfunction and urinary retention rarely complicate antireflux surgery. This is most commonly encountered after bilateral extravesical ureteral reimplantation.[37–39] Although urinary retention is usually self-limited, it has been reported to occur in up to 26% of these patients.[40] Several investigators have pursued the etiology of this phenomenon from an anatomic standpoint. Barrieras and colleagues found that by modifying their technique to minimize dissection below the ureteral hiatus, they were able to reduce the incidence of urinary retention.[39] They hypothesized that this technique limited injury to the autonomic nerve fibers coursing into the bladder in the region of the trigone. Leissner and colleagues went on to confirm this via cadaver dissections, which revealed the location of the pelvic plexus to be 1.5 cm dorsomedial to the distal ureter.[37]

Terminal branches from the plexus were identified coursing towards the bladder trigone in a delicate network surrounding the distal ureter. These branches could easily be damaged by dissection outside the plane of the mesoureter or by dissection dorsal and medial to the ureterovesical hiatus. These data support the theory that bladder dysfunction post-bilateral extravesical reimplantation may have a similar etiology to that following hysterectomy or APR: namely, efferent nerve denervation. Recently, the same group of investigators created an animal model of neurologic injury resulting from ureteral dissection at the ureteral hiatus, confirming their previous anatomic findings.[41] Unilateral or bilateral efferent nerve blockade was accomplished via Xylocaine (lidocaine (lignocaine)) injection at the ureterovesical junction, which resulted in complete abolishment of motor response to sacral anterior nerve root stimulation.

Radiation therapy

Radiation therapy (RT) kills neoplastic cells. Unfortunately, its curative potential is limited by its potential to damage normal tissues which lie within its path. For many years it was believed that peripheral nerves were relatively radioresistant and did not serve as 'dose-limiting' structures when planning a course of radiotherapy.[42] In the last decade, however, observation of post-irradiation brachial and lumbosacral plexopathies have made it clear that peripheral nerve damage may occur after sufficient dose.[43,44] These plexopathies will result in paresthesias and/or paralysis.[45] In cancer patients, radiation-induced cellular alterations may render peripheral nerves more sensitive to the ill effects of chemotherapy. Alternatively, chemotherapeutic agents may sensitize neural tissues to the effects of radiation.[46] Of note, there is often a lag period between treatment/exposure and the development of symptoms of neurologic injury. This is largely due to the major mechanism by which ionizing radiation causes cellular damage, i.e. destruction of DNA. If sublethal damage incurred by a cell is not repaired, death will occur when the damaged cell attempts to reproduce. When RT has been directed at the peripheral nervous system, cell death may occur months to years later due to slow reproductive cycles of glial and Schwann cells.[47] Peripheral nerve injury may also be incurred by radiation-induced damage to vascular endothelium, obliterating critical neural blood supply. Radiation-induced perineural fibrosis may also result in compression and ischemia of peripheral nerves. Although studies reporting direct radiation-induced injury to the pelvic peripheral nervous system are scarce, there are numerous studies documenting the indirect damage inflicted, inferred by reports of erectile and bladder dysfunction post-radiotherapy.[48–50] For the purposes of this discussion, we focus on radiation-induced peripheral neuropathies leading to bladder dysfunction.

The pelvis is a relatively confined space that contains closely approximated visceral organs, including the bladder, prostate, uterus, and rectosigmoid portions of the large intestine. As previously discussed, these organs are in close proximity to the autonomic and somatic nerves which innervate them. External beam RT designated for any one particular organ will therefore inevitably result in simultaneous radiation exposure to other vital structures, including blood vessels and peripheral nerves.

There have been successful attempts to limit radiation exposure to bystander tissues, including three-dimensional treatment plans, conformal radiation, stereotactic radiosurgery, and brachytherapy. Due to the anatomically close relationship between the pelvic viscera and their innervating nerves, however, it is likely that peripheral nerve exposure and subsequent injury will occur with any treatment modality implemented in the pelvis. In fact, Tait and colleagues did not find a significant difference in prevalence of urinary symptoms in patients receiving conformal vs conventional pelvic RT for the treatment of pelvic malignancies.[51] Even low-dose radiotherapy can inflict significant damage. Indeed, animal studies have revealed the threshold dose for peripheral neuropathy following RT is merely 15–20 Gy, well below the normal dose utilized for most pelvic malignancies.[52,53] Unfortunately, the same anatomic relationships that render peripheral nerves susceptible to injury during RT lead to difficulties in distinguishing if peripheral nerve injury alone is responsible for dysfunctional changes

within the LUT. The bladder and urethra themselves will often be incidentally exposed to RT (intentionally at times), resulting in direct radiation damage to microvascular, epithelial, and muscular components and anatomically mediated dysfunction.

Functional changes in the LUT have been reported after pelvic RT for the treatment of prostate, bladder, rectal, cervical, and uterine cancers.[51,54–57] Behr and colleagues performed urodynamic testing on 104 patients who received pelvic irradiation for cervical carcinoma with maximal follow-up of 10 years.[58] Sixty percent of patients developed *de-novo* urge incontinence related to detrusor instability concomitant with poor vesical compliance and diminished cystometric capacity. Whereas maximal urethral closure pressures were initially unchanged by irradiation, the risk for stress urinary incontinence (SUI) increased over time and was significant by 6 years post-therapy. This suggests the possibility for neurogenically mediated vesical and urethral dysfunction.

The delay in the development of SUI may be related to the gradual dying off of sympathetic and pudendal nerve supply to the urethral sphincteric mechanism. In agreement with this theory are the observations of Litwin and colleagues, who showed that the time course for decline in urinary function in patients who received RT differed from that of patients who underwent radical prostatectomy for prostate cancer. Patients who received RT experienced a gradual decline in urinary function and an increase in urinary bother from irritative symptoms with time up to 1 year post-therapy where symptoms approached the severity of patients who underwent radical prostatectomy.[55]

Severe urgency/frequency syndrome and urge incontinence in post-RT patients were also identified by Parkin and colleagues.[54] Hanfmann and colleagues noted a decrease in micturitional volumes to 70% of that observed before RT for prostate cancer by 6 weeks after therapy.[57] At surgical exploration, Sindelar and colleagues identified perineural fibrosis in pelvic nerve trunks in patients who received RT for treatment of pelvic sarcomas.[59] This finding suggests RT-mediated peripheral nerve injury as a viable source for LUT dysfunction. Michailov and colleagues perfomed muscle bath contractile studies on rat detrusor strips exposed to external beam radiation. An increase in basal tone was noted occurring simultaneously with a decreased sensitivity to acetylcholine-mediated contraction. These data infer a possible mechanism for end-organ neurogenic injury to result in the observed clinical effects of hypertonia, decreased functional capacity, and diminished micturitional pressure.[60] It is evident that more studies need to be performed to evaluate the effects and functional consequences of RT on pelvic peripheral nerves. From indirect evidence, however, it is apparent that radiation-mediated peripheral nerve injury has a role in post-RT bladder dysfunction.

Managing the patient with vesicourethral dysfunction related to peripheral nerve injury

As a general rule, treatment of vesicourethral dysfunction after peripheral nerve injury should be directed by the urodynamic findings. As the time course and completeness of recovery after surgery or radiotherapy are not predictable, conservative treatment should be implemented initially prior to any irreversible surgical endeavors. For the patient in urinary retention, clean intermittent catheterization (CIC) is preferable to a chronic indwelling Foley catheter. The presence or absence of bladder outlet obstruction as well as sphincteric integrity should be established to determine the potential beneficial or harmful effects of transurethral resection. In the case of the hypocontractile detrusor, CIC may be continued indefinitely until the return of bladder contractility. A period of at least 6 months should pass before considering any definitive surgical intervention in the patient with sphincteric incontinence or poor compliance, as the natural history of peripheral nerve injury suggests that function may return over time.

Summary

Iatrogenic injury to peripheral nerves innervating the LUT during the course of pelvic surgery or radiotherapy may result in significant vesicourethral dysfunction. Detailed knowledge of neuroanatomy and physiology of the bladder and urethra will help avoid these injuries in patients requiring these interventions. Should injury occur, urodynamic evaluation is key for the detection of concomitant pathology and planning management to restore vesicourethral function.

References

1. Chancellor MB, Yoshimura N. Physiology and pharmacology of the bladder and urethra. In: Walsh PC, Retik AL, Vaughan ED, et al, eds. Campbell's urology, 8th edn. Philadelphia: WB Saunders, 2002: 846–848.

2. de Groat WC, Vizzard MA, Araki I, Roppolo JR. Spinal interneurons and preganglionic neurons in sacral autonomic reflex pathways. In: Holstege G, Bandler R, Saper C, eds. The emotional motor system. Prog Brain Res 1996; 107:97.

3. de Groat WC, Booth AM. Physiology of the urinary bladder and urethra. Ann Intern Med 1980; 92:312.

4. Kihara K, de Groat WC. Sympathetic efferent pathways projecting to the bladder neck and proximal urethra in the rat. J Auton Nerv Syst 1997; 62:134.

5. Hollabaugh, RS, Steiner MS, Seller KD, et al. Neuroanatomy of the pelvis: implications for colonic and rectal resection. Dis Colon Rectum 2000; 43(10): 1390–1397.

6. Mundy AR. An anatomical explanation for bladder dysfunction following rectal and uterine surgery. BJU 1982; 54:501–504.

7. Strasser H, Ninkovic M, Hess M, et al. Anatomic and functional studies of the male and female urethral sphincter. World J Urol 2000; 8:324–329.

8. Burgos FJ, Romero J, Fernandez E, et al. Risk factors for developing voiding dysfunction after abdominoperineal resection for adenocarcinoma of the rectum. Dis Colon Rectum 1988; 31:682–685.

9. Kinn AC, Ohman U. Bladder and sexual function after surgery for rectal cancer. Dis Colon Rectum 1986; 29:43–48.

10. Aagaard J, Gerstenberg TC, Knudsen JJ. Urodynamic investigation predicts bladder dysfunction at an early state after abdominoperineal resection of the rectum for cancer. Surgery 1986; 99:564–568.

11. Gerstenberg TC, Neilsen ML, Clausen S, et al. Bladder function after abdominoperineal resection of the rectum for anorectal cancer: urodynamic investigation before and after operation in a consecutive series. Ann Surg 1980; 191:81.

12. Hojo K, Sawada T, Moriya Y. An analysis of survival and voiding, sexual function after wide iliopelvic lymphadenectomy in patients with carcinoma of the rectum, compared with conventional lymphadenectomy. Dis Colon Rectum 1989; 32:128–133.

13. Blaivas JG, Barbalias GA. Characteristics of neural injury after abdominoperineal resection. J Urol 1983; 129:84.

14. Seski JC, Diokno AC. Bladder dysfunction after radical abdominal hysterectomy. Am J Obstet Gynec 1977; 128:643.

15. Forney JP. The effect of radical hysterectomy on bladder physiology. Am J Obstet Gynec 1980; 138:374.

16. Parys BT, Woolfenden KA, Parsons KF. Bladder dysfunction after simple hysterectomy: urodynamic and neurological evaluation. Eur Urol 1990: 17:129–133.

17. Kirkegaard P, Hjortrup A, Sanders S. Bladder dysfunction after low anterior resection for mid-rectal cancer. Am J Surg 1981; 141:266.

18. Fowler JW, Bremner DN, Moffat LEF. The incidence and consequences of damage to the parasympathetic nerve supply to the bladder after abdominoperineal resection of the rectum for carcinoma. Br J Urol 1978; 50:95.

19. Yalla SV, Andriole GL. Vesicourethral dysfunction following pelvic visceral surgery. J Urol 1981; 32:503–509.

20. Norris JP, Staskin DR. History, physical examination, and classification of neurogenic voiding dysfunction. Urol Clin N Am 1996; 23(3):337–343.

21. Nickell K, Boone TB. Peripheral neuropathy and peripheral nerve injury. Urol Clin N Am 1996; 23(3):491–500.

22. Siroky MB, Sax DS, Krane RJ. Sacral signal tracing: the electrophysiology of the bulbocavernosus reflex. J Urol 1979; 122:661–664.

23. Simmons HT. Retention of urine after excision of the rectum. Br Med J 1938; 1:171.

24. McGuire EJ. Urodynamic evaluation after abdominoperineal resection and lumbar intervertebral disk herniation. Urology 1975; 6:63.

25. Hojo K, Vernava AM 3rd, Sugihara K, et al. Preservation of urine voiding and sexual function after rectal cancer surgery. Dis Colon Rectum 1991; 34:532–539.

26. Fishman IJ, Shabsigh R, Kaplan AL. Lower urinary tract dysfunction after radical hysterectomy for carcinoma of the cervix. Urology 1986; 28:462–468.

27. Fraser AC. The late effects of Wertheims's hysterectomy on the urinary tract. J Obstet Gynaec Br Commonw 1966; 73:1002–1007.

28. Tong XK, Huo RJ. The anatomical basis and prevention of neurogenic voiding dysfunction following radical hysterectomy. Surg Radiol Anat 1991; 13:145–148.

29. Smith PH, Ballantyne B. The neuroanatomical basis for denervation of the urinary bladder following major pelvic surgery. Br J Surg 1968; 55:929.

30. Iio S, Yoshioka S, Nishio S, et al. Urodynamic evaluation for bladder dysfunction after radical hysterectomy. Jpn J Urol 1993; 84(3):535–540.

31. Kilkku P, Hirvonen T, Gronoos M. Supra-vaginal uterine amputation vs. abdominal hysterectomy: the effects on urinary symptoms with special reference to pollakisuria, nocturia and dysuria. Maturitas 1981; 3:197–204.

32. Kuwabara Y, Suzuki M, Hashimoto M, et al. New method to prevent bladder dysfunction after radical hysterectomy for uterine cervical cancer. J Obstet Gyn Res 2000; 26(1):1–8.

33. Ficazzola MA, Nitti VW. The etiology of post-radical prostatectomy incontinence and correlation of symptoms with urodynamic findings. J Urol 1998; 160(4):1317–1320.

34. Winters JC, Appell RA, Rackley RR. Urodynamic findings in post-prostatectomy incontinence. Neurourol Urodynam 1998; 17:493–498.

35. Hubert J, Hauri D, Leuener M, et al. Evidence of trigonal denervation and reinnervation after radical retropubic prostatectomy. J Urol 2001; 165:111–113.

36. Columbo R, Bertini R, Salonia A, et al. Nerve and seminal sparing radical cystectomy with orthotopic urinary diversion for select patients with superficial bladder cancer: an innovative surgical approach. J Urol 2001; 165:51–55.

37. Leissner J, Allhoff EP, Wolff W, et al. The pelvic plexus and antireflux surgery: topographical findings and clinical consequences. J Urol 2001; 165(5):1652–1655.

38. Fung LCT, McLorie GA, Jain U, et al. Voiding efficiency after ureteral reimplantation: a comparison of extravesical and intravesical techniques. J Urol 1995; 153:1972.

39. Barrieras D, Lapointe S, Reddy PP, et al. Urinary retention after bilateral extravesical ureteral reimplantation: does dissection distal to the ureteral orifice have a role? J Urol 1999; 162:1197.

40. Zaontz MR, Maizels M, Sugar EC, et al. Detrusorraphy: extravesical ureteral advancement to correct vesicoureteral reflux in children. J Urol 1987; 138:947.

41. Seif C, Braun PM, Martinez Portillo FJ, et al. The risk of bladder denervation during antireflux surgery: a reliable neurophysiological model. J Urol 2002; 167(Suppl 4): 426.

42. Rubin P, Cassarett GW, eds. Central nervous system. In: Clinical radiation pathology. Philadelphia: WB Saunders, 1968:609–661.

43. Johnstone PAS, Wassermann EM, O'Connell PG, et al. Lumbosacral plexopathy secondary to hyperfractionated radiotherapy: a case presentation and literature review. Radiat Oncol Invest Clin Basic Res 1993; 1:126–130.

44. Olsen NK, Pfeiffer P, Johannsen L, et al. Radiation-induced brachial plexopathy; neurological follow-up in 161 recurrence-free breast cancer patients. Int J Radiat Oncol Biol Phys 1993; 26:43–49.

45. Esteban A, Traba A. Fasciculation-myokymic activity and prolonged nerve conduction block. A physiopathological relationship in radiation-induced brachial plexopathy. EEG Clin Neurophys 1993; 89(6):382–391.

46. Keime-Guibert F, Napolitano M, Delattre JY. Neurological complications of radiotherapy and chemotherapy. J Neurol 1998; 245: 695–708.

47. Posner JB. Side effects of radiation therapy. In: Posner JB, ed. Neurologic complications of cancer. Philadelphia: FA Davis, 1995:312.

48. Crook J, Esche B, Futter N. Effect of pelvic radiotherapy for prostate cancer on bowel, bladder and sexual function: the patient's perspective. Urology 1996; 47(3):387–394.

49. Incrocci L, Koos Slob A. Incidence, etiology, and therapy for erectile dysfunction after external beam radiotherapy for prostate cancer. Urology 2002; 60:107.

50. Nguyen LN, Pollack A, Zagars GK. Late effects after radiotherapy for prostate cancer in a randomized dose–response study: results of a self-assessment questionnaire. Urology 1998; 51(6):991–997.

51. Tait DM, Nahum AE, Meyer LC, et al. Acute toxicity in pelvic radiotherapy; a randomized trial of conformal versus conventional treatment. Radiother Oncol 1997; 42:121–136.

52. Kinsella TJ, DeLuca AM, Barnes M, et al. Threshold does for peripheral neuropathy following intraoperative radiotherapy (IORT) in a large animal model. Int J Radiat Oncol Biol Phys 1991; 20:697–701.

53. Johnstone PAS, DeLuca AM, Bacher JD, et al. Clinical toxicity of peripheral nerve to intraoperative radiotherapy in a canine model. Int J Radiat Oncol Biol Phys 1995; 32(4):1031–1034.

54. Parkin DE, Davis JA, Symonds RP. Long-term bladder symptomatology following radiotherapy for cervical carcinoma. Radiother Oncol 1987; 9(3):195–199.

55. Litwin MS, Pasta DJ, Yu J, et al. Urinary function and bother after radical prostatectomy or radiation for prostate cancer: a longitudinal, multivariate quality of life analysis from the cancer of the prostate strategic urologic research endeavor. J Urol 2000; 164(6):1973–1977.

56. Maier U, Ehrenbock PM, Hofbauer J. Late urological complications and malignancies after curative radiotherapy for gynecological carcinomas: a retrospective analysis of 10,709 patients. J Urol 1997; 158(3):814–817.

57. Hanfmann B, Engels M, Dorr W. Radiation-induced impairment of urinary bladder function. Assessment of micturition volumes. Strahlenther Onkolog 1998; 174(Suppl 3):96–98.

58. Behr J, Winkler M, Willgeroth F. Functional changes in the lower urinary tract after irradiation of cervix carcinoma. Strahlenther Onkolog 1990; 166(2):135–139.

59. Sindelar WF, Hoekstra H, Restrepo C, et al. Pathological tissue changes following intraoperative radiotherapy. Am J Clin Oncol 1986; 9(6):504–509.

60. Michailov MC, Neu E, Tempel K. Influence of x-irradiation on the motor activity of rat urinary bladder in vitro and in vivo. Strahlenther Onkolog 1991; 167(5):311–318.

21

Dementia and lower urinary tract dysfunction

Ryuji Sakakibara and Takamichi Hattori

Introduction

Urinary incontinence, dementia, and osteoporosis are major concerns in a geriatric population that has grown rapidly in recent decades. Of these three, urinary incontinence is very often associated with dementia, since both conditions originate from the same underlying disorder and urinary incontinence occurs secondarily from dementia. Urinary incontinence can result in medical morbidity, impaired self-esteem of the patient, caregiver's stress, early institutionalization of the patient, and considerable financial cost. However, incontinence in persons with dementia has received limited study. In some nursing home settings, incontinence may be accepted as the norm and approached with therapeutic nihilism, although it is a potentially treatable condition. This chapter reviews the current concepts on lower urinary tract dysfunction associated with dementia, with particular reference to its prevalence, etiology, mechanism, and management.

Prevalence

Prevalence rate of urinary incontinence

Of the lower urinary tract dysfunction in patients with dementia, most investigators have focused on the prevalence of urinary incontinence.[1–14] Many studies rely on both patient and family/caregiver reports, since patients with dementia may underreport the problem owing to their under-recognition, forgetfulness, and possible denial of the condition because of its embarrassing nature.

Prevalence rates varied considerably: from 11% to 90% of individuals with dementia had incontinence, which may depend on patient selection (Table 21.1). As expected, institutional samples had the highest prevalence (90%), with progressively lower rates reported for mixed institutional-community dwelling samples (around 40%) and individuals attending outpatient clinics and living at home (lowest prevalence of 11%).

The International Continence Society defines urinary incontinence as 'the involuntary loss of urine which is a social or hygienic problem and is objectively demonstrable.'[15] This definition implies a certain severity of incontinence, although many studies looked at the presence or absence of urinary incontinence.

Ouslander et al[7] found that 65% of incontinent subjects had fewer than three episodes per week, 11% had three–six episodes per week, and 24% had incontinence once a day or more. McLaren et al[14] found that 90% of incontinent subjects had at least one episode during the 3-week assessment period, 78% had one episode a week, and 40% had incontinence once a day. Thus, according to these studies, more than two-thirds of incontinent patients with dementia have at least one episode a week. This figure contrasts with general population surveys of elderly individuals, of whom about 5% have urine loss at least once a week.[16] According to Campbell et al[10] urinary incontinence was found in 53% of patients with dementia and in 13% of non-demented older individuals.

In post-stroke patients who were admitted for a rehabilitation program, Noto[12] found that urinary incontinence was present in 83% of patients with dementia and in 45% of non-demented patients. Institutional residents with dementia who were continent on admission were more likely to develop incontinence during a 12-month follow-up period, and incontinence was less likely to resolve in those individuals.[17,18] In addition, dementia is more prevalent in incontinent individuals than in those without. Palmer et al[17] and Ouslander et al[18] reported that 83% of incontinent nursing home residents had dementia compared with only 58% of continent residents. Thus, these community-based and institutional studies confirm the frequent association between urinary incontinence and cognitive impairment.

However, it should be emphasized that association does not imply causation. Many studies were performed irrespective of underlying disease, although it may considerably affect the prevalence rates of incontinence.

Table 21.1 *Prevalence of urinary incontinence in persons with dementia*

Study	Year	Setting	*n*	Mean age (years)	Dementia type	Rate of incontinence (%)	Reference
Teri	1989	Dementia clinic	56	71	AD	11	1
Teri	1988	Dementia clinic	127	77	AD	15	2
Teri	1990	Dementia clinic	106	77	AD	15	3
Swearer	1988	Dementia clinic	95	69	AD/MID/mixed	17	4
Udaka	1994	Neurology inpatients/outpatients	38	69	AD	21	5
Berrios	1986	Psychiatry outpatients	100	80	AD/MID/mixed	35	6
Ouslander	1990	Community	184	76	AD/MID/mixed	36	7
Rabins	1982	Psychiatry inpatients/outpatients	55	–	AD/MID/other	40	8
Burns	1990	Psychiatry inpatients/outpatients	178	80	AD	48	9
Campbell	1985	Random survey: home/institution	83	>64	–	53	10
Borrie	1992	Chronic care hospital	139	–	–	78	11
Noto	1994	Rehabilitation hospital	36	68	MID	83	12
Toba	1996	Chronic care hospital	867	>64	–	89	13
Mclaren	1981	Psychogeriatric inpatients	121	81	AD/MID	90	14

As expected, compared with multi-infarct dementia, Berrios[6] found that incontinence was more prevalent in Alzheimer's disease, which is the major etiology of severe cognitive decline. However, in dementia outpatient clinics, Teri et al[1-3] found urinary incontinence in only 11–15% of patients with Alzheimer's disease. On the contrary, Kotsuoris et al[19] found urinary incontinence in up to 50% of 84 outpatients with multi-infarct dementia. Thus, urinary incontinence in multiple cerebral infarction tends to appear earlier than in Alzheimer's disease. Of particular importance is that urinary incontinence in those patients was not always accompanied by dementia, and was often preceded by urinary frequency and urgency.[20] This implies that urinary incontinence in multiple cerebral infarction may have a different mechanism than in Alzheimer's disease, as will be discussed later.

Sex distribution

Among adults older than 60 years of age, urinary incontinence is twice as common in women as in men, reflecting anatomical differences in the urethra and the pelvic floor muscles that lead to stress urinary incontinence.[16] Alzheimer's disease also occurs more commonly in women. However, previous studies did not find a significant difference in the prevalence of incontinence between men and women with dementia.[6,7,9] On the contrary, Ouslander et al[18] reported that the prevalence of urinary incontinence was twice as high in males as in females, and Palmer et al[17] found that male gender increased the probability of urinary incontinence by 68% 1 year after admission to a nursing home. These results are in line with the findings that men have more rapid and severe mental and physical deterioration than women admitted to nursing homes.[17] The presence of prostatic hypertrophy predisposing to urinary overflow, and male predominance of multi-infarct dementia may explain these findings.[17,18]

Etiology

We now briefly discuss the underlying etiologies of both dementia and lower urinary tract dysfunction. However, in a clinical context, comorbidity of degenerative and vascular pathologies seems likely.

Alzheimer's disease

Alzheimer's disease is the most common cause of dementia in the elderly, and accounts for more than 50% of dementia patients.[21] The pathological hallmarks of this disease include senile plaques and neurofibrillary tangles. Axial and coronal slices of magnetic resonance imaging (MRI) scans often reveal atrophy of the cerebral cortex and the hippocampus; the latter accounts for memory impairment of the patients.

Dementia in Alzheimer's disease is characterized by loss of memory, intellectual dysfunction, disturbances in speech such as anomia (difficulty in word finding), and various types of apraxia and agnosia. In practice, dementia can be suspected by scores in a feasible test, i.e. mini-mental status examination (MMSE), when the subject gains less than 23 of 30 scores. Emotional disturbances include depression in about 25% of patients, and agitation and restlessness are also common. Motor signs are particularly rare early in the course of the illness, but, as the disease progresses, increased reflexes and parkinsonian syndrome may develop. Myoclonus is occasionally reported. Decreased motivation and initiative are also significant features. In most advanced cases, abulia (loss of psychomotor activity) and akinetic mutism occur. As discussed earlier, prominent urinary disturbances do occur in Alzheimer's disease but are uncommon in the early stage of the disease.

Multiple cerebral infarction

Multiple cerebral infarction is the second most common cause of dementia in the elderly, and, if dementia is the main problem, it is called a multi-infarct (vascular) dementia.[22] Cardinal features of multi-infarct dementia include history of stroke, stepwise deterioration, fluctuating course, focal neurological symptoms, parkinsonian syndrome with wide-based gait, emotional incontinence, and the presence of arteriosclerotic risk factors such as hypertension. Of these features, Kotsoris et al[19] found that urinary disturbance, noted in 50%, frequently preceded a development of dementia by 5 years and more. Similarly, gait disturbance, noted in 24%, preceded a development of dementia by 2 years and more. Even though two-thirds of men with urinary disturbance had been diagnosed with benign prostatic hypertrophy, urinary symptoms often persisted after prostatectomy. Fluid-attenuated inversion recovery (FLAIR) imaging of MRI scan is most sensitive for detecting and grading multiple cerebral infarction, particularly white matter changes. Sakakibara et al[20] classified MRI-defined white matter multi-infarction into grades 1–4, and found that urinary disturbance was more common than cognitive or gait disorders, particularly in patients with mild (grade 1) lesion. In addition, nocturnal urinary frequency was a more common and earlier feature than urinary incontinence (Figure 21.1).[26]

Therefore, it is likely that urinary disturbance is the initial manifestation in a number of multi-infarction patients.

Diffuse Lewy body disease

Diffuse Lewy body disease (DLBD) is a newly recognized entity, that is considered to be the second most common degenerative cause of dementia.[23] In particular, DLBD attracts growing attention since cognitive impairment of this disorder responds well to central cholinergic agents.[24] The name of DLBD is derived from pathology. Lewy bodies are cytoplasmic inclusion bodies, and appear to be widespread in the cerebral cortex and in the basal ganglia in this disorder. Lewy bodies have been shown to be the pathological hallmark of Parkinson's disease, but in Parkinson's disease Lewy bodies appear almost exclusively in the substantia nigra of the basal midbrain. Thus, clinical features of DLBD are characterized by a combination of dementia and parkinsonian syndrome, and visual hallucinations and fluctuation of the symptoms are common. Up to now, no urodynamic data are available in DLBD. However, Del-Ser et al[25] found that onset of urinary incontinence was significantly earlier in DLBD (3.2 years after dementia onset) than in Alzheimer's disease (6.5 years after dementia onset). Urinary incontinence is often associated with severe cognitive decline in Alzheimer's disease, but usually precedes severe mental failure in DLBD. A less common but significant feature of DLBD is widespread autonomic failure. In such cases, clinical presentations may mimic those of the Shy–Drager syndrome.

Other cerebral causes

Less common, but potentially treatable causes of dementia should be addressed. Normal pressure (communicating) hydrocephalus is such a disorder that occurs in the elderly.[27] Clinical features of this disorder are often indistinguishable from those of multi-infarct dementia – i.e. parkinsonian syndrome, urinary incontinence, and dementia – and the former two very often precede dementia. However, in established cases the level of consciousness tends to decline, which is rarely seen in multi-infarct dementia. MRI scans reveal the presence of disproportionally dilated cerebral ventricles with cortical pressure signs. CT (computed tomography)-ventriculography reveals a delayed disappearance (reflux) of contrast medium from lateral ventricles. A positive spinal tap test may predict successful outcome of shunt surgery. Chronic subdural hematoma is a cause of transient dementia and urinary incontinence. These signs usually appear several weeks after an episode of fall, though they are not always apparent in elderly individuals.

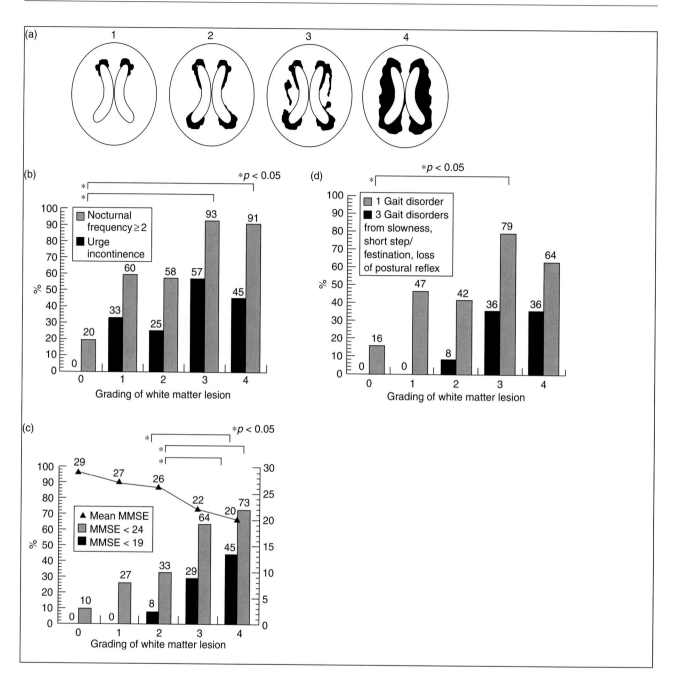

Figure 21.1

Cerebral white matter lesion and urinary dysfunction. (a) Schematic presentation of the grading of white-matter lesion on MRI (according to Brand-Zawadzki et al[26]). Grade 1: punctated foci of high signal intensity in the white matter immediately at the top of the frontal horns of the lateral ventricles. Grade 2: white-matter lesions were seen elsewhere but remained confined to the immediate subependymal region of the ventricles. Grade 3: periventricular as well as separate, discrete, deep white-matter foci of signal abnormality. Grade 4: discrete white-matter foci had become large and coalescent. (b) Urinary dysfunction and white-matter lesion on MRI. (c) Cognitive disorder and white-matter lesion on MRI. MMSE: mini-mental state examination. (d) Gait disorder and white-matter lesion on MRI.

One-side dominant pyramidal signs are common features, since this disease usually has laterality even though it occurs bilaterally. CT scans reveal crescent-like hematoma, particularly in the frontoparietal region.

Mechanism

In order to keep continence in the elderly, there needs to be:

1. the presence of a normal lower urinary tract with intact innervation for both urinary filling and voiding
2. an emotional ability to hold urine after having the first sensation and proper motivation to urinate in the toilet
3. a cognitive ability to know how to get to a toilet and how to adjust clothing
4. a mobile ability to reach the toilet with hand dexterity for disrobing
5. an absence of medications that adversely affect the lower urinary tract innervation or alertness
6. a proper environment, including access to toilets and lack of restraints.

It is very likely that incontinence in elderly demented patients is multifactorial, and often one factor relates to another.

Functional incontinence

Functional incontinence is a term for incontinence that is not derived from abnormality in the lower urinary tract or its innervation, but from decreased motivation, cognitive disability, and immobility. From the viewpoint of less mobile patients, toilet has as though gone far away as it used to be. For patients with cognitive decline, toileting may become a worry because of the difficulty of finding their way. But for others, toileting or even incontinence may no longer be a concern. Many studies have shown that severity of immobility and dementia are positively correlated with functional incontinence.[28] Of these, gait disorder may be an early and prominent feature in multiple cerebral infarction and DLBD, and may lead to functional incontinence and frequent falls, whereas it is very uncommon in the early stage of Alzheimer's disease. Characteristics of the parkinsonian gait in these diseases are slow, short-stepped gait with festination and postural instability. Wide-based ataxic gait often overlaps the short-stepped gait, particularly in cases of multiple cerebral infarction. The responsible sites for the gait disorder seem to be in the basal ganglia and in the medial frontal lobe, particularly the supplementary motor area or its pathways.

In addition, incontinence may develop because of confusion secondary to a superimposed delirium. Major depression occurs in up to 20% of patients with Alzheimer's disease, and the apathy, psychomotor retardation, and lack of initiative may also precipitate immobility. Resnick et al[29] performed regression analysis and found that cognitive impairment only doubled the risk of incontinence. Similarly, Jirovec and Wells[30] found that, in nursing home residents with dementia, immobility emerged as the best predictor of urinary incontinence. McGrother et al[31] found that 96% of subjects with dementia and incontinence also had dependence on getting to the toilet or dressing, and the combination of dementia and locomotor problems was 13 times more common among incontinent than continent individuals. The important implication of these findings is that, in those patients, improvement in initiative and mobility for toileting may well lead to a reduction of incontinence. In particular, treatment will be successful insofar as urinary sensation and incontinence are made aware of, and told to caregivers by persons with dementia.

Social and environmental factors also need to be considered. In some nursing home settings, diapers are automatically used for any patient, continent or not, and, if incontinence is found, balloon catheters are indwelled. Consequently, continence seems to be neither expected nor a high priority of care. In addition, toilet facilities may not be visible or easily accessible, thereby increasing the risk of incontinence. It should be mentioned that physical restraints can be iatrogenic causes of immobility. Behaviorally disturbed nursing home residents are more often restrained and unable to get to the toilet.

Drug-induced incontinence and retention

Drugs that may affect either the central nervous system or the lower urinary tract are potential causes of transient incontinence. In a study of 84 older, incontinent, female nursing home residents, Keister and Creason[31] found that 70% of subjects were taking a drug having the potential to cause incontinence. Antipsychotic medications, antidepressants, benzodiazepines, and sedatives are frequently used to treat agitation, insomnia, and depression, and may cause incontinence through increased confusion, sedation, parkinsonism, and immobility. Urinary retention and overflow may result from the anticholinergic side-effects of tricyclic antidepressants and antipsychotic medications.

Nocturnal polyuria

Nocturnal polyuria is a common reason for nocturia in the elderly, and is potentially treatable. Nocturnal polyuria in older individuals seem to be multifactorial. It may result from congestive heart failure or liver cirrhosis, but may also have a cerebral etiology. Cerebrovascular disease may cause nocturnal polyuria, particularly when it involves the hypothalamic region that contains arginine vasopressin (AVP) neurons. We had such patients, who lost circadian rhythm of plasma AVP, which normally rises at night. Diabetes is also a common cause of polyuria.

Stress urinary incontinence

It is important to evaluate for comorbid stress incontinence, since it is a very common condition due to pelvic floor weakness in older women, and is potentially treatable. In an older incontinent population, Payne[33] described that one-half of patients suffered from pure stress incontinence, 10–20% had pure urge incontinence, and the remaining patients had a mixed form. Resnick et al[34] noted that a significant proportion of women with dementia also had stress urinary incontinence. Although the reliability of diagnosing stress incontinence decreased with increasing severity of dementia, 80% of those with MMSE scores of 10–23 and 66% of those with scores of 9 or less were still able to perform a stress maneuver.

Detrusor hyperreflexia during filling

Although urodynamic study is a gold standard for examining lower urinary tract function, not many detailed studies have been made in cognitively impaired older subjects, because of the methodological (reliability) and ethical (feasibility and benefit) issues. To ensure accuracy of the urodynamic results, the tests are better performed by physicians with/without well-trained assistants, encouraging and communicating with the patients, particularly for assessing bladder capacity. In severely demented patients, we occasionally need to assume their urinary sensation from their facial and bodily expressions. Rectal pressure monitoring is a necessity to subtract pressure changes that come from unwanted body movements and strains. Sphincter electromyography (EMG) recording is a matter of controversy since it is considered a bit harmful, although it may provide us with important information when there are large post-void residuals. Considering these difficulties, there is an opinion that urodynamic testing should only be undertaken if empirical therapy has failed and other therapy approaches need to be tried, and if surgery is being considered. In addition, urodynamic testing has been considered as not a prerequisite for a pharmacological trial in patients with symptoms of overactive bladder.

Detrusor hyperreflexia (DH) or detrusor overactivity is urodynamically defined as an involuntary phasic increase in detrusor pressure >10 cmH$_2$O during fillings; it is commonly associated with decreased bladder volumes at first sensation and maximum desire to void. DH is observed in a significant proportion of cognitively intact older subjects. In those subjects, two major etiologies for DH have been proposed: central and peripheral. Peripheral etiology includes detrusor muscle change, which may increase with age, detected by electron microscopy.[35] Muscle cells from patients with DH *in vitro* have greater spontaneous contractile activity than those from normal detrusor, and greater sensitivity to electrical field stimulation and acetylcholine.[36] Attention has also been paid to men with outlet obstruction in which increased α-adrenergic receptors and morphological–biochemical changes of the detrusor muscles may lead to increased contractile activity and possible DH in the patient.[37] In such cases, surgical treatment of obstruction may lessen DH.

Central etiology is thought to be more significant. It is well known that cerebral diseases can lead to a loss of the brain's inhibitory influence on the spino-bulbo-spinal micturition reflex (Figure 21.2). The information that arises from the lower urinary tract reaches the pontine micturition center (PMC), which then activates the descending pathway to the sacral preganglionic neurons innervating the bladder.[38] The anteromedial frontal cortex is thought to be the higher center for micturition, since lesions of this area lead to DH and urinary retention; the latter occurs particularly in the initial phase. Recent positron emission tomography (PET) studies have shown that during bladder filling the frontal micturition center is tonically active together with activation in the basal ganglia and the pontine storage center that is located adjacent to the PMC.[39,40] Griffiths et al[40] studied 128 geriatric incontinent patients, one-half of them having dementia, showing that one-half the population had DH by videourodynamic study. In addition, single-photon emission computed tomography (SPECT) imaging showed that patients with DH had significant underperfusion in the right frontal lobe. Similarly, cognitively intact, community dwelling older individuals commonly show 'silent' multiple cerebral infarction by MRI scans.[20,42] Detailed examination reveals the presence of gait disorder, which is suggestive of the disease. Most of the individuals were continent, but often had nocturnal urinary frequency and urgency due in part to DH. According to Yu et al[28] in 133 incontinent female nursing home residents, 88% of them having dementia, urodynamic studies revealed normal bladder function in 41%, DH in 38%, stress incontinence in 16%, and overflow incontinence from outlet obstruction in 5%. Resnick et al[34] reported that 64% of nursing home individuals with dementia had DH compared with 47% of those who

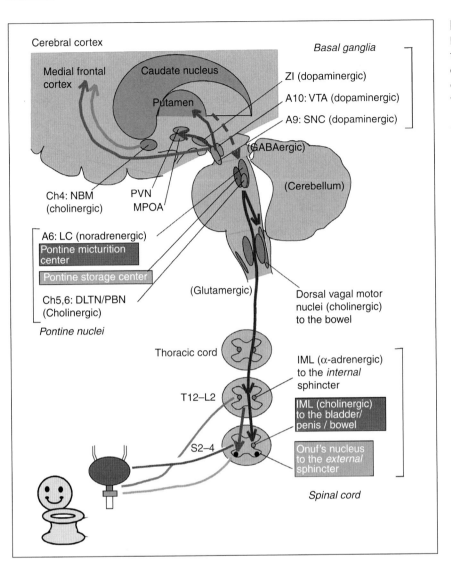

Figure 21.2
Neural mechanism as for urinary function. Brain diseases that cause dementia commonly affect the frontal cortex and the basal ganglia, both of which are relevant to neural control of micturition. Some deep brain structures may also contribute to micturition function such as nucleus basalis Mynert (NBM) (cholinergic) and ventral tegmental area (VTA) (dopaminergic) that send fibers to the frontal cortex.

were cognitively intact. In women, positive correlation was found between the presence of DH and dementia. These findings suggest a correlation between these two conditions, and that demented patients often have DH as a significant cause of incontinence.

Although not many studies have specified the types of dementia, Mori et al[43] examined 46 institutionalized dementia patients, comprising Alzheimer's disease in 31, multi-infarct dementia in 11, and both in 4. They found DH in 58% of Alzheimer's disease, in 91% of multi-infarct dementia, and in 50% of mixed type. Sugiyama et al[44] found DH in 40% of 20 patients with Alzheimer's disease. In particular, DH was noted in 8 of 13 incontinent patients and none of 7 continent patients.

Sphincter EMG revealed uninhibited sphincter relaxation (USR) in a patient. When USR occurs together with DH, incontinence becomes more prominent, which is thought to be a feature of cerebral diseases. The pathology of Alzheimer's disease involves the medial frontal lobe,

which receives various inputs from an other brain area. Of particular importance is the cholinergic pathway that originates from the nucleus basalis Mynert (Ch4 cell group). In experimental studies, lesions in this small nucleus give rise to DH, suggesting cortical cholinergic neurons have an inhibitory role on the micturition reflex.[45] Sakakibara et al[46] examined 19 patients with multi-infarct dementia. All patients had nocturnal frequency and urgency, and 70% had urinary incontinence of urge and stress types. Urodynamic studies revealed DH in 70% and a low compliance curve in 10%. Sakakibara et al[20] urodynamically studied 22 elderly subjects with white matter multi-infarction and 11 subjects without. DH was significantly more prevalent in those with white matter lesions (82%) than in those with normal MRI (9%). Although not statistically significant, USR was more common in subjects with white matter lesion. Thus, according to these reports, DH contributes to urinary frequency and urgency incontinence in multi-infarct dementia more than in Alzheimer's disease.

Impaired detrusor contractility during voiding

Resnick and Yalla[47] reported that a subgroup of incontinent elderly individuals with DH, of whom most were women, had impaired bladder contractility (DHIC) that led to post-micturition residuals (PMR) with an average volume of 95 ml. Although Eastwood and Lord[48] were not able to replicate these findings, Elbadawi et al[49] found that patients with DHIC could be differentiated from those with DH and normal contractility on the basis of detrusor ultrastructure. Another important finding by Resnick and Yella[47] was that sphincter EMG of the patients with DHIC did not show detrusor-sphincter dyssynergia. We previously performed pressure–flow analysis in 8 patients with Alzheimer's disease who had neither PMR nor detrusor-sphincter dyssynergia. However, the mean voiding pressure of the patients was 54 cmH$_2$O (range 20–101 cmH$_2$O) and 5 had weak detrusor.

Sakakibara et al[20] also found that persons with multi-infarction had PMR more commonly – 50% had an average volume of 93 ml – than those without (9%). Correctly diagnosing the impaired contractility group with urodynamic testing is of therapeutic importance, because such patients may be at risk of acute urinary retention if given anticholinergic medication.[47] Kuwabara et al[50] studied PMR volumes by portable echography (BV5000) in 82 institutionalized dementia patients, consisting of Alzheimer's disease in 45, multi-infarct dementia in 19, normal pressure hydrocephalus in 5, Pick's disease in 2, and other causes in 11. Eighty-three percent of the patients had urinary urgency or incontinence. They found PMR > 100 ml in 6 patients (8%), consisting of Alzheimer's disease in 5 and multi-infarct dementia in 1. However, the cause of large PMR in the patients was assumed to be drug-induced in 1, prostate hypertrophy in 1, frontal lobectomy for pre-existing schizophrenia in 1, and unknown in 2. Of comorbid conditions that may affect detrusor contractility, lumbar spondylosis and diabetic polyneuropathy are common in the elderly. Examination of the lower extremities for sensation and deep tendon reflexes may provide a cue to suspect these disorders. These issues are also a particular problem in patients who have undergone prostate hypertrophy for large PMR or retention, since impaired detrusor contractility during voiding is a significant factor that may lead to unsuccessful surgical outcome.[47]

Management

In general, management for lower urinary tract dysfunction in dementia patients needs to be individualized, and the risk/benefit ratio of these procedures, particularly invasive or irreversible treatments, needs to be carefully considered.

Treatment of transient causes

The first step of management is to identify and treat transient acute causes of incontinence. Acute causes may be recalled from the mnemonic 'DIAPERS' (Delirium, Infection, Atrophic vaginitis, Pharmaceuticals, Psychological, Endocrine, Restricted mobility, Stool impaction).[51] Some factors are derived from the dementing illness, but others are from the comorbid medical conditions, inappropriate environment, and medication. There is also an interrelationship between these factors. An elderly patient's delirium may be secondary to, for example, a pharmacological or infectious outcome.

Toileting/behavioral therapy

Toileting regimens (behavioral therapy) have been used to manage functional incontinence in elderly individuals. Patients with decreased motivation, cognitive disability, and gait disorder are highly likely to be incontinent. With prompted voiding, patients who have decreased motivation are asked on a regular schedule if they need toileting assistance, but are toileted only if they request assistance. Prompted voiding is usually combined with positive reinforcement, in the form of praise, for appropriate toileting requests and for dryness. On most occasions, patients require physical assistance with toileting because of comorbid gait disorder and cognitive disability. According to Skelly and Flint,[52] who carefully reviewed seven studies, when checked every 1–2 hours during waking hours, patients were dry 64% of the time at baseline on average. After treatment, this figure rose to 76%. This translated into a mean relative reduction of wet episodes of 32%. Better response to the treatment was obtained in less-demented patients, who could recognize the need to void, and had incontinence fewer than 4 episodes per 12-hour period. As expected, normal bladder function also predicted better response. With scheduled toileting, patients who have little or no motivation are toileted on a regular schedule (fixed schedule), usually every 2 hours, or a schedule that matches the patient's own voiding pattern (individualized schedule). Ouslander et al[53] examined the effects of a fixed, 2-hourly toileting schedule on 15 cognitively impaired patients with DH, of whom 53% needed physical assistance. Toileting significantly reduced the incidence of incontinence from 43% to 32%. Flint and Skelly[54] reported that 55% of ambulatory dementia patients became dry or had a significant improvement in incontinence with toileting schedule. However, Jirovec[55] reported that 6 weeks of scheduled toileting did not improve incontinence in a group of demented and dependent nursing home residents, although poor staff compliance with the toileting program contributed to the negative outcome. The results suggest that more severely demented, and less mobile individuals with bladder abnormalities are the least likely to benefit from toileting programs. There are cost/benefit studies that the labor costs of toileting programs may be higher than the savings in laundry costs to the nursing home.[56] However, carefully selecting patients who can most benefit from toileting regimens is one possible way of reducing conflict.

Environmental settings are also important for managing functional incontinence. Chaufreau-Rena et al[57] assessed whether enhanced visual cues, such as painting the toilet doors bright orange and displaying large pictures of a lady using a toilet, would have an impact on incontinence in severely demented women on a psychogeriatric ward. However, when environmental changes were the only treatment intervention, incontinence did not improve. Nevertheless, recommended toilet settings may include mobility aids such as hallway handrails, canes, walkers, and wheelchairs; easy toilet access and visibility; toilet facilities such as lighting, grab bars, and toilet seat height; automatic washing devices for the buttocks and lifting-up commodes; and, finally, the patient's easy disrobing. Also, if continence is to be maximized, alternatives to physical restraints need to be sought.

Medication

Cognitive impairment and decreased motivation

Although the etiology of Alzheimer's disease remains uncertain, the cognitive deficits in Alzheimer's disease patients are thought to be due, at least in part, to a decrease in cholinergic innervation of the cerebral cortex and the basal forebrain. Loss of cholinergic nerve terminals in Alzheimer's disease is detected *in vivo* by PET using acetylcholinesterase (AChE) activities. There are several central cholinomimetic agents, including donepezil hydrochloride and rivastigmine: both of them are central AChE inhibitors that decrease degradation of acetylcholine, thus increasing the concentration of acetylcholine in the synaptic cleft. These agents inhibit AChE selectively in the brain,[58] which reverses cognitive decline in mild-to-moderate Alzheimer's disease patients for at least 6–12 months.[59] Clinicians must be aware that these agents may cause gastrointestinal adverse effects. As mentioned above, a subgroup of Alzheimer's disease patients have urge incontinence and DH even in their early stage. Hashimoto et al[60] reported that 7% of the patients taking 5 mg/day of donepezil showed urinary incontinence as a potential initial adverse effect. However, we did not see such adverse effects in Alzheimer's disease patients by urodynamic studies. Cognitive impairment in patients with DLBD also responded well to central cholinergic agents.[24] In patients

with mild-to-moderate dementia, decreased motivation can be treated with 200–300 mg/day of amantadine hydrochloride. However, it has not been determined as to whether these drugs could ameliorate the domains of toileting and functional incontinence in disability scales. Aniracetam is a pyrrolidinone derivative, and is thought to facilitate cholinergic neurotransmission. In an open study of 52 senile post-stroke patients, some of whom had dementia, Kumon et al[61] found that 600 mg/day of aniracetam benefited 46% of the patients for their urinary and fecal incontinence.

Gait disorder

Gait disorder is a part of parkinsonian syndrome in multi-infarct dementia and DLBD, but is also mildly seen in Alzheimer's disease. Although levodopa seems not as effective as in Parkinson's disease, 200–300 mg/day of this drug (usually coupled with peripheral dopa-decarboxylase inhibitor) ameliorates gait disorder in dementia patients, and may be of benefit in treating functional incontinence. Levodopa is better prescribed with rehabilitation programs, since Jirovec[62] found that, in cognitively impaired nursing home residents, a daily exercise program designed to improve walking had a significant impact on reducing daytime incontinence. Physicians should also be aware of potential adverse effects of levodopa, such as postural hypotension and hallucinations. Although levodopa seems to ameliorate urinary urgency in early, untreated Parkinson's disease patients, it may augment DH in advanced cases with motor fluctuation.

Detrusor hyperreflexia

Medications used to treat DH include anticholinergic agents such as propantheline, oxybutynin, and propiverine, and smooth muscle relaxants such as flavoxate. Mori et al[43] performed urodynamic studies in 46 dementia patients, and found DH in 58% of Alzheimer's disease and 91% of multi-infarct dementia patients. An open trial with 20 mg/day of propiverine hydrochloride for 2 weeks was done irrespective of the presence of DH. They found that 40% of patients showed an increased bladder capacity or lessened frequency of incontinence. Both types of dementia groups responded almost equally, and patients with DH showed more satisfactory response.

Tobin and Brocklehurst[63] used a combination of propantheline bromide (15 mg/day) and flavoxate hydrochloride (200 mg/day) to treat urinary incontinence in a cognitively impaired nursing home population, of whom 95% were clinically diagnosed as overactive bladder. There was a significant reduction in nocturnal but not daytime incontinence compared with controls. Burgio et al[64] found that, in 197 cognitively intact elderly women with predominantly urge incontinence, either 7.5–15 mg/day of oxybutynin hydrochloride (68.5%) or behavioral treatment (80.7%) was more effective than placebo (39.4%) in randomized controlled trials. However, in dementia patients with DH, Zorzitto et al[65] did not find that 15 mg/day of propantheline was any more effective than placebo. When the dose of propantheline was increased to 30 mg, there was a statistically significant improvement, but the clinical benefit was outweighed by the presence of adverse effects in 50% of subjects.

Although DH seems to be the cause of urinary frequency and urgency incontinence in those patients, negative findings of the study contrast with the reported efficacy of anticholinergic medications in approximately 50% of cognitively intact, independently mobile older outpatients with incontinence.[66] Therefore, treatment for DH may be of benefit only in mild-to-moderate dementia without marked immobility. The use of medications with anticholinergic side-effects in older persons is a concern, particularly when there is a risk of exacerbating cognitive impairment. Although oxybutynin has been developed as a peripherally acting drug, recent research suggests that it has some adverse effects on cognitive function.[67] Other more common side-effects are dryness of the mouth and constipation.

Stress incontinence

Tricyclic antidepressants are commonly used to treat both DH and stress incontinence since they have both anticholinergic and α-adrenergic properties, the latter of which is expected to increase urethral tone. However, a randomized controlled study to examine the effect of a tricyclic on incontinence in an exclusively older group of patients did not find a statistically significant difference between imipramine hydrochloride (mean dose 54 mg) and placebo.[68] One has to exercise caution in using imipramine in the older person because of its sedative, hypotensive, and cardiac effects and the risk of falls. Alpha-adrenergic agonists such as midodrine hydrochloride have been shown to benefit some older women with stress incontinence.[66] The estrogen quinestradol was reported to be effective in reducing the frequency of incontinence in older women. However, prolonged estrogen therapy may increase the risk of endometrial carcinoma.

Outlet obstruction

Prazosin hydrochloride, a nonselective α_1-adrenergic antagonist, is effective in the symptomatic management of benign prostatic hypertrophy. However, adverse effects of α-adrenergic blockers may limit their use in frail elderly patients such as those with orthostatic hypotension. The proximal urethra has an abundance of α_{1A-D}-adrenergic receptors. In contrast, the vascular wall has an abundance of α_{1B} receptors, particularly in the elderly.[69] Prazosin may block both α_{1B} receptors in the vascular wall and α_{1A-D} receptors in the proximal urethra. Recently launched selective α_{1A-D}-adrenergic blockers, such as tamsulosin hydrochloride and naftopidil, are of choice because of fewer side-effects.

Nocturnal polyuria

Desmopressin is a potent analogue of AVP, and has been used to treat patients with nocturnal polyuria due probably to impaired circadian rhythm of the plasma AVP.[70] We prescribed 5 μg of intranasal desmopressin once a night in post-stroke patients who had impaired circadian AVP rhythm, and noted improvement of the nocturnal polyuria. This small dose of desmopressin is unlikely to cause adverse effects, even though hyponatremia and signs of cardiac failure should be checked regularly. A recently launched tablet form is feasible and may be of particular benefit.

Pelvic muscle exercises and biofeedback

Pelvic muscle exercises, sometimes combined with biofeedback, have been used successfully to treat stress incontinence in older women.[71] For the procedure to be effective, the patient must actively contract and relax pubococcygeal muscles up to 80 times a day for several months. However, Tobin and Brocklehurst[63] note that, because most of their patients have severe cognitive and physical deterioration, they were unable to cooperate with treatment for stress incontinence.

Electrical stimulation

In an uncontrolled trial, Lamhut et al[72] studied the effectiveness of electrical stimulation in nine incontinent female nursing home patients with DH. These patients had severe cognitive impairment, were bed bound, and were completely dependent in activities of daily living. They were treated with stimulation for 15 min twice a week for 8 weeks using a rectal probe. In this group of subjects, the treatment was not effective, and was associated with a 20% increase in the average number of incontinent episodes. Two patients were withdrawn from the study because of agitation associated with the procedure.

Surgery

Surgery has been used to treat benign outlet obstruction and stress incontinence in older patients, when conservative methods and medications have failed or are not appropriate.[73] In some frail older persons, these problems can be corrected, or at least improved, by newer, less strenuous surgical techniques that can be completed in a short period of time, including transurethral incision of the prostate (TUIP) and tension-free vaginal tapes (TVT). However, whether repair of these outlet lesions reliably restores continence in frail, demented individuals remains to be established.

Devices, pads, and catheters

Indwelling catheters are often used excessively and inappropriately in frail demented patients, even for a relief of incontinence, and are associated with a high rate of morbidity. Clean intermittent catheterization (CIC) is used to treat an underactive detrusor and other causes of urinary retention. The rate of symptomatic urinary tract infection and bladder stone formation is lower compared with indwelling catheters. However, it is often difficult to perform CIC in demented patients because of uncooperativeness, aggression, and agitation, and also increased demands on staff time. Indwelling catheterization should be restricted to persons who have urinary retention that cannot otherwise be treated, or to persons who are most severely demented with akinetic mutism, or as a short-term measure to allow for the healing of pressure sores. As one way of avoiding the use of catheters, absorbent pads and special undergarments are recommended for those patients whose incontinence has failed to respond to other treatment modalities.

Summary

Urinary incontinence is common in patients with dementia, and is more prevalent in demented than in non-demented older individuals. Since the etiology of incontinence is multifactorial, an assessment of factors within and outside the lower urinary tract is required in order to maximize continence in these patients. Patients with decreased motivation, cognitive disability, gait disorder, and detrusor hyperreflexia (DH) are highly likely to be incontinent. However, a careful clinical evaluation with a measurement of post-void residuals seems to be sufficient to guide treatment in most cases. Most research on the management of urinary incontinence in dementia patients has focused on toileting programs for functional incontinence and on drug treatments for DH. To date, the use of anticholinergic medications for DH is still under consideration, although many studies have employed severely demented cases. It is possible that, in less-impaired individuals who are aware of and able to tell the carer of their urinary sensation or incontinence, anticholinergic medication is of greater benefit. Prompted and scheduled toileting for patients with decreased motivation and immobility appears to be an effective approach in managing incontinence. In future, centrally acting drugs that can improve gait and cognitive function may become an option for the treatment of urinary incontinence in dementia patients.

References

1. Teri L, Borson S, Kiyak A, Yamagishi M. Behavioral disturbance, cognitive dysfunction, and functional skill; prevalence and relationship in Alzheimer's disease. J Am Geriatr Soc 1989; 37:109–116.

2. Teri L, Larson EB, Reifler BV. Behavioral disturbance in dementia of the Alzheimer's type. J Am Geriatr Soc 1988; 36:1–6.

3. Teri L, Hughes JP, Larson EB. Cognitive deterioration in Alzheimer's disease: behavioural and health factors. J Gerontol 1990; 45:P58–P63.

4. Swearer JM, Drachman DA, O'Donnell BF, Mitchell AL. Troublesome and disruptive behaviors in dementia. J Am Geriatr Soc 1988; 36:784–790.

5. Udaka F, Nishinaka K, Kameyama M, et al. Urinary dysfunction in dementia; 1. dementia of Alzheimer type. Voiding Disorder Digest 1994; 2:271–275.

6. Berrios GE. Urinary incontinence and the psychopathology of the elderly with cognitive failure. Gerontology 1986; 32:119–124.

7. Ouslander JG, Zarit SH, Orr NK, Muira SA. Incontinence among elderly community-dwelling dementia patients. J Am Geriatr Soc 1990; 38:440–445.

8. Rabins PV, Mace NL, Lucas MJ. The impact of dementia on the family. JAMA 1982; 248:333–335.

9. Burns A, Jacoby R, Levy R. Psychiatric phenomena in Alzheimer's disease. IV: Disorders of behaviour. Br J Psychiatry 1990; 157:S6–S94.

10. Campbell AJ, Reinken J, McCosh L. Incontinence in the elderly: prevalence and prognosis. Age Ageing 1985; 14:65–70.

11. Borrie MJ, Davidson HA. Incontinence in institutions: costs and contributing factors. Can Med Assoc J 1992; 147(3):322–328.

12. Noto H. Urinary dysfunction in dementia; 2. multi-infarct dementia. Voiding Disorder Digest 1994; 2:277–284.

13. Toba K, Ouchi Y, Orimo H, et al. Urinary incontinence in elderly inpatients in Japan; a comparison between general and geriatric hospitals. Aging Clin Exp Res 1996; 8:47–54.

14. McLaren SM, McPherson FM, Sinclair F, Ballinger BR. Prevalence and severity of incontinence among hospitalised, female psychogeriatric patients. Health Bull 1981; 39:157–161.

15. International Continence Society. Standardization of terminology of lower urinary tract function. Scand J Urol Nephrol 1988; 1(Suppl 14): 5–19.

16. Herzog AR, Fultz NH. Prevalence and incidence of urinary incontinence in community-dwelling populations. J Am Geriatr Soc 1990; 38:273–281.

17. Palmer MH, German PS, Ouslander JG. Risk factors for urinary incontinence one year after nursing home admission. Res Nurs Health 1991; 14:405–412.

18. Ouslander JG, Palmer MH, Rovner BW, German PS. Urinary incontinence in nursing homes: incidence, remission and associated factors. J Am Geriatr Soc 1993; 41:1083–1089.

19. Kotzoris H, Barclay LL, Kheyfets S, et al. Urinary and gait disturbances as markers for early multi-infarct dementia. Stroke 1987; 18:138–141.

20. Sakakibara R, Hattori T, Uchiyama T, Yamanishi T. Urinary function in elderly people with and without leukoaraiosis: relation to cognitive and gait function. J Neurol Neurosurg Psychiatry 1999; 67(5):658–660.

21. American Psychiatric Association. Diagnostic and statistical manual of mental disorders, 4th edn. Washington, DC: American Psychiatric Association Press, 1994.

22. Roman GC, Tatemichi TK, Erkinjuntti T, et al. Vascular dementia, diagnostic criteria for reaserch studies; report of the NINDS-AIREN International Workshop. Neurology 1993; 43:250–260.

23. McKieth IG, Galasko D, Kosaka K, et al. Consensus guidelines for the clinical and pathologic diagnosis of dementia with Lewy bodies (DLB); report of the consortium on DLB international workshop. Neurology 1996; 47:1113–1124.

24. McKieth IG, Del-Ser T, Spano P, et al. Efficacy of rivastigmine in dementia with Lewy bodies; a randomized, double-blind, placebo-controlled international study. Lancet 2000; 356(9247):2024–2025.

25. Del-Ser T, Munoz DG, Hachinski V. Temporal pattern of cognitive decline and incontinence is different in Alzheimer's disease and diffuse Lewy body disease. Neurology 1996; 46:682–686.

26. Brant-Zawadzki M, Fein G, Van Dyke C, Kiernan R, Davenport L, de Groot J. MR imaging of the aging brain; patchy white-matter lesions and dementia. Am J Neuroradiol 1985; 6(5):675-682.

27. Ahlberg J, Noren L, Blomstrand C, Wikkelso C. Outcome of shunt operation on urinary incontinence in normal pressure hydrocephalus predicted by lumbar puncture. J Neurol Neurosurg Psychiatry 1988; 51:105–108.

28. Yu LC, Rohner TJ, Kaltreider DL, et al. Profile of urinary incontinent elderly in long-term care institutions. J Am Geriatr Soc 1990; 38:433–439.

29. Resnick NM, Baumann M, Scott M, et al. Risk factors for incontinence in the nursing home: a multivariate study. Neurourol Urodyn 1988; 7:274–276.

30. Jirovec MM, Wells TJ. Urinary incontinence in nursing home residents with dementia: the mobility-cognition paradigm. Appl Nurs Res 1990; 3:112–117.

31. McGrother CW, Jagger C, Clarke M, Castleden CM. Handicaps associated with incontinence: implications for management. J Epidemiol Commun Health 1990; 44:246–248.

32. Keister KJ, Creason NS. Medications of elderly institutionalized incontinent females. J Adv Nurs 1989; 14:980–985.

33. Payne C. Epidemiology, pathophysiology and evaluation of urinary incontinence and overactive bladder. Urology 1998; 51(Suppl 2a):3–10.

34. Resnick NM, Yalla SV, Laurino E. The pathophysiology of urinary incontinence among institutionalized elderly persons. N Engl J Med 1989; 320:1–7.

35. Elbadawi A, Yalla SV, Resnick NM. Structural basis of geriatric voiding dysfunction. 3. Detrusor overactivity. J Urol 1993; 150:1668–1680.

36. Kinder RB, Mundy AR. Pathophysiology of idiopathic detrusor instability and detrusor hyper-reflexia; an in vitro study of human detrusor muscle. Br J Urol 1987; 60(6):509–515.

37. Elbadawi A, Yalla SV, Resnick NM. Structural basis of geriatric voiding dysfunction. 4. Bladder outlet obstruction. J Urol 1993; 150: 1681–1695.

38. de Groat WC, Booth AM, Yoshimura N. Neurophysiology of micturition and its modification in animal models of human disease. In: Maggi CA, ed. The autonomic nervous system: nervous control of the urogenital system, Vol 3. London: Horwood Academic Publishers, 1993:227–290; Griffiths D. Basics of pressure-flow studies. World J Urol 1995; 13:30–33.

39. Blok BFM, Holstege G. The central control of micturition and continence; implications for urology. BJU Int 1999; 83(Suppl 2):1–6.

40. Nour S, Svarer C, Kristensen JK, et al. Cerebral activation during micturition in normal men. Brain 2000; 123:781–789.

41. Griffiths DJ, McCracken PN, Harrison GM, et al. Cerebral etiology of urinary urge incontinence in elderly people. Age Ageing 1994; 23:246–250.

42. Kitada S, Ikei Y, Hasui Y, et al. Bladder function in elderly men with subclinical brain magnetic resonance imaging studies. J Urol 1992; 147:1507–1509.

43. Mori S, Kojima M, Sakai Y, Nakajima K. Bladder dysfunction in dementia patients showing urinary incontinence; evaluation with cystometry and treatment with propiverine hydrochloride. Jpn J Geriat 1999; 36:489–494.

44. Sugiyama T, Hashimoto K, Kiwamoto H, et al. Urinary incontinence in senile dementia of the Alzheimer type (SDAT). Int J Urol 1994; 1:337–340.

45. Komatsu K, Yokoyama O, Otsuka N, et al. Central muscarinic mechanism of bladder overactivity associated with Alzheimer type senile dementia. Neurourol Urodyn 2000; 4:539–540.

46. Sakakibara R, Hattori T, Tojo M, et al. Micturitional disturbance in patients with cerebrovascular dementia. Autonom Nerv Syst 1993; 30:390–396.

47. Resnick NM, Yalla SV. Detrusor hyperactivity with impaired contractile function. JAMA 1987; 257:3076–3081.

48. Eastwood H, Lord A. Are there two types of detrusor hyperreflexia? Neurourol Urodyn 1990; 9:415–416.

49. Elbadawi A, Yalla SV, Resnick NM. Structural basis of geriatric voiding dysfunction. 2. Ageing detrusor; normal versus impaired contractility. J Urol 1993; 150:1657–1667.

50. Kuwabara S, Naramoto C, Suzuki N, et al. Silent post-micturition residuals in elderly subjects with dementia; a study with ultrasound echography. Senile Dementia 1997; 11:417–421.

51. Resnick NM, Yalla SV. Current concepts; management of urinary incontinence in the elderly. New Engl J Med 1985; 313:800–815.

52. Skelly J, Flint AJ. Urinary incontinence associated with dementia. J Austr Geriat Soc 1995; 43:286–294.

53. Ouslander JG, Blaustein J, Connor A, Pitt A. Habit training and oxybutynin for incontinence in nursing home patients: a placebo controlled study. J Am Geriatr Soc 1988; 36:40–46.

54. Flint AJ, Skelly JM. The management of urinary incontinence in dementia. Int J Geriatr Psychiatry 1994; 9:245–246.

55. Jirovec MM. Effect of individualized prompted toileting on incontinence in nursing home residents. Appl Nurs Res 1991; 4:188–191.

56. Schnelle JF, Sowell VA, Hu TW, Traughber B. Reduction of urinary incontinence in nursing homes: Does it reduce or increase costs? J Am Geriatr Soc 1988; 36:34–39.

57. Chanfreau-Rona D, Bellwood S, Wylie B. Assessment of a behavioural programme to treat incontinent patients in psychogeriatric wards. Br J Clin Psychol 1984; 23:273–279.

58. Shinotoh H, Aotsuka A, Fukushi K, et al. Effect of donepezil on brain acetylcholinesterase activity in patients with AD measured by PET. Neurology 2001; 56:408–410.

59. Burns A, Rossor M, Hecker J, et al., the International Donepezil Study Group. The effects of donepezil in Alzheimer's disease; results from a multinational trial. Dementia and Geriatric Cognitive Disorders 1999; 10:237–244.

60. Hashimoto M, Imamura T, Tanimukai S, et al. Urinary incontinence; an unrecognised adverse effect with donepezil. Lancet 2000; 356:568.

61. Kumon Y, Sakaki S, Takeda S, et al. Effect of aneracetam on psychiatric symptoms after stroke. J New Remedies Clin 1997; 46:231–243.

62. Jirovec MM. The impact of daily exercise on the mobility, balance and urine control of cognitively impaired nursing home residents. Int J Nurs Stud 1991; 28:145–151.

63. Tobin GW, Brocklehurst JC. The management of urinary incontinence in local authority residential homes for the elderly. Age Ageing 1986; 15:292–298.

64. Burgio KL, Locher JL, Goode PS, et al. Behavioural vs drug treatment for urge urinary incontinence in older women; a randomized controlled trial. JAMA 1998; 280:1995–2000.

65. Zorzitto ML, Jewett MS, Fernie GR. Effectiveness of propantheline bromide in the treatment of geriatric patients with detrusor instability. Neurourol Urodyn 1986; 5:133–140.

66. Ouslander JG, Sier HC. Drug therapy for geriatric urinary incontinence. Clin Geriatr Med 1986; 2:789–807.

67. Donnellan CA, Fook L, McDonald P, Playfer JR. Oxybutynin and cognitive dysfunction. BMJ 1997; 315:1363–1364.

68. Castleden CM, Duffin HM, Gulati RS. Double-blind study of imipramine and placebo for incontinence due to bladder instability. Age Ageing 1986; 15:299–303.

69. Schwinn DA. Novel role for α1-adrenergic receptor subtypes in lower urinary tract symptoms. BJU Int 2000; 86(Suppl 2):11–22.

70. Cannon A, Carter PG, McConnel PG, Abrams P. Desmopressin in the treatment of nocturnal polyuria in the male. BJU Int 1999; 84:20–24.

71. Wells TJ, Brink CA, Diokno AC, et al. Pelvic muscle exercise for stress urinary incontinence in elderly women. J Am Geriatr Soc 1991; 39:785–791.

72. Lamhut P, Jackson TW, Wall LL. The treatment of urinary incontinence with electrical stimulation in nursing home patients: a pilot study. J Am Geriatr Soc 1992; 40:48–52.

73. Gillon G, Stanton SL. Long-term follow-up of surgery for urinary incontinence in elderly women. Br J Urol 1984; 56:478–481.

22

Pathologies of the basal ganglia (Parkinson's disease and Huntington's disease)

Satoshi Seki, Naoki Yoshimura, and Osamu Nishizawa

Introduction

It is well known that disorders of basal ganglia such as Parkinson's disease can affect lower urinary tract function. The basal ganglia are a group of anatomically closely related subcortical nuclei and have been implicated in a wide range of behavioral functions, including motor, cognitive, and emotional functions. The prominent involvement of the basal ganglia in motor control has been recognized in clinical and experimental investigations.[1,2] Damage to these nuclei does not cause weakness, but usually causes dramatic motor abnormalities, as well as lower urinary tract dysfunction. But the mechanisms that cause the clinical symptoms have not been completely clarified.

In this chapter an overview of the current concept of the contribution of the basal ganglia system to lower urinary tract function, as well as to general motor function, is given. Then, a review of the literature that describes lower urinary tract dysfunction in patients with disorders of the basal ganglia, such as Parkinson's disease and Huntington's disease, is provided.

Functional anatomy of the basal ganglia

The basal ganglia consists of several subcortical nuclei, including the striatum, the globus pallidus, the subthalamic nucleus, and the substantia nigra.

Striatum

Striatum, which consists of the caudate, the putamen, and the nucleus accumbens, is the main input structure of the basal ganglia. The caudate and putamen receive most of the afferents from the entire cerebral cortex, most probably using excitatory amino acids as transmitters; in this sense they are the doorway into the basal ganglia. The output neurons of the striatum use gamma-aminobutyric acid (GABA) as the principal transmitter,[3] co-localized with the neuropeptides enkephalin or substance P/dynorphin.[4–7]

Substantia nigra

The substantia nigra is divided into two parts: the substantia nigra pars compacta (SNpc) and the substantia nigra pars reticulata (SNpr). The SNpc receives input from the caudate and putamen and sends information right back. The SNpr also receives input from caudate and putamen but sends information outside the basal ganglia. SNpc neurons produce dopamine as a transmitter, which is important for the micturition reflex as well as for normal movement.

Globus pallidus

The globus pallidus is also divided into two parts: the globus pallidus externa (GPe) and the globus pallidus interna (GPi). Both receive input from the caudate and putamen, and both communicate with the subthalamic nucleus (STN).

Physiology and pathophysiology of motor dysfunction in Parkinson's disease

The study of the circuitry of the basal ganglia has mainly been focused on the control of motor function.[8] The current model of the organization of the basal ganglia was proposed in the 1980s.

Physiology of the basal ganglia

Cortical information that reaches the striatum is conveyed to the basal ganglia output structure (GPi–SNpr complex) via two pathways (Figure 22.1A). One is an inhibitory direct pathway from the striatum to the GPi–SNpr complex, which mainly uses inhibitory neurotransmitter, GABA. Another is an indirect pathway, which includes (1) an inhibitory projection from the striatum to the GPe, (2) an inhibitory projection from the GPe to the subthalamic nucleus (STN), and (3) an excitatory projection from the STN to the GPi–SNpr complex. These two inhibitory pathways (striato–GPe and GPe–STN) use GABA as a transmitter and the excitatory pathway (STN to GPi–SNpr complex) is activated by glutamate (Figure 22.1A).[9]

The information is then transmitted back to the cerebral cortex via the thalamus. The activity of spiny striatal neurons, which are the origin of the direct and indirect pathways, is modulated by dopamine released from nerve terminals of dopaminergic neurons in the SNpc.

Dopamine D_2 receptors are expressed in striatopallidal neurons in the indirect pathway, whereas D_1 receptors are located on neurons in the direct pathway (striatonigral/striatoentopeduncular neurons)[10] (Figure 22.1A). Dopamine is thought to inhibit neuronal activity through dopamine D_2 receptors in the indirect pathway and to excite neurons via dopamine D_1 receptors in the direct pathway (Figure 22.1A).

Thus, increased activity of the direct pathway is associated with facilitation of movement and activation of the indirect pathway is associated with inhibition of movement.

Pathophysiology of motor dysfunction in Parkinson's disease

Parkinson's disease (PD) is a chronic progressive neurological disease that is characterized by a decrease in spontaneous movements, gait difficulty, postural instability,

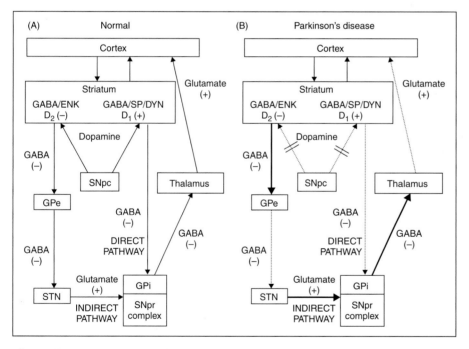

Figure 22.1

Simplified scheme of neural organization in the basal ganglia under (A) normal conditions and (B) in Parkinson's disease. (A) The striatum receives multiple afferent inputs from the cerebral cortex. The GPi–SNpr complex exerts a tonic GABAergic inhibitory output upon excitatory premotor neurons located in the thalamus. The direct pathway arises from striatal neurons that contain GABA plus peptides substance P (SP) or dynorphin (DYN) and project monosynaptically to the GPi–SNpr complex. The indirect pathway originates from striatal neurons that contain GABA and enkephalin (ENK). Its output is conveyed polysynaptically to the GPi–SNpr complex via GPe and STN. Dopamine increases neuronal activity in the direct pathway via D_1 receptor and inhibits neurons in the indirect pathway via D_2 receptor. Bradykinesia or akinesia observed in Parkinson's disease is thought to result from increased GABAergic inhibition of thalamic premotor neurons. (Thick and broken arrows indicate increased and decreased activity, respectively.) SNpr, substantia nigra pars reticulata; SNpc, substantia nigra pars compacta; GPe, globus pallidus externa; GPi, globus pallidus interna; STN, subthalamic nucleus; GABA, gamma-aminobutyric acid.

rigidity, and tremor. Depigmentation, neuronal loss, and gliosis of the substantia nigra, particularly in SNpc and locus ceruleus, are typical abnormalities found in the brain of patients with PD.

In Parkinson's disease, the normal inhibitory dopaminergic input to the indirect pathway is decreased, resulting in increased inhibition of GPe (Figure 22.1B). Because the GPe–STN pathway uses GABA as a transmitter, the STN becomes hyperactive. Hyperactivity of the STN results in increased activation of the GPi–SNpr complex, leading to decreased activity of the thalamus and its cortical projection areas. This increased output from the indirect pathway is enhanced further by a reduction in the GABA mediated by the direct pathway.

Physiology and pathophysiology of lower urinary tract dysfunction in Parkinson's disease

Dopaminergic systems and micturition reflex

Among the brain structures that regulate micturition, the globus pallidus has been reported to suppress spontaneous detrusor contractions in early studies,[11,12] and the subthalamus and substantia nigra can reportedly inhibit reflex bladder contractions. Electrical stimulation of the basal ganglia, including the SNpc, inhibits the micturition reflex in the cat.[13] In addition, this inhibition of the micturition reflex by stimulation of the substantia nigra was blocked by an injection of the D_1-selective antagonist SCH 23390 into the lateral ventricle, and also was mimicked by an intracerebroventricular application of the D_1-selective agonist SKF 38393.[13] Thus, it is thought that dopaminergic neurons originating in the SNpc inhibit the micturition reflex via central dopamine D_1 receptors. Furthermore, a recent study revealed that a D_1 dopaminergic antagonist (SCH 23390) facilitated the micturition reflex, whereas a D_1 agonist (SKF 38393) had no effect on the reflex bladder contractions in awake rats, suggesting that dopaminergic neurons originating in the substantia nigra tonically inhibit the micturition reflex through dopamine D_1 receptors under normal conditions (Figure 22.2A).[14]

Disruption of this tonic dopaminergic inhibition, by destroying the nigrostriatal pathway with the neurotoxin 1-methyl-4-phenyl-1,2,3,6-tetrahydropyridine (MPTP), produces Parkinson-like motor symptoms in monkeys accompanied by hyperreflexic bladders,[15–17] as reported in patients with PD. The detrusor overactivity was suppressed by stimulation of D_1-like receptors with SKF 38393 or pergolide (Figure 22.2B).[16,17] Thus, it is assumed that detrusor overactivity in patients with PD is due to activation failure of inhibitory mechanisms via dopamine D_1 receptors (Figure 22.2B).

While D_1 receptors mediate inhibition of the micturition reflex, stimulation of dopamine D_2 receptors facilitates the micturition reflex.[13,14,16–18] In awake rats, systemic application of a D_2 agonist (quinpirole) induced detrusor overactivity, which was blocked by a D_2 antagonist (remoxipride).[14] Similarly, systemic application of quinpirole induced detrusor overactivity in monkeys,[16,17] and treatment with bromocriptine, a D_2 receptor agonist, exacerbated urinary frequency in humans with Parkinson's disease.[19] However, since D_2 receptor-mediated facilitation of the micturition reflex was similarly found in normal and MPTP-induced parkinsonian monkeys,[16,17] and microinjection of dopamine to the pontine micturition center reduced bladder capacity and facilitated the micturition reflex in normal cats,[20,21] it is possible that D_2-like receptor-mediated effects on bladder function might be mediated by dopaminergic mechanisms in systems other than the nigrostriatal dopaminergic pathways (Figure 22.2A). On the other hand, nonselective dopamine agonists, such as apomorphine and levodopa, facilitate micturition reflex in experimental animals, possibly via dopamine D_2 receptors.[16,22,23]

A human study using single-photon emission computed tomography (SPECT) has also suggested that a reduction in the nigrostriatal dopaminergic neurons is related to the urinary disturbance in patients with PD.[24]

Clinical features of lower urinary tract dysfunction in patients with Parkinson's disease

Symptoms

Voiding dysfunction occurs in 35–70% of patients with PD[25] and most of these patients are diagnosed as PD for several years before the onset of urinary symptoms.[26] Bonnet et al have reported that the age at onset of urinary tract symptoms was 58.7 years and the symptoms began approximately 6 years after onset of parkinsonian motor symptoms.[27]

Storage symptoms, such as increased daytime frequency, nocturia, urgency, and urge urinary incontinence, are most commonly found in Parkinson's disease.[26–29] Patients also have voiding symptoms alone or a combination, although voiding symptoms that are secondary to PD are thought to be infrequent and moderate.[27] It should be noted that voiding function may be influenced by various types of

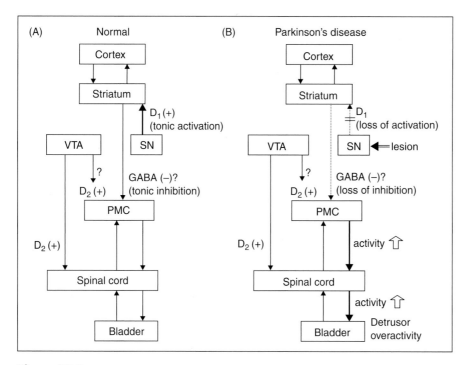

Figure 22.2
Hypothetical view of the relationship between the micturition reflex and dopaminergic systems (A) under normal conditions and (B) in Parkinson's disease. (A) Dopaminergic neurons originating in the substantia nigra pars compacta tonically activate dopamine D_1 receptors, leading to tonic inhibition of the pontine micturition center (PMC), probably through an activation of GABAergic inhibitory receptors. On the other hand, dopamine neurons arising from other brain areas such as the ventral tegmental area (VTA) might stimulate the micturition reflex via dopamine D_2 receptors in the PMC or the spinal cord. (B) In patients with Parkinson's disease, neuronal cell loss in the substantia nigra pars compacta produces a deficit of dopamine and causes a failure of an activation of inhibitory mechanisms via dopamine D_1 receptors. This failure may be induced by a loss of GABAergic inhibition upon PMC, resulting in detrusor overactivity. (Thick and broken arrows indicate increased and decreased activity, respectively.) GABA, gamma-aminobutyric acid.

treatments for the primary disease, PD, and that lower urinary tract dysfunction such as bladder outlet obstruction, which is common in the elderly, may coexist.

Several studies have also shown that the severity of urinary symptoms is related to the neurological disability or disease severity.[24,27,30,31] Araki and Kuno reported that international prostate symptom score (I-PSS) correlated well with disease severity in patients with PD.[30]

Bladder function

Neurogenic detrusor overactivity during filling phase[32] is most commonly found in urodynamic observations in patients with PD, ranging from 36% to 93%,[27–30,33–37] while bladder sensation is preserved. In the voiding phase, acontractile or underactive detrusor is also found (0–48%).[24,27–30,35,37] Because the incidence of detrusor overactivity with impaired contractile function increases with disease severity, it is possible that long-term detrusor overactivity may eventually lead to

deteriorated bladder contractile function at late stages of Parkinson's disease.[30]

Urethral function

Previous studies have shown some disagreement on urethral dysfunction induced by PD. Detrusor-sphincter dyssynergia in patients with PD has been reported in some studies,[30,35] but not in others.[28,29,36] This discrepancy may be caused by misinterpretation of electromyography (EMG) or the inclusion of patients with other neurological disorders. In addition, the presence of levodopa – which is most commonly used as a therapeutic agent for PD – at the time of study may affect these results.

However, it seems likely that impaired relaxation or delay in striated sphincter relaxation may exist in patients with PD.[28,37] Pavlakis et al introduced a term 'sphincter bradykinesia', which is characterized by a normal guarding reflex during the filling phase of the CMG and by failure of the striated sphincter to relax rapidly before detrusor contraction,[28] suggesting that bradykinesia is characteristic of PD and represents a manifestation of skeletal muscle hypertonicity involving perineal floor muscles.

Smooth muscle urethral sphincter dysfunction has not been reported in patients with PD.

Treatment

Various therapeutic options are available for voiding dysfunction in patients with PD, but it should be noted that these patients might have another cause leading to voiding dysfunction such as benign prostatic hyperplasia (BPH), which is common in the elderly. Christmas et al demonstrated that subcutaneous injection of apomorphine (nonselective dopamine receptor agonist) improved flow rate and reduced post-void residual in patients with PD, suggesting that bladder outlet obstruction secondary to BPH may be distinguished from voiding dysfunction secondary to PD.[33]

A high incidence of post-prostatectomy urinary incontinence has been reported by Staskin and coworkers. They reported that 28% of patients with PD who underwent transurethral prostatectomy (TUR-P) exhibited urinary incontinence and they concluded that poor or absent voluntary sphincter control was the major risk factor of incontinence following TUR-P in the parkinsonian patients.[38] However, Chandiramani and associates pointed out that a poor outcome following prostatic surgery may be due to the inadvertent inclusion of some men with multiple system atrophy (MSA),[26,39] which is a condition most frequently misdiagnosed, even by specialists, as Parkinson's disease.[40] The term 'multiple system atrophy' is synonymous with striatonigral degeneration (SND) when parkinsonism predominates, olivopontocerebellar atrophy (OPCA) when cerebellar signs predominate, and Shy–Drager syndrome when autonomic failure is dominant. Voiding disturbance in MSA is characterized by more incidence with urinary incontinence, significant post-void residual and worsening urinary control after urological surgery.[39,41]

Clinical studies, in which the effect of levodopa or apomorphine on bladder behavior in patients with PD was examined, have shown conflicting results. It is reasonable to assume that nonselective dopamine receptor agonists such as levodopa and apomorphine facilitate micturition reflex via dopamine D_2 receptors, resulting in worsening of detrusor overactivity. But some authors have demonstrated an improvement in detrusor overactivity with levodopa or apomorphine in some patients with PD and aggravation in others,[29,33] whereas Stocchi et al found no improvement of detrusor overactivity with apomorphine.[37] Metabolites of these agents or diversity of disease severity might have affected these results.

Huntington's disease

Huntington's disease (HD) is a degenerative disease with autosomal dominant inheritance characterized by progressive neuronal loss in the basal ganglia, especially in the caudate nucleus and cerebral cortex.[42] The exact mechanisms underlying neuronal death in HD are still unknown. Although the disease may begin at any time from childhood to old age (average age of onset is approximately 40 years), adult-onset HD is characterized by a triad of progressive motor, cognitive, and emotional symptoms.

There has been little investigation regarding urinary tract dysfunction in patients with HD. Wheeler et al reviewed the neurourological findings in 6 patients with HD who complained of lower urinary tract symptoms, and found that 4 of the patients had detrusor overactivity with a normal sphincter, while the remaining 2 patients exhibited no abnormal findings. Symptoms include urinary frequency, urgency, nocturia, and incontinence, and the onset of these symptoms was 6.1 years after the onset of HD.[43] A recent survey of 1283 symptomatic individuals with HD found that lower urinary tract symptoms occurred in the late stage of HD, typically more than 10 years after onset.[44]

Anticholinergic agents could be useful to alleviate urological symptoms. However, in patients with severe neurological disability, a permanent indwelling catheter or urosheath drainage may be required.

References

1. Flowers KA. Visual "closed-loop" and "open-loop" characteristics of voluntary movement in patients with Parkinsonism and intention tremor. Brain 1976; 99:269–310.

2. Evarts EV, Teravainen H, Calne DB. Reaction time in Parkinson's disease. Brain 1981; 104:167–186.

3. Kita H, Kitai ST. Glutamate decarboxylase immunoreactive neurons in rat neostriatum: their morphological types and populations. Brain Res 1988; 447:346–352.

4. Vincent SR, Hokfelt T, Christensson I, Terenius L. Dynorphin-immunoreactive neurons in the central nervous system of the rat. Neurosci Lett 1982; 33:185–190.

5. Vincent S, Hokfelt T, Christensson I, Terenius L. Immuno-histochemical evidence for a dynorphin immunoreactive striato-nigral pathway. Eur J Pharmacol 1982; 85:251–252.

6. Beckstead RM. Complementary mosaic distributions of thalamic and nigral axons in the caudate nucleus of the cat: double anterograde labeling combining autoradiography and wheat germ-HRP histochemistry. Brain Res 1985; 335:153–159.

7. Kanazawa I, Emson PC, Cuello AC. Evidence for the existence of substance P-containing fibres in striato-nigral and pallido-nigral pathways in rat brain. Brain Res 1977; 119:447–453.

8. Obeso JA, Rodriguez-Oroz MC, Rodriguez M, et al. Pathophysiology of the basal ganglia in Parkinson's disease. Trends Neurosci 2000; 23:S8–S19.

9. Levy R, Hazrati LN, Herrero MT, et al. Re-evaluation of the functional anatomy of the basal ganglia in normal and Parkinsonian states. Neuroscience 1997; 76:335–343.

10. Le Moine C, Bloch B. D1 and D2 dopamine receptor gene expression in the rat striatum: sensitive cRNA probes demonstrate prominent segregation of D1 and D2 mRNAs in distinct neuronal populations of the dorsal and ventral striatum. J Comp Neurol 1995; 355:418–426.

11. Lewin RJ, Dillard GV, Porter RW. Extrapyramidal inhibition of the urinary bladder. Brain Res 1967; 4:301–307.

12. Raz S. Parkinsonism and neurogenic bladder. Experimental and clinical observations. Urol Res 1976; 4:133–138.

13. Yoshimura N, Sasa M, Yoshida O, Takaori S. Dopamine D1 receptor-mediated inhibition of micturition reflex by central dopamine from the substantia nigra. Neurourol Urodyn 1992; 11:535–545.

14. Seki S, Igawa Y, Kaidoh K, et al. Role of dopamine D1 and D2 receptors in the micturition reflex in conscious rats. Neurourol Urodyn 2001; 20:105–113.

15. Albanese A, Jenner P, Marsden CD, Stephenson JD. Bladder hyperreflexia induced in marmosets by 1-methyl-4-phenyl-1,2,3,6-tetrahydropyridine. Neurosci Lett 1988; 87:46–50.

16. Yoshimura N, Mizuta E, Kuno S, et al. The dopamine D_1 receptor agonist SKF 38393 suppresses detrusor hyperreflexia in the monkey with parkinsonism induced by 1-methyl-4-phenyl-1,2,3,6-tetrahydropyridine (MPTP). Neuropharmacology 1993; 32:315–321.

17. Yoshimura N, Mizuta E, Yoshida O, Kuno S. Therapeutic effects of dopamine D1/D2 receptor agonists on detrusor hyperreflexia in 1-methyl-4-phenyl-1,2,3,6-tetrahydropyridine-lesioned parkinsonian cynomolgus monkeys. J Pharmacol Exp Ther 1998; 286: 228–233.

18. Kontani H, Inoue T, Sakai T. Dopamine receptor subtypes that induce hyperactive urinary bladder response in anesthetized rats. Jpn J Pharmacol 1990; 54:482–486.

19. Kuno S, Mizuta E, Yoshimura N. Different effects of D1 and D2 agonists on neurogenic bladder in Parkinson's disease and MPTP-induced parkinsonian monkeys. Mov Disord 1997; 12:

20. de Groat WC, Booth AM, Yoshimura N. Neurophysiology of micturition and its modification in animal models of human disease. In: Maggi CA, ed. The autonomic nervous system, Vol. 3, Nervous control of the urogenital system. London: Harwood Academic Publishers, 1993:227–290.

21. Roppolo JR, Noto H, Mallory BS, de Groat WC. Dopaminergic and cholinergic modulation of bladder reflexes at the level of the pontine micturition center in the cat. Soc Neurosci Abstr 1987; 13:733.

22. Ishizuka O, Pandita RK, Mattiasson A, et al. Stimulation of bladder activity by volume, L-dopa and capsaicin in normal conscious rats – effects of spinal alpha 1-adrenoceptor blockade. Naunyn Schmiedebergs Arch Pharmacol 1997; 355:787–793.

23. Sillen U, Rubenson A, Hjalmas K. Central cholinergic mechanisms in L-DOPA induced hyperactive urinary bladder of the rat. Urol Res 1982; 10:239–243.

24. Sakakibara R, Shinotoh H, Uchiyama T, et al. SPECT imaging of the dopamine transporter with [(123)I]-beta-CIT reveals marked decline of nigrostriatal dopaminergic function in Parkinson's disease with urinary dysfunction. J Neurol Sci 2001; 187:55–59.

25. Wein A. Neuromuscular dysfunction of the lower urinary tract and its management. In: Walsh PC, Retik AB, Vaughan C, Wein A, eds. Campbell's urology. Philadelphia: WB Saunders, 2002:931–1026.

26. Chandiramani VA, Palace J, Fowler CJ. How to recognize patients with parkinsonism who should not have urological surgery. Br J Urol 1997; 80:100–104.

27. Bonnet AM, Pichon J, Vidailhet M, et al. Urinary disturbances in striatonigral degeneration and Parkinson's disease: clinical and urodynamic aspects. Mov Disord 1997; 12:509–513.

28. Pavlakis AJ, Siroky MB, Goldstein I, Krane RJ. Neurologic findings in Parkinson's disease. J Urol 1983; 129:80–83.

29. Fitzmaurice H, Fowler CJ, Rickards D, et al. Micturition disturbance in Parkinson's disease. Br J Urol 1985; 57:652–656.

30. Araki I, Kuno S. Assessment of voiding dysfunction in Parkinson's disease by the international prostate symptom score. J Neurol Neurosurg Psychiatry 2000; 68:429–433.

31. Hattori T, Yasuda K, Kita K, Hirayama K. Voiding dysfunction in Parkinson's disease. Jpn J Psychiatry Neurol 1992; 46:181–186.

32. Abrams P, Cardozo L, Fall M, et al. The standardisation of terminology of lower urinary tract function: report from the Standardisation Sub-committee of the International Continence Society. Neurourol Urodyn 2002; 21:167–178.

33. Christmas TJ, Kempster PA, Chapple CR, et al. Role of subcutaneous apomorphine in parkinsonian voiding dysfunction. Lancet 1988; 2:1451–1453.

34. Sakakibara R, Hattori T, Uchiyama T, Yamanishi T. Videourodynamic and sphincter motor unit potential analyses in Parkinson's disease and multiple system atrophy. J Neurol Neurosurg Psychiatry 2001; 71:600–606.

35. Khan Z, Starer P, Bhola A. Urinary incontinence in female Parkinson disease patients. Pitfalls of diagnosis. Urology 1989; 33:486–489.

36. Gray R, Stern G, Malone-Lee J. Lower urinary tract dysfunction in Parkinson's disease: changes relate to age and not disease. Age Ageing 1995; 24:499–504.

37. Stocchi F, Carbone A, Inghilleri M, et al. Urodynamic and neurophysiological evaluation in Parkinson's disease and multiple system atrophy. J Neurol Neurosurg Psychiatry 1997; 62:507–511.

38. Staskin DS, Vardi Y, Siroky MB. Post-prostatectomy continence in the parkinsonian patient: the significance of poor voluntary sphincter control. J Urol 1988; 140:117–118.

39. Fowler CJ. Urinary disorders in Parkinson's disease and multiple system atrophy. Funct Neurol 2001; 16:277–282.

40. Quinn N. Parkinsonism – recognition and differential diagnosis. BMJ 1995; 310:447–452.

41. Beck RO, Betts CD, Fowler CJ. Genitourinary dysfunction in multiple system atrophy: clinical features and treatment in 62 cases. J Urol 1994; 151:1336–1341.

42. Feigin A, Zgaljardic D. Recent advances in Huntington's disease: implications for experimental therapeutics. Curr Opin Neurol 2002; 15:483–489.

43. Wheeler JS, Sax DS, Krane RJ, Siroky MB. Vesico-urethral function in Huntington's chorea. Br J Urol 1985; 57:63–66.

44. Kirkwood SC, Su JL, Conneally P, Foroud T. Progression of symptoms in the early and middle stages of Huntington disease. Arch Neurol 2001; 58:273–278.

23

Urinary dysfunction in multiple system atrophy

Ryuji Sakakibara, Clare J Fowler, and Takamichi Hattori

Introduction

Multiple system atrophy (MSA) is an uncommon but well-recognized disease entity that both neurologists and urologists may encounter. The term MSA was introduced by Graham and Oppenheimer in 1969, to describe a group of patients with a disorder of unknown cause affecting extrapyramidal, cerebellar, and autonomic pathways.[1] MSA includes the disorders previously called striatonigral degeneration (SND),[2] sporadic olivopontocerebellar atrophy (OPCA),[3] and the Shy–Drager syndrome.[4] The discovery in 1989 of glial cytoplasmic inclusions in the brain of patients with MSA[5] provided a pathological marker for the disorder (akin to Lewy bodies in idiopathic Parkinson's disease (IPD)), and confirmed that SND, OPCA, and the Shy–Drager syndrome are the same disease with differing clinical presentations. Immunocyto-chemistry showed that the glial cytoplasmic inclusions of MSA are ubiquitin-, tau-, and alpha-synuclein positive, possibly representing a cytoskeletal alteration in glial cells that results in neuronal degeneration.

MSA can be classified as MSA-P (parkinsonism predominant), or MSA-C (cerebellar predominant), according to the major motor deficit. Clinical differential diagnosis between MSA-P, the commonest clinical form, and IPD is difficult even for the specialists. However, lack of one-side dominance and resting tremor, poor response to levodopa, and rapid progression are all 'red flags' which raise the alert for a diagnosis of MSA.[6] MSA-C can mostly be distinguished from hereditary spinocerebellar ataxias, although some individuals with such disorders do not have apparent heredity. Autonomic failure (AF) is almost invariably present[7] and can be an initial manifestation (AF-MSA).[8] Autonomic failure occurs in other neurodegenerative diseases, i.e. a subset of patients with IPD (AF-PD), and pure autonomic failure (PAF), both now being considered as members of Lewy body diseases. This chapter reviews the current concepts of the urinary dysfunction in MSA, with particular reference to urinary symptoms, (video-)-urodynamic assessment and sphincter electromyography (EMG), and patient management.

Urinary symptoms

Urinary dysfunction and orthostatic hypotension

Of various symptoms due to AF (i.e. erectile dysfunction, urinary dysfunction, postural hypotension, or respiratory stridor), urinary dysfunction has been attracting less attention than postural hypotension, in patients with MSA, although it may result in recurrent urinary tract infection and be a cause of morbidity.[9] In addition, urinary incontinence results in impaired self-esteem of the patient, caregiver's stress, and considerable cost. Postural hypotension was pointed out first in AF-MSA, which turned out to be a marker of autonomic involvement in this disorder. Both of the original 2 patients discussed by Shy and Drager had urinary frequency, incontinence, and urinary retention.[4] Other variants (MSA-P and MSA-C) rarely develop orthostatic hypotension in their early stage. However, in the original reports, 3 of 4 patients with MSA-P showed voiding difficulty, retention, and urinary incontinence,[2] and both patients with MSA-C had voiding difficulty and urinary incontinence.[3] Thus, which is the more common and earlier autonomic feature in MSA?

In our previous study of 121 patients with MSA,[10] urinary symptoms (96%) were more common than orthostatic symptoms (43%) ($p < 0.01$) (Figure 23.1). The most frequent urinary symptom was difficulty of voiding in 79% of the patients, followed by nocturnal urinary frequency in 74%, and the other symptoms included sensation of urgency in 63%, urge incontinence in 63%, diurnal urinary frequency in 45%, enuresis in 19%, and urinary retention in 8%. In addition, the most frequent orthostatic symptom was postural faintness in 43%, followed by blurred vision in 38% and syncope in 19%. These figures are almost in accordance with those by Wenning et al,[11] who noted urinary incontinence in 71% and urinary retention in 27%, and postural faintness in 53% and syncope in 15% of 100 patients with MSA. In the 53 patients with both urinary and orthostatic symptoms, patients who had urinary

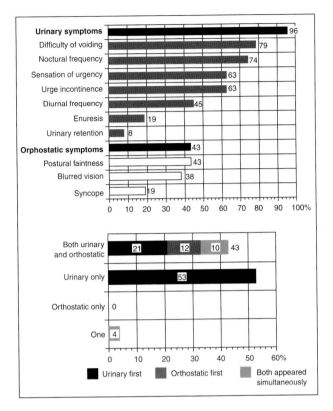

Figure 23.1
Urinary dysfunction and orthostatic hypotension in MSA.

symptoms first (48%) were more common than those who had orthostatic symptoms first (29%), and there were patients who developed both symptoms simultaneously (23%).[10] These findings indicate that urinary dysfunction is a more common and often earlier manifestation than orthostatic hypotension in MSA.

Urinary dysfunction and motor disorders

Looking at both urinary and motor disorders, approximately 60% of patients with MSA develop urinary symptoms either preceding or at the time of presentation with the motor disorder[9,10] (Figure 23.2). This figure indicates that many of these patients seek urological advice early in the course of their disease. Since the severity of the urinary symptoms is severe enough for surgical intervention, male patients with MSA may undergo urological surgery for prostatic outflow obstruction before the correct diagnosis has been made. The results of the surgery are often transient or unfavorable because of the progressive nature of this disease. Male erectile dysfunction (MED) is often the first presentation,[9,10] which may further precede the occurrence of urinary dysfunction in MSA. The urologist confronted with a patient showing these features should

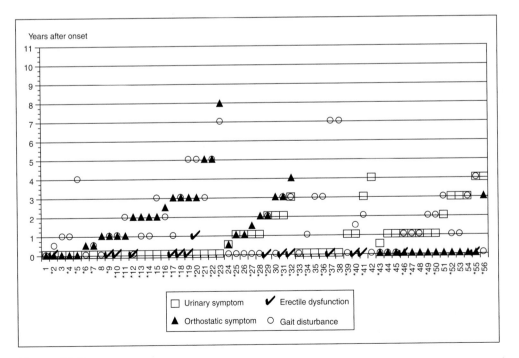

Figure 23.2
Autonomic and motor disorders in MSA.

be cautious of embarking on an operative approach. The neurologist encountering a patient with marked urinary symptoms might consider future investigation by brain magnetic resonance imaging (MRI) scan and sphincter EMG.

Since motor disorder of MSA mostly mimics that of IPD, urogenital distinction between these two diseases is worth considering, although a number of the earlier studies on 'Parkinson's disease and the bladder' might include patients with MSA. The prevalence rate of urinary dysfunction in MSA is more common than 58–71% of IPD,[10,12–14] and, similarly, that of urgency incontinence in MSA is more common than 33% of IPD. In addition, urinary dysfunction is never the initial presentation in IPD.

Urodynamic assessment

Since MSA is a neurodegenerative disease that affects multiple brain regions, patients with the disease may have a wide range of urodynamic abnormalities that change with progression of the illness.

Detrusor hyperreflexia and uninhibited external sphincter relaxation

Filling phase abnormalities included detrusor hyperreflexia in 33–100% and uninhibited external sphincter relaxation in 33% of MSA,[9,14–16] figures similar to those reported in IPD[10,12–16] (Figure 23.3). Detrusor hyperreflexia is urodynamically defined as involuntary phasic increase in detrusor pressure > 10 cmH$_2$O during bladder filling, which is

commonly associated with decreased bladder volumes at first sensation and maximum desire to void. It is detrusor hyperreflexia which seems to be the major cause of urgency incontinence in patients with MSA. But when coupled with uninhibited sphincter relaxation, incontinence may worsen.[17] It is well known that cerebral diseases can lead to a loss of the brain's inhibitory influence on the spino-bulbo-spinal micturition reflex. The information that arises from the lower urinary tract reaches the periaqueductal gray matter (PAG), then goes down to the pontine micturition center (PMC), an area identical or just adjacent to the locus ceruleus, which then activates the descending pathway to the sacral preganglionic neurons innervating the bladder.[18] The basal ganglia are thought to be one of the higher centers for micturition, since lesions of this area lead to detrusor hyperreflexia.[19,20] Recent positron emission tomography (PET) studies have shown that the hypothalamus, PAG, midline pons, and cingulate cortex are activated during urinary filling.[21] Central pathology of MSA includes neuronal loss of neuromelanin-containing cells in the locus ceruleus[22] as well as in the nigrostriatal dopaminergic system,[19] and to a lesser extent, the frontal cortex.[23,24] These areas seem to be responsible for the occurrence of detrusor hyperreflexia and uninhibited sphincter relaxation in MSA patients.

The responsible sites for the cardiovascular autonomic failure in MSA are mostly central, which is in contrast to the peripheral lesion in PAF.[7] However, 31–45% of the patients with MSA also revealed low compliance detrusor, which is defined as maximum bladder capacity/tonic detrusor pressure increase <20 ml/cmH$_2$O.[10] Low compliance detrusor is known to occur in patients with spina bifida, or in animals with experimental cauda equina lesion, most probably reflecting neuronal loss of bladder preganglionic neurons in the sacral cord and their fibers

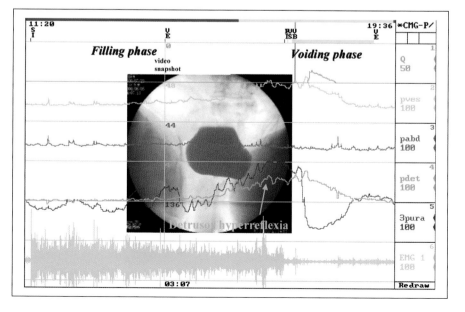

Figure 23.3
Detrusor hyperreflexia.

(pelvic nerve).[25,26] In addition, urodynamic study showed an increase in bladder volume at first sensation and/or bladder capacity, indicating impaired bladder sensation, in 12% of the patients.[10] Impaired bladder sensation may reflect pelvic and/or pudendal sensory neuropathy in MSA,[27] and these patients are best instructed to perform scheduled voiding, irrespective of their urinary sensation, to avoid overdistention injury of the bladder. Bethanechol test is the established method to detect lesions in the most peripheral site.[28] A minimum amount (2.5 mg) of bethanechol, a cholinergic agent, is injected subcutaneously, which is an amount that is not sufficient to evoke bladder contraction in normal subjects. However, when the bladder is denervated, cholinergic receptor densities in the postsynaptic membrane increase and result in abnormal detrusor pressure rise on bethanechol injection. Nineteen percent of MSA patients revealed the denervation supersensitivity of the detrusor.[10]

Impaired detrusor contractility and detrusor-sphincter dyssynergia

Incomplete bladder emptying is a significant feature in MSA. In fact, 47% of the patients with MSA had post-micturition residuals >100 ml, which was noted in none of the patients with IPD ($p < 0.01$).[14] Factors relevant to the voiding disorder in MSA include the urethral outlet and the detrusor. Pressure–flow analysis refers to the simultaneous monitoring of detrusor pressure and urinary flow, and

drawing the relation curve between these two (Figure 23.4). Although it was originally developed for diagnosing outlet obstruction due to prostatic hypertrophy,[29,30] pressure–flow analysis is useful for evaluating neurogenic voiding difficulty:[31] The AG number represents a grade of urethral obstruction, and an AG number >40 means outflow obstruction in men.[29] In MSA patients, the mean AG numbers (12 in women and 28 in men) were smaller than those in IPD (40 in women and 43 in men, respectively).[14] However, a subset of patients with MSA may have an obstructive pattern, the reason for which is unknown. Detrusor-external sphincter dyssynergia is a factor contributing to the neurogenic urethral relaxation failure,[31] which is noted in 47% of MSA patients.[14,32] Drugs used for alleviating parkinsonism and postural hypotension – i.e. levodopa and its metabolites such as norepinephrine (noradrenaline), and vasoconstricting drugs such as midodrine – may contract the bladder neck by stimulating alpha$_1$-adrenergic receptors.[33] Although there is no report of the incidence of detrusor-bladder neck dyssynergia[34] in MSA, alpha$_1$-adrenergic receptor antagonists benefited a subgroup of MSA patients by reducing post-micturition residuals.[35]

Pressure–flow analysis showed that a weak detrusor contraction during voiding in MSA (71% in women and 63% in men) is more common than that of IPD (66% in women and 40% in men, respectively).[14] Therefore, it is likely that impaired detrusor contractility accounts mostly for the voiding difficulty and the raised post-micturition residuals in MSA. A subset of patients with MSA have detrusor hyperactivity with impaired contractility during voiding;[36] the exact mechanism of this phenomenon has yet to be ascertained. However, it has been recognized that the

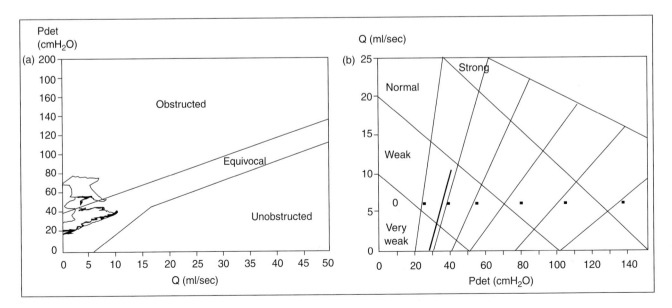

Figure 23.4
Two pressure–flow nomograms: (a) Abrams–Griffiths nomogram; (b) Schafer nomogram; Pdet: detrusor pressure; Q: urinary flow rate.

central mechanisms underlying bladder filling and voiding are distinct from each other; i.e. the area promoting micturition is located in the PMC and the frontal cortex, whereas that promoting urinary storage is in the pontine storage center, basal ganglia, and also the frontal cortex.[18] Lesions in these areas may cause a various combination of urinary filling and voiding disorders. In addition, repeated urodynamic studies in MSA patients showed that the cystometrogram changed from detrusor hyperreflexia to low compliance or atonic detrusor, and from negative to positive bethanechol supersensitivity.[10] In fact, as the disease progresses, symptoms may change from urinary urgency and frequency to those due to incomplete bladder emptying.[9] These findings suggest that the responsible sites of the bladder disorder may change from supra- to infranuclear during the course of the illness.

Nocturnal polyuria

Other than bladder disorders, patients with MSA may have nocturnal polyuria, which results in nocturnal urinary frequency and morning hypotension. In normal children over 7 years and adults, circadian release of arginine vasopressin (AVP) from the posterior pituitary gland into plasma has its peak during nighttime. This leads to a nocturnal decrease of urine formation, and the ratio of nighttime to daytime urine production is usually <1:2. This circadian rhythm can be impaired in congestive heart failure, nephrosis, and cirrhosis with ascites. However, postmortem study of the brain in patients with MSA indicated that there is a degeneration of AVP neurons in the suprachiasmatic nucleus,[37] which leads to an impaired circadian rhythm of plasma AVP concentration in MSA.[38,39] In addition, postural hypotension during daytime may also cause nocturnal polyuria in patients with MSA.[40] This is probably due to a combination of factors that include compensatory supine hypertension at nights, leading to increased glomerular filtration.

Sphincter electromyography and videourodynamics

Of particular importance is the group of anterior horn cells in the sacral spinal cord which project fibers to the external sphincters. They were first described by Onufrowicz in 1900, and hence became known as the 'Onuf's nucleus'. Postmortem studies in patients dying with MSA demonstrated a selective loss of anterior horn cells in Onuf's nucleus which are spared in amyotrophic lateral sclerosis.[43,44] Since in IPD the anterior horn cells of Onuf's nucleus are also spared, sphincter EMG can be

a means of distinguishing between MSA-P and IPD. The external (striated) urethral sphincter is a component in the maintenance of continence, and is innervated by the somatic pudendal nerve. The changes of chronic reinnervation which occur in the motor units of the external sphincter have been demonstrated by EMG.[41,42] Similar neurogenic changes have been demonstrated in the anal and urethral sphincters in MSA. As the anal sphincter is more superficial, needle EMG causes less discomfort and is therefore the preferred test. By varying the position of the needle electrode, 10 different motor units can be identified and the overall mean duration calculated. It is important to include, in the measurement of duration, the highly stable but low-amplitude late (satellite) components which may be separated from the initial part of the complex by an isoelectric period of several milliseconds (Figure 23.5). The control range of values for duration of motor units is wide,[42] but a mean duration of motor unit potentials >10 ms or more than 20% of motor unit potentials with a duration >10 ms are most sensitive for diagnosing chronic reinnervation.[45] Previous reports showed neurogenic motor unit potentials in 75–100% of patients with MSA[8,14–16,45] and in 0–17% of IPD.[14–16] Although denervation can be found in the other skeletal muscles in MSA, it occurs much earlier in the external sphincter muscles.[46]

Up to 40% of patients with MSA may have low resting urethral pressure,[9] which most probably reflects sphincter weakness. The resulting denervation of the urethral sphincter

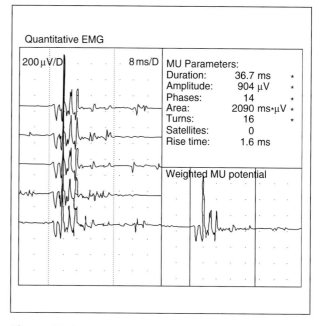

Figure 23.5
External sphincter EMG. A motor unit recorded from the anal sphincter of a patient with multiple system atrophy shows an abnormally prolonged duration (upper range of normal is less than 10 milliseconds) and stable low amplitude late components. (D = division; EMG = electromyography; MU = motor unit.)

together with detrusor hyperreflexia is a reason why urge incontinence is such a pronounced and early feature of MSA.[8] Sphincter weakness in MSA may also result in stress urinary incontinence, which occurs particularly in female patients.[47]

The bladder neck, also known as the internal (smooth) urethral sphincter, is another component in the maintenance of continence that is innervated by the sympathetic hypogastric nerve. Videourodynamic study is an established method to evaluate bladder neck function. It is a combination of visualizing the lower urinary tract simultaneously with EMG-cystometry, and urethral pressure at the external urethral sphincter can be obtained with visual guidance using a radiopaque marker. In normal subjects, the bladder neck is closed throughout the bladder filling to avoid leaking. However, an open bladder neck is found in 46–100% of MSA and in 23–31% of PD patients, and an open bladder neck at the start of bladder filling, even without the accompaniment of detrusor hyperreflexia, was noted in none of PD but in 53% of MSA patients ($p < 0.01$)(Figure 23.6).[14] Because open bladder neck is common in patients with myelodysplasia or lower thoracic cord lesion at T12–L2 (where sympathetic intermediolateral nuclei are located), and is reproduced by systemic or intraurethral application of alpha$_1$-adrenergic blockers,[48] it is likely that the open bladder neck reflects the loss of sympathetic innervation.

Management of urinary dysfunction

Detrusor hyperreflexia

The bladder is innervated by the parasympathetic pelvic nerve, and has an abundance of M$_{2/3}$ muscarinic receptors. Detrusor hyperreflexia may reflect increased micturition reflex either via the brainstem or the sacral cord, which can be treated with anticholinergic medication such as tolterodine, oxybutynin, propiverine, or propantheline. These drugs diminish the parasympathetic tone on bladder smooth muscle, and are usually tried in patients with urinary urgency and frequency. However, anticholinergic side-effects, such as a dry mouth (probably mediated by M$_3$ receptors) and constipation (M$_{2/3}$ receptors) in particular, may limit their use in a proportion of the patients. A subset of patients with MSA may develop mild cognitive decline in their advanced stage. Since use of anticholinergic drugs has a risk of cognitive impairment,[49] though much less common than its peripheral effects, we have to be careful to manage urinary dysfunction in such patients. Anticholinergic drugs do ameliorate urgency and frequency, but may also reduce bladder contractility during voiding.[8] Therefore, it should be better to measure post-void residuals regularly in the patients. If the residual urine volume exceeds 100 ml, the medication should be withdrawn or added with clean intermittent catheterization (CIC).

Whether centrally acting drugs, such as pergolide (dopaminergic D$_{1/2}$-receptor agonist) for parkinsonism, might ameliorate urinary dysfunction in MSA is not fully studied.[50] Early untreated IPD patients with mild urgency and frequency tend to benefit from levodopa (D$_{1/2}$) treatment. However, in advanced IPD patients with on-off phenomenon, levodopa may augment detrusor hyperreflexia.[51] Since D$_1$ selective stimulation inhibits the micturition reflex which D$_2$ selective stimulation facilitates, balance of these stimulations may explain the various effects of the drugs.

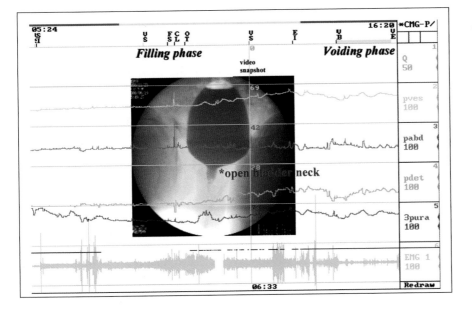

Figure 23.6
Open bladder neck.

Incomplete bladder emptying

More than a half of patients with MSA have urinary dysfunction either preceding or at the time of presentation with motor disorder. Since many of these patients develop incomplete bladder emptying, they may be misdiagnosed as having prostatic hypertrophy. In fact, the results of urological surgery are often unfavorable, since impaired detrusor contractility contributes more to the voiding difficulty than outflow obstruction. Therefore, it is important to avoid inappropriate urological surgery in patients with MSA,[52] and a conservative approach with medical measures to manage urinary problems can be effective.

An estimation of the post-void residual urine volume is a simple and useful test in patients with MSA as they may be unaware that their bladders do not empty completely. If the patient has a significant post-micturition residue and is symptomatic, this aspect of their problem should be managed by intermittent catheterization by the patients or caregivers. However, in patients with advanced disease and severe neurological disability, a permanent indwelling catheter, either transurethral or suprapubic, or urosheath drainage may be required.

Since incomplete bladder emptying in patients with MSA is mostly due to weak detrusor contraction, drugs acting on outflow obstruction are unlikely to benefit all patients. However, in some patients, alpha-adrenergic blockers may be effective in lessening post-void residual volumes, due probably to detrusor-sphincter dyssynergia.[35] Uro-selective blockers such as tamsulosin and naftopidil may be of choice because of fewer side-effects such as orthostatic hypotension. In contrast, the most commonly used drugs to treat postural hypotension in MSA are adrenergic agonists. However, administration of amezinium, an adrenergic drug, may increase post-void residuals compared to that before treatment in the patients.[33] Amezinium most probably stimulates the alpha receptors, both in the vascular wall (alpha$_{1B}$ receptors, particularly in the elderly[53]) and the proximal urethra (alpha$_{1A/D}$-adrenergic receptors).

Nocturnal polyuria

Nocturnal polyuria can be estimated by a frequency volume chart, when the ratio of nighttime to daytime urine production exceeds 1:2. Desmopressin is a potent analogue of AVP (hypertensive and antidiuretic effects: 100 vs 100 in AVP; 0.39 vs 1200 in desmopressin, respectively), and is used in the treatment of diabetes insipidus due to a loss of posterior pituitary AVP secretion. Mathias et al[39] used 2–4 μg of intramuscular desmopressin in patients with autonomic failure including MSA for ameliorating morning hypotension, which resulted from abnormal loss of body fluid during the nighttime. We also prescribed 5 μg of intranasal desmopressin once a night in the MSA patients with impaired circadian rhythm of AVP and nocturnal polyuria, with benefit. This small dose of desmopressin is unlikely to cause adverse effects. But hyponatremia and signs of cardiac failure should be checked for regularly. Tablet form is now available and may be more convenient for patient use.

Summary

Urinary dysfunction is a prominent autonomic feature in patients with MSA, which is more common (more than 90%) and occurs earlier than orthostatic hypotension in this disorder. Since the clinical features of MSA may mimic those of IPD, a distinctive pattern of urinary dysfunction in both disorders is worth looking at. In contrast to IPD, MSA patients have more marked urinary dysfunction, which consists of both urgency incontinence and post-void residuals >100 ml. Videourodynamic and sphincter EMG analyses are important tools to know the extent of these dysfunctions and assists in determining the management as well as the diagnosis of the disorders. The common finding in both disorders is detrusor hyperreflexia, which accounts for urinary urgency and frequency. However, detrusor-sphincter dyssynergia, open bladder neck at the start of bladder filling (internal sphincter denervation), and neurogenic sphincter EMG (external sphincter denervation) are all characteristic features of MSA. These features may reflect pathological lesions in the basal ganglia, pontine tegmentum, intermediolateral cell column, and the sacral Onuf's nucleus. During the course of the disease, the balance of pathophysiology changes from central to peripheral, with the predominance of bladder emptying disorder.

Since MSA is a progressive disorder and impaired detrusor contractility is common, it is important to avoid inappropriate urological surgery in the patients. A conservative approach with medical measures includes anticholinergics for urinary urgency and frequency, desmopressin for nocturnal polyuria, uro-selective alpha-blockers for voiding difficulty, and CIC for large post-void residuals.

References

1. Graham JG, Oppenheimer DR. Orthostatic hypotension and nicotinic sensitivity in a case of multiple system atrophy. J Neurol Neurosurg Psychiatry 1969; 32:28–34.

2. Adams RD, van Bogaert L, Eecken HV. Striato-nigral degeneration. J Neuropathol Exp Neurol 1964; 23:584–608.

3. Dejerine J, Thomas A. L'atrophie olivo-ponto-cérébelleuse. Nouvelle Iconographie de la Salpêtriére 1900; 13:30–70.

4. Shy GM, Drager GA. A neurological syndrome associated with orthostatic hypotension; a clinical-pathologic study. Arch Neurol 1960; 2:511–527.

5. Papp MI, Kahn JE, Lantos PL. Glial cytoplasmic inclusions in the CNS of patients with multiple system atrophy (striatonigral degeneration, olivopontocerebellar atrophy and Shy–Drager syndrome). J Neurol Sci 1989; 94:79–100.

6. Quinn N. Parkinsonism-recognition and differential diagnosis. BMJ 1995; 310:447–452.

7. Bannister R, Mathias CJ. Clinical features and investigation of the primary autonomic failure syndromes. In: Bannister R, Mathias CJ, eds. Autonomic failure, 3rd edn. Oxford: Oxford Medical Publications, 1992: 531–547.

8. The Consensus Committee of the American Autonomic Society and the American Academy of Neurology. Consensus statement on the definition of orthostatic hypotension, pure autonomic failure, and multiple system atrophy. Neurology 1996; 46:1470.

9. Beck RO, Betts CD, Fowler CJ. Genito-urinary dysfunction in Multiple System Atrophy: clinical features and treatment in 62 cases. J Urol 1994; 151:1336–1341.

10. Sakakibara R, Hattori T, Uchiyama T, et al. Urinary dysfunction and orthostatic hypotension in multiple system atrophy; which is the more common and earlier manifestation? J Neurol Neurosurg Psychiatry 2000; 68:65–69.

11. Wenning GK, Ben Shlomo Y, Magalhaes M, et al. Clinical features and natural history of multiple system atrophy – an analysis of 100 cases. Brain 1994; 117:835–845.

12. Christmas TJ, Chapple CR, Lees AJ, et al. Role of subcutaneous apomorphine in parkinsonian voiding dysfunction. Lancet 1998; Dec 24/31:1451–1453.

13. Fitzmaurice H, Fowler CJ, Richards D, et al. Micturition disturbance in Parkinson's disease. Br J Urol 1985; 57:652–656.

14. Sakakibara R, Hattori T, Uchiyama T, Yamanishi T. Videourodynamic and sphincter motor unit potential analyses in Parkinson's disease and multiple system atrophy. J Neurol Neurosurg Psychiatry 2001; 71:600–606.

15. Berger Y, Salinas JM, Blaivas JG. Urodynamic differentiation of Parkinson disease and the Shy–Drager syndrome. Neurourol Urodynam 1990; 9:117–121.

16. Stocchi F, Carbone A, Inghilleri M, et al. Urodynamic and neurophysiological evaluation in Parkinson's disease and multiple system atrophy. J Neurol Neurosurg Psychiatry 1997; 62:507–511.

17. Sand PK, Bowen LW, Ostergard DR. Uninhibited urethral relaxation; an unusual cause of incontinence. Obstet Gynecol 1986; 68: 645–648.

18. de Groat WC, Booth AM, Yoshimura N. Neurophysiology of micturition and its modification in animal models of human disease. In: Maggi CA, ed. The autonomic nervous system: nervous control of the urogenital system, Vol 3. London: Horwood Academic Publishers, 1993:227–290. Griffiths D. Basics of pressure-flow studies. World J Urol 1995; 13:30–33.

19. Yoshimura N, Mizuta E, Kuno S, et al. The dopamine D1 receptor agonist SKF 38393 suppresses detrusor hyperreflexia in the monkey with parkinsonism induced by MPTP. Neuropharm 1993; 32:315–321.

20. Sakakibara R, Fowler CJ. Cerebral control of bladder, bowel, and sexual function and effects of brain disease. In: Fowler CJ, ed. Neurology of bladder, bowel, and sexual function. Boston: Butterworth-Heinemann, 1999:229–243.

21. Aswal BS, Berkley KJ, Hussain I, et al. Brain responses to changes in bladder volume and urge to void in healthy men. Brain 2001; 124:369–377.

22. Daniel SE. The neuropathology and neurochemistry of multiple system atrophy. In: Bannister R, Mathias CJ, eds. Autonomic failure, 3rd edn. Oxford: Oxford Medical Publications, 1992:564–585.

23. Fujita T, Doi M, Ogata T, et al. Cerebral cortical pathology of sporadic olivopontocerebellar atrophy. J Neurol Sci 1993; 116:41–46.

24. Andrew J, Nathan PW. Lesions of the anterior frontal lobes and disturbances of micturition and defaecation. Brain 1964; 87:233–262.

25. Morgan C, Nadelhaft I, de Groat WC. Location of bladder preganglionic neurones within the sacral parasympathetic nucleus of the cat. Neurosci Lett 1979; 14:189–194.

26. Skehan AM, Downie JW, Awad SA. The pathophysiology of contractile activity in the chronic decentralized feline bladder. J Urol 1993; 149:1156–1164.

27. Blaivas JG. The neurophysiology of micturition; a clinical study of 550 patients. J Urol 1982; 127:958–963.

28. Lapides J, Friend CR, Ajemian EP, Reus WS. Denervation supersensibility as a test for neurogenic bladder. Surg Gyn Obst 1962; 114:241–244.

29. Abrams P. Objective evaluation of bladder outlet obstruction. Br J Urol 1995; 76(Suppl 1):11–15.

30. Shäfer W. Principles and clinical application of advanced urodynamic analysis of voiding dysfunction. Urol Clin North Am 1990; 17:553–566.

31. Sakakibara R, Fowler CJ, Hattori T, et al. Pressure-flow study as an evaluating method of neurogenic urethral relaxation failure. J Auton Nerv Syst 2000; 80:85–88.

32. Blaivas JG, Sinha HP, Zayed AAH, Labib KB. Detrusor-sphincter dyssynergia; a detailed electromyographic study. J Urol 1981; 125:545–548.

33. Sakakibara R, Uchiyama T, Asahina M, et al. Amezinium metilsulfate, a sympathomimetic agent, may increase the risk of urinary retention in multiple system atrophy. Clin Auton Res 2003; 13(1):51–53.

34. Schurch B, Yasuda K, Rossier AB. Detrusor bladder neck dyssynergia revisited. J Urol 1994; 152:2066–2070.

35. Sakakibara R, Hattori T, Uchiyama T, et al. Are alpha-blockers involved in lower urinary tract dysfunction in multiple system atrophy? A comparison of prazosin and moxisylyte. J Auton Nerv Syst 2000; 79:191–195.

36. Resnick NM, Yalla SV. Detrusor hyperactivity with impaired contractile function. JAMA 1987; 257:3076–3081.

37. Ozawa T, Oyanagi K, Tanaka H, et al. Suprachiasmal nucleus in a patient with multiple system atrophy with abnormal circadian rhythm of arginine vasopressin secretion into plasma. J Neurol Sci 1998; 154:116–121.

38. Ozawa T, Tanaka H, Nakano R, et al. Nocturnal decrease in vasopressin secretion into plasma in patients with multiple system atrophy. J Neurol Neurosurg Psychiatry 1999; 67:542–545.

39. Mathias CJ, Fosbraey P, DaCosta DF, et al. The effect of desmopressin on nocturnal polyuria, overnight weight loss, and morning postural hypotension in patients with autonomic failure. BMJ 1986; 293: 353–356.

40. Wilcox CS, Aminoff MJ, Penn W. Basis of nocturnal polyuria in patients with autonomic failure. J Neurol Neurosurg Psychiatry 1974; 37:677.

41. Fowler CJ, Kirby RS, Harrison MJG, et al. Individual motor unit analysis in the diagnosis of disorders of urethral sphincter innervation. J Neurol Neurosurg Psychiat 1984; 47:637–641.

42. Fowler CJ. Pelvic floor neurophysiology. In: Binnie C, ed. Clinical neurophysiology, Vol. 1. Oxford: Butterworth-Heinemann, 1995: 233–250.

43. Mannen T, Iwata M, Toyokura Y, Nagashima K. Preservation of a certain motor neurone group in amyotrophic lateral sclerosis: its clinical significance. J Neurol Neurosurg Psychiatry 1977; 4:464–469.

44. Sakuta M, Nakanishi T, Toyokura Y. Anal muscle electromyograms differ in amyotrophic lateral sclerosis and Shy–Drager syndrome. Neurology 1978; 28:1289–1293.

45. Palace J, Chandiramani VA, Fowler CJ. Value of sphincter electromyography in the diagnosis of multiple system atrophy. Muscle and Nerve 1997; 20:1396–1403.

46. Pramstaller PP, Wenning GK, Smith SJM, et al. Nerve conduction studies, skeletal muscle EMG, and sphincter EMG in multiple system atrophy. J Neurol Neurosurg Psychiatry 1995; 580:618–621.

47. Sakakibara R, Hattori T, Kita K, et al. Stress-induced urinary incontinence in patients with spinocerebellar degeneration. J Neurol Neurosurg Psychiatry 1998; 64:389–391.

48. Yamanishi T, Yasuda K, Sakakibara R, et al. The effectiveness of terazosin, an $\alpha 1$-blocker, on bladder neck obstruction as assessed by urodynamic hydraulic energy. BJU Int 2000; 85:249–253.

49. Donnellan CA, Fook L, McDonald P, Playfer JR. Oxybutynin and cognitive dysfunction. BMJ 1997; 315:1363–1364.

50. Yamamoto M. Pergolide improves neurogenic bladder in patients with Parkinson's disease. Movem Dis 1997; 12(Suppl):328.

51. Uchiyama T, Sakakibara R, Yamanishi T, Hattori T. An effect of l-dopa on micturition in patents with Parkinson's disease; a comparison of 'on' and 'off' periods. 30th Annual Meeting of International Continence Society, Tampere, Finland, September 2000.

52. Chandiramani VA, Palace J, Fowler CJ. How to recognize patients with parkinsonism who should not have urological surgery. Br J Urol 1997; 80:100–104.

53. Schwinn DA. Novel role for alpha 1-adrenergic receptor subtypes in lower urinary tract symptoms. BJU Int 2000; 86(Suppl 2): 11–22.

24

Multiple sclerosis

Line Leboeuf and Angelo E Gousse

Introduction

Multiple sclerosis (MS) is a complex, autoimmune relapsing–remitting disorder of the central nervous system (CNS) that results in disabling neurologic deficits. The etiology and pathogenesis of the disease are still unknown, but there is increasing evidence that the primary disease mechanism of MS is related to an autoimmune attack on the CNS myelin, although genetic, environmental, and viral factors have all been implicated. The clinical course of the disease is extremely variable and unpredictable from one individual to the other but voiding dysfunction is present in the majority of these patients at some point in time during the evolution of the illness. Not only does voiding dysfunction represent a considerable psychosocial burden to affected individuals but it also poses great challenges to the treatment team. In that regard, knowledge of the pathophysiology and clinical evolution of MS, as well as proper evaluation and individualized treatments, is essential to the urologist to prevent complications and increase the quality of life of these patients.

History and epidemiology of multiple sclerosis

We owe to Jean-Martin Charcot in 1868 the correlation between the clinical presentation of MS and its pathologic description.[1] However, the first identification of the lesions in MS was presented by Cruveilhier (1835) and Carswell (1838) 30 years earlier.[2]

The disease has an incidence of about 7 in 100,000 every year, with a prevalence of 120 per 100,000, and a lifetime risk of 1 in 400.[3] A clear gender difference exists, females being more commonly affected than men by a ratio of 2:1. Populations vary in their susceptibility to MS; the prevalence is approximately 1 per 1000 in Americans, and 2 per 1000 in northern Europeans. In contrast with Caucasians, MS is less common in Orientals.[4,5] Prevalence rates are also reported to be greatest at the extremes of latitudes in both the northern and southern hemispheres.[6] This uneven geographic distribution of the disease has been attributed to environmental factors but recent studies have demonstrated that genetic susceptibility may play a more important role in determining the prevalence of the disease in a particular location than was previously believed.[7] The risk of MS in monozygotic twins seems to be in favor of this argument; hence, the concordance rate for monozygotic twins is approximately 30% compared to 3–5% in dizygotic twins and 0.1–0.4% in non-twin siblings and the general population.[8] Multiple sclerosis is diagnosed most often between the ages of 20 and 50 years old, with pediatric and geriatric populations being rarely affected by the disease.[9,10]

Pathogenesis of multiple sclerosis

The pathologic hallmarks of multiple sclerosis are, as described by Charcot, the zones of acute focal inflammatory demyelination or plaques in the white matter of the brain and spinal cord. At the present time, the precise etiology of MS remains unknown, although numerous studies have implicated, alone or in combination, genetic, environmental, viral, and autoimmune factors. Growing experimental evidence points, however, toward an autoimmune mechanism for the chronic multifocal plaques from which the disease gets its name.

Immunopathology

The autoimmune attack on CNS myelin in MS leads to a loss of saltatory conduction and velocity in axonal pathways. The oligodendrocyte, which is primarily responsible for synthesis and maintenance of the myelin sheath around nerve axons in the CNS, is phagocytosed, and subsequently this event leads to demyelination. The resultant edema worsens the neurologic impairment. Chronic attacks will eventually lead to scarring of nerves, with associated severe and often permanent neurologic dysfunction.[3,9–11] The phenomenon of acute demyelination is believed to be the first event leading to neurologic dysfunction in MS. However, with successive offences, repetitive cell reactivity will isolate the nerve lesions, further reducing remyelination potential and the capacity of damaged nerves to accommodate cumulative deficits. This second phase seems to mark the transition from temporary to persistent neurologic deficit.[3]

Cell-mediated autoimmunity

The contribution of autoreactive T lymphocytes to the demyelinating process appears crucial.[12] In the peripheral circulation, T lymphocytes, activated by unknown mechanisms, will migrate through the blood–brain barrier, where they will be stimulated by binding of the T-cell receptor with class II major histocompatibility complex to the antigen on the surface of an antigen-presenting cell. Release of proinflammatory cytokines by the activated T lymphocytes will then enhance macrophage activity that may injure the myelin processes or oligodendroglial cells.[10]

Humoral and antibody-mediated autoimmunity

The association of T cells and antigen in the CNS activates B-lymphocyte cells, which subsequently differentiate into antibody-secreting plasma cells. The potential for damage from those antibodies resides in the opsonization of the autoimmune target and the activation of the complement membrane attack complex; all of these phenomena subsequently cause damage to myelin and the myelin oligodendrocyte glycoprotein (MOG).[13] Antibodies to MOG have been demonstrated within human MS lesions.[14]

Genetics

The question of genetic predisposition to MS has been raised by reports from twin and sibling studies. As previously mentioned, concordance rates between monozygotic twins are approximately 30%, compared with 5% for dizygotic twins and non-twin siblings.[8] It has also been found that the risk of MS for genetically unrelated family members living with an index case is the same as the risk in the general population.[15] Several chromosomal linkages have also been associated with multiple sclerosis, notably at the 1p, 6p, 10p, 17q, and 19q sites.[16] The disease seems to conform to the inheritance pattern of a polygenic disease.[17]

Although genetic predisposition seems to play a prominent role in the physiopathology of MS, at this time genetic factors are not yet clearly determined and explain only part of the susceptibility to MS. Lack of identification of a major susceptibility gene and the discordance rate of 70% between monozygotic twins despite identical genetic background remain to be explored.

Infectious agents

Multiple infectious agents have been proposed to be linked to the physiopathology of MS. Agents currently under investigation include Epstein–Barr virus (EBV), human herpesvirus 6 (HHV-6), and *Chlamydia pneumoniae*.[18] It has been proposed that a genetically susceptible individual could be exposed to an infectious agent at a critical time, leading subsequently to development of MS, with acute attacks possibly related to reactivation of the latent infection.[10] Also, autoimmune offence against self-antigens could be triggered by infectious agents that are antigenically similar to normal tissue.[19] Wandinger et al[20] have reported 100% EBV seropositivity for immunoglobulin G (IgG) antibodies in MS patients, compared with 90% IgG and 4% IgM in normal controls. Also, the same authors found that acute relapses of MS were associated with the presence of reactivation of EBV DNA within blood. Moreover, other investigators have found HHV-6 in actively demyelinating plaques.[21] The bacteria *Chlamydia pneumoniae* were cultured from the cerebrospinal fluid of 64% of MS patients and from 11% of controls.[22]

As these results have not been invariably confirmed by other laboratories at this time, most authors agree that more studies are necessary to delineate the mechanisms of action of those infectious agents and even more work is required to link these agents to the pathogenesis of MS.

Clinical presentation and course of multiple sclerosis

The neurologic symptoms and signs of MS reflect the location of the affected site within the CNS and are the consequences of demyelination on axons conduction (Figure 24.1). Involvement of the cerebrum can lead to cognitive, sensory, and motor impairment, with or without epilepsy and focal cortical deficits.[3] When assessed with magnetic resonance imaging (MRI), the cerebrum is almost always involved but usually most abnormalities cannot be linked to specific clinical symptoms.[23] Lesions of the optic nerve typically lead to painful loss of vision, whereas those of the cerebellum and brainstem may present with tremor, ataxia, vertigo, diplopia, and impaired speech

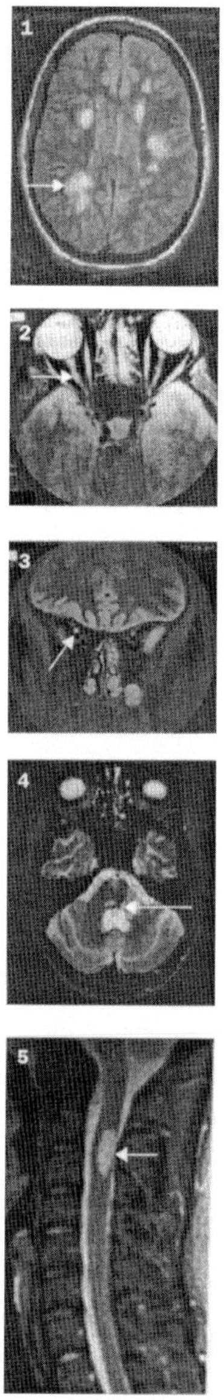

Figure 24.1

Lesion sites, syndromes, and symptomatic treatments in multiple sclerosis. T2-weighted magnetic resonance imaging (MRI) abnormalities (arrows) in the cerebrum (**1**), right optic nerve, longitudinal section, (**2**), transverse section (**3**), brainstem and cerebellar peduncle (**4**), and cervical spinal cord (**5**). TENS, transcutaneous electric nerve stimulation. Reproduced from Compston[8] with permission from *Journal of Neurology*.

Site	Symptoms	Signs	Treatment Established efficacy	Equivocal efficacy	Speculative
Cerebrum	Cognitive impairment	Deficits in attention, reasoning, and executive function (early); dementia (late)	–	–	–
	Hemi-sensory and motor	Upper motor neuron signs	–	–	–
	Affective (mainly depression)		Antidepressants	–	–
	Epilepsy (rare)		Anticonvulsants	–	–
	Focal cortical deficits (rare)		–	–	–
Optic nerve	Unitateral painful loss of vision	Scotoma, reduced visual acuity, color vision, and relative afferent pupillary defect	Low vision aids	–	–
Cerebellum and cerebellar pathways	Tremor	Postural and action tremor, dysarthria	–	–	Wrist weights, carbamazepine, isoniazid, beta-blockers, clonazepam, thalamotomy, and thalamic stimulation
	Clumsiness and poor balance	Limb incoordination and gait ataxia	–	–	–
Brainstem	Diplopia, oscillopsia	Nystagmus, internuclear, and other complex opthalmolplegias	–	–	Baclofen, gabapentin, isoniazid
	Vertigo		–	Prochloropherazine, cinnarizine	–
	Impaired speech and swallowing	Dysarthia and pseudo-bulbar palsy	Tricyclic anti-depressants	–	Speech therapy
	Paroxysmal symptoms		Carbamazepine, gabapentin	–	–
Spinal cord	Weakness Stiffness and painful spasms	Upper motor neuron signs Spasticity	– Tizanidine, baclofen, dantrolene, benzodiazepines intrathecal baclofen	– Botulinum toxin, IV corticosteroids	– Cannabinoids
	Bladder dysfunction		Anticholinergics and intermittent self catheterization, suprapubic catheterization	Desmopressin, intravescial capsaicin	Abdominal vibration, cranberry juice
	Erectile impotence		Sildenafil	–	–
	Constipation		Bulk laxatives, enemas	–	–
Other	Pain		Carbamazepine, gabapentin	Tricyclic anti-depressants, TENS	–
	Fatigue		Amantadine	Modafanil	4-aminopyridine, pemoline fluoxetine
	Temperature sensitivity and exercise intolerance		–	–	Cooling suit, 4-aminopyridine

and swallowing. The spinal cord is frequently affected with subsequent alterations of motor, sensory, and autonomic function, with or without bowel, bladder, and erectile dysfunction.[3,10] Other symptoms such as debilitating fatigue, paresthesias on neck flexion (Lhermitte's symptoms) and heat-exacerbated symptomatic worsening (Uthoff's symptom) may be present.[10] As many lesions can be clinically silent, other causes for symptom complex must be sought before considering the diagnosis of MS, all of which are beyond the scope of this chapter and are covered comprehensively elsewhere.[24]

Current accepted clinical diagnostic categories for MS present as follows: relapsing–remitting (RRMS), secondary progressive (SPMS), primary progressive (PPMS), and progressive–relapsing (PRMS).[25] Approximately 80% of patients present with RRMS, typically described as discrete clinical attacks followed by full recovery. RRMS is mostly encountered in the younger population. Years after onset, approximately 30–40% of RRMS patients will develop a more progressive chronic course characterized by progressive persistent deficits with or without acute clinical attacks; hence, it is termed secondary progressive MS. In 20% of

Table 24.1 *Factors of good and poor prognosis in multiple sclerosis (Adapted from Keegan and Noseworthy)*[10]

Good prognosis	Poor prognosis
Female gender	Male gender
Younger age of onset	Predominant cerebellar and motor involvement
Optic neuritis	
Sensory attacks	Incomplete resolution of attacks
Complete recovery from attacks	Progressive course from onset
Few attacks	Frequent early attacks
Long inter attacks interval	Short inter attacks interval

Reproduced from Compston[8] with permission from *Journal of Neurology*.

patients, the disease is primary progressive from onset, without clinically evident relapses.[26] Alternatively, these patients can later experience superimposed exacerbation of neurologic dysfunction, a condition referred to as PRMS.

Overall life expectancy from disease onset is estimated to be approximately 25 years, death being almost invariably caused by unrelated events. Due to the wide variety of clinical features and presentations, prognosis varies widely. Isolated sensory and visual symptoms have been associated with good prognosis and with complete recovery.[3] On the other hand, motor involvement with coordination and balance deficits have been linked with poorer prognosis. Clinical indicators of good and poor prognosis have been described by some authors[27] and are presented in Table 24.1.

Diagnosis of multiple sclerosis

Diagnosis of MS is based on clinical evidence of symptoms and is facilitated by paraclinical data: i.e. MRI, cerebrospinal fluid (CSF) analysis with oligoclonal bands, and visually evoked potentials (Figure 24.2).[23] A purely clinical diagnosis of MS is made upon the occurrence of two or more distinct attacks, affecting more than one anatomical site within the myelinated regions of the CNS (cerebral white matter, brain stem, cerebellar tracts, optic nerves, spinal cord). Also a single clinical attack with additional lesions discovered by paraclinical evidence can suggest the diagnosis.

MRI of the brain and spinal cord is the most sensitive investigational technique in the diagnosis of MS. More than 95% of patients with MS have T2-weighted white matter abnormalities, although these are not always diagnostic.[3] MRI can also help predict the risk of progression to clinically definite MS in a patient with a single episode; monosymptomatic patients with one or no brain MRI lesions are at low risk of developing a second clinical attack in the subsequent decade (15–20%) in contrast to patients with two or more cerebral MRI lesions, who are at high risk (85%) for a second attack over the same period.[28] However, imaging is most useful in the investigation of individuals with clinically isolated lesions or insidious progressive disease at a single site.

CSF protein electrophoresis shows oligoclonal IgG bands in more than 90% of cases of MS.[3] Its role in the pathogenesis of MS is unresolved but confirms the inflammatory nature of the underlying pathology, therefore excluding alternative explanations. Evoked potentials measure conduction along afferent CNS pathways following stimulation of a sensory receptor.[3] Abnormal conduction may identify a clinically occult demyelinated lesion and provide evidence in diagnostically difficult situations. Finally, before attributing the diagnosis of MS, the clinician must exclude other causes of focal or multifocal CNS disease.[24]

Neurologic effect of multiple sclerosis on the urinary tract

Neuroanatomy and neurophysiology of normal lower urinary tract

Bladder and sphincter function is considered a single physiologic unit whose purpose is the efficient, low-pressure storage and expulsion of urine. These rather discrete and simple functions are achieved through the complex coordination of the autonomic, somatic, and central nervous systems (Figure 24.3). The parasympathetic and sympathetic divisions of the autonomic nervous system produce, via their action through neurotransmitters and receptors in the bladder and urethral sphincter, bladder emptying and storage (Table 24.2). The somatic innervation of the lower urinary tract is provided by neurons in the spinal segment S2 to S4. Through the pudendal nerve these fibers activate contraction of the external urethral sphincter, producing retention of urine and continence.

Bladder function is also controlled by centers in the brainstem, as reported from mammalian animal experiments,[29] and later confirmed in human studies.[30] The so-called pontine micturition center provides coordination between the autonomic and somatic nervous systems involved in voiding, providing a 'switch' phenomenon between the storage and emptying phases of micturition. Higher control of micturition is located in the medial frontal cortex and the diencephalon; these regions are

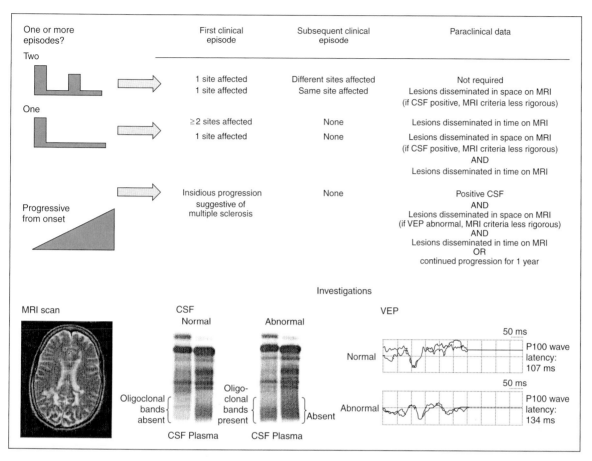

Figure 24.2

Criteria for diagnosis of multiple sclerosis. The principle is to establish that two or more episodes affecting separate sites within the central nervous system have occurred at different times, using clinical analysis or laboratory investigations. Dissemination in space based on MRI requires: any three features from (1) one gadolinium (Gd)-positive or nine T2 MRI lesions; (2) ≥1 infratentorial lesion; (3) ≥1 juxtacortical lesion; or (4) ≥3 periventricular lesions. If VEPs or CSF are positive, ≥ 2 MRI lesions consistent with multiple sclerosis are sufficient. Dissemination in time of MRI lesions requires: one Gd-positive lesion at >3 months after the onset of the clinical event; or a Gd-positive or new T2 lesion on a second scan repeated 3 months after the first. Patients having an appropriate clinical presentation, but who do not meet all of the diagnostic criteria, can be classified as having possible multiple sclerosis. MRI, magnetic resonance imaging; CSF, cerebrospinal fluid; VEP, visually evoked potential test. (Reproduced with permission Compston.[3])

responsible for voluntary control of the initiation and cessation of micturition. Detailed description of voiding and storage pathways are beyond the scope of this chapter and are comprehensively covered elsewhere in this book.

Suprasacral, sacral, and intracranial plaques' effects

Oppenheimer, in an autopsy study of patients with multiple lesions, demonstrated that almost all exhibited cervical spinal cord demyelination with marked involvement of lateral corticospinal and reticulospinal tracts. Moreover, the lumbar and sacral cord were involved in 40% and 18% of patients, respectively.[31] Because innervation of

the detrusor and external urethral sphincter is mediated via these lateral spinal tracts, and knowing the predilection of demyelinating plaques for the cervical spinal cord, most MS patients have lower urinary tract dysfunction. Litwiller et al have divided the effects of MS on the urinary tract as suprasacral, sacral, and intracranial.[11]

Suprasacral plaques

Interruption of the reticulospinal pathways between the pontine and sacral micturition centers may cause loss of synergistic activity between the urethral sphincter and the detrusor, possibly resulting in detrusor-external sphincter dyssynergia (DESD).[32] On the other hand, the lack of supraspinal suppression of autonomous bladder contraction may result from lesions in the corticospinal tract.

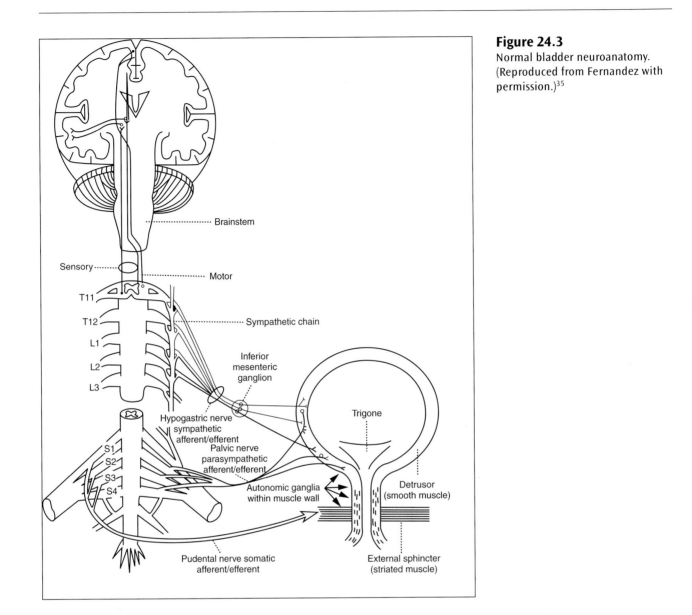

Figure 24.3
Normal bladder neuroanatomy.
(Reproduced from Fernandez with permission.)[35]

Table 24.2 *Innervation of the bladder (modified from Fernandez)[35]*

Division	Spinal cord	Nerve	Neurotransmitter	Receptor	Mechanism	Effect
Parasympathetic	S2 to S4	Pelvic	Acetylcholine	Muscarinic	Contraction of detrusor	Bladder emptying
					Relaxation of outlet (urethra)	Bladder emptying
Sympathetic	T10 to L2	Hypogastric	Norepinephrine	Beta	Relaxation of detrusor	Retention of urine
				Alpha	Contraction of outlet (urethra)	Retention of urine
Somatic	Efferent S2 to S4 Afferent S2 to S4	Pudendal	Acetylcholine	Nicotinic	Contraction of external sphincter	Retention of urine

Sacral plaques

Studies have demonstrated a 20% incidence of involvement of the sacral cord in autopsy patients.[33] Moreover, Mayo and Chetner reported that almost two-thirds of patients with sacral plaques had detrusor hypocontractility and 5% had areflexia.[34] Hence, it has been postulated that plaques located in the spinal afferents and efferents of the sacral reflex arc may inhibit bladder contraction and therefore result in impaired emptying or urinary retention.

Intracranial plaques

Intracranial plaques can be found in approximately 60–80% of patients;[11] their location involves any area of the white matter, but particularly the periventricular zone. In those patients affected with this type of lesion, the micturition reflex as well as the synergistic integration of bladder and urethral sphincter function remain intact. Micturition is thus physiologically unimpaired. However, perception of fullness and ability to inhibit bladder contraction are dependent on an alert and normally functioning sensorium. Intracranial plaques may result in loss of voluntary control of initiation or prevention of voiding. Disease in the supraspinal CNS may account for detrusor hyperreflexia.

Urologic symptoms associated with multiple sclerosis

Urologic symptoms in patients with MS are shown to vary greatly from study to study, their incidence ranging from 52% to 97%. The best-known series addressing urinary symptoms in MS are summarized in Table 24.3.[11,35,36] Frequency and urgency are the most frequent, manifested in 31–86% of patients, whereas incontinence and obstructive symptoms with or without urinary retention are reported in 34–72% and 2–49%, respectively.[11,35,36] Although lower urinary tract symptoms are frequent in the MS population, voiding problems are rarely the sole initial presentation of the disease:[32,37] only about 10% of patients present solely with voiding symptoms at the time of initial clinical manifestation of MS.[32,37,38]

Moreover, correlation between urologic symptoms and urodynamic evaluation has been reported unreliable as indicators of the extent of vesical dysfunction.[39–41] Koldewijn et al have demonstrated urodynamic evidence of urinary dysfunction in 100% of symptomatic patients and in 50% of asymptomatic ones.[39] Also, in another study, nearly half of the patients with elevated post-void residual (PVR) felt sensation of incomplete emptying as compared with nearly all patients expressing complaints of incomplete emptying had elevated PVR.[42] Some authors have postulated that the poor correlation between objective clinical findings and subjective symptoms may be explained by the chronicity of the disease and subsequent adaptation to the symptom complex. Failure or denial to recognize symptoms is another explanation.[43] Of upmost importance is the study of Bemelmens et al showing that MS patients without urologic symptoms can have urologic pathology. Hence, 52% of asymptomatic patients had anomalies on urodynamic evaluation, suggesting that the corticospinal and reticulospinal tracts are commonly involved at a subclinical level and that this involvement can be found quite early in the demyelinating process. Patients who deny urologic problems can still have significant urodynamically verifiable pathology.

Table 24.3 *Percentage of patients affected by symptoms of bladder dysfunction in multiple sclerosis (modified from Fernandez)*[35]

Study		No. of patients	Urgency	Frequency	Urge incontinence	Hesitancy	Retention
Sachs	1921	57	31	–	37	49	–
Langworthy	1938	97	54	33	34	40	–
Carter	1950	36	24	17	50	–	17
Miller	1965	321	60	50	36	33	2
Bradley	1973	90	86	60	–	28	20
Philp	1981	52	61	59	47	25	8
Goldstein	1983	86	32	32	49	–	–
Awad	1984	47	85	65	72	36	–
Gonor	1985	64	70	48	56	30	–
Betts	1992	170	85	82	63	49	–
Hennessey	1999	191	71	76	19	48	–

Finally, studies have reported that patients older than 50 years of age seem to be more bothered by bladder symptoms.[41] An explanation for this is the possible cumulative effect of other diseases causing bladder dysfunction such as benign prostatic hyperplasia (BPH), pelvic relaxation associated with stress incontinence, and longer duration of disease in older patients. No significant relationship between overall incidence of symptoms and gender exists, but men with MS have a higher incidence of obstructive symptoms and complications, possibly related to age-related changes in the prostate or severity of DESD in men.[39]

Recent studies have demonstrated that lower urinary symptoms were strongly related to disability status, as measured by the expanded disability status scale[39,41] with weaker relation to disease duration and age, as it was previously reported. The extent of pyramidal dysfunction also seems to be a strong predictor of urologic pathology.[44] Finally, the disease presentation may influence bladder function, as SPMS shows increased risk of bladder function deterioration.[44]

Urologic complications such as urinary tract infection (UTI), stones, renal impairment, incontinence, and deaths associated with lower urinary tract dysfunction in MS are decreasing as knowledge of the course of the disease, sophisticated evaluation, follow-up, and intermittent catheterization are becoming widespread. Although the incidence of MS is higher in women than in men, urologic complications occur more frequently in the latter, and about half of the affected men have DESD. It is believed that the high prevalence of incontinence in women may protect them by decreasing the risk of developing dangerously elevated intravesical pressures, hence impeding serious bladder or renal function.[43] Also, one has to be careful in attributing urologic symptoms in MS patients to their underlying neurologic disease, as common urologic disorders may coexist, mimic, or aggravate the neurologic dysfunction. Although only 7% of patients with MS will develop serious bladder or renal problems in the course of the disease, it is important to recognize the impact of morbidity from urologic symptoms, especially UTI and incontinence. These factors pose a great burden on the patients and every effort should be made to address them.

Evaluation of urinary tract dysfunction in patients with multiple sclerosis

History

Initial assessment of MS patients should include a comprehensive history and physical examination. The history aims to ascertain whether urologic symptoms exist and should begin by emphasis on description of irritative or obstructive symptoms and urinary incontinence. Temporal and spatial characterization of symptoms, use of a protective device, assessment of fluid intake, and quality of life should also be addressed.[11] One should also determine the presence or absence of urologic complications: upper or lower urinary tract infection, hematuria, and stones. Past medical and surgical history is mandatory, since urologic pathologies like BPH or stress incontinence are common in the older population and may confuse the neurourological profile. Medication should be noted, as many drugs may affect bladder function. Of particular importance is the young patient with unexplained urologic symptoms. In those patients, every effort should be made to elicit neurologic symptoms suggestive of MS, and prompt referral is mandatory.[11]

Physical examination

The genitourinary evaluation begins with an abdominal examination to ensure that there is no overt evidence of bladder distention. Careful inspection of external genitalia may reveal hypospadias or urethral erosion in patients with an indwelling catheter. Prostate and testicular palpation may aid in cancer screening and BPH detection. The pelvic examination should be performed to evaluate sensory and motor function of the pelvic floor and sacral dermatomes. Determination of the anal sphincter tone and reflex and perineal sensation may help to evaluate the presence of neurologic disease of the bladder since absent anal reflexes, lax anal tone, or absent perineal sensation may be associated with neurologic disease of the bladder. Also, pelvic evaluation is important to determine the presence of concomitant urethral hypermobility or vaginal prolapse, the latter itself being able to cause irritative or obstructive voiding symptoms.

A directed neurologic examination can not only help understand the extent of the disease but can also help to predict urologic dysfunction. For instance, investigators have noted an association between hyperactive deep tendons reflexes and DESD.[38] Betts et al have reported a high correlation between cerebellar signs such as ataxia and dysdiadochokinesis and detrusor areflexia.[42] Finally, as mentioned earlier, the degree of lower extremity motor dysfunction may be the best predictor of urologic and bladder dysfunction.[44]

After the preliminary history and physical examination, routine laboratory tests include urine analysis and culture and serum creatinine. Urinary tract infection is common in MS patients and has been reported in as many of 60% of patients.[43] Also, an elevated serum creatinine may herald renal insufficiency in an asymptomatic patient. A voiding diary may also be useful to objectively assess the voiding complaints and evaluate the extent of the incontinence problem.

Although the definite diagnosis of multiple sclerosis is based on clinical judgment, MRI is used routinely and is diagnostic in 70–95% of patients with clinically confirmed MS.[45] The most common MRI abnormality associated with MS, although nonspecific for the disease, is a focus of increased signal intensity on T2-weighted scans corresponding to a plaque demyelination.[46] However, many patients are found to have lesions on MRI without clinical evidence of the disease as reported in imaging studies of normal subjects.[47] Conversely, the absence of lesions on MRI does not exclude the diagnosis of MS, as illustrated in the criteria used for the diagnosis of the disease. Finally, there does not seems to exist any correlation between MRI findings and specific urodynamic parameters.[48]

Cerebrospinal fluid analysis and evoked responses provide additional evidence for the diagnosis of MS. However, although abnormal findings are common, no characteristic of these tests is specific, neither to the disease itself nor to the urological dysfunctions associated with it.

Koldewijn et al have reported an incidence of upper tract abnormalities of 7% in a study of 2076 patients with MS,[39] showing that upper tract deterioration is the exception rather than the rule. DESD, the presence of an indwelling catheter, and poor bladder compliance are risks factors that have been strongly linked to upper tract deterioration.[32,40] Although baseline radiographic assessment remains an integral part of initial evaluation, the low incidence of upper tract deterioration has led many urologists to abandon routine yearly upper tract imaging unless baseline studies are abnormal or there is a change in clinical status.[41]

Lower tract imaging seldom helps with the management of patients with MS. However, it may be beneficial to discriminate between neurogenic voiding and other lower urinary tract lesions in the genesis of voiding dysfunction.

Urodynamic evaluation

A thorough urodynamic evaluation is mandatory for effectively diagnosing urinary tract dysfunction and planning urinary tract management. The purposes of urodynamic testing are to determine and classify the type of voiding dysfunction and to identify risks factors such as DESD, decreased bladder compliance, and high detrusor filling pressures. All these factors are known to predispose to upper tract problems, including vesicourethral reflux, bladder and kidney stones, hydronephrosis, pyelonephritis, and renal insufficiency.

The incidence of abnormal urodynamic findings in patients with voiding symptoms and MS approaches 100%. The incidence of normal urodynamic findings in symptomatic patients, on the other hand, is approximately 10%, as revealed by a meta-analysis of 1900 patients[11] (Table 24.4). Bemelmans et al have addressed the particular situation of MS patients without urinary complaints; in their study, they demonstrated a 52% incidence of clinically silent urodynamic abnormalities.[49] This study stresses that even MS patients who deny urologic symptoms can have significant urodynamic pathology.

Three major patterns of urodynamic dysfunction have been described in MS patients and are reported in Table 24.4:

1. detrusor hyperreflexia without bladder outlet obstruction
2. detrusor hyperreflexia with outlet obstruction (DESD)
3. detrusor hypocontractility or areflexia.

Detrusor hyperreflexia without bladder outlet obstruction

The most common urodynamic abnormality in MS is detrusor hyperreflexia, which is manifested symptomatically by urinary urgency, frequency, nocturia, and incontinence (Figure 24.4). These findings correlate well with the high incidence of intracranial and cervical spinal plaques.[31] In a meta-analysis of 22 published series, Litwiller et al reported that 62% of patients had detrusor hyperreflexia on urodynamic findings.[11]

Detrusor hyperreflexia with bladder outlet obstruction

Detrusor hyperreflexia with DESD is the second most common urodynamic finding in patients with neurogenic bladder associated with MS (Figure 24.5) and is reported in 25% of patients.[11] The hyperreflexic contraction occurs without proper relaxation of the external urethral sphincter. DESD usually presents with obstructive symptoms and incomplete emptying, the latter being possibly related to sphincteric dysfunction or incomplete bladder contraction. As opposed to DESD in spinal cord patients, DESD in MS patients is rarely associated with upper tract dysfunction, suggesting that the hyperreflexia and extent of external sphincter spasms may be less severe than in spinal cord injury (SCI) patients.[39,50]

Detrusor hyporeflexia

Finally, detrusor hyporeflexia (Figure 24.6) is reported in approximately 20% of patients[11] and symptoms include straining or incapacity to void and/or overflow incontinence. Mayo and Chetner have reported that almost

Table 24.4 *Published series of urodynamic patterns in multiple sclerosis (modified from Litwiller et al)*[11]

Study		No. of patients	Hyperreflexia		DSD		Hyporeflexia		Normal	
			No.	%	No.	%	No.	%	No.	%
Anderson and Bradley	1973	52	33	(63)	16	(31)	21	(40)	2	(4)
Awad et al	1984	57	38	(66)	30	(52)	12	(21)	7	(12)
Beck et al	1981	46	40	(87)	–	(–)	6	(13)	–	(–)
Betts et al	1993	70	63	(91)	–	(–)	–	(–)	7	(10)
Blaivas et al	1979	41	23	(56)	12	(30)	16	(40)	2	(4)
Bradley et al	1973	99	58	(60)	20	(20)	40	(40)	1	(1)
Bradley	1978	302	127	(62)	–	(–)	103	(34)	10	(24)
Ciancio et al	2001	22	10	(45)	5	(23)	4	(18)	3	13
Eardley et al	1991	24	15	(63)	6	(27)	3	(13)	6	(25)
Goldstein et al	1982	86	65	(76)	57	(66)	16	(19)	5	(6)
Gonor et al	1985	64	40	(78)	8	(12)	13	(20)	1	(2)
Hinson and Boone	1996	70	44	(63)	15	(21)	20	(28)	6	(9)
Koldewijn et al	1995	212	72	(34)	27	(13)	32	(8)	76	(36)
Mayo and Chetner	1992	89	69	(78)	5	(6)	5	(6)	11	(12)
McGuire and Savastano	1984	46	33	(72)	21	(46)	13	(28)	0	(0)
Petersen and Pederson	1984	88	73	(83)	36	(41)	14	(16)	1	(1)
Philip et al	1981	52	51	(99)	16	(37)	0	(0)	1	(2)
Piazza and Diokno	1997	31	23	(74)	9	(47)	2	(6)	3	(9)
Schoenburg et al	1979	39	27	(69)	20	(5)	2	(6)	6	(15)
Sirls et al	1994	113	79	(70)	15	(28)	17	(15)	7	(6)
Summers	1978	50	26	(52)	6	(12)	6	(12)	9	(18)
Van Poppel and Baert	1987	160	105	(66)	38	(24)	38	(24)	16	(10)
Weinstein et al	1988	91	64	(70)	16	(18)	15	(16)	11	(12)
Total/Total No. (%)		1904	1204	(63.24)	378/1469	(25.73)	398	(20.9)	191	(10)

DSD, detrusor-sphincter dyssynergia; No., number.

two-thirds of patients with sacral plaques had detrusor hyporeflexia and 5% had detrusor areflexia.[34]

As neurologic patterns in MS are known to change over time, since the disease is dynamic and is characterized by exacerbations and remissions, changes in urodynamic patterns have also been reported. Changes in lower urinary tract function with time and in response to treatment can occur. No generalizations concerning patterns of changes can be drawn, but a significant proportion of patients (15–55%) will develop changes on urodynamic testing, undermining the need for repeat urodynamic studies, even in patients with persistent stable symptomatology.[51,52]

Management of urinary manifestations of multiple sclerosis

The aim of treatment of the neurogenic patient is management of lower urinary tract symptoms, prevention

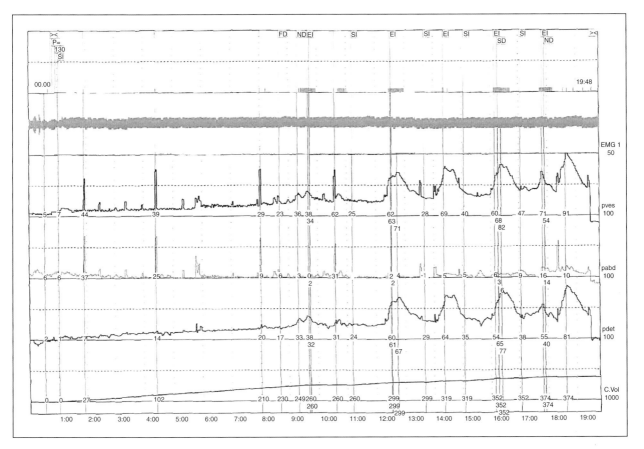

Figure 24.4
Detrusor hyperreflexia without bladder outlet obstruction.

of urinary tract infections, preservation of the upper urinary tract, and improvement of the quality of life. The choice of treatment should be based on a clear understanding of the pathology and on objective parameters, as well as on the patient's disability, autonomy, manual dexterity, and motivation. Since symptoms of MS can change over time due to its remission–exacerbation pattern, treatment modalities should preferably be reversible and permanent surgical procedures should be avoided as much as possible. Table 24.5 is a summary of the different options presented below.

Detrusor hyperreflexia without bladder outlet obstruction

Behavioral modifications and pelvic floor rehabilitation

Voiding symptoms can often be improved by simple behavioral manipulations, but the success of voiding mostly relies on the patient's motivation. Regular voiding may reduce hyperreflexic contraction by emptying the bladder before a critical state of filling is reached. Limitation of fluids may help prevent irritative symptoms, as well as avoidance of beverages such as coffee, tea, cola, and alcohol that may cause diuresis or irritation of the bladder. Although behavioral modification is a conservative treatment modality, objective evaluation should not be overlooked. Empirical treatment trials without proper evaluation should be avoided, as it may lead to improper care and complications.[11]

Suppression of an involuntary detrusor contraction by stimulation of the perineal musculature is the physiologic principle underlying pelvic floor rehabilitation. This modality has already been part of the treatment of many problems, such as stress incontinence, urgency, sexual dysfunction, and fecal incontinence. Pelvic floor rehabilitation has been reported to be of some value in the treatment of detrusor instability and urgency, by influencing the sacral micturition reflex and thus inhibiting detrusor hyperreflexia. De Ridder et al have noted a subjective improvement in 76.7% of patients,

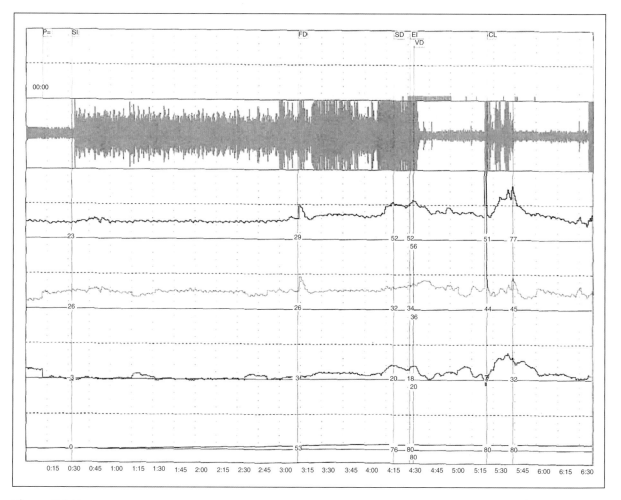

Figure 24.5
Detrusor hyperreflexia with bladder outlet obstruction.

with significant improvement in functional bladder capacity, frequency, and incontinence, as evaluated by urodynamic study.[53]

Clean intermittent catheterization and catheter drainage

Clean intermittent catheterization (CIC) is a simple and very effective treatment modality for neurogenic voiding dysfunction, either in patients with primary emptying difficulties or after pharmacologic therapy in patients with detrusor hyperreflexia.[40,43] Urodynamic evaluation is required to define bladder storage capabilities and to select the optimum catheterization interval. Chronic catheter drainage after pharmacologic therapy in patients with detrusor hyperreflexia should be considered only after all the treatment options have been evaluated.

Pharmacologic therapy

Since almost two-thirds of patients with MS have detrusor hyperreflexia, treatment often involves pharmacologic therapy to suppress uninhibited bladder contractions. Traditionally, oxybutynine chloride has been among the most widely used drugs. It binds competitively to the muscarinic receptor, thus suppressing bladder contractions. Response rates in MS patients have been reported in the range of 65–80%.[11] However, because of the anticholinergic profile of its side-effects – namely, decreased salivation, constipation, and blurred vision – discontinuation of treatment was reported in as many as 50% of patients.[54] Tolterodine, a potent antimuscarinic agent, was specifically developed for the treatment of the overactive bladder. It is a selective muscarinic receptor blocker with efficacy proven equivalent to oxybutynin but with a more favorable tolerability profile.[55] In certain patients with combined storage and emptying failure, CIC may be used in concert with anticholinergic therapy. In

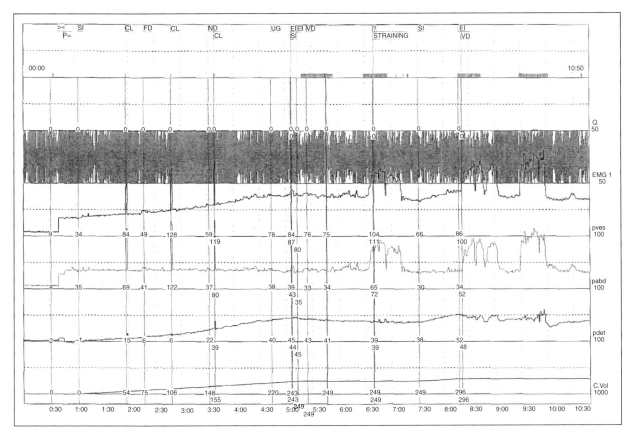

Figure 24.6
Detrusor hyporeflexia.

these patients, urinary retention is promoted by anticholinergics and the 'paralyzed' bladder is hence drained by CIC.

Intravesical instillation of oxybutynin is another treatment option for detrusor hyperreflexia, and is reported to alleviate side-effects of oral medication.[56,57] Capsaicin and resiniferatoxin, the newer intravesical agents, are thought to exert a selective neurotoxic action on axons of C sensory fibers. These fibers appear to play an important role in bladder reflex pathways following spinal cord insult. Intravesical capsaicin and resiniferatoxin are known to reduce the amplitude of hyperreflexic contractions and have been used in selective research centers for the treatment of intractable detrusor hyperreflexia.[58,59]

Nocturia and enuresis are common problems in MS and the effect of sleep disturbance may be detrimental to the patient's functional level. Desmopressin, a synthetic analogue of vasopressine, has been proven efficacious and safe in the management of these problems in that population.[60,61]

Surgical management

The role of surgical intervention in the management of patients with neurogenic dysfunction secondary to MS has

been reduced dramatically with the advent of CIC. As a general rule, non-operative treatment should be used as long as possible. As the course of the disease is dynamic and progressive, permanent procedures should be performed only after stabilization of the neurologic status and after all other conservative options have been exhausted. Evaluation of manual dexterity, disability, life expectancy, and social support should be undertaken as well as a thorough urodynamic characterization of the neurogenic voiding dysfunction.

Denervation procedures of the bladder have been reported for treatment of detrusor hyperreflexia and include selective dorsal rhizotomy, subtrigonal injection of phenol or alcohol, and bladder myotomy and transection. These techniques, although displaying good short-term results, have not proven to produce satisfactory long-term effects.[62]

Augmentation cystoplasty with or without a catheterizable limb (using the ileocecal valve or intussuscepted portion of the small bowel) is usually reserved for the patient with refractory detrusor hyperreflexia in whom all other non-operative options have failed. Bladder augmentation will allow attainment of large volumes of urine in the bladder with low-filling pressures. Excellent results can

Table 24.5 *Management options of MS patients based on urologic dysfunction*

Detrusor hyperreflexia without bladder outlet obstruction:
- Behavioral modification and pelvic floor rehabilitation
- Clean intermittent catheterization/catheter drainage
- Pharmacologic therapy
- Surgical management
    Denervation procedures
    Augmentation cystoplasty
- Neuromodulation
- Botulinum toxin

Detrusor hyperreflexia with bladder outlet obstruction:
- Clean intermittent catheterization/catheter drainage
- External sphincterotomy
- Augmentation cystoplasty
- Ileal conduit
- Cutaneous ileovesicostomy
- Neuromodulation
- Botulinum toxin

Detrusor hyporeflexia:
- Clean intermittent catheterization/catheter drainage
- Credé's maneuver (women)
- Urinary diversion

be expected in at least 80% of patients, but most will require CIC; thus, the ability to perform CIC is mandatory if one is to consider this type of procedure.[63,64] Careful evaluation of sphincteric competence may also obviate the need for a concomitant outlet procedure such as pubovaginal sling or sphincter prosthesis.

Neuromodulation

Sacral nerve stimulation (SNS) modulates dysfunctional voiding behavior in patients by a mechanism not fully understood but comprising detrusor inhibition via afferent and/or efferent stimulation of sacral nerves.[65] Although the Food and Drug Administration (FDA) approved indications for SNS are urge incontinence, urgency–frequency syndrome, and non-neurogenic urinary retention, sacral nerve stimulation has been evaluated as a reversible treatment option for neurogenic refractory urge incontinence related to detrusor hyperreflexia. Chartier-Kastler et al have reported a 43.6-month long-term efficacy of this technique in 7 out of 9 patients with urodynamically demonstrable detrusor hyperreflexia, with or without DESD.[66] Although sacral neuromodulation seems to be a promising therapy for neurogenic disease, further studies and long-term results with an extended cohort of SCI and MS patients are yet to be obtained.

Botulinum-A toxin

Botulinum-A toxin inhibits calcium-mediated release of acetylcholine vesicles at the neuromuscular junction, which results in reduced muscle contractility and atrophy at the injection site.[67] Injections into the detrusor muscle seem to be a safe conservative treatment for detrusor hyperreflexia in SCI patients. In a study of 21 patients, Schurch et al found that 19 of them underwent complete continence at 6 weeks and 11 out of 22 at 36 weeks.[68] However, to our knowledge, no study involving an MS population has been undertaken.

Detrusor hyperreflexia with bladder outlet obstruction

Behavioral modifications and pelvic floor rehabilitation

Pelvic floor spasticity and DESD are both predictors of poor prognosis, and behavioral modifications and pelvic floor rehabilitation should be reserved for mildly symptomatic patients. Some women may be guided in voiding by Credés maneuver, but this may put the upper urinary tract at risk.[40] Although the maneuver appears easier and less invasive, in women, with time, a significant number of patients develop daytime and nighttime frequency and stress incontinence. Consequently, CIC should be the method of choice.

Clean intermittent catheterization and catheter drainage

Patients with detrusor hyperreflexia have higher treatment failures and more upper tract damage.[32] The most reasonable treatment is CIC. The alternative, in the male, if he cannot perform CIC is external sphincterotomy, which is discussed below. The other alternative for both sexes is indwelling catheter but those patients, as mentioned earlier, have a higher incidence of upper tract changes.[32]

Pharmacologic therapy

Symptoms of neurogenic voiding dysfunction complicated by bladder outlet obstruction may be treated by alpha antagonists (terazosin, doxazosin, tamsulosin) or muscle relaxants (diazepam, baclofen, dantrolene). Alpha antagonists aim at blockage of the sympathetic receptors of the smooth muscle component of the proximal urethra and bladder neck, thereby decreasing the sphincter tone and relieving bladder outlet obstruction. These treatments have had mixed results in MS patients.[69] Commonly encountered side-effects include orthostatic hypotension, dizziness, and lassitude.

Surgical management

Patients with DESD are at higher risk of upper tract damage.[32] In those males who cannot be treated with conservative measures, outlet reducing procedures such as transurethral external sphincterotomy, self-expandable urethral stents, or balloon dilatation may be necessary. The conventional and most-used technique is external sphincterotomy, which typically involves transurethral incision of the external sphincter. These procedures allow for total urinary incontinence, which can afterward be managed by condom catheter drainage. They are best reserved for the patient with limited hand function for whom CIC is not an option or for patients who do not have caretakers that can provide this service.[70,71] The performance of supravesical diversion (ileal conduit) has decreased with the widespread acceptance of augmentation cystoplasty. The latter, constructed with or without a continent stoma, is the preferred method. These procedures should be reserved for patients with failure of conservative therapy who lack the fine motor skills to do CIC.[62] Cutaneous ileovesicostomy has been used successfully for storage or emptying abnormalities. In this procedure, a segment of ileum is used to construct a 'chimney' from the bladder to allow cutaneous drainage to an external collection device.[72] Such procedure should be reserved for individuals who cannot have CIC performed, either by themselves or by others, and who wish to avoid chronic indwelling catheter drainage.

Botulinum-A toxin

Phelan et al evaluated prospectively 22 SCI patients with DESD who were voiding by indwelling catheters or by CIC. After botulinum-A toxin injection in the external sphincter, all patients except 2 were able to void without catheterization.[67] For treatment of DESD, the duration of botulinum effect has been reported to be approximately 3 months for a single injection[68,73] but monthly intervals for 3 months resulted in clinical effects up to 9 months.[68] Hence, botulinum-A toxin may be an alternative to external sphincterotomy for men with neuropathic DESD. It produces a reversible chemical sphincterotomy, which avoids the risks associated with the surgical procedure. However, the main disavantage is the need for repeated injections to maintain results. This treatment has to be considered in cases of failure of more traditional conservative modalities and before definitive surgery. To our knowledge, no study has prospectively evaluated the effect of botulinum toxin on the MS population.

Neuromodulation

Chartier-Kastler et al have evaluated the use of SNS for patients with detrusor hyperreflexia. They implanted a sacral neurostimulator into 9 patients, of whom 5 had detrusor hyperreflexia with DESD. Four of these patients had improvement in frequency, volume voided, and urinary incontinence.[66] Long-term results have to be carefully evaluated, particularly in the light of an evolutive disease such as MS. However, it could become a minimally invasive therapy used in the armamentarium of modalities for the disease.

Detrusor hyporeflexia

Behavioral modifications and pelvic floor rehabilitation

In certain patients with high post-void residuals, behavioral modifications such as bladder emptying maneuvers (Credé), double-voiding, and Valsalva can all assist with bladder emptying. Also, timed voiding may also be helpful by avoidance of overdistention of the bladder. Pelvic floor stimulation in the hyporeflexic bladder has been proven to play a very limited role.[74]

Clean intermittent catheterization and catheter drainage

For some patients with more advanced disease and/or poor hand dexterity, catheterization may be a problem. These patients may require an indwelling catheter or suprapubic cystostomy. The latter is an attractive option as it has several advantages over a conventional indwelling catheter: urethral erosion and traumatic hypospadias may be avoided and personal hygiene and catheter care are simplified because of the accessibility of the catheter and its position remote from perineal or vaginal soilage. Also, the external genitalia can be free of foreign bodies and may render sexual activity possible.[62,74]

Chronic catheter drainage should be considered only after all the treatment options have been exhausted. The risks of bladder calculi, infection, and squamous cell carcinoma[74–76] should be weighed against the advantages for the patient.

Pharmacologic therapy

There is no proven pharmacologic therapy for detrusor hyporeflexia or areflexia. Bethanechol chloride, a cholinergic agonist, was used in the past but no prospective placebo-controlled trial has ever demonstrated its efficacy in MS.[77]

Surgical management

When MS patients present symptoms, have urologic complications, or cannot perform CIC, urinary diversion is to be considered. However, the risks and benefits of this major surgical procedure must be carefully evaluated, especially in those patients with advanced disease.

Neuromodulation

Detrusor areflexia or hyporeflexia, i.e. impaired detrusor function of neurogenic origin, as a cause of voiding dysfunction, is a contraindication for sacral neuromodulation therapy. Destruction of the peripheral innervation will not allow neuromodulation therapy to be effective.[65]

Conclusion

Urinary tract dysfunction is the fate of the majority of patients suffering from MS with the advancing course of their disease. Due to the poor correlation between subjective symptoms and objective parameters, a thorough evaluation of the urinary tract is mandatory in patients with and without urinary symptoms. Although many options exist for treatment of the neurogenic bladder, a stepwise approach with conservative and initially reversible therapy is important considering the waxing and waning course of the disease. Long-term follow-up aims at preserving renal function while minimizing symptoms and enhancing quality of life.

References

1. Charcot M. Histologie de la sclerose en plaques. Gaz Hop Paris 1868; 141:554.

2. McDonald WI. The dynamics of multiple sclerosis. The Charcot Lecture. J Neurol 1993; 240:28.

3. Compston A, Coles A. Multiple sclerosis. Lancet 2002; 359:1221–1231.

4. Shibasaki H, McDonald WI, Kurojwa Y. Racial modifications of clinical picture of multiple sclerosis: comparison between British and Japanese patients. J Neurol Sci 1981; 49:253–271.

5. Kira J, Kanai T, Nishimura Y, et al. Western versus Asian types of multiple sclerosis: immunogenetically and clinically distinct disorders. Ann Neurol 1996; 40:569–574.

6. Compston A. Risks factors for multiple sclerosis: race or place? J Neurol Neurosurg Psychiatry 1990; 53:821–823.

7. Poser CM. The epidemiology of multiple sclerosis: a general overview. Ann Neurol 1994; 36(S2):S180–S193.

8. Sadovnick A, Eberg G, Dyment D, Rish N, and Canadian Collaborative Study Group. Evidence for genetic basis of multiple sclerosis. Lancet 1996; 347:1728–1730.

9. Hinson JL, Boone TB. Urodynamics and multiple sclerosis. Urol Clin N Am 1996; 23(3):475–481.

10. Keegan BM, Noseworthy JH. Multiple sclerosis. Annu Rev Med 2002; 53:285–302.

11. Litwiller SE, Frohman EM, Zimmern PE. Multiple sclerosis and the urologist. J Urol 1999; 161:743–757.

12. Zhang J, Markovic-Plese S, Lacet B, et al. Increased frequency of interleukin 2-responsive T cells specific for myelin basic protein and proteolipid protein in peripheral blood and cerebrospinal fluid of patients with multiple sclerosis. J Exp Med 1994; 179:973–984.

13. Archelos JJ, Storch MK, Hartung HP. The role of B cells and autoantibodies in multiple sclerosis. Ann Neurol 2000; 47:694–706.

14. Genain CP, Cannella B, Hauser SL, Raine CS. Identification of autoantibodies associated with myelin damage in multiple sclerosis. Nat Med 1999; 5:170–175.

15. Ebers G, Sadovnick A, Rish N. Canadian Collaborative Study Group. A genetic basis for familial aggregation in multiple sclerosis. Nature 1995; 377:150–151.

16. Sawcer S, Meranian M, Setakis E, et al. A whole genome screen for linkage disequilibrium in multiple sclerosis confirms disease associations with regions previously linked to susceptibility. Brain 2002; 125:1337–1347.

17. Compston A. The genetic epidemiology of multiple sclerosis. Philos Trans R Soc Lond, B Biol Sci 1999; 354:1623–1634.

18. Hunter SF, Hafler DA. Ubiquitous pathogens – links between infection and autoimmunity in MS? Neurology 2000; 55:164–165.

19. Albert LJ, Inman RD. Molecular mimicry and autoimmunity. N Engl J Med 1999; 341:2068–2074.

20. Wandinger KB, Jabs W, Siekhaus A, et al. Association between clinical disease activity and Epstein–Barr virus reactivation in MS. Neurology 2000; 55:178–184.

21. Challoner P, Smith K, Parker J, et al. Plaque-associated expression of human herpesvirus 6 in multiple sclerosis. Pro Natl Acad Sci USA 1995; 92:7440–7444.

22. Sriram S, Stratton C, Yao S, et al. *Chlamydia pneumoniae* infection of the central nervous system in multiple sclerosis. Ann Neurol 1999; 46:6–14.

23. McDonald WI, Compston A, Edan G, et al. Recommended diagnostic criteria for multiple sclerosis: guidelines from the International Panel on the diagnosis of multiple sclerosis. Ann Neurol 2001; 50:121–127.

24. Weinshenker B, Lucchinetti C. Acute leukoencephalopathies: differential diagnosis and investigation. Neurologist 1998; 4:148–166.

25. Lublin FD, Reingold SC. Defining the clinical course of mutiple sclerosis: results of an international survey. Neurology 1996; 46:907–911.

26. Werring DJ, Bullmore ET, Toosy AT, et al. Recovery from optic neuritis is associated with a change in the distribution of cerebral response to visual stimulation: a functional magnetic resonance imaging study. J Neurol Neurosurg Psychiatry 2000; 68:441–449.

27. Weinshenker BG, Rice GPA, Noseworthy JH, et al. The natural history of multiple sclerosis: a geographically based study. III. Multivariate analysis of predictive factors and models of outcome. Brain 1991; 114:1045–1056.

28. O'Riordan JI, Thompson AJ, Kingsley DP, et al. The prognostic value of brain MRI in clinically isolated syndromes of the CNS. A 10-year follow-up. Brain 1998; 121:495–503.

29. Griffiths D, Holstege G, de Wall H, Dalm E. Control and coordination of bladder and urethral function in the brain stem of the cat. Neurourol Urodyn 1990; 9:63–82.

30. Blok B, Willemsen T, Holstege G. A pet study of brain control of micturition in humans. Brain 1997; 129:111–121.

31. Oppenheimer DR. The cervical cord in multiple sclerosis. Neuropathol Appl Neurobiol 1978; 4:151–162.

32. Blaivas JG, Barbalias GA. Detrusor external sphincter dyssynergia in men with multiple sclerosis: an ominous urologic condition. J Urol 1984; 131:91–94.

33. Philip T, Read DJ, Higson RH. The urodynamic characteristics of multiple sclerosis. Br J Urol 1981; 53:672–675.

34. Mayo ME, Chetner MP. Lower urinary tract dysfunction in multiple sclerosis. Urology 1992; 39:67–70.

35. Fernandez O. Mechanisms and current treatments of urogenital dysfunction in multiple sclerosis. J Neurol 2002; 249:1–8.

36. Hennessey A, Robertson NP, Swingker R, et al. Urinary, faecal and sexual dysfunction in patients with multiple sclerosis. J Neurol 1999; 246:1027–1032.

37. Beck RP, Warren KG, Whitman P. Urodynamic studies in female patients with multiple sclerosis. Am J Obstet Gynecol 1981; 139:273–276.

38. Goldstein I, Siroky MB, Sax DS, Krane RJ. Neurourologic abnormalities in multiple sclerosis. J Urol 1982; 128:541–545.

39. Koldewijn EL, Hommes OR, Lemmens AJG, et al. Relationship between lower urinary tract abnormalities and disease-related parameters in multiple sclerosis. J Urol 1995; 154:169–173.

40. McGuire EJ, Savastano JA. Urodynamic findings and long-term outcome management of patients with multiple sclerosis-induced lower urinary tract dysfunction. J Urol 1984; 132:713–715.

41. Sirls LT, Zimmern PE, Leach GE. Role of limited evaluation and aggressive medical management in multiple sclerosis: a review of 113 patients. J Urol 1994; 151:946–950.

42. Betts CD, D'Mellow MT, Fowler CJ. Urinary symptoms and the neurological features of bladder dysfunction in multiple sclerosis. J Neurol Neurosurg Psychiatry 1993; 56:245–250.

43. Chancellor MB, Blaivas JG. Urological and sexual problems in multiple sclerosis. Clin Neurosci 1994; 2:189–195.

44. Awad SA, Gajewski JB, Sogbein SK, et al. Relationship between neurological and urological status in patients with multiple sclerosis. J Urol 1984; 132:499–502.

45. Lee KH, Hashimoto SA, Hooge JP, et al. Magnetic resonance imaging of the head in the diagnosis of multiple sclerosis: a prospective 2-year follow-up with comparison of clinical evaluation, evoked potentials, oligoclonal banding, and CT. Neurology 1991; 41:657–660.

46. Goodkin DE, Rudick RA, Ross JS. The use of brain magnetic resonance imaging in multiple sclerosis. Arch Neurol 1994; 51:505–516.

47. Prineas JW, Barnard RO, Kwon EE, et al. Multiple sclerosis: remyelination of nascent lesions. Ann Neurol 1993; 33:137–151.

48. Kim YH, Goodman C, Omessi E, et al. The correlation of urodynamic findings with cranial magnetic resonance imaging findings in multiple sclerosis. J Urol 1998; 159:972–976.

49. Bemelmans BL, Hommes OR, Van Kerrebroek PEV, et al. Evidence for early lower urinary tract dysfunction in clinically silent multiple sclerosis. J Urol 1991; 145:1219–1224.

50. Gonor SE, Carroll DJ, Metcalfe JB. Vesical dysfunction in multiple sclerosis. Urology 1985; 25:429–431.

51. Wheeler JS Jr, Siroky MB, Pavlakis AJ, et al. The changing neurourologic pattern of multiple sclerosis. J Urol 1983; 130:1123–1126.

52. Ciancio SJ, Mutchnik SE, Rivera VM, Boone TB. Urodynamic pattern changes in multiple sclerosis. Urology 2001; 57:239–245.

53. De Ridder D, Vermeulen C, Ketelaer P, et al. Pelvic floor rehabilitation in multiple sclerosis. Acta Neurol Belg 1999; 99:61–64.

54. Thuroff JW, Bunke B, Ebner A, et al. Randomized, double-blind, multicenter trial on treatment of frequency, urgency and incontinence related to detrusor hyperactivity: oxybutynin versus propantheline versus placebo. J Urol 1991; 145:813–817.

55. Abrams P, Freeman R, Anderstrom C, Mattiasson A. Tolterodine, a new antimuscarinic agent: as effective but better tolerated than oxybutynin in patients with an overactive bladder. Br J Urol 1998; 81(6):801–810.

56. Madersbacher H, Jilg G. Control of detrusor hyperreflexia by the intravesical instillation of oxybutynine hydrochloride. Paraplegia 1991; 29:84–90.

57. Weese DL, Roskamp DA, Leach GE, Zimmern PE. Intravesical oxybutynin chloride: experience with 42 patients. Urology 1993; 41(6): 527–530.

58. de Ridder D, Chandiramani V, Dasgupta P, et al. Intravesical capsaicin as a treatment for refractory detrusor hyperreflexia: a dual center study with long-term follow up. J Urol 1997; 158:2087–2092.

59. Lazzeri M, Beneforti P, Spinelli M, et al. Intravesical resiniferatoxin for the treatment of hypersensitive disorder: a randomized placebo controlled study. J Urol 2000; 164:676–679.

60. Valiquette G, Herbert J, Meade-D'Alisera P. Desmopressin in the management of nocturia in patients with multiple sclerosis. Arch Neurol 1996; 53:1270–1275.

61. Eckford SD, Swami KS, Jackson SR, Abrams PH. Desmopressin in the treatment of nocturia and enuresis in patients with multiple sclerosis. Br J Urol 1994; 74(6):733–735.

62. Chancellor MB, Blaivas JG. Multiple sclerosis. Probl Urol 1993; 7(1):15–33.

63. Goldwasser B, Webster GD. Augmentation and substitution enterocystoplasty. J Urol 1986; 135:215–224.

64. Luangkhot R, Peng BCH, Blaivas JG. Ileocecocystoplasty for the management of refractory neurogenic bladder: surgical technique and urodynamic findings. J Urol 1991; 146:1340–1344.

65. Scheepens WA, van Kerrebroeck PEV. Indications and predictive factors. In: Udo J, Grunewald V, eds. New perspectives in sacral nerve stimulation. London: Martin Dunitz, 2002:89–98.

66. Chartier-Kastler E, Ruud Bosch JLH, Perrigot M, et al. Long-term results of sacral nerve stimulation (S3) for the treatment of neurogenic refractory urge incontinence related to detrusor hyperreflexia. J Urol 2000; 164:1476–1480.

67. Phelan MW, Franks M, Somogyi GT, et al. Botulinum toxin urethral sphincter injection to restore bladder emptying in men and women with voiding dysfunction. J Urol 2001; 165:1107–1110.

68. Schurch B, Stohrer M, Kramer G, et al. Botulinum-A toxin for treating detrusor hyperreflexia in spinal cord injured patients: a new

alternative to anticholinergic drugs? Preliminary results. J Urol 2000; 164:692–697.

69. O'Riordan JI, Doherty C, Javed M, et al. Do alpha-blockers have a role in lower urinary tract dysfunction in multiple sclerosis? J Urol 1995; 153:1114–1116.

70. Lockhart JL, Vorstman B, Weinstein D, Politano VA. Sphincterotomy failure in neurogenic bladder disease. J Urol 1986; 135:86–89.

71. Sauerwein D, Gross AJ, Kutzenberger J, Ringert RH. Wallstents in patients with detrusor-sphincter dyssynergia. J Urol 1995; 154:495–497.

72. Schwartz SL, Kennely MJ, McGuire EJ, Farber GJ. Incontinent ileovesicostomy urinary diversion in the treatment of lower urinary tract dysfunction. J Urol 1994; 152:99.

73. Schurch B, Hauri D, Rodic B, et al. Botulinum-A toxin as a treatment of detrusor-sphincter dyssynergia: a prospective study in 24 cord injury patients. J Urol 1996; 155:1023–1029.

74. Rashid TM, Hollander JB. Multiple sclerosis and the neurogenic bladder. Phys Med Rehab Clin N Am 1998; 9(3):615–629.

75. Broecker BH, Klein FA, Hackler RH. Cancer of the bladder in spinal cord injury patients. J Urol 1981; 125:196–197.

76. Bejany DE, Lockhart JL, Rhamy RK. Malignant vesical tumors following spinal cord injury. J Urol 1987; 138:1390–1392.

77. Finkbeiner AE. Is bethanechol chloride clinically effective in promoting bladder emptying? A literature review. J Urol 1985; 134:443–449.

Other diseases (transverse myelitis, tropical spastic paraparesia, progressive multifocal leukoencephalopathy, Lyme disease)

Tomáš Hanuš

Transverse myelitis

Previously, all lesions involving the spinal cord were termed myelitis. With improved understanding of the underlying neurophysiology, only true spinal inflammatory processes are now designated as myelitis. Myelitis is classified either by the duration of symptom progression (acute, subacute, or chronic) or by the etiology (viral, bacterial, parasitic, tuberculosis, and idiopathic). These disorders may selectively affect different parts of the nervous system, spinal cord, and meninges (meningomyelitis), or meninges and roots (meningoradiculitis). The inflammatory distribution is termed poliomyelitis when it is confined to the gray matter, and leukomyelitis if it is within the white matter. When the entire thickness of the spinal cord is involved, it is called transverse myelitis (TM). TM causes various neurological manifestations. Bladder dysfunction is common, and may be the only sequel. The neurological events during normal micturition that culminate in a detrusor contraction and urethral relaxation are integrated in the rostral brainstem in an area designated as the pontine micturition center. Any lesion within the spinal cord, such as trauma, multiple sclerosis, myelodysplasia, and myelitis, that causes disruption of this pathway may result in detrusor-external sphincter dyssynergia (DESD). If the disease process involves the sacral (S2 to S4) cord or roots, a lower motor neuron lesion may occur as well, with pudendal or parasympathetic dysfunction. When the thoracolumbar cord is affected, sympathetic dysfunction may occur. Urodynamic study is helpful in evaluating the bladder dysfunction and also in its management. Its characteristics and natural history, particularly in relation to neurological outcome, have also been described in a pediatric population in recent years, but it is a relatively rare condition in children. Some authors have reported that the recovery rate is generally complete. Long-term follow-up of urological function in all TM patients is recommended.

Ganesan and Borzyskowski[1] described the characteristics and course of urinary tract dysfunction after acute transverse myelitis (ATM) in 10 children, with ages ranging from 8 months to 16 years. They were studied with videourodynamics and followed up in a pediatric neuro-urology clinic. Nine of the 10 children had obstructive urinary tract symptoms at presentation and all went on to develop irritative urinary tract symptoms (frequency and urgency) about 1 month after the initial presentation. Videourodynamics showed a combination of irritative (detrusor hyperreflexia) and obstructive (detrusor-sphincter dyssynergia, or DSD) abnormalities in most patients, and enabled management to be specifically directed towards these. The patients' progress was followed up for a median duration of 36 months. All had residual bladder dysfunction, and only 4 were asymptomatic on treatment. The degree of recovery of bladder function was not related to the degree of motor recovery.

Cheng et al[2] assessed the long-term urological outcome of children with ATM. The medical records of children with ATM over the last 15 years were reviewed. The median age of the 5 children with ATM at the time of onset was 6 years (range = 2–12 years). The median length of follow-up was 5 years (2–10 years). Four children recovered completely from paraparesis; 2 had no urinary symptoms with normal micturition. However, videourodynamic studies 3 years after the acute onset revealed that 4 out of the 5 children, including 1 without any urinary symptom, suffered from residual bladder dysfunction – 2 from contractile neurogenic bladder and 2 from an intermediate type of neurogenic bladder.

Leroy-Malherbe et al[3] retrospectively studied the files of 21 children admitted at the mean age of 8 years 5 months (2 years to 14 years 8 months) for acute transverse myelopathy. Bladder sphincter dysfunction occurred in the first days of the disease in 85% of these patients. Abnormal perception of micturition was one of the most constant and specific symptoms. Anorectal function was also impaired. A complete regressive course was noted in 38% of patients, minor sequelae in 39%, and major sequelae beyond 6 months in 23%. No upper tract deterioration was noted after 3 years of follow-up. The factors for a favorable prognosis were early motor function recovery (especially recommencement of walking before 20 days) and early management of bladder dysfunction. Inability to void had a better prognosis than urinary incontinence. Early systematic bladder drainage in case of inability to void might be essential for an improved prognosis.

Gomes et al[4] described the clinical and urodynamic features of patients with voiding dysfunction secondary to myelopathy. *Schistosomiasis mansoni* is an endemic fluke infection in South America, the Caribbean, and Africa. In the USA and Europe, people may be infected mainly through travel to endemic areas and immigration of infected individuals. Clinical involvement of the spinal cord is a well-recognized complication of the disease. The typical manifestations are those of an ATM, with sudden onset of lower extremity neuropathy associated with bladder and bowel dysfunction. They reviewed the records and urodynamic studies of 14 consecutive patients – 10 men and 4 women, age range 23–49 years, with schistosomal myelopathy confirmed by cerebrospinal fluid (CSF) serology for *Schistosomiasis mansoni* – who were referred for evaluation of voiding dysfunction during a 2-year period. At the time of the urological evaluation, 9 patients had chronic neurological and urinary symptoms and 5 patients had recent onset of acute symptoms. Voiding function, history, urological complications, and outcomes after therapy for schistosomiasis were reviewed. Of the patients with acute disease (5 patients), the urological symptoms included urinary retention (3 patients) and incontinence (2 patients). Three patients had concurrent lower back pain and lower limb neurological deficits. Urodynamic studies were performed in 3 patients, and revealed bladder areflexia in 2 patients, with detrusor hyperreflexia and external sphincter dyssynergia in 1 patient. The patients were started on clean intermittent catheterization (CIC) and received praziquantel and corticosteroids. Praziquantel is used as an antiparaziticum– antihelminticum. Its efficiency is based on the suppression of the enzyme fumarate reductase in myofibril membranes and in neuromuscular synapses of parasites.

Three patients had complete resolution of their symptoms, 1 patient recovered normal voiding function, but the neurological deficits persisted, and one patient showed no clinical improvement. All patients with chronic schistosomal myelopathy presented with lower limb neurological deficits of varying degrees and urinary symptoms, including difficulty emptying the bladder (7 patients), urinary incontinence (6 patients), and urgency and frequency (2 patients). Laboratory and radiographic evaluation of patients with chronic disease revealed urinary tract infection in 5 patients, hydronephrosis in 2 patients, and bladder calculi in 2 patients.

Urological management consisted of antibiotics, CIC, anticholinergic medication, and stone removal, as appropriate. Conservative treatment failed in one patient who required ileocystoplasty. Schistosomal myelopathy is a potential cause of severe voiding dysfunction secondary to spinal cord disease. A high index of suspicion is paramount, because early medical intervention can abort the progression of neurological deterioration.

Kalita et al[5] evaluated micturition abnormalities in ATM and correlated them with evoked potentials, magnetic resonance imaging (MRI), and urodynamic findings. Of the 18 patients with ATM, aged 4–50 years, 15 had paraparesis and 3 quadriparesis. These ATM patients had a neurological evaluation with tibial somatosensory and motor evoked potential studies in the lower limbs. Spinal MRI and urodynamic studies were performed. Neurological outcome was determined on the basis of the Barthel index score at 6 months as poor, partial, or complete. In some patients, urodynamic studies were repeated at 6 and 12 months. Spinal MRI in 14 of the 18 patients revealed T2 hyperintense signal changes, extending for at least 3 spinal segments in 13; 1 patient had normal MRI. In the acute stage, 17 patients had a history of urinary retention and 1 patient had urge incontinence. On follow-up, at 6 months, 2 patients regained normal voiding, retention persisted in 6 patients, and storage symptoms developed in 10 patients, of whom 5 also had emptying difficulties. Urodynamic studies showed an areflexic or hypocontractile bladder in 10 patients, detrusor hyperreflexia with poor compliance in 2 patients, and DSD in 3 patients. Early abnormal urodynamic findings commonly persisted at the 6- and 12-month examinations. Persistent abnormalities included detrusor hyperreflexia, dyssynergia, and areflexic bladder. The urodynamic abnormalities correlated with muscle tone and reflex changes but not with sensory or motor evoked potentials, muscle power, MRI signal changes, sensory level, or 6-month outcome.

Sakakibara et al[6] reported on 10 patients with ATM. Seven had urinary retention, and the other 3 patients had difficulty voiding within 1 month from disease onset. Five of the patients with retention regained spontaneous voiding. After a mean follow-up period of 40 months, 9 patients still had urinary symptoms, including difficulty voiding in 5 patients and urinary frequency, urgency, and incontinence in 4 patients. Four patients had urinary symptoms as the sole sequel of ATM. Urodynamic studies performed on 9 patients revealed that all of the 3 patients with urge incontinence had detrusor hyperreflexia, all of the 4 patients with retention had an areflexic cystometrogram as well as sphincter hyperreflexia, and 3 of the 5 patients with voiding difficulty had DSD. An areflexic cystometrogram tended to change to a low-compliant bladder, followed by detrusor hyperreflexia or a normal cystometrogram. Analysis of the motor unit potentials of the external sphincter revealed that 2 of the 3 patients had high-amplitude or polyphasic neurogenic changes. Supranuclear as well as nuclear types of parasympathetic and somatic nerve dysfunctions seemed to be responsible for micturition disturbance in these ATM patients.

Chan et al[7] reported the case of a 63-year-old Chinese man who presented with tetraparesis and urinary incontinence.[7] The initial diagnosis was cord compression from cervical spondylosis. The patient relapsed 3 months after cervical laminectomy. The TM picture, left optic atrophy and suggestive brainstem evoked potentials, led to treatment of a presumptive demyelinating process. The presence of vitiligo, however, led to the detection of high titers of antinuclear antibodies (ANA) and the presence of anti-nonhistone antibodies. The patient was then diagnosed to have a lupus (systemic lupus erythematosus, SLE)-like disease, which was not fully evolved. He was prescribed pulsed cyclophosphamide and prednisolone with significant gains both neurologically and functionally up to 1 year of follow-up. That it can occur in men in the seventh decade of life heightens the need for awareness in our approach to the myelopathic patient.

In the following year Chan et al[8] published the clinical features of 9 lupus patients who presented with transverse myelopathy (TM) and ascertained functional outcomes when treated early with high-dose corticosteroids and/or cyclophosphamide. These 9 patients, who developed a total of 14 TM episodes, were studied retrospectively. All of them were female, and their ages ranged from 21 to 59 years. Nine episodes of paraparesis, 3 of tetraparesis, 1 of numbness, and 1 of neurogenic bladder were reported early in the diagnosis of SLE (median of 2 years). Neurogenic bowel and bladder and the presence of ANA and ds-DNA were invariable.

Berger et al[9] reported abnormal detrusor behavior in 6 TM patients. Computed tomography (CT) scans and myelograms were uninformative, and CSF studies were normal. Erythrocyte sedimentation rate (ESR) and complement levels were insensitive as markers of disease activity. The treatment regimens included pulses of methylprednisolone and/or cyclophosphamide, followed by prednisolone. The functional outcome was uniformly good with independent ambulation in all except 3 patients (who needed assistive devices), and improvement of motor scores. Acute hospital stays were short (range of 3–45 days), while only 2 patients were referred for inpatient rehabilitation. Bladder abnormalities persisted despite motor recovery.

Six men and 2 women with a history of TM and persistent lower urinary tract symptoms underwent neuro-urological evaluation: 4 patients were neurologically intact, while the remainder had residual neurological deficits. Urodynamic studies revealed DSD in 6 patients. Two patients had detrusor hyperreflexia, of whom 1 patient also had an incompetent sphincter. Erectile or ejaculatory dysfunction was reported by 3 men. The study concluded that prolonged bladder and sexual dysfunction caused by spinal cord inflammatory insult, may persist despite systemic neurological recovery. Therefore, bladder management guided by initial and follow-up urodynamics is recommended.

The clinical symptoms of ATM and the urodynamic findings in ATM are summarized in Tables 25.1 and 25.2, respectively.

Table 25.1 *Clinical symptoms at the time of diagnosis of ATM*

Author	No. of patients	Urgency	Urge incontinence	Urinary retention	Obstruction and voiding
Ganesan and Borzyskowski[1]	10	9	–	–	–
Cheng et al[2]	5	–	–	–	2
Leroy-Malherbe et al[3]	21	–	–	–	–
Gomes et al[4]	14	–	2	3	–
Kalita et al[5]	18	–	1	17	–
Sakakibara et al[6]	10	–	–	7	3
Berger et al[9]	6	–	–	–	–

Table 25.2 *Urodynamic findings in ATM*

Author	No. of patients	Hyperreflexia	Areflexia	Dyssynergia (DSD)	Sphincter incompetence
Gomes et al[4]	3	–	2	1	–
Kalita et al[5]	15	2	10	3	–
Berger et al[9]	6	2	–	6	1

Tropical spastic paraparesis

Human T-cell lymphotropic virus type 1-associated myelopathy.

Etiopathogenesis and epidemiology

Tropical spastic paraparesis (TSP) is a condition associated with and probably caused by T-cell lymphotropic virus type l (HTLV-I).[10,11] HTLV-I is a retrovirus with affinity for CD-4 cells.

It is a common cause of paraparesis in the West Indies,[12] where it was formerly known as Jamaican neuropathy or myelopathy, and in the southern islands of Japan, where it is called HTLV-I-associated myelopathy or HAM.[13] But it is also found widely in the tropics and subtropics, and in immigrants to northern Europe from endemic areas.[11,14]

Pathology

Pathologically, there is meningomyelitis with demyelination and axonal loss, particularly affecting the corticospinal tracts. These findings are most marked in the low thoracic and upper lumbar regions.[11,12,15]

Symptomatology

This infection may give rise to a broad spectrum of disorders, including T-cell leukemia/lymphoma, myelopathy/tropical spastic paraparesis complex (M/TSP), and, to a lesser extent, uveitis, arthritis, polymyositis, and peripheral neuropathy. M/TSP is a progressive chronic myelopathy characterized by spasticity, hyperreflexia, muscle weakness, and sphincter disorders. Much less frequently it may precede, or give rise to, a cerebellar syndrome with ataxia and intention tremor. The widespread nature of the pathological changes within the nervous system results in a complex variety of urodynamic and neurophysiological features. Gait disturbance is the main symptom of HAM, but bladder dysfunction is one of the major characteristic symptomatologies, as these patients complain frequently of urinary disturbances.

Fujiki et al[16] reported the case of a 75-year-old woman with HAM presenting with cerebellar signs. She was admitted because of walking unsteadiness, which initially appeared 3 years previously with gradual worsening. Neurological examination revealed limb and truncal ataxia, cerebellar-type dysfunction of eye movement, pyramidal signs, diminished vibration sense, and neurogenic bladder. Anti-HTLV-I antibody titers in serum and CSF were markedly elevated. MRI revealed abnormal signals in cerebral white matter, mild cerebellar atrophy, and thoracic cord atrophy. Cerebellar signs and symptoms, the initial and main neurological manifestations in this patient, were improved by steroid therapy. This case was considered unique among HAM, because the cerebellum was the main site of the lesions.

The presence of a cerebellar syndrome or neuropathy of uncertain origin, in endemic areas, should lead to the inclusion of HTLV-I infection in the differential diagnosis, even in the absence of pyramidal symptoms or defined M/TSP. Maternal seropositivity supports the hypothesis of mother–daughter transmission during lactation. Anti-HTLV-I antibody and anti-T-lymphocyte (ATL)-like cells can be present in the peripheral blood of patients with HAM.

A clinical case with a cerebellar syndrome and peripheral neuropathy as manifestations of HTLV-I infection was described by Carod-Artal et al.[17] This described a 13-year-old girl who presented with a neurological syndrome which had started with tremor of the head and limbs, ataxia, dysmetria, frequent falls, and sphincter disorders. During the $2\frac{1}{2}$ years that she had had this illness, she had developed spastic paraparesis of the legs and had repeated urinary infections. Serology of blood and CSF was positive for HTLV-I by ELISA (enzyme-linked immunosorbent assay) and confirmed by Western blot. Electromyography (EMG) showed predominantly axonal sensomotor neuropathy. A neurogenic bladder was detected on functional urodynamic studies. On MRI there was moderate atrophy of the thoracic spinal cord, and slight alterations of the subcortical white matter.

Urodynamic findings

The condition is characterized by progressive paraparesis associated with back pain and micturition disturbances. While there have been many reports concerning the clinical and immunological features of this condition, little attention has been paid to the bladder dysfunction which commonly accompanies it. Most patients show urodynamic evidence of detrusor hyperreflexia and DSD.[18] The finding of supranuclear voiding dysfunctions seems to be in accordance with the known pathological lesions of this disease.

Sakiyama et al[19] evaluated the symptoms and urodynamic examinations of 21 untreated HAM patients: although 2 patients (11%) had no urinary symptom, 19 patients (89%) suffered from dysuria, pollakiuria, incontinence, or urgency. The combination of irritative and obstructive urinary disturbance was a characteristic symptom in HAM patients. In 3 patients, the urinary symptoms preceded the gait disturbance, the main symptom of HAM. In a urodynamic study overactive bladder was found in 14 patients (66%), although 3 patients (15%) showed underactive or acontractile bladder with disturbance of urinary sensation. No abnormal urethral pressure profile (UPP) measurements were recorded, but DSD was revealed frequently by EMG. This typical dysfunction of HAM patients was thought to be caused by destruction of the lateral column of the spinal cord.

Eardley et al[20] reported clinical features, urodynamic results, and neurophysiological findings in 5 patients with urinary symptoms related to TSP. All their patients had typical neurological findings of TSP with a spastic paraparesis associated with a variable amount of sensory loss in the lower limbs. All patients had irritative urinary symptoms (frequency, nocturia, or urgency) and in all but 1 patient there was associated urge incontinence. Three patients had normal coordinated sphincter relaxation. Cystometrograms revealed bladder capacities ranging from 125 to 275 ml. Filling pressures were normal in 3 patients, ranging from 6 to 10 cmH$_2$O, and elevated to 26 cmH$_2$O in 1 woman. All patients had involuntary detrusor contractions with a pressure of 40–84 cmH$_2$O during voiding. The patients were aware of the involuntary detrusor contractions, which they sensed as an urge to void that could not be aborted. On voiding cystourethrography 1 woman with symptoms for more than 10 years had severe trabeculation and 2 patients had bladder diverticula. Of the 5 patients, 4 had urinary symptoms simultaneously with other neurological symptoms, while urinary symptoms developed 2 years later in the other patient.

Voiding dysfunction was also evaluated in 26 patients (9 males and 17 females) with HAM by Yamashita and Kumazawa.[21] Of these 26 patients, 22 (85%) had difficulty urinating, 15 (58%) had urinary frequency, and 9 (35%) had urge incontinence. Cystograms disclosed trabeculated bladder in 5 patients, vesicoureteral reflux in 3 patients, and bladder neck obstruction in 5 patients. In 25 patients (96%), urodynamic studies showed detrusor hyperreflexia with normal urethral function during storage. Of these, 17 patients, had detrusor underactivity with DSD during micturition. One patient had normal detrusor function during storage and detrusor areflexia during voiding.

In 1991, Imamura et al[22] performed clinical surveys and urodynamic examinations on 25 untreated patients with HAM. Although 4 patients (16%) were entirely aware of their urinary symptoms, the onset of urinary symptoms preceded other pyramidal symptoms in 6 patients (24%). All patients suffered from dysuria: the cause of dysuria was thought to be mainly DESD, but in some patients an

underactive detrusor and poor opening of the bladder neck at voiding were also causes of the dysuria.

Again, in 1994, Imamura[23] evaluated 50 cases of untreated HAM by urodynamic studies to clarify the nature of the urinary disturbances and to find out suitable urological treatment. Both irritative and obstructive symptoms coexisted in these HAM patients. Thirty-eight percent of the patients experienced only urinary symptoms throughout the affected period; their main cause of frequency was detrusor hyperreflexia at the filling phase, which was found in 58% of patients. However, decreased effective bladder capacity due to a large amount of residual urine was possibly another cause of frequency. DSD was the main cause of difficult voiding, but in some cases an underactive detrusor at the voiding phase was also implicated. Hydronephrosis was observed in only 5 kidneys, although as many as 30 out of 46 patients (65.2%) showed bladder deformities. Seventeen patients (34%) had urinary tract infection at first visit. As daily activity was disturbed, mean residual urine volume, the incidence of detrusor hyperreflexia, and DSD were all increased. Medical treatment was effective to relieve the subjective symptoms, but urodynamic examination did not necessarily review improvement. Intermittent catheterization was needed and was successful in 64% of all cases.

Walton and Kaplan[24] presented their urodynamic findings in 4 female patients and 1 male patient with TSP. Of the 5 patients, 4 presented with DESD, and 1 had detrusor hyperreflexia with coordinated sphincter contraction.

Hattori et al[25] reported their findings from micturitional histories and urodynamic studies in 5 patients with HAM. Histories showed that all patients had obstructive as well as irritative micturitional symptoms, and, in 4 patients, their micturitional symptoms appeared from disease onset. Urodynamic studies revealed that 4 patients had residual urine volume (average 170 ml), all had detrusor hyperreflexia, 2 patients had DSD, and none presented neurogenic changes in external urethral sphincter EMG. The findings of supranuclear-type voiding dysfunctions seemed to be in accordance with the known pathological lesions of this disease.

Matsumoto et al[26] performed clinical and electrophysiological studies in 9 HAM cases. Spastic paraparesis and neurogenic bladder were present in 8 patients; sensory disturbances were detected only in 4 patients. The conduction velocities of the posterior tibial and sural nerves were reduced in 2 patients. Median nerve somatosensory nerve potentials (SSEP) revealed a delay of N11, N13, N14, and N20 peak latencies and an increase of N9–N20, N13–N14, and N13–N20 interpeak latencies. Electrophysiological studies are the most accurate indicators of diffuse involvement not only of the central motor and sensory pathways but also of the peripheral nervous system.

The urodynamic findings in TSP are summarized in Table 25.3.

Table 25.3 *Urodynamic findings in TSP*

Author	No. of patients	Hyperreflexia	Areflexia	Dyssynergia (DSD)
Eardley et al[20]	5	–	–	5
Walton and Kaplan[24]	5	1	–	4
Hattori et al[25]	5	5	–	2

Complications

Lower urinary symptoms associated with HAM/TSP are common, but have been regarded as 'neurogenic' due to spinal involvements. In some cases, these symptoms are persistent, progressive, and not directly correlated with the severity of other neurological symptoms of the lower spinal cord. These findings prompted Nomata et al[27] to locate organic lesions in the lower urinary tract and to correlate them with HTLV-I infection. Among 35 HAM patients with lower urinary symptoms, they found 4 patients with persistent and progressive symptoms, 3 patients with contracted bladder, and another patient with persistent prostatitis. Histological or cytological examinations indicated local lymphocytic infiltrations in the lower urinary tract in all cases: 3 by bladder infiltration, and the other by a high concentration of lymphocytes in expressed prostatic secretions. Of the 3 patients whose urinary samples were available, 2 showed significant increases in the concentration of urinary anti-HTLV-I antibody of IgA class. The urinary IgA antibody of the third patient was not elevated, but the sample had been obtained after resection of the affected bladder. None of the control cases showed significant anti-HTLV-I IgA antibody in urine except for a case of gross hematuria due to chemotherapy directed against adult T-cell leukemia. The authors suggested inclusion of these processes into the spectrum of complications for HAM/TSP. The elevated excretion of anti-HTLV-I of IgA class in urine may be an indicator of these complications. There is a tendency for urinary dysfunction to become worse as the primary disease progresses.

Treatment

Idiopathic or HTLV-I-associated progressive spastic paraparesis does not have a clear treatment. Cartier et al[28] assessed the effects of a medication containing cytidine monophosphate, uridine triphosphate, and vitamin B12 in the treatment of progressive spasticity. Patients with the disease were randomly assigned to receive Nucleus CMP forte (containing disodium cytidine monophosphate 5 mg, trisodium uridine triphosphate 3 mg, and hydroxycobalamin 2 mg) three times a day or placebo for 6 months. Gait, spasticity, degree of neurogenic bladder, and somatosensitive evoked potentials were assessed during treatment. Forty-six patients aged 25–79 years were studied: 24 were female and 29 were HTLV-I positive. Twenty-two patients were treated with the drugs and the rest with placebo. Gait and spasticity improved in 7 of 22 patients receiving the drug and in one of 24 receiving placebo ($p < 0.05$). Neurogenic bladder improved in 10 of 22 patients receiving the drug and in 4 of 24 patients receiving placebo (NS). SSEPs improved in 4 of 7 patients treated with the drug and in 2 of 7 patients treated with placebo. The medication caused a modest improvement in patients with progressive spastic paraparesis and was free of side-effects.

Harrington et al[29] used danazol for the treatment of urinary incontinence in TSP with an 84% success rate. They reported an impressive reduction in urinary frequency and incontinence in 7 consecutive women with TSP who were given danazol 200 mg three times daily. All 7 women had HTLV-I antibodies in CSF and peripheral blood, and HTLV-I infection was further confirmed by polymerase chain amplification. All 7 women had urinary frequency, incontinence, and spastic paraparesis of the legs; they could walk short distances but only 1 woman could do so unassisted. Danazol is a mild anabolic agent with attenuated virilizing effects and has been used extensively in diseases that affect women such as endometriosis and idiopathic thrombocytopenic purpura. Side-effects include fatigue, weight gain, symptomless increases in liver enzymes, and amenorrhea. Danazol also has immunomodulatory effects and is effective in autoimmune blood diseases. Autoimmune factors may play a role in TSP but this does not explain the impressive relief of incontinence noted in their 7 patients.

Saito et al[30] reported 4 patients (3 females and 1 male) diagnosed by neurologists to have HAM with spastic gait disturbance and increased titer of antibody to HTLV-I. They complained of urge incontinence, bed wetting, difficulty in micturition, and/or pollakisuria. Urodynamically, severe uninhibited detrusor contractions were observed in 3 patients; on the other hand, detrusor contractility was completely lost in the other patient. In all patients, bladder sensation was well-preserved. Corticosteroids and interferon could not improve their urological symptoms. CIC relieved urinary incontinence in 3 patients who had a significant amount of residual urine. The authors believed that HAM in patients suffering from severe voiding difficulty is a good indication for CIC.

Namima et al[31] presented 2 case reports with HAM. Patient 1 (a 24-year-old female) had complained of slowly progressing urinary incontinence (since age 14) and gait disturbance (since age 18). A marked pyramidal disorder was observed, and anti-HTLV-I antibody (1:640) was present in her peripheral blood. She was diagnosed as having HAM. Repeated urodynamic studies revealed exacerbation of overactive bladder and DSD with disease progressing. Patient 2 (a 48-year-old male) had complained of gait disturbance (since age 32) and progressive urinary hesitancy (since age 46). Physical examination revealed a marked pyramidal disorder. Anti-HTLV-I antibody (1:200) and ATL-like cells were present in his peripheral blood. He was diagnosed as having HAM. Voiding cystourethrography demonstrated abnormal bladder wall changes. Urodynamic studies revealed overactive bladder and marked DSD. Medications based on adrenocortical steroids and standard urological care have improved urinary symptoms in both cases.

Conclusions

In summary, TSP is a spinal cord disorder caused by the retrovirus HTLV-I. Patients commonly have urinary complaints that usually begin simultaneously with complaints of extremity weakness. This process must be distinguished from multiple sclerosis. Eighty percent of TSP patients with urinary complaints have DSD. Thus, it seems prudent to aggressively evaluate patients with TSP who have urinary symptoms. These patients are at high risk for DESD and should undergo urodynamic evaluation before instituting appropriate therapy. This is particularly true in men with TSP to prevent the potentially deleterious effects of untreated and unrecognized DESD on the upper tract. HAM patients must be carefully followed up by urologists to prevent urinary tract deterioration.

Progressive multifocal leukoencephalopathy

Two widespread human polyomaviruses, BK virus (BKV) and JC virus (JCV), establish latency in the urinary tract, and can be reactivated in AIDS. JCV might cause progressive multifocal leukoencephalopathy, but although up to 60% of AIDS patients excrete BKV in their urine, there have been few reports of BKV-related renal and/or neurological diseases.

Bratt et al[32] investigated by polymerase chain reaction (PCR) approximately 400 CSF samples from immunosuppressed individuals with neurological symptoms for the presence of polyomaviruses at the Gay Men's Health Clinic in Sweden. BKV could be demonstrated in the brain, CSF, eye tissues, kidneys, and peripheral blood mononuclear cells. BKV DNA has, so far, only been found in 1 case. They also analyzed the brain, eye tissue, CSF, urine, and peripheral blood mononuclear cells by nested PCR for polyomavirus DNA. Macroscopic and microscopic examinations were performed of the kidney and brain postmortem. Immunohistochemical stainings for two BKV proteins, VP1 and agnoprotein, were performed on autopsy material and virus-infected tissue culture cells. Although reports of BKV infections in the nervous system are rare, there is now evidence of its occurrence in immunocompromised patients, and the diagnosis should be considered in such cases with neurological symptoms and signs of renal disease. The diagnosis is simple to verify and is important to establish.

Lyme disease

Manifestations of what we now call Lyme disease (LD) were first reported in the medical literature in Europe in 1883. Over the years, various clinical signs of this illness have been noted as separate medical conditions: acrodermatitis, chronica atrophicans, lymphadenosis benigna cutis, erythema migrans, and lymphocytic meningoradiculitis (Bannwarth's syndrome). However, these diverse manifestations were not recognized as indicators of a single infectious illness until 1975, when LD was described following an outbreak of apparent juvenile arthritis, preceded by a rash, among residents of Lyme, Connecticut.

LD is an infection caused by *Borrelia burgdorferi* – a type of bacterium called a spirochete – that is carried by deer ticks. An infected tick can transmit the spirochete to the humans and animals it bites. Untreated, the bacterium travels through the bloodstream, establishes itself in various body tissues, and can cause a number of symptoms, some of which are severe.

LD manifests itself as a multisystem inflammatory disease that affects the skin in its early, localized stage, and spreads to the joints, nervous system, and, to a lesser extent, other organ systems in its later, disseminated stages. If diagnosed and treated early with antibiotics, LD is almost always readily cured. Generally, LD in its later stages can also be treated effectively, but because the rate of disease progression and individual response to treatment varies from one patient to the other, some patients may have symptoms that linger for months or even years following treatment. In rare instances, LD causes permanent damage.

Symptoms

The early symptoms of LD can be mild and easily over-looked. Persons who are aware of the risk of LD in their communities and who do not ignore the sometimes subtle early symptoms are most likely to seek medical attention and treatment early enough to be assured of a full recovery. The first symptom is usually an expanding rash (erythema migrans, EM), which is thought to occur in 80–90% of all LD cases.

As the LD spirochete continues to disseminate through the body, a number of other symptoms can occur, including severe fatigue, a stiff aching neck, and peripheral nervous system (PNS) involvement, such as tingling or numbness in the extremities or facial palsy (paralysis).

The more severe, potentially debilitating symptoms of later-stage LD, may occur weeks, months, or, in a few cases, years after a tick bite. These can include severe headaches, painful arthritis and swelling of the joints, cardiac abnormalities, and CNS involvement leading to cognitive (mental) disorders.

Common symptoms seen in various stages of LD:

- Early localized (acute) stage: solid red or bull's-eye rash, usually at the bite site; swelling of the lymph glands near the tick bite; generalized aches; and headache.
- Early disseminated stage: two or more rashes not at the bite site; migrating pains in joints/tendons; headache; stiff aching neck; facial palsy (facial paralysis similar to Bell's palsy); tingling or numbness in the extremities; multiple enlarged lymph glands; abnormal pulse; sore throat; changes in vision; fever of 100–102°F; and severe fatigue.
- Late stage: arthritis (pain/swelling) of one or two large joints; disabling neurological disorders (disorientation; confusion; dizziness; short-term memory loss; inability to concentrate, finish sentences, or follow conversations; mental 'fog'); numbness in arms/hands or legs/feet.

It was observed that the urinary tract may be involved in two respects in the course of LD: (1) voiding dysfunction may be part of the neuroborreliosis and (2) the spirochete may directly invade the urinary tract. Several neurological manifestations of LD, both central and peripheral, have been described. Associated neurological symptoms fall broadly into three syndromes: encephalopathy, polyneuropathy, and leukoencephalitis.

Experimental observations

Schwan et al[33] experimentally infected white-footed mice, *Peromyscus leucopus*, in the laboratory with *B. burgdorferi*, the causative agent of LD. After the mice were infected by intraperitoneal or subcutaneous inoculation or by tick bite, attempts were made to culture spirochetes from the urinary bladder, spleen, kidney, blood, and urine. Spirochetes were most frequently isolated from the bladder (94%), followed by the kidney (75%), spleen (61%), and blood (13%).

No spirochetes were isolated from the urine. Tissue sectioning and immunofluorescence staining of the urinary bladder demonstrated spirochetes within the bladder wall. The results demonstrate that cultivation of the urinary bladder is very effective at isolating *B. burgdorferi* from experimentally infected white-footed mice and that culturing this organ may be productive when surveying wild rodents for infection with this spirochete.

Pavia et al[34] demonstrated the efficacy of an evernimicin (SCH27899) *in vitro* and in an animal model of LD. The minimum inhibitory concentrations (MIC) of evernimicin at which 90% of *B. burgdorferi* patient isolates were inhibited ranged from 0.1 to 0.5 μg/ml. Evernimicin was as effective as ceftriaxone against *B. burgdorferi* in a murine model of experimental LD. As assessed by culturing the urinary bladders of infected C3H mice, no live *Borrelia* isolates were recoverable following antibiotic treatment.

These same authors[34] also collected 34 small mammals in the vicinity of Ljubljana and tested them for the presence of *B. burgdorferi sensu lato* by PCR of urinary bladder tissues, using universal flagellin primers and species-specific rRNA primers. Seventeen small mammals (50%) were found to be positive, and 7 animals were infected with 2 species of *B. burgdorferi sensu lato* simultaneously. The most commonly found species was *B. afzelii* ($n = 14$), followed by *B. burgdorferi sensu stricto* ($n = 7$) and *B. garinii* ($n = 3$), as determined by species-specific primers. The authors concluded that PCR is a rapid and reliable method to detect infection with *B. burgdorferi sensu lato* in small mammals.

Previous studies by Czub et al[35] have demonstrated that the urinary bladder is a consistent source for isolating the LD spirochete *B. burgdorferi* from both experimentally infected and naturally exposed rodents. They examined histopathological changes in the urinary bladder of different types of rodents infected experimentally with Lyme spirochetes, including BALB/c mice (*Mus musculus*), nude mice (*M. musculus*), white-footed mice (*Peromyscus leucopus*), and grasshopper mice (*Onychomys leucogaster*). The animals were inoculated intraperitoneally, subcutaneously, or intranasally with low-passaged spirochetes, high-passaged spirochetes, or phosphate-buffered saline. They were killed at various times after inoculation, and approximately one-half of each urinary bladder and kidney was cultured separately in BSK-II medium while the other half of each organ was prepared for histological examination. Spirochetes were cultured from the urinary bladder of all 35 mice inoculated with low-passaged spirochetes, whereas spirochetes could not be isolated from any kidneys of the same mice. The pathological changes observed most frequently in the urinary bladder of the infected mice were the presence of lymphoid aggregates, vascular anomalies, including an increase in the number of vessels and thickening of the vessel walls, and perivascular infiltrates. The results demonstrate that nearly all individuals (93%) of the four types of mice examined had a cystitis associated with spirochetal infection. The heart can also be severely affected in humans with LD, causing conduction defects and, rarely, heart failure. Although immunodeficient and young mice may develop cardiac lesions, cultivation of *B. burgdorferi* from cardiac tissues of experimentally infected animals has not been reported previously.

Goodman et al[36] infected Syrian hamsters with *B. burgdorferi 297* and found a marked tropism of the spirochete for myocardial and urinary tract tissues: 56 of 57 hearts (98%) and 52 of 58 bladders (90%) were culture-positive. The cardiac infection was persistent and could be documented in 21 of 22 hearts (96%) cultured from days 28–84 post-infection. The urinary tract was also a site of persistent infection in most animals, with 18 of 23 bladders (78%) being culture-positive from days 28–84. The persistence of spirochetes was specific for the heart and bladder, as indicated by negative cultures of specimens from the liver and spleen in which only 1 of 23 cultures was positive from days 28–84. Because of the high isolation rates, tropism, and persistence that we found for *B. burgdorferi* in the hamster heart and bladder, these sites might be useful and important for the cultivation of spirochetes in experimental studies that evaluate the efficacies, both of candidate vaccines in preventing infection and of antibiotics in eradicating organisms from privileged sites. In addition, the clear demonstration of persistent cardiac infection with *B. burgdorferi* may provide a useful model for studying the pathogenesis of cardiac LD.

Clinical observations

EM rash, which may occur in up to 90% of reported cases, is a specific feature of LD, and treatment should begin immediately. Even in the absence of EM rash, diagnosis of early LD should be made solely on the basis of symptoms and evidence of a tick bite, not blood tests, which can often give false results if performed in the first month after initial infection (later on, the tests are considered more reliable). If early symptoms are undetected or ignored, it is recommended to use ELISA and Western-blot blood tests. These tests are considered more reliable and accurate when performed at least 1 month after initial infection, although no test is 100% accurate.

If there are neurological symptoms or swollen joints, in addition, a PCR test can be done via a spinal tap or withdrawal of synovial fluid from an affected joint. This test amplifies the DNA of the spirochete and will usually indicate its presence.

Since the possibility of asymptomatic infection with *B. burgdorferi* had been suggested by a positive serology in healthy subjects, Karch et al[37] hypothesized that these subjects might excrete borrelial DNA sequences in urine, as happens in patients with Lyme borreliosis. They found borrelial sequences by nested PCR in urine samples from 3 of 13 healthy *B. burgdorferi* antibody-positive adults, but not from 79 antibody-negative healthy controls. After therapy with doxycycline, the urine samples were repeatedly negative for *B. burgdorferi* DNA. The authors concluded that urinary excretion of borrelial DNA sequences may occur in seropositive healthy subjects during asymptomatic infection. Demonstration of such sequences in urine must be interpreted cautiously and may not necessarily prove a borrelial cause of disease.

Druschky et al[38] reported on a 57-year-old patient suffering from the typical symptoms of normal-pressure hydrocephalus (NPH), including gait disturbance, urinary incontinence, and mental deterioration. CSF analysis established the diagnosis of chronic active Lyme neuroborreliosis with lymphocytic pleocytosis and intrathecal *B. burgdorferi* antibody production. After several weeks of intravenous antibiotic treatment, normalization of the CSF parameters as well as a clear improvement of clinical symptoms were observed so that surgical shunting was no longer indicated. Interference with subarachnoid CSF flow may be a possible cause of the observed symptomatic NPH in a patient with chronic Lyme neuroborreliosis.

Aberer et al[39] reported the case of a 38-year-old male patient with coexisting acrodermatitis chronica atrophicans, lichen sclerosus et atrophicus, and recurrent diabetic metabolic disorders since 9 years. Serologically, IgG antibodies against *B. burgdorferi* could be detected. Unmoving, winded structures, morphologically resembling borreliae could be demonstrated in urine sediment by dark field microscopy. Additionally, tubulointerstitial nephritis was diagnosed by the presence of dysmorphic hematuria, pathological polyacrylamide gel electrophoresis, and elevated α_1- and β_2-microglobulin in urine. The authors suggested that the excreted spirochete-like structures were borreliae, which may be the putative infectious agent for the development of lichen sclerosus et atrophicus in the genital area.

In 1993, Chancellor et al[40] described 7 patients with neuroborreliosis who also had lower urinary tract dysfunction. Urodynamic evaluation revealed detrusor hyperreflexia in 5 patients and detrusor areflexia in 2 patients. Neurological and urological symptoms in all patients were slow to resolve and convalescence was protracted.

Treatment

Early treatment of LD (within the first few weeks after initial infection) is straightforward and almost always results in a full cure. Treatment begun after the first 3 weeks will also likely provide a cure, but the cure rate decreases the longer treatment is delayed.

Doxycycline, amoxicillin, and Ceftin (cefuroxime axetil) are the oral antibiotics most highly recommended for treatment of all but a few symptoms of LD. A 4-week course of oral doxycycline is just as effective in treating late LD, and much less expensive, than a similar course of intravenous ceftriaxone unless neurological or severe cardiac abnormalities are present. If these symptoms occur, immediate intravenous treatment is recommended.

Conservative bladder management, including CIC guided by urodynamic evaluation, is recommended. Chancellor et al[41] published the first report of urinary retention as the initial clinical presentation of LD. Paralysis and urinary retention resolved with intravenous ceftriaxone antibiotic.

Olivares et al[42] reported a case of ATM related to Lyme neuroborreliosis that presented with isolated acute urinary retention and no lower-extremity impairment. This case, documented by urodynamic and electrophysiological investigations, partially resolved after 6 weeks of intravenous ceftriaxone, affording removal of the indwelling catheter. Alpha-blocker therapy was needed for 3 months, until the complete normalization of urodynamic and electrophysiological records. This case study indicates that whenever urinary retention is associated with ATM or occurs alone, the patient should be investigated for LD. Relapses of active LD and residual neurological deficits are common. Urologists practicing in areas endemic for LD need to be aware of *B. burgdorferi* infection in the differential diagnosis of neurogenic bladder dysfunction.

References

1. Ganesan V, Borzyskowski M. Characteristics and course of urinary tract dysfunction after acute transverse myelitis in childhood. Dev Med Child Neurol 2001; 43:473–475.

2. Cheng W, Chiu R, Tam P. Residual bladder dysfunction 2 to 10 years after acute transverse myelitis. J Paediatr Child Health 1999; 35:476–478.

3. Leroy-Malherbe V, Sebire G, Hollenberg H, et al. Neurogenic bladder in children with acute transverse myelopathy. Arch Pediatr 1998; 5:497–502.

4. Gomes CM, Trigo-Rocha F, Arap MA, et al. Schistosomal myelopathy: urologic manifestations and urodynamic findings. Urology 2002; 59:195–200.

5. Kalita J, Shah S, Kapoor R, Misra UK. Bladder dysfunction in acute transverse myelitis: magnetic resonance imaging and neurophysiological and urodynamic correlations. J Neurol Neurosurg Psychiatry 2002; 73:154–159.

6. Sakakibara R, Hattori T, Yasuda K, Yamanishi T. Micturition disturbance in acute transverse myelitis. Spinal Cord 1996; 34:481–485.

7. Chan KF, Kong KH, Boey ML. Great mimicry in a patient with tetraparesis: a case report. Arch Phys Med Rehabil 1995; 76:391–393.

8. Chan KF, Boey ML. Transverse myelopathy in SLE: clinical features and functional outcomes. Lupus 1996; 5:294–299.

9. Berger Y, Blaivas JG, Oliver L. Urinary dysfunction in transverse myelitis. J Urol 1990; 144:103–105.

10. Gessain A, Barin F, Vernant JC, et al. Antibodies to human T-lymphotropic virus type-1 in patients with tropical spastic paraparesis. Lancet 1985; (8452):407–410.

11. Cruickshank JK, Rudge P, Dalgleish AG, et al. Tropical spastic paraparesis and human T cell lymphotropic virus type 1 in the United Kingdom. Brain 1989; 112:1057–1090.

12. Montgomery RD, Cruickshank EK, Robertson WB, et al. Clinical and pathological observations on Jamaican neuropathy. A report of 206 cases. Brain 1964; 87:425–460.

13. Roman GC, Roman LN. Tropical spastic paraparesis. A clinical study of 50 patients from Tumaco (Columbia) and review of the worldwide literature features of the syndrome. J Neurol Sci 1988; 87:121–125.

14. Gout O, Gessain A, Bolgert F, Saal F, et al. Chronic myelopathies associated with human T-cell lymphotropic virus type-1. A clinical serological and immunovirological study of ten patients in France. Arch Neurol 1989; 46:255–260.

15. Iwasaki Y. Pathology of chronic myelopathy associated with HTLV1 infection (HAM/TSP). J. Neurol Sci 1990; 96:103–123.

16. Fujiki N, Oikawa O, Matsumoto A, Tashiro K. A case of HTLV-I associated myelopathy presenting with cerebellar signs as initial and principal manifestations. Rinsho-Shinkeigaku 1999; 39:852–855.

17. Carod-Artal FJ, Del-Negro MC, Vargas AP, Rizzo I. Cerebellar syndrome and peripheral neuropathy as manifestations of infection by HTLV-I human T-cell lymphotropic virus. Rev Neurol 1999; 29:932–935.

18. Shibasaki H, Endo C, Kuroda Y, et al. Clinical picture of HTLV-1 associated myelopathy. J Neurol Sci 1988; 87:15–24.

19. Sakiyama H, Nishi K, Kikukawa H, Ueda S. Urinary disturbance due to HTLV-1 associated myelopathy. Nippon Hinyokika Gakkai Zasshi 1992; 83:2058–2061.

20. Eardley I, Fowler CJ, Nagendran K, et al. The neurourology of tropical spastic paraparesis. Br J Urol 1991; 68:598–603.

21. Yamashita H, Kumazawa J. Voiding dysfunction: patients with human T-lymphotropic-virus-type-1-associated myelopathy. Urol Int 1991; 47 (Suppl 1):69–71.

22. Imamura A, Kitagawa T, Ohi Y, Osame M. Clinical manifestation of human T-cell lymphotropic virus type-I-associated myelopathy and vesicopathy. Urol Int 1991; 46:149–153.

23. Imamura A. Studies on neurogenic bladder due to human T-lymphotropic virus type-I associated myelopathy (HAM). Nippon Hinyokika Gakkai Zasshi 1994; 85:1106–1115.

24. Walton GW, Kaplan SA. Urinary dysfunction in tropical spastic paraparesis: preliminary urodynamic survey. J Urol 1993; 150:930–932.

25. Hattori T, Sakakibara R, Yamanishi T, et al. Micturitional disturbance in human T-lymphotropic virus type-1-associated myelopathy. J Spinal Disord 1994; 7:255–258.

26. Matsumoto SC, Nakasato O, Kataoka, A, et al. Myelopathy associated with HTLV-1: clinical electrophysiologic study. Neurologia 1993; 8:291–294.

27. Nomata K, Nakamura T, Suzu H, et al. Novel complications with HTLV-1-associated myelopathy/tropical spastic paraparesis: interstitial cystitis and persistent prostatitis. Jpn J Cancer Res 1992; 83:601–608.

28. Cartier L, Castillo JL, Verdugo R. Effect of the Nucleus CMP forte in 46 patients with progressive spastic paraparesis. Randomized and blind study. Rev Med Chil 1996; 124:583–587.

29. Harrington WJ Jr, Sheramata W, Cabral L. Danazol for urinary incontinence in tropical spastic paraparesis. Lancet 1992; 339 (8789):368.

30. Saito M, Kato K, Kondo A, Miyake K. Neurogenic bladder in HAM (HTLV-I associated myelopathy). Hinyokika Kiyo 1991; 37:1005–1008.

31. Namima T, Sohma F, Imabayashi K, et al. Two cases of neurogenic bladder due to HTLV-1 associated myelopathy (HAM). Nippon Hinyokika Gakkai Zasshi 1990; 81:475–478.

32. Bratt G, Hammarin AL, Grandien M, et al. BK virus as the cause of meningoencephalitis, retinitis and nephritis in a patient with AIDS. AIDS 1999; 13:1071–1075.

33. Schwan TG, Burgdorfer W, Schrumpf ME, Karstens RH. The urinary bladder, a consistent source of *Borrelia burgdorferi* in experimentally infected white-footed mice (*Peromyscus leucopus*). J Clin Microbiol 1988; 26:893–895.

34. Pavia CS, Wormser GP, Nowakowski J, Cacciapuoti A. Efficacy of an evernimicin (SCH27899) *in vitro* and in an animal model of Lyme disease. Antimicrob Agents Chemother 2001; 45:936–937.

35. Czub S, Duray PH, Thomas RE, Schwan TG. Cystitis induced by infection with the Lyme disease spirochete, *Borrelia burgdorferi*, in mice. Am J Pathol 1992; 141:1173–1179.

36. Goodman JL, Jurkovich P, Kodner C, Johnson RC. Persistent cardiac and urinary tract infections with *Borrelia burgdorferi* in experimentally infected Syrian hamsters. J Clin Microbiol 1991; 29:894–896.

37. Karch H, Huppertz HI, Bohme M, et al. Demonstration of *Borrelia burgdorferi* DNA in urine samples from healthy humans whose sera contain *B. burgdorferi*-specific antibodies. J Clin Microbiol 1994; 32:2312–2314.

38. Druschky K, Stefan H, Grehl H, Neundorfer B. Secondary normal pressure hydrocephalus. A complication of chronic neuroborreliosis. Nervenarzt 1999; 70:556–559.

39. Aberer E, Neumann R, Lubec G. Acrodermatitis chronica atrophicans in association with lichen sclerosus et atrophicans: tubulo-interstitial nephritis and urinary excretion of spirochete-like organisms. *Acta Derm Venereol* 1987; 67:62–65.

40. Chancellor MB, McGinnis DE, Shenot PJ, et al. Urinary dysfunction in Lyme disease. J Urol 1993; 149:26–30.

41. Chancellor MB, Dato VM, Yang JY. Lyme disease presenting as urinary retention. J Urol 1990; 143:1223–1224.

42. Olivares JP, Pallas F, Ceccaldi M, et al. Lyme disease presenting as isolated acute urinary retention caused by transverse myelitis: an electrophysiological and urodynamical study. Arch Phys Med Rehabil 1995; 76:1171–1172.

26

Cerebrovascular accidents, intracranial tumors, and urologic consequences

Adam J Flisser and Jerry G Blaivas

Definition, epidemiology, management

Cerebrovascular accident (CVA), or stroke, is the clinical manifestation of ischemia or infarction of brain tissue due to hemorrhage or arterial occlusion. CVA is a leading cause of medical morbidity and mortality, representing the third most common cause of death in the United States,[1] and accounting for 1 of every 14.3 deaths in the United States in 1999, and 4–5% of deaths in patients 35–74 years of age in Canada, Germany, and the United Kingdom.[2] In addition, cerebrovascular accidents carry a significant medical morbidity, with 15–30% of patients who survive a CVA becoming permanently disabled. Of stroke survivors, 20–25% die within a year and 14% will suffer additional CVAs within the first year. The cost of treatment for stroke patients is billions of dollars annually ($3.6 billion in the United States in 1998), and accounts for 4% of the National Health Service budget of the UK.[2,3]

Risk factors for CVAs include age, hypertension, cardiac disease, atrial fibrillation, and vascular disease associated with diabetes mellitus or hypercholesterolemia.[4] Multiple potential etiologies are common, due to the coexistence of advanced age, cardiac and vascular disease, and metabolic disorders; as many as 22% of stroke patients will have more than one risk factor,[5] and 38% of patients who experience recurrent stroke will have a different etiology for their secondary event.[6]

The acute management of CVA is primarily aimed at achieving medical stability while preventing exacerbation of the vascular injury.[4] After an acute change in a patient's neurologic status, assessment of the patient's airway, breathing, and circulation should be followed by serum glucose testing. The differential diagnosis includes stroke, transient ischemic attack, seizure, tumor, migraine, and metabolic and infectious processes. Cranial imaging by non-contrast computed tomography (CT) will differentiate hemorrhage, tumor, and acute ischemia, and will allow

therapy to be appropriately directed against the pathology. Hemorrhage may be controlled by medical and surgical intervention. The acute management of ischemic stroke may salvage ischemic brain tissue that has not yet suffered infarction; the patient's blood pressure should be maintained unless it in itself poses a medical risk, such as with concurrent myocardial infarction. In the early post-CVA period, cerebral edema can cause clinically significant mass effects, and can require corrective medical or surgical intervention. Thrombolytic therapies, including aspirin, heparin, and tissue plasminogen activator, which carry the risk of intracranial hemorrhage, can improve functional outcomes in selected patients who meet clinical criteria.[7,8]

The primary medical impact of CVA is due to the serious sensory and motor deficits that can result from brain injury; however, urologic consequences are a significant cause of morbidity.

Urologic impact

Urinary incontinence and stroke are intimately related. Due to the risk factors for CVA, specifically age, CVA is most common in a subset of the population that already has a higher prevalence of urinary incontinence (25–44%).[9–11] In the elderly population in general, and especially in those who are institutionalized, comorbidities such as cardiac and vascular disease are also frequently encountered.

Urinary incontinence is also a potential consequence of CVA. Numerous studies have shown rates of incontinence of 50–70% immediately following CVA,[12–14] with persistent incontinence in 15–30% of patients. Studies have suggested that approximately 70% of survivors of hemispheric strokes will suffer transient urinary incontinence.[12] In another series of patients, 51% of stroke survivors experienced urinary incontinence within the first year, with 15% remaining incontinent thereafter.[13] Brittain et al meta-analyzed studies of stroke patients that included 2800 patients, finding an incidence of incontinence of 32–79% on admission for CVA, and 25% at the time of discharge.[15]

Marinkovic and Badlani reviewed studies on voiding and sexual dysfunction in men and women after CVA,[16] finding evidence of depression, decreased libido, physical limitations, and overall sexual dissatisfaction in patients following CVA.

Disability and death associated with incontinence after cerebrovascular accident

Borrie et al prospectively studied 151 patients with new CVA, of whom 17% had pre-existing incontinence: 60% of the survivors were incontinent after 1 week, with 42% of the survivors still incontinent at 1 month after CVA; there was a significant association between the presence of incontinence and the presence of severe motor defect, mental impairment, and impaired mobility.[17] Barer reviewed 362 stroke victims, concluding that severity of incontinence was itself an independent predictor of worse outcome after CVA.[14]

Anderson et al[18] noted that incontinent stroke survivors had a relative risk of 1-year mortality of 3.9; Nakayama et al[19] found that the mortality after CVA was only 7% in continent stroke survivors, compared with 52% in incontinent stroke survivors. Matthews and Oxybury[20] and Jiminez and Morgan[21] also identify incontinence as an important risk factor for mortality due to CVA. Wade and Hewer suggested that incontinence predicted a poor outcome more reliably than did a history of impaired consciousness in the early stages of stroke.[22] Taub and colleagues found the presence of initial incontinence to predict disability at 3 and 12 months with a specificity of 78%.[23]

In addition to the association of severe CVA and incontinence, incontinence after stroke may have an important effect on the post-discharge care and management of the patient. van Kuijik et al studied 143 stroke patients, and found that, in contrast to aphasia, cognitive impairment, and proprioceptive deficits, the presence of incontinence was significantly associated with discharge to a nursing facility.[24] The presence of incontinence may even lead caregivers to recommend institutionalization in this group of patients.[15,25,26] Other research has not found an association between incontinence and discharge destination, while supporting the negative effect of urinary incontinence on a patient's functional independence.[27] Thus, the presence of incontinence has important implications for the stroke patient's prognosis, disposition, and care.

Cerebrovascular accident and incontinence: pathophysiology

Not all incontinence following CVA is directly related to neurologic injury to the micturition pathways. Gelber et al enumerated three mechanisms to account for incontinence after CVA, comprising disruption of the micturition pathways, general impairment from motor and cognitive deficits, and overflow incontinence unrelated to the CVA itself.[28] This helps to explain the transience of acute incontinence following CVA; as patients who do not suffer from specific urologic injury recover cognitive and physical function, their incontinence will resolve. Incontinence that is not intrinsically related to neuro-urologic causes can also result after a frontal lobe CVA that decreases a patient's awareness of, or concern about, voiding and maintenance of continence.

For patients with urinary incontinence resulting from their neurologic injury, the precise urologic impact of a CVA depends on the location of the injury, the extent of the damage, and the role of the affected area. In the normal individual, continence and voiding are governed by reflex arcs that travel from the bladder to the pons and that are integrated with volitional pathways originating in the cortex, connecting the bladder to the sensorimotor cortex through the pudendal nucleus located in the lower spinal cord.[29–31]

Cranial imaging and the neuro-urology of micturition

Attempts to correlate urodynamic findings with the specific location of brain injury are ongoing. In general, detrusor hyperreflexia is thought to result from the interruption of suprapontine inhibitory tracts. Studies have suggested that the region of bladder control includes the superomedial portion of the frontal lobe and the genu of the corpus callosum, which are connected through the basal ganglia to the pontine mesencephalic reticular formation.[32] Blok and colleagues performed positron emission tomography (PET) scans on normal subjects before and during normal micturition, demonstrating increased blood flow to regions of the pons, hypothalamus, and inferior frontal gyrus on the right side[33] during voiding and during unsuccessful attempts to void, in areas analogous to the 'pontine micturition center', L-region, and M-region, found through invasive techniques to be present in the cat.[34–36] Kuroiwa et al noted that injury to areas of the right cerebral hemisphere was associated with the symptom of urge incontinence.[37]

In a series of 33 patients imaged by CT scan after CVAs Khan et al found that those with lesions that spared the cerebral cortex and internal capsule were able to maintain normal control of the urinary sphincter.[38]

Burney et al prospectively studied 60 patients, attempting to correlate the location of CVA to the urologic impact of the stroke, and confirmed that most of the patients with injury to the frontoparietal lobes and internal capsule suffered from detrusor hyperreflexia and lacked volitional control of the external sphincter. Almost half of the patients in that series suffered from retention and overflow incontinence, which occurred in conjunction with injuries to the internal capsule, basal ganglia, thalamus, pons, cerebellum, and frontoparietal lobes.[39]

Neuro-urologic effects of cerebrovascular accident

Acute disruption of CNS micturition pathways sometimes results in a period of detrusor areflexia and 'cerebral shock'. The mechanism is unknown. The bladder is typically acontractile and normal urinary sphincter tone generally prevents incontinence, except when overflow incontinence ensues, a finding in as many as 21% of patients.[28] Detrusor areflexia is seen commonly in the initial post-CVA period, but resolves in most patients. Kong and Young found urinary retention in 29% of CVA patients within 4 weeks of stroke to be significantly associated with cognitive impairment, diabetes mellitus, aphasia, and urinary tract infection. By the time of discharge, 96% of these patients were able to void spontaneously;[40] however, longer periods of acontractility have been observed.[41] van Kuijik and colleagues observed incontinence after ischemic stroke in a series of 143 patients in a 6-month period, and found an incidence of incontinence of 29/1000 persons per month in patients whose average entry into the study was 5–6 weeks following their stroke. Without treatment, the incidence of recovering continence was 146/1000 persons per month.[24]

After the acute period of cerebral shock, the most common urodynamic finding in patients after CVA is detrusor hyperreflexia with coordinated sphincter function. Detrusor-external sphincter dyssynergia (DESD) is not seen after CVA unless there is another spinal lesion present. Some patients with detrusor hyperreflexia have uncoordinated contractions of the sphincter that may be confused with DESD; many authors have termed this pseudodyssynergia.[29,39,42,43] This phenomenon is believed to be a conscious or subconscious effort on the part of the patient to prevent incontinence by contracting the sphincter during the involuntary detrusor contraction.

Badlani et al noted detrusor hyperreflexia in 46% of patients after CVA.[44] Khan and colleagues[38] observed detrusor hyperreflexia in patients with injury to the cerebral cortex, internal capsule, basal ganglia, and thalamus, and

confirmed the findings of Tsuchida et al,[41] who observed hyperreflexia after CVA affecting the frontal lobe or internal capsule. Krimchansky et al examined 17 patients in a post-traumatic vegetative state; 100% had hyperreflexic bladders, but no patient exhibited dyssynergia.[45]

Detrusor areflexia is also a common finding.[38,46] Badlani et al found the incidence of detrusor areflexia to be 20% in their series.[44] The presence of large residual urine volumes after CVA[47] can result in a higher rate of urinary tract infection; however, it is possible that pre-existing prostatic obstruction or diabetes raises the apparent incidence of this problem following stroke.

Clinical findings and management

In order to determine the appropriate urologic management after CVA, a thorough history and physical examination are essential, as therapy should be tailored to patients' underlying pathophysiology as well as to their capacity for understanding, awareness, concern, and motivation for treatment. Furthermore, the patient's premorbid urologic health should be determined if possible, as this will have a significant impact on the patient's potential for functional recovery. Problems such as bladder overactivity or large residual volumes may be attributable to pre-existing pathology.

After CVA, an acute phase of days to weeks is followed by a variable recovery period that in time leads to a stable clinical state (Figure 26.1).

Acute stage

Immediately after stroke the patient may require an indwelling catheter until he is clinically stable, but intermittent catheterization is preferable.[48] Thereafter, there are four possibilities – normal micturition, urinary retention, incontinence, or other lower urinary tract symptoms. No matter which of these conditions ensues, we recommend obtaining a post-void residual urine measurement for baseline (for the patient who appears to be voiding normally), or to help in management (for the patient who is incontinent or has urinary retention).

Incontinence

In the acute stage, incontinence is usually due to detrusor hyperreflexia or infection, but urinary retention with overflow is not uncommon. Infection should be treated with culture-specific antibiotics and, if incontinence persists, further management depends upon the symptoms,

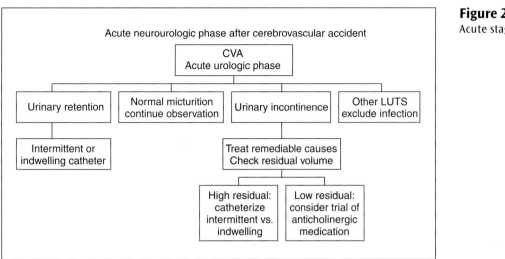

Figure 26.1
Acute stage.

examination, and post-void residual urine. It is usually possible by history and examination to determine whether the incontinence is due to overactive bladder or sphincteric weakness. The latter is not very common, but should be excluded by history and examination with a full bladder. If the incontinence appears to be due to overactive bladder, attention is first turned to remediable causes such as inattention, confusion, apathy, delirium, restricted mobility, and fecal impaction.[49] If residual urine is minimal, a trial of anticholinergic medications is reasonable. If residual urine volume is found to be high, intermittent catheterization or an indwelling catheter may be necessary to empty the bladder and control the incontinence.

Urinary retention

Urinary retention may be due to either detrusor areflexia or urethral obstruction. Urethral obstruction is almost always a premorbid condition and the neurologic insult is the 'straw that broke the camel's back'. In the acute stage, urinary retention is ideally managed with intermittent catheterization, but in many instances this is not practical, and an indwelling catheter will be required.

Other lower urinary tract symptoms

Other lower urinary tract symptoms (LUTS) include storage symptoms (urinary frequency, urgency, nocturia, and pain) and voiding symptoms (dysuria, hesitancy, weak stream, and intermittency). For those with storage symptoms, urinary tract infection is the most common cause. Once infection has been excluded, a stepwise evaluation is made to diagnose other common conditions such as BPH and prostate cancer in men, and pelvic organ prolapse and atrophic vaginitis in women. Sometimes after stroke patients complain of severe LUTS, particularly urgency or

a constant feeling of the need to void, for which no cause can be found. We believe that some of these patients suffer from a kind of bladder paresthesia resulting from CVA.

Recovery stage

From a clinical perspective, the recovery stage is present for as long as the patient continues to show neurologic improvement. This may last days, weeks, months, and sometimes even years. During the recovery stage, patients are best managed empirically. Irreversible or surgical therapies should not generally be considered until the patient is medically and neurologically stable. As a general rule, the recovery stage as defined here lasts about 1 year. It is during this period that we recommend urodynamic investigation to determine the patient's post-stroke urologic baseline and to coordinate urologic therapy (Figure 26.2).

Detrusor hyperreflexia

The initial treatment of detrusor hyperreflexia, with or without concomitant urethral obstruction or impaired contractility, is anticholinergic medication in conjunction with behavior modification (Figures 26.3 and 26.4). When residual urine is clinically problematic, self-intermittent catheterization (SIC) may be necessary. The presence of residual urine, even with urethral obstruction, is not in itself an absolute contraindication to anticholinergic medications, or an indication for intermittent catheterization. Rather, in many instances, it is possible to accept large residual urine volumes as long as the patient does not develop urinary retention, clinical infections, stones, or renal impairment. Careful urologic surveillance of the patient is mandatory in these cases. Of course, the ideal treatment and care may not

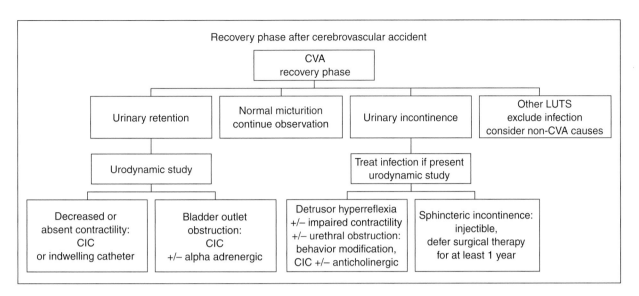

Figure 26.2
Recovery stage.

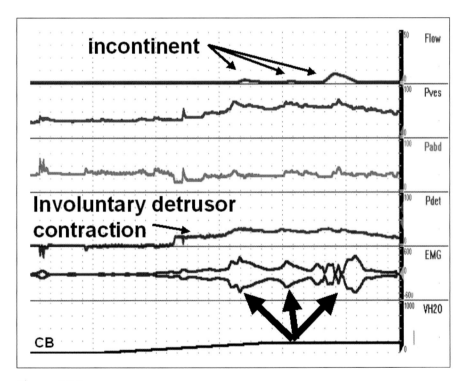

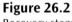

Figure 26.3
Videourodynamic study (VUDS) of a 68-year-old woman who sustained a CVA one year prior to presentation, with resulting right hemiparesis. Her chief complaint was urinary frequency, urgency, and urge incontinence, worst during sleep hours. Voiding diary showed a 24 hour voided volume of 2250 ml, 14 voids, a maximum voided volume of 360 ml and nocturnal polyuria.
During filling there was an involuntary detrusor contraction at a bladder volume of 220 ml. She perceived the contraction as an urge to void and voluntarily contracted her sphincter, evidenced by the increased EMG activity (large arrows). She was able to momentarily prevent incontinence, but she was unable to abort the detrusor contraction and eventually incontinence ensued. She was successfully treated with a program of behavior modification, anticholinergics and furosemide 6 hours before bedtime.
Flow = uroflow (ml/s), Pves = bladder pressure (cmH$_2$O), Pabd = abdominal pressure, Pdet = detrusor pressure, EMG = electromyography, VH$_2$O = infused volume of water (ml). (Courtesy of JG Blaivas, MD.)

be possible because of neurologic deficits that make SIC impractical, or because of limitations in medical resources that undermine optimal patient care. In these cases, regrettably, an indwelling catheter may be the best alternative.

Sphincteric incontinence

Sphincteric incontinence in the recovery phase after CVA is due to pre-existing sphincter dysfunction; it is not a consequence of the stroke itself. Treatment should be guided by the functional status and motivation of the patient. Injectible therapy such as collagen or synthetic materials used as bulking agents for the bladder neck, while usually a temporary solution, can provide symptomatic relief for the patient and allows deferring definitive treatment during the patient's rehabilitation, but is not usually considered unless the patient is highly motivated and has severe incontinence. Timed voiding and moderate fluid restriction can decrease the morbidity of sphincteric incontinence by keeping bladder volumes artificially low. In patients in

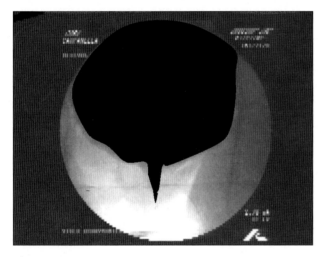

Figure 26.4
Fluoroscopic image during voiding of the patient depicted in Figure 26.3. (Courtesy of Jerry G. Blaivas, MD.)

whom this cannot be accomplished, indwelling catheters, absorbent pads or diapers, and condom catheters all provide potential solutions to the problem of incontinence.

Urinary retention

SIC is the treatment of choice in cases of retention associated with poor or absent detrusor contractility as well as in cases of urethral obstruction. In addition, α-adrenergic agonists may be clinically useful. In men presenting with acute urinary retention unrelated to stroke, α-blockers increased the proportion of subjects who could void spontaneously 24 h after the initiation of therapy.[50] Indwelling catheters are indicated only when other therapies are not feasible.

Stable stage

The stable stage is defined by the absence of further evidence of neurologic improvement and can make its appearance as long as 1 or 2 years after the stroke. Treatment guidelines assume that the patient is not going to make any further neurologic recovery, but, of course, most patients are still at risk for further cerebrovascular events and many still require anticoagulation therapy (Figure 26.5).

Urinary incontinence

The management is the same as in patients without CVA; however, the increased surgical risks in patients with neurologic deficits and with medical risk factors for CVA must be considered, as well as the relative difficulty of self-catheterization in this group of patients should SIC become necessary. In patients who suffer from refractory urge incontinence due to detrusor hyperreflexia and who fail conservative therapies, augmentation cystoplasty can be a potential solution,[51] and continence rates as high as 89% have been reported.

Figure 26.5
Stable stage.

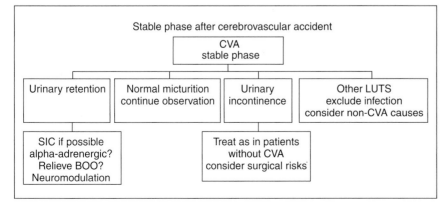

Urinary retention

When urinary retention is due to absent or impaired detrusor contractility the most reasonable treatment is SIC, but in many stroke patients this is not practical because of the neurologic deficit and many are relegated to an indwelling catheter. In men, empiric prostate resection or incision or other outlet-reducing procedures may be considered. Sacral neuromodulation is an emerging technique that may be helpful in patients with neurogenic bladder who have failed first-line therapies for either detrusor hyperreflexia or urinary retention;[52] however, its utility in stroke patients remains to be proven.[53]

Other lower urinary tract symptoms

In men, coexisting prostatic obstruction poses a most difficult problem (Figures 26.6 and 26.7). Detrusor hyperreflexia is a common finding in post-prostatectomy stroke patients,[54] and postoperative incontinence is a serious risk. Lum and Marshall enumerated several risk factors for poor outcome from prostatic resection,[55] including surgery within 1 year of CVA, bilateral hemispheric involvement, and advanced neurologic deficits. Staskin et al found that abnormal voluntary sphincter control was a significant risk factor for post-prostatectomy incontinence in patients suffering from Parkinson's disease and prostatic obstruction

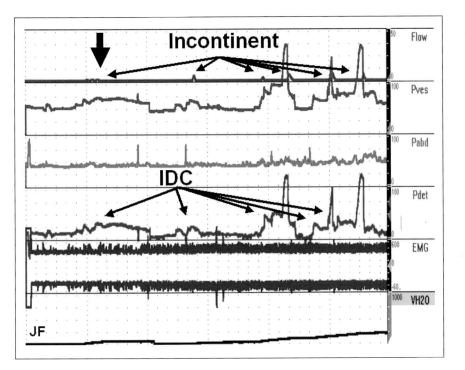

Figure 26.6
VUDS of a 75-year-old man with benign prostatic hypertrophy and prostatic urethral obstruction who suffered a CVA one year prior to the study. His chief complaints were urinary urgency and nocturia. VUDS showed involuntary detrusor contractions during filling, associated with severe urges to void. He was able to contract the sphincter, temporarily preventing incontinence, but could not abort the detrusor contraction and was incontinent. The EMG tracing shows artifactual AC interference. Flow = uroflow (ml/s), Pves = bladder pressure (cm H_2O), Pabd = abdominal pressure, Pdet = detrusor pressure, EMG = electromyography, VH_2O = infused volume of water (ml). (Courtesy of J.G. Blaivas, MD.)

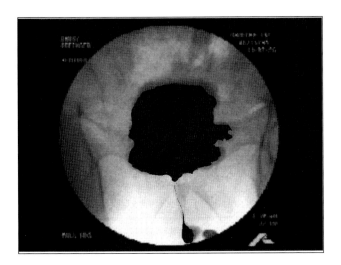

Figure 26.7
Fluoroscopic image during voiding of the patient depicted in Figure 26.6 showing prostatic urethral obstruction. (Courtesy of J.G. Blaivas, MD.)

who underwent transurethral prostatectomy.[43] For these reasons, we believe that surgery to relieve urinary retention or irritative symptoms should not be performed until urodynamic testing confirms bladder outlet obstruction. The type of detrusor overactivity and the patient's degree of awareness and control may have prognostic implications,[56] but no studies have yet been done to document this. Alpha-adrenergic blockers used in the treatment of benign prostatic hyperplasia may have a role in decreasing the risk of urinary retention; however, studies are ongoing.

Intracranial neoplasms

Intracranial tumors, through mass effect or in association with hemorrhage, have the same potential as CVA to disrupt the normal mechanisms of voiding. Lang et al reported urinary retention in two patients who had intracranial lesions that compressed the frontal cortex.[57] Fowler reviewed the studies of Maurice-Williams[58] and Mochizuki and Saito,[59] which have contributed to identification of frontal areas of the brain as essential for normal urinary control.

References

1. US Department of Health. Births and deaths: United States, 1995. Monthly vital statistics report. 1996; 45(3):Suppl 2.

2. American Heart Association. 2002 heart and stroke statistical update. Dallas, Texas: American Heart Association, 2001.

3. Isard PA, Forbes JF. The cost of stroke to the National Health Service in Scotland. Cerebrovasc Dis 1992; 2:47–50.

4. Smith WS, Hauser SL, Easton JD. Cerebrovascular diseases. In: Braunwald E, Hauser SL, Fauci AS, et al, eds. Harrison's principles of internal medicine. 15th edn. New York: McGraw-Hill, 2001: 2369–2391.

5. Caplan LR. Multiple potential risks for stroke. JAMA 283(11): 1479–1480.

6. Yamamoto H, Bogousslavsky J. Mechanism of second and further strokes. J Neurol Neurosurg Psychiatry 1998; 64:771–776.

7. Moonis M, Fisher M. Considering the role of heparin and low-molecular-weight heparins in acute ischemic stroke. Stroke 2002; 33(7):1927–1933.

8. Meschia JF, Miller DA, Brott TG. Thrombolytic treatment of acute ischemic stroke. Mayo Clin Proc 2002; 77(6):542–551.

9. Peet SM, Castleden CM, McGrother CW. Prevalence of urinary and faecal incontinence in hospitals and residential and nursing homes for older people. BMJ 1995; 311:1063–1064.

10. Tobin GW, Brocklehurst JC. The management of urinary incontinence in local authority residential homes for the elderly. Age Ageing 1986; 14:292–298.

11. Palmer MH, German PS, Ouslander JG. Risk factors for urinary incontinence one year after nursing home admission. Residential Nursing Health 1991; 13:405–412.

12. Redding MJ, Winter SW, Hochrein SA, et al. Urinary incontinence after unilateral hemispheric stroke: a neurologic epidemiologic perspective. J Neurorehab 1987; 1:25.

13. Brocklehurst JC, Andrews K, Richards B, Laycock PJ. Incidence and correlates of incontinence in stroke patients. J Am Geriatric Soc 1985; 33:540–542.

14. Barer DH. Continence after stroke: useful predictor or goal of therapy? Age Ageing 1989; 18:183–191.

15. Brittain KR, Peet SM, Potter JF, Castleden CM. Prevalence and management of urinary incontinence in stroke survivors. Age and Ageing 1999; 28:509–511.

16. Marinkovic SP, Badlani G. Voiding and sexual dysfunction after cerebrovascular accidents. J Urol 2001; 165:359–370.

17. Borrie MJ, Campbell AJ, Caradoc-Davies TH, Spears GFS. Urinary incontinence after stroke: a prospective study. Age and Ageing 1986; 15:177–181.

18. Anderson CS, Jamrozik KD, Broadhurst RJ, et al. Predicting survival for 1 year among different subtypes of stroke. Stroke 1994; 25:1935–1944.

19. Nakayama H, Jorgenson HS, Pedersen PM, et al. Prevalence and risk factors of incontinence after stroke: the Copenhagen stroke study. Stroke 1997; 28:58–62.

20. Matthews WB, Oxybury JM. Prognostic factors in stroke. In: Ciba Foundation Symposium, No. 34. Amsterdam: Elsevier, 1975:1–279.

21. Jimenez J, Morgan PG. Predicting improvement in stroke patients referred for inpatient rehabilitation. Can Med Assoc J 1979; 121:1481–1484.

22. Wade DT, Hewer RL. Outlook after acute stroke: urinary incontinence and loss of consciousness compared in 532 patients. Quart J Med 1985; 56:601–608.

23. Taub NA, Wolfe CD, Richardson E, et al. Predicting the disability of first-time stroke sufferers at 1 year. 12 month follow-up of a population-based cohort in Southeast England. Stroke 1994; 25:352–357.

24. van Kuijik AA, van der Linde H, van Limbeek J. Urinary incontinence in stroke patients after admission to a postacute inpatient rehabilitation program. Arch Phys Med Rehabil 2001; 82:1407–1411.

25. Ouslander JG, Kane RL, Abrass IB. Urinary incontinence in elderly nursing home patients. JAMA 1982; 248:1194–1198.

26. Noekler LS. Incontinence in elderly cared for by family. Gerontologist 1987; 27:194–200.

27. Gross JC. Urinary incontinence and stroke outcomes. Arch Phys Med Rehabil 2000; 81:22–27.

28. Gelber AG, Good DC, Laven LJ, Verhulst SJ. Causes of urinary incontinence after stroke: a prospective study. Age Ageing 1986; 15:177–181.

29. Blaivas JG. The neurophysiology of micturition: a clinical study of 550 patients. J Urol 1982; 127:958–963.

30. Bradley WE, Timm GW, Scott FB. Innervation of the detrusor muscle and urethra. Urol Clin N Am 1974; 1:3.

31. Chancellor MB, Yoshimura N. Physiology and pharmacology of the bladder and urethra. In: Walsh PC, ed. Campbell's urology, 8th edn. Philadelphia: WB Saunders, 2002:813–886.

32. Gosling J. Anatomy (physical and neural) of the lower urinary tract. In: Schick E, Corcos J, eds. Neurogenic bladder, adults and children. New York: Marcel Dekker, 2003.

33. Blok BFM, Willemsen ATM, Holstege G. A PET study on brain control of micturition in humans. Brain 1997; 120:111–121.

34. Holstege G, Griffiths D, de Wall H, Dalm E. Anatomical and physiological observations on supraspinal control of bladder and urethral sphincter muscles in the cat. J Comp Neurol 1986; 250:449–461.

35. Griffiths D, Holstege D, de Wall H, Dalm E. Control and coordination of bladder and urethral function in the brain stem of the cat. Neurourol Urodyn 1990; 9:63–82.

36. Fowler CJ. Neurological disorders of micturition and their treatment. Brain 1999; 122:1213–1231.

37. Kuroiwa Y, Tohgi H, Ono S, Itoh M. Frequency and urgency of micturition in hemiplegic patients: relationship to hemisphere laterality of lesions. J Neurol 1987; 234:100–102.

38. Khan Z, Starer P, Yang WC, Bhola A. Analysis of voiding disorders in patients with cerebrovascular accidents. Urology 1990; 35:265–270.

39. Burney TL, Senapati M, Desai S, Choudhary ST, Badlani GH. Effects of cerebrovascular accident on micturition. Urol Clin North Am 1996; 23(3):483–490.

40. Kong KH, Young S. Incidence and outcome of poststroke urinary retention: a prospective study. Arch Phys Med Rehabil 2000; 81(1):136–143.

41. Tsuchida S, Hiromitsu N, Yamaguchi O, et al. Uroydnamic studies on hemiplegic patients after cerebrovascular accident. Urology 1983; 21:315–318.

42. Wein AJ, Barrett DM. Etiologic possibilities for increased pelvic floor electromyographic activity during cystometry. J Urol 1982; 127:949–952.

43. Staskin DS, Vandi Y, Siroky, MB. Postprostatectomy incontinence in the Parkinsonian patient: the significance of poor voluntary sphincter control. J Urol 1988; 140(1):117–118.

44. Badlani GH, Vohra S, Motola JA. Detrusor behavior in patients with dominant hemispheric strokes. Neurourol Urodynam 1991; 10:119–123.

45. Krimchansky BZ, Sazbon L, Heller L, et al. Bladder tone in patients in post-traumatic vegetative state. Brain Inj 1999; 12(11):899–903.

46. Feder M, Heller L, Tadmor R, et al. Urinary continence after stroke: association with cytometric profile and computerized tomography findings. Eur Neurol 1987; 27:101–105.

47. Garrett VE, Scott JA, Costich J, et al. Bladder emptying assessment in stroke patients. Arch Phys Med Rehab 1989; 70:41–43.

48. Lloyd LK, Kuhlemeir LV, Fine PR, et al. Initial bladder management in spinal cord injury: does it make a difference? J Urol 1986; 135:523–527.

49. Resnick NM. Geriatric incontinence. Urol Clin N Am 1996; 23(1):55–75.

50. McNeill SA, Daruwala PD, Mitchell IDC, et al. Sustained-release alfuzosin and trial without catheter after acute urinary retention: a prospective, placebo-controlled trial. BJU Int 1999; 84:622–627.

51. Chartier-Kastler EJ, Mongiat-Artus P, Bitker MO, et al. Long-term results of augmentation cystoplasty in spinal cord injury patients. Spinal Cord 2000; 38(8):490–494.

52. Chartier-Kastler EJ, Bosch JLHR, Perrigot M, et al. Long-term results of sacral nerve stimulation (S3) for the treatment of neurogenic refractory urge incontinence related to detrusor hyperreflexia. J Urol 2000; 164:1476.

53. Jonas U, Grunewald V, eds. New perspectives in sacral nerve stimulation. London: Martin Dunitz, 2002.

54. Khan Z, Bhola A. Prostatism and male urinary incontinence. Semin Urol 1987; 5:108–113.

55. Lum SK, Marshall VR. Results of prostatectomy in patients following a cerebrovascular accident. Br J Urol 1982; 54:186–189.

56. Flisser AJ, Walmsley K, Blaivas JG. Urodynamic classification of patients with symptoms of overactive bladder. J Urol 2003; 169(2):529–534.

57. Lang EW, Chesnut RM, Hennerici M. Urinary retention and space-occupying lesions of the frontal cortex. Eur Neurol 1996; 36:43–47.

58. Maurice-Williams RS. Micturition symptoms in frontal tumours. J Neurol Neurosurg Psychiatry 1974; 37:431–436.

59. Mochizuki H, Saito H. Mesial frontal lobe syndromes: correlations between neurological deficits and radiological localizations [Review]. Tohoku J Exp Med 1990; 161(Suppl):231–239.

27

Intervertebral disc prolapse

Erik Schick and Pierre E Bertrand

Introduction

Intervertebral disc prolapse causes direct neurologic damage by mechanical compression of the spinal cord or the nerve roots emerging from it. This damage is proportional to the severity and length of compression on these structures. Table 27.1 summarizes the consequences of these events. The chances for recovery are inversely proportional to the duration and degree of neural compression.[1] Figures 27.1 and 27.2 outline the structure of a normal nerve cell and Figure 27.3 illustrates the patterns of injury.

The most frequent site of disc herniations is lumbar, followed by cervical and thoracic spine; some are asymptomatic. By age 60, nearly one-third of asymptomatic patients have one or more herniated lumbar discs.[2] About 90% of symptomatic herniated discs occur at the L4–L5 or L5–S1 level,[3] and 90% inside the spinal canal.[4] A strong correlation was observed between the level of herniation and age: lumbar disc herniation is more cranially localized in older patients.[5] In the cervical spine C6–C7 is the site of 60–70% of herniated discs, and C5–C6 accounts for 20–30%.[6] About 15% of asymptomatic adults have

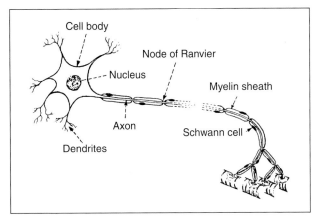

Figure 27.1

Structure of the nerve cell and axon. Each axon represents an elongation of the nerve cell – lying within the central nervous system, e.g. anterior horn cell, or in an outlying ganglion, e.g. dorsal root ganglion. The cell body maintains the viability of the axon, being the center of all cellular metabolic activity. (Reproduced with permission from Lindsay KW, Bone I, Callander R. Neurology and neurosurgery illustrated, 2nd edn. London: Churchill Livingstone, 1991.)

Table 27.1 *Nerve lesions according to the severity and length of compression*			
Compression	Consequences	Recovery	Pathology
Short and mild	Nerve impulse blocked	Almost immediate	Local ischemia
Moderate	Nerve impulse blocked	Several weeks; depends on remyelinization	Local demyelinization axon preserved (Figure 27.3A)
Local, progressive, chronic	Progressive decrease in motor impulse transmission	Depends on degree of remyelinization	Segmental demyelinization, between Ranvier's node, at the site of compression and its vicinity
Severe, but temporary	Section of nerve fibers	Depends on axonal regeneration in Schwann's cell tube	Wallerian degeneration distally (Figure 27.3B)
Severe and chronic	Section of nerve fibers	None; Schwann's cell tube remains blocked by compression; retrograde axonal degenerescence	Wallerian degeneration (Figure 27.3C)

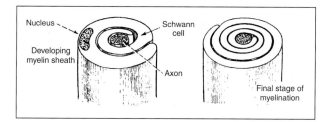

Figure 27.2
Many axons are surrounded by an insulation of myelin, which is enveloped by the Schwann cell membrane. Myelin is a protein–lipid complex. The membrane of the Schwann cell 'spirals' around the axon, and results in the formation of a multilayer myelin sheath. All axons have a cellular sheath – Schwann cell – but not all axons are myelinated. (Reproduced with permission from Lindsay KW, Bone I, Callander R. Neurology and neurosurgery illustrated, 2nd edn. London: Churchill Livingstone, 1991.)

thoracic disc herniation in magnetic resonance imaging (MRI) studies.[7] On the other hand, symptomatic thoracic disc herniations represent only 0.25–0.57% of all symptomatic disc herniations.[7,8]

Cervical spine

There is no mention in the literature of urethrovesical dysfunction associated with disc herniation at the level of the cervical spine.

Thoracic spine

Stillerman et al[9] analyzed their own series of 82 symptomatic herniated thoracic discs in 71 patients, and made an extensive review of the recent literature (from 1986 to 1997). Among the 71 patients they operated on, they noted bladder dysfunction in 24% (17 out of 71), with urgency being the most common complaint. The incidence of bladder/bowel dysfunction in the reviewed literature was somewhat higher, 35% (72 out of 208). The review did not mention the type of bladder dysfunction encountered.

Lumbar spine: cauda equina syndrome

As 95% of disc prolapses are in the lumbar and lumbosacral region, we focus our discussion mainly on this region. Figure 27.4 illustrates the interrelation between two lumbar vertebrae. Presentation of lumbar disc prolapses can be divided into two categories: those with major symptoms other than urologic (sciatic neuralgia, cauda

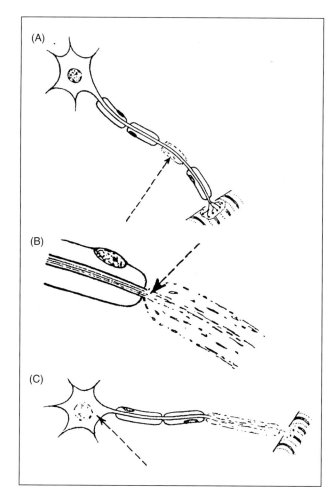

Figure 27.3
Patterns of injury. (A) Segmental degeneration. Scattered destruction of the myelin sheath occurs without axonal damage. The primary lesion affects the Schwann cell. (B) Wallerian degeneration. Degeneration of axon distally following its interruption. The axon disintegrates and the myelin brakes up into globules. Regeneration of nerve is possible because the basement membrane of the Schwann cell survives and acts as a skeleton along which the axon regrows. (C) Distal axonal degeneration. Damage to the cell body or to the axon will affect the viability of the axon, which will 'die back' from the periphery. Loss of the myelin sheath occurs as a secondary event. Recovery is slow because the axon must regenerate. When the cell body is destroyed no regrowth will occur. (Reproduced with permission from Lindsay KW, Bone I, Callander R. Neurology and neurosurgery illustrated, 2nd edn. London: Churchill Livingstone, 1991.)

equina syndrome, etc.) and those showing only urologic manifestations (vesicourethral dysfunction).

The level of termination of the spinal cord, the conus medullaris, is between T12 and L1–L2, most frequently at the mid-portion of L1.[10] The descending nerve bundles run posterior to the lumbar vertebral bodies until they exit the spinal canal, and are called cauda equina. Central

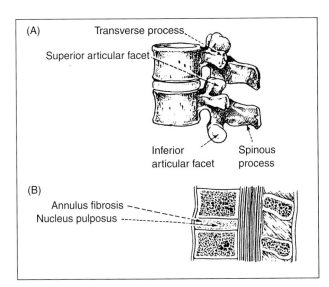

Figure 27.4
(A) Interrelation between two lumbar vertebrae.
(B) Intervertebral discs act as shock absorbers for the bony spine. A tough outer layer, the annulus fibrosis, surrounds a softer central nucleus pulposus. Discs degenerate with age, the fluid within the nucleus pulposus gradually drying out. Disc collapse produces excessive strain on the facet joints, i.e. the superior and inferior articulatory processes of each vertebral body, and leads to degeneration and hypertrophy. (Reproduced with permission from Lindsay KW, Bone I, Callander R. Neurology and neurosurgery illustrated, 2nd edn. London: Churchill Livingstone, 1991.)

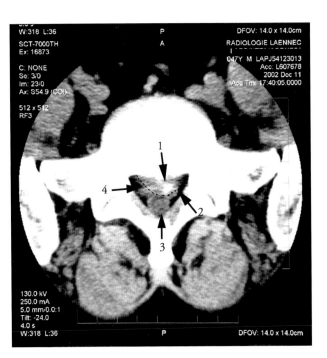

Figure 27.5
Central protrusion of a lumbar disc resulting in a stenosis of the spinal canal of at least 50%. (1) Prolapsed disc; (2) compression of the S1 nerve root at the left; (3) compression of the cauda equina by the central herniation of the intervertebral disc; (4) normal S1 nerve root at the right side. (Courtesy of Dr Mario Séguin.)

protrusion of the disc occurs in 1–15% of cases and fibers of the cauda equina can thus be compressed[11] (Figure 27.5). Cauda equina syndrome is characterized by low-back pain, perineal sensory loss (saddle anesthesia), bilateral sciatic motor weakness of the lower extremities, or chronic paraplegia, with loss of voluntary control of both anal and urethral sphincter, and of sexual responsiveness.[12,13] The earliest case of cauda equina syndrome was described by Jonathan Hutchinson in 1889 and was secondary to manipulation of the lumbar spine under general anesthesia.[14] Most disc prolapses occur at the L4–L5 or L5–S1 level and, when central, they can affect nerve roots exiting at S2–S4 sacral levels, interfering with normal vesicourethral function (Figures 27.6 and 27.7).

Jennet[15] estimates that in the majority of lumbar disc prolapses the cauda equina is involved. This opinion is challenged by others. In a series of 121 patients operated on by Tay and Chacha[16] only 8 patients presented with compression of the cauda equina. In a large series of 1972 patients who underwent lumbar discoidectomy, as reported by Nielsen et al,[17] only 26 (1.32%) presented with cauda equina syndrome.

Nerve bundles of the cauda equina contain parasympathetic and somatic fibers. The clinical presentation is often dominated by the effects of compression of the somatic fibers. This may explain why vesicourethral and rectal dysfunctions have been studied less frequently. Classically, vesicourethral dysfunction in this syndrome is estimated to have a frequency rate of 1–16%.[15,18–27] Rosomoff et al[28] were the first to include cystometry in the routine preoperative evaluation of patients with disc prolapse. They found a 96% incidence of hypotonic bladder. Andersen and Bradley[29] studied urethral and bladder innervation in 8 patients with protruded lumbar disc documented by myelography and found detrusor areflexia in all of them. Among the 30 patients with lumbar disc disease reported by Mosdal et al,[30] 18 patients had lower urinary tract symptoms; six patients had areflexic bladder and 13 patients had hyposensitive and/or hypotonic detrusor. These data suggest that a significant proportion of patients with symptomatic lumbar disc prolapse will also have bladder dysfunction, even if lower urinary tract disturbances are not the predominant symptoms.

A relatively small number of patients with disc prolapse will not have symptoms related to somatic nerve compression, and will become clinically manifest exclusively by urinary symptoms. These cases are of particular interest for the urologist, aware of the neurologic bases for lower urinary tract symptoms.

Jennet[15] was first to suggest that urinary retention might be the only symptom of a prolapsed disc, followed by

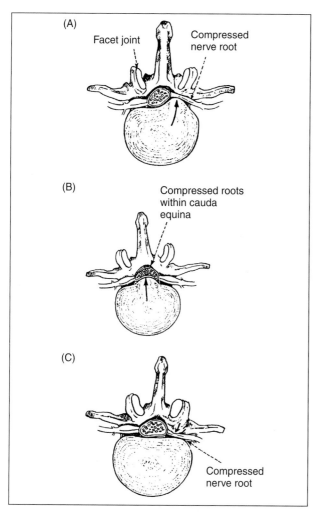

Figure 27.6
(A) Lateral disc protrusion. (B) Central disc protrusion compressing the cauda equina. (C) Hypertrophied facet joint. (Reproduced with permission from Lindsay KW, Bone I, Callander R. Neurology and neurosurgery illustrated, 2nd edn. London: Churchill Livingstone, 1991.)

Gangai[31] 10 years later. Emmett and Love[32,33] analyzed in detail the urologic manifestations of disc prolapse. Subsequently, several other case reports or small series have been published.[34–43] It is worthwile to note that in these reports females often outnumbered males.[36,40]

Urinary symptoms

Only a small number of patients will report urinary symptoms spontaneously. A more probing questionnaire, however, will reveal lower urinary tract disturbances in many patients.[38,44] No pathognomonic urinary symptom exists for lumbar disc prolapse. The most frequent symptom is acute or chronic urinary retention.[16,32,34,39,44–47]

Irritative symptoms sometimes precede urinary retention.[32,45] Dysuria,[30,36,38–40] disappearance of normal desire to void,[38–40,45] decreased flow,[38,41] urinary incontinence related to stress,[38,46] or by overflow[40] have also been described.

Urologic investigations

Cystoscopy

A number of observations can be made in a patient with lumbar disc prolapse:

1. a decrease or absence of sensation during the passage of the instrument through the urethra and less discomfort with movement of the instrument or touching of the trigone
2. a sensation of hypogastric fullness rather then real desire to void during bladder filling
3. the absence of bladder wall trabeculation, even in the presence of a large residual urine.

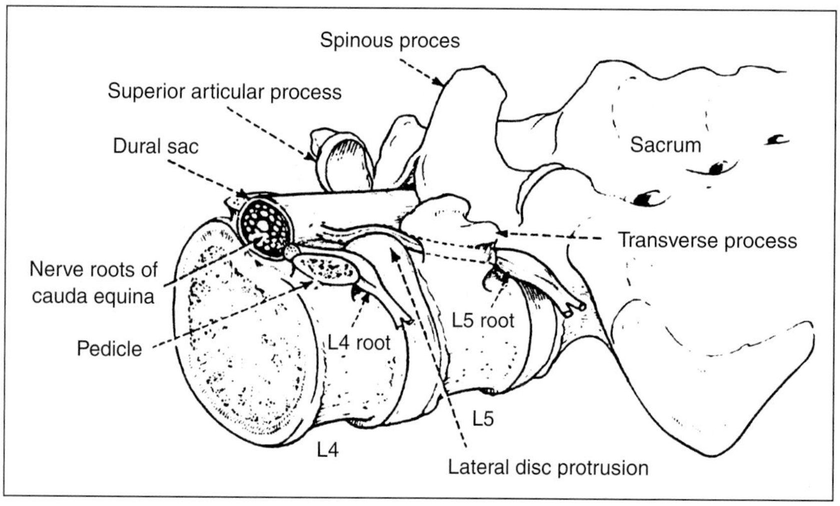

Figure 27.7
Lateral disc herniations usually compress the nerve root exiting through the foramen below the affected level, e.g. an L4–L5 disc lesion will compress the L5 root. Large disc protrusions or a free fragment may compress any adjacent root. (Reproduced with permission from Lindsay KW, Bone I, Callander R. Neurology and neurosurgery illustrated, 2nd edn. London: Churchill Livingstone, 1991.)

This triade should evoke the possibility of a lumbar disc prolapse as the cause of urinary symptoms,[32,33,37] even with a negative neurologic examination. Susset et al[41] reported a case of partial bladder denervation secondary to a disc prolapse in which mild bladder wall trabeculation was present and desire to void preserved.

Urodynamics

This is probably the best diagnostic tool to evaluate visceral innervation originating from the lumbosacral spine. Rosomoff[48] suggested that cystometry was the best test to diagnose cauda equina lesions. This opinion has been challenged by few. Emmett and Love[32] reported that cystoscopy can give the same, and sometimes more, diagnostic information than does cystometry. According to Cheek et al[39] urodynamics are more useful in the postoperative period to document treatment outcome, mainly because before treatment it cannot distinguish between an areflexic neurogenic bladder and a decompensated, non-contractile bladder resulting from chronic overdistention.

Experimental animal studies suggest that the cystometrogram is only sensitive to severe compression of the cauda equina. Detrusor areflexia appears to occur with blockage of axoplasmic flow and early sensory changes occur with neurovenous congestion.[49]

Detrusor areflexia develops in approximately 25% of patients with lumbar intervertebral disc protrusion. In cauda equina syndrome, cystometry is similar to that of a neurogenic areflexic bladder. Capacity is significantly increased;[27,36,38,48,50,51] during the filling phase the curve is flat, hypotonic,[36,48,50] and the first desire to void is delayed or abolished.[30,36,38,46,48,50] During voiding the detrusor is hypocontractile.[29,36,38,46,48] It should be noted, however, that in a few, well-documented lumbar disc prolapses, bladder capacity and filling phase were normal.[30,36]

Jones and Moore[45] were first to describe the coexistence of lumbar disc prolapse and bladder hyperreflexia. In a series of 81 patients with neurogenic bladder secondary to disc prolapse or spinal degeneration, 22 patients had hyperreflexic bladders.[52] Mosdal et al[30] described an identical case and Hellström et al[53] added 3 other cases. In these cases there was usually no post-void residual urine, and bladder sensitivity was normal. Hyperreflexia was not secondary to outflow obstruction but presumably due to 'irritation of the nerve root'.[52]

Shin et al[54] studied 50 patients with complete cauda equina injury. Bladder compliance was decreased in 28% (14/50) and normal in 72% (36/50). Detrusor hyperreflexia was observed in 6 out of the 14 patients with low-compliant bladder, but none in the normal-compliant group. Hyperreflexia disappeared with the normalization of compliance and capacity. These authors concluded

that low compliance appeared to be the main cause of hyperreflexia.

Norlèn[55] reported α-adrenergic activity in the bladder of cats who underwent parasympathetic denervation. The same phenomenon was observed in humans as well. This α-adrenergic activity can be responsible for detrusor contractions during the filling phase which can be misinterpreted as being true hyperreflexia due to parasympathetic activity.

It is interesting to observe that bladder compliance is normal in areflexic bladders secondary to disc prolapse.[46] This is in contrast with the areflexic bladder resulting from trauma or myelodysplasia, where compliance is often decreased.

Murnaghan et al[56] transsected the cauda equina in monkeys and obtained low-compliant bladders. The compliance of these bladders could be improved by administration of phentolamine and emepromium bromide.[55] This suggests that the decreased compliance was of neurogenic origin, due to both α-adrenergic and cholinergic activities.

The areflexic bladder, as observed in disc protrusion, has a normal compliance. This areflexia is thus not motor in origin – as in the experiences of Murnaghan et al,[56] or reported by Sandri et al[57] – but secondary to lesions of the sensory fibers of the bladder, or to incomplete lesions of the parasympathetic preganglionic fibers.[46] The bethanechol supersensitivity test is positive in 100% of areflexic and low-compliant bladders from other causes, but it is significantly less positive in those when areflexia is secondary to lumbar disc prolapse. This suggests that in the latter situation motor impairment is not primary, but a consequence of sensory impairment.[58] The injury to the muscle fibers of these large decompensated bladders probably results from chronic overdistention and not from a direct neurologic lesion.[47]

Bladder dysfunction, primarily sensitive and secondarily motor in nature, explains the urinary symptoms encountered and the observations made during urodynamic testing (Table 27.2).

Flowmetry

Few authors have studied free flowmetry in lumbar disc prolapse. As expected, in the majority of cases the maximum and mean flows are decreased.[29,30,38,39,41] Kontturi[38] established a relation between the degree of nerve compression and the decrease in mean flow. This, however, does not seem to be the rule, because Andersen and Bradley[29] and Mosdal et al[30] reported that 50% of their patients had normal flowmetry. Sometimes the flow curve undulates, suggesting Valsalva maneuvers during micturition.[30,39]

Table 27.2 *Usual urologic manifestations of cauda equina syndrome*

	Compression of the sensory fibers of the sacral roots	Consequences of the motoricity of the detrusor
Endoscopy	Hyposensitivity of the urethra and the trigone Bladder proprioception delayed or abolished Cystoscopic capacity increased	Bladder wall without trabeculations Increased post-void residual urine
Cystometry	Proprioception (B_1) delayed or abolished Cystometric capacity increased	Bladder wall compliance normal Hypo- or contractile detrusor
Free flowmetry		Maximum flow rate and mean flow rate decreased
Urethral pressure profilometry		Maximum urethral closure pressure normal or decreased (depends on pudendal nerve injury)
Electrophysiology	Sensory threshold of penis (or clitoris) altered	Bulbocavernosus (or clitorido-anal) reflex latency increased or abolished Denervation (to various extent) of pelvic floor muscles

Urethral pressure profilometry

Kontturi[38] found a normal sphincteric tone in every patient. He was unable to establish any relation between urethral pressure profile (UPP) parameters and the severity of neural injury as demonstrated clinically or radiologically on myelography. He noted, however, that in the group of patients with the most severe neurological impairment, sphincter tonus was abnormally high in patients with urinary retention and the sphincter was hypotonic in those patients with urinary incontinence.

McGuire[59] analyzed UPP in 6 patients with disc prolapse. Proximal urethral pressure was normal, an expected finding since herniated lumbar discs do not interfere with hypogastric plexus activity. McGuire also noted a decrease in tone at the membraneous urethra in 2 patients in whom electromyographic activity was poor in the striated sphincter. Chuang et al[51] reported on 14 patients who had lesions below the conus medullaris and had anal sphincter abnormalities. All the patients showed a significant decrease in maximum urethral closure pressure, which suggested injury to the pudendal nerve by the protruded disc.

Electromyography

Electromyographic (EMG) activity of the pelvic floor was not studied systematically in this patient population. Andersen and Bradley[29] could not register any electrical activity in 1 of 18 patients. Fanciullacci et al[46] analyzed 22 patients and found no electrical activity in 16 patients and an abnormal EMG in 6 patients.

Electromyelography

Susset et al[41] found an increased bulbocavernosus latency time in their patients. Urethroanal reflex was perturbed in two-thirds of the patients studied by Andersen and Bradley,[29] as well as by Fanciullacci et al.[46] These observations suggest an alteration in the somatic segmental innervation of the vesicourethral unit. The sensory threshold of the penis (or clitoris) was often altered.[46]

Table 27.2 summarizes the urologic manifestations of cauda equina syndrome.

Postoperative results

When conservative measures fail, the treatment of herniated discs is surgical, with excision of the disc(s).

The evaluation of immediate and long-term results is difficult because subjective improvement does not necessarily match functional recuperation, as demonstrated by urodynamics and electrophysiologic studies.[39] Several authors reported significant improvement, even complete recovery, of preoperative lower urinary tract symptoms.[16,28,30,32,34,36,37,41,47,60] Scott,[26] however, found no noticeable improvement, especially when perianal anesthesia persisted.

Urodynamic evaluation can return to normal.[35,38,41,59] Recovery of vesical function is poor or even nonexistent when neurologic signs, particularly perianal anesthesia, remain.[26–38] Perianal anesthesia is considered the most important prognostic indicator.[50] However Hellström et al[53] reported 3 patients with persistant bilateral perianal anesthesia and a contractile detrusor. Gleave et al[47] found no relation between bladder recovery and persisting saddle anesthesia. Seventy nine percent of their patients had no urinary symptoms, but 78% remained with perianal sensory deficit. (These patients, however, did not have a urodynamic evaluation.) For several authors, detrusor areflexia has a tendency to remain permanent.[29,46] Fanciullacci et al[46] demonstrated that

the afferent branch of the pudendal reflex arc is more vulnerable than its efferent branch. This might explain why perianal anesthesia rarely recovers. Detrusor recovery is not proportional to the dimension of the disc prolapse.[61]

Opinions are divided as to what extent this pathology should be considered as a surgical emergency. Some researchers[17,53,62–64] advocate rapid decompression because it improves the chances of detrusor recovery. Other researchers[15,47,50,65,66] found no relation between the delay to surgery and normalization of bladder function. One possible exception could be decompression in an acute episode within the first 6 hours, the limit of time for axone ischemia to become irreversible.[47] In all reported series, such rapid intervention is exceptional.

Short-term recovery of bladder function is often poor after lumbar disc surgery; indeed, the recovery of bladder function may be very slow, taking months to years.[66,67] From the urologic point of view, these patients need careful long-term follow-up.

Conclusions

Intervertebral disc prolapse of the lumbar spine compressing the cauda equina can lead to urethrovesical dysfunction. In the great majority of cases it results in

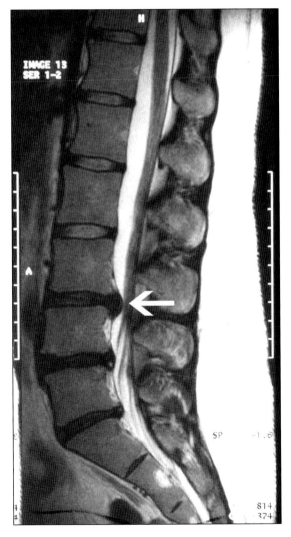

Figure 27.8
Magnetic resonance image (sagittal plane) of a sequestered discal fragment (arrow). Note the difference on MRI of the degenerated disc at the L3–L4 level, compared with normal intervertebral discs at more proximal levels. (Courtesy of Dr Marie-Christine Roy.)

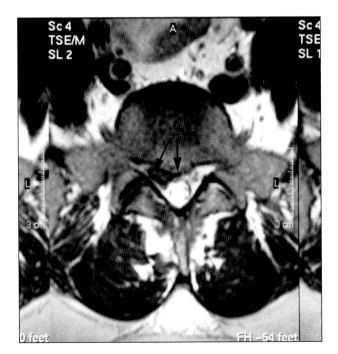

Figure 27.9
Magnetic resonance image (transverse plane). Right lateral protrusion of the herniated intervertebral disc: (1) disc fragment on the right side; (2) mid-line exophytic growth. (Courtesy of Dr Mario Séguin.)

an areflexic detrusor. This areflexia is secondary to an impairment of the afferent, sensitive, branch of the sacral reflex arc which, in turn, influences its efferent, motor branch. The distal urethral sphincteric mechanism is usually intact.

There exists a particular form of lumbar disc protrusion, that is well documented in the literature – about 100 cases published, the majority in females – in which the only clinical symptom is urinary retention. The desire to void is modified, with the patient describing hypogastric fullness. Physicians should suspect this condition when the bladder has a huge capacity, a significant post-void residual urine, no bladder wall trabeculation, and a hyposensitive urethra and trigone during cystoscopy. Urodynamics will demonstrate a flat curve during the filling phase and an increased bladder wall compliance. The first desire to void is delayed, or even abolished. Electrophysiologic studies show an increased bulbocavernosus (or clitoridoanal) latency time. Radiologic exploration, preferably MRI, should confirm the clinical diagnosis (Figures 27.8 and 27.9).

Treatment is the surgical removal of the protruded disc. There is no concensus in the literature on the degree of urgency of this condition. Common sense dictates rapid intervention, when possible. Complete recovery of urethrovesical function may take months, or even years. An extended follow-up is indicated.

References

1. Spinner M, Spencer PS. Nerve compression lesions of the upper extremity. A clinical and experimental review. Clin Orthop 1974; 104:46–67.

2. Boden SD, Davis DO, Dina TS, et al. Abnormal magnetic-resonance scans of the lumbar spine in asymptomatic subjects. A prospective investigation. J Bone Joint Surg Am 1990; 72:403–408.

3. Williams AL, Haughton VM. Disc herniation and degenerative disc disease. In: Newton TH, Potts DG, eds. Modern neuroradiology, Vol. 1, Computed tomography of the spine and spinal cord. 1983; 213–249.

4. Siebner HR, Faulhauer K. Frequency and specific surgical management of far lateral lumbar disc herniations. Acta Neurochir (Wien) 1990; 105:124–131.

5. Dammers R, Koehler PJ. Lumbar disc herniation: level increases with age. Surg Neurol 2002; 58:209–212.

6. Russell EG. Cervical disc disease. Radiol 1990; 177:313–325.

7. Williams MP, Cherryman GR, Husband JE. Significance of thoracic disc herniation demonstrated by MR imaging. J Comput Assist Tomogr 1989; 13:211–214.

8. Awwad EE, Martin DS, Smith KR Jr, Baker BK. Asymptomatic versus symptomatic herniated thoracic discs: their frequency and characteristics as detected by computed tomography after myelography. Neurosurgery 1991; 28:180–186.

9. Stillerman CB, Chen TC, Couldwell WT, Zhang W, Weiss MH. Experience in the surgical management of 82 symptomatic herniated thoracic discs and review of the literature. J Neurosurg 1998; 88: 623–633.

10. Toribatake Y, Baba H, Kawahara N, et al. The epiconus syndrome presenting with radicular-type neurological features. Spinal Cord 1997; 35:163–170.

11. Goldman HB, Appell RA. Lumbar disc disease. In: Appell RA, ed. Voiding dysfunction. Totowa, NJ: Humana, 2000:149–162.

12. Orendacova J, Cizkoca D, Kafka J, et al. Cauda equina syndrome. Prog Neurobiol 2001; 64:613–637.

13. Wein AJ. Neuromuscular dysfunction of the lower urinary tract and its management. In: Walsh P, Retik AB, Vaughan ED Jr, Wein AJ, eds. Campbell's urology, 8th edn. Philadelphia: WB Saunders, 2002: 931–1026.

14. Silver JR. The earliest case of cauda equina syndrome caused by manipulation of the lumbar spine under general anesthetic. Spinal Cord 2001; 39:51–53.

15. Jennet WB. A study of 25 cases of compression of the cauda equina by prolapsed intervertebral disc. J Neurol Neurosurg Psychiatry 1956; 19:109–116.

16. Tay EC, Chacha PB. Midline prolapse of a lumbar intervertebral disc with compression of the cauda equina. J Bone Joint Surg Br 1979; 61-B:43–46.

17. Nielsen B, de Nully M, Schmidt K, Iversen-Hansen RI. A urodynamic study of cauda equina syndrome due to lumbar disc herniation. Urol Int 1980; 35:167–170.

18. Mixter WJ, Barr JS. Rupture of the intervertebral disc with involvement of the spinal canal. New Engl J Med 1934; 211:210–215.

19. Dandy WB. Serious complications of ruptured intervertebral disc. JAMA 1942; 119:474–477.

20. Ver Brugghen A. Massive extrusions of the lumbar intervertebral disc. Surg Gyn Obstet 1945; 81:269–277.

21. Waris W. Lumbar disc herniation. Acta Chir Scand 1948 (Suppl 140): 1–134.

22. O'Connell JE. Protrusion of the lumbar intervertebral discs. A clinical review based on 500 cases treated by excision of the protrusion. J Bone Joint Surg Br 1951; 33-B:8–30.

23. Eyre-Brook AL. A study of late results from disc operations. Br J Surg 1952; 39:289.

24. Shephard RH. Diagnosis and prognosis of cauda equina syndrome produced by protrusion of lumbar disc. Br Med J 1959; 2: 1434–1439.

25. Wilson PJ. Cauda equina compression due to intrathecal herniation of an intervertebral disk: a case report. Br J Surg 1962; 49:423–426.

26. Scott PJ. Bladder paralysis in cauda equina lesions from disc prolapse. J Bone Joint Surg 1965; 47-B:224–235.

27. Aho AJ, Auranen A, Pesonen K. Analysis of cauda equina symptoms in patients with lumbar disc prolapse. Preoperative and follow-up clinical and cystometric studies. Acta Chir Scand 1969; 135:413–420.

28. Rosomoff HL, Johnson JD, Gallo AE, et al. Cystometry in the evaluation of nerve root compression in the lumbar spine. Surg Gyn Obstet 1963; 117:263–270.

29. Andersen JT, Bradley WE. Neurogenic bladder dysfunction in protruded lumbar disc and after laminectomy. Urology 1976; 8:94–96.

30. Mosdal C, Iversen P, Iversen-Hansen R. Bladder neuropathy in lumbar disc disease. Acta Neurochir (Wien) 1979; 46:281–286.

31. Gangai M. Acute urinary obstruction secondary to neurologic diseases. J Urol 1966; 95:805–808.

32. Emmett JL, Love JG. Urinary retention in women caused by asymptomatic protruded lumbar disc: report of 5 cases. J Urol 1968; 99:597–606.

33. Emmett JL, Love JG. Vesical dysfunction caused by protuded lumbar disc. J Urol 1971; 105:86–91.

34. Malloch JD. Acute retention due to intervertebral disc prolapse. Br J Urol 1965; 37:578.

35. Yarxley RP. Note on urinary retention due to intervertebral disc prolapse. Br J Urol 1966; 38:324–325.

36. Ivanovici F. Urine retention: an isolated sign in some spinal cord disorders. J Urol 1970; 104:284–286.

37. Ross JC, Jameson RM. Vesical dysfunction due to prolapsed disc. Br Med J 1971; 3:752–754.

38. Kontturi M. Investigations into bladder dysfunction in prolapse lumbar intervertebral disc. Ann Chir Gynaecol Fenn Suppl 1968; 162:1–53.

39. Cheek WR, Anchondo H, Raso E, Scott B. Neurogenic bladder and lumbar spine. Urology 1973; 2:30–33.

40. Dan N, Golovsky D, Sharpe D. Urinary retention and intervertebral disc protrusion. Med J Aust 1980; 2:258–260.

41. Susset JG, Peters ND, Cohen SI, Ghonhem GM. Early detection of neurogenic bladder dysfunction caused by protruded lumbar disc. Urology 1982; 20:461–463.

42. Hsu CH. Herniated disk: an obscure cause of neurogenic bladder in males. Kans Med 1996; 97:16–17.

43. Sylvester PA, McLoughlin J, Sibley GN, et al. Neuropathic urinary retention in the absence of neurological signs. Postgrad Med J 1995; 71:747–748.

44. Kontturi M, Harviainen S, Larmi TK. Atonic bladder in lumbar disc herniation. Acta Chir Scand Suppl 1966; 357:232–235.

45. Jones DL, Moore T. The types of neuropathic bladder dysfunction associated with prolapsed lumbar intervertebral discs. Br J Urol 1973; 45:39–43.

46. Fanciullacci F, Sandri S, Politi P, Zanollo A. Clinical, urodynamic and neurophysiological findings in patients with neuropathic bladder due to a lumbar intervertebral disc protrusion. Paraplegia 1989; 27:354–358.

47. Gleave JR, Macfarlane R. Prognosis for recovery of bladder function following lumbar central disc prolapse. Brit J Neurosurg 1990; 4:205–209.

48. Rosomoff HL. The neurogenic bladder of lumbar disc syndromes. Trans Am Neurol Assoc 1964; 89:249–251.

49. Delamarter RB, Bohlman HH, Bodner D, Biro C. Urologic function after experimental cauda equina compression. Cystometrograms versus cortical-evoked potentials. Spine 1990; 15:864–870.

50. Kostuik JP, Harrington I, Alexander D, et al. Cauda equina syndrome and lumbar disc herniation. J Bone Joint Surg Am 1986; 68:386–391.

51. Chuang TY, Cheng H, Chan RC, et al. Neurourologic findings in patients with traumatic thoracolumbar vertebra junction lesions. Arch Phys Med Rehabil 2001; 82:375–379.

52. Jameson RM. Urological management in non-traumatic paraplegia: disc protrusions, multiple sclerosis and spinal metastasis. Paraplegia 1976; 13:228–234.

53. Hellström P, Kortelainen P, Kontturi M. Late urodynamic findings after surgery for cauda equina syndrome caused by a prolapsed lumbar intervertebral disc. J Urol 1986; 135:308–312.

54. Shin JC, Park CI, Kim HJ, Lee IY. Significance of low compliance bladder in cauda equina injury. Spinal Cord 2002; 40:650–655.

55. Norlèn L, Dahlstrom A, Sundin T, Svedmyr N. The adrenergic innervation and adrenergic receptor activity of the feline urinary bladder and urethra in the normal state and after hypogastric and/or parasympathetic denervation. Scand J Urol Nephrol 1976; 10:177–184.

56. Murnaghan GF, Gowland SP, Rose M, et al. Experimental neurogenic disorders of the bladder after section of the cauda equina. Br J Urol 1979; 51:518–523.

57. Sandri SD, Fanciullacci F, Zanollo A. Pharmacologic tests in low compliance areflexic bladders. Proc 15th Annual Meeting ICS, London, 1987:162.

58. Sandri SD, Fanciullacci F, Politi P, Zanollo A. Urinary disorders in intervertebral disc prolapse. Neurourol Urodyn 1987; 6:11–19.

59. McGuire EJ. Urodynamic evaluation after abdomino-perineal resection and lumbar intervertebral disc herniation. Urology 1975; 6:63–70.

60. Rosomoff HL, Johnston JD, Gallo HE, et al. Cystometry as an adjunct in the evaluation of lumbar disc syndromes. J Neurosurg 1970; 33:67–74.

61. Robinson RG. Massive protrusions of lumbar discs. Br J Surg 1965; 52:858–865.

62. Dinning TA, Schaeffer HR. Discogenic compression of the cauda equina: a surgical emergency. Aust NZ J Surg 1993; 63:927–934.

63. Kennedy JG, Soffe KE, McGrath A, et al. Predictors of outcome in cauda equina syndrome. Eur Spine J 1999; 8:317–322.

64. Shapiro S. Medical realities of cauda equina syndrome secondary to lumbar disc herniation. Spine 2000; 25:348–351.

65. Gleave JR, Macfarlane R. Cauda equina syndrome: what is the relationship between timing of surgery and outcome? Br J Neurosurg 2002; 16:325–328.

66. Leroi AM, Berkelmans I, Rabehenoina C, et al. Results of therapeutic management of vesico-urethral and anorectal disorders in 20 patients with cauda equina syndrome. Neurochirurgie (Paris) 1994; 40:301–306.

67. Chang HS, Nakagawa H, Mizuno J. Lumbar herniated disc presenting with cauda equina syndrome. Long-term follow-up of four cases. Surg Neurol 2000; 53:100–104.

28

Spinal and cord tumors

Jacques Corcos and Rafael Glickstein

Introduction

The most common spinal tumors are extradural metastasis from another primary neoplasia. Primary spinal cord tumors are infrequent, representing only 10–15% of all primary central nervous system (CNS) lesions. In the pediatric population, astrocytomas are the most persistent tumors. In adults, neurofibromas, meningiomas, ependymomas, and astrocytomas are the most commonly found lesions.[1]

Spinal tumors are usually classified according to their origin and topography. Okuyama et al[2] categorized spinal metastasis as, first, extradural lesions arising either from a bony metastasis on a vertebra or from a lesion in the peridural space. Both lesions give cord compression symptoms. Intradural carcinomatosis, the second category of spinal metastasis, evokes cord irritative symptoms. The last but rare category comprises intramedullary metastasis.[2,3]

Primary spinal neoplasias are classified as extramedullary–intradural and intramedullary lesions. Extramedullary–intradural tumors are essentially meningiomas and neurofibromas/schwannomas. Intramedullary lesions are most frequently astrocytomas, ependymomas, and, rarely, hemangioblastomas or lipomas.[4]

Clinical presentation

Besides the frequent bladder or external sphincter dysfunction secondary to these tumors, pain, motor and sensory disturbances, bowel, and sexual dysfunctions are often

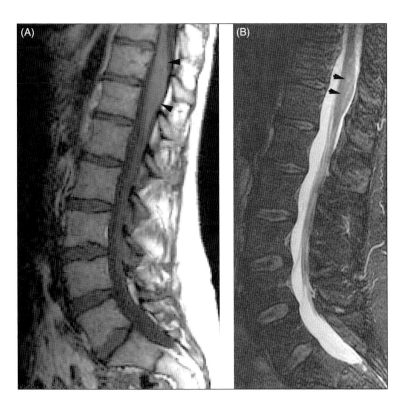

Figure 28.1
Ependymoma. Sagittal T1 (A) and T2 (B) MRI of the lumbar spine demonstrates heterogeneous mass lesion (arrows) of the distal cord extending to the conus medullaris. This mass represents an ependymoma.

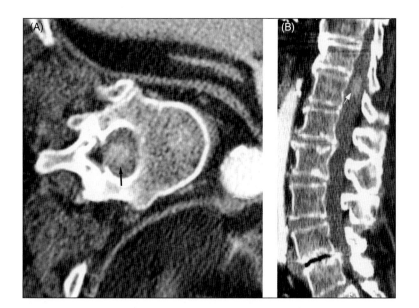

Figure 28.2
Intramedullary metastasis. Infused axial CT (A) and reconstructed sagittal (B) imaging of the lumbar spine on a patient with a pacemaker and a clinical history of breast carcinoma demonstrates enhancing mass lesion corresponding to intramedullary metastatic lesion.

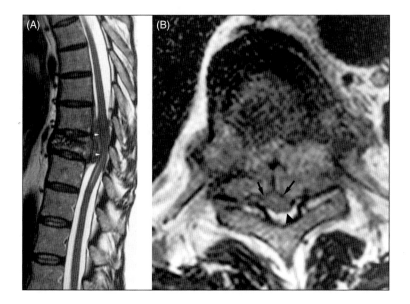

Figure 28.3
Cord compression due to epidural metastasis. Sagittal (A) and axial (B) T2 MRI of the thoracic spine demonstrates cord compression at the T7 level due to epidural mass (arrows) and associated pathological fracture due to metastasis of bladder carcinoma. Note early syringomyelia of the distal cord.

associated symptoms. According to Copeman,[5] the reasons for consulting are back pain in 68%, lower limb weakness in 61%, and urinary retention in 36% of these patients. Barron et al[3] found back pain in 75%, motor or sensitive nerve compression symptoms in 68%, and urinary retention in 39% of such cases. Pain is typically worse at night and aggravated by maneuvers that increase intracranial pressure such as straining or coughing. Nerve compression leads to reduced sensation of pain and extreme temperatures, long track signs, weakness, constipation, and retention as well as sphincteric deficiency in cauda equina syndromes. The lower the lesion the more frequent are the urinary symptoms. Hattori et al[6] reported that 93% of cases with lesions at L1 or lower presented with urinary

retention or irritative bladder symptoms. Similar observations were made by Campbell.[7]

Clinical diagnosis

Characteristics of pain and neurological deficits or irritative symptoms are key elements of the clinical diagnosis. Physical examination may reproduce the pain by vertebral palpation and confirm the neurological findings of decreased pain and/or temperature sensation, muscle weakness, modified lower limb reflexes, diminished anal tone, and bulbo (or clitorido) cavernous reflex. Suprapubic palpation of a vesical globe may incriminate urinary retention.

Urinary symptoms as first presentation of a spinal cord tumor are rare.[8] Sloof et al[9] reviewed 301 cases of spinal cord tumors and found only 2.6% revealed by urinary or bowel symptoms. This confirmed the frequency reported by Campbell[7] (20%) but was much higher than the results of Barron et al[3] who reported 38% of prostate cancer bony metastases revealed by a urinary retention.

Imaging

Suspicions of bony metastases can be confirmed by plain film of the spine showing either hyperdensity typical of an osteoblastic lesion, or hypodensity and destruction typical of an osteoclastic lesion.

Nuclear bone scan is extremely useful for screening of non-symptomatic metastasis or to detect early lesions. Bone scans are not specific to the lesion type (primary, secondary, benign, infection, etc.) and have to be interpreted in the clinical context.

Magnetic resonance imaging (MRI) is the radiographic technique of choice in the evaluation of spinal tumoral lesions. Multiplanar imaging with different MRI techniques can assess the precise anatomical location, extent of the pathological processes, and correct relationship with other anatomical structures.

The classification of intramedullary, intradural, or extradural lesions based on myelograms can be better evaluated by MRI. With signal characteristics, location, and relationship of the lesion, it is often possible to be certain of the case histology. Nevertheless, computed tomography (CT) scans or myelograms are still useful when MRI scanning is contraindicated because of metallic cerebral clips, pacemakers, etc.

Treatment

It is not the focus of this chapter to detail the specific treatment of tumoral lesions. Surgery, radiation therapy, hormonotherapy, bisphosphonates, and chemotherapy are used alone or combined in the treatment of primary and secondary tumors.

Urological treatment of the lower urinary dysfunction provoked by these lesions depends on the type of dysfunction.[6] Urinary retention is usually managed by clean intermittent catheterization (CIC). When medical management fails with myorelaxant agents such as baclofen and botulinum toxin injections, detrusor-sphincter dyssynergia is usually managed by CIC as far as symptoms are present (mainly retention and/or high pressure voiding). Overactive bladders are usually treated with anticholinergics. Other treatment modalities such as botulinum toxin, intravesical instillation, neuromodulation, etc., can also be proposed.

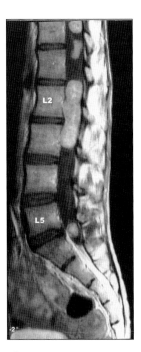

Figure 28.4
Multiple neurofibromas. Infused sagittal T1-weighted MRI of the lumbar spine showing multiple intradural enhancing mass lesions corresponding to neurofibromas on a patient with neurofibromatosis type II.

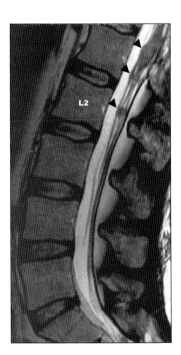

Figure 28.5
Intraconal and intradural extramedullary metastatic lesion. Sagittal T2 MRI of the lumbar spine demonstrates intraconal and cauda equina nodules (arrows) from primitive neuroectodermal tumor.

However, no experience with their use in the treatment of neurogenic bladder secondary to spinal cord tumor has been reported, and one must consider the prognosis of the tumor when choosing the best therapeutic approach.

References

1. Preston-Martin S. Epidemiology of primary CNS neoplasms. Neurol Clin 1996; 14:273–290.

2. Okuyama T, Suzuki S, Ono K, et al. Metastatic spinal tumor involving the spinal cord. An analytical study on a series of 12 cases verified by myelography and/or autopsy. Bull Tokyo Med Dent Univ 1969; 16:187–209.

3. Barron KD, Hirano A, Araki S, Terry RD. Experience with metastatic neoplasms involving the spinal cord. Neurology 1959; 9:91.

4. Preston-Martin S. Epidemiology of primary CNS neoplasms. Neurol Clin 1996; 14:273–290.

5. Copeman MC. Presenting symptoms of neoplastic spinal cord compression. J Surg Oncol 1988; 37:24–25.

6. Hattori T, Yasuda K, Sakakibara R, Yamanishi T, Kitahara H, Hirayama K. Micturitional disturbance in tumors of the lumbosacral area. J Spinal Disord 1992; 5(2):193–197.

7. Campbell EW Jr. Bladder dysfunction related to lesions of the spinal cord. South Med J 1967; 60:364–366.

8. Gunasekera WS, Richardson AE, Seneviratne KN, Eversden ID. Clinical correlation of urodynamic findings in patients with localized partial lesions of the spinal cord and cauda equina. Surg Neurol 1984; 21:148–154.

9. Sloof JL, Hernohas JW, McCarty CS. Primary intramedullary tumours of the spinal cord and filum terminal. Philadelphia: WB Saunders, 1964.

29

Spinal cord injury and cerebral trauma

Jerzy B Gajewski

Introduction

Disturbances of micturition are very common with head and spinal cord injuries. The range of bladder symptoms caused by neurological lesions is wide and determined by whether the lesion primarily affects supraspinal control, the pontine–sacral neural circuit, or the sacral nerves and whether these lesions are predominantly motor or sensory, or both. The role of this innervation in bladder physiology is the key to understanding bladder dysfunction in head trauma and spinal cord injury.

Neuroanatomy

The function of the lower urinary tract is storage of urine and emptying when socially accepted. This is controlled and coordinated by the neurological system. Micturition is a coordinated contraction of the detrusor muscle of the bladder and relaxation of the proximal (smooth muscle of the bladder neck and urethra) and distal (striated muscle) external urethral sphincters following release of cortical inhibition. Control of micturition is localized in the cortical, pontine, and sacral centers connected by a neural circuit that extends from the cortex through the pons to the sacral cord.[1,2] The cortical areas influencing bladder control include the limbic lobes and paracentral lobules from which fibers pass to the pons and downward in the corticospinal tracts to the anterior and lateral horn cells at S2–4. In rat locus ceruleus may be involved in arousal, which is mediated by bladder distention.[3]

Human positron emission tomography (PET) scans have shown two distinct cortical areas involved in micturition and contraction of the pelvic floor[4] (Figure 29.1). The right prefrontal cortex showed increased activity during micturition and during attempts to voluntarily inhibit voiding. The anterior cingulated gyrus activity is decreased during inhibition of voiding. Voluntary contraction of the female pelvic floor causes increased activity in superomedial precentral gyrus (part of the primary motor cortex).[5]

Basal ganglia, hypothalamus, and cerebellum all modulate function of the lower urinary tract through the pontine micturition center (PMC).

Coordination of the detrusor contraction and sphincter relaxation is mainly done by the PMC located in the brainstem. Normally, the external sphincter activity increases during bladder distention, then ceases when a bladder contraction occurs. In the cat, there appears to be a spinal neural organization that can mediate coordinated activity in the bladder preganglionic neurons and pudendal interneuron pools independently from the PMC.[6,7]

There seem to be two centers in the pontine region; first, the PMC, which is responsible for emptying, is located in the nucleus ceruleus alpha (Lca) M region, and, secondly, the pontine urine storage facilitator center (PUSFC), which is located in the nucleus locus subceruleus (Lsc) L region.[8,9] PET study in healthy men and women confirmed the presence of the L region and the M region (Figure 29.2).[3,4] Experimental study on cats showed that the ascending projection from the lumbosacral region transmitted information from the bladder to the periaqueductal gray (PAG) and initiated voiding by triggering the M region of the PMC (Figure 29.3).[10] Facilitatory and inhibitory influences from the cortical and subcortical centers are exerted on this neural circuit, with the overall effect being inhibitory. Normal micturition is believed to involve a spino-bulbo-spinal reflex activation of parasympathetic preganglionic neurons (to the bladder) and inhibition of pudendal motoneurons – Onuf's nucleus (to the striated urethral sphincter).[11,12] PMC projection to the Onuf's nucleus is not direct and may involve interneurons in sacral intermediomedial (IMM) cell columns.[13] Afferent (sensory) and efferent (motor) nerve fibers connect the bladder and urethra to the sacral and thoracolumbar segments. Interneurons involved in bladder reflexes are located in the region of the sacral parasympathetic nucleus (SPN), the dorsal commissure (DCM), and superficial laminae of the dorsal horn.[14,15] In cats, Aδ fibers comprise the peripheral afferent pathway involved in the reflex.[16–18] Sensory fibers subserving proprioception and muscle stretch sensation from the lower urinary tract travel in

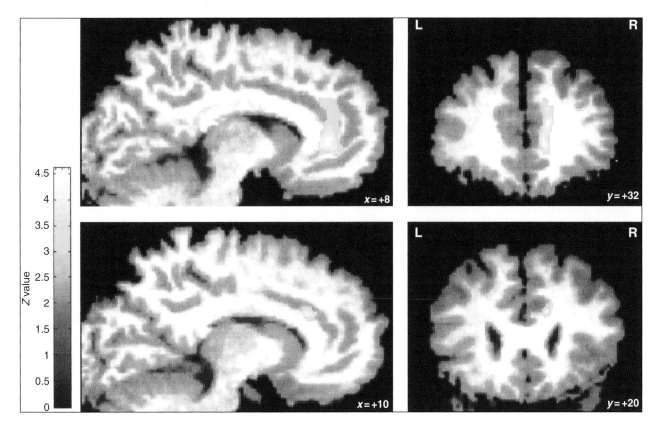

Figure 29.1

Top: significant differences in rCBF in the anterior cingulated gyrus, comparing successful micturition with voluntary withholding of urine (scan 2 − scan 1; average of 10 subjects). *Bottom*: significant differences in rCBF in the anterior cingulated gyrus, comparing unsuccessful micturition with voluntary withholding of urine (scan 2 − scan 1; average of 7 subjects). Uncorrected threshold of $p < 0.001$. (Reproduced with permission from Block[4].)

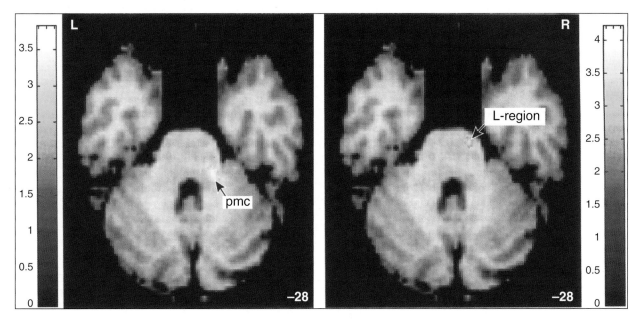

Figure 29.2

Left: significant differences in rCBF in the right dorsal pontine tegmentum (indicated by pmc = pontine micturition center) after the comparison between conditions 'successful micturition' (scan 2) and 'empty bladder' (scan 3). *Right*: significant differences in rCBF in the right ventral pontine tegmentum (indicated by L-region) after the comparison between conditions 'successful micturition' (scan 2) and 'empty bladder' (scan 3). The threshold used for display is uncorrected ($p < 0.005$). The number −28 refers to the distance in millimeters relative to the horizontal plane through the anterior and posterior commissures (z direction). The numbers on the color scale refer to the corresponding Z scores. Areas with significant activity are superimposed on the average MRI scan (from 6 normal subjects) and have been transformed stereotactically to fit a standard atlas. L = left side of the brain; R = right side. (Reproduced with permission from Block[5].)

the pelvic, hypogastric, and pudendal nerves to the sacral (S2, 3, and 4) and thoracolumbar (T11–L2) cord. Sensory impulses of touch, pain, and fullness from bladder mucosa travel via pelvic nerves. Most of these fibers are thin Aδ-myelinated axons and some are unmyelinated C-fiber axons. Most Aδ-myelinated axons connect to mechano-receptors in the detrusor (cats) and are involved in the normal micturitional reflex.[19] C fibers in the pelvic nerve do not transmit impulses from the bladder distention or contraction and are 'silent';[20] they have been found to be sensitized by intravesical chemical irritation (Figure 29.4). Some other reports indicated that both C fibers and Aδ-myelinated neurons can be silent.[21] Sensory impulses of temperatures and distention, particularly from the trigone, pass centrally in sympathetic nerves (hypogastric nerves and/or sacral sympathetic chain) and are relayed to the cortex for conscious awareness through the dorsal columns and spinothalamic tracts. This conscious awareness produces the feeling of bladder fullness, the desire to void, or pain.

Motor fibers pass distally along the same paths. The parasympathetic system via pelvic nerves exerts a con-tractile effect on detrusor muscle (muscarinic receptors). Parasympathetic preganglionic motoneurons are located in the S2–S4 segments in humans[22] and S1–S3 in cats[23] and reside in the sacral intermediolateral (IML) cell group. Parasympathetic neurons (nitric oxide) also mediate relaxation of the urethral smooth muscles during voiding.[24] The sympathetic system, via hypogastric nerves and sympathetic chain, innervates smooth muscles of the bladder (β receptors), bladder neck, and urethra (α_1 receptors). Human sympathetic preganglionic motoneurons are located in the lumbar intermediolateral area at the level of the L1–L4 cord.[22] The somatic system, via pudendal nerves (nicotinic receptors), controls the external striated urethral sphincter (rhabdosphincter). Although the pontine–sacral neural circuit for micturi-tion can function autonomously, it is controlled after infancy by higher inhibitory influences from the brain, which are under conscious, or at least precon-scious, control.[25]

Normally, the bladder will fill with urine slowly, stretching the detrusor muscle to accommodate a larger volume with low pressure. This bladder property is called compliance and depends on both neural and non-neural factors. During storage, parasympathetic activity is low, allowing the detrusor muscle to relax. Simultaneously, sympathetic activity is high, causing the smooth muscle of the bladder neck and urethra to contract. Sympathetic activity also inhibits parasympathetic ganglia (α_2 recep-tors) and relaxes detrusor directly (β receptors). Somatic activity increases with increased bladder volume, allow-ing the rhabdosphincter to remain contracted. When the bladder contains 400–500 ml of urine, there is cortical awareness of a desire to void. Micturition is initiated by

voluntary inhibition of the rhabdosphincter activity followed by deinhibition of the bladder reflexes. Parasympathetic activity increases and sympathetic and somatic activity decreases, allowing the detrusor to con-tract against little resistance and the bladder empties completely.

Central nervous system neuropharmacology

Catecholamines

Pelvic preganglionic and pudendal motoneuron areas in the sacral spinal cord receive catecholamine projections from pontine centers.[26,27] Thus, it would be expected that bladder and sphincter reflexes would be affected by adrenergic influences. Dorsal horn interneurons are sub-ject to descending modulation from the raphe magnus and locus ceruleus, implying mediation by a primary amine.[28] Alpha$_2$ agonists selectively suppress noxious inputs to dorsal horn projection neurons.[29] Whether the selective effect is also expressed on visceral inputs to such cells, or onto other cells in visceral spinal pathways, is unknown. The influence of norepinephrine (noradrena-line) on motor function may be due to a widespread action on interneurons in the ventral horn.[30] Central α adrenoceptors do influence somatic and viscerosomatic reflexes related to the external sphincter in animals[31–33] and probably in man.[34] It has been suggested that dorsal horn neurons can exhibit different or additional afferent inputs after spinal transection.[35] Anatomic plasticity of spinal synaptic contacts may underlie this phenomenon. Alpha$_2$ agonists also have a beneficial effect on bladder-sphincter dyssynergia[32] and on spasticity associated with spinal injury.[36]

Serotonin

The raphe magnus, raphe obscurus, and raphe pallidus provide the serotonergic innervation of the spinal cord.[37] The descending serotonergic projection consists of myelinated and unmyelinated fibers traveling in the dor-solateral funiculus.[38] Serotonin (5-hydroxytryptamine or 5-HT) is released in the dorsal horn by stimulation within the nucleus raphe magnus.[39] Multiple 5-HT-receptor subtypes have been located in the spinal cord.[40–42] Serotonin is considered as an inhibitory modu-lator of micturition at the spinal level.[43,44] Both a sero-tonergic agonist and a precursor inhibit bladder contractions in rats.[45] A 5-HT antagonist (methysergide) decreases the volume threshold of the micturition reflex

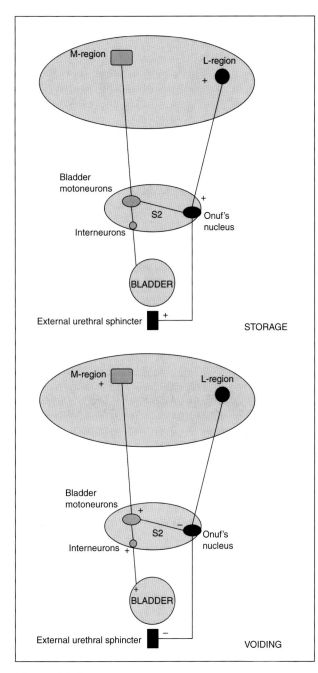

Figure 29.3
Arrangement of the sacro–pontine axis.

in cats.[46] At the supraspinal level, however, in normal conscious rats, 5-HT receptors can enhance the micturition reflex induced by bladder filling.[47]

Gamma aminobutyric acid

Gamma aminobutyric acid (GABA) is known to be involved in supraspinal control of micturition reflex.

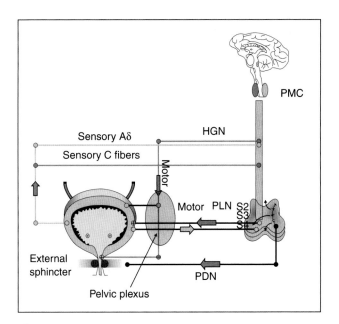

Figure 29.4
Innervation of the lower urinary tract. PMC, pontine micturition center; PDN, pudendal nerve (somatic); HGN, hypogastric nerve (sympathetic); PLN, pelvic nerve (parasympathetic).

GABA or GABA agonist suppresses reflex bladder activity and increases voiding threshold when injected into the brainstem, and the GABA antagonists have an opposite action. It appears that there is a tonic GABAergic supraspinal inhibition of the micturition reflex.[48,49]

Opioid peptides

Opioid peptides and related drugs are well-known modulators of nociception. They also influence somatic reflex mechanisms by a spinal action.[50] The pharmacology of opioids is complicated by the existence of several receptor types and subtypes[51] and the three major opioid receptor types – μ, δ, and κ – are present in the spinal cord.[52,53] Although there is evidence that there are at least two subtypes of κ receptor,[54] appropriately selective blocking drugs are available only for the κ_1 subtype.

Immunohistochemistry in the sacral spinal cord has demonstrated that both the parasympathetic nucleus (preganglionic neurons of the pelvic nerve) and Onuf's nucleus (motoneuron pool of the pudendal nerve to the external sphincter) are richly innervated by opioid-containing nerve terminals.[55] However, the details of the opioid pharmacology in these two areas differ.

The susceptibility of bladder function to depression by opioid peptides or morphine is well known in both animals and man.[56–62] The depression may be reversed by opioid antagonists or by increasing bladder pressure (i.e. bladder contraction can be obtained), but the volume threshold is increased.[60,62,63] Pharmacological analysis in animals has indicated that, at the spinal cord level, the inhibition of micturition is attributable to activation of δ-opioid receptors.[64] However, in man the involvement of μ-opioid receptors cannot be discounted due to the activity of epidural morphine.[57] It should be noted that epidural pentazocine, a κ-opioid agonist, does not produce urinary retention.[65] Also, it has been shown that while μ or δ opioids suppress micturition, they do not inhibit reflex-evoked pudendal nerve activity.[66,67] On the other hand, pudendal nerve activity is suppressed by ethylketocyclazocine, a fairly selective κ-opioid agonist.[67] The presence of opioid receptor subtypes selectively associated with different components of the sacral spinal mechanisms for bladder and sphincter control may make it possible to differentially affect the components.

Head injury
Coma

Head injury can cause temporary dysfunction (coma) or permanent lesion. Unconsciousness after cerebral injury relates to compression, hemorrhage, or ischemia. The brainstem can be displaced downwards or the temporal lobe herniates through the tentorial opening. Classification of the different stages of coma is best described by the Glasgow Scale.[68] The lesion has to be at the level of the midbrain and thalamus or higher to produce coma.[69] In most cases of coma, spontaneous micturition is possible and there seems to be some perception of bladder fullness in lighter stages.[70] Because only the suprapontine area is affected, coordination between the detrusor and sphincter remains. Voiding is synergistic, with no residual. Most of the patients, however, showed decreased detrusor compliance. An indwelling Foley catheter, which patients usually have, may cause detrusor irritation and may explain increased stiffness of the bladder. Lack of sympathetic inhibition of bladder activity by the cerebrum, as in progressive autonomic and multiple system failure,[71,72] can be another explanation. In some comatose patient, however, there is temporary bladder retention. It is not clear if this is related to bladder overstretching immediately after the accident or to active cerebral bladder inhibition. The possibility of temporary pontine shock similar to spinal shock cannot be excluded.

Suprapontine neurogenic detrusor overactivity

If the amount of cortical inhibition running in descending pathways is reduced by a suprapontine injury, there will be diminished awareness of bladder fullness, with diminished ability to inhibit the micturition reflex. This results in an uninhibited detrusor contraction, with synergistic relaxation of the proximal and distal sphincter. Animal studies showed that injury above the inferior colliculus eliminated the inhibitory effect on the micturition center, whereas a lesion below this point abolished the normal micturition reflex.[73] Human PET study showed that the control areas of micturition are mostly located on the right side of the brain (Figure 29.5).[4,74] Some clinical reports indicate that urge incontinence is more commonly associated with right-sided damage.[75] Other clinical observations suggest that unilateral right cortical lesions (prefrontal damage) produce transient dysfunction, whereas bilateral lesions produce permanent dysfunction.[76]

Experimental results indicate that supraspinal nitric oxide has an important role in bladder overactivity after cerebral infarction but it does not affect normal micturition in rats. This finding suggests a central mechanism sensitive to nitric oxide for bladder overactivity after cerebral infarction.[77]

During the filling phase, when the bladder contains a comparatively small volume of urine, inhibition of the suprapontine reflex arc will fail and the detrusor muscle will contract. There is no resistance from the urethra because of adequate relaxation of the sphincters due to the preserved sacro-pontine reflex arc. Patients with suprapontine detrusor overactivity will complain of frequency, urgency, and incontinence and, in severe cases, lack of sensory or motor control of the micturition reflex. They have no residual urine and thus are not prone to bladder infections.

Urodynamic studies may show early (small-volume) detrusor contractions, no detrusor-sphincter dyssynergia (the sphincter relaxes during detrusor contraction), and voiding without residual (Figure 29.6).

Spinal cord injury
Classification

The most comprehensive classification is that developed by the American Spinal Injury Association (ASIA) (Figure 29.7). It utilizes examination of dermatomes and myotomes to determine the level and completeness of the

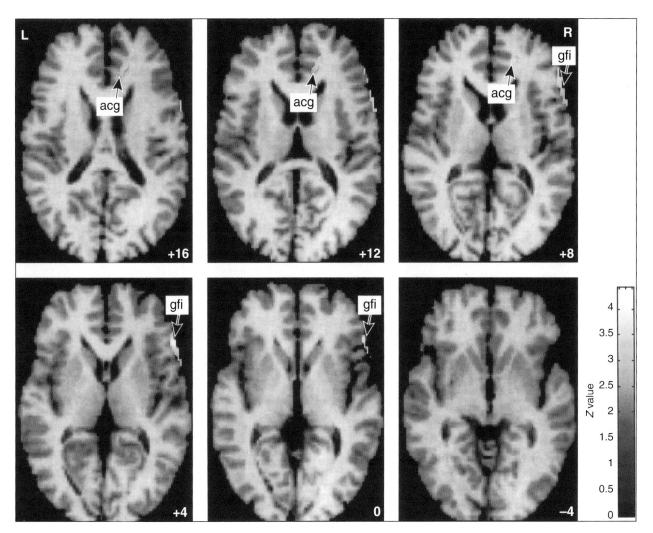

Figure 29.5
Significant differences in rCBF in the cortical areas after the comparison between the conditions 'successful micturition' (scan 2) and 'urine withholding' (scan 1). Note the activation of the right anterior cingulated gyrus (acg) in z planes +8 to +16, and the right inferior frontal gyrus (gfi) in z planes 0 to +12. (Reproduced with permission Block[5].)

sensory and motor functions and distinguishes four classes of spinal cord injury based on the Frankel system and five clinical syndromes:

- *Central cord syndrome* is a result of hemorrhagic necrosis of the central gray matter and some of the medial white matter and is most commonly due to hyperextension injury. More caudal fibers of the corticospinal and spinothalamic tract are localized in the spine more lateral, and hence are better protected from the central necrosis; consequently, arms are more affected than legs. Bladder dysfunction is also less common.

- *Brown-Séquard syndrome* is a rare unilateral cord condition which can result from penetrating injury or asymmetric disc herniation. It presents as ipsilateral motor weakness and sense impairment of fine touch and position and contralateral sensory impairment of

pain and temperature. Bladder dysfunction in the pure condition is uncommon.

- *Anterior cord syndrome* is characterized by injury to the anterior aspects of the cord, with preservation of the posterior columns and dorsal horns. There is a motor deficit and loss of pain and temperature sensation below the level of the injury.

- *Conus medullaris and cauda equina syndrome* result from damage to the conus and spinal nerve roots, leading to flaccid paraplegia and sensory loss. Sacral reflexes can be partially or totally lost.

The bladder in 'spinal shock'

Following an acute spinal cord injury (the first 2 weeks to 3 months) at a level above the sacral segments, the central synapses between the afferent and efferent arms of the

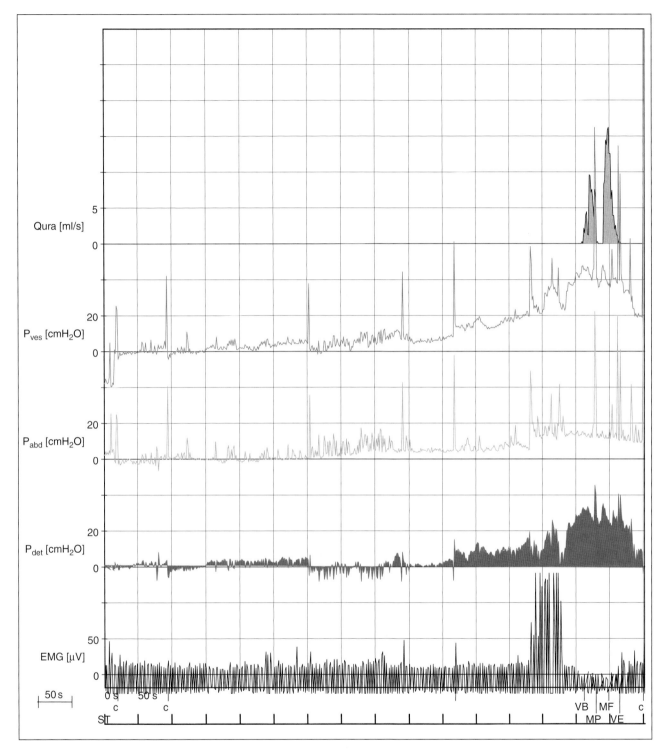

Figure 29.6

Pressure–flow study in the patient with a suprapontine lesion. The patient has no sensation; however, voiding is coordinated between the detrusor (P_{det}) and external sphincter EMG. EMG activity decreases during detrusor contraction. Qura, flow rate; P_{ves}, bladder pressure; P_{abd}, abdominal pressure.

micturition reflex will be rendered inactive. The mechanism of the spinal shock is unclear and may relate to lack of supraspinal facilitation or to total depression of the interneuronal activity due to release of inhibitory transmitters.

The detrusor will be paralyzed (acontractile detrusor), and there will be no conscious awareness of bladder fullness. However, the bladder neck and proximal urethra remains closed and the bladder will continue to distend because the

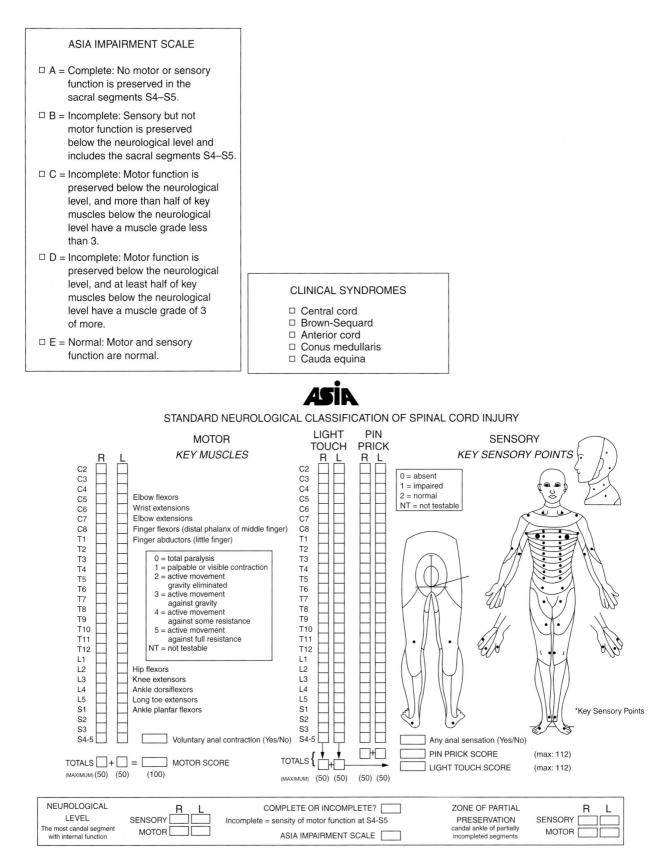

Figure 29.7
Classification developed by the American Spinal Injury Association (ASIA).

reflex arc does not function. The resulting retention of urine is followed by dribbling incontinence as a consequence of an overflow. Infection resulting from the large amount of residual urine may become a serious recurrent problem. The only reflex activity which is preserved or returns almost immediately is anal and bulbocavernosus reflex. Bladder reflex activity recovers usually within 2–3 months. It has been shown that sacral root stimulation during spinal shock facilitates recovery of the reflex activity of the detrusor.[78] We have also found that perineal and urethral stimulation is necessary for recovery of bladder reflex activity in spinally transected cats.[79]

Upper motor neuron lesion

Suprasacral neurogenic detrusor overactivity

This follows the stage of spinal shock resulting from a *cord injury above the S1 level.* Reflex bladder function eventually occurs in experimental animals and in man after suprasacral cord injury. This function is different from normal in that:

- it involves different afferent fibers (C fibers in the cat)[16]
- bladder contractions are poorly sustained[80]
- the urethra and bladder become discoordinated[81]
- previously 'irrelevant' stimuli influence the bladder[11] and/or external sphincter activity.[82]

Consciousness of bladder sensation may not be totally absent but voluntary inhibition of the micturition reflex arc is lost. The initial retention of urine with accompanying overflow incontinence during the stage of spinal shock gives way to the effects of an augmented reflex arc and results in a small, spastic, and overactive bladder. The bladder empties incompletely because of the dyssynergic contraction of the external sphincter, reflex inhibition from the dyssynergic sphincter, and primary detrusor failure (discoordinated contraction). Overall, this alteration in central organization results in a high voiding pressure, residual urine, and incontinence. These subsequently lead to recurrent infection, hydronephrosis, and finally to renal failure. In some instances of an incomplete suprasacral lesion, synergistic relaxation of the external sphincter is preserved. In these patients, given time, reflex bladder contraction in response to skin stimulation may be learned, thus allowing the patient some voluntary control.

Afferent fibers

Normal micturition reflex involves Aδ-fiber afferents. Only in inflammatory states are C-fiber afferents involved (chemosensitivity). After spinal cord injury C-fiber afferents mediate (mechanosensitivity) the abnormal sacral segmental bladder reflex.[16,83] The mechanism of this change from chemosensitivity to mechanosensitivity of C fibers is unclear.

Detrusor underactivity

The normal micturition reflex is controlled by spinal (sacral) and supraspinal centers.[84] After suprasacral spinal cord injury some reflex bladder function persists. However, the bladder contractions are ineffective and poorly sustained[80] and the urethra and bladder become uncoordinated.[32] It has been assumed that poor detrusor function is primarily due to reflex inhibition from the dyssynergic sphincter.[85] There are suggestions that primary detrusor failure might also be of significance.[86] In some instances of cervical and high thoracic spinal cord injury (10–20%) detrusor acontractility and external sphincter denervation is present, indicating a distinct and separate lesion in the sacral area.[87–89]

Detrusor-sphincter dyssynergia (internal and external)

Pons coordinate the micturition reflex. Any lesion between the sacral and pontine level may produce discoordinated voiding, which results in increased external sphincter activity during detrusor contraction. Detrusor-sphincter dyssynergia (DSD) correlates with a completeness but not the level of the upper motor neuron lesion.[90] DSD is responsible for the bladder outlet obstruction and, in combination with neurogenic detrusor overactivity, for high, sustained intravesical pressure, which is the most common cause of upper tract complications in spinal cord injury.[91,92] Diagnosis of DSD is based on electromyography (EMG) recording during cystometography (CMG) and voiding. There is an increased EMG activity during bladder contraction. In true DSD, increased EMG activity correlates with an ascending portion of the detrusor contraction curve, as opposed to dysfunction voiding, in which the EMG increase is more random (Figure 29.8).[93] Normal constant increase in the activity of the external urethral sphincter during bladder filling before contraction is called guarding reflex.[90] This reflex is lost in patients with complete upper motor neuron lesion and correlates well with DSD.[94]

The sympathetic system controls the bladder neck and proximal urethra from T10 to L2 spinal cord segments.[95] A spinal cord lesion above T10 removes supraspinal inhibitory control of the sympathetic vesicourethral neurons, resulting in bladder neck functional obstruction (smooth muscles dyssynergia).[96] Urologic manifestations of smooth muscle dyssynergia are the same as

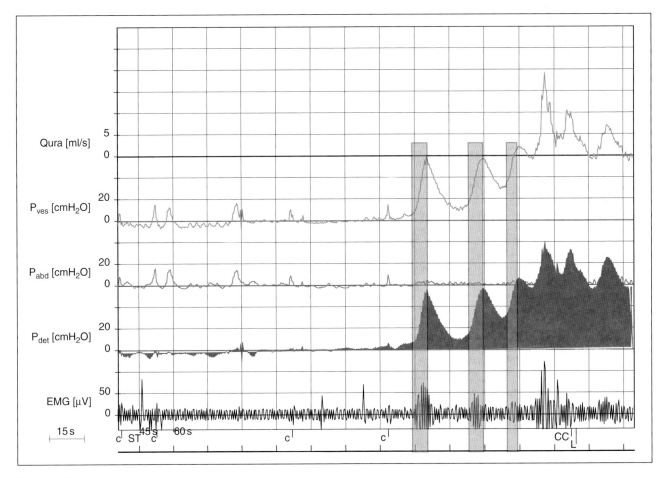

Figure 29.8
Pressure–flow study in the patient with a suprasacral complete lesion. The patient has detrusor-sphincter dyssynergia (DSD). Increase in external sphincter EMG activity is during the ascending phase of detrusor contraction (P_{det}) – shaded area. There is no urine flow because of severe bladder outlet obstruction due to DSD. Qura, flow rate; P_{ves}, bladder pressure; P_{abd}, abdominal pressure.

with detrusor-external sphincter dyssynergia. Outflow obstruction is at the level of the bladder neck and proximal urethra and adds to the obstruction at the level of the external sphincter.[97]

Abnormal reflex activity after spinal injury

Bladder activity can be influenced not only by its own sensory inputs but also by those from the colon and anal sphincter[98] and from somatic structures (e.g. perineum).[99] Visceral afferents can also have effects on somatic reflexes, particularly polysynaptic ones.[99] Sacral spinal interneurons appear to be one site for these interactions. After acute suprasacral spinal transection, the external urethral sphincter quickly recovers its response to bladder distention. However, the absence of the normal suppression of this reflex during bladder contraction creates inefficient voiding. In chronic suprasacral spinal injury, previously

'irrelevant' stimuli to penis, perineal skin, etc., can cause bladder contraction[11,99] and/or external sphincter activity[82] in both man and animals.

The 'skin–CNS–bladder reflex', in animal experiments, is effective in initiating bladder contractions after acute transection of the lumbar spinal cord. It is suggested that somatic motor axons can innervate bladder parasympathetic ganglion cells and thereby transfer somatic reflex activity to the bladder smooth muscle.[100]

Autonomic dysreflexia

In the patient with a neurologic midthoracic or higher spinal lesion, autonomic dysreflexia may occur.[101,102] These syndromes are secondary to loss of supraspinal inhibitory control of a thoracolumbar sympathetic outflow and result from massive discharge of the sympathetic system. Systemic manifestation of the autonomic dysreflexia

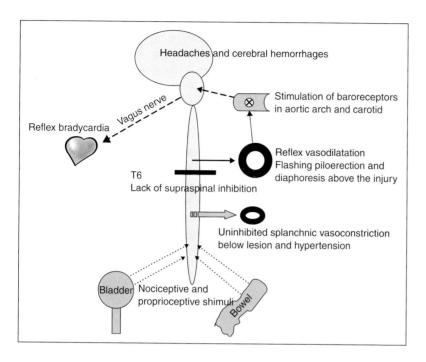

Figure 29.9
Autonomic dysreflexia.

(usually with lesion above T6) includes sweating below and cutaneous flushing above the level of the neurologic lesion, pounding headache, nasal congestion, and piloerection.[103,104] Splanchnic vasoconstriction occurs rapidly, causing hypertension which may be life threatening due to intracranial hemorrhage. There is a paradoxical bradycardia, mediated through vagus nerves (Figure 29.9). Autonomic dysreflexia can be triggered by noxious stimulus below the level of the spinal cord injury, and includes bladder distention, urologic manipulations, constipation, and skin irritation.[105] The severity of the dysreflexia depends on the sprouting of myelinated and unmyelinated primary afferents below the injury. Although there is no evidence that sprouting reaches directly autonomic or motor neurons, an increased pool of interneurons contributes to exaggerated autonomic reflexes (dysreflexia).[106] An animal study showed that blocking intraspinal sprouting minimized dysreflexia.[107]

Lower motor neuron lesion

Spinal cord injury to the *sacral paths at S1–4* results in parasympathetic decentralization of the bladder detrusor and somatic denervation of the external urethral sphincter and loss of some afferent pathways. In a complete lesion, conscious awareness of bladder fullness will be lost and the micturition reflex is absent. Some pain sensation can be preserved because the hypogastric (sympathetic) nerve is intact.

Bladder

Parasympathetic decentralization results in degeneration and regeneration changes in the muscle cells of the bladder detrusor as well as in their innervating axons[108] and that can account for the abnormal physiologic and pharmacologic behavior observed. In the chronic decentralized human and feline bladder, an increase in adrenergic innervation to the detrusor has been reported.[109–111] This results in the outgrowth of sympathetic fibers in the detrusor and the conversion of their functional role from β-adrenoreceptor-mediated relaxation to α-adrenoreceptor-mediated contraction.[109,110,112] This change in sympathetic function appeared only after complete lesions.[112] On the other hand, deGroat and Kawatani[113] postulated that unilateral parasympathetic preganglionic denervation of the detrusor leads to a reinnervation of the denervated cholinergic ganglions by sympathetic preganglionic pathways. This new pathway provides a means for eliciting excitatory bladder muscle responses.

It has been suggested that an altered sympathetic pathway could explain the decrease in detrusor compliance associated with lower motor neuron (LMN) lesions in monkeys[114] and dogs.[115] McGuire and Morrissey[114] demonstrated in monkeys that complete intradural sacral rhizotomy produced hypertonic areflexic bladder, whereas selective dorsal root damage produced hypotonic areflexic detrusor. Further studies showed that α-adrenergic blockade partially reversed the effect of chronic denervation on detrusor compliance in these animals[116] and in dogs.[115] Gunasekera et al[117] reported decreased bladder compliance in more than half of patients with acquired LMN lesions. More than 70% of patients with myelodysplasia have bladders with low compliance.[118] In our study[119] of patients with LMN lesions, all of which were on intermittent catheterization, we could not demonstrate any changes in detrusor compliance, regardless of whether the lesion was complete or incomplete. This is in agreement with a laboratory study[120] in which compliance was not decreased 3 months after sacral root injury in cats. These findings imply that ongoing activity from the sacral cord or pelvic afferent nerve traffic is not required for the maintenance of normal detrusor compliance in this situation. The role of the sympathetic system, however, in the parasympathetically decentralized bladder detrusor is still unclear.

The chronic complete parasympathetically decentralized bladder develops supersensitivity to muscarinic stimulants[121] which can be demonstrated as a marked increase in the intravesical pressure, in response to subcutaneous bethanechol. In partial LMN lesions, supersensitivity was not detected in rats[122] or dogs.[123] Using an alternative way of performing the bethanechol test (reduction in threshold dose of bethanechol rather than an increase in bladder pressure used as an indicator), El-Salmy et al[124] demonstrated supersensitivity of the detrusor in cats with partial sacral rhizotomies. In our study,[119] patients with complete or incomplete lesions responded to bethanechol injection with bladder pressure increase, although the more dramatic response was seen in patients with complete lesions. These findings dispute the validity of the bethanechol test in differentiating between complete and incomplete lesions.

Urethra and external urinary sphincter

Urethra is mainly innervated by the sympathetic system and only sparsely by the parasympathetic system. Maximum urethral pressure (MUP) values were low, however, in our patients[119] when compared with our normal values or other[125] standards. There was no significant difference between complete and incomplete lesions. Mattiasson et al[126] also reported that MUP was significantly lower in patients with parasympathetic decentralization than in volunteers. Loss of somatic innervation to the external sphincter may account for this finding. Phentolamine had little effect on MUP in our study in contrast to the finding in volunteers with normal lower urinary tracts.[125] There is a possibility that sympathetic influence over urethral closure pressure has been lost in this situation. Other researchers have reported variable urethral pressure profile responses to α-adrenergic blockers in LMN lesions.[127] In a complete LMN lesion due to somatic denervation of the external sphincter, striated muscle activity is abnormal. EMG is characterized by individual action potentials which are of increased amplitude and duration, and are polyphasic with

some abnormal spontaneous activity in the form of positive waves and fibrillation potentials.[128] Conscious control is lost; however, some muscle tone is preserved. Narrowing in the region of the external urethral sphincter is not an uncommon finding. Proposed mechanisms include:

- fibrosis of the urethral sphincter[129]
- sympathetic dyssynergia[130]
- denervation supersensitivity[131] or autonomic reinnervation of the rhabdosphincter.[132]

Bladder neck and proximal urethra

Bladder neck and proximal urethra receive a dual cholinergic and adrenergic innervation from the pelvic and hypogastric nerve, respectively.[112,133–135] Laboratory studies have demonstrated a predominance of α-adrenergic receptors in that area.[136–138] Normally, the bladder neck should remain closed except during voiding.[139] Neurogenic and non-neurogenic factors influence competence of the bladder neck. The hydromechanical effect of Credé's maneuver has been shown to reduce proximal urethral closure pressure in cats with a sacral injury.[140] It is not clear if an open bladder neck in an LMN lesion is a primary neurologic defect or is secondary to associated detrusor dysfunction (increased stiffness or autonomous waves) or treatment. There are conflicting reports regarding what neurologic lesion causes an open bladder neck.[118,141,142] McGuire and Wagner[142] found that a complete, isolated sacral decentralization of the parasympathetic and pudendal nerves did not result in an open bladder neck, which conflicts with our results.[119] We have shown that bladder neck incompetence is related to completeness of the LMN lesion and that α-sympathetic blockade (phentolamine) had an effect on the bladder neck closing mechanism only in incomplete lesions. The data imply that, in addition to sympathetic function, some sacral root activity takes part in the maintenance of bladder neck closure, either through efferent parasympathetic activity or by providing an afferent link to a sympathetic reflex. Kirby et al[143] found the bladder neck open in all patients with pelvic nerve injury or cauda equina lesion. Open bladder neck was also found in almost 90% of children with myelodysplasia.[118] Extensive autonomic system damage (after A-P resection) was found to be associated with open bladder neck, probably due to sympathetic denervation.[144] However, a contribution from the increased intravesical pressure cannot be ruled out.

Neurogenic bladder dysfunction is more common than was previously diagnosed. A recent report by Ahlberg et al[145] showed that up to 82% of 'idiopathic bladder' dysfunction has pathologic neurologic findings, which indicates that patients with voiding dysfunction should be considered to have a neurologic underlying condition unless proven otherwise.

References

1. Barrington FJF. The effect of lesions of the hind- and mid-brain on micturition in the cat. Quart J Exp Physiol 1925; 15:81–102.

2. Bradley WE, Teague CT. Spinal cord representation of the peripheral neural pathways of the micturition reflex. J Urol 1969; 101:220–223.

3. Imada N, Koyama Y, Kawauchi A, et al. State dependent response of the locus caeruleus neurons to bladder distention. J Urol 2000; 164(5):1740–1744.

4. Block BFM, Willemsen ATM, Holstege G. A PET study on the brain control micturition in humans. Brain 1997; 120:111–121.

5. Block BFM, Sturms LM, Holstege G. Brain activation during micturition in women. Brain 1998; 121:2033–2042.

6. Shefchyk SJ. The effect of lumbosacral deafferentation on pontine micturition centre-evoked voiding in the decerebrate cat. Neurosci Lett 1989; 99:175–180.

7. Fedirchuk B, Shefchyk SJ. Effects of electrical stimulation of the thoracic spinal cord on bladder and external urethral sphincter activity in the decerebrate cat. Exp Brain Res 1991; 84:635–642.

8. Griffiths D, Holstege G, Dalm E, de Wall H. Control and coordination of the bladder and urethral function in the brainstem of the cat. Neurourol Urodyn 1990; 9:63–82.

9. Nishizawa O, Sugaya K. Cat and dog: higher centre of micturition. Neurourol Urodyn 1994; 13:169–179.

10. Block BFM, de Weerd H, Holstege G. Ultrastructural evidence for a paucity of projections from the lumbosacral cord to the pontine micturition centre or M-region in the cat: a new concept for organization of micturition reflex with the periaqueductal gray as central relay. J Comp Neurol 1995; 359:300–309.

11. De Groat WC, Ryall RW. Reflexes to sacral parasympathetic neurones concerned with micturition in the cat. J Physiol (Lond) 1969; 200:87–108.

12. Blaivas JG. The neurophysiology of micturition: a clinical study of 550 patients. J Urol 1982; 127:958–963.

13. Holstege G, Griffiths D, De Wall H, Dalm E. Anatomical and physiological observation on supraspinal control of bladder and urethral sphincter muscles in the cat. J Comp Neurol 1986; 250: 449–461.

14. De Groat WC, Araki I, Vizzard MA, et al. Developmental and injury induced plasticity in micturition reflex pathway. Behav Brain Res 1998; 92:127–140.

15. Nadelhaft I, Vera PL. Neurons in the rat brain and spinal cord labeled after pseudorabies virus injected into the external urethral sphincter. J Comp Neurol 1996; 375:502–517.

16. De Groat WC, Nadelhaft I, Milne RJ, et al. Organization of the sacral parasympathetic reflex pathways to the urinary bladder and large intestine. J Auton Nerv Syst 1981; 3:135–160.

17. De Groat WC. Neuropeptides in pelvic afferent pathways. Experientia 1987; 43:801–813.

18. De Groat WC. Spinal cord projections and neuropeptides in visceral afferent neurons. Prog Brain Res 1986; 67:165–187.

19. Habler HJ, Janig W, Koltzenburg M. Myelinated primary afferents of the sacral spinal cord responding to slow filling and distension of the cat urinary bladder. J Physiol 1993; 463:449–460.

20. Habler HJ, Janig W, Koltzenburg M. Activation of unmyelinated afferent fibers by mechanical stimuli and inflammation of the urinary bladder in the cat. J Physiol 1990; 425:545–562.

21. Morrison JFB. The activation of bladder wall afferent nerves. Exp Physiol 1998; 84:131–136.

22. Pick J. The autonomic nervous system: morphological, comparative, clinical and surgical aspects. Philadelphia: Lippincott, 1970.

23. Morgan C, Nadelhaft I, De Groat WC. Location of bladder preganglionic neurons within the sacral parasympathetic nucleus of the cat. Neurosci Lett 1979; 14:189–194.

24. Bennett BC, Kruse MN, Roppolo JR, et al. Neural control of urethral outlet activity *in vivo*. Role of nitric oxide. J Urol 1995; 153:2004–2009.

25. De Groat WC. Anatomy and physiology of the lower urinary tract. Urol Clin N Am 1993; 20:383–401.

26. Westlund KN, Coulter JD. Descending projections of the locus coeruleus and subcoeruleus/medial parabrachial nuclei in monkey: axonal transport studies and dopamine-β-hydroxylase immunocytochemistry. Brain Res Rev 1980; 2:235–264.

27. Kojima M, Matsuura T, Kimura H, et al. Fluorescence histochemical study on the noradrenergic control to the anterior column of the spinal lumbosacral segments of rats and dog, with special reference to motoneurons innervating the perineal striated muscles (Onuf's nucleus). Histochem 1984; 81:237–241.

28. Willis WD. Descending control of spinal cord nociceptive neurons. Prog Sens Physiol 1982; 3:77.

29. Fleetwood-Walker SM, Mitchell R, Hope PJ, Molony V, Iggo A. An α2 receptor mediates the selective inhibition by noradrenalin of nociceptive responses of identified dorsal horn neurones. Brain Res 1985; 334(2):243–254.

30. Jordan LM, McCrea DA, Steeves JD, Menzies JE. Noradrenergic synapses and effects of noradrenalin on interneurons in ventral horn of the cat spinal cord. Can J Physiol Pharmacol 1977; 55(3):399–412.

31. Gajewski JB, Downie JW, Awad SA. Experimental evidence for a central nervous system site of action in the effect of alpha-adrenergic blockers on the external urinary sphincter. J Urol 1984; 133:403–409.

32. Galeano C, Jubelin B, Carmel M, Ghazal G. Urodynamic action of clonidine in the chronic spinal cat. Neurourol Urodyn 1986; 5:475–492.

33. Downie JW, Bialik GJ. Evidence for a spinal site of action of clonidine on somatic and viscerosomatic reflex activity evoked on the pudendal nerve in cats. J Pharmacol Exp Ther 1988; 246:352–358.

34. Nordling J, Meyhoff HH, Hald T. Sympatholytic effect on striated urethral sphincter. Scand J Urol Nephrol 1981; 15:173–180.

35. Brenowitz GL, Pubols LM. Increased receptive field size of dorsal horn neurons following chronic spinal cord hemisections in cats. Brain Res 1981; 216:45–59.

36. Tuckman J, Chu DS, Petrillo CR, Naftchi NE. Clinical trial of an alpha-adrenergic receptor stimulant drug (clonidine) for treatment of spasticity in spinal cord injured patients. In: Naftchi NE, ed. Spinal cord injury. New York: SP Medical and Scientific Books, 1982:133–137.

37. Jones SL, Light AR. Serotoninergic medullary raphespinal projection to the lumbar spinal cord in the rat: a retrograde immunohistochemical study. J Comp Neurol 1992; 322:599–610.

38. Westlund KN, Lu Y, Coggeshall RE, Willis WD. Serotonin is found in myelinated axons of the dorsolateral funiculus in monkeys. Neurosci Lett 1992; 141:35–38.

39. Abhold RH, Bowker RM. Descending modulation of dorsal horn biogenic amines as determined by in vivo dialysis. Neurosci Lett 1990; 108:231–236.

40. Laporte AM, Koscielniak T, Ponchant M, et al. Quantitative autoradiographic mapping of 5-HT3 receptors in the rat CNS using [125I]Iodo zacopride and [3H]Zacopride as radioligands. Synapse 1992; 10:271–281.

41. Seybold VS. Distribution of histaminergic, muscarinic and serotonergic binding sites in cat spinal cord with emphasis on the region surrounding the central canal. Brain Res 1985; 342:291–296.

42. Pubols LM, Bernau NA, Kane LA, et al. Distribution of 5-HT1 binding sites in cat spinal cord. Neurosci Lett 1992; 142:111–114.

43. McMahon SB, Morrison JFB. Factors that determine the excitability of parasympathetic reflexes to the bladder. J Physiol (Lond) 1982; 332:35–43.

44. Thor KB, Blitz-Siebert A, Helke CJ. Autoradiographic localization of 5HT1 binding sites in autonomic areas of the rat dorsomedial medulla oblongata. Synapse 1992; 10(3):217–227.

45. Steers WD, de Groat WC. Effects of m-chlorophenylpiperazine on penile and bladder function in rats. Am J Physiol 1989; 257:R1441–1449.

46. Espey MJ, Downie JW, Fine A. Effect of 5-HT receptor and adrenoceptor antagonists on micturition in conscious cats. Eur J Pharm 1991; 195:301–304.

47. Ishizuka O, Gu B, Igawa Y, et al. Role of supraspinal serotonin receptors for micturition in normal conscious rats. Neurourol Urodyn 2002; 21:225–230.

48. Sillen U, Rubenson A, Hjalmas K. Central cholinergic mechanisms in L-DOPA induced hyperactive urinary bladder of the rat. Urol Res 1982; 10:239–243.

49. Yoshimura N, Sasa M, Yoshida O, Takaori S. Dopamine D-1 receptor mediated inhibition of micturition reflex by central dopamine from substantia nigra. Neurourol Urodyn 1992; 11:535–545.

50. Zeigelgansberger W. Opioid actions on mammalian spinal neurons. Int Rev Neurobiol 1984; 25:243.

51. Wood PL. Multiple opiate receptors: support for unique mu, delta and kappa sites. Neuropharmacology 1982; 21:487–497.

52. Morris BJ, Herz A. Distinct distribution of opioid receptor types in rat lumbar spinal cord. Naunyn-Schmiedeberg's Arch Pharmacol 1987; 336:240–243.

53. Traynor JR, Wood MS. Distribution of opioid binding sites in spinal cord. Neuropeptides 1987; 10:313–320.

54. Wollemann M, Benyhe S, Simon J. The kappa-opioid receptor: evidence for different subtypes. Life Sci 1993; 52:599–611.

55. Glazer E, Basbaum A. Leucine enkephalin: localization in and axoplasmic transport by sacral parasympathetic preganglionic neurons. Science 1980; 208:1479–1481.

56. Gustafsson LL, Schildt B, Jacobsen K. Adverse effects of extradural and intrathecal opiates: report of a nationwide survey in Sweden. Br J Anaesth 1982; 54:479–486.

57. Rahwal N, Mollefors K, Axelsson K, et al. An experimental study of urodynamic effects of epidural morphine and of naloxane reversal. Anesth Analg 1983, 62:641–647.

58. De Groat WC, Kawatani M, Hisamitsu T, et al. The role of neuropeptides in the sacral autonomic reflex pathways of the cat. J Autonom Nerv Syst 1983, 7:339–350.

59. Jubelin B, Galeano C, Ladouceur D, et al. Effect of enkephalin on the micturition cycle of the cat. Life Sci 1984, 34:2015–2027.

60. Dray A, Metsch R. Inhibition of urinary bladder contractions by spinal action of morphine and other opioids. J Pharmacol Exp Ther 1984; 231:254–260.

61. Hisamitsu T, De Groat WC. The inhibitory effect of opioid peptides and morphine applied intrathecally and intracerebroventricularly on the micturition reflex in the cat. Brain Res 1984; 298:51–65.

62. Bolam JM, Robinson CJ, Hofstra TC, Wurster RD. Changes in micturition volume thresholds in conscious dogs following spinal opiate administration. J Autonom Nerv Syst 1986; 16:261–277.

63. Herman RH, Wainberg MC, delGiudice PF, Willscher MK. The effect of a low dose of intrathecal morphine on impaired micturition reflexes in human subjects with spinal cord lesion. Anesthesiology 1988; 69:313–318.

64. De Groat WC, Kawatani M. Neural control of the urinary bladder: possible relationship between peptidergic inhibitory mechanisms and detrusor instability. Neurourol Urodyn 1985; 4:285–300.

65. Kalia PK, Madan R, Saksena R, et al. Epidural pentazocine for postoperative pain relief. Anesth Analg 1983; 62:949–950.

66. Dray A, Metsch R. Spinal opioid receptors and inhibition of urinary bladder motility in vivo. Neurosci Lett 1984; 47:81–84.

67. Thor KB, Hisamitsu T, Roppolo JR, et al. Selective inhibitory effects of ethylketocyclazocine on reflex pathways to the external urethral sphincter of the cat. J Pharmacol Exp Ther 1989; 248:1018–1025.

68. Born JD, Hans P, Albert A, Bonnal J. Interobserver agreement in assessment of motor response and brain stem reflexes. Neurosurgery 1987; 20:513–517.

69. Benoit G, Al-Youssef I, Richard F, Jardin A. Neuroanatomical study of micturition. Ann Urol Paris 1986; 20:158–165.

70. Wyndaele JJ. Urodynamics in comatose patients. Neurourol Urodyn 1990; 9:43–52.

71. Kirby RS. Autonomic failure and the role of the sympathetic nervous system in the control of the lower urinary tract function. Clin Sci 1986; 70 (Suppl 14):45s–50s.

72. Shy GM, Drager GA. A neurological syndrome associated with orthostatic hypotension a clinical-pathologic study. Arch Neurol (Chicago) 1960; 2:511–527.

73. Tang PC. Levels of brain stem and diencephalon controlling micturition reflex. J Neurophysiol 1955; 18:583–595.

74. Blok BFM, Sturms LM, Holstege G. Brain activation during micturition in women. Brain 1998; 121:2033–2042.

75. Kuroiwa Y, Tohgi H, Ono S, Itoh M. Frequency and urgency of micturition in hemiplegic patients: relationship to hemisphere laterality of lesions. J Neurol 1987; 234:100–102.

76. Mochizuki H, Saito H. Mesial frontal lobe syndrome: correlations between neurological deficits and radiological localizations. Tohoku J Exp Med 1990; 161(Suppl):231–239.

77. Kodama K, Yokoyama O, Komatsu K, et al. Contribution of cerebral nitric oxide to bladder overactivity after cerebral infarction in rats. J Urol 2002; 167:391–396.

78. Hassuna M, Li JS, Sawan M, et al. Effect of early bladder stimulation on spinal shock: experimental approach. Urology 1992; 40:563–573.

79. Downie JW, Espey MJ, Gajewski JB. Contribution of perineal stimulation to the emergence of distension-evoked bladder contractions in spinal cats. Society for Neuroscience Meeting, San Diego, CA, 1995.

80. Blaivas JG. The neurophysiology of micturition: a clinical study of 550 patients. J Urol 1982; 127:958–963.

81. Galeano C, Jubelin B, Germain L, Guenette L. Micturitional reflexes in chronic spinalized cats: the underactive detrusor and detrusor-sphincter dyssynergia. Neurourol Urodyn 1986; 5:45–63.

82. Downie JW, Awad SA. The state of urethral musculature during the detrusor areflexia after spinal cord transection. Invest Urol 1979; 17:55–59.

83. De Groat WC, Kawatani M, Hisamitsu T, et al. Mechanisms underlying the recovery of urinary bladder function following spinal cord injury. J Auton Nerv System 1990; 30:S71–S77.

84. Barrington FJF. The nervous mechanism of micturition. Quart J Exp Physiol 1914; 8:33.

85. Yalla SV, Blunt KJ, Fam BA, et al. Detrusor-urethral sphincter dyssynergia, J Urol 1977; 118:1026–1029.

86. Griffiths DJ. Residual urine, underactive detrusor function and the nature of detrusor/sphincter dyssynergia. Neurourol Urodyn 1983; 2:289–294.

87. Dimitrijevic MR, Larsson LE, Lehmkuhl D, Sherwood AM. Evoked spinal cord and nerve root potentials in human using a non-invasive recording technique. Electroencephalogr Clin Neurophysiol 1978; 45:331–340.

88. Beric A, Dimitrijevic MR, Light JK. A clinical syndrome of rostal and caudal spinal injury: neurological, neurophysiological and urodynamic evidence for occult sacral lesion. J Neurol Neurosurg Psychiatry 1987; 50(5):600–606.

89. Beric A, Light JK. Correlation of bladder dysfunction and lumbosacral somatosensory evoked potential S wave abnormality in spinal cord injured patients. Neurourol Urodyn 1988; 7:131–140.

90. Siroky MB, Krane RJ. Neurologic aspects of detrusor sphincter dyssynergia, with reference to the guarding reflex. J Urol 1982; 127:953–957.

91. McGuire EJ, Savastano JA. Long term follow-up of spinal cord injury patients managed by intermittent catheterization. J Urol 1983; 129:775–776.

92. Wang SC, McGuire EJ, Bloom DA. A bladder pressure management system for myelodysplasia – clinical outcome. J Urol 1988; 140:1499–1502.

93. Rudy DC, Woodside JR. Non-neurogenic neurogenic bladder. The relationship between intravesical pressure and external sphincter electromyogram. Neurourol Urodyn 1991; 10:169–176.

94. Rud DC, Awad SA, Downie JW. External sphincter dyssynergia: an abnormal continence reflex. J Urol 1988; 140:105–110.

95. De Groat WC, Lalley PM. Reflex firing in the lumbar sympathetic outflow to activation of vesical afferent fibres. J Physiol 1972; 226:289–309.

96. Schurch B, Yasuda K, Rossier AB. Detrusor bladder neck dyssynergia revisited. J Urol 1994; 152:2066–2070.

97. Awad SA, Downie JW, Kiruluta HG. Alpha-adrenergic agents in urinary disorders of proximal urethra. Part II. Urethral obstruction due to "sympathetic dyssynergia". Br J Urol 1978; 50:336–339.

98. Floyd K, Hick VE, Morrison JF. The influence of visceral mechanoreceptors on sympathetic efferent discharge in the cat. J Physiol Lond 1982; 323:65–75.

99. Sato A, Sato Y, Sugimoto H, Terui N. Reflex changes in the urinary bladder after mechanical and thermal stimulation of the skin at various segmental levels in cats. Neuroscience 1977; 2:111–117.

100. Xiao CG, De Groat WC, Godec CJ, et al. "Skin-CNS-bladder" reflex pathway for micturition after spinal cord injury and its underlying mechanisms. J Urol 1999; 162:936–942.

101. Head H, Riddoch G. The autonomic bladder, excessive sweating and some other reflex conditions, in gross injuries of the spinal cord. Brain 1917; 40:188–.

102. Guttmann L, Whitteridge D. Effects of bladder distention on autonomic mechanisms after spinal cord injuries. Brain 1947; 70:361.

103. Rossier A, Bors E. Urological and neurological observations following anesthetic procedures for bladder rehabilitation of patients with spinal cord injuries. I. Topical anesthesics. J Urol 1962; 87:876.

104. Perkash I. An attempt to understand and to treat voiding dysfunction during rehabilitation of the bladder in spinal cord injury patients. J Urol 1976; 115:36–40.

105. Yalla SV. Spinal cord injury. In: Krane RJ, Siroky MB, eds. Clinical neuro-urology. Boston: Little, Brown and Company, 1979; 229–243.

106. Krenz NR, Weaver LC. Sprouting of primary afferent fibers after spinal cord transection in the rat. Neuroscience 1998; 85:443–458.

107. Krenz NR, Meakin SO, Krassioukov AV, Weaver LC. Neutralizing intraspinal nerve growth factor blocks autonomic dysreflexia caused by spinal cord injury. J Neurosci 1999; 19:7405–7414.

108. Elbadawi A, Atta MA, Franck JI. Intrinsic neuromuscular defects in the neurogenic bladder. I. Short-term ultrastructural changes in muscular innervation of the decentralized feline border base following unilateral sacral ventral rhizotomy. Neurourol Urodyn 1984; 3:93–113.

109. Sundin T, Dahlstrom A, Norlen LJ, Svedmyr N. The sympathetic innervation and adrenoreceptor function of the human lower urinary tract in the normal state and after parasympathetic denervation. Invest Urol 1977; 14:322–328.

110. Norlen LJ, Dahlstrom A, Sundin T, Svedmyr N. The adrenergic innervation and adrenergic receptor activity of the feline urinary bladder and urethra in the normal state and after hypogastric and/or parasympathetic denervation. Scan J Urol Nephrol 1976; 10:177–184.

111. Atta MA, Franck I, Elbadawi A. Intrinsic neuromuscular defects in the neurogenic bladder. II. Long-term innervation of the unilaterally decentralized feline bladder base by regenerated cholinergic, increased adrenergic and emergent probable "peptidergic" nerves. Neurourol Urodyn 1984; 3:185–200.

112. Sundin T, Dahlstrom A. The sympathetic innervation of the urinary bladder and urethra in the normal state and after parasympathetic denervation at the spinal root level. An experimental study in cats. Scan J Urol Nephrol 1973; 7:131–149.

113. deGroat WV, Kawatani M. Reorganization of sympathetic preganglionic connections in cat bladder ganglia following parasympathetic denervation. J Physiol 1989; 409:431–449.

114. McGuire EJ, Morrissey SG. The development of neurogenic vesical dysfunction after experimental spinal cord injury or sacral rhizotomy in non-human primates. J Urol 1982; 128:1390–1393.

115. Ghoniem GM, Regnier HC, Biancani P, et al. Effect of bilateral sacral decentralization on detrusor contractility and passive properties in dog. Neurourol Urodyn 1984; 3:23–33.

116. McGuire EJ, Savastano JA. Effect of alpha-adrenergic blockade and anticholinergic agents on the decentralized primate bladder. Neurourol Urodyn 1985; 4:139–142.

117. Gunasekera WSL, Richardson AE, Seneviratne KN, Eversden ID. Significance of detrusor compliance in patients with localized partial lesions of the spinal cord and cauda equina. Surg Neurol 1983; 20:59–62.

118. McGuire EJ, Woodside JR, Borden TA, Weiss RM. Prognostic value of urodynamic testing in myelodysplastic patients. J Urol 1981; 126:205–209.

119. Gajewski JB, Awad SA, Heffernan LPH, et al. Neurogenic bladder in lower motor neuron lesion: long-term assessment. Neurourol Urodyn 1992; 11:509–518.

120. Skehan AM, Downie JW, Awad SA. Control of bladder stiffness in normal and chronic decentralized feline bladder. J Urol 1993; 149:1165–1173.

121. Lapides J, French CR, Ajemian EP, Reus WF. A new method for diagnosis of the neurogenic bladder. Univ Mich Med Bull 1962; 28:166.

122. Carpenter FG, Rubin RM. The motor innervation of the rat urinary bladder. J Physiol 1967; 192:609–617.

123. Diokno AC, Davis R, Lapides J. Urecholine test for denervated bladders. Invest Urol 1975; 13:233–235.

124. El-Salmy S, Downie JW, Awad SA. Bladder and urethral function and supersensitivity to subcutaneously administered bethanechol in cats with chronic cauda equina lesions. J Urol 1985; 134: 1011–1018.

125. Donker PJ, Ivanovici F, Neach EL. Analysis of the urethral pressure profile by means of electromyography and the administration of drugs. Br J Urol 1972; 44:180–193.

126. Mattiasson A, Andersson K-E, Sjogren C. Urethral sensitivity to alpha-adrenoceptor stimulation and blockade in patients with parasympathetically decentralised lower urinary tract and in healthy volunteers. Neurourol Urodyn 1984; 3:223–233.

127. Clarke SJ, Thomas DG. Characteristics of the urethral pressure profile in flaccid male paraplegics. Br J Urol 1981; 53:157–161.

128. Blaivas JG. A critical appraisal of specific diagnostic techniques. In: Krane RJ, Siroky MB, eds. Clinical neuro-urology. Little, Brown and Company, 1979; 69–109.

129. Bauer SB, Labib KB, Dieppa RA, Retik AB. Urodynamic evaluation of the boy with myelodysplasia. Urology 1977; 10:354–362.

130. Awad SA, Downie JW. Sympathetic dyssynergia in the region of the external sphincter: a possible source of lower urinary tract obstruction. J Urol 1977; 118:636–640.

131. Parsons KF, Turton MB. Urethral supersensitivity and occult urethral neuropathy. Br J Urol 1980; 52:131–137.

132. Elbadawi A, Atta MA. Intrinsic neuromuscular defect in the neurogenic bladder. V. Autonomic re-innervation of the male feline rhabdosphincter following somatic denervation by bilateral sacral ventral rhizotomy. Neurourol Urodyn 1986; 5:65–85.

133. Kluck P. The autonomic innervation of the human urinary bladder, bladder neck and urethra. A histochemical study. Anat Rec 1980; 198:439–447.

134. Elbadawi A. Neuromorphological basis of vesicourethral function I. Histochemistry, ultrastructure and function of intrinsic nerves of the bladder and urethra. Neurourol Urodyn 1982; 1:3–50.

135. Awad SA, Downie JW, Kiruluta HG. Alpha adrenergic agents in urinary disorders of the proximal urethra. Part I. Sphincteric incontinence. Br J Urol 1978; 50:332–335.

136. Awad SA, Downie JW. The adrenergic component in the proximal urethra. Urol Int 1977; 32:192–197.

137. Nergardh A. The functional role of adrenergic receptors in the outlet region of the bladder. An in vitro and in vivo study in the cat. Scand J Urol Nephrol 1974; 8:100–107.

138. Caine M, Raz S, Zeigler M. Adrenergic and cholinergic receptors in prostate, prostatic capsule and bladder neck. Br J Urol 1975; 47:193–202.

139. Stephenson TP, Wein AJ. The interpretation of urodynamics. In: Mundy AR, Stephenson TP, Wein AJ, eds. Urodynamics: principles, practice and application. London: Churchill-Livingstone, 1984: 93–115.

140. Flood HD, Downie JW, Awad SA. Urethral function after chronic cauda equina lesions in cats. I. The contribution of the mechanical factors and sympathetic innervation to proximal sphincter dysfunction. J Urol 1990; 144:1022–1028.

141. Barbalias GA, Blaivas JG. Neurologic implication of the pathologically open bladder neck. J Urol 1983; 129:780–782.

142. McGuire EJ, Wagner FC. The effects of sacral denervation on bladder and urethral functions. Surg Gynecol Obstet 1977; 144:343–346.

143. Kirby RS, Flower C, Gilpin S, et al. Non-obstructive detrusor failure. A urodynamic, electromyographic, neurohistochemical and autonomic study. Br J Urol 1983; 55:652–659.

144. Blaivas JG, Barbalias GA. Characteristics of neural injury after abdominoperineal resection of the rectum. J Urol 1983; 129:84–87.

145. Ahlberg J, Edlund C, Wikkelsö C, et al. Neurological signs are common in patients with urodynamically verified "Idiopathic" bladder overactivity. Neurourol Urodyn 2002; 21:65–70.

30

Cerebral palsy, cerebellar ataxia, AIDS, phacomatosis, neuromuscular disorders, and epilepsy

Mark W Kellett and Ling K Lee

Introduction

In previous chapters, authors have described neurological disorders that are frequently associated with, or produce characteristic neurogenic bladder disturbances. In this chapter the authors review a number of miscellaneous conditions in which neurogenic disorders of the bladder may infrequently occur, either as a manifestation of the primary disease, or sometimes as a complication of disease treatment. Although urinary disturbance is well recognized in many of the conditions discussed, in others, such as neuromuscular disorders, cases are rare and reports are largely anecdotal.

Cerebral palsy

Cerebral palsy is becoming increasingly common as more premature low birthweight infants are surviving in neonatal intensive care units and are prone to insults to their central nervous system. Adverse events such as infection, cerebrovascular accident, or anoxia, in the prenatal and perinatal period can permanently damage areas in the brain which lead to the non-progressive disorders of motor function seen in cerebral palsy. The most common manifestation is muscle spasticity (70–80%), with athetoid, hypotonic, and ataxic motor disorders making up the rest. Intellectual capacity is directly related to the severity of physical impairment. The combination of mental, neurological, and physical handicap means urinary symptoms and incontinence are commoner in patients with cerebral palsy.

Roijen et al[1] sent a continence questionnaire to the parents of 601 children (ages between 4 and 18 years old) with cerebral palsy and received a response from 459 (76%). The prevalence for primary urinary incontinence in this study was 23.5%. Daytime continence usually preceded nocturnal continence and 85% of children gained nocturnal continence within the year of achieving daytime continence.

In this study, 96% of all cerebral palsy children with normal intelligence (IQ > 65) were continent, demonstrating the importance of comprehension and communication skills for continence training. The ability to achieve continence was related to the extent of both physical and mental handicap (Table 30.1) and, not surprisingly, children with spastic tetraplegia and low intelligence (IQ < 65) were the least likely to become continent. The majority of children with cerebral palsy (89%) who were continent became so before 12 years old, and a small minority would continue to gain control spontaneously into their late teens.

Although urinary incontinence is the commonest reason for a urological referral (Table 30.2), a significant number of patients with cerebral palsy have other lower urinary tract symptoms.[2–5] Over a 7-month period, McNeal et al[5] interviewed 50 patients (between 8 and 29 years old) with cerebral palsy who attended outpatient clinics and actively sought out symptoms of urinary dysfunction. More than one-third (36%) had two or more urinary symptoms,

Table 30.1 *The percentage of children aged 6 years old with cerebral palsy (CP) of different severity who were continent compared to normally developing children*[1]

At age 6 years old	Percent continent
Normally developing	92
Spastic hemiplegia	80
Spastic diplegia	84
Spastic tetraplegia	54
CP with IQ > 65	80
CP with IQ < 65	38
Spastic tetraplegia with IQ < 65	33

prompting referral for further urological assessment. In reality, the overall incidence of lower urinary tract symptoms could be higher, as McNeal's study excluded patients with IQs < 40. Mayo[3] found an unusually high incidence of voiding difficulty in 17 of the 33 patients who underwent videocystometrogram. The patients predominantly had difficulty initiating a urinary stream and two adult patients were using catheters for urinary retention. His group of patients was older (10 patients >20 years old, 3 patients >55 years old) and Mayo postulated that obstructive symptoms might become more prevalent as patients with cerebral palsy progress into adult life. This, he felt, was due to lack of voluntary control over a 'spastic' pelvic floor.

A hyperreflexic bladder (involuntary contractions during bladder filling in the presence of a known neurological disorder) consistent with an upper motor neuron injury was the commonest urodynamic finding in symptomatic patients with cerebral palsy[2-6] (Table 30.3). Symptoms of urgency and frequency appear to correlate well with an overactive detrusor. Mayo demonstrated hyperreflexia in 14 of the 16 patients with urge ± incontinence compared to only 8 out of the 17 patients with voiding difficulties. Reduced bladder capacity was also a common finding, and occasionally a noncompliant bladder with end-fill instability was found to be

responsible for the patient's symptoms. A voiding study was more difficult to obtain, bearing in mind that a proportion of patients were wheelchair-bound and had learning disabilities. Therefore, it is difficult to estimate the incidence of detrusor underactivity or bladder outlet obstruction in patients with cerebral palsy. Excluding two patients who were in retention and one with detrusor-sphincter dyssynergia, Mayo found the remaining 14 of 17 patients with voiding difficulties had low post-void residual volumes and none had significant trabeculation to suggest obstruction. During urodynamic evaluation on 57 children with cerebral palsy, Decter et al also carried out electromyography (EMG) on the external sphincter using needle electrodes. They identified 11 patients with incomplete lower motor neuron injury to the sphincter. This was defined as a partially denervated sphincter which, when stimulated, has a reduced number of motor units recruited to contract, but whose amplitude and duration of action potential may be increased during voiding simulating dyssynergia.[4] However, Decter et al did not comment as to whether these patients had outflow obstruction. Although uncommon, the finding of detrusor-sphincter dyssynergia and lower motor neuron lesions (acontractile bladder) implies that the perinatal injury that caused the abnormal neurology in cerebral palsy may also involve the

Table 30.2 *The distribution of the common lower urinary tract symptoms in patients with cerebral palsy undergoing urological assessment. Some patients had multiple symptoms*

	McNeal et al[5]	Decter et al[4]	Mayo[3]	Reid and Borzyskowski[2]
Number of patients	50	57	33	27
Symptoms:				
Incontinence[a]	54%	86%	48%	74%
Urgency	18%			37%
Frequency		51%		56%
Dribbling	6%			
Hesitancy/voiding difficulties		3.5%	46%	11%
Retention		2%	6%	7%

[a]Incontinence includes urge/stress/day and/or enuresis.

Table 30.3 *Urodynamic findings on patients with cerebral palsy*

	McNeal et al[5]	Decter et al[4]	Drigo et al[6]	Mayo[3]	Reid and Borzyskowski[2]
Number of patients	13	57	9	33	27
Hyperreflexic	4 (31%)	35 (61%)	9 (100%)	22 (67%)	21 (78%)
End-fill instability	2 (15%)				
Detrusor-sphincter dyssynergia		7 (17%)	2 (22%)	1 (3%)	5 (19%)
Acontractile bladder		1			2

spinal cord. The incidence of vesicoureteric reflux on videourodynamics varied from 1.8% to 35%,[2–4,6] but none of the authors comment on renal impairment or the presence of reflux nephropathy.

Given the risk of upper tract damage in neurogenic voiding dysfunction, Brodak et al[7] prospectively screened on sonography 90 patients (age 1–25 years old) with or without urological symptoms in an attempt to determine if urinary tract screening was necessary for patients with cerebral palsy. On first ultrasound, seven of the 90 patients had renal abnormalities, which were hydronephrosis in three, renal asymmetry in two, and non-visualization in two. On a follow-up ultrasound, only two of the three had persistent hydronephrosis and had ultrasound evidence of a neurogenic bladder, i.e. marked bladder wall trabeculation and/or resolution of hydronephrosis following catheterization. The authors concluded that routine urinary tract screening was not justified because urinary tract abnormalities were only detected in 2% of patients studied.

Patients with cerebral palsy are more prone to urinary tract infections[8] (UTIs) and should be investigated with ultrasound imaging of kidneys, bladder, and post-micturition residual volume. A plain kidney, ureter, and bladder (KUB) X-ray is useful although renal tract stones are uncommon.[9] In the presence of abnormalities, further evaluation with videourodynamics, micturating cystourethrography, renogram, etc., should be performed. Decter et al[4] found that all six children with UTIs (single episode or recurrent) in their study had radiological and urodynamic abnormalities, four had detrusor-sphincter dyssynergia, and one had chronic retention due to detrusor failure (one other was not specified). In contrast, Reid and Borzyskowski's study[2] involved 13 patients with a history of UTIs but vesicoureteric reflux was demonstrated in only one patient who had hyperreflexia and detrusor-sphincter dyssynergia.

Treatment is primarily with anticholinergic drugs for hyperreflexic bladders and patients with symptoms of urge and frequency. Post-micturition bladder residuals should then be closely monitored, as clean intermittent catheterization may be necessary with increasing residuals. Prophylactic antibiotics are used for UTIs and reflux nephropathy. Adrenergic drugs may be effective for a weak bladder neck causing stress incontinence.[2] Mayo advocated muscle relaxants (e.g. diazepam, baclofen) for his patients with voiding difficulties due to spasticity of their pelvic floor muscles.[3] Using a combination of medication and behavioral modification (e.g. frequent voiding schedule), Decter et al[4] were able to improve the incontinence in 21 of the 27 cerebral palsy patients (78%) who had adequate follow-up data. Cerebral palsy patients with detrusor-sphincter dyssynergia are most at risk of developing hydronephrosis and renal deterioration, and should have long-term upper tract monitoring. In these patients with worsening renal function and in whom intermittent catheterization is not a realistic alternative, a vesicostomy or urinary diversion (ileal conduit or continent diversion)

should be performed.[2–4,10] Long-term catheterization for neuropathic bladders is generally not recommended because of the high complication rates of stone formation, urinary bypassing, and upper tract dilation.[11,12]

Selective sacral dorsal rhizotomy for controlling lower limb spasticity in cerebral palsy patients may result in a lower motor neuron lesion of the bladder. Abbott et al noted urinary retention in 7% of the 200 patients who underwent this procedure, although it was transient in all but one of the 13 patients.[13] Houle et al demonstrated an increase in bladder capacity ($p < 0.005$) by carrying out pre- and postsacral rhizotomy urodynamic studies in 13 patients.[14] The resultant improved bladder storage and better mobility enabled some patients to become continent, and Sweetser et al found that the patients with milder forms of spasticity were most helped by this procedure.[14,15]

Cerebellar and spinocerebellar disorders

In cerebellar ataxia, the cerebellum and/or the pathways connecting the cerebellum with other parts of the nervous system undergo progressive, premature neuronal death and atrophy. The result is a heterogeneous spectrum of motor abnormalities, which is manifested in an abnormal broadbased gait, incoordination, tremor, dysarthria, and motor and autonomic dysfunction. The etiology in many cases is an underlying genetic abnormality of which Friedreich's ataxia is the commonest and accounts for at least 50% of hereditary ataxias. The non-hereditary ataxias can present acutely, subacutely, or can also have a chronic course. The nature and extent of urinary disturbances depend on the site of involvement in the central nervous system. In isolated cerebellar disorders urinary disturbance is generally absent.[17] More frequently the degenerative neuropathological process affects multisystems, including the brainstem, cerebrum, and spinal cord, in which case urinary symptoms are more likely.

In patients with spinocerebellar ataxia, urinary symptoms most commonly manifest as incontinence and urgency. Among 195 patients (aged between 8 and 54 years) with hereditary spinocerebellar ataxia, Chami et al found 23% had urgency and 6% had urinary incontinence.[16] Reports on urodynamic findings in patients with ataxia are limited (Table 30.4) and in some the authors have found it difficult to classify the bladder disturbance.[16–18] Detrusor hyperreflexia appears to be the most common finding, which is not surprising as the cerebellum and basal ganglia are important in influencing the cerebral–brainstem loop that facilitates the coordinated voluntary control of the voiding reflex. Detrusor–sphincter dyssynergia and acontractility are less common and correlate with the extent of neuronal damage in the spinal cord. In Chami's paper, 36 of the 55 patients who had urodynamic studies had no urinary problems, and although 23 (64%) had normal urodynamic

Table 30.4 *Urodynamic findings in patients with cerebellospinal ataxia*

	Leach et al[17]	Vezina et al[18]	Chami et al[16]
Number of patients	15	17	55
Hyperreflexia	8 (53%)	7 (41%)	14 (25%)
Detrusor-sphincter dyssynergia	3 (6%)	6 (37%)	
Detrusor acontractility	4 (27%)		9 (16%)

studies, detrusor hyperreflexia and detrusor acontractility were found in six and two patients, respectively.[16]

Treatment for urgency and urge incontinence in patients with ataxia ideally should be specific to the urodynamic findings. However, the likelihood is an underlying hyperreflexic bladder and these patients could be treated empirically with anticholinergics if they do not carry large residual volumes. Patients with underactive detrusor can be treated with intermittent catheterization. Leach et al successfully treated their three patients with sphincter dyssynergia with a combination of α-sympathetic blockade (phenoxybenzamine), diazepam, and baclofen.[17]

Non-hereditary ataxias with a multitude of etiologies – e.g. alcohol intoxication, neurosarcoidosis, superficial siderosis – can present acutely or subacutely, with urinary incontinence as a common co-presenting symptom.[19–23] Urodynamic studies are not commonly performed in the investigation of such patients, but when they have been carried out a hyperreflexic bladder has typically been identified.[19,20,23] Treatment will depend on the etiology and prognosis of the underlying condition. In some cases improvements in urinary control will occur as the underlying disease responds to specific treatment.[19,20,23]

Human immunodeficiency virus infection and acquired immunodeficiency syndrome

LUTS in the well HIV-positive patient is uncommon and, if present, is usually due to UTI.[24] However, at the time of seroconversion to HIV, the patient may experience a variety of neurological syndromes, including acute urinary retention and sacral sensory loss.[28] Impaired micturition becomes more common with disease progression and can occur as part of a global neurological dysfunction or due to infection.[24–27] Hermieu et al[26] undertook urodynamics and neurological evaluation in 39 HIV-positive patients presenting with LUTS. A urodynamic abnormality, either an overactive or underactive detrusor or detrusor-sphincter

dyssynergia, was identified in 87% of patients. Of these, 61% had AIDS-related neurological problems such as cerebral toxoplasmosis, HIV demyelination disorders, motor dysfunction, and AIDS-related dementia. This heralded a poor prognosis, as 43% in this group died after 2–24 months (mean 8 months). Detrusor failure due to a lower motor lesion is uncommon and is usually caused by malignancy or infection such as herpes. These patients should be taught clean intermittent self-catheterization. Long-term indwelling catheters are best avoided in HIV-infected patients because of their vulnerability to *Staphylococcus aureus* bacteremia. CMV polyradiculopathy is very rare but eminently treatable and reversible if caught early.[28] The patient presents with back and sciatica pain with bladder or bowel dysfunction. A lumbar puncture is performed and the diagnosis is made by finding a polymorphonuclear cell-predominant pleocytosis and by confirming the presence of cytomegalovirus (CMV) using polymerase chain reaction (PCR) in the cerebrospinal fluid.

Phacomatosis

Phacomatoses encompass a number of disorders characterized by various neurocutaneous abnormalities.[29] Minor features are often present from birth, but, with age, neoplasia can often develop. Bladder disorders are unusual in many of these conditions, but the reported cases are discussed below. In some phacomatoses, such as tuberose sclerosis, bladder disorders have not been reported. Neurogenic bladder abnormalities have most commonly been reported in neurofibromatosis.

Neurofibromatosis

Type 1 (von Recklinhausen's disease)

There are numerous reports of various neurofibromatosis type 1 associated tumors affecting the urinary system and particularly the bladder. They are usually derived from nerves of the pelvic, vesical, and prostatic plexuses[30] and include benign, and less commonly, malignant neurofibromas,[30–50] paragangliomas,[51] and other occasional malignant tumors.[52] They should be suspected when patients with neurofibromatosis develop any urinary symptoms, as they may present in a multitude of ways. Lower urinary tract symptoms, enuresis, flank pain, incontinence, or symptoms related to urinary tract obstruction may occur, but in addition localized pain, low back pain, and lower limb dysesthesia can occur.[53] These symptoms may result from the tumor size[54] and/or neurogenic involvement.[55–57]

A conservative management approach to tumors causing urinary symptoms has been suggested due to likely damage to adjacent organs on attempted extirpation. However, careful follow-up is necessary to detect signs of upper tract obstruction, which may be a sign of tumor progression or malignant transformation.[54]

Type 2 (central type)

Neurofibromatosis type 2, and related conditions such as spinal schwannomatosis,[58] may also lead to upper motor neuron syndromes when tumors such as schwannomas, neurofibromas, meningiomas, or hamartomas[59] damage the spinal cord.[60–64] Neurofibromas or schwannomas,[64,65] or other tumors,[66] may involve the conus or cauda equina. In such cases, a mixture of upper and/or lower motor neuron bladder symptoms could occur. The typical presentation of conus and cauda equina lesions and the effects on the bladder have been described in earlier chapters.

Cobb syndrome

Cobb syndrome is a rare neurocutaneous syndrome manifest by cutaneous nevi and spinal angiomas within the same metaphere.[67] Wakabayashi et al[68] recently reported an 8-year-old boy presenting with difficulty initiating micturition, constipation, low back pain, and a mild spastic paraparesis. Multiple angiokeratomas were present over dermatomes of the cervical region and lower sacral region on the right and over the lumbar and sacral areas on the left. Multiple angiomas were present in the cervicothoracic spinal cord and conus medullaris, with evidence of bleeding from an upper thoracic angioma that had probably produced his presenting symptoms. The boy's symptoms gradually improved without surgical intervention. This phenotype most closely resembles Cobb syndrome, but unusually the boy also had cerebral angiomas that are rare in this condition.

Klippel–Trénaunay–Weber syndrome

In Klippel–Trénaunay–Weber syndrome intracranial and intraspinal angiomas may occur in association with hypertrophy of skeletal muscles and visceral involvement.[69–71] Urinary symptoms would be expected if symptomatic spinal cord pathology occurred due to pressure or bleeding from large spinal angiomas. Kojima et al[72] reported one such case with a nevus flammeus, varices, hypertrophy, and elongation of the left leg. She presented with a progressive paraparesis and urinary retention due to an extensive spinal arteriovenous malformation extending from T11 to L2. The arteriovenous malformation was treated surgically with an initial deterioration in bladder function; however, 6 months later, her motor function improved to the preoperative state and the bladder dysfunction disappeared.

Various other non-neurogenic genitourinary manifestations may occur in Klippel–Trénaunay syndrome. They tend to occur in the more severe cases and usually involve cutaneous vascular malformations of the trunk, pelvis, and genitalia, sometimes with intra-abdominal and intrapelvic extension of the vascular malformations.[73]

Proteus syndrome

Proteus syndrome has numerous manifestations. It is characterized by massive tissue overgrowth and asymmetry. Frequent features include partial gigantism of hands and feet, nevi, and hemihypertrophy, as well as other multisystem involvement.[29] Neurogenic bladder symptoms are not a reported feature of this condition,[29] but urinary tract involvement may occur. In one case presenting with renal tract stones, left-sided ureterovesical reflux was found on the same side as hemihypertrophy. The authors postulated that the unilateral involvement was a feature related to hemihypertrophy;[74] however, similar cases have not been reported to further corroborate this. In another case, leiomyoma of the urinary bladder occurred.[75]

Neurocutaneous melanosis

Neurocutaneous melanosis is a form of phakomatosis in which there is a proliferation of melanocytes in skin and meninges. The most common skin lesion is a giant pigmented hairy nevus, but diffuse pigmentation can also occur. Infiltration of the pia and arachnoid by melanocytes can usually be seen macroscopically. There is an approximately 2–13% risk of malignant change in skin and a 50% risk of malignant change in the meninges. Typical neurological abnormalities include hydrocephalus (probably due to vascular obstruction of the fourth ventricle), epilepsy, intracranial hemorrhage, cranial nerve palsies, and psychiatric disturbance. Neurogenic bladder has not been a feature, except in one case reported by Sawamura et al.[76] The 13-year-old subject of their report presented with signs attributable to a large right frontal malignant leptomeningeal melanoma. Amongst his other clinical features was a neurogenic bladder, although, as there was no direct spinal involvement from the neurocutaneous melanosis, it was more likely to be attributable to his coexisting spina bifida. In 28 additional cases reviewed from the literature, neurogenic bladder disturbance was not reported, suggesting that it is unlikely to be a disease feature.[76]

Neuromuscular disorders

Neuromuscular junction disorders

Myasthenia gravis

Myasthenia gravis is an autoimmune disorder due to the presence of antiacetylcholine receptor antibodies that bind to the nicotinic cholinergic receptors at the motor endplate of the neuromuscular junction. It typically affects striated muscle, causing weakness with fatigability. In 15% of patients its effects are confined to the ocular and facial muscles, causing ptosis and diplopia; however, more generalized weakness occurs in the majority of the remaining patients. Although the antibodies act on nicotinic cholinergic receptors, antibodies have also been demonstrated against muscarinic cholinergic receptors.

Bladder disturbance attributable to myasthenia gravis is unusual, but a number of individual case reports have been published.[77–81] The clinical, urodynamic, and neurophysiological findings in these cases are summarized in Table 30.5. The bladder dysfunction in all cases resembled a lower motor neuron pattern with variable degrees of detrusor areflexia/atonia. In the patient reported by Sandler et al,[81] the voiding dysfunction was complete and prolonged and the patient required long-term intermittent catheterization. Unfortunately, the authors do not report on the response of the original myasthenia gravis symptoms. In other patients, urinary symptoms have responded to medical therapy directed at the myasthenia gravis.[78,80] In some rare cases, voiding dysfunction may be the initial presenting symptom,[77,79] and in others may be associated with an exacerbation of generalized myasthenia gravis.[79,81] The detrusor muscle is predominantly under the control of the parasympathetic nervous system with muscarinic innovation. Detrusor failure suggests involvement of acetylcholine receptor antibodies at muscarinic receptors on the detrusor muscle itself or in the pelvic ganglia. The fluctuation in severity related to drug treatment of myasthenia gravis suggests a causal relationship in some cases.

Table 30.5 *The clinical, urodynamic, and neurophysiological findings of myasthenia gravis (MG) patients with bladder disturbance*

References	Age Gender	Myasthenia characteristics	Urinary symptoms	Urodynamic and EMG[a] findings
78	59 Female	Generalized MG	Difficulty voiding Incomplete bladder emptying Frequency Severity related to treatment with pyridostigmine	Normal bladder capacity (430 ml) Normal filling sensation Atonic detrusor (pressure <8 cmH$_2$O) during attempted void Voiding by abdominal pressure with poor flow and interrupted flow pattern
79	31 Female	Generalized MG	Stress incontinence Bladder neck suspension 8 months before MG diagnosed Associated with deterioration in MG condition	Open bladder neck Inability to sustain pelvic floor contraction Bladder hyperreflexia
80	20 Female	Seronegative Generalized MG	'Urinary disturbance' Symptoms responded to treatment with steroids and thymectomy	Atonic bladder
77	Elderly Male	Generalized MG	Urgency and urge incontinence Uncontrollable flatus and fecal incontinence on sneezing and coughing	Detrusor hyporeflexia
81	39 Female	Seropositive Generalized MG	Incontinence followed by retention with constipation at time of myasthenic crisis	Bladder capacity 662 ml Areflexic detrusor Unable to generate detrusor contraction and unable to void EMG – low-intensity discharges during bladder filling

[a]EMG, electromyography.

Urinary symptoms in myasthenia gravis have also been reported in male patients who have undergone prostatic surgery. Greene et al reported six men with bladder outflow obstruction who underwent a transurethral resection of the prostate (TURP) and subsequently developed urinary incontinence. They hypothesized that of the resection had led to some form of injury to the external sphincter that had already been compromised by the underlying myasthenia gravis. They therefore recommended an incomplete resection in order to leave distal tissue that they felt would prevent trauma to the sphincter. They later reported a seventh man with myasthenia gravis who underwent an incomplete resection who initially remained dry, but 3 months later developed urge incontinence.

Subsequently, Wise et al found that incontinence after TURP was associated with the use of blended current, and that patients treated with either high-frequency unblended current, partial proximal resection, or open prostatectomy remained dry.[82] Unfortunately, urodynamic or EMG studies were not made in these cases and, therefore, the pathophysiological mechanism is unclear. However, Khan and Bhola[83] reported another patient who remained continent after an open prostatectomy. Preoperative EMG of the external urinary sphincter revealed fatigability and abnormal motor units, suggesting an underlying neurogenic weakness of the continence mechanism. They postulated that electrical current could further damage this mechanism, possibly by damaging residual acetylcholine receptors.[83]

Lambert–Eaton myasthenic syndrome

Lambert–Eaton myasthenic syndrome (LEMS) is characterized by muscle weakness as well as autonomic dysfunction; it is associated with small cell lung cancer in approximately 60% of cases and is often associated with the presence of anti-P/Q-type voltage-gated calcium channel antibodies.[84–86] Dysautonomia is frequent in LEMS and involves cholinergic and adrenergic systems,[87–91] but neurogenic bladder involvement is rare.

In one series of 50 patients, autonomic symptoms occurred in 80% of patients, with dry mouth and impotence being the most frequently experienced symptoms, followed by constipation, blurred vision, and sweating abnormalities; there were no reports of bladder dysfunction.[88] Another study involving 30 patients had similar findings.[89] Bladder dysfunction has been reported in five cases,[87,92,93] although detailed features, including urodynamic findings, have only been reported in one case.[93] In this report, Satoh et al[93] describe a 71-year-old Japanese woman with neurophysiologically and serologically confirmed Lambert–Eaton myasthenic syndrome. She was initially treated with anticholinesterase drugs, corticosteroids, and plasma exchange. Four years after presentation her condition deteriorated and she was unable to stand or

walk. She complained of a dry mouth and urinary frequency greater than 15 times per day. Urodynamic studies consisting of uroflowmetry, cystometry, and urethral pressure recordings were made before and after treatment with 3,4-diaminopyridine. Maximum urinary flow rate was decreased at 12.8 ml/s, suggestive of an underactive detrusor. Bladder emptying was reasonable, with post-void residual urine volumes of 37, 170, and 70 ml on three separate measurements. After treatment with 10 mg of 3,4-diaminopyridine, muscle weakness and dry mouth dramatically improved and this was associated with reduced urinary frequency. Post-treatment anal sphincter EMG and detrusor and abdominal pressures also increased markedly during voiding; and the maximum urine flow rate normalized from 12.8 to 17.9 ml/s. However, detrusor underactivity is not usually associated with urinary frequency, although the patient's urinary symptom improved with better detrusor contractility.

Detrusor muscle pressure and abdominal muscle pressure were reduced in voiding, which suggests that the neurogenic bladder was caused by defective neurotransmission in both autonomic detrusor muscle and skeletal abdominal muscle. Furthermore, the response to 3,4-diaminopyridine suggests that the neurogenic bladder was directly attributable to the dysautonomia of Lambert–Eaton myasthenic syndrome. The authors speculated that this was due to the action of anti-P/Q-type voltage-gated calcium channel antibodies on the bladder. In support of this theory, they cite a number of animal studies suggesting an important role for these antibodies in mediating neurotransmitter release in the urinary bladder of mice, rats, and guinea pigs.[91,94,95]

Muscular dystrophies

Myotonic dystrophy

Myotonic dystrophy is a disorder characterized by myotonia (sustained contraction of muscle in response to electrical or percussive stimuli) and dystrophy (progressive loss of skeletal muscle with fibrosis and fatty infiltration). However, it is a multisystem disorder, with the most prominent manifestations in skeletal muscle, cardiac conduction system, brain, smooth muscle, and lens. It is inherited as an autosomal dominant trait with variable penetrance and phenotypic expression, and it demonstrates the phenomena of anticipation with worsening of the disease in subsequent generations. The genetic mutation primarily responsible for the autosomal dominant inheritance of myotonic dystrophy is a variable triplet repeat (CTG) that is located on chromosome 19 in the 3′ untranslated region of a gene with protein kinase domains named myotonin protein kinase.[96]

Smooth muscle abnormalities are well recognized in myotonic dystrophy but predominantly affect the gastrointestinal tract. Urinary tract dysfunction is much less commonly encountered.[97] Clinically, urinary retention without evidence of additional pathological changes was noted in a number of early reports.[98–100] Bundschu et al,[101] described two brothers with myotonic dystrophy who developed dilatation of the renal pelvis, ureter, and bladder due to presumed smooth muscle involvement. In a subsequent study involving nine patients, Orndahl et al[102] found bladder function to be normal in all cases assessed using cystometrograms. However, symptomatic bladder dysfunction has been reported in two more recent systematic studies involving 16 patients:[103,104] urinary symptoms were reported in six of the 16 patients, with urinary urgency, frequency, and stress incontinence being the predominant complaints; symptoms often occurred at a young age. Urodynamic investigation revealed reduced urethral pressures and abnormal motor units in the external sphincter. There was a suggestion that, in women in particular, pelvic floor muscle involvement may have been contributory.

Pathological changes in reported cases have been variable. The bladder was reported to be normal in one autopsied case;[105] however, in another case, Harvey et al[98] found slight vacuolization of the bladder smooth muscle syncytium and an increased number of nuclei. Furthermore, Pruzanski and Huvos,[106] in another autopsy study, demonstrated muscle degeneration in the bowel and bladder. Histology of the bladder showed separation of myofibrils by edematous fibrous tissue, variation in muscle fiber size and shape, and longitudinal myofibers showed break up with hypereosinophilia. Fibrous tissue replacement, as seen in the bladder of the latter case, is frequently seen in skeletal muscles of patients with myotonic dystrophy. However, it should be noted that this patient also had evidence of prostatic hyperplasia with some trabeculation of the bladder wall, and thus the significance of these pathological changes is uncertain.[106]

Limb-girdle muscular dystrophy

Limb-girdle muscular dystrophies (LGMD) are a group of genetically heterogeneous disorders that share similar presenting features.[107] Their classification is based on mode of inheritance and chromosomal localization; currently, 11 limb-girdle dystrophies can be defined by gene product, but identification of others is likely soon.[107,108] Limb-girdle dystrophies occur in both sexes, with onset between the second and sixth decade, usually in late childhood or early adulthood, although onset can occur at almost any age. Weakness in many cases begins in the pelvic girdle musculature, then spreads to the pectoral muscles, although the reverse is not unusual.

The various phenotypes have been widely characterized and urinary symptoms are unusual. However, Dixon et al[109] has reported a 48-year-old woman with clinical, laboratory, and neurophysiological evidence of LGMD with urinary symptoms that appeared to be related to the presence of LGMD. The patient was nulliparous and had originally developed stress incontinence at the age of 12 years when jumping. This progressed over subsequent years until it was present on coughing and walking. Videocystometrogram showed marked bladder descent and stress incontinence with no detrusor instability and normal urethral sphincter EMG. Histology of pelvic floor muscles revealed changes consistent with LGMD: large variability of fiber size with hypertrophied and atrophic fibers and type 1 fiber predominance, frequent internal nuclei, and disruption of the myofibrillar pattern. Unfortunately, at the time this report was made, it was impossible to identify the specific phenotype, although it may represent a subtype with early and predominant involvement of pelvic muscles. Although not directly neurogenic in etiology, the weak pelvic floor muscles led to abnormal positioning of the vesicourethral junction, which was the most likely cause of the incontinence in this case.

Duchenne's muscular dystrophy

Duchenne's muscular dystrophy (DMD) is an X-linked disorder that is the most common muscular dystrophy in children. It is characterized by progressive weakness of skeletal muscle with onset in early childhood. The disorder is caused by loss-of-function mutations of an extremely large gene located on the X-chromosome (Xp21). The protein product of the gene, dystrophin, is absent or markedly deficient. Dystrophin is a cytosolic protein associated with the external membrane of skeletal, cardiac, and smooth muscle cells and of some neurons. Lack of dystrophin ultimately leads to a chronic necrotizing myopathy with marked muscle wasting. The disease progresses over 20 years and is always associated with an inability to walk.[110]

Despite the fact that most patients with DMD have normal sphincter function, some patients will experience urinary incontinence. It is not uncommon for a short period of urinary and bowel incontinence to occur around the age of 12 years, as the child becomes wheelchair-dependent. This appears unrelated to structural pathology such as increasingly severe scoliosis, and is thought to be a manifestation of depression. It usually resolves within a few months.[111]

Neurogenic bladder disorders do also occur, albeit unusually. In one retrospective study from the Mayo Clinic in Rochester, 33 patients with DMD, born between 1953 and 1983 and followed during their second decade of life, were studied. Urinary disturbance was described in only two of the 33 cases (6%); it occurred relatively late in the disease course, and in both cases was manifest by urinary retention. In one 12-year-old boy, acute urinary retention occurred several weeks following surgery for correction of scoliosis.

In the other case, acute urinary retention appeared while undergoing an excretory cystourethrogram for nephrolithiasis. Although this settled, acute retention recurred several months later. Detailed urodynamic studies were not reported and the authors were unclear about the significance of these findings in view of the associated events.[112]

In another study, Caress et al[113] identified seven boys with DMD who had undergone urodynamic tests at the Children's Hospital of Boston during the years 1978–1994. The clinical, urodynamic, and neurophysiological findings are summarized in Table 30.6. Five of the boys complained of urinary incontinence and two had difficulty initiating voiding consistent with urinary retention. Five of the boys had undergone a spinal fusion procedure, and in two of these there was a temporal relationship between their spinal fusion surgery and the onset of urinary dysfunction, similar to the case reported by Boland et al.[112] In one of these boys acute urinary retention and left lateral thigh and testicular numbness occurred immediately following his T4–L5 spinal fusion. In another boy, bladder and bowel incontinence was associated with paraplegia and a T10 sensory level following a spinal fusion procedure. None of the other six patients had upper motor neuron signs, although the severe muscle wasting and weakness could have obscured subtle signs.

Sacral reflexes were preserved in all of the patients and bladder contractions were of normal or high pressures in all but one child. Urodynamic studies and EMG were abnormal in six cases, with five out of six exhibiting upper motor neuron dysfunction. There was no clear pattern of bladder size or post-void residual urine volume in this group, but uninhibited contractions were a frequent finding (4/5), as was bladder/sphincter dyssynergia (3/5). One patient had normal reflexes but enlarged motor units suggestive of

reinnervation and was classified as having lower motor neuron dysfunction. This 11-year-old had a normal capacity bladder, an initial post-void residual urine volume of 250 ml.[113] Despite the advanced disease course in most of the cases, unlike the previous case with LGMD,[109] there was no evidence of myopathic motor units or abnormal spontaneous activity in the pelvic floor muscles. Furthermore, bladder pressures generated during voiding or during uninhibited contractions were normal or elevated, suggesting that no significant detrusor myopathy was present.[113]

The upper motor neuron lesions in these cases, and in the case of Boland and colleagues,[112] are most likely to be due to progressive scoliosis or complications of surgical treatment, or both. The temporal nature of urinary disturbance to a surgical procedure in at least three of nine reported cases suggests a direct causal relationship. In the other cases that had undergone surgery, the lack of a clear temporal relationship does not exclude a similar mechanism. Caress and colleagues also postulate that upper motor neuron dysfunction could result from the action of DMD on the central nervous system.[113] Dystrophin is present in the normal brain and its presumed absence in DMD patients may be related to the cognitive deficiencies seen in many affected individuals; thus, they suggest that an absence of dystrophin in the brain or spinal cord could account for the upper motor neuron findings. However, they conclude that it is an unlikely explanation, as there are no other upper motor neuron signs and it would be unlikely to cause isolated bladder/sphincter dyssynergy.[113]

The treatment of bladder disturbance in these cases followed standard therapy and all patients were subsequently treated with anticholinergic medicines or clean intermittent catheterization or both.

Table 30.6 *Clinical features and neurophysiological findings in seven patients with Duchenne's muscular dystrophy (adapted from Caress et al[113])*

Patient	Age	History of spinal fusion	Symptoms	Urodynamics/ urethral EMG	Detrusor-sphincter dyssynergy	Uninhibited contractions	Motor unit appearance
1	17	Yes	Retention	Normal	No	No	Normal
2	14	Yes	Urgency, incontinence	UMN	No	Yes	Normal
3	11	Yes	Voiding difficulty	LMN	No	No	Long duration
4	17	Yes	Incontinence, frequent UTIs	UMN	Yes	Yes	Normal
5	8	No	Incontinence	UMN	No	Yes	Normal
6	16	?	Urgency, UTI, incontinence	UMN	Yes	Yes	Normal
7	16	Yes	Incontinence	UMN	Yes	Yes	Normal

EMG, electromyography; LMN, lower motor neuron; UMN, upper motor neuron; UTIs, urinary tract infections.

Epilepsy

Urinary incontinence is a common and well-recognized feature of epileptic seizures. Indeed, inquiry into loss of continence during seizures or blackouts is a routine aspect of history taking. Incontinence during episodes of loss of consciousness is, however, not diagnostic of seizures, and must always be considered along with other ictal features because incontinence can also occur in other disorders, causing loss of consciousness, even simple faints.

Seizures are symptoms of cerebral dysfunction, resulting from paroxysmal hyperexcitable and/or hypersynchronous discharges of neurons involving the cerebral cortex. Epilepsy is defined as a disorder characterized by recurrent epileptic seizures. The clinical manifestations are extremely variable and depend on the cortical areas involved. The International Classification of Epileptic Seizures divides the clinical manifestations into partial seizures, which begin in a part of one hemisphere, and generalized seizures, which begin in both hemispheres simultaneously. The signs and symptoms of simple partial seizures are determined by the function of the cortical area involved and are divided by the International Classification into motor, sensory, autonomic, and psychic phenomena.[114]

Urinary symptoms occurring with seizures include urgency and incontinence. During typical absence seizures, pressure recordings with catheterization reveal increased intravesicular pressure secondary to detrusor muscle contraction.[115] Enuresis following generalized tonic-clonic seizures is due to relaxation of the external sphincter.[116] During absence status, urinary incontinence occurs as a result of either micturitional automatism or neglect. Isolated ictal enuresis is rare. The exact frequency of incontinence in different seizure types is not known.

The urinary system is primarily under the control of the autonomic nervous system. It is not surprising, therefore, that seizures involving the autonomic nervous system are associated with incontinence, usually with other symptoms that are often more prominent. Autonomic seizures are well recognized and often arise from mesiobasal limbic, frontal, orbital, or opercular regions. There is likely to be rapid spread of seizure activity in to hypothalamic areas, further contributing to autonomic symptoms. Autonomic seizures are more common in the presence of impairment of consciousness, but may also occur with apparently fully preserved awareness and responsiveness.[117–119] Symptoms in autonomic seizures include vomiting, pallor, flushing, sweating, piloerection, pupil dilatation, borborygmi, and incontinence. These may occur as simple partial seizures or sometimes as an aura prior to complex partial or secondary generalized seizures. However, they must be distinguished from secondary effects of other seizure types (e.g. complex partial or generalized tonic-clonic seizures) that cause autonomic signs as a later feature.[117]

Autonomic symptoms and signs are present in all generalized tonic-clonic seizures and in most complex partial and absence attacks. Collectively, autonomic phenomena comprise an important and substantial portion of partial seizure symptoms, representing approximately one-third of all simple partial seizures.[118–120] The majority of these are referable to the epigastrium. Other types of autonomic seizures are uncommon.

Autonomic symptoms are particularly prominent in the so-called Panayiotopoulos syndrome (early-onset benign childhood seizures with occipital spikes).[121,122] Cardinal features of this condition include infrequent partial seizures that consist of a combination of autonomic and behavioral disturbances, vomiting, deviation of the eyes, often with impairment of consciousness that can frequently progress to convulsions. It is common for one or more of the symptoms to either predominate, or in other cases to be absent. Thus, autonomic disturbances of pallor and sweating, alone or together with behavioral disturbances (mainly irritability), may predominate, particularly in the early stages of the ictus.[123–126] Incontinence of urine and sometimes feces can occur with other autonomic or behavioral features even in nocturnal seizures. Incontinence occurs in about 10% of cases, usually when consciousness is impaired even without convulsions. Seizures are typically long, often lasting for 5 or more minutes and, in 40% for hours consistent with partial status epilepticus. The condition is considered benign with an excellent prognosis. About half of all patients only have a single attack, and in the majority of the remainder spontaneous remission occurs within a few years. For this reason antiepileptic drug treatment is rarely used.

Urinary frequency and incontinence has also been reported as an adverse reaction to antiepileptic medication. Incontinence is an unusual side-effect of carbamazepine and valproic acid,[127] and was reported in a single case during a clinical trial of gabapentin;[128] however, details of the urinary disturbance and outcome are not available. More recently, Gil-Nagel et al[129] reported urinary incontinence in three of their 394 cases treated with gabapentin at their tertiary referral center. The clinical details of the three cases are summarized in Table 30.7. Gabapentin-related incontinence included isolated urinary incontinence in one case with temporal lobe epilepsy and severe double incontinence in two cases with secondary generalized epilepsy. The problem persisted as long as patients were taking the drug and disappeared soon after it was discontinued or the dose was reduced. The three patients had medically refractory seizures and two adults had signs of generalized or multifocal neurological dysfunction, including mental retardation and hemiplegia. Incontinence did not appear to be related to seizure activity in any patient and video-EEG recordings in one patient corroborated this. Unfortunately, urodynamic assessment was not undertaken in any of the cases, and, therefore, the physiological

Table 30.7 *Urinary disturbances associated with gabapentin treatment*[129]

Age Gender	Seizure type	Neurological status	Urinary disturbance	Gabapentin dose	Other antiepileptic drugs	Outcome
43 Male	Secondary GTCS Atypical absence tonic	'Mental retardation' Secondary to perinatal hypoxic ischemic brain injury	Daily bladder and rectal incontinence unrelated to seizures	600 mg t.i.d.	Carbamazepine 600 mg/day Phenytoin 300 mg/day	Incontinence resolved on reducing dose to 300 mg b.i.d.
34 Female	Secondary GTCS Complex partial	Congenital hemiplegia	Weekly bladder and rectal incontinence unrelated to seizures	1800 mg/day	Phenytoin 250 mg/day Phenobarbital 180 mg/day	Resolved when dose reduced to 300 mg/day prior to discontinuation
12 Male	Complex partial	Hyperactivity and tics Convulsive status epilepticus age 4 years	Daily urinary incontinence unrelated to seizures	200 mg t.i.d.	Valproate 500 mg b.i.d.	Resolved 2 days after gabapentin stopped

b.i.d., twice a day; t.i.d., three times a day; GTCS: generalized tonic-clonic seizures.

mechanism for the incontinence is unclear. However, the authors postulated that because gabapentin is distributed in most organs and tissues, it could act at one or more sites involving not only the brain and spinal cord but also the gastrointestinal and urinary tracts. Gabapentin enhances the action of glutamate dehydrogenase and is a weak inhibitor of GABA transaminase and may therefore modulate glutamate and GABA. Both these neurotransmitters are involved in the regulation of micturition in the central nervous system. Thus, incontinence could be related to the effect of gabapentin in the cortex, interfering with the inhibition that the frontal lobe exerts on the pontine micturition center. It is possible that pre-existing damage to the cerebral cortex acted as a substrate for the development of gabapentin-induced incontinence.

Treatment of incontinence related to epilepsy primarily involves optimization of antiepileptic drug treatment, or other therapies, to minimize the frequency and severity of seizures. However Harari and Malone-Lee[130] reported beneficial effects of oxybutynin in one patient with epilepsy. The 30-year-old man was invariably incontinent during seizures and also at night on occasions. On the assumption that incontinence was due to hyperreflexic detrusor contractions during seizures the authors prescribed oxybutynin at a dose of 5 mg twice daily. On this dose, he remained continent despite further seizures.

From the earlier discussion it can be seen that incontinence in seizures has many potential mechanisms. In this case detrusor hyperreflexia may have been prominent; however, oxybutynin may not be as effective if other mechanisms are operating, particularly if incontinence is a feature of autonomic seizures themselves.

References

1. Roijen LE, Postema K, Limbeek VJ, Kuppevelt VH. Development of bladder control in children and adolescents with cerebral palsy. Develop Med Child Neurol 2001; 43(2):103–107.

2. Reid CJ, Borzyskowski M. Lower urinary tract dysfunction in cerebral palsy. Arch Dis Child 1993; 68(6):739–742.

3. Mayo ME. Lower urinary tract dysfunction in cerebral palsy. J Urol 1992; 147(2):419–420.

4. Decter RM, Bauer SB, Khoshbin S, et al. Urodynamic assessment of children with cerebral palsy. J Urol 1987; 138(4 Pt 2):1110–1112.

5. McNeal DM, Hawtrey CE, Wolraich ML, Mapel JR. Symptomatic neurogenic bladder in a cerebral-palsied population. Develop Med Child Neurol 1983; 25(5):612–616.

6. Drigo P, Seren F, Artibani W, et al. Neurogenic vesico-urethral dysfunction in children with cerebral palsy. Ital J Neurolog Sci 1988; 9(2):151–154.

7. Brodak PP, Scherz HC, Packer MG, Kaplan GW. Is urinary tract screening necessary for patients with cerebral palsy? J Urol 1994; 152(5 Pt 1):1586–1587.

8. Moulin F, Quintart A, Sauvestre C, et al. [Nosocomial urinary tract infections: retrospective study in a pediatric hospital]. Arch Pediatr 1998; 5(Suppl 3):274S-278S.

9. Kroll P, Martynski M, Jankowski A. [Staghorn calculi of the kidney and ureter as a urologic complication in a child with cerebral palsy]. Wiadomosci Lekarskie 1998; 51(Suppl 3):98–101.

10. Connolly B, Fitzgerald RJ, Guiney EJ. Has vesicostomy a role in the neuropathic bladder? Z Kinderchir 1988; 43(Suppl 2):17–18.

11. Honda N, Yamada Y, Nanaura H, et al. Mesonephric adenocarcinoma of the urinary bladder: a case report. Hinyokika Kiyo 2000; 46(1):27–31.

12. Tan PK, Edmond P. Longterm indwelling urethral catheterization for neuropathic bladders – an audit. J R Coll Surg Edinb 1994; 39(5):307–309.

13. Abbott R, Johann-Murphy M, Shiminski-Maher T, et al. Selective dorsal rhizotomy: outcome and complications in treating spastic cerebral palsy. Neurosurgery 1993; 33(5):851–857; discussion 857.

14. Houle AM, Vernet O, Jednak R, et al. Bladder function before and after selective dorsal rhizotomy in children with cerebral palsy. J Urol 1998; 160(3 Pt 2):1088–1091.

15. Sweetser PM, Badell A, Schneider S, Badlani GH. Effects of sacral dorsal rhizotomy on bladder function in patients with spastic cerebral palsy. Neurourol Urodyn 1995; 14(1):57–64.

16. Chami I, Miladi N, Ben Hamida M, Zmerli S. [Continence disorders in hereditary spinocerebellar degeneration. Comparison of clinical and urodynamic findings in 55 cases]. Acta Neurologica Belgica 1984; 84(4):194–203.

17. Leach GE, Farsaii A, Kark P, Raz S. Urodynamic manifestations of cerebellar ataxia. J Urol 1982; 128(2):348–350.

18. Vezina JG, Bouchard JP, Bouchard R. Urodynamic evaluation of patients with hereditary ataxias. Can J Neurol Sci 1982; 9(2):127–129.

19. Sakakibara R, Hattori T, Uchiyama T, Yamanishi T. Micturitional disturbance in a patient with neurosarcoidosis. Neurourol Urodyn 2000; 19(3):273–277.

20. Carod-Artal FJ, del Negro MC, Vargas AP, Rizzo I. [Cerebellar syndrome and peripheral neuropathy as manifestations of infection by HTLV-1 human T-cell lymphotropic virus]. Revista de Neurologia 1999; 29(10):932–935.

21. Nakane S, Motomura M, Shirabe S, et al. [A case of superficial siderosis of the central nervous system – findings of the neuro-otological tests and evoked potentials]. No to Shinkei – Brain & Nerve 1999; 51(2):155–159.

22. Fujiki N, Oikawa O, Matsumoto A, Tashiro K. [A case of HTLV-I associated myelopathy presenting with cerebellar signs as initial and principal manifestations]. Rinsho Shinkeigaku – Clinical Neurology 1999; 39(8):852–855.

23. Sakakibara R, Hattori T, Yasuda K, et al. Micturitional disturbance in Wernicke's encephalopathy. Neurourol Urodyn 1997; 16(2):111–115.

24. Gyrtrup HJ, Kristiansen VB, Zachariae CO, et al. Voiding problems in patients with HIV infection and AIDS. Scand J Urol Nephrol 1995; 29(3):295–298.

25. Zeman A, Donaghy M. Acute infection with human immunodeficiency virus presenting with neurogenic urinary retention. Genitourin Med 1991; 67(4):345–347.

26. Hermieu JF, Delmas V, Boccon-Gibod L. Micturition disturbances and human immunodeficiency virus infection. J Urol 1996; 156(1):157–159.

27. Menendez V, Valls J, Espuna M, et al. Neurogenic bladder in patients with acquired immunodeficiency syndrome. Neurourol Urodyn 1995; 14(3):253–257.

28. So YT, Olney RK. Acute lumbosacral polyradiculopathy in acquired immunodeficiency syndrome: experience in 23 patients. Ann Neurol 1994; 35(1):53–58.

29. Baraister M. Neurocutaneous disorders. In: Baraister M, ed. The genetics of neurological disorders, 3rd edn. Oxford: Oxford University Press, 1997:85–101.

30. Hintsa A, Lindell O, Heikkila P. Neurofibromatosis of the bladder. Scand J Urol Nephrol 1996; 30(6):497–499.

31. Hulse CA. Neurofibromatosis: bladder involvement with malignant degeneration. J Urol 1990; 144(3):742–743.

32. Nyholm HC. [Neurofibromatosis with bladder localization]. Ugeskr Laeger 1980; 142(37):2426–2427.

33. Kramer SA, Barrett DM, Utz DC. Neurofibromatosis of the bladder in children. J Urol 1981; 126(5):693–694.

34. Aygun C, Tekin MI, Tarhan C, et al. Neurofibroma of the bladder wall in von Recklinghausen's disease. Int J Urol 2001; 8(5):249–253.

35. Miller WB Jr, Boal DK, Teele R. Neurofibromatosis of the bladder: sonographic findings. J Clin Ultrasound 1983; 11(8):460–462.

36. Kargi HA, Aktug T, Ozen E, Kilicalp A. A diffuse form of neurofibroma of bladder in a child with von Recklinghausen disease. Turk J Pediatr 1998; 40(2):267–271.

37. Jensen A, Nissen HM. Neurofibromatosis of the bladder. Scand J Urol Nephrol 1976; 10(2):157–159.

38. Torres H, Bennett MJ. Neurofibromatosis of the bladder: case report and review of the literature. J Urol 1966; 96(6):910–912.

39. Winfield HN, Catalona WJ. An isolated plexiform neurofibroma of the bladder. J Urol 1985; 134(3):542–543.

40. Merksz M, Toth J, Kiraly L. Neurofibromatosis of the bladder. Int Urol Nephrol 1985; 17(1):53–59.

41. Gold BM. Neurofibromatosis of the bladder and vagina. Am J Obstet Gynecol 1972; 113(8):1055–1056.

42. Dahm P, Manseck A, Flossel C, et al. Malignant neurofibroma of the urinary bladder. Eur Urol 1995; 27(3):261–263.

43. Rober PE, Smith JB, Sakr W, Pierce JM Jr. Malignant peripheral nerve sheath tumor (malignant schwannoma) of urinary bladder in von Recklinghausen neurofibromatosis. Urology 1991; 38(5):473–476.

44. Borden TA, Shrader DA. Neurofibromatosis of bladder in a child: unusual cause of enuresis. Urology 1980; 15(2):155–158.

45. Pycha A, Klingler CH, Reiter WJ, et al. Von Recklinghausen neurofibromatosis with urinary bladder involvement. Urology 2001; 58(1):106.

46. Carlson DH, Wilkinson RH. Neurofibromatosis of the bladder in children. Radiology 1972; 105(2):401–404.

47. Maneschg C, Rogatsch H, Bartsch G, Stenzl A. Treatment of giant ancient pelvic schwannoma. Tech Urol 2001; 7(4):296–298.

48. Mimata H, Kasagi Y, Ohno H, et al. Malignant neurofibroma of the urinary bladder. Urol Int 2000; 65(3):167–168.

49. Sharma NS, Lynch MJ. Intrapelvic neurilemmoma presenting with bladder outlet obstruction. Br J Urol 1998; 82(6):917.

50. Salvant JB Jr, Young HF. Giant intrasacral schwannoma: an unusual cause of lumbrosacral radiculopathy. Surg Neurol 1994; 41(5):411–413.

51. Burton EM, Schellhammer PF, Weaver DL, Woolfitt RA. Paraganglioma of urinary bladder in patient with neurofibromatosis. Urology 1986; 27(6):550–552.

52. Reich S, Overberg-Schmidt US, Leenen A, Henze G. Neurofibromatosis 1 associated with embryonal rhabdomyosarcoma of the urinary bladder. Pediatr Hematol Oncol 1999; 16(3):263–266.

53. Dominguez J, Lobato RD, Ramos A, et al. Giant intrasacral schwannomas: report of six cases. Acta Neurochirurg 1997; 139(10):954–959; discussion 959–960.

54. Chakravarti A, Jones MA, Simon J. Neurofibromatosis involving the urinary bladder. Int J Urol 2001; 8(11):645–647.

55. Clark SS, Marlett MM, Prudencio RF, Dasgupta TK. Neurofibromatosis of the bladder in children: case report and literature review. J Urol 1977; 118(4):654–656.

56. Daneman A, Grattan-Smith P. Neurofibromatosis involving the lower urinary tract in children. A report of three cases and a review of the literature. Pediatr Radiol 1976; 4(3):161–166.

57. Cheng L, Scheithauer BW, Leibovich BC, et al. Neurofibroma of the urinary bladder. Cancer 1999; 86(3):505–513.

58. Evans DG, Mason S, Huson SM, et al. Spinal and cutaneous schwannomatosis is a variant form of type 2 neurofibromatosis: a clinical and molecular study. J Neurol Neurosurg Psychiatry 1997; 62(4):361–366.

59. Brownlee RD, Clark AW, Sevick RJ, Myles ST. Symptomatic hamartoma of the spinal cord associated with neurofibromatosis type 1. Case report. J Neurosurg 1998; 88(6):1099–1103.

60. Chaparro MJ, Young RF, Smith M, et al. Multiple spinal meningiomas: a case of 47 distinct lesions in the absence of neurofibromatosis or identified chromosomal abnormality. Neurosurgery 1993; 32(2):298–301; discussion 301–302.

61. Babjakova L, Jurkovic I, Krajcar R, Kocan P. [Multiple intracranial and intraspinal meningiomas in the neurocristopathy (phacomatosis) type of neurofibromatosis]. Ceskoslovenska Patologie 2000; 36(4):150–155.

62. Kawsar M, Goh BT. Spinal schwannoma as a cause of erectile dysfunction with urinary incontinence and groin and testicular pain. Int J STD AIDS 2002; 13(8):584–585.

63. Honda E, Hayashi T, Goto S, et al. [Two different spinal tumors (meningioma and schwannoma) with von Recklinghausen's disease in a case]. No Shinkei Geka – Neurological Surgery 1990; 18(5):463–468.

64. Mizuo T, Ando M, Azima J, et al. [Manifestation of mictional disturbance in four cases of von Recklinghausen's disease]. Hinyokika Kiyo – Acta Urologica Japonica 1987; 33(1):125–132.

65. Caputo LA, Cusimano MD. Schwannoma of the cauda equina. J Manipul Physiol Ther 1997; 20(2):124–129.

66. Acharya R, Bhalla S, Sehgal AD. Malignant peripheral nerve sheath tumor of the cauda equina. Neurolog Sci 2001; 22(3):267–270.

67. Kissel P, Dureurx JB. Cobb syndrome. Cutaneomeningospinal angiomatosis. In: Bruyn GW, Vinken PJ, eds. Handbook of clinical neurology. New York: North Holland; 1972; 14:429–445.

68. Wakabayashi Y, Isono M, Shimomura T, et al. Neurocutaneous vascular hamartomas mimicking Cobb syndrome. Case report. J Neurosurg 2000; 93(1 Suppl):133–136.

69. Klippel M, Trénaunay P. Du naevus variquex osteo-hypertropique. Arch Genet Med 1900; 3:641–672.

70. Weber FP. Angioma formation in connection with hypertrophy of limbs and hemihypertrophy. Br J Dermatol 1907; 19:231–235.

71. Weber FP. Hemangioectatic hypertrophy of limbs. Congenital phlebarteriectasia and so-called congenital varicose veins. Br J Child Dis 1918; 15:13–17.

72. Kojima Y, Kuwana N, Sato M, Ikeda Y. Klippel–Trénaunay–Weber syndrome with spinal arteriovenous malformation – case report. Neurologia Medico-Chirurgica 1989; 29(3):235–240.

73. Furness PD 3rd, Barqawi AZ, Bisignani G, Decter RM. Klippel–Trénaunay syndrome: 2 case reports and a review of genitourinary manifestations. J Urol 2001; 166(4):1418–1420.

74. Ben Becher S, Bouaziz A, Harbi MM, et al. [Protee syndrome associated with renal lithiasis and vesico-ureteral reflux]. Archives Francaises de Pediatrie 1993; 50(7):599–601.

75. Horie Y, Fujita H, Mano S, et al. Regional Proteus syndrome: report of an autopsy case. Pathol Int 1995; 45(7):530–535.

76. Sawamura Y, Abe H, Murai H, et al. [An autopsy case of neurocutaneous melanosis associated with intracerebral malignant melanoma]. No to Shinkei – Brain & Nerve 1987; 39(8):789–795.

77. Berger AR, Swerdlow M, Herskovitz S. Myasthenia gravis presenting as uncontrollable flatus and urinary/fecal incontinence. Muscle Nerve 1996; 19(1):113–114.

78. Christmas TJ, Dixon PJ, Milroy EJ. Detrusor failure in myasthenia gravis. Br J Urol 1990; 65(4):422.

79. Howard JFJ, Donovan MK, Tucker MS. Urinary incontinence in myasthenia gravis: a single fibre electromyographic study. Ann Neurol 1992; 32:254 [Abstract].

80. Matsui M, Enoki M, Matsui Y, et al. Seronegative myasthenia gravis associated with atonic urinary bladder and accommodative insufficiency. J Neurol Sci 1995; 133(1–2):197–199.

81. Sandler PM, Avillo C, Kaplan SA. Detrusor areflexia in a patient with myasthenia gravis. Int J Urol 1998; 5(2):188–190.

82. Wise GJ, Gerstenfeld JN, Brunner N, Grob D. Urinary incontinence following prostatectomy in patients with myasthenia gravis. Br J Urol 1982; 54(4):369–371.

83. Khan Z, Bhola A. Urinary incontinence after transurethral resection of prostate in myasthenia gravis patients. Urology 1989; 34(3):168–169.

84. Newsom-Davis J. Lambert–Eaton myasthenic syndrome. Current Treat Options Neurol 2001; 3(2):127–131.

85. Sanders DB. The Lambert–Eaton myasthenic syndrome. Adv Neurol 2002; 88:189–201.

86. Vincent A, Lang B, Newsom-Davis J. Autoimmunity to the voltage-gated calcium channel underlies the Lambert–Eaton myasthenic syndrome, a paraneoplastic disorder. Trends Neurosci 1989; 12(12):496–502.

87. Khurana RK, Koski CL, Mayer RF. Autonomic dysfunction in Lambert–Eaton myasthenic syndrome. J Neurol Sci 1988; 85(1):77–86.

88. O'Neill JH, Murray NM, Newsom-Davis J. The Lambert–Eaton myasthenic syndrome. A review of 50 cases. Brain 1988; 111(Pt 3):577–596.

89. O'Suilleabhain P, Low PA, Lennon VA. Autonomic dysfunction in the Lambert–Eaton myasthenic syndrome: serologic and clinical correlates. Neurology 1998; 50(1):88–93.

90. Waterman SA. Autonomic dysfunction in Lambert–Eaton myasthenic syndrome. Clin Auton Res 2001; 11(3):145–154.

91. Waterman SA, Lang B, Newsom-Davis J. Effect of Lambert–Eaton myasthenic syndrome antibodies on autonomic neurons in the mouse. Ann Neurol 1997; 42(2):147–156.

92. Henriksson KG, Nilsson O, Rosen I, Schiller HH. Clinical, neurophysiological and morphological findings in Eaton Lambert syndrome. Acta Neurol Scand 1977; 56(2):117–140.

93. Satoh K, Motomura M, Suzu H, et al. Neurogenic bladder in Lambert–Eaton myasthenic syndrome and its response to 3,4-diaminopyridine. J Neurol Sci 2001; 183(1):1–4.

94. Frew R, Lundy PM. A role for Q type Ca^{2+} channels in neurotransmission in the rat urinary bladder. Br J Pharmacol 1995; 116(1):1595–1598.

95. Houzen H, Hattori Y, Kanno M, et al. Functional evaluation of inhibition of autonomic transmitter release by autoantibody from Lambert–Eaton myasthenic syndrome. Ann Neurol 1998; 43(5):677–680.

96. Roses AD, Chang L. Myotonic dystrophy. In: Gilman S, ed. MedLink neurology. San Diego: MedLink Corporation, 2002. Available at www.medlink.com.

97. Harper PS. Smooth muscle in myotonic dystrophy. In: Harper PS, ed. Major problems in neurology, 37: myotonic dystrophy, 3rd edn. London: WB Saunders, 2001: 91–108.

98. Harvey JC, Sherbourne DH, Siegel CI. Smooth muscle involvement in myotonic dystrophy. Am J Med 1965; 39:81–90.

99. Kohn NN, Faires JS, Chiu VSW. Unusual manifestations due to involvement of involuntary muscles in dystrophia myotonica. New Engl J Med 1964; 271:1179.

100. Pruzanski W. Myotonic dystrophy – a multisystem disease: report of 67 cases and a review of the literature. Psychiatr Neurol 1965; 149:302.

101. Bundschu HD, Hauger W, Lang HD. [Myotonic dystrophy (urological features and histochemical findings in muscle) (author's transl)]. Deutsche Medizinische Wochenschrift 1975; 100(24):1337–1341.

102. Orndahl G, Kock NG, Sundin T. Smooth muscle activity in myotonic dystrophy. Brain 1973; 96(4):857–860.

103. Bernstein IT, Andersen BB, Andersen JT, et al. Bladder function in patients with myotonic dystrophy. Neurol Urodyn 1992; 11:219–223.

104. Sakakibara R, Hattori T, Tojo M, et al. Micturitional disturbance in myotonic dystrophy. J Auton Nerv Sys 1995; 52(1):17–21.

105. Black WC, Ravin A. Studies in dystrophia myotonica. Arch Pathol 1947; 44:176.

106. Pruzanski W, Huvos AG. Smooth muscle involvement in primary muscle disease. I. Myotonic dystrophy. Arch Pathol Lab Med 1967; 83(3):229–233.

107. Bushby KM. Making sense of the limb-girdle muscular dystrophies. Brain 1999; 122(Pt 8):1403–1420.

108. Bushby K. The limb-girdle muscular dystrophies. Eur J Paediatr Neurol 2001; 5(5):213–214.

109. Dixon PJ, Christmas TJ, Chapple CR. Stress incontinence due to pelvic floor muscle involvement in limb-girdle muscular dystrophy. Br J Urol 1990; 65(6):653–654.

110. Acsadi G. Duchenne muscular dystrophy. In: Gilman S, ed. MedLink Neurology. San Diego: MedLink Corporation, 2002. Available at www.medlink.com.

111. Brooke MH. Muscular dystrophies: Duchenne muscular dystrophy. In: Brooke MH, ed. A clinicians view of neuromuscular diseases, 2nd edn. Baltimore: Williams and Wilkins, 1986: 117–154.

112. Boland BJ, Silbert PL, Groover RV, et al. Skeletal, cardiac, and smooth muscle failure in Duchenne muscular dystrophy. Pediatr Neurol 1996; 14(1):7–12.

113. Caress JB, Kothari MJ, Bauer SB, Shefner JM. Urinary dysfunction in Duchenne muscular dystrophy. Muscle & Nerve 1996; 19(7):819–822.

114. Epilepsy Commission on Classification and Terminology of the ILAE. Proposal for revised clinical and electroencephalographic classification of epileptic seizures. Epilepsia 1981; 22:489–501.

115. Gastaut H, Batini C, Broughton R, et al. Polygraphic study of enuresis during petit mal absences. Electroencephalogr Clin Neurophysiol 1964:616–626.

116. Gastaut H, Broughton R, Roger J, Tassinari C. Generalized non-convulsive seizures without local onset. In: Vinken P, Bruyn G, eds. Handbook of clinical neurology. New York, 1974; 15:130–144.

117. Liporace JD, Sperling MR. Simple autonomic seizures. In: Engel JJ, Pedley TA, eds. Epilepsy: the comprehensive CD-ROM. Philadelphia: Lippincott, Williams and Wilkins, 1999.

118. Gupta AK, Jeavons PM, Hughes RC, Covanis A. Aura in temporal lobe epilepsy: clinical and electroencephalographic correlation. J Neurol Neurosurg Psychiatry 1983; 46(12):1079–1083.

119. Palmini A, Gloor P. The localizing value of auras in partial seizures: a prospective and retrospective study. Neurology 1992; 42(4): 801–808.

120. Devinsky O, Kelley K, Porter RJ, Theodore WH. Clinical and electroencephalographic features of simple partial seizures. Neurology 1988; 38(9):1347–1352.

121. Panayiotopoulos CP. Autonomic seizures and autonomic status epilepticus specific to childhood. Arch Pediatr Adolesc Med 2002; 156(9):945.

122. Weig S. Panayiotopoulos syndrome: a common and benign childhood epileptic syndrome. In: Panayiotopoulos CP, ed. J Neurol Sci 2002; 202(1–2):99.

123. Panayiotopoulos CP. Early-onset benign childhood occipital seizure susceptibility syndrome: a syndrome to recognize. Epilepsia 1999; 40(5):621–630.

124. Panayiotopoulos CP. Extraoccipital benign childhood partial seizures with ictal vomiting and excellent prognosis. J Neurol Neurosurg Psychiatry 1999; 66(1):82–85.

125. Panayiotopoulos CP. Benign childhood epileptic syndromes with occipital spikes: new classification proposed by the International League Against Epilepsy. J Child Neurol 2000; 15(8):548–552.

126. Panayiotopoulos CP. Panayiotopoulos syndrome. Lancet 2001; 358(9275):68–69.

127. Physicians Desk Reference, 5th edn. Montvale: Medical Economics Company, 1996.

128. Handforth A, Treiman DM. Efficacy and tolerance of long-term, high-dose gabapentin: additional observations. Epilepsia 1994; 35(5):1032–1037.

129. Gil-Nagel A, Gapany S, Blesi K, et al. Incontinence during treatment with gabapentin. Neurology 1997; 48(5):1467–1468.

130. Harari D, Malone-Lee JG. Oxybutynin and incontinence during grand mal seizures. Br J Urol 1991; 68(6):658.

Part IV

Evaluation of neurogenic bladder dysfunction

31

Clinical evaluation: history and physical examination

Gary E Lemack

Introduction

The starting point for any new patient with neurologic disease that is referred with lower urinary tract (LUT) complaints is a thorough history and physical examination. While more exact and specific means are often necessary to pinpoint the nature of bladder dysfunction in such patients, a directed, though thorough history and physical examination are essential to defining which patients require more costly and invasive testing, and which can be followed with alternative strategies. The ongoing refinement of urodynamic testing certainly has permitted the precise characterization of bladder dysfunction in patients with severe neurogenic disorders, but failing to know what questions to ask and what signs to observe can lead to erroneous diagnoses and inappropriate testing. The focus of this chapter will be on obtaining as much information as possible on the initial visit by directed questioning and a focused examination, so as to be able to discern what testing, if any, is necessary on future visits.

History
Nature of neurologic disease

Most, though not all patients, will come already with a known neurologic disease. In patients with progressive conditions, it is useful to establish the onset of symptoms – often not the same as the timing of diagnosis – as well as recent changes in symptom severity, as this information may clearly influence treatment recommendations. Even patients with a presumably fixed neurologic condition, such as spinal cord injury (SCI) or myelomeningocele, may have symptomatic deterioration (i.e. due to development of a syrinx), and therefore any recent changes in sensory or motor function should be directly questioned. Often, patients or their caregivers will have tremendous insight

into the medical condition and will, for example, know the Hoehn and Yahr stage of their Parkinson's disease, which can be useful in predicting the severity of bladder dysfunction and prospects for further deterioration.[1] Patients with multiple sclerosis may give a history of recurrent flares in conjunction with worsening urinary symptoms, which should signal an investigation for recurrent urinary infections as a possible source.

In patients with more recent acute events, such as cerebrovascular accident, information about the stroke location and the recovery since the event can be useful, since stroke location can impact on prognosis.[2] Patients with history of back surgery (often several procedures) should be questioned as to the vertebral level of the surgery, and for the presence of ongoing sensory deficit.

Current treatments should also be documented, with particular attention to medications. Medications with properties that can affect the bladder outlet (typically with either α-agonist or α-antagonist properties) or detrusor contractility (typically those with anticholinergic properties) should be recorded, along with narcotic and skeletal muscle relaxant use.

Nature of lower urinary tract symptoms

Duration of symptoms

The timing of onset of urinary symptoms is a crucial piece of information to obtain during history taking. In slowly progressive diseases, such as multiple sclerosis, a clear date of onset will be impossible to establish, though a general assessment of the time course over which the symptoms worsened is essential. In some patients, the date of onset will be quite clear, though often, as is the case in patients with cerebrovascular accidents, the presence of pre-existing symptoms may be difficult to discern. Still, the clear temporal relationship of a particular urinary symptom with an event is strong evidence of a causal relationship, which can be further supported by urodynamic testing. A patient with SCI and stable LUT function who suddenly develops new incontinence may need to have repeated spinal cord imaging, whereas a patient with slowly improving urinary urgency following a stroke can often be safely followed with noninvasive monitoring.

Previous urologic history

Patients will often come referred with a diagnosis of recurrent urinary tract infections, but precisely documenting the offending organism and its sensitivities is essential to discovering its source. Failure to clear an ongoing infection (persistence) and repeated bouts of new infections imply different etiologies. Clearly, the method of bladder management will affect the susceptibility to infection, and the use of indwelling or intermittent catheterization should be documented. Additionally, the duration of each catheter use before change, and cleaning technique used (intermittent catheterization) should be recorded, as well as a careful reassessment of catheterization technique. A history of previous bladder, prostate, or upper tract surgery must be carefully detailed, and operative notes of complex reconstructions reviewed.

Current urinary symptoms

Lower urinary tract symptoms (LUTS) should be carefully assessed at the time of initial presentation. Patients should be questioned for the presence or progression of urinary urgency, frequency, and nocturia, in addition to other symptoms typically associated with disorders of bladder filling. Often, a 2- or 3-day voiding diary (see Chapter 33) can be of tremendous help in establishing micturition frequency and voided volumes.[3,4] In general, greater than 8 voids per day is considered abnormal, though clearly this finding is nonspecific. Urinary frequency may represent detrusor overactivity, impaired bladder capacity, excessive urine production (polyuria), impaired bladder emptying, urinary infection, stone disease, inflammatory bladder conditions, as well as many other possible etiologies.

LUTS typically associated with the voiding such as urinary hesitancy, straining, loss of stream, and interrupted urine flow are also important to establish. A staccato type of voiding pattern (choppy, interrupted pattern) can be a warning sign indicating detrusor-sphincter dyssynergia, and should prompt a more thorough evaluation, including urodynamic testing. Excessive straining, too, is nonspecific and could represent detrusor failure or bladder outlet obstruction, and therefore should also prompt urodynamic testing in patients with known neurologic disease.

Incontinence, when present, should be characterized fully. Stress incontinence, occurring with increases in intra-abdominal pressure, and most frequently associated with physical activity, coughing, straining, and sneezing, should be assessed for severity, approximate time of onset, and degree of progression. During history taking, incontinence may be assessed by pad usage (nonspecific) and questionnaire response, although questionnaire response may not be a reliable indicator of severity of stress-related leakage.[5,6] Several validated questionnaires are available in men[7] and women,[8] though few were specifically designed for use in patients with neurogenic bladder conditions.[9]

Urge incontinence – which is thought to be due to detrusor overactivity, rather than pelvic floor hypermobility or intrinsic sphincteric weakness alone, as is the case with stress leakage – may be best assessed by a voiding diary and pad usage. Typical symptoms include the sudden, uncontrollable urge to urinate, nighttime leakage episodes, and, sometimes, leakage during intercourse. This is the most common pattern among patients with multiple sclerosis, cerebrovascular accident, and Parkinson's disease, among whom the urodynamic finding of neurogenic detrusor overactivity is quite common.

Patients with overflow incontinence may present with constant low-grade dribbling, recurrent urinary infections, or, at times, renal insufficiency due to the presence of significantly elevated post-void residuals. In most instances, overflow incontinence is due to detrusor failure or severe bladder outlet obstruction. Patients in the spinal shock phase of SCI will typically present with this pattern (due to detrusor areflexia), which will often persist in those with lower lumbar and sacral cord injuries. Patients with continuous incontinence – which may be due to ureteral ectopy, fistula formation, or occasionally a scarred, fixed urethra – will report constant urinary drainage, often with very infrequent voids due to the lack of urine accumulation in the bladder.

Non-genitourinary review of systems

An assessment of bowel function is imperative, as often bowel and bladder dysfunction parallel one another in patients with neurologic conditions. In patients with SCI, the nature of bowel program should be established (i.e. digital stimulation, suppository use, etc.). The presence of fecal incontinence, tenesmus, chronic constipation, or obstipation should also be recorded.

A sexual history is also quite important, as sexual dysfunction is also extremely common among men and women with neurologic conditions.[10,11] Women may report lack of desire (loss of libido) or inability to have intercourse secondary to vaginal pain or dryness, or due to enhanced vaginal sensitivity (hyperesthesia), particularly in the case of multiple sclerosis. Men may report erectile dysfunction often secondary to altered penile sensation. Ejaculatory disturbances due to these changes in sensation (leading to either premature or delayed ejaculation), or bladder neck dysfunction (retrograde ejaculation) are also not uncommon. Patients with sympathetic outflow interruption, such as those with complete spinal cord lesions, will often experience anejaculation. In such instances, vibratory stimulation to the penis or electrical stimulation applied transrectally can often result in successful ejaculation.

Physical examination
Neurologic assessment

A brief neurologic examination is essential when first evaluating patients with presumed neurovesical dysfunction. Mental status should be assessed, as significant cognitive dysfunction and memory disturbances have been independently associated with abnormal toileting behavior. An appreciation of past and present intellectual capacity may also provide insight into the progression of LUT disorders, as well as guide the degree of complexity of treatment strategies. Both motor strength and sensory level should be determined, as distribution of motor and sensory disturbances can often predict LUT dysfunction.[12]

There should also be a thorough evaluation of both cutaneous and motor reflexes at the time of the initial encounter. The bulbocavernosus reflex, which is elicited by gently squeezing the glans penis in men or gentle compression of the clitoris against the pubis in women and simultaneously feeling for an anal sphincter contraction (by placing a finger in the rectum), assesses the integrity of the S2–S4 reflex arc. The anal reflex, which assesses integrity of S2–S5, can be checked by applying a pinprick to the mucocutaneous junction of the anus and evaluating for anal sphincter contraction. The cremasteric reflex may be somewhat less reliable, but assesses sensory dermatomes supplied by L1–L2.

Muscle motor reflexes should also be routinely evaluated. The most common of these are the biceps reflex (assesses C5–C6), patellar reflex (L2–L4), and Achilles (ankle) reflex (L5–S2). Evidence of an upper motor neurologic injury would include spasticity of the involved skeletal muscle, heightened response to reflex testing, and an upgoing toe on gentle stroking of the plantar surface of the foot (positive Babinski's sign).

General issues

Mode of ambulation and recent progression of ambulatory disturbances should be assessed at the initial visit. Clearly, the degree of physical independence of the patient, particularly as it relates to the ability to get to the toilet, often affects the degree of urge-related leakage episodes. Additionally,

certain patients who are non-ambulatory may have great difficulty with self-urethral catheterization. Should that be the case, an abdominal catheterizable stoma may be a more reasonable option in the appropriately selected patient.

Hand function in patients with cervical SCI, and particularly the ability to grasp firmly between the thumb and index or middle finger, must be carefully judged in patients who may require intermittent catheterization following treatment. However, it is no longer mandatory that patients have use of both hands prior to such an intervention, as single-unit catheter/collection systems have become commercially available.

An evaluation of the skin, particularly in the gluteal region should be carried out, as localized skin and subcutaneous infections as well as more severe skin breakdown are not uncommon among patients with restricted mobility. Such issues will need to be addressed before major reconstructive procedures are considered. Some patients may also have intrathecal pumps in place and their location, as well as that of their tubing, should be assessed prior to surgical endeavors.

Pelvic examination

Pelvic examination should be carried out to assess for vaginal estrogenization (noting a loss of lubrication, rugation, and blanching of the mucosal surface), and pelvic prolapse. One should also observe for urine loss (either spontaneous or induced by Valsalva's maneuver or cough). An assessment of the urethra is essential in both men and women, particularly those with chronic indwelling catheters, as traumatic hypospadias in men and bladder neck erosion in women may require surgical repair. A careful examination of sensation of the genitalia may provide insight into the nature of sexual dysfunction, as both hypo- and hyperesthesia have been described among patients with neurologic conditions. A rectal examination should assess for sphincter tone and for stool impaction, as chronic constipation may aggravate voiding dysfunction. In men, the prostate should be examined for areas of tenderness or fluctuance, since prostatitis and prostatic abscesses are not uncommon among men with severe neurovesical dysfunction, particularly those with chronic indwelling catheters.

Conclusion

As a starting point to a complete assessment of the neurourologic patient, a thorough history and physical examination are essential. Data obtained during this initial interview will determine when more invasive testing is necessary, and provide guidance as to the most appropriate treatment strategies for any given patient.

References

1. Lemack GE, Dewey RB, Roehrborn CG, et al. Questionnaire-based assessment of bladder dysfunction in patients with mild to moderate Parkinson's disease. Urology 2000; 56:250–254.

2. Khan Z, Starer P, Yang YC, Bhola A. Analysis of voiding disorders in patients with cerebrovascular accidents. Urology 1990; 32:265–270.

3. Wyman JF, Choi SC, Harkins SW, et al. The urinary diary in evaluation of incontinent women: a test–retest analysis. Obstet Gynecol 1988; 71:812–817.

4. Groutz A, Blaivas JG, Chaikin DC, et al. Noninvasive outcome measures of urinary incontinence and lower urinary tract symptoms: a multicenter study of micturition diary and pad tests. J Urol 2000; 164:698–701.

5. Lemack GE, Zimmern PE. Predictability of urodynamic findings based on the Urogenital Distress Inventory questionnaire. Urology 1999; 54:461–466.

6. Harvey MA, Kristjansson B, Griffith D, Versi E. The Incontinence Impact Questionnaire and the Urogenital Distress Inventory: a revisit of their validity in women without a urodynamic diagnosis. Am J Obstet Gynecol 2001; 185:25–31.

7. Barry MJ, Fowler FJ Jr, O'Leary MP, et al., and the Measurement Committee of the American Urological Association. The American Urological Association symptom index for benign prostatic hyperplasia. J Urol 1992; 148:1549–1557.

8. Uebersax JS, Wyman FF, Shumaker SA, et al. Short forms to assess life quality and symptom distress for urinary incontinence in women: the incontinence impact questionnaire and urogenital distress inventory. Neurourol Urod 1995; 14:131–139.

9. Sakakibara R, Shinotoh H, Uchiyama T, et al. Questionnaire-based assessment of pelvic organ dysfunction in Parkinson's disease. Auton Neurosci Bas Clin 2001; 92:76–85.

10. Lundberg PO, Hutler B. Female sexual dysfunction in multiple sclerosis: a review. Sex Dis 1996; 14:65–72.

11. Aisen ML, Sanders AS. Sexual dysfunction in neurologic disease: mechanisms of disease and counseling approaches. Am Urolog Assoc Update Ser 1998: 17:274–279.

12. Betts CD, D'Mellow MT, Fowler CJ. Urinary symptoms and the neurological features of bladder dysfunction in multiple sclerosis. J Neurol Neurosurg Psychiatry 1993; 56(3):245–250.

32

Quality of life assessment in neurogenic bladder

Patrick Marquis

Introduction

Normal bladder function requires coordinated interaction of sensory and motor components of both the somatic and autonomic nervous systems. The micturition reflex is a finely tuned neurological event that requires integration of most levels of the nervous system to regulate voiding function, so that damage to any one of the many neurological mechanisms involved affects urination. In particular, bladder contraction and reflex control depends on an intact neural axis – specifically, an undamaged sacral spinal cord together with its afferent and efferent connections.[1] Spinal cord injury (SCI), by contrast, generally results in absent sensation below the level of the lesion and, although patients with upper motor neuron lesions can have a local reflex of bladder contraction, it is often opposed by smooth and striated muscle dyssynergia in the sphincters controlling bladder voiding. Neurogenic bladder problems are therefore a near universal feature of spinal cord injury.

In the United States alone, there are at present estimated to be 200,000 patients with SCI and the number increases by about 10,000 per year.[2] According to De Vivo et al[3] the commonest causes of SCI are road accidents (45%), falls (22%), acts of violence (16%), and sports trauma (13%); 82% of victims are male, with a mean age of 31 years. This, self-evidently, represents a dramatic loss of healthy productive years for the individuals and major adaptation for their families, as well as a significant socioeconomic burden.

Spinal cord injury is serious in all cases, but the degree of resultant disability depends on the site of the injury along the spine. Five decades ago, treatment was largely aimed at keeping patients alive during the immediate post-injury period. When acute SCI management had improved to the point where survival was likely, the focus of treatment shifted to preventing the long-term medical complications which subsequently appeared, with urinary disorders being reported in one 25-year prospective study as the leading cause of death in SCI patients up to the mid 1970s.[4] Two decades later, a 13-member Department of Health expert panel reported that diseases of the urinary system had become only the fifth most common primary or secondary cause of death in SCI patients but that 80% or patients reported a urinary tract infection by their 16th year post-injury.[5] Nowadays, respiratory problems are regarded as the major cause of death in SCI patients, together with accidents and suicide, but urinary disorders remain a significant secondary cause of death and a major cause of morbidity.[6–8]

In practice, the impact of traumatic SCI is even greater than the usually drastic functional and mobility effects on the patients themselves, since it normally extends to sudden and fundamental changes in roles and relationships which affect uninjured family members.[9–11] The outcome and resolution of the shift in relationships between the injured and uninjured family members can profoundly affect how the SCI person reacts to and comes to terms with their injury, which in turn can affect their rehabilitation and ultimate ongoing quality of life (QoL). It follows that successful SCI treatment may also provide benefits which extend beyond patients themselves, to alter the QoL of the affected family members.

Patient quality of life

SCI sufferers are affected both physically and psychologically during the acute injury phase, during the process of adjustment after injury, and by their ongoing life situation once their medical situation has stabilized. Siösteen et al assessed the quality of life of 56 SCI patients in three subgroups ranked according to functional ability:[12] C6 tetraplegics, wheelchair-dependent paraplegics and ambulant paraplegics were assessed according to various functional and emotional criteria to arrive at an estimate of sickness impact profile (SIP) in both physical and psychological dimensions, the hospital anxiety and depression scale (HAD), and a mood activity checklist (MACL). Quality of life was self-assessed on both a visual analogue scale (VAS) and by means of 18 specific questionnaire points.

Sweden has extensive social and legislative support structures for disabled persons which are probably superior to those available in many other countries, and which could be expected to improve the lot of SCI patients as a result. Nevertheless, the authors found that disability severity had particular impacts on home and kitchen management and on mobility in the neighborhood. In their view, however, these impacts were partly explained by patient choice in obtaining help with some aspects of daily living in order to concentrate their own energies on other aspects, such as self-care or socializing, plus external factors such as architectural impediments that curtailed outdoor mobility and access. This was borne out by the finding that engagement in social and recreational activities, physical training, and private transport were not restricted by more severe disability.

Mental well-being and perceived overall QoL seemed to be influenced much more by engagement in social activities and the ability to drive adapted cars than they were by the degree of physical dysfunction. However, a cause and effect relationship is much harder to establish, since it may be that either patients with little depression or high levels of satisfaction with their lives are more likely to engage in these activities, or participation in itself might benefit mental well-being and perceived quality of life. Age and age at injury were negatively correlated to activity levels in all areas – especially social activities – but again this may be due more to the possibility that older persons are generally less able to cope with major life changes than younger persons with more energy and the motivation to find new goals and interests.

Overall, in this Swedish study, despite considerable group differences in levels of physical functioning, over 80% of subjects were gainfully employed or engaged in studies, and most had active leisure time. They reported normal or close to normal mood states and QoL perceptions, which shows that despite their often profoundly changed physical circumstances, it is entirely possible for SCI patients to lead satisfying and productive lives in the community, if extensive societal support and stimulation are available. Few societies provide the level of support found in Sweden, however, and it may be that familial adaptation and QoL, as well as that of the patient, are compromised when such support is lacking.

Family influences

Since the impact of SCI normally extends beyond patients themselves, McGowan and Roth studied the relationships between functional independence, perceived family functioning, and duration of disability in 41 non-institutionalized post-traumatic SCI families.[13] How SCI patients relate to their families can influence the emotional effects of their injury[14,15] and, as a result, the extent and course of their rehabilitation.[16,17] In fact the family's ability to adjust successfully is critical, but sudden permanent disability in one member places great strain on the whole family unit[18] so that communication patterns can change,[19] along with levels of emotional intimacy[16,20] and role identification.[21] In cases of poor treatment outcomes in SCI rehabilitation, investigation of the family context may be vital for a proper understanding of what has happened and how best to improve matters.[22]

The nature of the SCI patient–family interaction changes over time, from the initial acute crisis through to the necessary longer-term adjustment. It seems reasonable to assume therefore that family QoL likewise varies over time and that the estimation of QoL needs to take the time course of the family process into account. Family members may eventually become resentful despite at first seeming supportive, especially if rehabilitation progresses less well than expected. Despite some evidence that duration of disability may be correlated to greater acceptance of SCI,[23] some patients may actually regress in their acceptance of SCI disability over time[24] and in any case it may take years for some patients and families to fully accept their altered circumstances. McGowan and Roth's study worked with post-rehabilitation SCI patients and families. They found that SCI patients with higher levels of self-initiation of activities, social involvement, and overall levels of independence (which are all associated with improved QoL) perceived their family environment as affectively responsive, openly communicative, and clear in the delineation of role responsibilities.

Quality of life measurement in spinal cord injury

Various authors have used a range of instruments in an attempt to measure QoL in SCI patients. The Short-Form 36-item questionnaire (SF-36)[25] is a widely used and validated instrument for assessing QoL in illnesses as varied as diabetes, migraine, and heart disease. It has been used to measure QoL in urinary disorders[26,27] but is not an SCI-specific instrument. Other instruments such as the SIP have been employed in related disorders[28] but it is also not an SCI-specific instrument and, in addition, these instruments are less sensitive to changes in single patients with a specific condition, having been developed for the study of whole populations.

A review of the general medical literature (Medline, 1997) and a QoL specialist database, OLGA[29] revealed that although 13,000 articles were identified using the keyword 'QoL', only 20 were on SCI and none were specifically on urinary disorders in SCI. A recent Medline literature research confirmed this finding, with less than 18 articles identified using 'urogenic bladder' and 'QoL' as key words from 1996 to 2002. Most of the researches studied the QoL related to the underlying conditions such as SCI or multiple sclerosis. Very few focus on the specific QoL issues related to urinary disorders.[30–44]

Several validated QoL questionnaires have been specifically developed for urinary disorders in both men and women, but these are specific for urgency and mixed incontinence. Questionnaires relevant to men only include examples such as the benign prostate hypertrophy (BPH) health-related quality of life.[45] But none of these questionnaires was developed to assess all types of urinary disorder in a way that is specific to SCI or multiple sclerosis populations. Indeed, these questionnaires, even though specific to urinary disorders are not relevant to assess the impact of neurogenic bladder on QoL. A meta-analysis of 3710 articles on QoL and SCI between 1983 and 1992 reported:[46] 'because of limited rigour of research design and poor validity of measurements, conclusion about the ability of rehabilitative care to improve the quality of life for spinal cord injured persons could not be drawn from the studies reviewed'. The authors concluded that 'QoL research with SCI persons needs to be better designed and should include more uniform and valid criteria'.

Furthermore, the challenge researchers have to face when attempting to assess the QoL of patients with neurogenic bladder is to understand the specific burden of the urinary disorders in relation to the overall QoL impact of the underlying condition such as SCI or multiple sclerosis.

In order to overcome some of these shortcomings and provide a highly relevant measurement instrument, Costa et al undertook a series of patient interviews which resulted in an extensive list of relevant concepts that were subsequently developed into a highly relevant questionnaire to assess urinary disorders in SCI.[47]

Development and validation of a specific quality of life questionnaire to assess the impact of urinary disorders in spinal cord injury patients

A multidisciplinary scientific committee, consisting of urologists, rehabilitators, epidemiologists, and QoL experts, was convened with the intention of developing and validating a questionnaire to evaluate the extent to which urinary disorders specifically affect the QoL of SCI patients. The questionnaire could be used in international multicenter studies or to monitor the patient's care. The group opted for the sequential development approach, in which the questionnaire would be developed and validated in one language, followed by translation into other languages, with further linguistic and psychometric validation. The questionnaire was developed and validated in French, before being translated into English.

By interviewing patients and reviewing the literature, a range of QoL problems and concerns relevant to SCI patients with urinary disorders were identified and phrased in patient-relevant wording. Paraplegic, tetraplegic, or conus medullaris syndrome patients were interviewed. The interviews consisted of one section on the impact of functional impairment and one section about specific problems related to urinary dysfunction. This double-component structure was aimed at identifying and separating problems due to functional impairment from those caused by urinary disorders.

The initial exhaustive list of concepts extracted from the interviews led to the generation of questions based on the exact patient speech wording. These questions were analyzed for content validity by the committee and through face-to-face interviews with patients. Patients were asked if the questions were easy to understand, relevant, and if any important questions were missing from the questionnaire. The resulting questionnaire contained 84 questions, which were grouped into four broad issues: limitations (26 items), constraints (27 items), fears (18 items), and feelings (13 items). The questionnaire was designed to be patient-administered or interviewer-administered, depending on the degree of handicap.

The questionnaire generated through patient interviews was used in a cross-sectional validation study in 300 French patients with varying degrees of disability. Patients also completed a 56-item generic questionnaire, the Subjective Quality of Life Profile (SQLP).[48,49] This questionnaire offers two advantages over the well-known generic instruments like the SF-36. First, the SQLP does not measure functional status related to normality or ability to perform physical activities like walking or climbing stairs (which are irrelevant in most SCI patients). Instead, it uses items related to functional status to ask about the quality and the extent to which subjects are satisfied, or not, with their ability to perform activities like going where they want when alone, moving around at home, or playing sports, if any. In addition, the SQLP allows the user to generate targeted questions to supplement the core questionnaire. These questions were generated using the same questionnaire format in the areas of autonomy, social interaction, material comfort, sexual relationships, and adaptation of living.

An item reduction was performed on each scale whereby, in order to be retained, an item had to satisfy several psychometric criteria, as well as passing scientific committee review of its perceived relevance and importance. This yielded a list of questions, which was subsequently reduced after iterative analysis to a final 30-item questionnaire, assessing the specific impact of urinary problems (Specific IUP) grouped into four scales: limitations

Table 32.1 *Abbreviated content of the specific section of the Qualiveen™ questionnaire*

Scale	Item	Abbreviated item content
Limitations (9 items)	1	Bothered by urine leaks during the day
	2	Bothered by urine leaks at night
	3	Bothered by incontinence pads
	4	Bothered by a set timetable to pass urine during activities
	5	Bothered by time spent passing urine
	6	Bothered because nights are disturbed
	7	Bothered when traveling
	8	Bothered by personal hygiene problems when away
	9	Bladder problems complicate life
Constraints (8 items)	10	Able to go out without planning in advance
	11	Give up going out
	12	Be more dependent due to bladder problems
	13	Life regulated by bladder problems
	14	Plan everything
	15	Think about taking a change (clothes/incontinence pads)
	16	Wear incontinence pads as a precaution
	17	Be careful about quantity of fluid you drink
Fears (8 items)	18	Smell of urine
	19	Have urinary infections
	20	Bladder problems worsening
	21	Disturb partner at night
	22	Urine leaks during sexual intercourse
	23	Side-effects from drugs
	24	Skin problems
	25	Money problems due to expenses related to bladder problems
Feelings (5 items)	26	Feel ashamed because of bladder problems
	27	Loss of self-respect because of bladder problems
	28	Conceal bladder problems
	29	Questioning looks from others regarding time spent in toilets
	30	Worry because of bladder problems

Qualiveen is a registered trade mark of Coloplast A/S, Humlebaek, DK-3050, Denmark.

(9 items), constraints (8 items), fears (8 items), and feelings (5 items). The abbreviated content is shown in Table 32.1.

The psychometric properties of the reduced questionnaire were then assessed, including internal consistency, test–retest reliability, and clinical validity. The clinical validity was confirmed by testing hypotheses about the behavior of scores of the QoL instrument in various clinical situations, such as the overall degree of difficulty urinating, the derived satisfaction or dissatisfaction with urination, and the time spent urinating.[50]

Key findings from a specific quality of life questionnaire

Perrouin-Verbe et al have collated data from 400 SCI patients.[51] They self-administered the 30-item specific impact of urinary problems (Specific IUP) questionnaire, plus an additional 9-item general quality of life (General QoL) section derived from the SQLP. The questionnaire was named Qualiveen™ (registered trade mark of Coloplast A/S, Humlebaek, DK-3050, Denmark).

Scores range from 0 to 4 for the Specific IUP questionnaire, with 0 indicating no impact of urinary disorders on QoL (no limitations, or constraints or fears or negative feelings) and 4 indicating a high specific impact on QoL (greatest limitation, constraints, fears or negative feelings) and from -2 to $+2$ for the General QoL index, with negative values indicating poor QoL, positive values indicating good QoL, and 0 indicating neutral position (neither bad nor good).

The relationship between the specific scales of the Specific IUP and the General QoL index were studied using the Pearson correlation coefficient. Values between 0.40 and 0.60 were expected to mean that deterioration of the Specific IUP could lead to impairment in the general QoL.

Clinical validity was assessed by a number of comparisons of QoL scores in subgroups according to different sociodemographic and clinical criteria (gender, age, type of lesion, concomitant pathology, total incontinence, help at home, treatment for urinary problems, urinary tract infections, time since injury, mode of urination, time taken to urinate, use of protective devices or collectors). Kruskal–Wallis or Wilcoxon tests were used for group comparisons.

Results

The 400 SCI patients consisted mainly of men (72.5%), with an average age of 40 years, most of whom were living with a partner (59.0%) and receiving help at home (57.5%). More than half (52.2%) of the participants in the reference group were paraplegic and more than one-quarter (27.2%) were tetraplegic. The most frequently encountered methods of urination were self-catheterization (41.2%), percussion (27.7%), and abdominal straining or Credé's maneuver (22.5%). More than half the population wore protective or urine collection devices (52.2%); 58.8% reported having had a urinary infection in the previous 30 days, 30.2% had undergone surgery for urinary problems, and 44.7% of respondents were on treatment for their urinary problems. Table 32.2 shows that the Specific IUP scales were negatively correlated with the General QoL index, indicating that the higher the impact of urinary problems, the lower the General QoL, which confirmed the hypotheses. Correlations were statistically significant ($p < 0.001$).

Similarly, an increase in the score of the Specific IUP leads to an impairment in the General QoL, as shown in Figure 32.1: patients reporting lower scores, indicating low impact of urinary disorders (quartile 1), had a higher General QoL than patients reporting moderate scores (quartiles 2 and 3). Patients reporting the highest impact of urinary disorders (quartile 4) had the lowest General QoL.

Other key findings were found:

- Differences were observed between men and women for each of the specific scores but not for the General QoL index (not statistically significant). Women had higher limitations, constraints, and negative feelings and higher Specific IUP than men, indicating more specific QoL impairment. Women therefore tended to be more concerned about the limitations imposed by their urinary disorder, such as having to wear protective devices, spending a long time urinating, and problems experienced with personal hygiene while away from home. Men, on the other hand, reported more fears, such as a higher tendency to be concerned about smelling of urine, having bladder infections, or urine leaks.
- The General QoL index decreased consistently with age ($p \leq 0.0001$) but age didn't seem to influence the specific impact of urinary disorder on QoL.
- Specific QoL scores didn't reveal significant differences between the types of lesion, although tetraplegic patients reported higher levels of constraints and fears. Quality of life was particularly impaired in the early years post-injury, as patients reported more limitations and negative feelings, as well as poorer general QoL compared with those with older injuries.
- Patients requiring help at home reported both lower Specific and General QoL.
- The existence of concomitant pathologies affected QoL and gave higher scores in all four dimensions of the Specific IUP, as well as lower General QoL scores.
- The time taken to urinate affected both Specific and General QoL greatly. Patients who spent more than 10 min urinating reported higher limitations, constraints, and negative feelings. No difference was observed for the level of fears. The General QoL was also most severely affected in patients taking more than 10 min to urinate.
- Concerning the mode of urination, patients catheterized by someone else presented significantly worse values for the limitations and the constraints dimensions. Thus, ability to self-catheterize as opposed to requiring catheterization by others had an important impact on the General QoL: the latter presenting the lowest General QoL scores.

Table 32.2 *Correlation of Specific IUP scores, Specific IUP index, and the General QoL*

	Limitations	Constraints	Fears	Feelings	SIUP index	GQoL index
Limitations	1.00					
Constraints	0.65	1.00				
Fears	0.58	0.52	1.00			
Feelings	0.63	0.53	0.50	1.00		
SIUP index	0.87	0.81	0.78	0.82	1.00	
GQoL index	−0.45	−0.48	−0.33	−0.51	−0.54	1.00

$p < 0.001$ (Pearson's correlation coefficients).

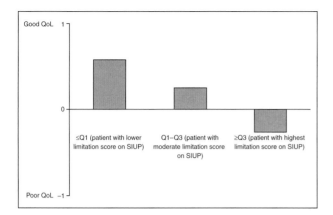

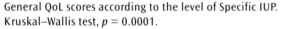

Figure 32.1
General QoL scores according to the level of Specific IUP.
Kruskal–Wallis test, $p = 0.0001$.

- Conversely, the use of protective devices or collectors had significant negative consequences on every dimension of the QoL.
- Patients who were completely incontinent had significantly higher constraints, feelings, and fears, indicating poorer Specific QoL although this itself did not reach significance.
- Patients undergoing treatment for urinary problems had significantly higher limitations, constraints, and fears than patients who were not being treated for urinary problems. For the feelings dimension the difference was non-significant. The difference in the General QoL index scores of these patients was not significant. Similarly, the effect of urinary tract infection was not reflected in the General QoL index score, although patients with urinary tract infections had significantly higher scores in all SIUP scales except for the feelings dimension.

Overall, the process followed to create the questionnaire has allowed the development of an instrument relevant to a broad range of SCI patients. It is the first specific instrument developed and shown to be reliable and valid in this population and has the added benefit of being supported by data generated in 400 SCI patients with varying degrees of disability, age, and gender.

These data can be considered as a reference which should be of great benefit to clinicians and health-related quality of life researchers. Knowing the baseline scores of a reference population should give a context to users of the questionnaire and allow them to interpret scores by comparison with those reference data – especially in judging whether scores are lower, higher, or similar to those in the same type of patients, and in judging the benefits of an intervention. This is particularly important in the case of disease-specific questionnaires, where comparison with normal data in a general population is inappropriate.

Summary

Most patients with a traumatic SCI subsequently develop urological problems, often due to bladder dysfunction brought about by the impaired nervous control caused by the spinal injury. Thankfully, today's improved urological care of neurogenic bladder means that life-threatening urinary tract complications leading to renal insufficiency or kidney failure now cause few deaths amongst SCI patients. It remains true, however, that SCI urological complications result in significant morbidity and can have drastic effects on the quality of life of SCI patients. Existing and emerging therapies need to be evaluated not simply in terms of their effect on bladder function or control per se but also in terms of any change in overall QoL that such therapeutic effects may bring about.

Treatment of neurogenic bladder may include one or more physical, neurological, behavioral, or pharmacological modalities, some of which can be difficult to compare directly. Consequently, the assessment of patient QoL is arguably one of the most relevant and perhaps reliable ways of measuring and comparing real-world clinical benefits. In order to fulfill this potential validation role, however, it is important to develop QoL instruments which are themselves robust, so that observed effects can safely be related to the treatment under investigation, rather than variability in the QoL measure employed.

Importantly, the occurrence of neurogenic bladder after SCI affects not only patients themselves but also their families or social contacts, who may find themselves suddenly thrust into an unexpected pseudo-nursing role, just as they and the patient are having to come to terms with the dramatic change in circumstances arising from the injury. An effective QoL instrument should help to quantify some of these effects and any changes brought about by existing or investigational therapies.

The SF-36 instrument and similar QoL measures have been used in many diseases, including SCI, but while they can quantify general health-related quality of life in SCI, they do not measure the specific impact of urological SCI problems such as neurogenic bladder. A reliable and validated specific questionnaire such as the Qualiveen, by contrast, can distinguish between patients with varying degrees of disability. References scores are available for a large population of SCI patients with different levels of urinary dysfunction, thus providing physicians and researchers with a context for the results from future studies.

This type of questionnaire is required to monitor patient QoL, providing a more comprehensive overview of patient's care, complementary to traditional clinical parameters. This questionnaire can also be used in clinical studies to assess the effect of interventions and treatments. The responsiveness of the questionnaire to change over time has not yet been investigated and this will be the subject of future research. Also, its validity in multiple sclerosis has to be assessed.

References

1. Wein AJ. Neuromuscular dysfunction of the lower urinary tract and its treatment. In: Campbell's urology, 7th edn. Philadelphia: WB Saunders, 1998:953–1006.

2. Stover SL, Fine PR, eds. Spinal cord injury: the facts and figures. Birmingham: University of Alabama at Birmingham, 1986.

3. De Vivo MJ, Richards JS, Stover SL, Go BK. Spinal cord injury: rehabilitation adds life to years. West J Med 1991; 154:602–606.

4. Hackler R. A 25 year prospective mortality in the spinal cord injured patient; comparison with the long term living paraplegia. J Urol 1977; 117:486–493.

5. Agency for Health Care Policy and Research. Prevention and management of urinary tract infections in paralyzed persons: summary, evidence report/technology assessment number 6. Silver Spring, MD: Agency for Health Care Policy and Research, US Department of Health and Human Services, 1999.

6. Stover SL, Fine PR. Epidemiology and economics of spinal cord injury. Paraplegia 1987; 25:225–231.

7. De Vivo MJ, Black KJ, Stover SL. Causes of death during the first 12 years after spinal cord injury. Arch Phys Med Rehabil 1993; 74:248–254.

8. Whiteneck GG, Charlifue SW, Frankel HL, et al. Mortality, morbidity and psychosocial outcomes of persons spinal cord injured more than 20 years ago. Paraplegia 1992; 30:617–630.

9. Bartol G. Psychological needs of the spinal cord injured person. J Neurosurg Nurs 1978; 10:171–175.

10. Bishop DS, Epstein NB, Baldwin LM. Disability: a family affair. In: Freeman DS, Trute B, eds. Treating families with special needs. Alberta, Canada: Alberta Association of Social Workers, 1982.

11. Hohman NGW. Psychological aspects of treatment and rehabilitation of the spinal cord injured person. Clin Orthop Rel Res 1975; 112:81–88.

12. Siösteen A, Lundqvist C, Blomstrand C, et al. The quality of life of three functional spinal cord injury subgroups in a Swedish community. Paraplegia 1990; 28:476–488.

13. McGowan MB, Roth S. Family functioning and functional independence in spinal cord injury adjustment. Paraplegia 1987; 25:357–365.

14. Harris P, Patel SS, Greer W, Naughton JAL. Psychological and social reactions to acute spinal paralysis. Paraplegia 1973; 2:132–136.

15. Klein RF, Dean A, Bogdonoff MD. The impact of illness upon the spouse. J Chronic Dis 1967; 20:241–248.

16. Bracken MB, Shepard MJ. Coping and adaptation following acute spinal cord injury: a theoretical analysis. Paraplegia 1980; 18:74–85.

17. Dinsdale SM, Lesser AL, Judd F. Critical psycho-social variables affecting outcome in a regional spinal cord center. Proc Vet Admin Spinal Cord Injury Conf 1971; 18:193–196.

18. Steinglass P, Temple S, Lisman SA, Reiss D. Coping with spinal cord injury: the family perspective. Gen Hosp Psych 1982; 4:259–264.

19. Rohrer K, Adelman B, Puchett J, et al. Rehabilitation in spinal cord injury: use of a patient–family group. Arch Phys Med Rehab 1980; 61:225–229.

20. Cleveland M. Family adaptation to the traumatic spinal cord injury of a son or daughter. Soc Wk in Health Care 1979; 4:459–471.

21. Shellhase LJ, Shellhase FE. Role of the family in rehabilitation. Soc Casework 1972; 11:544–550.

22. Trieschman RB. Spinal cord injuries: psychological, social and vocational adjustment. New York: Pergamon Press, 1980.

23. Woodrich F, Patterson JB. Variables related to acceptance of disability in persons with spinal cord injuries. J Rehab 1980; 3:26–39.

24. Rosensteil AK, Roth S. Relationship between cognitive activity and adjustment in four spinal-cord injured individuals: a longitudinal investigation. J Human Stress 1982; 3:35–43.

25. Ware JE, Snow KK, Kosinski M, Gandek M. SF-36 health survey. Manual and interpretation guide. Boston New England Medical Center: The Health Institute, 1993.

26. Sand PK, Staskin D, Miller J, et al. Effect of urinary control insert on quality of life incontinent women. Int Urogynecol J 1999; 10(2):100–105.

27. Fuhrer MJ, Rintala DH, Hart KA, et al. Relationship of life satisfaction to impairment, disability and handicap among persons with spinal cord injury living in the community. Arch Phys Med Rehab 1992; 73:552–557.

28. Schurmans JR, Weerman PC, Bosch JL, et al. Quality of life in heterotopic and orthotopic neobladder reconstruction: a comparison. Acta Urol Belg 1995; 63(3):55–58.

29. Erickson P, Scott J. The on-line guide to quality of life assessment (OLGA): resource for selecting quality of life assessments. In: Walker S, Rosser RM, eds. Quality of life assessments: key issues in the 1990s. Dordrecht: Kluwer Academic Publisers, 1993:221–232.

30. Lowe JB, Furness PD 3rd, Barqawi AZ, Koyle MA. Surgical management of the neuropathic bladder. Sem Pediatr Surg 2002; 11(2):120–127.

31. Fernandez O. Mechanisms and current treatments of urogenital dysfunction in multiple sclerosis. J Neurol 2002; 249(1):1–8.

32. Zorzon M, Zivadinov R, Monti Bragadin L, et al. Sexual dysfunction in multiple sclerosis: a 2-year follow-up study. J Neurol Sci 2001; 187(1–2):1–5.

33. Kachourbos MJ, Creasey GH. Health promotion in motion: improving quality of life for persons with neurogenic bladder and bowel using assistive technology. Sci Nursing 2000; 17(3):125–129.

34. Yavuzer G, Gok H, Tuncer S, et al. Compliance with bladder management in spinal cord injury patients. Spinal Cord 2000; 38(12):762–765.

35. Weld KJ, Dmochowski RR. Effect of bladder management on urological complications in spinal cord injured patients. J Urol 2000; 163(3):768–772.

36. Kumar H, Cauchi J, MacKinnon AE. Periurethral Goretex sling in lower urinary recontruction. Eur J Pediatr Surg 1999; 9(suppl 1):33–34.

37. Rashid TM, Hollander JB. Multiple sclerosis and the neurogenic bladder. Phys Med Rehab Clin N Am 1998; 9(3):615–629.

38. Westgren N, Levi R. Quality of life and traumatic spinal cord injury. Arch Phys Med Rehab 1998; 79(11):1433–1439.

39. Bakke A, Malt UF. Psychological predictors of symptoms of urinary tract infection and bacteriuria in patients treated with clean

intermittent catheterization: a prospective 7-year study. Eur Urol 1998; 34(1):30–36.

40. Vaidyananthan S, Soni BM, Brown E, et al. Effect of intermittent urethral catheterization and oxybutynin bladder instillation on urinary continence status and quality of life in a selected group of spinal cord injury patients with neuropathic bladder dysfunction. Spinal Cord 1998; 36(6):409–414.

41. Sutton MA, Hinson JL, Nickell KG, et al. Continent ileocecal augmentation cystoplasty. Spinal Cord 1998; 36(4):246–251.

42. Stohrer M, Kramer G, Goepel M, et al. Bladder autoaugmentation in adult patients with neurogenic voiding dysfunction. Spinal Cord 1997; 35(7):456–462.

43. Kuo HC. Clinical outcome and quality of life after enterocystoplasty for contracted bladders. Urolog Int 1997; 58(3):160–165.

44. Wielink G, Essink-Bot ML, van Kerrebroeck PE, et al. Sacral rhizotomies and electrical bladder stimulation in spinal cord injury. 2. Cost-effectiveness and quality of life analysis. Dutch Study Group on sacral anterior root stimulation. Eur Urol 1997; 31(4):441–446.

45. Lukacs B, Leplege A, MacCarthy C, Comet D. Construction and validation of a BPH-specific health-related quality of life scale including evaluation of sexuality. Proc Am Urol Ass 1995; 153(Suppl):320A.

46. Evans RL, Hendricks RD, Connis RT, et al. Quality of life after spinal cord injury: a literature critique and meta-analysis (1983–1992). J Am Paraplegia Soc 1994; 17:60–66.

47. Costa P, Perrouin-Verbe B, Colvez A, et al. Quality of life in spinal cord injury patients with urinary difficulties: development and validation of Qualiveen. Eur Urol 2001; 39:107–113.

48. Dazord A, Astolfl F, Guisti P, et al. Quality of life assessment in psychiatry: the Subjective Quality of Life Profile (SQLP) – first results of a new instrument. Community Ment Health J 1998; 34:525–535.

49. Guérin P, Dazord A, Cialdella Ph, et al. Le questionnaire "Profil de la Qualité de la Vie Subjective". Premiers éléments de validation. Thérapie 1991; 46:131–138.

50. Bergner M, Rothman ML. Health status measures: an overview and guide for selection. Ann Rev Public Health 1987; 8:191–210.

51. Perrouin-Verbe B, Amarenco G, Marquis P, et al. Quality of life related to urinary disorders in spinal cord injury patients. Use of the specific questionnaire Qualiveen: study of 400 patients. Submitted to Arch Phys Med Rehab.

33

The voiding diary

Martine Jolivet-Tremblay and Pierre E Bertrand

Introduction

Since the advent of urodynamic studies in clinical practice, urologists have tried to analyze voiding habits to better define lower urinary tract symptoms (LUTS). The bladder being an 'unreliable witness', diagnosis based solely on clinical symptoms was revealed to be inadequate.

The voiding diary is a well-known diagnostic tool for this purpose and it is now a component of every serious investigation. Unfortunately, it is still frequently overlooked by some, even if it is one of the simplest noninvasive tests to evaluate the function of the lower urinary tract (LUT). The patients complete it at home and/or at work, and it offers the advantage of assessing the severity of LUTS in their customary environment. By filling out the voiding diary, patients become active participants in the diagnostic process and their degree of motivation can be assessed.

The first studies published on voiding diaries concerned only urinary incontinence. However, since the end of the 1980s the voiding diary has become a widely accepted tool in the investigation of voiding dysfunctions, including obstructive uropathy, urinary tract infection, vesicoureteral reflux, and neurogenic bladder dysfunction.

The voiding diary is now a crucial part of most research protocols and has become an important criteria in the indication of treatments, such as injection of Botox (botulinum toxin A–hemagluttinin complex) or implantation of neurostimulation/neuromodulation devices.

Definition and terminology
The Abrams–Klevmark classification

Abrams and Klevmark[1] have described four different voiding diaries in a laudable effort to standardize the terminology. This classification is based on the type and amount of information contained in each of them (Table 33.1). The charts give objective information on the number of voidings, the distribution of voiding between daytime and nighttime, and each voided volume. The charts can also be used to record episodes of urgency and leakage and the number of incontinence pads used. The frequency–volume chart is not only useful in the assessment of voiding disorders but also in treatment follow-up.

Table 33.1 *Voiding diaries: the Abrams–Klevmark classification*

Frequency chart	Frequency–severity chart	Frequency–volume chart	Urinary diary
Number of voidings + Number of incontinence episodes	Number of voidings + Number of incontinence episodes + Number of pads used	Time of each voiding + Volume of each voiding + Time of each incontinent episode	Time of each voiding + Volume of each voiding + Time of each incontinent episode + Types of drinks, foods, activities related to LUTS

Reproduced with modifications from Jolivet-Tremblay M, Schick E. The voiding diary. In: Corcos J, Schick E, eds. The urinary sphincter. New York: Marcel Dekker, 2001: 262.
LUTS, lower urinary tract symptoms.

The frequency chart

In this very simple chart only the number of micturitions and the number of incontinence episodes are registered per 24 hours. This limited information does not include urinary volume or the degree of incontinence.

The frequency–severity chart

In this chart, the number of micturitions and episodes of incontinence will be noted plus the number of pads used or cloths changed. This diary is a better evaluation of the severity of incontinence. However, it does not provide information on urinary volume or quantity of urine lost.

The frequency–volume chart

This type of voiding diary is the most widely used by urologists. It provides the maximum of information. Although it demands some effort on the part of the patient, it is an investment in his welfare. The time and the volume of urine voided at each micturition plus the number and the timing of each incontinent episode are registered on a chart. From this, the 24-hour diuresis, the frequency of micturition, the functional capacity of the bladder, and daytime diuresis, compared with nocturnal diuresis, etc., can be calculated. This type of voiding diary, however, does not provide information on fluid intake or its distribution through a 24-hour period.

The urinary diary

This is the most elaborate and complicated form of voiding diary. Besides its role as a frequency–volume chart, it also provides information on the types and number of beverages and foods taken every day. The patient also notes any activities related to LUTS. This type of chart is very onerous to the patient and is often difficult to analyze for the physician. It is mostly used in research protocols. Under normal circumstances, knowledge of fluid intake is not absolutely necessary since it generally parallels total diuresis.

The International Continence Society classification

In a recent report[2] a subcommittee of the International Continence Society suggested three types of diaries (Table 33.2):

1. *micturition time chart*, which records only the times of micturitions, day and night, for at least 24 h
2. *frequency–volume chart*, which records the volumes voided as well as the times of micturitions, day and night, for at least 24 h
3. *bladder diary*, which records the times of micturitions, voided volumes, incontinence episodes, pad usage, and other information such as fluid intake, the degree of urgency, and the degree of incontinence.

Rationale for the voiding diary

Routine use of the voiding diary in the investigation and follow-up of patients with LUTS will fulfill four objectives:

1. The voiding diary leads to an objective measurement of the patient's subjective complaints in a familiar environment. Patient perception of voiding habits may be misleading. For example, McCormack et al[3] studied 88 consecutive patients in whom urinary frequency was evaluated by a questionnaire at the first visit. This

Table 33.2 *Voiding diaries: the ICS classification*

Micturition time chart	Frequency–volume chart	Bladder diary
Times of micturition (minimum 24 hours)	Times of micturitions (minimum 24 hours) + Volumes voided at each micturition	Times of micturitions + Volumes voided at each micturition + Incontinence episodes + Pad usage, fluid intake, degree of urgency, degree of incontinence

was compared with the frequency obtained by analyzing the frequency–volume chart filled out by the patient for 7 consecutive days. A very wide discrepancy was noted between subjectively estimated frequency and chart-determined frequency.

2. It can help the physician to identify the etiology of the patient's LUTS.
3. As previously mentioned, when taking an active role in the elaboration of his voiding calendar, the patient becomes a participant to the diagnosis and treatment of the urological problem. This may serve as a measure of his motivation to get well.
4. The voiding diary is also an important tool in the follow-up of a medical treatment or a specific surgery. Siltberg et al[4] estimated that the voiding diary provided the best tool for follow-up in the treatment of the urge syndrome. It is now of common use in many clinical research protocols.

Data extracted from the voiding diary

Important parameters about the frequency of micturition and the number of episodes of incontinence can be extracted by careful examination of the data in the voiding diary. It also provides an accurate estimate of total diuresis in a 24-hour period. Nowadays, in the majority of urodynamic laboratories, all the parameters can be entered into a computer and, using a simple software program, a more precise and detailed analysis may be done. This kind of computer program, like the one developed in our laboratory, calculates the following parameters: the mean voided volume per micturition (ml), the frequency (units), the diuresis (ml/min), the mean interval between micturitions (min), and the voided volume during a specific period of the day (ml). All these parameters are calculated separately for daytime and nighttime. The rising micturition is the first daytime voiding registered in the software. This first voided volume is considered part of nocturnal diuresis and is treated as such by the computer program. It is assumed that daytime lasts 16 h (960 min) and nighttime 8 h (480 min). Therefore, the amount of urine voided during the day is divided by 960 and during the night by 480, to give the day and night diuresis in milliliters per minute. Further analysis produces two more parameters: output per 24 h (ml), which is the total voided volume during a 24-hour period, and the ratio between nighttime and daytime diuresis. In addition, the computer prints out the number of days analyzed, the number of incontinence episodes occurring during this period, and the number of micturitions for which volume was not measured by the patient. The computer program is designed to automatically correct daytime and nighttime diuresis as well as

Table 33.3 *Basic data provided by software*

Parameter	Normal	1 SD
Day:		
Mean voided volume (ml)	2.37	67
Frequency	5.63	1.26
Diuresis (ml/min)	1.11	0.35
Corrected diuresis (ml/min)	1.11	0.35
Interval between micturitions (min)	222	60
Output (ml)	1005	497
Corrected output (ml)	1005	497
Night:		
Mean voided volume (ml)	379	132
Frequency	0.08	0.16
Diuresis (ml/min)	0.84	0.27
Corrected diuresis (ml/min)	0.84	0.27
Interval between micturitions (min)	454	50
Output (ml)	409	130
Corrected output (ml)	409	130
Output in 24 hours (ml)	1473	386
Corrected output in 24 hours (ml)	1473	386
Diuresis ratio (night/day)	0.81	0.30

Reproduced with modifications from Jolivet-Tremblay M, Schick E. The voiding diary. In: Corcos J, Schick E, eds. The urinary sphincter. New York: Marcel Dekker, 2001: 264.

the total volume voided (output per day, output per night, output per 24 h) for micturitions when volume was not measured. The mean voided volume is calculated from all recorded volumes. This mean volume is then substituted for each missing micturition volume to give the corrected output. The diuresis ratio (night/day) is derived from this corrected diuresis.[5]

To facilitate interpretation of the patient's data, the computer will print out the normal value for each parameter, along with the standard deviation (SD) and the standard normal deviation (Z-value), which is the number of SDs an observation lies away from the mean. A Z-value of 2.00 or more suggests a significant deviation from the mean[6] (Table 33.3).

Furthermore, this software is able to print a graph of the mean voided volumes over a 24-hour period as a function of time.

We have used this computer program in our urodynamic laboratory for almost 20 years, analyzing more than 2000 frequency–volume diaries.

Normal values

To determine valuable information from the parameters of the voiding diary, it is essential to know normal values.

However, surprisingly, very little data are available concerning the normal values of voiding diaries. This is an important issue because baseline values are needed to compare data from patients with different LUTS.

Children

Normal values are difficult to obtain in children, and data in the literature are sparse. Bloom et al[7] analyzed the voiding habits of 1192 children without a history of urinary tract infection. They obtained a mean frequency of about 4–5 micturitions per day. Data were obtained by questionnaire, and no frequency–volume chart was filled out.

Mattsson[8] studied 206 children, aged 7–15 years, considered asymptomatic. All of them completed a 24-hour frequency–volume chart. They voided 2–10 times a day, but 95% of them had a voiding frequency of 3–8. About 10% voided once during the night. Voided volume varied greatly, the morning voiding being the largest, and the last voiding before bedtime, the smallest. Single voided volume varied between 20 and 800 ml, with total volumes over 24 h between 325 and 2100 ml. Wan et al[9] estimated that voiding frequency for normal children was approximately 6 times daily. They used a frequency chart on which urine volume could be measured, but this was not mandatory. They found the diary particularly useful in infrequent voiding. Hellström et al,[10] studying the micturition habits of 3556 7-year-old children, found that the frequency of micturition was 3–7 per day among those without symptoms of bladder disturbance and without previous urinary tract infection.

Esperanca and Gerrard[11] determined urinary frequency in 297 normal children aged 4–14 years. The average frequency for 4 year olds was 5.3 micturitions, whereas for 12 year olds it was 4.8.

Bower et al[12] constructed nomograms for mean maximum voided volume, mean voided volume, and mean minimum voided volume for specific age groups using data obtained from 322 incontinent children, aged 6–11 years, who completed a 2-day frequency–volume chart. They noted a wide variation of voided volumes, very much as Mattsson and Lindström did in normal children.[13] Based on all these findings, frequency–volume charts by themselves seem to be an unsuitable screening tool for children.

Females

There are abundant data published about normal values on the frequency–volume charts in women. Several authors[4,5,14–16] have established normal values for healthy women. Comparison of these data is given in Table 33.4.

Table 33.4 *Data obtained from frequency–volume charts of normal females*

	Boedker et al[42] (n = 123)	Larsson and Victor[14] (n = 151)	Siltberg et al[4] (n = 151)	Saito et al[15] (n = 20)[a]	Kassis and Schick[5] (n = 33)
Mean voided volume (day) in ml				179	237 (± 67)
Mean voided volume (night) in ml		} 250 (±79)	} 240	230	379 (± 132)
Mean frequency (day)				6.8	5.63 (± 1.26)
Mean frequency (night)	} 5.7	} 5.8 (± 1.41)	} 5.5	0.5	0.08 (± 0.16)
Diuresis in ml/min (day)					1.11 (± 0.35)
Diuresis in ml/min (night)					0.84 (± 0.27)
Excreta in ml (day)				1149	1.005 (± 497)
Excreta in ml (night)				234	409 (± 130)
Diuresis per 24 hours in ml	1350	1430 (± 487)	1350	1272	1473 (± 386)
Night diuresis					
Day diuresis					0.81 (± 0.30)
Functional capacity in ml		460 (± 174)	450		

Reproduced with permission from Jolivet-Tremblay M, Schick E. The voiding diary. In: Corcos J, Schick E, eds. The urinary sphincter. New York: Marcel Dekker, 2001:266.

[a]Also includes normal males.

It was in studies done on women that authors began to analyze diurnal and nocturnal data separately. The first results were obtained by Saito et al[15] and Kassis and Schick.[5] This distiction is important because nighttime diuresis may exceed daytime diuresis and be responsible for nocturia, especially in the elderly.

On this particular subject, according to Saito et al[15] an increase in urine volume during the night can be induced by three physiological events related to aging. First, the circadian rhythm of antidiuretic hormone or atrial natriuretic hormone secretion may be abnormal.[17] Second, the glomerular filtration rate or renal plasma flow may be altered because of a reduction in the concentrating ability of the distal tubules. Finally, an impaired cardiovascular system may not be able to supply sufficient amounts of blood to the kidneys during waking hours, creating edema in the lower extremities, which becomes mobilized in the supine position.

The calculated ratio of night over day diuresis can draw attention to one of these phenomena, which is important to recognize, because its logical consequence, nocturia, has nothing to do with a vesicourethral pathology (such as outflow obstruction, unstable bladder function, etc.).

Males

For men, no precise data concerning reference values for frequency–volume charts are published to our knowledge. The study already quoted by Saito et al[15] included males and females, but did not separate them in two subgroups. One reason for this lack of data may be the difficulty in defining the clinical characteristics of a normal male without LUTS. This 'normality' probably changes with age.

Recent data from the literature suggest that in men with LUTS suggestive of BPH, the urodynamically proven obstruction is the most important factor influencing voided volumes, cystometric capacity, and residual urine volume. By contrast, voiding frequency is not significantly influenced, because patients with small voided volumes minimize their fluid intake.[18] Using a 3-day frequency–volume chart Blanker et al[19] showed that the average volume per void declined with advancing age. Nocturnal voiding frequency seems to be indicative of nocturnal urine production, but nocturnal urine production is only a modest discriminator for increased nocturnal voiding frequency. These observations indicate that in daily practice the use of nocturnal urine production to explain nocturnal voiding frequency is of little value.[20] It should also be noted that in a recent large population-based study of 1688 men, circadian urine production could only be demonstrated in men younger than 65.[21]

Duration of the chart

There are no clear guidelines in the literature on the minimum number of days necessary to produce a reliable diary. A wide range of 1–14 days exists. The gold standard for now is probably 7 days. Abrams[22] recommended a 7-day chart, Barnick and Cardozo[23] a 5-day chart, Sommer et al[24] a 3-day chart, and Larsson and Victor[14] a 48-hour chart.

Barnick and Cardozo[23] compared a 5-day chart with a 1-day chart in a group of 150 women attending a urodynamic clinic. They found a significant correlation between the two sets of results with $p < 0.0001$.

Wyman et al[25] studied a 2-week diary in 55 incontinent women, and compared the first week with the second week. They concluded that a 1-week diary is sufficient to assess the frequency of micturition and incontinence episodes. The 7-day diary can consequently be considered as the gold standard for voiding diaries. This has recently been confirmed by Homma et al.[26]

Gisolf et al[27] reported on reliability of data obtained from the 24-hour frequency–volume charts of 160 men with LUTS secondary to BPH. Their study suggested that the 24-hour chart compared favorably to 3 days or more charts and concluded that the 1-day chart provided sufficient insight into voiding habits of this group of patients. According to Matthiessen et al,[28] nocturia secondary to nocturnal polyuria can be detected by a 3-day frequency–volume chart in men with LUTS suggestive of BPH. van Melick et al[29] analyzed 2- or 3-day charts of 98 females with urodynamically proven motor urge incontinence and concluded that a single 24-hour chart is sufficient to gain insight into these patients' voiding habits. Locher et al[30] focused on the number of incontinence episodes in a group of 214 community-dwelling women, aged 40–90 years. Based on the number of days necessary to obtain an internal consistency of 0.90 for Cronbach's alpha, they estimated that a 7-day frequency–volume chart is needed to provide a stable and reliable measurement of the frequency of incontinence episodes. Nygaard and Holcomb[31] compared two 7-day diaries completed at 4-week intervals by 138 stress urinary incontinent women. They observed a good correlation for the number of incontinence episodes between the two diaries (0.831), and the results of the first 3-day diaries correlated well with the last 4-day diaries. They concluded that a 3-day diary is an appropriate outcome measure for clinical trials evaluating treatments for stress incontinence, but a 7-day diary is preferable when the number of incontinence episodes is considered. Fitzgerald and Brubaker[32] introduced a new variable in the analysis of voiding diaries: the number of micturitions per liter of intake. They estimated that this represents the most stable measure to compare two 24-hour charts.

Recently Schick et al[33] compared the standard 7-day chart to various lengths of frequency–volume charts analyzing 14 parameters. Overall results showed that a 4-day diary is almost identical to the 7-day diary. However, when the number of incontinence episodes was considered of primary importance, a 5-day diary was preferable. This reduction in duration made compliance to the voiding diary easier for the patient.

How we do it

Patients are invited to fill out a 4-day frequency–volume chart in which diurnal and nocturnal voiding is clearly identified. The patient is specifically asked to register the time and volume of each voiding as well as the time of each incontinence episode. When, for some reason, the patient is unable to measure a voided volume, he notes only the time, and puts an 'X' instead of the volume. Volume can be expressed in milliliters (ml) or in fluid ounces (fl oz), but should remain uniform throughout the chart. The back of the chart offers simple instructions for completion, with examples for the patient.

It is clinically proven that patients easily understand the elaboration of the frequency–volume chart. More than 95% of our patients fill out the chart correctly. At the beginning we offered lenghty explanations to every patient. But, with time, written instructions proved to be clear enough to forego verbal explanations. The chart can be sent out by mail, fax, or even e-mailed, so that the patient arrives for a visit with complete frequency–volume information.

Reliability of the voiding diary

To be reliable, frequency–volume charts must be filled out correctly. In an effort to verify their accuracy, Palnaes Hansen and Klarskov[34] studied 18 subjects who noted their fluid intake and voided volumes and collected 24-hour urine samples for three consecutive days. They concluded that self-reported frequency–volume chart data are valid and useful for patients with voiding symptoms.

Barnick and Cardozo[23] studied 106 consecutive patients who received a 5-day frequency–volume chart by mail, to be filled out before their physical examination. Only 40% of them completed the chart correctly for the full 5 days.

Robinson et al[35] compared two 7-day diaries in 278 incontinent women. The first was completed with minimal instructions, the second after receiving extensive instructions. They concluded that a 7-day diary remained a reliable tool to assess urinary symptoms, even if patients received minimal instructions on filling out the chart.

According to our own experience, more that 1000 patients correctly completed the frequency–volume chart without extensive verbal instructions. The fact that we allow our patients to use milliliters or fluid ounces for volume measurements is probably helpful, because older people are less familiar with the metric system. Bailey et al[36] presented results similar to our own, with most patients completing the chart correctly before their first visit.

The frequency–volume chart as a diagnostic tool

The possibility of using the frequency–volume chart as a diagnostic tool is very tempting because of its simplicity and noninvasiveness. Several authors explored this possibility. Larsson and Victor[37] compared the frequency–volume charts of 81 stress-incontinent patients with those of 151 asymptomatic women. Interestingly, all three parameters (total voided volume, frequency, and largest single voided volume) differed statistically between the two groups; however, because of marked overlapping, the frequency–volume chart was judged an unreliable diagnostic tool for stress incontinence.

Larsson et al[38] analyzed the frequency–volume chart in bladder instability, compared it with a group of women without other LUTS, and related it to cystometric findings, to evaluate the quantitative aspects of urgency incontinence. A 2-day period on a 7-day chart was evaluated. None of the parameters of the frequency–volume chart (frequency of micturition, mean voided volume, largest single voided volume, and variability in voided volumes) were useful in differentiating between motor urgency and normal voiding habits. Moreover, no correlation was found between any of the data from the frequency–volume chart and the filling phase of urodynamic studies (first desire to void, bladder volume at first unstable contraction, bladder capacity, and bladder volume at first leakage). The authors concluded that frequency–volume charts didn't help in differential diagnosis, but that mean voided volume represented a good measure of the severity of detrusor instability symptoms.

In another study, Fink et al[39] compared the 24-hour frequency–volume chart in stress-incontinent and urge-incontinent women. When applying logistic regression to these two groups, the frequency of micturition during nighttime was the parameter that best discriminated between these medical conditions. Mean voided volume (over the 24-hour period) showed the highest differentiating power with $p < 0.0001$, but the large overlap between groups limited the value of the frequency–volume chart for differential diagnosis.

More recently, Siltberg et al[4] proposed a nomogram on which the frequency of micturition was plotted against the range of voided volumes. According to these authors, this plot could be used to select the degree of certainty (with 10% intervals for probability) of having motor urgency incontinence vs stress incontinence. Tincello and Richmond[40] tested this nomogram in 216 patients: for detrusor instability, it had a sensitivity of 52% and a specificity of 70%; for genuine stress incontinence, the sensitivity and specificity were 66% and 65%, respectively. They concluded that formal cystometric evaluation was necessary in incontinent females because the nomogram did not provide enough diagnostic information.

These observations are not really surprising. It seems simplistic to attempt characterization of such different complex physiopathological entities as continence and voiding with a single parameter: in this case, the frequency–volume chart. Nonetheless, this diagnostic tool remains an important element in our understanding of patient symptomatology and still one of the first tests to choose because it is easy to complete and it can be repeated later to assess the results of therapy.

Interpretation of frequency–volume charts

In our department, the computer software we described above analyzes every frequency–volume chart filled out by a patient. The most important parameters in the clinical setting are the frequency of micturition (day and night), 24-hour urinary output, the ratio of nighttime diuresis to daytime diuresis, and the mean voided volume (day and night). The hour-by-hour distribution is also very helpful.

Normal frequency–volume chart

Table 33.5 represents the results of a 3-day frequency–volume chart filled out by a 42-year-old lady who was referred because of incontinence. Three voided volumes were not recorded, representing 14.29% of the total number of micturitions during this 3-day period. The 24-hour corrected urinary output was within normal limits (1462 ml; Z-value: (0.03)), as well as the night/day diuresis ratio (0.73; Z-value: (0.28)). Daytime frequency (7.00; Z-value: 1.09) and nighttime frequency (0.00; Z-value: (0.50)) were almost within normal limits. Figure 33.1 illustrates the graphic representation of voidings and the mean voided volumes during a 24-hour period. The greatest single voided volume (480 ml), which represents in this example the daytime functional bladder capacity, was registered at 07:00 h. No micturition occurred between midnight and 07:00 h, and between 13:00 h and 16:00 h.

Table 33.5 *Normal frequency–volume chart (for details see text)*

Parameter	Patient's data (±1 SD)	Normal (±1 SD)	Z-value
Day:			
Mean voided volume (ml)	187 (72)	237 (±67)	(0.75)
Voiding frequency	7.00 (0.00)	5.63 (±1.26)	1.09
Diuresis (ml/min)	0.97	1.11 (±0.35)	(0.39)
Corrected diuresis (ml/min)	1.17	1.11 (±0.35)	0.17
Interval between micturitions (min)	192 (601)	222 (±60)	(0.50)
Output (ml)	935 (92)	1005 (±497)	(0.14)
Corrected output (ml)	1122 (92)	1005 (±497)	0.24
Maximal voided volume (ml)	480		
Night:			
Mean voided volume (ml)	340 (18)	379 (±132)	(0.30)
Voiding frequency	0.00	0.08 (±0.16)	(0.50)
Diuresis (ml/min)	0.71	0.84 (±0.27)	(0.49)
Corrected diuresis (ml/min)	0.71	0.84 (±0.27)	(0.49)
Interval between micturition (ml)	480 (0)	454 (±50)	0.52
Output (ml)	340 (102)	409 (±130)	(0.53)
Corrected output (ml)	340 (102)	409 (±130)	(0.53)
Maximal voided volume (ml)	0.00		
Output in 24 hours (ml)	1275	1473 (±386)	(0.51)
Corrected output in 24 hours (ml)	1462	1473 (±386)	(0.03)
Diuresis ratio (night/day)	0.73	0.81 (±0.3)	(0.28)

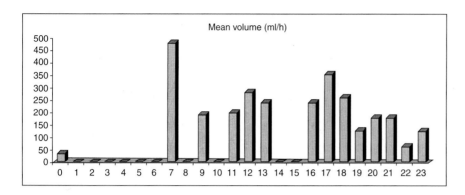

Figure 33.1
Graphic representation of a normal frequency–volume chart.

Increased 24-hour output (polyuria)

This type of voiding diary is relatively common and can be seen in patients with unbalanced diabetes or simple potomania of different magnitude.

This 45-year-old female consulted with symptoms suggestive of mixed urinary incontinence. She reported voiding about 20 times a day and 4–6 times at night. She complained of a sensation of incomplete emptying. Endoscopy revealed a bladder capacity of 300 ml and a post-void residual urine of 120 ml. The bladder wall was trabeculated, grade II. Gynecological examination showed a grade II anterior vaginal wall prolapse, resulting from a lateral defect. The Q-tip test demonstrated a 25° urethral mobility (normal <30°). No urinary incontinence could be observed during cough in the supine position. On multichannel urodynamics, bladder capacity was 750 ml and the first desire to void occurred at 262 ml. Bladder wall compliance was normal. Maximum urethral closure pressure was 65 cmH$_2$O and the cough leak-point pressure was negative. No uninhibited detrusor contractions could be detected during the filling phase, but a strong post-void contraction was registered which, in view of the clinical symptoms, was considered as a manifestation of unstable bladder.

The frequency–volume chart (Table 33.6) showed a tremendous increase in the corrected 24-hour urinary output (12,591 ml!) with a normal night/day diuresis ratio (0.91; Z-value: 0.33). Daytime voiding frequency was 18.71, not because of a decrease in mean voided volumes (494 ml; Z-value: 3.83), but due to an important daytime diuresis (8746 ml; Z-value: 15.58). Nighttime diuresis was even more pronounced (3845 ml; Z-value: 26.43). In spite of this, voiding frequency was increased to a lesser degree (3.00; Z-value: 18.25), mainly because the mean nocturnal voided volume also increased (961 ml; Z-value: 4.41). The mean hourly voided volume (Figure 33.2) reflects the difference in mean voided volumes for nighttime and daytime.

Nocturnal polyuria

A 69-year-old female consulted because of urgency and increased frequency. She claimed hourly micturitions during the day and 5–6 voidings each night. She was enuretic until the age of 9. Endoscopy revealed grade II bladder trabeculation associated with a cystoscopic capacity of 400 ml. Urodynamic study demonstrated an unstable bladder with the first uninhibited contraction occurring at 60 ml. Cystometric capacity was 175 ml and the first desire to void occurred at 62 ml.

Her 7-day frequency–volume chart (Table 33.7) showed a slight increase in the 24-hour corrected output (1961 ml; Z-value: 1.15), but a significantly increased night/day ratio (4.66; Z-value: 12.84). Her daytime frequency was somewhat increased (7.43; Z-value: 1.43), but clearly less than the claimed frequency reported during the initial interview. Note that the decreased mean daytime voided volume (99 ml; Z-value: (2.06)) is not very different from the bladder volume at the first desire to void (62 ml) and the appearance of the first uninhibited detrusor contraction (60 ml). The chart confirms the significantly increased nighttime frequency (5.14; Z-value: 31.64), accompanied by a decreased mean voided volume (208 ml; Z-value: (1.29)).

On the graphical representation (Figure 33.3) one can easily see the predominantly nocturnal diuresis with the maximal functional capacity (325.31 ml) occurring during the second part of the night (04:00 h).

Sensory urgency

A 73-year-old female patient complained of stress urinary incontinence but also experienced incontinence episodes which were not associated with stress or urgency. Cystometric capacity was 800 ml with no post-void residual urine. Her bladder was stable on multichannel urodynamics. Abdominal leak-point pressure was estimated between

Table 33.6 *Increased 24-hour output (polyuria) (for details see text)*

Parameter	Patient's data (±1 SD)	Normal (±1 SD)	Z-value
Day:			
Mean voided volume (ml)	494 (205)	237 (±67)	3.83
Voiding frequency	18.71 (1075)	5.63 (±1.26)	10.38
Diuresis (ml/min)	8.82	1.11 (±0.35)	22.02
Corrected diuresis (ml/min)	9.11	1.11 (±0.35)	22.86
Interval between micturitions (min)	56 (222)	222 (±60)	(2.77)
Output (ml)	8464 (864)	1005 (±497)	15.01
Corrected output (ml)	8746 (1086)	1005 (±497)	15.58
Maximal voided volume (ml)	1350		
Night:			
Mean voided volume (ml)	961 (212)	379 (±132)	4.41
Voiding frequency	3.00 (0.00)	0.08 (±0.16)	18.25
Diuresis (ml/min)	8.01	0.84 (±0.27)	26.56
Corrected diuresis (ml/min)	8.01	0.84 (±0.27)	26.56
Interval between micturition (ml)	120 (185)	454 (±50)	(6.68)
Output (ml)	3845 (617)	409 (±130)	26.43
Corrected output (ml)	3845 (617)	409 (±130)	26.43
Maximal voided volume (ml)	1380		
Output in 24 hours (ml)	12,309	1473 (±386)	28.07
Corrected output in 24 hours (ml)	12,591	1473 (±386)	28.80
Diuresis ratio (night/day)	0.91	0.81 (±0.3)	0.33

Table 33.7 *Nocturnal polyuria (for details see text)*

Parameter	Patient's data (±1 SD)	Normal (±1 SD)	Z-value
Day:			
Mean voided volume (ml)	99 (48)	237 (±67)	(2.06)
Voiding frequency	7.43 (1.18)	5.63 (±1.26)	1.43
Diuresis (ml/min)	0.56	1.11 (±0.35)	(1.57)
Corrected diuresis (ml/min)	0.66	1.11 (±0.35)	(1.28)
Interval between micturitions (min)	177 (436)	222 (±60)	(0.75)
Output (ml)	537 (190)	1005 (±497)	(0.94)
Corrected output (ml)	635 (145)	1005 (±497)	(0.74)
Maximal voided volume (ml)	295.74		
Night:			
Mean voided volume (ml)	208 (64)	379 (±132)	(1.29)
Voiding frequency	5.14 (0.83)	0.08 (±0.16)	31.64
Diuresis (ml/min)	2.61	0.84 (±0.27)	6.54
Corrected diuresis (ml/min)	2.67	0.84 (±0.27)	6.77
Interval between micturition (ml)	80 (209)	454 (±50)	(7.48)
Output (ml)	1251 (103)	409 (±130)	6.47
Corrected output (ml)	1280 (156)	409 (±130)	6.70
Maximal voided volume (ml)	325.31		
Output in 24 hours (ml)	1787	1473 (±386)	0.81
Corrected output in 24 hours (ml)	1916	1473 (±386)	1.15
Diuresis ratio (night/day)	4.66	0.81 (±0.3)	12.84

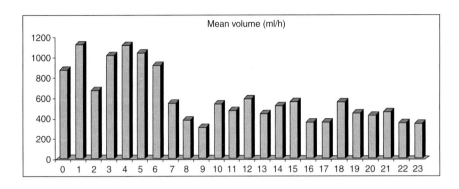

Figure 33.2
Graphic representation of the frequency–volume chart of a patient with an increased 24-hour output (polyuria).

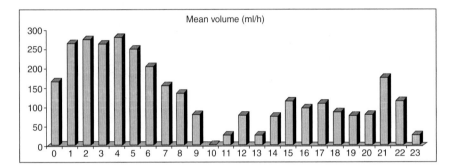

Figure 33.3
Graphic representation of the frequency–volume chart of a patient with significant nocturnal polyuria.

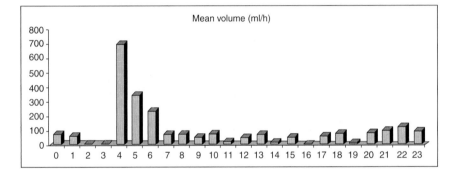

Figure 33.4
Graphic representation of the frequency–volume chart of a patient with sensory urgency.

100 and 150 cmH$_2$O, a grade III urethral incompetence,[41] explaining the clinical symptom of stress urinary incontinence.

Her 7-day frequency–volume chart (Table 33.8) demonstrated a 24-hour corrected urine output (1784 ml; Z-value 0.81) within normal limits. There was some degree of nocturnal polyuria (693 ml; Z-value: 2.18). Mean urinary frequency was 14.14 during daytime and 1.86 during nighttime, with mean voided volumes of 83 and 243 ml, respectively (Figure 33.4). The functional bladder capacity was 395.74 ml in daytime and 709.77 ml during the night. This significant difference between mean voided volumes in the absence of an unstable bladder suggested sensory urgency.

Effect of neuromodulation

A 29-year-old female was investigated because of significant increase in day and night urinary frequency,

associated with urgency, but she did not complain of incontinence. She claimed daytime voidings every 20 min and about 15 micturitions per night. Endoscopy was unremarkable, the cystoscopic capacity being 250 ml. Multichannel urodynamics failed to reveal uninhibited detrusor contractions during the filling phase. Cystometric capacity was 220 ml and the first desire to void occurred at a 42 ml volume in the bladder. The urethra was hypertonic (maximal urethral closing pressure: 104 cmH$_2$O).

The 7-day frequency–volume chart (Table 33.9) showed a normal 24-hour corrected urine output (1267 ml; Z-value: (0.53)) and a normal night/day diuresis ratio (0.50; Z-value: (1.04)). There was a very important decrease in the mean daytime (40 ml; Z-value: (2.94)) and nighttime (50 ml; Z-value: (2.49)) voided volumes. The voiding frequency was 25.57 during the day, and 4.71 during the night. The functional bladder capacity was 110.00 ml and 80.00 ml, respectively. Graphic representation exhibits almost constant mean voided volumes throughout the 24-hour period (Figure 33.5).

Table 33.8 *Sensory urgency (for details see text)*

Parameter	Patient's data (±1 SD)	Normal (±1 SD)	Z-value
Day:			
Mean voided volume (ml)	83 (63)	237 (±67)	(2.30)
Voiding frequency	14.14 (1.55)	5.63 (±1.26)	6.76
Diuresis (ml/min)	0.90	1.11 (±0.35)	(0.59)
Corrected diuresis (ml/min)	1.14	1.11 (±0.35)	0.08
Interval between micturitions (min)	92 (413)	222 (±60)	(2.17)
Output (ml)	866 (256)	1005 (±497)	(0.28)
Corrected output (ml)	1092 (237)	1005 (±497)	0.17
Maximal voided volume (ml)	295.74		
Night:			
Mean voided volume (ml)	243 (197)	379 (±132)	(1.03)
Voiding frequency	1.86 (0.35)	0.08 (±0.16)	11.11
Diuresis (ml/min)	1.44	0.84 (±0.27)	2.24
Corrected diuresis (ml/min)	1.44	0.84 (±0.27)	2.24
Interval between micturition (ml)	168 (203)	454 (±50)	(5.72)
Output (ml)	693 (243)	409 (±130)	2.18
Corrected output (ml)	693 (243)	409 (±130)	2.18
Maximal voided volume (ml)	709.77		
Output in 24 hours (ml)	1559	1473 (±386)	0.22
Corrected output in 24 hours (ml)	1784	1473 (±386)	0.81
Diuresis ratio (night/day)	1.60	0.81 (±0.3)	2.63

Table 33.9 *Pre-neuromodulation (for details see text)*

Parameter	Patient's data (±1 SD)	Normal (±1 SD)	Z-value
Day:			
Mean voided volume (ml)	40	237 (±67)	(2.94)
Voiding frequency	25.57	5.63 (±1.26)	15.83
Diuresis (ml/min)	0.98	1.11 (±0.35)	(0.37)
Corrected diuresis (ml/min)	1.02	1.11 (±0.35)	(0.25)
Interval between micturitions (min)	41	222 (±60)	(3.02)
Output (ml)	943	1005 (±497)	(0.13)
Corrected output (ml)	983	1005 (±497)	(0.04)
Maximal voided volume (ml)	110		
Night:			
Mean voided volume (ml)	50	379 (±132)	(2.49)
Voiding frequency	4.71	0.08 (±0.16)	28.96
Diuresis (ml/min)	0.49	0.84 (±0.27)	(1.30)
Corrected diuresis (ml/min)	0.59	0.84 (±0.27)	(0.92)
Interval between micturition (ml)	102	454 (±50)	(7.04)
Output (ml)	234	409 (±130)	(1.34)
Corrected output (ml)	284	409 (±130)	(0.96)
Maximal voided volume (ml)	80.00		
Output in 24 hours (ml)	1177	1473 (±386)	(0.77)
Corrected output in 24 hours (ml)	1267	1473 (±386)	(0.53)
Diuresis ratio (night/day)	0.50	0.81 (±0.3)	(1.04)

Dramatic changes were observed in the different parameters of the frequency–volume chart during percutaneous nerve stimulation (Table 33.10). Despite an increase in the corrected 24-hour urinary output (1623 ml; Z-value: 0.39), the night/day ratio did not change (0.43; Z-value: 0.39). The mean daytime voided volume increased significantly (184 ml; Z-value: (0.79)), as did the mean nighttime voided volume (219 ml; Z-value: (1.21)). Nocturia almost completely disappeared (0.29; Z-value: 1.29), as can also be seen in Figure 33.6. (Note the difference in the y-axis scale between Figures 33.5 and 33.6.) Daytime frequency was reduced by 60% (8.29;

Z-value: 2.11). Functional bladder capacity also increased significantly.

Conclusion

This overview of the literature on voiding diaries as well as our own experience leads us to the following conclusions.

Frequency–volume charts are an invaluable and indispensable tool in the investigation of LUTS patients and in understanding their symptoms. Interpretation of the

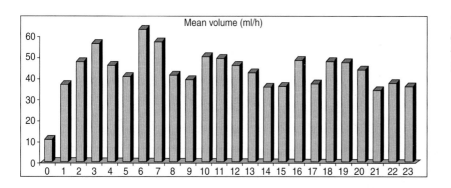

Figure 33.5
Graphic representation of the frequency–volume chart of a patient before testing for neuromodulation.

Table 33.10 *Per-neuromodulation (for details see text)*			
Parameter	Patient's data (±1 SD)	Normal (±1 SD)	Z-value
Day:			
Mean voided volume (ml)	184 (73)	237 (±67)	(0.79)
Voiding frequency	8.29 (1.67)	5.63 (±1.26)	2.11
Diuresis (ml/min)	1.21	1.11 (±0.35)	0.27
Corrected diuresis (ml/min)	1.40	1.11 (±0.35)	0.82
Interval between micturitions (min)	153 (506)	222 (±60)	(1.15)
Output (ml)	1158 (371)	1005 (±497)	0.31
Corrected output (ml)	1342 (371)	1005 (±497)	0.68
Maximal voided volume (ml)	400.00		
Night:			
Mean voided volume (ml)	219 (15)	379 (±132)	(1.21)
Voiding frequency	0.29 (1.70)	0.08 (±0.16)	1.29
Diuresis (ml/min)	0.52	0.84 (±0.27)	(1.18)
Corrected diuresis (ml/min)	0.59	0.84 (±0.27)	(0.94)
Interval between micturition (ml)	420 (660)	454 (±50)	(0.68)
Output (ml)	250 (134)	409 (±130)	(1.22)
Corrected output (ml)	281 (199)	409 (±130)	(0.98)
Maximal voided volume (ml)	200.00		
Output in 24 hours (ml)	1408	1473 (±386)	(0.17)
Corrected output in 24 hours (ml)	1623	1473 (±386)	0.39
Diuresis ratio (night/day)	0.43	0.81 (±0.3)	(1.26)

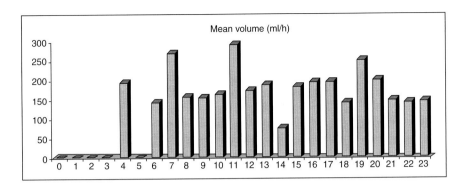

Figure 33.6
Graphic representation of the frequency–volume chart of the same patient as in figure 33.5, but during neuromodulation.

results is greatly simplified by simple computer software. The commercial unavailability of such software may explain why these charts are not more popular. Now, in many research protocols, small user-friendly computers are used to ease the completion of frequency–volume charts.

Normal values for women are well known. However, more research should be done to study voiding diaries in children. Reference values for men are desperately needed.

Although the 7-day diary is currently considered the gold standard, comparative studies have begun to determine whether the minimum number of days for a frequency–volume chart completion could be less than 7 and still maintain reliability.

The voiding diary is a precious diagnostic tool, but it cannot guarantee a precise diagnosis. Because of the complex nature of LUT dysfunction, it has become evident that frequency–volume charts will never replace urodynamic studies.

In addition to their value as a diagnostic tool, frequency–volume charts play an important role in evaluating the success of a surgical intervention (i.e. neuromodulation) or during follow-up of medical therapy.

In summary, the frequency–volume chart, although frequently overlooked, is a simple, objective, and noninvasive test for evaluating the function of the lower urinary tract.

References

1. Abrams P, Klevmark B. Frequency-volume charts: an indispensable part of lower urinary tract assessment. Scand J Urol Nephrol Suppl 1996; 179:47–53.

2. Abrams P, Cardozo L, Fall M, et al. The standardisation of terminology of lower urinary tract function: report from the standardisation sub-committee of the International Continence Society. Neurourol Urodyn 2002; 21:167–178.

3. McCormack M, Infante-Rivard C, Schick E. Agreement between clinical methods of measurement of frequency- and functional bladder capacity. Br J Urol 1992; 69:17–21.

4. Siltberg H, Larsson G, Victor A. Frequency/volume chart: the basic tool for investigating urinary symptoms. Acta Obstet Gynecol Scand 1997; 76(Suppl 166):24–27.

5. Kassis A, Schick E. Frequency-volume chart pattern in a healthy female population. Br J Urol 1993; 72:708–710.

6. Duncan RC, Knapp RG, Miller MC III. Introductory biostatistics for the health sciences. New York: John Wiley & Sons, 1977.

7. Bloom DA, Seeley WW, Ritchey ML, McGuire EJ. Toilet habits and continence in children: an opportunity sampling in search of normal parameters. J Urol 1993; 149:1087–1090.

8. Mattsson SH. Voiding frequency, volumes and intervals in healthy schoolchildren. Scand J Urol Nephrol 1994; 28:1–11.

9. Wan J, Kaplinsky R, Greenfield S. Toilet habits of children evaluated for urinary tract infection. J Urol 1995; 154:797–799.

10. Hellström AL, Hanson E, Hansson S, et al. Micturition habits and incontinence in 7-year-old Swedish school entrant. Eur J Pediatr 1990; 149:434–437.

11. Esperanca M, Gerrard JW. Nocturnal enuresis: studies in bladder function in normal children and enuretics. Can Med Ass J 1969; 101:324–327.

12. Bower WF, Moore KH, Adams RD, Shepherd RB. Frequency–volume chart data from incontinent children. Br J Urol 1997; 80:658–662.

13. Mattsson S, Lindström S. Diuresis and voiding pattern in healthy schoolchildren. Br J Urol 1995; 76:783–789.

14. Larsson G, Victor A. Micturition patterns in a healthy female population, studied with a frequency/volume chart. Scand J Urol Nephrol (Suppl 114) 1988; 114:53–57.

15. Saito M, Kondo A, Kato T, Yamada Y. Frequency-volume charts comparison of frequency between elderly and adult patients. Br J Urol 1993; 72:38–41.

16. Bodega A, Lendorf A, H-Nielsen A, Ghahn B. Micturition pattern assessed by the frequency/volume chart in a healthy population of men and women. Neurourol Urodynam 1989; 8:421–422.

17. Matthiesen TB, Rittig S, Norgaard JP, et al. Nocturnal polyuria and natriuresis in male patients with nocturia and lower urinary tract symptoms. J Urol 1996; 156:1292–1299.

18. Van Venrooij GE, Eckhardt MD, Boon TA. Data from frequency-volume charts versus maximum free flow rate, residual volume, and voiding cystometric estimated urethral obstruction grade and detrusor contractility in men with lower urinary tract symptoms suggestive of benign prostatic hyperplasia. Neurourol Urodyn 2002; 21:450–456.

19. Blanker MH, Groeneveld FP, Bohnen AM, et al. Voided volumes: normal values and relation to lower urinary tract symptoms in elderly men: a community-based study. Urology 2001; 57:1093–1098.

20. Blanker MH, Bernsen RM, Bosch JL, et al. Relation between nocturnal voiding frequency and nocturnal urine production in older men: a population-based study. Urology 2002; 60:612–616.

21. Blanker MH, Bernsen RM, Ruud Bosch JL, et al. Normal values and determinants of circadian urine production in older men: a population-based study. J Urol 2002; 168:1453–1457.

22. Abrams P. Urodynamics, 2nd edn. London: Springer-Verlag, 1997.

23. Barnick C, Cardozo L. Unpublished data quoted by Barnick C. In: Cardozo L, ed. Urogynecology. London: Churchill Livingstone, 1997:101–107.

24. Sommer P, Bauer T, Nielsen KK, et al. Voiding patterns and prevalence of incontinence in women. A questionnaire survey. Br J Urol 1990; 66:12–15.

25. Wyman JF, Choi SC, Harkins SW, et al. The urinary diary in evaluation of incontinent women. A test-retest analysis. Obstet Gynecol 1988; 71:812–817.

26. Homma Y, Ando T, Yoshida M, et al. Voiding and incontinence frequencies: variability of diary data and required diary length. Neurourol Urodyn 2002; 21:204–209.

27. Gisolf KW, van Venrooij GE, Eckhardt MD, Boon TA. Analysis and reliability of data from 24-hour frequency-volume charts in men with lower urinary tract symptoms due to benign prostatic hyperplasia. Eur Urol 2000; 38:45–52.

28. Matthiessen TB, Rittig S, Mortensen JT, Djurhuus JC. Nocturia and polyuria in men referred with lower urinary tract symptoms, assessed using a 7-day frequency-volume chart. BJU Int 1999; 83:1017–1022.

29. Van Melick HH, Gisolf KW, Ecjhardt MD, et al. One 24-hour frequency-volume chart in a woman with objective urinary motor urge incontinence is sufficient. Urology 2001; 58:188–192.

30. Locher JL, Goode PS, Roth DL, et al. Reliability assessment of the bladder diary for urinary incontinence in older women. J Gerontol A Biol Sci Med Sci 2001; 56:M32–M35.

31. Nygaard I, Holcomb R. Reproducibility of the seven-day voiding diary in women with stress urinary incontinence. Int Urogynecol J Pelvic Floor Dysfunc 2000; 11:15–17.

32. Fitzgerald MP, Brubaker L. Variability of 24-hour voiding diary variables among asymptomatic women. J Urol 2003; 169:207–209.

33. Schick E, Jolivet-Tremblay M, Dupont C, et al. Frequency-volume chart: the minimum number of days required to obtain reliable results. Neurourol Urodyn 2003; 22:92–96.

34. Palnaes Hansen C, Klarskov P. The accuracy of the frequency-volume chart: comparison of self-reported and measured volumes. Br J Urol 1998; 81:709–711.

35. Robinson D, McGlish DK, Wyman JF, et al. Comparison between urinary diaries completed with and without intensive patient instructions. Neurourol Urodynam 1996; 15:143–148.

36. Bailey R, Shepherd A, Trike B. How much information can be obtained from frequency-volume charts? Neurourol Urodynam 1990; 9:382–385.

37. Larsson G, Victor A. The frequency-volume chart in genuine stress incontinent women. Neurourol Urodynam 1992; 11:23–31.

38. Larsson G, Abrams P, Victor A. The frequency-volume chart in detrusor instability. Neurourol Urodynam 1991; 10:533–543.

39. Fink D, Perucchini D, Schaer GN, Haller U. The role of the frequency-volume chart in the differential diagnosis of female urinary incontinence. Acta Obstet Gynecol Scand 1999; 78:254–257.

40. Tincello DG, Richmond DH. The Larsson frequency/volume chart is not a substitute for cystometry in the investigation of women with urinary incontinence. Int Urogynecol J Pelvic Floor Dysfunct 1998; 9:391–396.

41. Schick E. The objective assessment of the resistance of the female urethra to stress: a scale to establish the degree of urethral incompetence. Urology 1985; 26:518–526.

42. Boedker A, Lendorf A, H-Nielsen A, Ghahn B. Micturition pattern assessed by the frequency/volume chart in a healthy population of men and women. Neurourol Urodyn 1989; 8:421–422.

34

The pad test

Martine Jolivet-Tremblay and Erik Schick

Introduction

Incontinence is not easy to quantify from patient interviews or clinical examinations.[1] Urinary incontinence, as defined by the International Continence Society (ICS) in 1988 is involuntary urine loss that is a social or hygienic problem.[2] This definition has been recently modified[3] to state simply that 'urinary incontinence is the complaint of any involuntary leakage of urine'. This modification became necessary because the previous definition related to a complaint on quality of life issues. Quality of life instruments have been and are being developed in order to assess the impact of both incontinence and other lower urinary tract symptoms on patients.[4] The importance of this condition, as perceived by the patient, differs widely from one individual to another. Some patients cannot accept the loss of a few drops of urine happening only during some specific, often limited, circumstance, whereas others wear diapers for years before seeking medical advice.

The role of the pad-weighing test is to quantify urine loss. It is the best available instrument for this purpose. However, it does not evaluate the impact a given degree of incontinence has on the patient's quality of life. The Urodynamic Society recommended the use of the pad-weighing test in the pre-treatment evaluation of incontinent patients as well as their post-treatment evaluation at each follow-up visit.[5] However, the Urodynamic Society did not specify the type of pad test to be used. On the other hand, the Agency for Health Care Policy and Research of the US Department of Health and Human Services did not mention the pad test for the identification and evaluation of urinary incontinence.[6] It is a tool that can be used for specific issues during the diagnostic process.

Discrimination between continence and incontinence

Because perineal pads absorb perspiration, vaginal discharge, etc., results should be interpreted with caution. It is important to determine an upper limit of weight gain by a pad in continent subjects before interpreting pad test results.

Many authors have investigated this issue (Table 34.1). Usually, the extra-urinary weight increase will be directly proportional to the length of the test. In the protocol described by Hahn and Fall,[7] the length of the exercise program is very brief. Each and every gram of increase in the pad weight is considered a urine loss. Continent patients show no pad weight increase at the end of the test. Conversely, Griffiths et al,[8] investigating elderly patients for 10 days, considered a diagnosis of urinary incontinence only if pad weight exceeded 10 g per 24 hours.

The majority of authors estimate that during a 1-hour test the upper limit of pad weight gain in continent subjects is close to 1 g, whereas during a 24-hour test it is between 4 and 10 g, with an upper limit of 15 g in 24 hours. According to these authors, a weight gain of more than 1 g in a single pad or 8 g in 24 hours may be considered significant. It should be remembered, nonetheless, that weight gains less than the above-mentioned limits do not exclude incontinence, and supplementary investigations may be necessary to confirm the diagnosis.[9]

Nygaard and Zmolek[10] carefully assessed the reproducibility of three comparable exercise protocols, their relationship with voided volume, and Pyridium® (phenazopyridine) staining in 14 continent volunteers. The average pad weight gain during these three sessions was 3.19 g ($\pm$ 3.16 g), with a range of 0.1–12.4 g. Because of the huge difference between subjects, they were unable to find a distinct cut-off value differentiating continence from incontinence. Similar experiences have been reported by others.[11] Adding Pyridium® (phenazopyridine) did not improve the specificity of the test.

Types of pad tests

Pad tests can primarily be divided into two groups: qualitative tests and quantitative tests.

Table 34.1 *Discrimination between continence and incontinence*

Length of test	Authors	Suggested value for continence	Comments
No time limit	Hahn and Fall[7]	0 g	–
40 min	Martin et al[53]	<2 g	(with 75% of cystometric capacity)
1 hour	Kroman-Andersen et al[43] Sutherst et al[1] Versi and Cardozo[54] Ali et al[48]	≤1 g 1 g <0.94 g <0.5 g	– – – –
2 hours	Walsh and Mills[55]	1.2 g ($\forall$1.35 g)/2 hours	
24 hours	Mouritzen et al[51] Lose et al[49] Versi et al[47] Griffiths et al[8]	<5 g/24 hours 4 g/24 hours 7.13 g ($\forall$4.32 g)/24 hours ≤10 g/24 hours	(max: 8 g) (95% upper confidence level <15)

Reproduced with permission from Schick E, Jolivet-Tremblay M. Detection and quantification of urine loss: the pad-weighing test. In: Corcos J, Schick E, eds. The urinary sphincter. New York: Marcel Dekker, 2001:276.

Qualitative tests

The qualitative test uses a substance to color urine orange: e.g. phenazopyridine (Pyridium), 200 mg three times a day. The patient is invited to wear hygienic pads and replace them periodically during normal daily activities. The degree of coloration on the pads is an assessment of incontinence.[12] This test is especially beneficial to document an insignificant urine loss which, however, may be quite bothersome for the patient, or when vaginal secretions cannot be differentiated easily from urinary incontinence.

A further approach has been suggested by Mayne and Hilton,[13] who compared the distal urethral electrical conductance test (DUEC) with weighed perineal pads and discovered that the DUEC was extremely sensitive at detecting leakage (sensitivity 97%). Janez et al[14] reported similar observations.

Quantitative tests

One of the initial efforts to quantify urine loss, interestingly, involved an electric device, the so-called Urilos system, designed by James et al.[15] It incorporates a pad containing dry electrodes. The urinary electrolytes alter the capacitance of the aluminum strip electrodes in the pad proportionally to the quantity of urine. Stanton and co-workers[16,17] investigated this device in greater detail. They noticed problems with reproducibility in different groups. In a group of 26 women exhibiting symptoms of urinary incontinence with a negative stress test 9 proved leakage. In a further group of 30 patients with symptoms of stress incontinence, one-third had a negative clinical stress test, but presented leakage with the Urilos system. Eadie et al[18]

concluded that the system was beneficial to confirm patient histories, in spite of the fact that it was laborious to achieve a quantitative measure of urine loss, particularly for volumes greater than 50 ml when the error range reached 35%. Presumably because of a lack of reliability, this device never gained wide acceptance.

A more efficient approach to the quantification of urine loss is to weigh perineal pads after different lengths of time during which patients are requested to execute standardized activities. This approach has resulted in a relatively large number of publications in which authors have experimented with various test durations, with or without different exercise protocols, in an attempt to define the optimal combination of reproducibility, reliability, and practicality.[19]

Patient populations
Children

Rare reports can be found in the literature on the use of pad tests in the pediatric population.

Hellström et al[20] compared a 2-hour pad test on the ward (with standardized activities and provoked diuresis) with a 12-hour pad test completed in the home environment. Both tests were similar in the detection of urine loss (68 and 70%, respectively), but the detection rate increased in about 10% of the 105 patients when fluid provocation was included in the home pad test.

Imada et al[21] studied 23 incontinent children with a 1-hour pad test, as recommended by the ICS,[1] and compared the results with an interval test during which the pad was utilized between three successive voidings and then weighed. They concluded that the interval test validates the clinical symptoms more appropriately than the 1-hour test. They advocated the former for the objective evaluation of urinary incontinence in children.

Adults

Many reports on the pad-weighing test for adults have been published in the literature: they vary mainly in the length of time the pad was employed. The short tests last 1 or 2 hours,[22–31] and are generally associated with a standardized exercise or activity program, but there can also be no time limit imposed with only an exercise protocol to follow.[7,32,33] The longer tests go from 12 hours up to 10 days.[8,34–38] Various authors compared tests of different lengths[29–31] or tests done in different environments.[39]

Exercise protocol without a fixed time schedule

The provocative pad test designed by Hahn and Fall[7] involved a sequence of exercises with the bladder filled to half of its cystometric capacity. The test–retest correlation was good ($r = 0.940$). The test takes about 20 min to complete. In control groups of clinically continent females, urine loss at the end of the exercise schedule was 0 g. They advocated the use of this test in incontinent females. However, because urge symptoms emerge at irregular intervals and sometimes in particular situations in patients with bladder instability, a test of longer duration, for example 24 hours, seems to be more reliable.

Mayne and Hilton,[32] after filling the bladder with 250 ml of normal saline solution, compared a short pad test program with a 1-hour test in the same population. They could not find a notable difference between the two protocols.

Miller et al[33] suggested the paper towel test to quantify urine loss associated with stress. After three deep coughs, the authors estimated the amount of urine loss by the wet area on a tri-folded paper towel placed on the perineal region. They found the test to be simple, with good test–retest reliability. They recommended its use for losses less than 10 ml because the paper towel becomes saturated with volumes exceeding 15 ml.

More recently, Persson et al[40] proposed a rapid perineal pad test with a standardized bladder volume (300 ml) and a standardized physical activity of only 1 min. They found the test reproducibility and feasibility acceptable, making it suitable for follow-up studies.

The 1-hour test

The 1-hour test is the most extensively studied, since it was recommended by the Standardisation Committee of the ICS.[1]

Several authors have examined the reproducibility and reliability of this test. Klarskov and Hald[25] found the test to

be reproducible and reliable when compared with subjective daytime incontinence. Jorgensen et al[28] advocated its reproducibility, particularly when bladder volume at the beginning of the test and diuresis during the test were taken into consideration ($r = 0.93$; $p < 0.0001$). When the test was achieved with a standardized bladder volume, the test–retest results were even superior ($r = 0.97$; $p < 0.001$), although personal variations of up to ± 24 g were noted.[30]

Mayne and Hilton[32] accomplished the test with 250 ml of fluid in the bladder. Lose et al[26] filled the bladder up to 50% of its cystometric capacity, whereas Kinn and Larsson[41] favored 75%.

The sensitivity of the test (i.e. the proportion of patients with incontinence who have a positive result) varies between 58 and 81%. Its positive predictive values (i.e. the probability of a patient with a positive test being incontinent), which is more relevant to clinical practice, is over 90%. The false-negative rate (i.e. incontinent patients with a negative pad test), nonetheless, is quite high (19–56.8%) (Table 34.2).

More recently Simons et al[42] compared two 1-hour tests performed with natural diuresis, 1 week apart. They concluded that, with similar bladder volumes, the test–retest reliability was clinically inadequate, as the first and second pad test could differ by -44 to $+66$ g.

It appears that the 1-hour test proposed by the ICS is not optimal, and its reliability is weak.[43] This can be improved when bladder volume at the beginning and during the test is known and standardized.

The 2-hour test

Some authors proposed extending the test to 2 hours because they felt that its exactitude might be improved. The patient is asked to drink a given amount of water as quickly as feasible at the beginning of the first hour to induce a constant level of diuresis. The pad test itself starts at the second hour and involves a fixed exercise protocol. Richmond et al[31] studied two groups of incontinent patients who were submitted to the same protocol, except that the exercise sequence varied. They found that the sequence in which exercises were accomplished did not affect the overall identification of incontinent patients. They estimated that the ideal length of the test was 2 hours. Haylen et al[44] reached the same conclusions. Eadie et al,[45] comparing the 2-hour pad test with the Urilos system, demonstrated that the 2-hour test did not produce reproducible results, and confirmed that it was difficult to obtain quantitative measures of urine loss with the Urilos system.

The 12-hour test

When medium- or long-term pad tests are examined, it is important to ensure that no significant evaporation takes place between the end of the test and the time the

Table 34.2 *Short-term pad test*

Authors	Sensitivity (%)	False-negative rate (%)	PPV (%)	NPV (%)	Comments
Anand et al[56]	70	30	92	53	Patients with LUTS
	81	19	91	72	Patients with SUI
Janez et al[57]	–	39.4	–	–	No fixed bladder volume
Cardozo and Versi[58]	68	32	91	48	No fixed bladder volume
Schüssler et al[59]	–	56.8	–	–	Fixed bladder volume
Jorgensen et al[28]	68	32	–	–	–
Lose et al[49]	58	42	–	–	Fixed bladder volume

PPV, positive predictive value; NPV, negative predictive value; LUTS, lower urinary tract symptoms; SUI, stress urinary incontinence.
Reproduced with permission from Schick E, Jolivet-Tremblay M. Detection and quantification of urine loss: the pad-weighing test. In: Corcos J, Schick E, eds. The urinary sphincter. New York: Marcel Dekker, 2001:279.

pads are weighed. In an evaporation test, the mean weight loss of the pads, placed in a hermetically closed plastic container, is 0.2 g (0.1–0.3) after 24 hours, irrespective of the water volume in the pad. Mean weight loss after 48 hours and 6 days is 0.4 g (0.2–0.7 g) and 0.8 g (0.5–1.2 g), respectively.[46] Versi et al[47] noted no difference in weight after 1 week, and less than a 5% change in weight after 8 weeks (with the upper 95% confidence limit of less than a 10% loss).

The 12-hour test has not been investigated on its own, but has been compared with the 1-hour test by Ali et al,[48] who estimated that the 1-hour pad test on the ward was characteristic of the importance of urinary loss that patients encountered in their home environment. Thus, a 12-hour prolongation was not considered to add clinically relevant information to that obtained during the 1-hour test.

The 24-hour test

This test was examined in detail by Rasmussen et al[46] and found to be reproducible when there are only modest changes in physical activity and diuresis. With extreme reduction of fluid intake or excessive activity, differences in urine loss may be noted. Lose et al[49] compared this test with the 1-hour test. Among 31 stress or mixed incontinent women, 58% were categorized as incontinent with the 1-hour test and 90% with the 24-hour home test. They stated that the 24-hour test is effective as a discriminating tool for incontinence, but that its reproducibility is too low to be useful in scientific studies.

Versi et al[47] examined the 24- and 48-hour tests. Test–retest analysis demonstrated a strong correlation, with coefficients of 0.90 and 0.94, respectively. The reproducibility of the two time schedules was good, suggesting no additional benefit of a prolonged 48-hour test compared with a 24-hour schedule.

Assessing the test–retest reliability of 24-, 48-, and 72-hour pad tests, Groutz et al[50] found that the 24-hour pad test was a reliable instrument for defining the degree of urinary loss. Longer test duration increased reliability, but was associated with decreased patient compliance.

Similar conclusions were made by Mouritzen et al,[51] who compared the 1-, 24-, and 48-hour tests. They concluded that the 1-hour test underestimated the degree of incontinence and related less with clinical parameters than did the 24-hour test. On the other hand, the 24-hour test was as informative as the 48-hour test, making the latter obsolete.

Considering these studies, the 24-hour pad test is considered by many as the gold standard for the quantification of urinary incontinence.

The 48-hour test

The reproducibility of the 48-hour test appeared to be satisfactory ($r = 0.90$) and equivalent with the 1-hour test. Nevertheless, there was no relationship between these two tests ($r = 0.10$) according to Victor and Åsbrink.[52] Ekelund et al[37] showed this test can be successfully carried out in the patient's home, even with elderly women.

The elderly

Elderly patients represent a particular challenge to clinicians trying to quantify urine loss. There is a high incidence of urge incontinence among these patients. Also, some of them have notable mental impairment, making the completion of the test difficult. Finally, a number of these patients are unable to perform any formally designed exercise program.

Griffiths et al[8,34,35] studied the pad test thoroughly in the geriatric community. They established that physical examination often failed to show leakage in incontinent patients. The patient's voiding diary and the 1-hour pad weighing test were often discordant and impractical. In their hands, the 24-hour pad test proved to be the best method to demonstrate and quantify incontinence. Combining this noninvasive test with invasive urodynamics, these authors identified the type of urinary incontinence in 100 elderly patients. They found that the 24-hour test had sufficient reproducibility and good sensitivity (88%) for detecting urine loss, which was mainly nocturnal urge incontinence. Its quantity depended, however, on the preceding evening's fluid intake and on nocturia. They concluded that nocturnal toileting and evening liquid limitation could diminish nocturnal incontinence by a tiny, but profitable, proportion of older patients with extreme urge incontinence.

O'Donnell et al[38] described a procedure which helps nursing personnel to recognize, grade, and register incontinence severity while supervising several patients. This procedure, however, has not been verified for its reproducibility.

Conclusion

From a clinician's perspective, the pad-weighing test is beneficial when the quantity of urine loss is a significant element of management decisions. It is useful in distinguishing urinary incontinence from excessive perspiration or vaginal secretions. In this respect, a 1-hour test, or even a briefer one may be satisfactory. Under these circumstances, the test must be accomplished with a known bladder volume in order to provide reliable and objective information about the patient's condition.

For scientific and research purposes, the 24-hour pad test should be adopted, since it has good reproducibility, is simple to perform, and is done in the patient's own environment. It is better suited to detect and quantify urine loss secondary to urge incontinence than the 1-hour test. The 24-hour test should be used, along with other parameters, to assess success rates following various treatment modalities.

References

1. Sutherst JR, Brown MC, Richmond D. Analysis of the pattern of urine loss in women with incontinence as measured by weighing perineal pads. Br J Urol 1986; 58:272–278.

2. Abrams P, Blaivas JG, Stanton SL, Andersen JT. The standardisation of terminology of lower urinary tract function. Scand J Urol Nephrol (Suppl 114) 1988:5–19.

3. Abrams P, Cardozo L, Fall M, et al. The standardisation of terminology of lower urinary tract function: Report from the Standardisation sub-committee of the International Continence Society. Neurourol Urodyn 2002; 21:167–178.

4. Corcos J, Beaulieu S, Donovan J, et al., and members of the Symptom and Quality of Life Assessment Committee of the First International Consultation on Incontinence. Quality of life assessment in men and women with urinary incontinence. J Urol 2002; 168:896–905.

5. Blaivas JG, Appell RA, Fantl JA, et al. Standards of efficacy for evaluation of treatment outcomes in urinary incontinence: recommendations of the Urodynamic Society. Neurourol Urodyn 1997; 16:145–147.

6. Fantl JA, Newman DK, Colling J, et al. Urinary incontinence in adults: acute and chronic management. Clinical Practice Guideline No. 2, 1996 Update. Rockville, MD: Department of Health and Human Services. Public Health Service, Agency for Health Care Policy and Research. AHCPR Publication 96-0682, March 1996.

7. Hahn I, Fall M. Objective quantification of stress urinary incontinence: a short, reproducible, provocative pad-test. Neurourol Urodyn 1981; 10:475–481.

8. Griffiths DJ, McCracken PN, Harrison GM, Gormley EA. Relationship of fluid intake on voluntary micturition and urinary incontinence in geriatric patients. Neurourol Urodyn 1993; 12:1–7.

9. Siltberg H, Victor A, Larsson G. Pad weighing test, the best way to quantify urine loss in patients with incontinence. Acta Obstet Gynecol Scand (Suppl) 1997; 166:28–32.

10. Nygaard I, Zmolek G. Exercise pad testing test in continent exercisers: reproducibility and correlation with voided volume, pyridium staining and type of exercise. Neurourol Urodyn 1995; 14:125–129.

11. Ryhammer AM, Djurhuus JC, Laurberg S. Pad testing in incontinent women: a review. Int Urogynecol J Pelvic Floor Dysfunc 1999; 10:111–115.

12. Iselin CE, Webster GD. Office management of female urinary incontinence. Urol Clin N Am 1998; 25:625–645.

13. Mayne CJ, Hilton P. The distal urethral electric conductance test: standardization of method and clinical reliability. Neurourol Urodyn 1988; 7:55–60.

14. Janez J, Rudi Z, Mihelic M, et al. Ambulatory distal urethral electric conductance testing coupled to a modified pad test. Neurourol Urodyn 1993; 12:324–326.

15. James ED, Flack FC, Caldwell KP, Martin MR. Continuous measurement of urine loss and frequency in incontinent patient. Preliminary report. Br J Urol 1971; 43:233–237.

16. Stanton SL. Urilos: the practical detection of urine loss. Am J Obstet Gynecol 1977; 128:461–463.

17. Robinson H, Stanton SL. Detection of urinary incontinence. Br J Obstet Gynecol 1981; 88:59–61.

18. Eadie AS, Glen ES, Rowan D. The Urilos recording nappy system. Br J Urol 1983; 55:301–303.

19. Soroka D, Drutz HP, Glazener CM, et al. Perineal pad test in evaluating outcome of treatments for female incontinence: a systematic review. Int Urogynecol J Pelvic Floor Dysfunc 2002; 13:165–175.

20. Hellström AL, Andersen K, Hjälmås K, Jodal U. Pad test in children with incontinence. Scand J Urol 1986; 20:47–50.

21. Imada N, Kawauchi A, Tanaka Y, Watanabe H. The objective assessment of urinary incontinence in children. Br J Urol 1998; 81(Suppl 3):107–108.

22. Sutherst J, Brown M, Shawer M. Assessing the severity of urinary incontinence in women by weighing perineal pads. Lancet 1981; 1:1128–1129.

23. Murray A, Price R, Sutherst J, Brown M. Measurement of the quantity of urine lost in women by weighing perineal pads. Proc International Continence Society, Leiden, 1982:243–244.

24. Wood P, Murray A, Brown M, Sutherst J. Reproducibility of a one-hour urine loss test (pad test). Proc International Continence Society, Aachen, 1983; II:515–517.

25. Klarskov P, Hald T. Reproducibility and reliability of urinary incontinence assessment with a 60 min test. Scand J Urol Nephrol 1984; 18:293–298.

26. Lose G, Gammelgaard J, Jorgensen TJ. The one-hour pad-weighing test: reproducibility and the correlation between the test result, the start volume in the bladder and the diuresis. Neurourol Urodyn 1986; 5:17–21.

27. Christensen SJ, Colstrup H, Hertz JB, et al. Inter- and intra-departmental variations of the perineal weighing test. Neurourol Urodyn 1986; 5:23–28.

28. Jorgensen L, Lose G, Andersen JT. One-hour pad weighing test for objective assessment of female urinary incontinence. Obstet Gynecol 1987; 69:39–42.

29. Lose G, Rosenkilde P, Gammelgaard J, Schroeder T. Pad-weighing test performed with standardised bladder volume. Urology 1988; 32:78–80.

30. Donnellan SM, Duncan HJ, MacGregor RJ, Russel JM. Prospective assessment of incontinence after radical retropubic prostatectomy: objective and subjective analysis. Urology 1997; 49:225–230.

31. Richmond DH, Sutherst RJ, Brown MC. Quantification of urine loss by weighing perineal pads. Observations on the exercise regimen. Br J Urol 1987; 59:224–227.

32. Mayne CJ, Hilton P. Short pad test: method and comparison with 1-hour test. Neurourol Urodyn 1988; 7:443–445.

33. Miller J, Ashton-Miller JA, Delancey JOL. The quantitative paper towel test for measuring stress related urine loss. Proc International Continence Society, Yokohama, 1997:43–44.

34. Griffiths DJ, McCracken PN, Harrison GM. Incontinence in the elderly: objective demonstration and quantitative assessment. Br J Urol 1991; 67:467–471.

35. Griffiths DJ, McCracken PN, Harrison GM, Gormley EA. Characteristics of urinary incontinence in elderly patients studied by 24-hour monitoring and urodynamic testing. Age Aging 1992; 21:195–201.

36. Ryhammer AM, Laurberg S, Djurhuus JC, Hermann AP. No relationship between subjective assessment of urinary incontinence and pad test weight gain in a random population sample of menopausal women. J Urol 1998; 159(3):800–803.

37. Ekelund P, Bergstrom H, Milson I, et al. Quantification of urinary incontinence in elderly women with the 48-hour pad test. Arch Gerontol Geriatr 1988; 7:281–287.

38. O'Donnell PD, Finkbeiner AE, Beck C. Urinary incontinence volume measurement in elderly male inpatients. Urology 1990; 35:499–503.

39. Wilson PD, Mason MV, Herbison GP, Sutherst JR. Evaluation of the home pad test for quantitative incontinence. Br J Urol 1989; 64:155–157.

40. Persson J, Bergqvist CE, Wolner-Hanssen P. An ultra-short perineal pad-test for evaluation of female stress urinary incontinence treatment. Neurourol Urodyn 2001; 20:277–285.

41. Kinn A, Larsson B. Pad test with fixed bladder volume in urinary stress incontinence. Acta Obstet Gynecol Scand 1987; 66:369–372.

42. Simons AM, Yoong WC, Buckland S, Moore KH. Inadequate repeatability of the one-hour pad test: the need for a new incontinence outcome measure. Br J Obstet Gynecol 2001; 108:315–319.

43. Kroman-Andersen B, Jakobsen H, Andersen J. Pad-weighing tests: a literature survey on test accuracy and reproducibility. Neurourol Urodynam 1989; 8:237–242.

44. Haylen BT, Fraser MI, Sutherst JR. Diuretic response to fluid load in women with urinary incontinence; optimum duration of pad test. Br J Urol 1988; 62:331–333.

45. Eadie AS, Glen ES, Rowan D. Assessment of urinary loss over a two-hour test period: a comparison between Urilos recording nappy system and the weighed perineal pad method. Proc International Continence Society, Innsbruck, 1984:94–95.

46. Rasmussen A, Mouritzen L, Dalgaard A, Frimond-Moller C. Twenty-four hour pad weighing test: reproducibility and dependency activity level and fluid intake. Neurourol Urodynam 1994; 13:261–265.

47. Versi E, Orrego G, Hardy E, et al. Evaluation of the home pad test in the investigation of female urinary incontinence. Br J Obstet Gynaecol 1996; 103:162–167.

48. Ali K, Murray A, Sutherst J, Brown M. Perineal pad weighing test: comparison of one hour ward pad test with twelve-hour home pad test. Proc International Continence Society, Aachen, 1983; I:380–382.

49. Lose G, Jorgensen L, Thunedborg P. 24-hour home pad weighing test versus 1-hour ward test in the assessment of mild stress incontinence. Acta Obstet Gynecol Scand 1989; 68:211–215.

50. Groutz A, Blaivas JG, Chaikin DC, et al. Noninvasive outcome measures of urinary incontinence and lower urinary tract symptoms: a multicenter study of micturition diary and pad tests. J Urol 2000; 164:698–701.

51. Mouritzen L, Berild G, Hertz J. Comparison of different methods for quantification of urinary leakage in incontinent women. Neurourol Urodyn 1989; 8:579–587.

52. Victor A, Åsbrink AS. A simple 48-hour test for quantification of urinary leakage in incontinent women. Proc International Continence Society, London, 1985:507–508.

53. Martin A, Halaska M, Voigt R. Our experience with modified pad weighing test. Proc International Continence Society, Halifax, 1992:233–234.

54. Versi E, Cardozo L. One hour single pad test as a simple screening procedure. Proc International Continence Society, Innsbruck, 1984:92–93.

55. Walsh JB, Mills GL. Measurement of urinary loss in elderly incontinent patients. A simple and accurate method. Lancet 1981; 1:1130–1131.

56. Anand D, Versi E, Cardozo L. The predictive value of the pad test. Proc International Continence Society, London, 1985:290–291.

57. Janez J, Plevnik S, Vrtacnik P. Short pad test versus ICS pad test. Proc International Continence Society, London, 1985:386–387.

58. Cardozo L, Versi E. The use of a pad test to improve diagnostic accuracy. Proc International Continence Society, Boston, 1986:367–369.

59. Schüssler B, Hesse U, Horn J, Lentsch P. Comparison of two clinical methods for quantification of stress urinary incontinence. Proc International Continence Society, Boston, 1986:563–565.

35

Endoscopic evaluation of neurogenic bladder

Jacques Corcos and Erik Schick

Introduction

Urethrocystoscopy is not useful in the initial evaluation of neurogenic bladders, but becomes very instrumental in the assessment of lower urinary tract complications. Urethrocystoscopy cannot, by any means, give information on lower urinary tract function. For example, external sphincter contractions and relaxation observed during voluntary movement do not reflect the real functional value of this complex unit. Another classic example is the examination of endoscopic aspects of the bladder neck, which cannot replace functional studies for the evaluation of its opening and closing.

Urethrocystoscopy helps in the appraisal of urethral and bladder anatomical anomalies, most of the time secondary to complications such as urethral strictures, trabeculations, bladder stones, and diverticula. The aim of this chapter is to review these different aspects with some illustrations.

Equipment

Different companies offer different types and sizes of extremely well-designed, rigid urethrocystoscopes (Figure 35.1), some with fixed lens (12–70°), others with exchangeable lens (0°, 30°, 70°, 120°). The choice of lens depends on the segment of urinary tract that we want to study: 0 or 30° for the urethra and 70 or 120° for the bladder in general.

Since sensitivity is often not a problem in neurogenic bladder patients, rigid urethrocystoscopes are often preferred. They give a much better optical field than flexible cystoscopes (Figure 35.2) and allow various manipulations through a bigger working channel (irrigation, washing, small stone extraction, etc.). Flexible cystoscopes are extremely useful in men with preserved sensitivity, and the test is usually painless. In our experiences we do not use any local anesthetic, but only lubricating jelly. Others prefer to inject 2% Xylocaine (lidocaine (lignocaine)) jelly transurethrally 2–4 min before the procedure. One of the biggest advantages of these cystoscopes is the possibility of introducing them in a supine as well as in a sitting position. Because of their deflection abilities, they allow a retrograde view of the bladder neck as well as the complete exploration of diverticula, whatever the position.

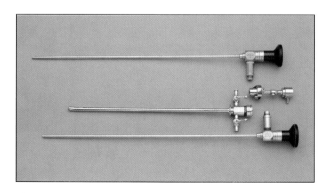

Figure 35.1
Rigid cystoscope.

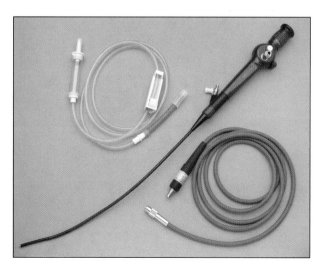

Figure 35.2
Flexible cystoscope.

Technique

Most of the time, the patient is installed in the lithotomy position, but, as mentioned earlier, a supine or a sitting position can be used with a flexible cystoscope.

After the usual disinfection of the genitalia with a non-alcoholic solution, draping creates a sterile field around the genitalia.

Once the patient is informed of the beginning of the examination, the cystoscope, lubricated with sterile jelly, is very gently introduced into the meatus. A global view of the urethra permits the confirmation of penile urethra integrity in men. The cystoscope is then pushed forward into the membranous urethra, making the external sphincter visible. This concentric muscle closes the urethra, and can usually be passed by gentle pressure on the cystoscope. The prostatic urethra is then observed, and the anatomy of the prostate noted, mainly the size of the lateral lobe and the presence or absence of a median lobe.

Once into the bladder, the technique is slightly different, depending on the type of cystoscope. With a rigid cystoscope, we normally use a 70° or 120° lens. The instrument will have only in–out and rotating motions, allowing a complete view of the bladder without bending the unit, which may cause unnecessary pain and discomfort. With a flexible cystoscope, the same in–out motion is applied, but the rotation motion is replaced by deflections of the instrument's tip, which gives a complete view of the bladder wall. Observation of the ureteral orifices, urine efflux from these orifices, and exploration of bladder diverticula may be necessary.

Washing, biopsies, etc., are performed at that time if indicated. Once the test is completed, the instrument is gently withdrawn after emptying of the bladder (when using a rigid instrument).

Drinking up to 6–8 glasses of water per day for 3 days is usually recommended and the patient is discharged. No antibiotics are required unless the patient has a heart artificial valve or it is considered necessary by the physician.

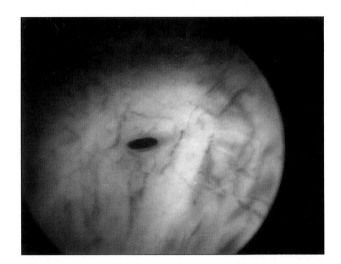

Figure 35.3
Urethral stricture.

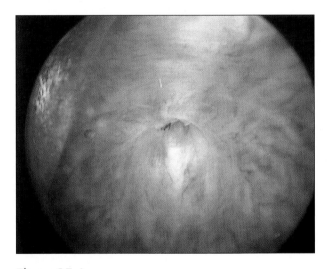

Figure 35.4
Urethral stricture.

Urethrocystoscopic findings

Urethral abnormalities

Urethral strictures

Indwelling catheters, multiple endoscopic manipulations, intermittent catheterizations, and neurogenic trophicity changes lead to frequent urethral strictures and false passages (Figures 35.3 and 35.4).

Strictures can be short and sometimes easy to break just with the cystoscope, or solid, long and tight enough to not allow the cystoscope to pass through. Neglected, they can generate urethral diverticula and urethroscrotal and urethrocutaneous fistulae.

Bladder neck cystoscopic evaluation

The degree of opening of the neurogenic bladder neck cannot be adequately evaluated by cystoscopy. False results can be induced by irrigation flow. These changes are dynamic and not anatomical. They should be evaluated by video urodynamic or simple voiding cystogram.

However, after bladder neck incision or resection to decrease bladder neck resistance, bladder neck strictures can be easily seen by cystoscopy, but, here again, their real impact on bladder function can be assessed only by voiding cystogram.

Endoscopic evaluation of urethral stents

Some specialized centers no longer perform incisional sphincterotomies, preferring endoluminal stents instead (i.e. Urolume – AMS). The techniques and results with these stents are detailed in Chapter 53.

It is usually easy to introduce a flexible cystoscope through these stents, which 'disappear' completely after a few months since the device is epithelialized through and in-between its pores: 90–100% of epithelialization of the stent has been demonstrated in 47.1% of cases 3 months after insertion, and in 87.7% of cases 12 months after insertion.

Mild epithelial hyperplasia can occur (34–44.4%) after stent insertion and may look like an obstructed urethra. Much less frequently, these strictures are severe (3.1%), requiring urethrotomy and sometimes insertion of a second stent at the same level as the first.[1]

Occasionally, however, and even several years later, part of the stent may remain visible, but usually does not cause any problems. Calcifications of the stents are rare. No stone formation has been reported.[1]

Structural bladder anomalies

The well-balanced bladder of a compliant patient looks normal (Figure 35.5) most of the time. However, it may show significant changes because of patient noncompliance with intermittent catheterization, medication, etc., or these treatments may have no effect.

Bladder wall abnormalities

Often associated with chronic infections but also often not related to any obvious disease, cystitis glandularis (Figure 35.6) and cystitis follicularis (Figure 35.7) can be found during systematic cystoscopic evaluation.

Bladder wall trabeculations

There is no consensus in the literature regarding the significance of bladder wall trabeculations (Figures 35.8–35.11).

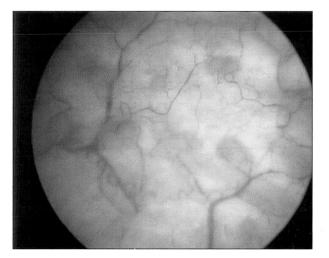

Figure 35.6
Cystitis glandularis.

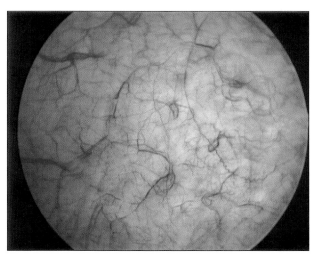

Figure 35.5
Normal bladder mucosa.

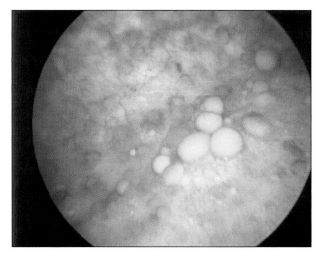

Figure 35.7
Cystitis follicularis.

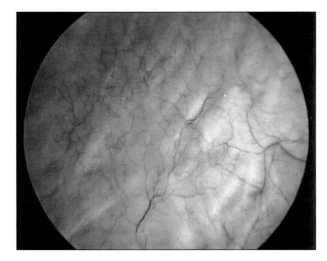

Figure 35.8
Trabeculation grade 1.

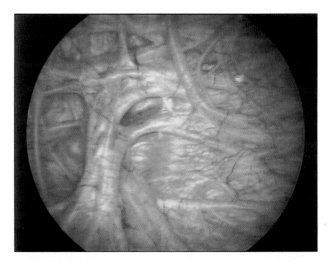

Figure 35.10
Trabeculation grade 3.

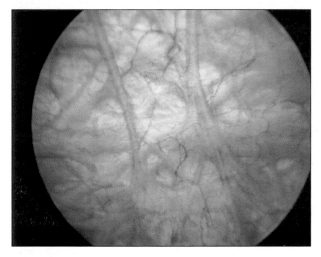

Figure 35.9
Trabeculation grade 2.

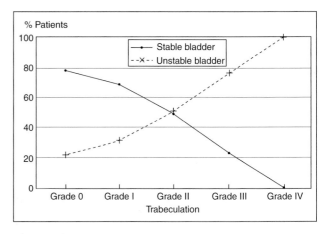

Figure 35.11
Trabeculation grade 4.

O'Donnell[2] suggested that they could be related to high bladder pressure.[1] To Brocklehurst,[3] McGuire,[4] Shah,[5] and O'Reilly[6] they are secondary to an infravesical obstruction. More authors believe that trabeculations reflect bladder overactivity and uninhibited contractions. Schick and Tessier[7] studied the correlation between endoscopic aspects of bladder walls and urodynamic parameters in 220 women. They concluded that there is a close correlation between trabeculation grade and the percentage of unstable bladders (Figure 35.12).

Ureteral orifices

High bladder pressure, recurrent infections, and changes in bladder wall thickness may provoke alterations in the shape of the ureteral orifices. In some cases, they can look

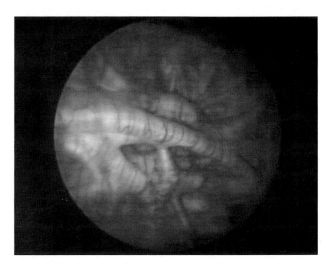

Figure 35.12
Correlation between the trabeculation grade and percentage of unstable bladders.

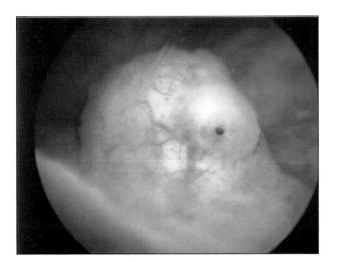

Figure 35.13
Ureterocele.

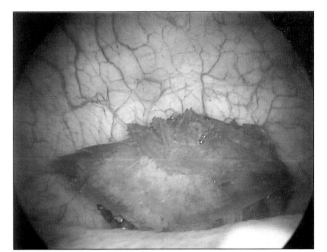

Figure 35.14
Bladder stone.

wide open. Their appearance cannot preclude the efficacy of the intramural ureteral valve mechanism and the presence of reflux. Reflux can be diagnosed only by cystogram with a contrast agent or a radioisotopic fluid. Ureterocele can have variable sizes (Figure 35.13).

Tumors, stones, and foreign bodies

Bladder stones

Usually secondary to infections, bladder stones are very frequent findings in neurogenic patients. They must be suspected in cases of recurrent *Proteus mirabilis* infections, increased spasticity or incontinence, elimination of small calcified fragments, etc. They are easy to diagnose by cystoscopy, and sometimes can be crushed for removal in the same set-up. Their aspects are extremely variable, from small, round, single or multiple stones to huge 'egg-like' stones (Figures 35.14 and 35.15).

Bladder tumors

Patients with chronic indwelling catheters must undergo annual cystoscopic bladder evaluation, which is the only way (with cytology) to detect suspicious lesions such as bladder carcinoma. Usually, these lesions start at the level of the trigone, where the catheter and the balloon lie down. In these patients, there is almost always a small reddish area which is difficult to differentiate from an early carcinoma (Figure 35.16). Biopsy of these lesions is a simple way of reassuring the physician and patient. Bladder tumors can

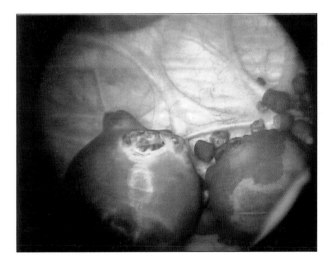

Figure 35.15
Bladder stone.

be located anywhere in the bladder and have different aspects, but most frequently papillary (Figure 35.17). Much less frequent are urethral tumors (Figure 35.18).

Foreign bodies

Foreign bodies are rare. Not infrequently, hairs can be found in patients with intermittent catheterization. Sometimes, they start to be calcified, and always have to be removed. Even less frequent are iatrogenic foreign bodies. Pieces of Foley catheter balloons or sutures from urological or non-urological procedures are eroded into the bladder (Figure 35.19 and 35.20).

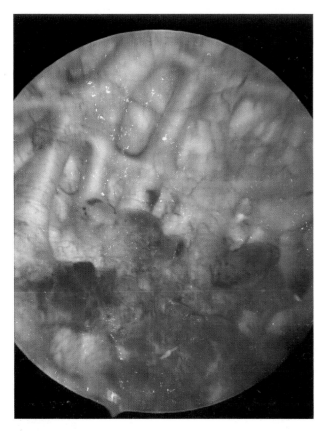

Figure 35.16
Mucosal catheter reaction.

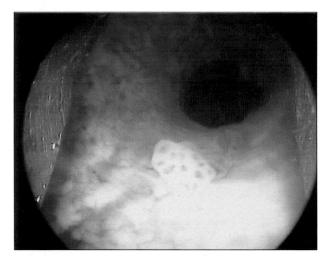

Figure 35.18
Urethral papillary tumor.

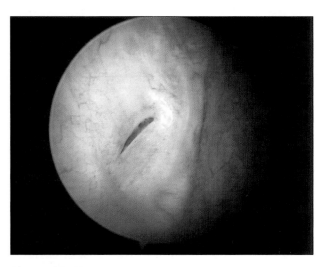

Figure 35.19
Stitch eroding the bladder wall.

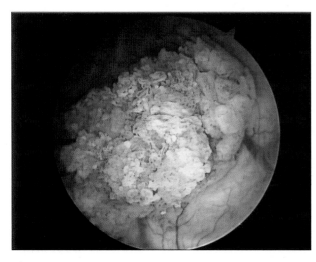

Figure 35.17
Bladder papillary tumor (partially calcified).

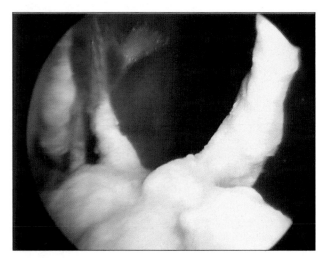

Figure 35.20
Calcified stitch into the bladder.

Conclusion

Urethrocystoscopy must be part of the regular evaluation of neurogenic bladders. It often allows us to understand the patient's worsening lower urinary tract function. Until now, and for most of the changes and abnormalities found by cystoscopy, no other test can replace it with the same accuracy and reliability.

References

1. Rivas DA, Chancelor MB. Sphincterotomy and sphincter stent prosthesis. In: Corcus J, Schick E, eds. The urinary sphincter. New York: Marcel Dekker, 2001:565–582.

2. O'Donnell P. Water endoscopy. In: Rax S, ed. Female urology. Philadelphia: WB Saunders, 1983:51–60.

3. Brocklehurst JC. The genito-urinary system. In: Brocklehurst JC, ed. Textbook of geriatric medicine and gerontology. New York: Churchill Livingstone, 1978:306–325.

4. McGuire EJ. Normal function of lower urinary tract and its relation to neurophysiology. In: Libertino IA, ed. Clinical evaluation and treatment of neurogenic vesical dysfunction. International perspectives in urology. Baltimore: Williams & Wilkins, 1984:1–15.

5. Shah PJR. Clinical presentation and differential diagnosis. In: Fitzpatrick JM, Krane RJ, eds. The prostate. Edinburgh: Churchill Livingstone, 1989:91–102.

6. O'Reilly PH. The effect of prostatic obstruction on the upper urinary tract. In: Fitzpatrick JM, Krane RJ, eds. The prostate. Edinburgh: Churchill Livingstone, 1989:111–118.

7. Schick E, Tessier J. Trabéculation de la paroi vésicale chez la femme: que signifie-t-elle? Presented at the 18th Annual Congress of the Association des Urologues du Québec, Montréal, November 1993.

36

Imaging techniques in the evaluation of neurogenic bladder dysfunction

Walter Artibani and Maria A Cerruto

In the evaluation of neurogenic bladder dysfunction, imaging techniques have the following goals and roles:

- they can suggest a neurogenic etiology in voiding disorders
- they can assess the central nervous system (CNS) in order to confirm and identify the neurogenic lesion, and to relate level and type of neurogenic lesion to bladder dysfunction
- they can evaluate the morphological status of the lower and upper urinary tract.

Imaging techniques suggesting a neurogenic etiology

Lumbosacral spine X-rays

Lower urinary tract (LUT) dysfunction in children, and more rarely in young adults, can be the expression of an underlying spinal dysraphism. In the majority of cases, abnormalities of the gluteosacral region and/or legs and foot are visible (e.g. small dimples, tufts of hair, subcutaneous lipoma, dermal vascular malformations, one leg shortness, high arched foot or feet). However, in some cases these abnormalities may be minimal or absent. A careful evaluation of the anteroposterior and lateral film of the lumbosacral spine can identify vertebral anomalies commonly associated with nervous system anomalies.[1–5]

Sacral agenesis involves the congenital absence of part or all of two or more sacral vertebrae. The absence of two or more sacral vertebrae always implies the presence of a neurogenic bladder dysfunction (Figures 36.1 and 36.2).[6,7]

The significance of spina bifida occulta can vary. Simple failure to fuse the laminae of the 4th and 5th lumbar vertebrae is unlikely to be important, but when the spinal canal

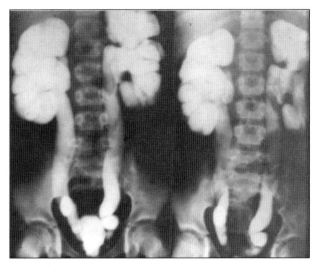

Figure 36.1
Sacral agenesis. Cystography: small retracted bladder and bilateral grade V vesicoureteric reflux.

is noticeably widened, there may be cord involvement (diastematomyelia, tethered cord syndrome).[8]

Open bladder neck and proximal urethra at rest

Open bladder neck and proximal urethra at rest, during the storage phase, can be observed during cystography, videourodynamics, or bladder ultrasonography, both in patients with and without neurologic diseases.

Distal spinal cord injury has been associated with an open smooth sphincter area, but whether this is due to sympathetic or parasympathetic decentralization or defunctionalization is still unclear.[9]

A relative incompetence of the smooth sphincter area may also result from interruption of the peripheral reflex

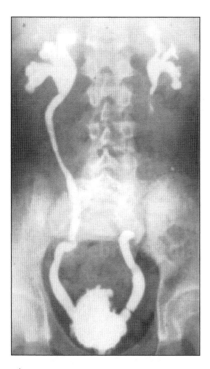

Figure 36.2
Sacral agenesis. Cystography: small sacculated bladder and bilateral grade III vesicoureteric reflux.

arc, which is very similar to the dysfunction observed in the distal spinal cord injury. Twenty-one out of 54 patients with spinal stenosis were found to have an open bladder neck at rest.[10,11]

In a review of 550 patients,[12] 29 out of 33 patients with an open bladder neck had neurologic diseases. Although the association was more commonly seen in patients with thoracic, lumbar, and sacral lesions, when compared to cervical and supraspinal lesions the difference was not significant. Damage of sympathetic innervation to the bladder was also frequently observed in patients undergoing major pelvic surgery, such as abdominal perineal resection of the rectum.

Patients with myelodysplasia showed an inordinately high incidence of open bladder neck (10 out of 18 patients, vs 19 out of 290 with different neurologic disorders).

Patients with sacral agenesis are included in the larger category of myelodysplastic patients and suffer from open bladder neck with areflexic bladder.

Shy–Drager syndrome is a Parkinson-like status with peripheral autonomic dysfunction. Detrusor hyperreflexia is usually found in association with an open bladder neck at rest and a denervated external sphincter.[13]

Peripheral sympathetic injury results in an open bladder neck and proximal urethra from damaged α-adrenergic innervation to the smooth muscle fibers of the bladder neck and proximal urethra.[14] Although it can occur as an isolated injury, this is usually associated with partial detrusor denervation and preservation of sphincter electromyographic (EMG) activity.

The loss of bladder neck closure suggests an autonomic neural deficit. The site and nature of the requisite deficit is unclear. Most authors agree on the importance of the sympathetic system in maintaining the integrity of the bladder neck,[15–19] although some authors have suggested the possible role of parasympathetic innervation.[20,21]

Open bladder neck at rest in children or in women with no neurologic diseases can represent a different disorder, either related to a congenital anomaly or secondary to an anatomical pelvic floor defect. Stanton and Williams[22] described an abnormality in girls with both diurnal incontinence and bed-wetting, based primarily on micturating cystourethrography, in which the bladder neck was wide open at rest. Murray et al[23] reported the 'wide bladder neck anomaly' in 24.5% of the girls (35) and 9.3% of the boys (10) amongst 251 children (143 girls and 108 boys) undergoing videourodynamics for the assessment of non-neuropathic bladder dysfunction (mainly daytime incontinence). The authors considered this anomaly as congenital and made the hypothesis that wide bladder neck anomaly in girls may provide a basis for the development of genuine stress incontinence in later life.

Chapple et al[24] reported that 21% of 25 totally asymptomatic women they investigated by transvaginal ultrasound had an open bladder neck at rest. Versi[25] found a 21% prevalence of open bladder neck at rest in 147 women visiting a urodynamic clinic and suggested that the finding is of little consequence.

Open bladder neck is a key point in defining type III stress incontinence according to the classification of Blaivas and Olsson.[26] This classification is based on history, imaging, and urodynamics, and distinguishes five diagnostic categories of stress incontinence. Incontinence type III is diagnosed by the presence of open bladder neck and proximal urethra at rest in the absence of any detrusor contraction suggesting an intrinsic sphincter deficiency. The proximal urethra no longer functions as a sphincter. There is obvious urinary leakage, which may be gravitational in nature or associated with minimal increase in intravesical pressure.

In pelvic fracture with membranous urethral distraction defects, when cystography (and/or cystoscopy) reveals an open bladder neck before urethroplasty, the probability of postoperative urinary incontinence may be significant, although the necessity of a simultaneous (or sequential) bladder neck reconstruction is controversial.[27–29]

In summary, when observing an open bladder neck and proximal urethra at rest, during the storage phase, whatever imaging technique is used, it may be worthwhile to evaluate the possibility of an underlying autonomic neural deficit (occult spinal dysraphism, sacral agenesis, post-surgery peripheral neural damage, Shy–Drager syndrome). Previous pelvic trauma or female gender can lead to a different perspective.

In the case of a manifest diagnosed neurogenic disease, open bladder neck and proximal urethra stand for various pathophysiologic situations and require a thorough urodynamic investigation in order to be correctly interpreted (e.g. sympathetic damage, associated detrusor-sphincter dyssynergia, previous endoscopic manipulation).

Imaging techniques assessing the central nervous system

Imaging of the central nervous system, otherwise known as neuroimaging, is a valuable aid in the diagnosis of a variety of CNS diseases which may cause LUT dysfunctions. Computed tomography (CT), magnetic resonance imaging (MRI), single-photon emission computed tomography (SPECT), and positron emission tomography (PET) have been used and reported.

When LUT symptoms are just part of the many symptoms caused by a CNS disease, the diagnosis is made on clinical grounds and neuroimaging is carried out only to confirm it. In rare cases, LUT symptoms are the only presenting symptoms of an underlying neurologic disorder and neuroimaging is instrumental in the diagnosis.

The literature shows an endless list of rare neurologic conditions presenting with different symptoms, including LUT symptoms, in which CT scan, MRI, SPECT, and PET imaging were carried out to identify the underlying CNS disease.

After a cerebrovascular accident, the urodynamic behavior of the lower urinary tract has been correlated to CT pictures of the brain.[30,31]

The presence of significant cerebral lesions has been clearly demonstrated by CT, MRI, or SPECT in the absence of clinical neurologic symptoms and signs in patients complaining of urge incontinence.[32] This can be particularly significant in elderly patients. Griffiths et al,[33] studying 48 patients with a median age of 80 years, reported that the presence of urge incontinence was strongly associated with depressed perfusion of the cerebral cortex and midbrain as determined from the SPECT scan.

Kitaba et al,[34] using MRI, reported subclinical lesions in the brain in 40 out of 43 men more than 60 years old who complained of urinary storage symptoms; of these 40 patients, 23 (57.5%) had detrusor hyperreflexia.

In spinal cord injured patients, CNS MRI can detect unsuspected cerebral or spinal lesions (ischemic and hemorrhagic areas, syringomyelia, spinal compression, spinal stenoses) which provide explanations for the possible discrepancy between the clinically assessed level of neurologic lesion and the urodynamically observed LUT dysfunction.

Spinal MRI is instrumental in diagnosing a tethered cord syndrome, as a primary disorder due to dural adhesions or as the outcome of previous surgical manipulation of the distal spinal cord.

PET studies provide information on specific brain structures involved in micturition in humans. In men and women who are able to micturate during scanning, an increase in regional blood flow was shown in the dorsomedial part of the pons close to the 4th ventricle, the pontine micturition center (PMC). PET studies carried out in both men and women also showed an activation of the mesencephalic periacqueductal gray (PAG) area during micturition. Based on experiments on cats, this area is known to project specifically to PMC and its stimulation elicits complete micturition. Experimental interruption of fibers from the PAG to the PMC results in a low-capacity bladder. PET studies during micturition in humans also showed an increased regional blood flow in the hypothalamus, including the preoptical area, which in cats can elicit bladder contractions.[35–37]

The present functional neuroimaging technology shows great potential to improve our knowledge of nervous functional anatomy in relation to vesicourethral function and dysfunction.

Imaging techniques of the lower and upper urinary tract in neurogenic bladder

Imaging of the lower urinary tract

Imaging of the lower urinary tract in neurogenic bladder dysfunctions aims at visualizing the morphology of the bladder and urethra, locating infravesical obstruction, vesicoureteric reflux, diverticula, fistula, and stones, providing a reasonable assessment of residual urine, and demonstrating leakage.

Bors and Comarr[38] described in detail the use of (video)-cystourethrography, with natural or retrograde filling, with or without ice-cooled contrast medium: the use of ice-cooled contrast medium – iced cystourethrography – can be useful in some suprasacral neurogenic patients in order to elicit detrusor reflex and voiding. Changes are detectable in the urethra (diverticula and fistulae at the level of penoscrotal junction, or a patulous urethra) and in the bladder (smooth overdistended bladder, trabeculation, wide open bladder neck, bladder asymmetry, 'Christmas Tree' bladder, thickened bladder wall, vesicoureteric reflux, paraureteric diverticula, bladder diverticula) (Figure 36.3). It is worthwhile to reread their description.

In expert hands ultrasonography can provide similar information. Color flow Doppler in combination with conventional B-mode sonography, has recently been

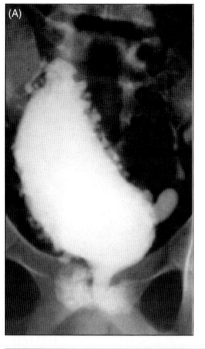

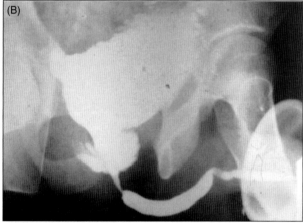

Figure 36.3
Myelomeningocele. Cystourethrography: (A) anteroposterior
projection – 'Christmas tree' bladder, paraureteral
diverticulum and grade I left vesicoureteric reflux, wide open
bladder neck and proximal urethra, intraprostatic ducts
visualization; (B) oblique projection during micturition –
narrowed membranous urethra.

shown to be effective for detection and follow-up of
vesicoureteric reflux in the neurogenic bladder, as an alternative to cystourethrography.[39]

LUT imaging by ultrasonography or cystourethrography
can be performed as a separate test, but it is better performed
at the time of urodynamic study (videourodynamics).[40]
Videourodynamics is generally regarded as the 'gold standard' in the evaluation of LUT tract dysfunction. However,
whether urodynamic and imaging testing should be
performed simultaneously or on separate occasions is still

controversial. Urodynamic examinations must be repeated
several times to obtain reproducibility. The more parameters
are studied, the more complicated the examination becomes,
with a correspondingly higher risk of bias. Nevertheless,
simultaneous videomonitoring along with tracings of detrusor pressure and possibly of EMG sphincter activity, are
important means to make sure that the imaging is performed
at the appropriate times so that the morphological features
can be related to the various functional states.

Severe bladder trabeculation with diverticula and pseu-
dodiverticula, vesicoureteric reflux, wide bladder neck, and
proximal urethra, and narrowing at the level of the membranous urethra can suggest, mainly in children, the
presence of neurogenic LUT dysfunction (occult spinal
dysraphism, non-neurogenic neurogenic bladder) even in
the absence of neurogenic symptoms and signs.[41–43] In
these cases imaging abnormalities indicate the need for
urodynamic evaluation, electrophysiological tests, and
CNS imaging.

Residual urine evaluation can be worthwhile in neurogenic LUT dysfunctions. Residual urine is defined by the
International Continence Society (ICS) as the volume of
fluid remaining in the bladder immediately following
completion of micturition.[44] Residual urine is usually
referred to as an absolute value, but it can be measured also
as a percentage of bladder capacity.

The measurement of post-void residual urine (PVR) can
be performed by invasive or noninvasive means: invasive
means are in-and-out catheterization and endoscopy; noninvasive means are transabdominal ultrasonography and
radioisotope studies.

In-and-out catheterization is indicated as the gold
standard for the measurement of PVR. Its invasiveness is
not an issue in patients who are or will be in a regimen of
intermittent catheterization. This method is subject to
inaccuracies if the person performing the catheterization is
not fully instructed as to the procedures and techniques to
assure complete emptying (moving the catheter in and out
slowly, twisting it, suctioning with syringe, suprapubic
pressure), especially in cases of bladder diverticula and
vesicoureteric reflux.[45] Stoller and Millard[46] showed inaccuracies in 30% of 515 male patients evaluated by full-time
urological nurses with a mean difference between the initial and the actual residual volume of 76 ml in 30% of inaccurate assessments. After further training by the nurses,
inaccurate assessments were reduced to 14%, with a mean
difference of 85 ml.

Before the era of ultrasonography, PVR was measured
noninvasively by the phenolsulfonphthalein excretion
test[47] or with isotopes.[48] These tools have now been practically abandoned.

Ultrasonography is the least-invasive method of determining the PVR. There are several methods for this measurement, which are based on transverse and longitudinal
ultrasound bladder imaging. Using either of three parameters

(length, height, width) or the surface area in the transverse image and the length obtained in the longitudinal image, various volume formulae for a spherical or an ellipsoid body are utilized to estimate the bladder volume. Currently, no single formula can be indicated as the best to calculate bladder volume.

Several studies report sufficient accuracy in the ultrasound estimation of PVR.[49–55] The intra-individual variability of PVR is high from day to day and even within a 24-hour period. This was reported in men with benign prostatic hypertrophy (BPH) by Birch et al[56] and by Bruskevitz et al.[57] Griffiths et al[58] examined the variability of PVR among 14 geriatric patients (mean age 77 years), measured by ultrasound at three different times of the day during each of two visits at 2–4 week intervals. Within-patient variability was large (SD 128 ml) because of a large systematic variation with time of the day, with greatest volumes in early morning. The inherent random variability of the measurement was much smaller (SD 44 ml).

There are no data with regard to PVR variability in neurogenic bladders. The factors influencing the variability of PVR measurement are voiding in unfamiliar surroundings, voiding on command with a partially filled or overfilled bladder, the interval between voiding and the estimation of residual (it should be as short as possible), the presence of vesicoureteric reflux or bladder diverticula.

Recently, portable scanners have been introduced, with automatic measurement of bladder volume. In a prospective comparison,[59] where 100 measurements of PVR by portable ultrasound were compared with measurements by catheterization, the mean absolute error of the scanner was 52 ml. For volumes below 200 and 100 ml, the error was 36 and 24 ml, respectively. The portable scanner appears to be a valid alternative to in-and-out catheterization.

Imaging of the upper urinary tract

Neurogenic bladder dysfunction, primarily in the case of low bladder compliance or detrusor-sphincter dyssynergia or chronic retention with incontinence, can undermine urine transport through the ureterovesical junction from the kidneys to the bladder, resulting in hydronephrosis and renal damage. The relationship between high bladder storage pressure and renal deterioration has been well established by McGuire et al in a cohort of myelodysplastic children, showing that a detrusor leak point pressure >40 cmH$_2$O is detrimental to the upper urinary tract function.[60] Renal impairment is usually detectable at various stages by imaging of the kidneys and/or renal function tests.

Upper tract imaging is advisable at baseline and during follow-up in all cases of neurogenic bladder dysfunction, and most of all in urodynamic situations with high risk of renal damage (high bladder pressure and inefficient voiding, with or without vesicoureteric reflux and infection).

The upper tract imaging modalities most commonly used include ultrasonography, intravenous urography (IVU), isotope scanning, CT scanning, and MRI.

Ultrasonography is an excellent tool for imaging of the upper urinary tract. It is noninvasive, and successful imaging of the kidneys is independent of renal function. Ultrasound can be used to assess many features of renal anatomy, including renal size and growth, hydronephrosis, segmental anomalies, stones, and tumors. In the evaluation of the patient with neurogenic LUT dysfunction, the detection of hydronephrosis is extremely important and may be a marker for a badly managed LUT. Because ultrasonography cannot predict function or degree of obstruction or reflux, other imaging modalities are often used after hydronephrosis is initially diagnosed by ultrasound. Ultrasound is an excellent tool to follow the degree of hydronephrosis or the response to treatment over time.

IVU is the original radiographic examination of the upper urinary (and lower) tract. Successful examination is dependent upon adequate renal function. Renal dysfunction, obstruction, congenital anomalies, fistula, stones, and tumors may be detected.

In some neurogenic patients, both kidney ultrasonography and IVU can be difficult to perform and interpret due to chronic constipation, excessive bowel gas, severe kyphoscoliosis or other spinal deformities, and the presence of internal fixation devices.

Isotopes are used primarily to examine functional characteristics of the upper urinary tract. Isotope scanning can be used to evaluate renal morphology and location. Renography is used to examine the differential function of the two kidneys as well as how they drain. There are many physiological factors and technical pitfalls that can influence the outcome, including the choice of radionuclide, timing of diuretic injection, state of hydration and diuresis, fullness or back pressure from the bladder, varying renal function, and compliance of the collecting system. Diuresis renography with bladder drainage is recommended when obstructive upper tract uropathy is suspected.[61–63]

CT scanning provides useful information about the anatomy of the upper urinary tract. Information can be independent of renal function; however, the addition of intravenous contrast can highlight specific anatomic characteristics (dependent upon renal function). CT scanning can be used as an alternative to ultrasonography or IVU, and in many cases provides additional information, although at a higher cost.

MRI offers some of the same benefits as CT in the evaluation of the upper urinary tract. Magnetic resonance urography is gaining popularity as an alternative to IVU, allowing multiplanar imaging and avoiding the intravenous injection of contrast media and the use of ionizing radiation. Its use in patients with neurogenic bladder due to spina dysraphism with gross spinal deformity has been shown to be valuable and effective, even in the presence of gross spinal deformity.[64]

Conclusions

Upper urinary tract imaging, by means of ultrasonography or MRI urography, is recommended at baseline and during follow-up, as needed, in neurogenic LUT dysfunctions. Their implementation is mandatory when low bladder compliance and chronic retention with/without incontinence indicate a high risk of renal impairment.

In the evaluation of the LUT, the simultaneous performance of imaging and urodynamics (videourodynamics) is the gold standard.

Some morphological findings at cystourethrography or ultrasonography – such as open bladder neck and proximal urethra at rest, heavily thickened sacculated and trabeculated asymmetric bladder, and membranous urethral narrowing – can have clinical and diagnostic relevance in raising the suspicion of a neurogenic disease, even in the absence of clear neurologic symptoms and signs.

Lumbosacral spine X-rays, followed when needed by MRI, have specific indications in children and young adults with suspected neurogenic LUT dysfunction, with or without gluteosacral stigmata.

CNS imaging should be considered when a neurologic disorder is suspected on the basis of clinical, imaging, and neurophysiological findings.

Functional neuroimaging by PET is going to provide new insight into the functional anatomy of CNS related to vesicourethral function and dysfunction. Neuroimaging can cover the gap between clinical neurologic level assessment and the type of vesicourethral dysfunction.

References

1. Anderson FM. Occult spinal dysraphism: a series of 73 cases. Pediatrics 1975; 55:826.

2. Flanigan RF, Russel DP, Walsh JW. Urologic aspects of tethered cord. Urology 1989; 33:80.

3. Kaplan WE, McLone DG, Richards I. The urologic manifestations of the tethered spinal cord. J Urol 1988; 140:1285.

4. Kondo A, Kato K, Kanai S, Sakakibara T. Bladder dysfunction secondary to tethered cord syndrome in adults: is it curable? J Urol 1986; 135:313.

5. Scheible W, James HE, Leopold GR, Hilton SW. Occult spinal dysraphism in infants: screening with high-resolution real-time ultrasound. Radiology 1983; 146:743.

6. Jacobson H, Holm-Bentzen M, Hage T. Neurogenic bladder dysfunction in sacral agenesis and dysgenesis. Neurol Urodyn 1985; 4:99.

7. Boemers TM, VanGool JD, DeJorg TPVM, Bax KMA. Urodynamic evaluation of children with caudal regression syndrome (caudal dysplasia sequence). J Urol 1994; 151:1038–1040.

8. Tarcey PT, Hanigan WC. Spinal dysraphism. Use of magnetic resonance imaging in evaluation. Clin Pediatr 1990; 29:228–233.

9. Artibani W, Andersen JT, Gaiewsky JB, et al. Imaging and other investigations. In: Abrams P, Cardozo L, Khoury S, Wein A, eds. Incontinence. 2nd International Consultation on Incontinence, 2001. Plymbridge Distributors, 2001:427–434.

10. Wein AJ. Pathophysiology and categorization of voiding dysfunction. In: Campbell's urology, 8th edn. Philadelphia: WB Saunders, 2002: 887–899.

11. Webster GD, Guralnick ML. The neurourologic evaluation. In: Campbell's urology, 8th edn. Philadelphia: WB Saunders, 2002: 900–930.

12. Barbalias GA, Blaivas JG. Neurologic implications of the pathologically open bladder neck. J Urol 1983; 129(4):780.

13. Salinas JM, Berger Y, De La Roche RE, Blaivas JG. Urological evaluation in the Shy–Drager syndrome. J Urol 1986; 135(4):741.

14. Blaivas JG, Barbalias GA. Characteristics of neural injury after abdominoperineal resection. J Urol 1983; 129(1):84.

15. de Groat WC, Steers WD. Autonomic regulation of the urinary bladder and sexual organs. In: Loewry AD, Spyers KM, eds. Central regulation of the autonomic functions, 1st edn. Oxford: Oxford University Press, 1990:313.

16. Nordling J. Influence of the sympathetic nervous system on lower urinary tract in man. Neurourol Urodyn 1983; 2:3.

17. Woodside JR, McGuire EJ. Urethral hypotonicity after suprasacral spinal cord injury. J Urol 1979; 121(6):783.

18. McGuire EJ. Combined radiographic and manometric assessment of urethral sphincter function. J Urol 1977; 118(4):632.

19. McGuire EJ. The effects of sacral denervation on bladder and urethral function. Surg Gynecol Obstet 1977; 144(3):343.

20. Nordling J, Meyhoff HH, Olesen KP. Cysto-urethrographic appearance of the bladder and posterior urethra in neuromuscular disorders of the lower urinary tract. Scand J Urol Nephrol 1982; 16(2):115.

21. Gosling JA, Dixon JS, Lendon RG. The autonomic innervation of the human male and female bladder neck and proximal urethra. J Urol 1977; 118(2):302.

22. Stanton SL, Williams D. The wide bladder neck in children. Br J Urol 1973; 45:60.

23. Murray K, Nurse D, Borzykowski M, Mundy AR. The congenital wide bladder neck anomaly: a common cause of incontinence in children. Br J Urol 1987; 59(6):533.

24. Chapple CR, Helm CW, Blease S, et al. Asymptomatic bladder neck incompetence in nulliparous females. Br J Urol 1989; 64(4):357.

25. Versi E. The significance of an open bladder neck in women. Br J Urol 1991; 68(1):42.

26. Blaivas JG, Olsson CA. Stress incontinence: classification and surgical approach. J Urol 1988; 139:737.

27. MacDiamis S, Rosario D, Chapple CR. The importance of accurate assessment and conservative management of the open bladder neck in patients with post-pelvic fracture membranous urethral distraction defects. Br J Urol 1995; 75:65.

28. Isekin CE, Webster GD. The significance of the open bladder neck associated with pelvic fracture urethral distraction defects. J Urol 1999; 162:347.

29. Shivde SR. The significance of the open bladder neck associated with pelvic fracture urethral distraction defects. J Urol 2000; 163:552.

30. Tsuchida S, Noto H, Yamaguchi O, Itoh M. Urodynamic studies in hemiplegic patients after cerebrovascular accidents. Urology 1983; 21:315.

31. Khan Z, Starer P, Yang WC, Bhola A. Analysis of voiding disorders in patients with cerebrovascular accidents. Urology 1990; 32:256.

32. Andrew J, Nathan PW. Lesions of the frontal lobes and disturbances of micturition and defecation. Brain 1964; 87:233–262.

33. Griffiths DJ, McCracken PN, Harrison GM, McEwan A. Geriatric urge incontinence: basic dysfunction and contributory factors. Neurourol Urodyn 1990; 9:406–407.

34. Kitada S, Ikel Y, Hasui Y, et al. Bladder function in elderly men with subclinical brain magnetic resonance imaging lesions. J Urol 1992; 147:1507–1509.

35. Blok BFM, Willemsen ATM, Holstege G. A PET study on brain control of micturition in human. Brain 1997; 120:111.

36. Blok BFM, Holdstege G. The central control of micturition and continence: implications for urology. Br J Urol Int 1999; 83(suppl 2):1.

37. Nour S, Svarer C, Kristensen JKL, et al. Cerebral activation during micturition in normal men. Brain 2000, 123:781–789.

38. Bors E, Comarr AE. Neurological urology, physiology of micturition, its neurological disorders and sequelae. Karger 1971:157.

39. Papadaki PJ, Vlychou MK, Zavras GM, et al. Investigation of vesicoureteral reflux with colour Doppler sonography in adult patients with spinal cord injury. Eur Radiol 2002; 12:366–370.

40. Webster DG, Kreder KJ. The neurourologic evaluation. In: Campbell's urology, 7th edn. Philadelphia: WB Saunders, 1998:927–952.

41. Hinman F. Urinary tract damage in children who wet. Pediatrics 1974; 54:142.

42. Allen TD. The non-neurogenic bladder. J Urol 1977; 117:232.

43. Williams DI, Hirst G, Doyle D. The occult neuropathic bladder. J Pediatr Surg 1975; 9:35.

44. ICS Standardization of terminology of lower urinary tract function. Neururol Urodyn 1998; 7:403.

45. Purkiss SF. Assessment of residual urine in men following catheterisation. Br J Urol 1990; 66(3):279.

46. Stoller ML, Millard RJ. The accuracy of a catheterized residual urine. J Urol 1989; 1741:15.

47. Ruikka I. Residual urine in aged women and its influence on the phenolsulfonphthaleine excretion test. Gerontol Clin 1963; 5:65–71.

48. Mulrow PJ, Huvos A, Buchanan DL. Measurement of residual urine with I-131-labeled Diodrast. J Lab Clin Med 1961; 57:

49. Piters K, Lapin S, Bessman AN. Ultrasonography in the detection of residual urine. Diabetes 1979; 28:320–323.

50. Pedersen JF, Batrum RJ, Grytter C. Residual urine detection by ultrasonic scanning. Am J Roentgenol Radium Ther Nucl Med 1975; 125:474–478.

51. Griffiths CJ, Muray A, Ramsden PD. Accuracy and repeatability of bladder volume measurement using ultrasonic imaging. J Urol 1986; 136:808.

52. Beacock CJM, Roberts EE, Rees RWM, Buck AC. Ultrasound assessment of residual urine. A quantitative method. Br J Urol 1985; 57:410–413.

53. West KA. Sonocystography. A method for measuring residual urine. Scand J Urol Nephrol 1967; 1:68.

54. McLean GK, Edell SL. Determination of bladder volumes by gray scale ultrasonography. Radiology 1978; 128:181–182.

55. Widder B, Kornhuber HH, Renner A. Restharnmessung in der ambulanten Versorgung mit einem Klein-Ultraschallgerat. Dtsch Med Wochen-schr 1983; 108:1552.

56. Birch NC, Hurst G, Doyle PT. Serial residual volumes in men with prostatic hypertrophy. Br J Urol 1998; 62:571.

57. Bruskewitz RC, Iversen P, Madsen PO. Value of post-void residual urine determination in evaluation of prostatism. Urology 1982; 20:602.

58. Griffiths DJ, Harrison G, Moore K, McCracken P. Variability of post-void residual urine volume in the elderly. Urol Res 1996; 24(1):23–26.

59. Ding YY, Sahadevan S, Pang WS, Choo PW. Clinical utility of a portable ultrasound scanner in the measurement of residual urine volume. Singapore Med J 1996; 37(4):365–368.

60. McGuire EM, Woodside JR, Borden TA. Prognostic value of urodynamic testing in myelodysplastic patients. J Urol 1981; 126:205–209.

61. Conway JJ. "Well-tempered" diuresis renography: it's historical development, physiological and technical pitfalls, and standardized technique protocol. Semin Nuclear Med 1992; 22:74–84.

62. Hvistendahl JJ, Pedersen TS, Schmidt F, et al. The vesico-renal reflex mechanism modulates urine output during elevated bladder pressure. Scand J Urol Nephrol 1997; 186(31 suppl):24.

63. O'Reilly PH. Diuresis renography. Recent advances and recommended protocols. Br J Urol 1992; 69:113–120.

64. Shipstone DP, Thomas DG, Darwent G, Morcos SK. Magnetic resonance urography in patients with neurogenic bladder dysfunction and spinal dysraphism. BJU Int 2002; 89:658–664.

37

Normal urodynamic parameters in children

Steven P Lapointe and Diego Barrieras

Introduction

Urodynamic examination yields invaluable information about lower urinary tract function in infants and children. First developed in adults, the techniques have been used in children extensively, using the same terminology and definitions as in adult urodynamics. The computers and devices used for evaluation of lower urinary tract function in children are similar to those used in adults, with appropriate catheter sizes according to age. Most importantly, these types of investigations are best performed by a physician or nurse who is specialized in the care of children. Caregivers must ensure that the results obtained do not reflect apprehension. The urodynamic team has to handle the child with care and patience, keeping a playful mood, distracting the child's attention from the surrounding environment, and following the pace set by the child to alleviate the pressure of performance. A center dedicated to children's care can accomplish this more easily, but with appropriate attention to these differences, children can be accommodated in an adult-oriented facility as well.

When evaluating a child with suspected lower urinary tract dysfunction, a detailed history should be obtained. The past medical history, especially previous urinary tract surgery or disease, and neurological status are relevant. The present medical history should include details about urinary tract infection, trauma, voiding pattern, incontinence, urgency, frequency, and urinary stream appearance; all are important. Bowel habits should be noted. To complete the history, we have found that recording a voiding diary gives objective data that can be repeated in the follow-up and involves the child and his parents in his care. Physical examination should include abdominal and genitalia examination, lumbosacral spine examination, and a brief neurological examination.

Because of the invasive and stressful nature of a complete urodynamics in children, uroflowmetry should be performed as an initial investigation of lower urinary tract dysfunction, except for children who present with diagnosed conditions such as spinal dysraphism or posterior valves. Uroflowmetry has been popularized as a study of lower urinary tract obstruction, mainly for benign prostatic hyperplasia (BPH).[1,2] Although the first reports on the use of uroflowmetry in children date back to the 1950s,[3] it had become a widespread tool by the 1980s.[4–7] Williot et al coupled measurement of uroflowmetry to post-void residual volume assessment using biplanar ultrasound.[7] They stated that the combination of dynamic flow analysis and accurate bladder residual volume assessment proved to be a simple yet comprehensive appraisal of the physiology of the lower urinary tract. These studies have several advantages that make them almost ideal for the pediatric population (see Table 37.1). They are noninvasive, physiological, and can be repeated as frequently as necessary.

Indications for uroflowmetry

Uroflowmetry has multiple applications in children of both sexes. It can be used in any clinical situation with suspected lower urinary tract dysfunction, even though it is not a highly specific diagnostic tool.[8] It has semiological value and gives important information as a screening method, helping diagnosis and/or leading to more elaborate testing (full urodynamics), particularly in evaluating voiding dysfunction and urinary tract infection. The studies can be used as a follow-up tool to assess the result of

Table 37.1 *Advantages and disadvantages of uroflowmetry in children*

Advantages	Disadvantages
Simple to perform	Not etiologic
Simple equipment	Less reproducible than in adults
Noninvasive	Children need to be toilet trained
Physiologic	
Can be repeated	
Low cost	

Table 37.2 *Indications for uroflowmetry in children*

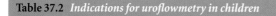

- Urgency, frequency syndrome

- Urinary tract infection

- Incontinence (except isolated nighttime incontinence)

- Dysfunctional voiding syndrome

- Non-neurogenic neurogenic bladder (Hinman/Allen syndrome)

- Vesicoureteric reflux before and after surgical correction

- Neurogenic bladder

- Infravesical obstruction (urethral valves, urethral or meatal stenosis)

- Follow-up in hypospadias surgery and other urethral reconstruction

- Biofeedback method for bladder retraining

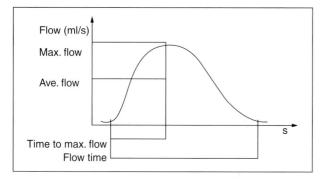

Figure 37.1
Normal uroflowmetry parameters.

surgical treatment, especially after hypospadias repair or in long-term follow-up of posterior urethral valve surgery. It is also very useful in following medical treatment, especially in bladder retraining for dysfunctional voiding and non-neurogenic neurogenic bladder.[9,10] In comparing multiple studies in the same patient, it is important to recognize that uroflowmetry in children is not as reproducible as in adults.[8,9] Consequently, the trend observed during successful studies has more diagnostic value.

Current indications for performing uroflowmetry in children are listed in Table 37.2.

The parameters obtained from uroflowmetry are identical to those in adults (Figure 37.1).

Technical aspects and pitfalls

To obtain optimal results from uroflowmetry, the voiding condition should be as close to normal as possible.

This is true in adults and it is even more important in children.[5,6] Children, especially under the age of 6, differ from older children and adults in the sense that they are usually less motivated, less patient, more apprehensive, and have limited understanding of what is going to happen.[6] The post-void residual volume can be determined by ultrasound using a mathematical model for calculation that considers the bladder to be a rectangular box. This equipment is readily available and cost-effective. Using a sagittal and a transverse view, two measures of bladder diameter are taken, and from these the volume in milliliters is generated. This technique is simple, noninvasive, accurate, and reproducible.[7] It should be noted that it has a slight tendency to overestimate the residual volume when compared to urethral catheterization.[8] Finally, like any ultrasonic technique it is operator-dependent, but this technique is easy to learn for those involved in urodynamic testing.

Interpretation of uroflowmetry

The availability of nomograms for analysis of uroflow data has been helpful in providing 'relative' data for size and weight, while recognizing that their absolute interpretation can be misleading.[4, 10–13] However, there are general principles that guide the interpretation of the uroflowmetry data in children. As in adults, the results obtained are an integration of detrusor contractility and urethral resistance.[5] We believe that the shape of the flow curve is the most important feature of uroflowmetry, followed by maximal flow rate. Interestingly, the shape of the normal flow curve in children is the same as in adults and is a bell-shaped curve (Figure 37.2A) in more than 90% of normal children, even if the voided volume is under 100 ml.[5,10,11] With low or high voided volumes the shape of the curve has a tendency toward a more plateau appearance. There are three frequently encountered shapes. The staccato shape (Figure 37.2B) is indicative of either abnormal sphincter relaxation, and may be a reflection of dysfunctional voiding as in the non-neurogenic neurogenic bladder, unsustained bladder contraction, or abdominal straining. Children with dysfunctional voiding often benefit from bladder retraining, in which case uroflowmetry and nomograms can be used as a method of biofeedback. A plateau-shaped (Figure 37.2C) curve may be normal but can indicate infravesical obstruction, especially if associated with a low maximal and average flow rates. In such a case, depending on history and physical examination, further diagnostic tests may be indicated. For example, a voiding cystogram would permit diagnosing posterior urethral that sometimes is present at an older age. It should also be noted that after hypospadias surgery uroflowmetry curves are references, and should be available in the laboratory.[4,10,11] From a practical standpoint, the maximal flow rate has more value than the average flow rate and has a linear relationship with the voided volume.[6] The maximal flow rate should equal the square root of the voided volume[6] (Q_{max} = square root of voided volume). For example, with a voided volume of 100 ml the maximal expected flow rate should be 10 ml/s and with a voided volume of 225 ml it should be 15 ml/s. Most often when these values are low, they are associated with a plateau-shaped curve.

Uroflowmetry and electromyography recordings

The residual volume estimate may provide conflicting results after uroflowmetry. When analyzing post-void residual volume in children, one should consider the fear and anxiety that might be involved on behalf of the child. However, we believe that, as a screening tool, a normal flow rate coupled with a complete emptying (0 ml) excludes the likelihood of serious underlying abnormalities.[2,7,13] On the contrary, defining what is a clinically significant residual volume is difficult in the face of an anxious child, and its value as a single diagnostic measure, grading of severity, or prognosis of urologic abnormality is poor. With young children, an isolated post-void residual volume measure without symptoms may merely reflect the child's apprehension. We would not ascribe any significance to it. Thus, we routinely use simultaneous electromyography (EMG) recordings with perineal patch electrodes to further discriminate normal children from patients with abnormal voiding pattern due to dysfunctional voiding or to underlying neurogenic bladder.

Treatment and further evaluation are then tailored according to the findings. If a child with no anatomical anomalies presents with clinical symptoms, high residual volume, or dyssynergia on cutaneous EMG recording, we would proceed with bladder and bowel management programs. Should the latter fail, despite simultaneous bladder-oriented pharmacotherapy, we would proceed with urodynamic studies. If a child presents with anatomical abnormalities during evaluation and an abnormal EMG–uroflowmetry, then we would proceed directly towards full urodynamic evaluation.

In summary, the noninvasive nature of EMG-coupled uroflowmetry and post-void residual assessment by ultrasound make them ideal in screening and follow-up of children. Their relative simplicity and ease of performance add to their wide application. The results of these studies are not highly specific but, when interpreted in the light of the clinical history, physical findings, and eventually other diagnostic studies, they give important

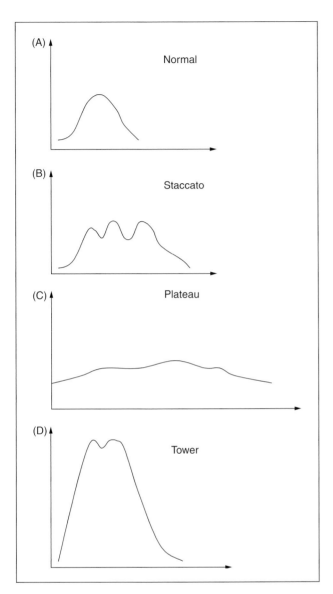

Figure 37.2
Normal and abnormal uroflowmetry curves.

those of a plateau type with low maximal and average flow rates. The physician should only be concerned when there is a trend towards worsening over successive studies.[14] A tower-shape curve (Figure 37.2D) is usually associated with a high maximal flow rate and is believed to be reflective of dysfunctional voiding. It is more frequently encountered in girls and is often referred to as 'supervoiders'.

One has to be critical when looking at these results. Artifacts, mostly caused by misdirection of the stream, will change the shape of the curve, as well as the numerical values generated.[5]

The maximal and average flow rates closely correlate with voided volume, which is dependent on the age and size of the child. Again, the nomograms are helpful as information in establishing a diagnosis, especially in dysfunctional voiding or Hinman/Allen syndrome, and elaborating a treatment plan and following its results (e.g. during bladder retraining as a feedback, and following hypospadias surgery).

Some children require more extensive urodynamic studies. Indications include abnormal curve pattern associated with detrusor-sphincter dyssynergia (DSD) on cutaneous EMG, abnormal flow rate with daytime urinary incontinence, and chronic or recurrent bacteriuria that is refractory to bladder and bowel management. Clear indications for complete urodynamics as the initial test include patients with suspected infravesical obstruction such as posterior valves, overt or suspected neurogenic bladder dysfunction, and treatment failures of vesicoureteral reflux.

Only a few studies have looked at normal urodynamics in children. Sillen et al[15] evaluated bladder function in healthy neonates and infants using free voiding studies with a 4-hour voiding observation and subsequent urodynamics studies. They showed that voiding in the healthy neonate is characterized by small, frequent voids of varying volume. Thirty percent of the cases presented an interrupted voiding pattern, which seemed to be an immature phenomenon since it was seen in 60% of preterm neonates and disappeared completely before the age of toilet training. They theorized that there exists a physiological DSD, which may explain the frequent postvoid residual observed in the young.[16,17] Along with the small caliber of the urethra, this can also explain the observed high voiding pressure. They observed some bladder hyperactivity on cystometric evaluation, as patients exhibited premature voiding contractions after only a few milliliters of filling volume with leakage of urine. Characteristics of the normal neonate micturition thus include physiological DSD, low bladder capacity, and high voiding pressure, associated with some detrusor hyperactivity.

Their findings are challenging the concept that neonates display simply a normal voiding reflex and that regulation of micturition in neonates involves higher neuronal pathways.

Another study from Sweden evaluated urodynamics in normal infants and children.[6] One of the most important statements of this study was that a tense and apprehensive child will not produce reliable urodynamic data. Studies should be done in an appropriate setting with an experienced urodynamicist. Their study also showed that inhibition of the detrusor improves during the first 5 years of life. Development of normal voiding pattern evolves as adequate proprioception of the bladder improves, allowing the child to have a better control on micturition. To this maturational process we should add the new concept of improvement of physiological DSD with age, as suggested by the study of Sillen et al.[15]

Urodynamic studies
Bladder capacity

Hjälmås observed that most urodynamic variables are age-dependent.[6] Several formulae have been proposed in the literature to assess normal bladder capacity in children (see Table 37.3). However, the most urodynamically sound formula was described by Houle et al,[20] as they evaluated 69 normal children, measuring total bladder capacity (ml), full resting pressure (cmH$_2$O), as well as the volume (ml) and the percentage of the total bladder capacity stored at detrusor pressures of less than 10, 20, 30, and 35 cmH$_2$O. According to their results, minimal acceptable total bladder capacity for age can be estimated by 16(age) + 70 in ml, which was derived using criteria for safe storage characteristics of the bladder in children. Table 37.3 summarizes some of these mathematical formulae.

Bladder compliance

Normal compliance in children has been established somewhat arbitrarily. The minimally acceptable value for bladder compliance during bladder filling has been set at 10 ml/cmH$_2$O.[21] Values above this level can be considered normal. Other researchers[22] have further stratified compliance as being poor <10 ml/cmH$_2$O, moderate between 10 and 20 ml/cmH$_2$O and mild between 21 and 30 ml/cmH$_2$O. The clinical relevance to such classification has yet to be determined.

It is important to remember that, as observed in adults, compliance may be influenced by the rate of bladder filling, which should be at a rate corresponding to 10% of the expected bladder capacity per minute. Compliance should be evaluated at regular intervals during cystometric recording (25–50–75%) as opposed to only at final capacity, since loss in compliance that occurs early in the filling phase puts the upper tract at higher risk than changes noted only near the end of the cystometric curve.[21]

Uninhibited contractions are recorded in the same way as in the adult; i.e. any appreciable detrusor contraction, especially if it causes urine leakage or urgency. (Since this chapter discusses only normal urodynamics in children, detrusor leak point pressure or abdominal leak point pressure will not be discussed, as they do not occur in the normal child.)

Voiding pressures

Hjälmås, in his study,[6] described intravesical pressures that are lower in girls than in boys, and lower in infants than in older children, but intravesical pressure does not vary with

Table 37.3 *Normal values for complete urodynamic studies in children*

Urodynamic characteristic	Normal value in children
Uroflow	Maximal flow rate = square root of the voided volume[6]
Bladder capacity (ml)	Houle et al:[20] 16 (age (years)) + 70 Koff:[18] (age (years) + 2) × 30 Kaefer et al:[19] (2 × age (years) + 2) × 30 (child <2 years old) (age (years) divided by 2 + 6) × 30 (child >2 years old) Hjälmås:[6] 30 + (age (years) × 30)
Uninhibited contractions	Any appreciable detrusor contraction
Bladder compliance	>10 ml/cmH$_2$O[21]
Voiding pressures	Infant male: median 100 cmH$_2$O[15] Infant female: median 70 cmH$_2$O[15] 1–3 years old child male: 70 cmH$_2$O[6] 1–3 years old child female: 60 cmH$_2$O[23] 7 years and older: similar to adult
Post-void residual (limited reliability)	Infant: 1 void/4 hour complete, median PVR 4–5 ml up to 2 years old: 4–5 ml[17] 3 years old and up: 0 ml

age. However, he mentioned that bladder pressure recordings represent the most important source of error when examining children. He strongly emphasized that the examination has to be performed in a kind, friendly, and relaxed atmosphere. Median pressure measurements in male infants of more then 100 cmH$_2$O and 60–70 cmH$_2$O in females have been observed. In children 1–3 years of age, voiding pressure can be 70 cmH$_2$O in males[6] and 60 cmH$_2$O in females.[23] After the age of 7, values tend toward those of adults.

Post-void residual

Post-void residual urine has been studied, but to date only a few studies have presented significant data as to what represents normal post-void residual urine. It is recognized that infants do not empty their bladder at each void,[17] but they seem to empty their bladder completely at least once during a 4-hour observation period.[15] Residual urine using a 4-hour observational protocol has been reported to be minimal (4–5 ml) up to age 2.[17,24] Residual urine should be 0 ml at 3 years and older.[24] Caution should be used when post-void residual urine is considered as a significant factor in diagnosis, as many children may present fear and anxiety at the time of observation.

A summary of normal urodynamic values in children is presented in Table 37.3.

References

1. Gleason DM, Lattimer JK. The pressure flow study: a method for measuring bladder neck resistance. J Urol 1962; 87:844.

2. Abrams PH, Griffiths DJ. The assessment of prostatic obstruction from urodynamics measurements and from residual urine. Br J Urol 1979; 51(2):129–134.

3. Scott RJ, McIlhaney JS. The voiding rates in normal children. J Urol 1959; 82:224.

4. Churchill BM, Gilmour RF, Williot P. Urodynamics. Pediatr Clin North Am 1987; 34:1133–1157.

5. Jorgensen JB, Jensen KM. Uroflowmetry. Urol Clin North Am 1996; 23:237–242.

6. Hjälmås K. Urodynamics in normal infants and children. Scand J Urol Nephrol Suppl 1988; 114:20–27.

7. Williot P, McLorie GA, Gilmour RF, Churchill BM. Accuracy of bladder volume determinations in children using a suprapubic ultrasonic bi-planar technique. J Urol 1989; 141:900–902.

8. Meunier P, Mollard P, Nemoz-Behncke C, Genet JP. [Urodynamic exploration in functional micturition disorders in children]. Arch Pediatr 1995; 2:483–491.

9. Ewalt DH, Bauer SB. Pediatric neurourology. Urol Clin N Am 1996; 23(3):501–509.

10. Segura CG. Urine flow in children: a study of flow chart parameters based on 1361 uroflowmetry tests. J Urol 1997; 157:1426–1428.

11. Jensen KM, Nielsen KK, Jensen H, et al. Urinary flow studies in normal kindergarten- and schoolchildren. Scand J Urol Nephrol 1983; 17:11–21.

12. Gaum LD, Wese FX, Liu TP, et al. Age related flow rate nomograms in a normal pediatric population. Acta Urol Belg 1989; 57:457–466.

13. Wese FX, Gaum LD, Liu TP, et al. Body surface related flow rate nomograms in a normal pediatric population. Acta Urol Belg 1989; 57:467–474.

14. Jayanthi VR, McLorie GA, Khoury AE, Churchill BM. Functional characteristics of the reconstructed neourethra after island flap urethroplasty. J Urol 1995; 153:1657–1659.

15. Sillen U. Bladder function in healthy neonates and its development during infancy. J Urol 2001; 166:2376–2381.

16. Roberts DS, Rendell B. Postmicturition residual bladder volumes in healthy babies. Arch Dis Child 1989; 64:825–828.

17. Sillen U, Solsnes E, Hellstrom AL, Sandberg K. The voiding pattern of healthy preterm neonates. J Urol 2000; 163:278–281.

18. Koff SA. Estimating bladder capacity in children. Urology 1983; 21:248.

19. Kaefer M, Zurakowski D, Bauer SB, et al. Estimating normal bladder capacity in children. J Urol 1997; 158:2261–2264.

20. Houle AM, Gilmour RF, Churchill BM, et al. What volume can a child normally store in the bladder at a safe pressure? J Urol 1993; 149:561–564.

21. Gilmour RF, Churchill BM, Steckler RE, et al. A new technique for dynamic analysis of bladder compliance. J Urol 1993; 150:1200–1203.

22. Horowitz M, Combs AJ, Shapiro E. Urodynamics in pediatric urology. In: Nitti VW, ed. Practical urodynamics. Philadelphia: WB Saunders, 1998:254–269.

23. Wen JG, Tong EC. Cystometry in infants and children with apparent voiding symptoms. Br J Urol 1998; 81:468–473.

24. Jansson UB, Hanson M, Hanson E, et al. Voiding pattern in healthy children 0 to 3 years old: a longitudinal study. J Urol 2000; 164:2050–2054.

38

Evaluation of neurogenic bladder dysfunction: basic urodynamics

Christopher E Kelly and Victor W Nitti

Classification of neurogenic voiding dysfunction

The main objective in assessing patients with suspected neurogenic lower urinary tract (LUT) dysfunction is to determine what effect the neurologic disease has on the entire urinary tract so that treatment can be implemented to relieve symptoms and prevent upper and lower urinary tract damage. The functional classification system described by Wein (Figure 38.1) is a useful framework with which to conceptualize neurogenic voiding dysfunction and provides a basis for the discussion of various diagnostic and treatment modalities.[1] This simple and practical system can be easily applied to our diagnostic criteria (e.g. urodynamics). Of equal importance is the fact that treatment options can be chosen based on this system. The functional classification system is based on the simple concept that the LUT has two basic functions: storage of adequate volumes of urine at low pressures, and voluntary and complete evacuation of urine from the bladder. For normal storage and emptying to occur there must be proper and coordinated functioning of the bladder and bladder outlet (bladder neck, urethra, external sphincter). Hence, neurogenic LUT dysfunction can be classified under the following rubrics: 'failure to store', 'failure to empty', or a combination thereof. Abnormalities in LUT function may be the result of bladder dysfunction, bladder outlet dysfunction, or a combined dysfunction. Figure 38.2 summarizes how neurologic disease can adversely affect the bladder and/or the bladder outlet, causing storage and emptying dysfunction.

Prior to our discussion, it is important to emphasize that symptoms do not always indicate the magnitude to which the disease is affecting the urinary tract, especially in neurologic disorders. Serious urinary tract damage can result in the absence of symptoms. It is also vital to realize that

---

Functional classification:

1. Emptying abnormality (failure to empty)
2. Storage abnormality (failure to store)
3. Emptying and storage abnormality

Anatomic abnormality:

1. Bladder dysfunction
2. Bladder outlet dysfunction
3. Bladder and bladder outlet dysfunction

Figure 38.1
Functional classification of voiding disorders.

Failure to store

A. Bladder dysfunction:
   • Neurogenic detrusor overactivity
   • Impaired compliance

B. Bladder outlet dysfunction:
   • Neurogenic intrinsic sphincter deficiency

Failure to empty

A. Bladder dysfunction:
   • Detrusor underactivity
   • Acontractile detrusor

B. Bladder outlet dysfunction:
   • Detrusor-external sphincter dyssynergia
   • Bladder neck dyssynergia

Figure 38.2
Effects of neurologic disease on storage and emptying function.

patients with neurologic disease are at risk for developing the same urologic and gynecologic problems as persons of the same age without neurologic disease.[2] For example, just because a women has had a cerebrovascular accident does not exclude her from having stress urinary incontinence. And, lastly, the clinician should remember that neurologic lesions may be 'complete' or 'incomplete'. Hence, urologic manifestations of neurologic disease may not always be predictable. A complete neuro-urologic evaluation of patients with neurogenic voiding dysfunction is therefore important.

In this chapter we will discuss the evaluation of patients with neurogenic LUT dysfunction with urodynamics. Prior to this discussion, a working knowledge of the neurophysiology of micturition is essential. This topic is covered in Chapter 6. Additionally, the effect of particular neurologic diseases on lower urinary tract function is covered elsewhere in the book.

Assessment of patients with neurogenic lower urinary tract dysfunction

History and physical examination

Any patient with obvious or suspected neurogenic voiding LUT dysfunction deserves a neurologic work-up. Controversy exists as to how often patients should be reassessed urologically. We recommend that patients be reviewed at least annually, and the complete work-up be repeated if significant changes occur in the neurologic status or LUT signs or symptoms.

Prior to urodynamic testing a complete history and physical examination are imperative. A thorough understanding of the patient's condition and symptoms are essential so that urodynamic investigations can be 'customized' to answer questions relevant to that particular patient. Initial evaluation of patients with suspected neurogenic LUT dysfunction should include a thorough history of the patient's general health and neurologic disease. It is important to understand how the neurologic disease affects daily activities, whether it affects other systems, and whether its course is stable or changing. In patients who do not have a history of neurologic disease (i.e. occult neurologic disease), it is important to carefully and directly question them even about their more subtle neurologic complaints.[2]

A standard and complete urologic examination should be performed on all patients with suspected neurogenic LUT dysfunction. A good general neurologic examination to assess sensation, strength, dexterity, and mobility is essential, as all of these can affect treatment of neurogenic LUT dysfunction. A specific and comprehensive evaluation of the sacral nerve (S2–S4) reflex arc is critical. A digital rectal examination will establish rectal tone and control. The bulbocavernosus reflex and perianal sensation should also be assessed. Finally, lower extremity spasticity along with patellar and ankle reflexes should be evaluated.

Laboratory studies

Basic serum and urine tests, including renal function tests and serum electrolytes, should be performed. Urinalysis and urine culture are essential, particularly in patients with an increased risk for developing urinary tract infections: those with chronic indwelling catheters, on intermittent self-catheterization, or those carrying high post-void residual volumes.

Noninvasive urodynamic assessment

Noninvasive studies such as uroflowmetry and measurement of post-void residual urine can be readily performed to give an initial assessment of the patient's ability to empty the bladder. While nonspecific for underlying dysfunction, uroflowmetry is often used as a screening test for voiding dysfunction and as a means for selecting patients for more sophisticated urodynamic studies. It also provides an objective way to monitor the emptying in patients who have specific diagnoses and are followed with observation or specific therapy.

Since the upper urinary tract in neurogenic voiding dysfunction can be adversely affected by secondary reflux, ascending infection, hydronephrosis, or stones, a baseline study is recommended. A renal ultrasound or intravenous pyelogram can be used to assess for hydronephrosis or stones. Bladder ultrasound provides an excellent modality to rule out bladder stones, which are reported in over 30% of patients with indwelling catheters.[3] When suspected, vesicoureteral reflux can be assessed by a voiding cystourethrogram or as part of a videourodynamic evaluation. When more detailed information on renal function is required, such as obstruction or cortical scarring, a nuclear renogram is obtained.

Although it is an invasive technique, a few words on cystourethroscopy are important. It is indicated in those with indwelling catheters on a yearly basis. Besides evaluating for bladder calculi, epithelial changes can be detected. These patients carry a 5% lifetime risk of developing squamous cell carcinoma of the bladder.[4–6]

Urodyamics

Multichannel urodynamic evaluation is the mainstay of evaluation in patients with neurogenic LUT dysfunction. The goals of urodynamic testing in patients with neurologic disease are:

1. To provide documentation of the effect of neurologic disease on the LUT.
2. To correlate the patient's symptoms with urodynamic events.
3. To assess for the presence of urologic risk factors associated with urologic complications: detrusor striated sphincter dyssynergia (DESD), impaired bladder compliance, sustained high-pressure detrusor contractions, and vesicoureteral reflux.

The urodynamic evaluation consists of several components, including the uroflowmetry, cystometrogram (CMG), abdominal pressure monitoring, electromyography (EMG), and voiding pressure–flow studies. Simultaneous fluoroscopic imaging of the entire urinary tract during urodynamics (i.e. videourodynamics) can be helpful in cases of known or suspected neurogenic voiding dysfunction. It is not unusual to repeat a study several times in order to fulfill the above goals.

Cystometrogram

The filling CMG is used to mimic the bladder's filling and storage of urine while the pressure–volume relationship within the bladder is recorded. It is best to fill the bladder at a rate of 30 ml/min or less. In our experience, faster filling rates can exaggerate urodynamic observations. Important bladder parameters with respect to neurologic disease are bladder sensation, the presence of involuntary detrusor contractions (IDC), compliance (storage pressures), and cystometric capacity. IDCs associated with neurologic disease are referred to as neurogenic detrusor overactivity according to the International Continence Society (Figure 38.3).[7] The magnitude, or pressure, of IDCs is often determined by the amount of resistance provided by the bladder outlet. For example, in cases of high outlet resistance such as DESD or anatomical obstruction, detrusor pressure with IDC can be quite high, whereas in cases of low outlet resistance, the IDC pressure is often low with subsequent incontinence. Neurogenic detrusor overactivity is caused by lesions above the sacral micturition center, including the spinal cord and brain. Simply stated, the inhibition of the spinal micturition reflex from suprapontine centers is blocked.

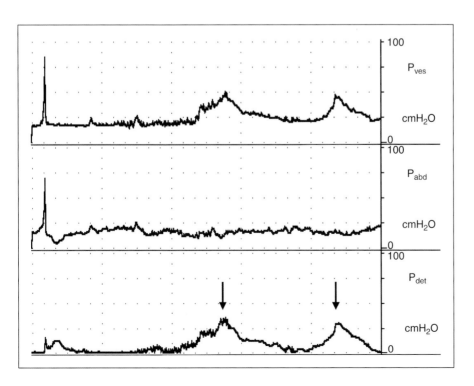

P_{ves}

cmH_2O

P_{abd}

cmH_2O

P_{det}

cmH_2O

Figure 38.3

Filling phase of a urodynamic study in a 68-year-old woman with urge incontinence after cerebrovascular accident. Note the involuntary detrusor contractions (arrows). There is a rise in total bladder pressure (P_{ves}) and detrusor pressure (P_{det}), but no change in abdominal pressure (P_{abd}).

There are several very important points regarding involuntary contractions:

1. The clinician must be absolutely sure that the contraction is indeed involuntary. Sometimes a patient may become confused during the study and actually void as soon as he feels the desire.
2. It is extremely important to determine whether or not a patient's symptoms are reproduced during the involuntary contraction. However, in cases of neurologic disease, IDCs can occur with symptoms and should not be discounted.
3. The volume at which contractions occur and the pressure of the contractions should be recorded.
4. It is often worthwhile to repeat the CMG at a slower filling rate if the patient experiences uncharacteristic symptoms (e.g. incontinence or spasms) or detrusor activity.
5. If the patient experiences incontinence during an involuntary contraction (urge incontinence), this should be noted. Sometimes the involuntary contraction will bring on involuntary voiding to completion (precipitant micturition).[8]

Compliance is defined as the change of volume for a change in detrusor pressure and is calculated by dividing the volume change (ΔV) by the change in detrusor pressure (ΔP_{det}) during that change in bladder volume. It is expressed in milliliters per centimeter H_2O (ml/cmH_2O). The spherical shape of the bladder as well as the viscoelastic properties of its components contribute to its excellent compliance, allowing storage of progressive volumes of urine at low pressure. When the pressure begins to rise with increasing volumes, compliance is decreased or 'impaired'. Impaired compliance is not uncommon in neurogenic voiding dysfunction and is potentially hazardous. The degree of impaired compliance in neurogenic voiding dysfunction is often dependent on outlet resistance. However, poor compliance can also occur with chronically catheterized bladders. Impaired compliance leads to high bladder storage pressures. The calculated value of compliance is probably less important than the actual bladder pressure during filling. This is because the compliance value can change, depending on the volume over which it is calculated. This is probably why compliance, despite being a well-known and accepted parameter, is rarely reported in terms of a discrete or well-defined value in the urologic literature.

Normal compliance has been difficult to establish. Toppercer and Tetreault evaluated a group of normal asymptomatic women and women with stress incontinence and found mean compliance to be 55.71 ± 27.37.[9] If two standard deviations are used, normal would be between 1 and 110 ml/cmH_2O. When compliance is calculated as a single point on the pressure–volume curve it becomes a 'static' property. Gilmour et al point out that this oversimplifies the concept of compliance and may lead to potentially erroneous conclusions.[10] For example, an abrupt and potentially dangerous rise in pressure may occur as compliance rapidly decreases.

However, the value for compliance will be very different, depending on whether it is calculated over the entire filling volume or over the volume in which the change in pressure actually occurred. McGuire and associates have shown that sustained pressures of 40 cmH_2O or greater during storage can lead to upper tract damage.[11] Storage pressures in this

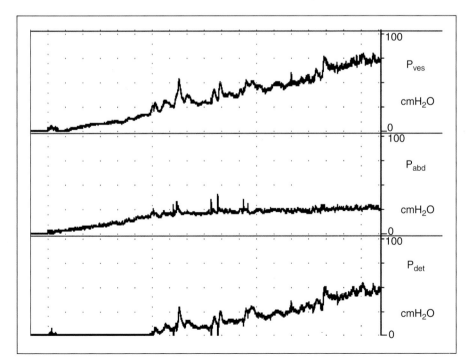

Figure 38.4

Impaired compliance in a 35-year-old male with a T8 spinal cord injury. Note that there is an initial rise in both total vesical pressure (P_{ves}) and abdominal pressure (P_{abd}), but the P_{ves} and, thus, the detrusor pressure (P_{det}) continue to rise to pressures exceeding 40 cmH_2O.

range are dangerous, regardless of the volume in the bladder or calculated compliance value (Figure 38.4). In poorly compliant bladders in children, Churchill and associates have suggested determining compliance between initial filling and the point at which detrusor pressure exceeds 35 cmH$_2$O.[10] More recently, these investigators have applied the concept of dynamic compliance and argue that the amount of time spent with bladder compliance less than 10 ml/cmH$_2$O (an empirically derived value) will strongly influence upper tract deterioration.[12]

We would certainly agree that prolonged high-pressure storage is an ominous urodynamic finding, independent of any discrete value of compliance. One must remember that compliance may be dependent on filling rate during a urodynamic study; overly rapid filling rates may produce erroneously lower compliance values. Lastly, neurogenic detrusor overactivity can mimic impaired compliance. Two methods of differentiating these two entities are (1) stopping the infusion rate and, if necessary, (2) having the patient perform a sustained Kegel maneuver to suppress possible involuntary contractions. Involuntary detrusor contractions can also occur in the face of impaired compliance (Figure 38.5).

Storage parameters – leak point pressures

During the filling portion of the cystometrogram, urinary storage can also be assessed. Assessment of storage is important because patients with neurogenic bladders often have issues pertaining to urinary incontinence and/or storage pressures. Urinary leakage can be secondary to a bladder dysfunction (neurogenic detrusor overactivity or impaired compliance) and/or a sphincteric dysfunction (e.g. intrinsic sphincter deficiency). The bladder, or detrusor,

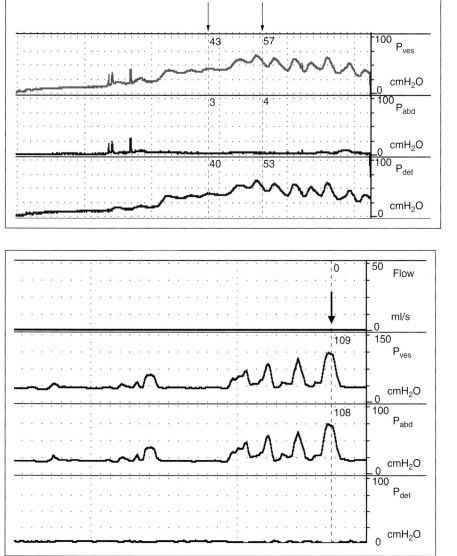

Figure 38.5
Involuntary detrusor contractions occurring in the face of impaired compliance in a teenage girl with myelomeningocele. The left arrow indicates where detrusor pressure equals and then exceeds 40 cmH$_2$O. The right arrow indicates where leakage occurs – at a bladder leak point pressure of 53 cmH$_2$O. P$_{ves}$, total vesical pressure; P$_{det}$, detrusor pressure; P$_{abd}$, abdominal pressure.

Figure 38.6
Urodynamic tracing of a female patient with stress incontinence. Tracing shows progressive Valsalva maneuvers until leakage occurs (arrow) at an abdominal pressure of 109 cmH$_2$O, which is the abdominal leak point pressure (ALPP). Note that there is no rise in detrusor pressure. P$_{ves}$, total vesical pressure; P$_{det}$, detrusor pressure; P$_{abd}$, abdominal pressure.

leak point pressure (DLPP) test measures the detrusor pressure required to cause urinary incontinence in the absence of increased abdominal pressure. The DLPP is a direct reflection of the amount of resistance provided by the external sphincter. The higher the bladder outlet resistance (e.g. as in detrusor-sphincter dyssynergia), the higher the DLPP. High storage pressures and high DLPP are potentially dangerous to upper urinary tracts (Figure 38.5). Knowledge of the DLPP is useful because it allows the clinician to determine the volume at which detrusor pressure reaches dangerous levels.

Urinary leakage secondary to sphincteric dysfunction can be measured by the abdominal or Valsalva leak point pressure (ALPP).[13] The ALPP is an indirect measure of the ability of the urethra to resist changes in abdominal pressure as an expulsive force.[14] Clinically, it is used to determine the

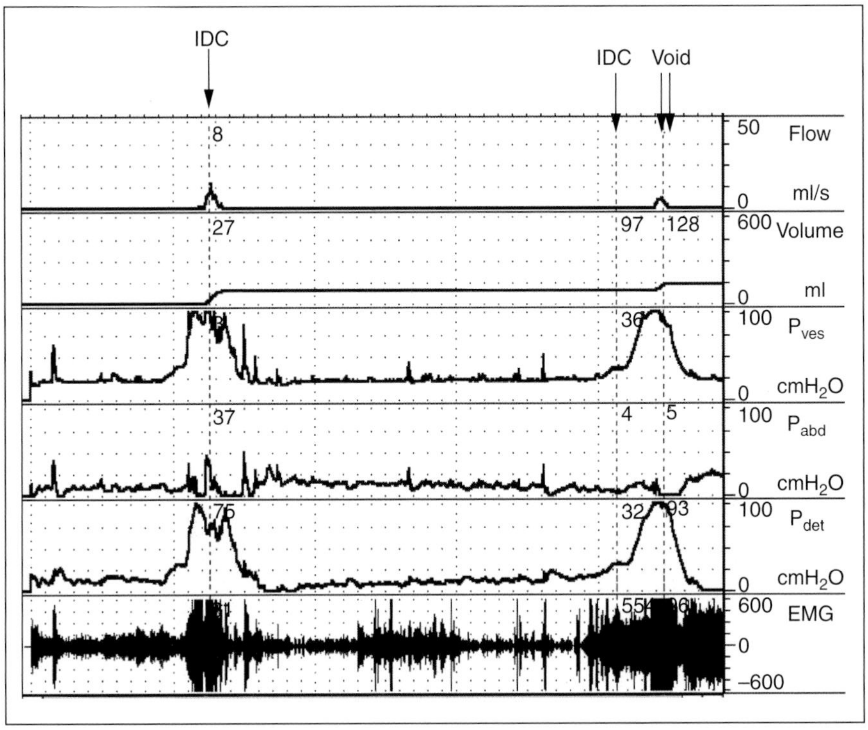

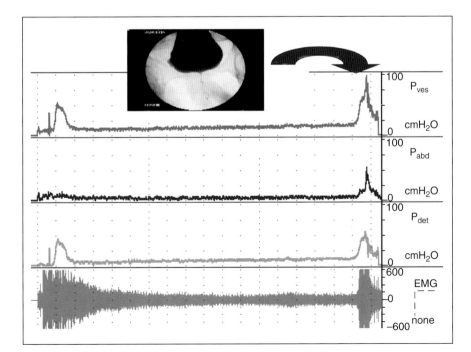

Figure 38.7
Urodynamic tracing of an 18-year-old woman with frequency, urgency, and urge incontinence who was diagnosed with a tethered cord. Note the involuntary detrusor contraction (IDC, arrow) associated with high-volume urine loss as registered in the flow meter. There is increased sphincter activity, as demonstrated by increased electromyograph (EMG) activity consistent with detrusor-external sphincter dyssynergia (DESD). On the second fill there is again an IDC, but this time the patient is instructed to void (double void). Note that there is increased EMG activity throughout the IC and 'voluntary void'. Detrusor pressures with IDCs are quite high because of the resistance of the contracting striated sphincter. P_{ves}, total vesical pressure; P_{det}, detrusor pressure; P_{abd}, abdominal pressure.

Figure 38.8
Detrusor-external sphincter dyssynergia (DESD) and detrusor-internal sphincter dyssynergia in a 35-year-old male with a high cervical spinal cord injury. There are two IDCs with associated increased electromyograph (EMG) activity consistent with DESD. However, the fluoroscopic picture taken at the time of the second IDC shows an incompletely opened bladder neck consistent with detrusor-internal sphincter dyssynergia. This patient underwent a striated sphincterotomy as well as a bladder neck incision to facilitate emptying and lower pressures. P_{ves}, total vesical pressure; P_{det}, detrusor pressure; P_{abd}, abdominal pressure.

presence of stress urinary incontinence and the degree of sphincter incompetence (Figure 38.6). Normally, there is no physiologic abdominal pressure that should cause incontinence, and therefore there is no 'normal ALPP'. Unlike the DLPP, an elevated ALPP does not indicate potential danger to the kidneys.

Voiding phase

As important as filling and storage is the voiding or emptying phase, known as micturition. Prior to urodynamic

assessment, one must determine how the patient voids. If voiding is voluntary, the strength and duration of the detrusor contraction is assessed. Detrusor contractility may be impaired in particular types of neurologic disease, particularly with lower motor neuron or denervating lesions. This can cause impaired contractility or areflexia.

Aside from detrusor contraction, outlet resistance can be measured while voiding. Although the most common cause of outlet resistance in neurogenic voiding dysfunction is DESD, bladder outlet obstruction can occur anywhere distal to the bladder. Several nomograms and formulas exist to categorize pressure–flow relationships in terms of non-obstructed, obstructed, or equivocal.[15–19] It is important to

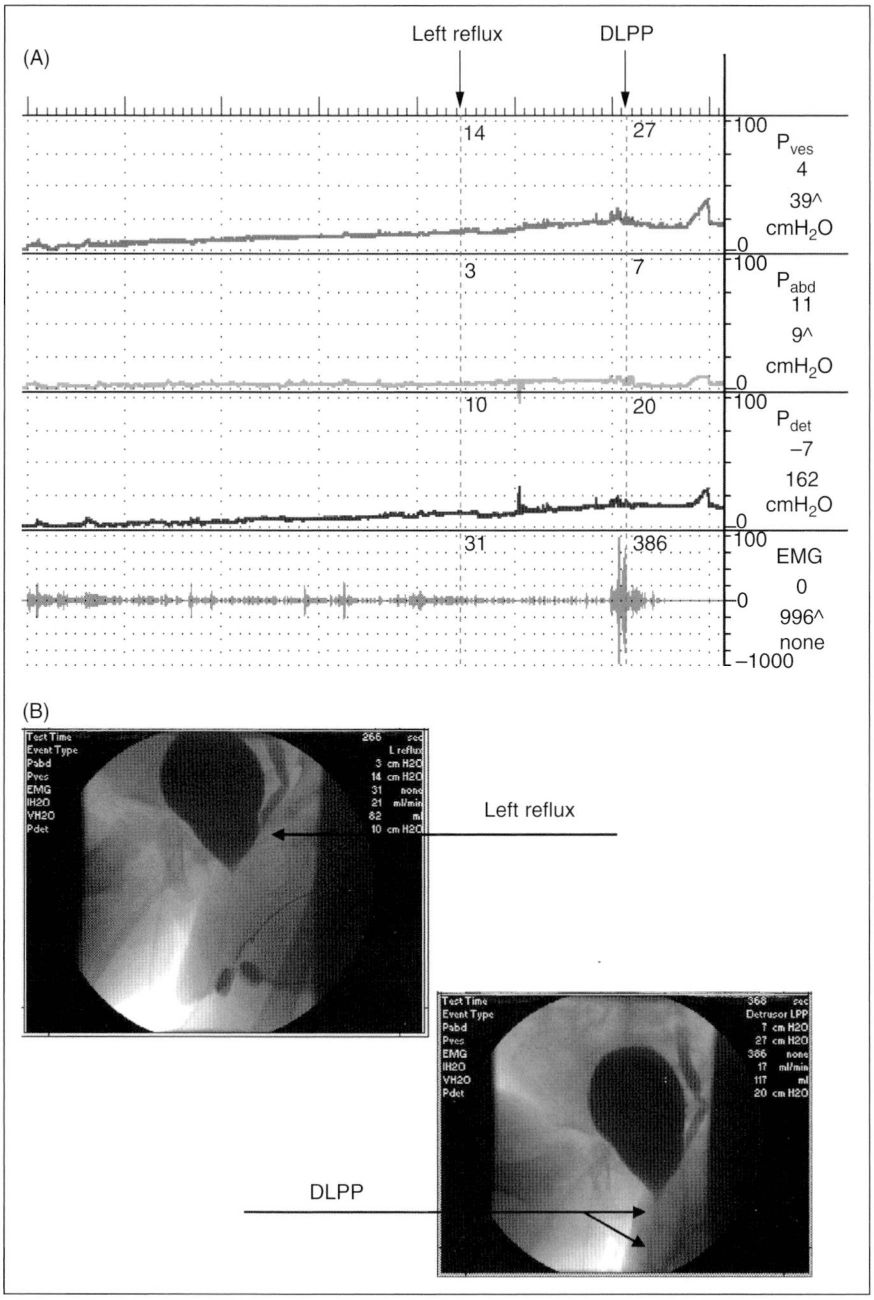

Figure 38.9
Videourodynamic study in a 3-year-old boy with myelomeningocele who is on anticholinergic medication but remains wet between catheterizations. There is mild left hydronephrosis on renal ultrasound. P_{ves}, total vesical pressure; P_{det}, detrusor pressure; P_{abd}, abdominal pressure. EMG, electromyography.
(A) This study shows that leakage occurs as a result of impaired compliance: bladder leak point pressure (DLPP) = 20 cmH$_2$O.
(B) Video portion shows left vesicoureteral reflux occurring at a relative low detrusor pressure of 10 cmH$_2$O (upper left arrow), and confirms the DLPP of 20 cmH$_2$O (lower right arrow).

note that interpretation of bladder outlet obstruction during urodynamics should be performed at the point at which the patient was told to void. If the patient has an involuntary bladder contraction and empties the bladder prematurely, this pressure–flow relationship should not be misinterpreted as being equivalent to normal physiologic voiding.

Electromyography during urodynamics permits the urologist to evaluate the striated sphincter function during micturition. Often, surface patch electrodes are used, but needle electrodes permit more accurate placement and more accurate recording. Normally, voluntary voiding is preceded by a complete relaxation of the striated sphincter. Detrusor-external sphincter dyssynergia refers to obstruction to the outflow of urine during bladder contraction caused by involuntary contraction of the striated sphincter during an IDC.[20,21] It is secondary to a neurologic lesion and is not associated with a learned voiding dysfunction such as dysfunctional voiding. DESD results in a functional obstruction that usually affects emptying, and ultimately leads to high storage pressures secondary to impaired compliance and incomplete emptying. True DESD is seen in patients with suprasacral spinal lesions (Figure 38.7). Depending on the level of the lesion, patients also may develop detrusor-internal sphincter dyssynergia. In such cases the bladder fails to open appropriately with a bladder contraction due to autonomic dysfunction. It typically occurs in lesions above T10. Detrusor-internal sphincter dyssynergia is best diagnosed by videourodynamics (Figure 38.8).

Videourodynamics

Videourodynamics, or simultaneous fluoroscopic monitoring of the urinary tract during urodynamics, is the most comprehensive and accurate way of assessing neurogenic lower urinary tract dysfunction (Figures 38.8 and 38.9).[22] During the evaluation of filling and storage, videourodynamics allows for the determination of vesicoureteral reflux and the pressure at which this occurs. Moreover, assessment of the DLPP or ALPP is facilitated as fluoroscopy is often more sensitive than direct observation in determining urinary leakage. Videourodynamics also permits the radiographic evaluation of the bladder neck during filling and anatomic abnormalities such as bladder and urethral diverticula and fistula. During the voiding phase, fluoroscopy permits an accurate determination of the site of obstruction when high-pressure/low-flow states exist. Videourodynamics also provides an excellent way of evaluating sphincter behavior during voiding, especially in cases where EMG tracing is imperfect or equivocal. Videourodynamics is the definitive test to determine the presence of detrusor-internal sphincter dyssynergia by the lack of opening of the bladder neck on fluoroscopy during a detrusor contraction. Using fluoroscopy

with EMG can help make the diagnosis of detrusor-internal and detrusor-external sphincter dyssynergia.[23]

Conclusion

In patients with known neurologic disease, careful urodynamic evaluation may be necessary to gauge any deleterious effect on the urinary tract, to determine the etiology of LUT symptoms, and to screen for any urologic risk factors. Often times, urodynamics are necessary for the asymptomatic patient because the effects of the disease on the urinary tract can be 'silent'. Patients without a history of neurologic disease whose urologic evaluation is suspicious for neurogenic LUT dysfunction should be evaluated for occult neurologic disease.

References

1. Wein AJ. Classification of neurogenic voiding dysfunction. J Urol 1981; 125:605.

2. Nitti VW. Evaluation of the female with neurogenic voiding dysfunction. Int Urogynecol J 1999; 10:119–129.

3. Bunts RC. Management of urological complications in 100 paraplegics. J Urol 1958; 79:733–736.

4. Bejany BE, Lockhart JL, Rhamy RK. Malignant vesical tumors following spinal cord injury. J Urol 1987; 138:1390–1392.

5. Bickel A, Culkin J, Wheeler J. Bladder cancer in spinal cord injury patients. J Urol 1991; 146:1240–1241.

6. Broecker BH, Klein FA, Hackler RH. Cancer of the bladder in spinal cord injury patients. J Urol 1981; 125:196–197.

7. Abrams P, Cardozo L, Fall M, et al. The standardization of terminology of lower urinary tract function. Neurourol Urodynam 2002; 21:167–178.

8. Nitti VW. Cystometry and abdominal pressure monitoring. In: Nitti VW, ed. Practical urodynamics. Philadelphia: WB Saunders, 1998:38–51.

9. Toppercer A, Tetreault JP. Compliance of the bladder: an attempt to establish normal values. Urology 1979; 14:204.

10. Gilmour RF, Churchill BM, Steckler RE, et al. A new technique for dynamic analysis of bladder compliance. J Urol 1993; 150:1200.

11. McGuire EM, Woodside JR, Borden TA. Prognostic value of urodynamic testing in meylodysplastic children. J Urol 1981; 126: 205.

12. Churchill BM, Gilmour PE, Williot P. Urodynamics. Ped Clin NA 1987; 34:1133.

13. McGuire EJ, Fitzpatrick CC, Wan J, et al. Clinical assessment of urethral sphincter function. J Urol 1993; 150:1452–1454.

14. McGuire EJ, Cespedes RD, O'Connell HE. Leak point pressures. Urol Clin N Am 1996; 23:253–262.

15. Abrams PH, Griffiths DJ. Assessment of prostate obstruction from urodynamic measurements and from residual urine. Br J Urol 1979; 51:129–134.

16. Schafer W. Principles and clinical application of advanced urodynamic analysis of voiding function. Urol Clin N Am 1990; 17:553–566.

17. Abrams P. Bladder outlet obstruction index, bladder contractility index and bladder voiding efficiency; three simple indices to define bladder voiding function. BJU Int 1999; 84:14–15.

18. Blaivas JG, Groutz A. Bladder outlet obstruction nomogram for women with lower urinary tract symptomatology. Neurourol Urodyn 2000; 19:553–564.

19. Lemack GE, Zimmern PE. Pressure flow analysis may aid in identifying women with outflow obstruction. J Urol 2000; 163(6):1823–1828.

20. Blaivas JG, Singa HP, Zayed AAH, Labib KB. Detrusor-external sphincter dyssynergia. J Urol 1981; 125:541–544.

21. Blaivas JG, Singa HP, Zayed AAH, Labib KB. Detrusor-external sphincter dyssynergia: a detailed EMG study. J Urol 1981; 125:545–548.

22. Blavais JG. Videourodynamic studies. In: Nitti VW, ed. Practical urodynamics. Philadelphia: WB Saunders, 1998:78–93.

23. Watanabe T, Chancellor MB, Rivas DA. Neurogenic voiding dysfunction. In: Nitti VW, ed. Practical urodynamics. Philadelphia: WB Saunders, 1998:142–155.

39

Urodynamics in infants and children

Kelm Hjälmås and Ulla Sillén

Introduction

Urodynamics in infants and children is basically the same procedure as in adults and shares the same techniques and objectives. There is, however, one fundamental difference: *the patient is a child*. Essentially, this means two things. First, a child harbors intuitive fear for any unknown procedure but is, at the same time, largely unresponsive to rational argumentation about the nature of and the need for the examination. Second, the child is a growing individual, increasing in weight 20-fold from infancy to puberty. This means that for children there exists no single set of 'normal' urodynamic variables but rather a continuum of each variable, depending on and correlating to the age and the body size of the individual.

This chapter will concentrate on those two aspects: first, on how to prepare, inform, reassure, encourage, and comfort the child before and during the urodynamic examination; second, how to report the expected range of 'normal' values for urodynamic variables from infancy to adolescence.

Historical notes on urodynamics in infants and children

It is hard to understand why bladder function in children did not receive any attention from medical scientists until the mid-20th century. Before that time, it seems to have been understood, without a trace of critical thinking, that almost all children had bladders that worked perfectly well, regarding both storage and evacuation of urine. If a functional disturbance such as incontinence was indeed noted, traditional wisdom suggested that it was due to psychological problems within the child and/or the family. In contrast, we are now aware that non-neurogenic bladder-sphincter dysfunction in children is caused by delayed maturation (most often genetically determined)

of the central nervous system (CNS) bladder control. Psychological problems in an incontinent child are a consequence of the bladder dysfunction, not the other way round, with few exceptions.

From 1959 onwards, the first urodynamic studies on normal and pathological bladder function in infants and children came into print.[1–9] A rapidly increasing number of studies followed, once it became clear that at age 7 years as many as 10% of children have non-neurogenic disturbance of bladder/sphincter function. Knowledge surfaced that bladder dysfunction plays a major role not only for urinary incontinence but also, even more importantly, for the creation and persistence of vesicoureteral reflux (VUR) and urinary tract infection (UTI), with the accompanying risk for deterioration of renal function.[10] Children with *neurogenic* bladder dysfunction (NBD) due to myelodysplasia and other disorders of the CNS were exposed to the same risk to an even larger degree. Surprisingly, however, this fact did not become obvious until the late 1960s, when it was finally understood that the devastating UTIs and the frequent progress of bacterial resistance during antibiotic therapy in myelomeningocele children was caused by inadequate bladder emptying, leaving post-void residual behind. Regular and low-pressure bladder evacuation with the aid of clean intermittent catheterization (CIC), introduced by Jack Lapides in 1972, led to a dramatic reduction in the rate and severity of UTIs in this patient group and even resulted in disappearance of reflux in many patients.[11]

Development of bladder function

The normal development of lower urinary tract function from infancy to adolescence has to be reviewed before describing the urodynamic procedures and techniques used in children and what results to expect. This is necessary in order to understand the dynamic nature of the urodynamic variables in the growing individual.

Bladder function during infancy has previously been regarded as automatic, with voiding induced by a constant volume in the bladder[12] and without cerebral influence. During the last decade it has been shown convincingly that the brain is already involved in the voiding reflex from birth. This is best illustrated by the finding that in the majority of cases newborn babies wake up or show signs of arousal before voiding.[13,14] This means that the reflex pathway connection to the cerebral cortex is anatomically already developed in this age group; however, voiding is neither conscious nor voluntary – the infant is only disturbed by the signal. Both maturation and probably training are needed for the voidings to be conscious and voluntary.

Neonates and infants void at varying bladder volumes during infancy and this is contrary to the belief that the voiding reflex is a simple spinal reflex elicited by a constant bladder volume. This has been shown in free voiding studies of both pre-term[15] and full-term infants[13] in whom bladder volume initiating voiding varies from 30% to 100% of functional bladder capacity. The reason for this variation is unknown, but the bladder volume initiating micturition is higher after a period of sleep.

The infant's voiding is also characterized by a physiological form of detrusor-sphincter dyscoordination, which has been shown in free voiding studies as interrupted voidings and increase in post-void residual urine (Figure 39.1).[16] This phenomenon has also been observed in urodynamic studies as an intermittent increase in the electromyographic (EMG) activity of the pelvic floor during voiding, concomitant with fluctuations in voiding detrusor pressure (Figure 39.2).[14,17] A longitudinal study of free voidings from birth to age 3 years revealed that the suggested dyscoordination disappears successively, and is not seen after potty-training age.[13] Another important observation in the study by Jansson et al[13] is the increase in post-void residual urine during the first couple of years of life. The reason for the incomplete emptying in infancy is probably the physiological form of dyscoordination discussed above, with interruption of the urine stream before the bladder is empty. However, with the acquisition of continence the residual volume decreased in this group of healthy children and the ability to empty the bladder was complete at the age of 3.

In the longitudinal study of free voidings by Jansson et al[13] it was also observed that bladder capacity was almost unchanged during the first two years of life but showed a steep increase at the time the child gets dry (see Figure 39.6). A similar accelerated increase in bladder capacity which is age related has also been noted in other studies.[12,18] This increased bladder capacity has been considered as a prerequisite for both day- and nighttime continence. Conversely, continence during night has been considered to be obtained only after achievement of day dryness.[19,20] The reason for this increase in bladder capacity has previously only been discussed in terms of general maturation.

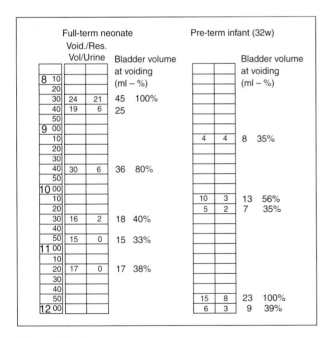

Figure 39.1
Four-hour voiding observation in a full-term neonate and a pre-term infant (gestation age 32 weeks) showing varying bladder volumes initiating voiding (the sum of voided volume and residual urine). The volumes vary between 33% and 100% of the highest volume in the bladder (= the bladder capacity) during the observation. Note the interrupted voiding seen once in the full-term and twice in the pre-term infant.

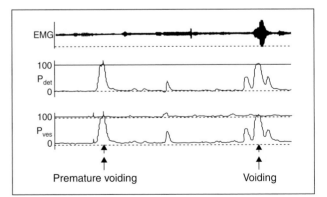

Figure 39.2
Cystometric recording in a non-refluxing newborn sibling of a child with vesicoureteral reflux (VUR). Note the premature voiding contraction after infusion of 5 ml with leakage of urine. Voiding after a total filling of 30 ml of saline shows an increase of electromyographic (EMG) activity of the pelvic floor and concomitant fluctuation in detrusor voiding pressure.

Acquisition of bladder control

Development of bladder control was earlier supposed to begin at 1 year of age and often to be fully developed by age 4.5 years. It was described by Muellner as 'a maturation which could not be influenced by training'. Another factor which was considered important was the doubling of bladder capacity between 2 and 4.5 years of age.[12,21] These statements about maturation, combined with the improvement in the quality of disposable napkins, have contributed to a more liberal view about what age potty-training should be started. In fact, during the last decades, potty-training has been regarded as unnecessary due to the belief that physical maturation should dictate when a child becomes dry. It is quite clear from other areas, however, that training can accelerate maturation.

Potty-training was instituted early before the era of disposable napkins. Some authors have reported bladder control much earlier than nowadays,[19,20] whereas others have not been able to show such a connection.[22]

If bladder control only means to void on the potty when the child is put there by the parent regularly or when the child indicates a need to void, it can be obtained early. The degree of maturation needed for such basic training is probably already present during the first year of life.[23] The goal of potty-training, to obtain full social bladder control, cannot be achieved solely with the early potty-training dicussed above. The prerequisites for success are influenced both by physical maturation and the child's interest in this task as well as by support from adults, routines, and parental expectations. Most children may stay dry in their usual milieu around the age of 2. However, the child has to reach at least 3.5–4 years of age to become mature enough to be able to cope with every aspect of their own toileting (including taking off and on clothes, flushing the toilet, closing the door, etc.).

The markedly improved emptying after potty-training, discussed above, is very interesting, since it is something that can be used in the treatment of incomplete emptying in this age group, through institution of potty-training earlier than what is common.

Indications for urodynamics in children

The indications for urodynamics in infants and children are the same as for adults: namely, suspicion of neurogenic or non-neurogenic bladder dysfunction or structural outflow obstruction. Thus, they include neurogenic bladder, gross vesicoureteral reflux (particularly in infants), recurrent UTIs, uroflow/residual measurement suggesting infravesical obstruction, and urinary incontinence (including nocturnal enuresis) that has been refractory to conventional treatment (urotherapy and drugs) for at least 1 year.

Neurogenic bladder dysfunction, whether suspected or established, is the most important of these indications. It should be said up front that cystometry in a patient with neurogenic bladder has to be repeated regularly during the patient's lifetime. In a child, cystometry should be performed at least once yearly because neurogenic bladder in the child is a dynamic disorder that is prone to change and then most often deterioration. The common cause is tethering of the spinal cord, which occurs in 75% of myelomeningoceles and in 100% of lipomyelomeningoceles.[24]

Age-related aspects

The investigation must be adapted to the child's needs!

In urology textbooks in the past, it could be read that 'cystometry cannot be performed in children younger than 7 years of age'. In one circumstance this statement was true: namely, when a young child was referred to a urodynamic laboratory that was used to examine adult patients only. Non-prepared children who hesitated to enter the laboratory and thereby upset the time schedule were looked upon as disturbing and irrational patients – which children certainly are if not treated according to their own needs! Children *are* irrational, sensitive, and skeptical towards all kinds of medical technology. Thus their need for information, patience, and loving care cannot be emphasized too much. The stress felt by a tense child during a urodynamic examination may very well generate results suggesting bladder dysfunction (overactive bladder and/or sphincter) even if that same child in a safe and relaxed mood would have shown completely normal urodynamic findings.

Ideally, the child should be prepared for what will be coming by being shown around the laboratory the day before the examination and given a summary in everyday language of what is going to happen (Figure 39.3). Several of these children have already undergone voiding cystography and may have unpleasant memories of the catheterization, so this topic has to be touched upon with great care.

During the examination, the child is handled in a relaxed and patient way. Even young children should be handled with respect for their personal integrity. As much as possible, the procedure should be performed 'as in play'. A video with popular cartoons has been a great asset in our laboratory and has helped children to overlook frightening equipment in the room (Figure 39.4). However, nothing can substitute for an experienced nurse or laboratory assistant who loves to take care of children.[25,26]

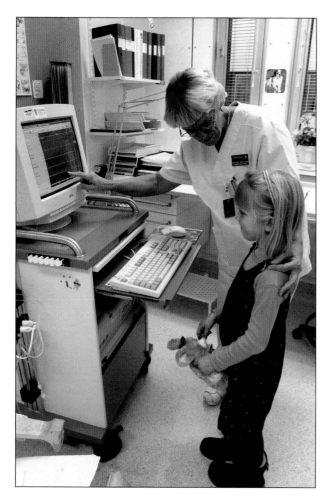

Figure 39.3
Child familiarizing herself with the urodynamic laboratory while receiving information from the laboratory assistant the day before the actual investigation.

Sedation

Exceptionally, when a child expresses outspoken anxiety for the procedure, in particular the catheterization, sedation with midazolam may be an option.[27] We have no experience with using midazolam (Dormicum®, Roche) in urodynamic studies but have used the drug for several years when performing voiding cystourethrography (VCUG).[28] In these studies the drug does not seem to affect bladder/sphincter function in any way, but placebo-controlled, randomized studies have not yet been performed. The sedation is satisfactory and side-effects very rare. The drug company only offers Dormicum for intravenous use. However, in our practise, we use the intravenous preparation for oral or rectal administration and have noticed the same sedative efficacy without added side-effects. For *oral administration*, Dormicum 5 mg/ml is used in the dosage 0.3–0.5 mg per kg body weight, max. 7.5 mg, mixed in a small amount of juice or cola. Effective sedation occurs within 15–30 min and the

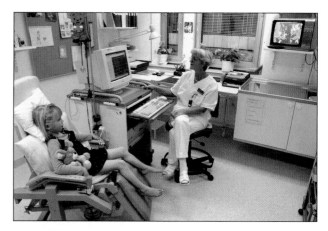

Figure 39.4
Cystometry is not necessarily a distressful experience, especially when an interesting video is running.

duration of sedation is 30–50 min. Dormicum 1 mg/ml is used for *rectal administration* in the dosage 0.2–0.3 mg per kg body weight, max. 5 mg. Effective sedation occurs within 10–20 min and duration of sedation is 30–50 min. Observe that pulse oximeter, suction apparatus, and equipment for ventilation should be at hand. If the child falls asleep, secure free airways. The child should be supervised for at least 1 h 30 min before leaving for home.[28] Midazolam for sedation of a child going through a urodynamic investigation may be a good option in the future once placebo-controlled, randomized studies have been performed.

Age

Infants below 1 year of age pose very few problems during urodynamic investigation. They are simply too young to be afraid of the procedure. The most problematic age group are children aged 2–4 years who are old enough to feel scared but too young to understand the reasons for the examination.

Children with neurogenic bladder generally accept the urodynamic investigation without much problems. It is easier for these children to accept and for the staff to perform the procedure than is the case for children with intact lower urinary tract sensation.

Urodynamic methodology
Noninvasive urodynamics
Uroflow

Measurement of the urinary flow rate, including assessment of the shape of the flow curve, is a very useful investigative tool in children with non-neurogenic bladder/sphincter dysfunction but has a very limited value in neurogenic bladder patients. The simple reason is that a child with neurogenic bladder is only exceptionally able to perform a formal micturition.

Post-void residual urine (assessed with ultrasound)

This procedure is mandatory and should be repeated frequently in all children with neurogenic bladder. In infants and small children, who are not treated with CIC, the 4-hour voiding observation is used to investigate emptying ability.[16] The child uses a napkin during the test and voidings are indicated by a gossip strip or a light signal. Voided volume is measured by weighing the napkin after each voiding and post-void residual urine is checked by ultrasonography. Since post-void residual urine varies also in healthy babies with complete emptying only occasionally, the investigation has to include a 4-hour period and not only isolated voidings.

Post-void residual urine should also be checked in patients on CIC to make sure that the catheterization is performed in a correct and efficient way. Some children tend to withdraw the catheter too early. Others may get a dislocation of the bladder when growing up, necessitating a change of body position during CIC in order to achieve complete emptying.

Pad test

To estimate and follow urinary leakage between voidings or catheterizations during daily activity, the pad test is the most appropriate investigation, including hourly change of pads that are weighed to get the leakage volume. The leakage volume and frequency are important parameters to follow at least once a year, since changes can indicate tethering. It is also important as an indicator of the efficacy of treatment with anticholinergic medication.

Pelvic electromyography using cutaneous electrodes

Pelvic EMG for registration of pelvic floor activity during cystometry will sometimes detect neuromuscular activity even in patients with neurogenic bladder, but it will be difficult or impossible to find out from which portion of the pelvic floor muscles the signals emanate. Therefore, in many instances, the EMG will not deliver any clinically useful information. Nevertheless, cutaneous EMG should be performed as routine in order to keep up the competence of the urodynamic laboratory.

Invasive urodynamics: traditional cystometry

Invasive urodynamics is synonymous with cystometry (with the possible addition of EMG using needle electrodes).

Frequently asked questions (FAQs) regarding cystometric techniques

At which points of time should infants and children with neurogenic bladder dysfunction be examined with cystometry? The literature provides strong evidence that CIC in congenital NBD should be started as soon as possible in infancy,[29,30] because there is an obvious risk of deterioration of bladder function already in infancy as well as later in childhood.[31,32] Frequent and regular follow-up of bladder function (cystometry at least once a year) is mandatory, in particular during the first 6 years of life.[33]

Gas or fluid filling of the bladder? Gas should not be used.

Fluid-filled or transducer tip catheters for pressure measurement? For obvious reasons, transducer tip catheters must be used for natural fill (ambulatory) cystometry. When traditional cystometry is performed in the laboratory, however, they are too fragile, too expensive, and too difficult to calibrate for regular use. A fluid-filled pressure measurement system should be the standard here.

Transurethral or suprapubic catheters? Double-lumen transurethral catheters are ideal for infants and children with neurogenic bladder. Most of these patients have limited or absent urethral sensation. Moreover, the possible obstruction caused by the transurethral catheter is of minor importance in this patient group, since it is hardly ever possible to perform a formal pressure–flow measurement.

What filling rate should be used? The rate at which fluid is instilled in the bladder influences bladder wall dynamics, thus capacity, intravesical pressure, and compliance.[34] High filling rates create an artificial situation, with continuous pressure rise. Therefore, filling rates have to be standardized and not allowed to exceed physiological filling rates during maximal diuresis. The recommended rate is 1/20 (5%) of the patient's expected bladder capacity per minute, since in a healthy individual the bladder will be filled to capacity in 20 min during maximal diuresis. The patient's expected bladder capacity can be assessed from a diary in which the parents note the CIC volumes for a couple of days. The largest volume should be chosen (excluding the first morning voiding). Alternatively (particularly in severe incontinence with small CIC volumes), the expected bladder capacity in children 3 years of age and above can be calculated from the simple rule-of-thumb equation:

$$\text{Expected bladder capacity (ml)} = 30 + (\text{age in years} \times 30)$$

An alternative rule of thumb is that 1% of the body weight approximately predicts a child's bladder capacity. A 3-year-old would be expected to have a bladder capacity around 120 ml, so a filling rate of 6 ml/min should be used.

How many filling cycles are needed? In non-neurogenic cases, two. Even if the child seems to be at ease during the examination, the first filling is experienced by the child as more stressful than the following ones. Detrusor and/or sphincter overactivity is therefore more commonly seen during the first filling. The second filling will already reflect the urodynamic status of the bladder in a reliable way. Additional fillings don't need to be done because they produce similar findings to the second one.[9] However, in children with neurogenic bladder a single filling may be sufficient because lower urinary tract sensation is impaired and psychological mechanisms hardly influence bladder/sphincter function.

When to stop filling in a patient unable to feel a desire to void? This is the common situation in patients with NBD. The infusion should be finished when any of the following occurs:

1. strong urgency
2. micturition
3. feeling of discomfort
4. high basic detrusor pressure (>40 cmH$_2$O)
5. large infused volume ($>150\%$ of the expected bladder capacity unless the CIC diary has shown larger volumes at CIC)
6. rate of urinary leakage $\geq$ rate of infusion.

When is the bladder cooling test (formerly Bors ice water test) indicated in the urodynamic investigation of infants and children with established or suspected NBD? In every case, as a general rule. It has been shown that neurologically normal infants and children exhibit a positive bladder cooling test (BCT) during the first 4 years of life, whereas the test is negative in children older than 6 years.[35] In infants and children with NBD, a negative BCT before age 4 demonstrates a lesion of the sacral reflex arch, whereas a positive BCT in children older than 6 years indicates a lesion of inhibiting suprasacral spinal pathways.[36] The BCT is performed after finishing the traditional cystometry. The reactivity of the detrusor is first checked with body-warm saline infused rapidly in an amount corresponding to one-third of the cystometric bladder capacity. If this infusion does not elicit any

significant detrusor contraction, the bladder is emptied and the same amount (one-third of bladder capacity) of cold (around 4°C) saline is infused rapidly. A positive test is defined as a detrusor contraction within 1 min with detrusor pressure ≥ 30 cmH$_2$O.

How to measure leak point pressure – and what is its value? The ideal way of measuring leak point pressure (LPP) is to note the detrusor pressure at the moment when leakage of urine is observed, during cystometry. This means that the laboratory assistant would have to monitor the patient's genital area continuously, which is seldom possible. Instead, the flowmeter is often used to indicate leakage; but it is then important to make adjustments for the time delay between pressure registration and the flowmeter deflection, in particular when leakage occurs in connection with a phasic detrusor contraction. It is assumed that LPP >40 cmH$_2$O in children with NBD suggests an increased risk for development of renal damage. This assumption makes sense, because maintained *intravesical* pressure above 30–40 cmH$_2$O is certainly associated with an increased incidence of VUR and upper tract dilatation.[37] Thus, an assessment of LPP should be routinely included in the urodynamic evaluation of a child with NBD.

What is the role of electromyography in the urodynamic evaluation of children with neurogenic bladder dysfunction? 'Quantitative' EMG using perineal surface electrodes (Ag/AgCl) will not always produce clinically valuable information in this patient group. It can be argued, however, that the EMG activity should be registered routinely in order to maintain competence in the urodynamic laboratory.

How should intra-abdominal pressure be measured? Ideally, with a transducer tip catheter inserted into the left fossa of the abdominal cavity, a method which does not cause any complications even during extended use for natural fill cystometry.[38] The second-best choice is to measure *prevesical* pressure in a minute pool of saline in the cavum Retzii between the bladder and the abdominal wall.[39] The common method, though, is to measure *intrarectal* pressure, hoping that it will represent intra-abdominal pressure. It does not, of course; at best, it gives a general idea about the extravesical pressure environment in which the bladder is working. However, the intrarectal pressure is easily accessible with a catheter passed through the anus. This fact – together with a solid chunk of urodynamic tradition – and, additionally, the invasive nature of the two first-mentioned options, helps to propagate intrarectal pressure as the standard for assessing perivesical pressure. The rectal catheter should be open-ended and continuously and slowly (3 ml/h) perfused with saline to prevent blocking by feces. It is important to check pressure transmission by asking the patient to strain or cough or by applying pressure on the suprapubic area. Be aware that the rectal catheter will sometimes transmit pressure peaks generated by spontaneous rectal contractions, something that may result in false-negative detrusor pressure readings. Thus, detrusor pressure calculated as intravesical minus intrarectal pressure is not always a reliable urodynamic variable.

Invasive urodynamics: videocystometry

Performing cystometry and fluoroscopic monitoring of the bladder and urethra at the same time no doubt increases the diagnostic accuracy of the urodynamic procedure, e.g. by allowing determination of bladder pressure at the moment when VUR occurs. The combined examination is also of value in patients with high-grade VUR where a common problem is to decide how much of the infused volume corresponds to bladder capacity and how much is stored in the refluxing systems. It can thus be said that some clinical questions will not be possible to answer without concurrent use of cystometry and X-ray. Therefore, videocystometry has become a standard urodynamic procedure for children with NBD (and other diagnoses) in many centers. However, videocystometry has its disadvantages. The most important of these is that videocystometry makes the examination even more complex by introducing additional machinery face to face to the (possibly) bewildered child. Even well-prepared and cooperative children may have difficulties in adapting to a highly sophisticated procedure. Since the child patient needs significant modification of the cystometric techniques compared to the adult, it can be questioned whether increasing the level of investigative sophistication is the right way to go. In our institution we have, so far, limited the use of videocystometry to clinical research (e.g. congenital reflux, posterior urethral valves) and to the occasional child with difficult-to-understand bladder problems where the combination of cystometry and imaging has sometimes helped us to arrive at the correct diagnosis.

Invasive urodynamics: natural fill (ambulatory) cystometry

Natural fill cystometry differs from traditional laboratory cystometry by (1) allowing the patient to be mobile, i.e. not restricting him to the laboratory chair, and (2) using the patient's own diuresis as the filling medium of the bladder. In both adults and children significant differences have been found between values obtained by artificial and natural filling urodynamics, respectively. Especially, steeper pressure rise and larger voided volumes were observed during and after artificial filling, whereas voiding pressures were found to be higher after natural filling. The natural fill cystometry also seems to be more sensitive in detecting detrusor instability than the traditional, artificial filling method.[40] The lower incidence of detrusor instability and the greater voided volumes found on traditional cystometry probably reflect an inhibition of detrusor function because of the relatively fast artificial filling.

In neurogenic bladders in adults, important differences were noted between conventional and natural fill cystometry. High increases in pressure registered during artificial filling, interpreted as low compliance of the bladder wall, were not reproduced during natural fill cystometry but rather replaced by phasic detrusor activity. Natural filling disclosed a combination of greater residual urine volumes, greater resting pressures, and greater phasic activity in patients with upper tract dilatation.[41]

In infants and children, results obtained by conventional cystometry and natural fill cystometry have shown the same differences as in adults regarding both non-neurogenic and neurogenic bladder dysfunction. The two methods were compared in a group of 17 children (mean age 6.8 years) with various urological disorders.[42] As in adults, the natural fill study yielded lower voided volumes, a less steep pressure rise on filling, and higher detrusor pressures during micturition. Additionally, natural fill urodynamics revealed detrusor instability in more patients than did the conventional cystometry.

The studies cited recorded bladder and rectal pressure for time periods ranging between 4 and 6 hours. In a study from our institution[38] we took full advantage of the ambulatory, natural fill method by extending the recording time to a mean of 20 hours. It was thus possible to compare the bladder behavior between day and night, which yielded interesting results. Also, the small patients were truly ambulatory since they were carrying the recording device in a backpack. There was no disruption of the child's normal activities and the children seemed almost completely unaware that they were subjected to a sophisticated investigation of their bladder function. Sixteen boys aged 1.4–6 years (mean age 3.4) with endoscopically resected posterior urethral valves (at a mean age of 3.6 months) were studied. All the boys had detrusor instability in the daytime but the bladders became stable during sleeping hours. At natural fill cystometry, voiding detrusor pressure was higher and functional bladder capacity much lower during the day than at night. Dissimilarities noted between natural fill and conventional cystometry were the same as found in all other studies.

A couple of studies have compared natural fill with conventional cystometry in children with neurogenic bladder. In 2 of 11 children with myelodysplasia (mean age 10 years) more phasic detrusor activity and higher pressure amplitudes were found during 6 h of natural fill cystometry.[43] In another study of 20 children (age 6–11 years) with neurogenic bladder, natural fill cystometry (mean duration 12 hours) discovered detrusor overactivity in 45% of the children in contrast to traditional cystometry in the same children where half had been judged to have normal bladder function and the other half low-compliance bladders.[44]

In conclusion, natural fill cystometry in infants, children, and adults shows a lower pressure rise during filling, a higher incidence of detrusor overactivity, a higher detrusor pressure on micturition, and a lower voided volume than is found at conventional cystometry. It cannot be excluded that 'low compliance neurogenic bladder' might sometimes turn out to be an investigational artifact due to the unphysiological high rate of artificial bladder filling, since studies in both children and adults have shown the rapid rise of pressure during artificial filling being replaced by phasic detrusor overactivity.[41,44] Natural fill urodynamics does not use artificial filling, and it causes minimal psychological trauma, especially important for the pediatric patient, so it no doubt delivers the more authentic reflection of true bladder physiology. However, data on natural fill cystometry in children with neurogenic bladder are still sparse, and, before replacing traditional with natural fill urodynamics, additional studies are needed. In particular, it will be necessary to find out how decreased distensibility of the bladder wall is presenting itself in the natural fill studies. Increase of basal detrusor pressure above 20–30 cmH$_2$O is seldom seen during natural fill but has been interpreted as an important sign of poor compliance when seen in traditional cystometry and found to be associated with dilatation of the upper tracts and deterioration of renal function. Since the rapid rise of basal detrusor pressure may be looked upon as a significant finding, it is still too early to appoint natural fill urodynamics to be the future golden standard in the investigation of neurogenic bladders in children, even if the possibility remains that natural fill may lead to profound reassessment of the urodynamic neurogenic pathophysiology.

Evaluation of urodynamic results

What are we looking for?

As in adult urodynamics, *the four C's*:

- capacity (of the bladder reservoir)
- contractility (of the detrusor and sphincter)
- compliance (of the bladder wall)
- continence.

And, in addition:

- lower urinary tract sensation
- evacuation (as reflected by absence or presence of post-void residual).

Normal urodynamic variables in infants and children

In infants and children, it goes without saying that normal values differ widely from the adult ones; and that, in growing individuals, variables such as bladder capacity vary according to the age and size of the child.

Bladder capacity

Increase of bladder capacity is not linear to age or weight during the first years of life. There are two periods when the increase is accelerated. The first is during the first months of life. In free voiding studies of pre-term infants in gestation week 32, median bladder capacity was 12 ml[15] (Figure 39.5) and in similar studies of full-term babies 3 months of age median capacity was 52 ml[13] (Figure 39.6). The capacity is almost unchanged at 1 and 2 years of age (67 and 68 ml, respectively). At 3 years of age, on the other hand, the median capacity is 123 ml, meaning a doubling during the third year of life (see Figure 39.6).[13]

The first step in increase of bladder capacity is thus around birth and is a fourfold increase, which should be compared with the increase in body weight, which is only three-fold. The second step is at the age of toilet-training when gaining control over voidings. The main stimulant for this second increase in bladder capacity can be suggested to be due to the fact that the child starts to get dry at

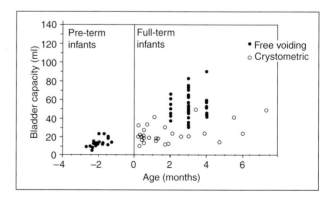

Figure 39.5
Age vs bladder capacity as measured in free voiding studies in both pre-term[15] and full-term[13] infants, and at cystometry in full-term infants.[17]

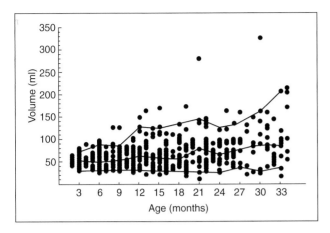

Figure 39.6
Bladder capacity vs age in a longitudinal study of free voidings in infants and children aged 0–3 years, investigated every 3rd month. The lines indicate the 5th, 50th, and 95th percentiles.[13]

night, which means higher overnight bladder volumes. Indications for such a connection are the finding that high overnight bladder volumes have been shown to be responsible for development of high bladder capacity in patients with VUR[45] and also in boys with posterior urethral valves.[38] Overnight bladder volume has also been shown to be the determinant for functional bladder capacity in healthy children after potty-training.[46]

The relationship between free voiding and cystometric capacity changes during the first years of life. In the neonatal period, cystometric capacity[17] is lower as compared to free voiding capacity[13] (see Figure 39.5), whereas after the infant year the opposite is seen. This can be partly attributed to the fact that older children postpone voiding at cystometry due to fear of voiding with a catheter in the bladder and of the unfamiliar situation of the assessment. This fear cannot be expected in the neonatal child and voiding is thus not postponed for this reason. Another possible explanation for the low cystometric capacity in the neonatal period might be the overactivity suggested by Bachelard et al, shown as an ease to induce detrusor contractions prematurely in catheter investigations.[17]

Even if development of bladder capacity during the first years of life is not linear, we suggest that a linear formula is used for calculation of expected bladder capacity for age as a simple rule of thumb. We have chosen to use:

Expected bladder capacity (ml) = 30 + (age in years $\times$ 30)[25]

since this linear increase in capacity is very similar to the nonlinear increase in capacity as described by Jansson et al[13] investigating children longitudinally from birth to age 3 years in free voiding studies (see Figure 39.6).

According to the International Continence Society (ICS), the term 'functional bladder capacity' should no longer be used because of difficulties of definition, and it should be replaced with 'voided volume'. Children void widely different volumes during the same day, sometimes when they feel a desire to void but quite often because their mothers tell them to go to the toilet.[46] The common way to decide a child's bladder capacity is to keep a voiding diary (frequency–volume chart) for 2 days and select the largest voiding volume, excluding the first morning voidings that rather represent nocturnal bladder capacity. For children on CIC, the same method is used to define the child's approximate bladder volume.

Measured capacity less than 65% of the calculated value is believed to denote a bladder which is *small for age*, whereas a measured volume that is more than 150% of the calculated value may denote a bladder that is *large for age*.[25]

Detrusor contractility

Storage phase. It has been shown during recent years that instability is rarely seen in infants[14,17] which is contrary to the earlier concept of instability as a normal phenomenon in this age group.[9] The lack of unstable contractions during filling has been shown in natural fill cystometry,[14] which is an investigation that is sensitive when it comes to identification of instability. This lack of instability during filling has also been observed in standard cystometric investigations of healthy infants, including a study of siblings of children with reflux.[17]

In infants with bladder dysfunction, on the other hand, instability during filling is common, such as those with posterior urethral valves[38] and neurogenic bladder.[31] Therefore, instability can probably be used to diagnose bladder dysfunction in this age group just like in older children.

During the first months of life, on the other hand, there seems to be another form of overactivity, which was observed in 20% of the children as an isolated detrusor contraction after only a few milliliters of filling at cystometry and, with leakage of urine, looked at as a premature voiding contraction.[17] Bladder capacity in these age groups urodynamically registered was also low,[17] and was much lower than that seen after free voidings.[13] These findings taken together indicate that the voiding reflex can easily be elicited in this age group, in the cystometric investigations, by a catheter in the bladder and infusion of saline (see Figure 39.2). This overactivity vanishes after a few months and, simultaneously, bladder capacity increases. The phenomenon does not seem to have anything to do with instability, since instability is seldom seen in infants,[14,17] but can rather be looked upon as an immature behavior of the detrusor muscle.[47,48]

Voiding phase. Voiding detrusor pressure is probably higher during early infancy compared to that seen in older children. Bachelard et al[17] and Wen and Tong[49] investigated infants considered to have normal low urinary tract with conventional cystometry using a urethral catheter. The pressure levels registered in these studies were very different; median 127 vs mean 75 cmH$_2$O. One explanation of the different results may be the age of the infants studied, which was median 1 month and 6 months, respectively. Yeung et al also found high voiding pressure levels in small infants.[42] However, it should be noted that they used natural fill cystometry, which gives higher pressure levels than standard cystometry.

Female infants have significantly lower pressures at voiding compared with males and only slightly higher than those of older girls (Table 39.1).

This difference in voiding detrusor pressure between males and females must be attributed to the difference in anatomy, with the long narrow urethra in male infants allowing higher outflow resistance and inducing higher voiding pressure. Thus, the standards for voiding pressure in healthy infants are imprecise and can be a median of more than 100 cmH$_2$O in males and 60–70 cmH$_2$O in females (see Table 39.1). In children 1–3 years of age median voiding pressures have been reported to be 70 cmH$_2$O in males[9] and 60 in females.[49]

High voiding pressure in infants is correlated with low bladder capacity. This further explains the above-described differences in voiding pressure levels in the studies by Wen and Tong[49] and Bachelard et al.[17] In the latter study, the infants were younger and thus had lower capacity.

Any discernible peak in the detrusor pressure recording during the filling phase is a pathological finding, but in order to avoid recording artifacts it may be prudent to allow only for peaks with a duration of >10 s and amplitude of >10 cmH$_2$O. In neurogenic bladder urodynamics, one should keep in mind that traditional cystometry seems to suppress phasic detrusor activity and exaggerate the rise of basic pressure (giving the impression of low compliance) compared with natural fill cystometry.[41,44]

Variables to register. Variables to register comprise the following:

- Number of phasic contractions and their duration and amplitude together with the infused volume when they occurred. Note subjective reaction, if any.

- Basic detrusor pressure at start and end of filling (excluding a possible sharp terminal rise of pressure). Avoid to include phasic contractions.
- Detrusor pressure at start of significant leakage (LPP) and the infused volume when leakage occurred.
- Absence or presence of a coordinated detrusor micturition contraction. In the case of a micturition contraction, any detrusor pressure above 100 cmH$_2$O is to be regarded as pathological in children, denoting outflow obstruction or detrusor overactivity, or both. In infant boys, higher values may be normal.

Bladder cooling test. Variables to register are:

- outcome: positive (detrusor contraction >30 cmH$_2$O) or negative (30 cmH$_2$O)
- maximal detrusor pressure, registered in cmH$_2$O.

Sphincter contractility

In children with neurogenic bladders, EMG registration will not always produce any information about urethral sphincter activity. When the EMG recording seems unreliable, indirect evidence will have to do. Leak point pressure >40 cmH$_2$O denotes either neurogenic sphincter overactivity or a sphincter with intact innervation. Likewise, the finding of intravesical pressures well above 40 cmH$_2$O without any detectable leakage of urine suggests detrusor-sphincter dyssynergia or, alternatively, a normal sphincter contracting to prevent leakage (guarding reflex).

Compliance of the bladder wall

The concept of compliance characterizes the distensibility of the bladder wall during the reservoir phase. A subnormal compliance value denotes increase of bladder wall stiffness due to change of wall structure or a tonic detrusor contraction and is a risk factor for development of upper tract damage. Compliance is expressed as the volume (ml) that the bladder can accommodate with a resulting pressure increase of 1 cmH$_2$O. It is calculated from a middle segment of the detrusor pressure registration up to 30 cmH$_2$O, avoiding phasic contractions. A 'normal' value for compliance in adults has not been validated but it is generally felt that it should be more than 20 ml/cmH$_2$O, e.g. that basic pressure increase up to an adult bladder volume of 400 ml should be 20 cmH$_2$O or less from empty to full bladder. But we will encounter problems trying to apply this value of compliance to the wide range of bladder volumes in children. For example, a child with a bladder capacity of 100 ml (which would be normal in a 3-year-old child) and a 20 cmH$_2$O pressure

Table 39.1 *Voiding detrusor pressure in infants*

	Mean voiding detrusor pressure (cmH$_2$O)	
References	Males	Females
Yeung et al[42]	117	75
Bachelard et al[17]	127	72
Wen and Tong[49]	75	60

increase from empty to full bladder will give a compliance value of 5 ml/cmH$_2$O, a value which would be clearly pathological in an adult. An adjustment must be done to make values comparable between children and adults. It has been suggested that the lowest acceptable value of compliance in a child should be 1/20 (5%) of the child's normal capacity per cmH$_2$O, a calculation that would be compatible with the lowest limit of 'normal' compliance, 20 ml/cmH$_2$O, in adults. Then, a compliance of 5 ml/cmH$_2$O at a bladder capacity of 100 ml would be within the normal range.

Safe capacity. Instead of calculating compliance in order to characterize the reservoir properties of the bladder wall, we use the concept of 'safe capacity' at our institution. The bladder volumes at 20 cmH$_2$O and 30 cmH$_2$O base line detrusor pressure are registered. The 20 cmH$_2$O value stands for a truly safe and the 30 cmH$_2$O a borderline value for compliance at reservoir capacity.

Continence

Cystometry of a child is not only a laboratory investigation but also allows for a careful and prolonged clinical observation of the child. In addition to the urodynamic results produced by the cystometry, this observation provides important information regarding the child's reactions to bladder filling and, not least, in which situations and at which bladder volumes leakage of urine can be noted.

Lower urinary tract sensation

From age 4 onwards, it is possible to extend the clinical observation during cystometry by asking the child whether he feels the catheter being introduced and if he experiences any sensation from the bladder during filling. Some degree of urethral sensation is not seldom present in children with neurogenic bladder, whereas bladder sensation is most often absent or very weak. Discomfort or pain at end filling when the bladder has become filled to capacity is probably elicited from functional sensory nerve endings in the peritoneum partly covering the bladder. When the child signals discomfort (in small children seldom verbally, but rather by being anxious, crying, or moving restlessly), infusion should be discontinued. The cystometry protocol should include the soft data obtained regarding sensation.

Bladder evacuation

Infants do not empty the bladder at every voiding,[13,15,16,49,51] but, characteristically one voiding during 4 hours is complete, according to results from the 4-hour observations. This is seen both in pre-term infants (gestation week 32)[15] and neonates, and during the first years of life.[13] The residual urine during 4 hours is more or less constant from the neonatal period until just before the age of 2 years; median 4–5 ml.[13,15,16] During the third year, when gaining control over voidings, on the other hand, the emptying of the bladder becomes complete, so that the median residual urine is 0 ml.[13]

In healthy children above 3–4 years of age, the bladder empties completely at each voiding. Five milliliters in post-void residual may be accepted due to the unavoidable time delay from the end of voiding until the bladder can be examined with ultrasound; 5–20 ml is borderline and is an indication for repeating the ultrasound. In schoolgirls treated for bacteriuria, recurrence was significantly more common in those with post-void residual urine greater than 5 ml.[52] In children with NBD, assessing post-void residual urine by aspiring through the bladder catheter may not always yield reliable results due to the common dislocation of the base of the neurogenic bladder, so a check with ultrasound is strongly recommended. Ultrasound to determine residual urine should also be performed frequently on all children on CIC for the same reason.

Conclusions

The free voiding pattern in the neonatal period is characterized by small, frequent voidings (one voiding per hour) with volumes that vary intra-individually and leave residual urine most of the time. The incomplete emptying is suggested to be due to a physiological form of dyscoordination. Towards potty-training age the emptying improves, and, at that time (third year), the bladder capacity also doubles. Voiding during quiet sleep is rarely seen, even in the neonatal infant, meaning that the child shows signs of arousal at voiding.

Bladder instability is rarely seen in urodynamic studies of young infants, although premature voiding contractions are seen in the neonatal period, with leakage of urine after only a few milliliters of filling. This latter increased reactivity of the detrusor muscle is also suggested to be responsible for the cystometric small bladder capacity in this age group and the high voiding pressure levels.

Classification of neurogenic bladder dysfunction in infants and children

A classification of neurogenic bladder in spina bifida children was suggested by van Gool.[53] As can be seen in Table 39.2, a simple but clinically useful classification can be created from the urodynamic data. Detrusor and sphincter are classified as underactive or overactive, so the neurogenic dysfunction can be categorized in four main groups. Two of these display underactive sphincter with incontinence as the major clinical problem, and the two others have overactive sphincter with outflow obstruction and deficient bladder emptying as their main clinical characteristics. It should be added, however, that about 5% of children with myelomeningocele display normal bladder function at cystometry, in particular those who have their spinal cord anomaly in a high position (cervical, thoracic, or high thoracolumbar) (Figure 39.7).

Table 39.2 *Four patterns of bladder-sphincter dysfunction in children with myelomeningocele*[53]

Sphincter	Detrusor		Clinical correlate
	Underactive	Overactive	
Underactive	35	42	Incontinence
Overactive	13	42	Outflow obstruction

Examples of common urodynamic patterns in neurogenic bladder dysfunction in children

The most ominous urodynamic pattern, threatening the integrity of the kidneys, is dyssynergia between detrusor and sphincter. The micturition detrusor contraction is counteracted by sphincter contractions, leading to poor evacuation of the bladder, as seen in a 4-year-old boy with lumbosacral myelomeningocele (Figure 39.8).

Almost equally dangerous for the renal health is the pattern with an underactive or paretic detrusor, low compliant bladder wall, and overactive sphincter (Figure 39.9). The child attempts, without much success, to empty the bladder by forceful contractions of the abdominal muscles. As in the previous case, a regular, carefully performed CIC program is absolutely essential in order to avoid UTIs, reflux, and renal damage in this 4-year-old boy with lumbosacral myelomeningocele.

The pattern is often not as clear-cut as in the two previous cases. In the next example, the detrusor is overactive and there is borderline compliance (Figure 39.10).

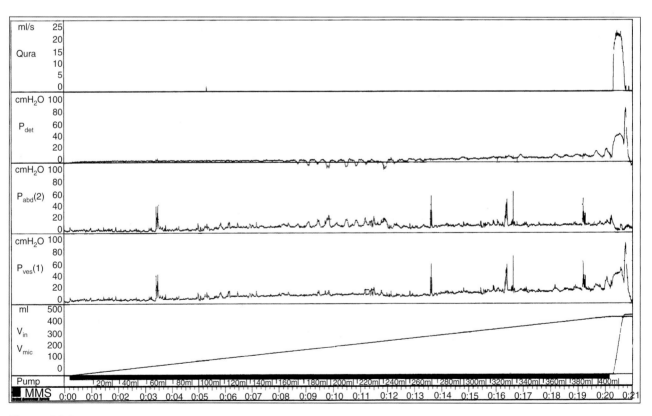

Figure 39.7
Normal cystometry in a 4-year-old boy with high thoracolumbar myelomeningocele.

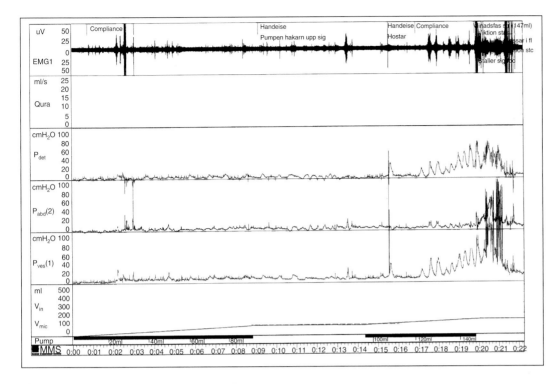

Figure 39.8
Normal compliance, discrete detrusor overactivity, and micturition contraction forcefully counteracted by sphincter contraction, thus pronounced dyssynergia, in a 4-year-old boy with lumbosacral myelomeningocele.

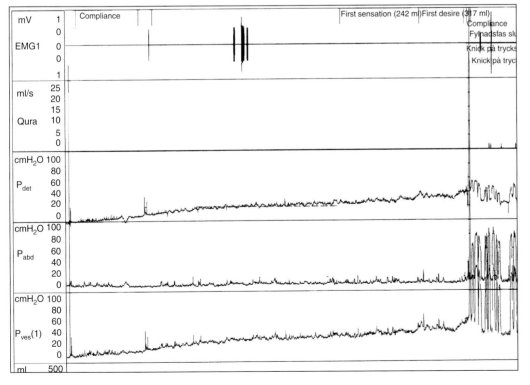

Figure 39.9
Detrusor underactivity, low bladder wall compliance, and poor effect of straining, suggesting sphincter overactivity, in a 4-year-old boy with lumbosacral myelomeningocele.

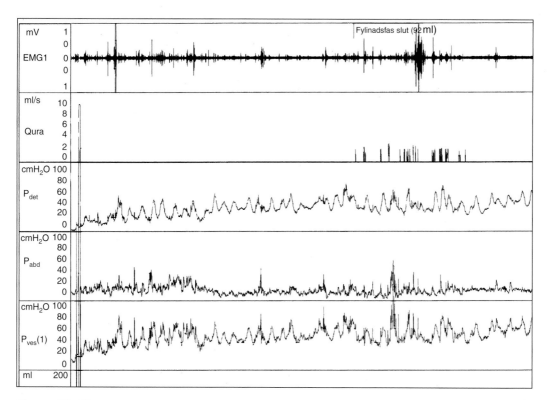

Figure 39.10

Example of cystometry which is not readily elucidated in a 9-month-old boy with lumbosacral myelomeningocele. Detrusor overactivity and borderline bladder wall compliance, but what about the sphincter behavior? Electromyography (EMG) may indicate a somewhat overactive pelvic floor, but there are, on the other hand, rather frequent mini-micturitions and a larger one at the end of the registration ('START MIKT').

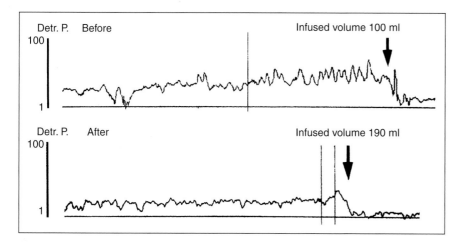

Figure 39.11

Intravesical oxybutynin may efficiently inhibit detrusor overactivity in a 5-year-old girl with lumbosacral myelomeningocele. Detrusor pressure and compliance become normal and capacity nearly doubles after intravesical instillation of 5 mg of oxybutynin.

The sphincter may also be somewhat overactive, as judged from the EMG; but, on the other hand, there are several small micturitions and a larger one at the end of the registration. This patient, with lumbosacral myelomeningocele, is only 9 months old, so there may remain an element of physiological immaturity in the urodynamic pattern.

The final example, a 5-year-old girl with lumbosacral myelomeningocele (Figure 39.11), depicts the beneficial effect on detrusor overactivity that is often attained with the use of detrusor-relaxing drugs (in this case, oxybutynin 5 mg twice daily administered intravesically). As can be seen, both phasic and tonic (compliance!) detrusor contractility normalizes.

References

1. Scott R Jr, McIlhaney JS. The voiding rates in normal male children. J Urol 1959; 82:244.

2. Zatz LM. Combined physiologic and radiologic studies of bladder function in female children with recurrent urinary tract infections. Invest Urol 1965; 3:278.

3. Whitaker J, Johnston GS. Estimation of urinary outflow resistance in children: simultaneous measurement of bladder pressure, flow rate and exit pressure. Invest Urol 1969; 7:127.

4. Palm L, Nielsen OH. Evaluation of bladder function in children. J Pediatr Surg 1967; 2:529.

5. Starfield B. Functional bladder capacity in enuretic and non-enuretic children. J Pediatr 1967; 70:777.

6. Gierup HJW. Micturition studies in infants and children. Intravesical pressure, urinary flow and urethral resistance in boys without infravesical obstruction. Scand J Urol Nephrol 1970; 3:217.

7. Kroigaard N. The lower urinary tract in infancy and childhood. Micturition cinematography with simultaneous pressure-flow measurement. Acta Radiol 1970; (suppl):300:3–175.

8. O'Donnell B, O'Connor TP. Bladder function in infants and children. Br J Urol 1971; 43:25.

9. Hjalmas K. Micturition in infants and children with normal lower urinary tract. A urodynamic study. Scand J Urol Nephrol 1976; (suppl)37.

10. Gool JD van, Kuijter RH, Donckerwolcke RA, et al. Bladder-sphincter dysfunction, urinary infection and vesico-ureteral reflux with special reference to cognitive bladder training. Contrib Nephrol 1985; 39:190.

11. Lindehall B, Claesson I, Hjalmas K, Jodal U. Effect of clean intermittent catheterisation on radiological appearance of the upper urinary tract in children with myelomeningocele. Br J Urol 1991; 67:415–419.

12. Muellner SR. Development of urinary control in children. JAMA 1960; 172:1256–1260.

13. Jansson UB, Hanson M, Hanson E, et al. Voiding pattern in healthy children 0 to 3 years old: a longitudinal study. J Urol 2000; 164:2050–2054.

14. Yeung C, Godley M, Ho C, et al. Some new insights into bladder function in infancy. Br J Urol 1995; 76:235–240.

15. Sillén U, Sölsnes E, Hellström A-L, Sandberg K. The voiding pattern of healthy preterm neonates. J Urol 2000; 163:278.

16. Holmdahl G, Hanson E, Hanson M, et al. Four-hour voiding observation in healthy infants. J Urol 1996; 156:1809–1812.

17. Bachelard M, Sillén U, Hansson S, et al. Urodynamic pattern in asymptomatic infants: siblings of children with vesicoureteral reflux. J Urol 1999; 162:1733.

18. Zerin M, Chen E, Ritchey M, Bloom D. Bladder capacity as measured at voiding cystourethrography in children: relationship to toilet training and frequency of micturition. J Urol 1993; 187:803.

19. Bakker E, Wyndaele JJ. Change in the toilet-training of children during the last 60 years: the cause of an increase in lower urinary tract dysfunction? BJU Int 2000; 86:248.

20. Brazelton TB. A child-oriented approach to toilet training. Pediatrics 1962; 29:121.

21. Klackenberg G. A prospective longitudinal study of children. Data on psychic health and development up to 8 years of age. Acta Paediatr Scand Suppl. 1971; 224:1–239.

22. Largo R, Molinari L, von Siebenthal K, Wolfensberge U. Does a profound change in toilet-training affect development of bowel and bladder control? Dev Med Child Neurol 1996; 38:1106–1116.

23. Marten W, deVries MD, deVries PNP. Cultural relativity of toilet training readiness: a perspective from East Africa. Pediatrics 1977; 60:170–177.

24. Shurtleff DB. 44 years experience with management of myelomeningocele: presidential address, Society for Research into Hydrocephalus and Spina Bifida. Eur J Pediatr Surg 2000; 10 (suppl 1):5–8.

25. Hjälmås K. Urodynamics in normal infants and children. Scand J Urol Nephrol 1988; (suppl) 114:20–27.

26. Swithinbank L, O'Brien M, Frank D, et al. The role of paediatric urodynamics revisited. Neurourol Urodyn 2002; 21:439–440.

27. Bozkurt P, Kilic N, Kaya G, et al. The effects of intranasal midazolam on urodynamic studies in children. Br J Urol 1996; 78:282–286.

28. Stokland E, Andreasson S, Jacobsson B, Jodal U, Ljung B. Sedation with midazolam for voiding cystourethrography in children: a randomized double-blind study. Pediatr Radiol 2003; 33(4):247–249.

29. Tanikaze S, Sugita Y. Cystometric examination for neurogenic bladder of neonates and infants. Hinyokika Kiyo 1991; 37:1403–1405.

30. Agarwal SK, McLorie GA, Grewal D, et al. Urodynamic correlates or resolution of reflux in meningomyelocele patients. J Urol 1997; 158:580–582.

31. Sillén U, Hanson E, Hermansson G, et al. Development of the urodynamic pattern in infants with myelomeningocele. Br J Urol 1996; 78:596–601.

32. Bauer SB. The argument for early assessment and treatment of infants with spina bifida. Dialog Pediatr Urol 2000; 23(11):2–3.

33. Tarcan T, Bauer S, Olmedo E, et al. Long-term follow up of newborns with myelodysplasia and normal urodynamic findings: is follow up necessary? J Urol 2001; 165:564–567.

34. Klevmark B. Natural pressure-volume curves and conventional cystometry. Scand J Urol Nephrol 1999; (suppl 201):1–4.

35. Geirsson G, Lindstrom S, Fall M, et al. Positive bladder cooling test in neurologically normal young children. J Urol 1994; 151:446–448.

36. Gladh G, Lindstrom S. Outcome of the bladder cooling test in children with neurogenic bladder dysfunction. J Urol 1999; 161:254–258.

37. Flood HD, Ritchey ML, Bloom DA, et al. Outcome of reflux in children with myelodysplasia managed by bladder pressure monitoring. J Urol 1994; 152:1574–1577.

38. Holmdahl G, Sillen U, Bertilsson M, et al. Natural filling cystometry in small boys with posterior urethral valves: unstable bladders become stable during sleep. J Urol 1997; 158:1017–1021.

39. Bjerle P. Relationship between perivesical and intravesical urinary bladder pressures and intragastric pressure. Acta Physiol Scand 1974; 92:465–473.

40. Robertson A, Griffiths C, Ramsden P, Neal D. Bladder function in healthy volunteers: ambulatory monitoring and conventional urodynamic studies. Br J Urol 1994; 73:242–249.

41. Webb RJ, Griffiths CJ, Ramsden PD, Neal DE. Ambulatory monitoring of bladder pressure in low compliance neurogenic bladder dysfunction. J Urol 1992; 148:1477–1481.

42. Yeung C, Godley M, Duffy P, Ransley P. Natural filling cystometry in infants and children. Br J Urol 1995; 75:531–537.

43. De Gennaro M, Capitanucci ML, Silveri M, et al. Continuous (6 hour) urodynamic monitoring in children with neuropathic bladder. Eur J Pediatr Surg 1996; 6(suppl 1):21–24.

44. Zermann DH, Lindner H, Huschke T, Schubert J. Diagnostic value of natural fill cystometry in neurogenic bladder in children. Eur Urol 1997; 32:223–228.

45. Sillén U, Hellström A-L, Sölsnes E, Jansson U-B. Control of voidings means better emptying of the bladder in children with congenital dilating VUR. BJU Int 2000; 85(suppl 4):13.

46. Mattsson SH. Voiding frequency, volumes and intervals in healthy school children. Scand J Urol Nephrol 1994; 28:1–11.

47. Sugaya K, de Groat WC. Influence of temperature on activity of the isolated whole bladder preparation of neonatal and adult rats. Am J Physiol Regul Integr Comp Physiol 2000; 278:238.

48. Zderic SA, Sillén U, Liu G-H, et al. Developmental aspects of bladder contractile function: evidence for an intracellular calcium pool. J Urol 1993; 150:623.

49. Wen JG, Tong EC. Cystometry in infants and children with no apparent voiding symptoms. Br J Urol 1998; 81:468.

50. Roberts DS, Rendell B. Postmicturition residual bladder volumes in healthy babies. Arch Dis Child 1989; 64:825–828.

51. Gladh G, Persson D, Mattsson S, Lindstrom S. Voiding patterns in healthy newborns. Neurourol Urodyn 2000; 19:177–184.

52. Lindberg U, Bjure J, Haugstvedt S, Jodal U. Asymptomatic bacteriuria in schoolgirls. III. Relation between residual urine volume and recurrence. Acta Paediatr Scand 1975; 64:437–440.

53. Van Gool J. Spina bifida and neurogenic bladder dysfunction: a urodynamic study. Thesis. Utrecht: Uitgeverij Impress, 1986:154.

40

Electrophysiological evaluation: basic principles and clinical applications

Simon Podnar and Clare J Fowler

Introduction

Electrophysiological methods record bioelectrical potentials generated by excitable cell membranes. When applied in a clinical setting to recordings from nerves and skeletal muscle these tests are often referred to as clinical neurophysiological investigations. Clinical neurophysiological methods are well-established, and have been used in clinical practice for almost half a century.

Neurophysiological techniques have so far been applied in the pelvic floor mostly for research purposes, but they have also been proposed for everyday diagnostics in selected groups of patients. The WHO Consensus on Incontinence stated that electrophysiological assessment is useful in selected patients with suspected peripheral nervous system lesions such as lower motor neuron (LMN) lesions, patients with multiple system atrophy (MSA), and also in women with urinary retention.[1]

The emphasis of this chapter is on clinically useful and 'established' electrophysiological tests, which are of diagnostic value in individual patients with neurogenic bladders. Concentric needle electromyography (CNEMG) and bulbocavernosus reflex (BCR) testing will be discussed in detail. Other tests not considered to be of clinical value in the diagnosis of individual patients will be only briefly described. For more detailed description of these research-type clinical uroneurophysiological tests,[1] reference to other reviews is recommended.[1,2]

Electrophysiological tests in assessment of patients

General remarks

A particular diagnostic test should be considered in a patient when the information it may provide will significantly affect further treatment and/or clarify prognosis. Clinical neurophysiological findings consistent with the diagnosis of 'a neurogenic bladder' can be found in patients with established diagnosis of neurological disease but in these circumstances add little to the case. However, in patients being investigated for bladder symptoms of suspected neurological origin, neurophysiological tests may reveal evidence of neural damage and thus point to neurological diagnosis.[3]

Basically, in neurological disease affecting the bladder, two main patterns of abnormalities can be found: the LMN and the upper motor neuron (UMN) pattern (see below), which are, respectively, due to lesions of the anterior horn cell or alpha motor neuron, spinal root, and peripheral nerve in the case of an LMN lesion (Figure 40.1) or due to

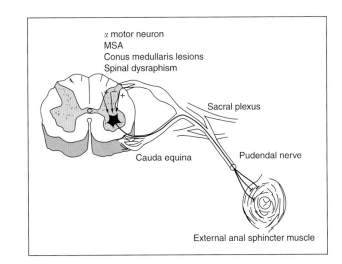

Figure 40.1
The sacral reflex arc. The sacral spinal cord, with sensory (afferent) root entering posteriorly, and motor (efferent) root leaving anteriorly, is shown. Although not shown here, below the lower end of the spinal cord (conus medullaris) lumbar and sacral spinal roots travel for several segments within the spinal canal before leaving it (cauda equina). An enlarged alpha motor neuron with facilitatory (+) and inhibitory (−) suprasegmental influences is also shown. MSA, multiple system atrophy.

damage of suprasegmental pathways in the central nervous system in the case of UMN lesions. Neurological examination is very valuable in helping to make the distinction between these two conditions. In very general terms a UMN lesion would be expected to be associated with detrusor overactivity, whereas an LMN lesion would be associated with bladder atonia (hyporeflexia), although this rule is by no means hard and fast.

Electrophysiological tests can be understood as an extension of the clinical neurological examination. The tests are seldom useful in patients with a completely normal neurological examination, and are helpful only in patients in whom specific neurological lesions are suspected.[3] In general, neurophysiological tests may be used to elucidate those findings summarized in Table 40.1. Some of these properties are relevant when applied to the striated muscle of the pelvic floor.

Other physiological tests to evaluate bladder disorders (measurement of post-void residual, uroflow, cystometry, etc.) are different in that they test function and, as a consequence, can be regarded as complementary. Similarly, neurophysiological tests are complementary to imaging studies – such as ultrasound, computer tomography (CT), and magnetic resonance imaging (MRI) – of the lower urinary tract. Neurophysiological tests, however, have limitations (Table 40.2).

Clinical assessment before electrophysiological evaluation

Selected patients with urinary disorders should be referred to specialists, who will perform a focused clinical examination of the lower urinary tract and anogenital region. To document and quantify patients' complaints, and obtain additional data, functional investigations (measurement of post-void residual, uroflow, cystometry) and imaging studies might be considered. A neural lesion would be suspected, particularly when bowel and sexual dysfunction accompany urinary dysfunction, and it

Table 40.1 *Unique information provided by electrophysiological tests. Normal clinical neurological examination and appropriate electrophysiological testing (see Method column) document preserved neural integrity, and other causes for the pelvic floor dysfunction should be sought. On the other hand, the electrophysiological test abnormality in appropriate clinical setting supports and documents the clinical diagnosis of a neurogenic lesion. The electrophysiological tests can then often help to provide information about severity, localization, and type (mechanism) of the lesion. These factors are crucial for the assessment of prognosis.*

Information	Structure	Method	Finding
Integrity preserved	The lower motor neuron	CNEMG	Absent spontaneous denervation activity; continuous MUP firing during relaxation
	Lower and upper motor neuron	CNEMG	Dense IP on voluntary activation
	Sacral reflex arc	CNEMG	Dense IP on reflex activation (touch)
		Sacral reflex response	Brisk BCR of normal latency
	Somatosensory pathways	Pudendal SEP	Normal shape and latency of responses
Localization of lesions	Root vs plexus/nerve	CNEMG	Paravertebral denervation activity in neighboring myotomes
		SNAP	Normal (penile) SNAP with impaired (penile) skin sensation
Severity of lesions	Complete vs partial	CNEMG	Profuse spontaneous denervation activity; absent MUPs
	Severe vs moderate	Sacral reflex response	BCR absent
Type of lesion	Conduction block vs axonotmesis	CNEMG	Absent/sparse spontaneous denervation activity
	Axonotmesis vs neurotmesis	CNEMG	Appearance of nascent MUPs after complete muscle denervation

BCR, bulbocavernosus reflex; CNEMG, concentric needle electromyography; IP, interference pattern; MUP, motor unit potential; SEP, somatosensory evoked potentials; SNAP, sensory nerve action potential.

Table 40.2 *The limitations of electrodiagnostic tests*

Limitations	Reason	Comments
Uncomfortable		Without significant risks
Difficult localization	• Multiple lesions • Proximal peripheral sacral lesions	Proximal lesion 'masks' distal on CNEMG, and distal lesion masks proximal on SNAP testing Paravertebral muscles are absent in the lower sacral segments
Timing of investigation	• Few abnormalities before several weeks post injury • Less pronounced pathological signs after a few months	
Tests do not reflect the function of the whole structure studied	Low correlation with function	No electrophysiological parameter validated to measure weakness

CNEMG, concentric needle electromyography; SNAP, sensory nerve action potential.

is then that uroneurophysiological evaluation would be considered.[3]

At the beginning of each uroneurophysiological evaluation, a focused history of the patient's complaints needs to be taken, including questions about urinary, anorectal, and sexual (dys)function. History of low back pain irradiating to legs, and numbness and tingling on the posterior part of thighs, buttocks, and in the perineal region will point to a cauda equina lesion (Chapters 27, 28). In older patients, inquiry about general slowness, disordered gait, tremor, and autonomic dysfunction (orthostatic hypotension, etc.) should be made to reveal extrapyramidal disorders such as Parkinson's disease (see Chapter 22). Dissemination of neurological symptoms in time and in neurological location (blurred vision, difficult gait, urinary and fecal urgency, etc.) suggests a diagnosis of demyelinating disease of the central nervous system (multiple sclerosis) (see Chapter 24). For research purposes the use of standardized questionnaires for anorectal,[4,5] urinary,[6,7] and sexual[8,9] (dys)function is recommended.

As a minimum, at the beginning of each electrophysiological evaluation a brief neurological examination should also be performed, looking for signs of pyramidal (UMN) and peripheral nervous system (LMN) lesions (particularly in lower limbs), and also for extrapyramidal and cerebellar signs. Examination of the anogenital region should in this setting include assessment of anal sphincter tone during rest, squeeze, and push, sensation of touch and pinprick in the perineal/perianal area, and eliciting of the BCR and anal reflex (bilaterally). If uroneurophysiological tests are to be performed, a detailed explanation of the aims and methods of the electrodiagnostic evaluation should be given to the patient.

Innervation of the pelvic structures

The nervous system is divided into two motor systems (the somatic and the autonomic), and the (somato)sensory system (Figure 40.2). Within a particular anatomical system we can distinguish central and peripheral parts. The central part includes the motor and sensory pathways contained within the brain and spinal cord (the central nervous system). The central nervous system also contains, at different levels, interneuronal systems, which are important in neural 'integrative functions' (e.g. sacral spinal interneurons in the BCR arc[10]).

The motor system comprises a UMN (i.e. all neurons participating in the supraspinal motor control), an LMN (innervating muscles and glands), and muscle. Cell bodies of the UMN lie in the motor cortex and other gray matter (nuclei) of the brain (including some brainstem nuclei) and connect directly or via interneurons to the LMNs of the spinal cord (and cranial motor nerve nuclei in the brainstem). The LMNs lie either in the anterior horns of

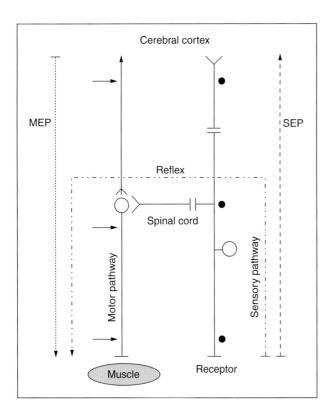

Figure 40.2
Components of the somatic sensory and somatic motor systems
and the electrophysiological tests that evaluate them. Arrows
on the motor (left) side indicate different stimulation sites
(from above) of motor cortex, spinal roots, and peripheral
nerves (terminal motor latency test). Small circles on the
sensory (right) side indicate different recording sites (from
below) from peripheral nerve (sensory nerve action potential,
SNAP), spinal roots/cord, and somatosensory cortex. (Note that
for SNAP recording both distal stimulation and proximal
recording[82] or reverse[83] could be employed.) In addition,
concentric needle electromyography (CNEMG) and single fiber
electromyography (SFEMG) assess the lower motor neuron and
muscle. Kinesiological EMG evaluates the integrity of upper
motor neuron and neurocontrol reflex arcs. MEP, motor
evoked potential; SEP, somatosensory evoked potential.
(Redrawn with permission from Vodušek DB.)[58]

Somatic lower motor neurons of the sacral spinal cord

The α motor neurons of the sphincter (Onuf's) nucleus are
somewhat smaller than those innervating limb and trunk
skeletal muscles. Like other motor neurons, which innervate striated muscle, they lie in the anterior horn of the
spinal cord. Their axons are of large diameter and myelinated to allow rapid conduction of impulses and travel to
the periphery in the cauda equina, the sacral plexus, and the
pudendal nerves (see Figure 40.1). Within the muscle,
the motor axon tapers and then branches to innervate
muscle fibers. Each motor neuron innervates a number of
muscle fibers – this constitutes the motor unit (MU). The
innervation of healthy muscle is such that fibers that are
part of the same MU are unlikely to be adjacent to one
another but are scattered in checkerboard pattern. The
diameter of the muscle area innervated by each lower
sacral α motor neuron (MU territory) is probably smaller
than the corresponding area in limb or trunk muscles.

Primary sensory neuron

Sensory receptors are the most peripheral part of the
somatic and autonomic sensory neurons. Receptors code
mechanical or chemical stimuli into bioelectrical activity –
i.e. nerve action potentials which traverse the peripheral
axon (within peripheral nerves and the sacral plexus), cell
body within the spinal ganglion, and the central axon of
the peripheral sensory neuron (within the cauda equina).
In the spinal cord the central axon branches, with segmental branches contributing in the reflex arc, and central
branches (within dorsal column) conveying sensory information to the brain. Both somatic and visceral parts of the
sensory system are organized in this way.

The simplified model of the neuromuscular system
includes also the autonomic system, which is divided into
sympathetic and parasympathetic parts.

Physiological principles of electrophysiological testing

An excitable membrane and transmission of traveling
action potentials are characteristic of nerve and muscle
cells. This bioelectrical activity is the substrate for function
of the nervous tissue (i.e. transmission of information) and
precedes the function of the muscle (i.e. contraction). It is
this bioelectrical activity which makes possible the application of electrodiagnostic methods.

To obtain the information about the bioelectrical
activity of muscle, nerve, spinal roots, spinal cord, and

the gray matter of the spinal cord (the somato-motor
nuclei) or in the lateral horns of the spinal cord (the autonomic nuclei): the first innervate skeletal muscle, and the
latter smooth muscle and glands.

The somatosensory system can be divided into a peripheral part (receptors and the sensory input into the spinal
cord) and a central part (ascending pathways in the spinal
cord and above). Sensory fibers from the skin and those
accompanying axons from α motor neurons are called
somatic afferents. Those accompanying autonomic
(parasympathetic or sympathetic) fibers are called visceral
afferents.

brain, recordings from these structures are necessary. All clinical neurophysiological recordings are extracellular. The electrodes may be near (i.e. intramuscular needle or wire electrodes), or distant from the source of bioelectrical activity (i.e. surface electrodes applied over the skin). The spread of the electrical field through tissues from the generators obeys physical laws of volume conduction. From muscle, both the ongoing (spontaneous) and elicited (willfully, reflexly, by nerve depolarization) activity can be recorded. From most of the other nervous structures (nerves, spinal roots, spinal cord), recording of the spontaneous bioelectrical activity can not be measured. To explore these structures, electrical (and less often magnetic or mechanical) stimulation is applied, and the propagated bioelectrical activity recorded at some distance along the nervous pathways. The electrophysiological responses obtained on stimulation are compound action potentials produced by simultaneous activation of populations of biological units (neurons, axons, muscle fibers of MUs).

Classification of electrophysiological tests

A functional classification of the electrophysiological tests consists of (see Figure 40.2):

- tests evaluating the somatic motor system (electromyography, EMG; terminal motor latency measurements, and motor evoked potentials, MEP)
- tests evaluating the sensory system (sensory neurography, somatosensory evoked potentials, SEP)
- methods assessing reflexes (BCR)
- tests assessing functioning of the sympathetic (sympathetic skin response, SSR) and parasympathetic autonomic nervous systems.

Such a 'logical' classification is preferable to a historical classification.

Uroneurophysiological tests that are of diagnostic value in individual patients with neurogenic bladder

Electromyography

Kinesiological electromyography

The aim of the kinesiological EMG is to assess patterns of individual muscle activity during various maneuvers (i.e. EMG activity patterns of pelvic floor muscle during bladder filling and voiding). It is usually not called kinesiological EMG, although this would be preferable to distinguish it from other EMG methods.

Various types of surface or intramuscular (needle or wire) electrodes can be used for recording of the kinesiological EMG signal. Bioelectrical activity will typically be sampled from a single intramuscular detection site. As motor unit potential (MUP) parameters are not analyzed, it can be recorded with a less-sophisticated apparatus than other types of EMG, even if intramuscular electrodes are used for recording. There is no commonly accepted standardized technique. When using surface electrodes there are problems related to the validity of the signal (e.g. artifacts and also contamination from other muscles). In contrast, with intramuscular electrodes in large pelvic floor muscles, there are questions as to whether the whole muscle is properly represented by the measured signal. Little is known about the normal activity patterns of different pelvic floor and sphincter muscles: urethral sphincter (US), urethrovaginal sphincter, the external anal sphincter (EAS) muscle, different parts of the levator ani, etc. It is generally assumed that they all act in a coordinated fashion (as one muscle), but differences have been demonstrated even between the intra- and peri-US in normal women.[11] Coordinated behavior is frequently lost in abnormal conditions, as has been shown for the levator ani, the US, and the EAS.[21]

The normal (kinesiological) sphincter EMG shows continuous activity of MUPs at rest, which may be increased voluntarily or reflexly. Such activity of low-threshold MUs[13] has been recorded for up to 2 hours[14] and even after subjects have fallen asleep during the examination.[15] Such activity can also be recorded in many but not all detection sites of the levator ani[16] and of the deeper EAS muscle.[17,18] The US and the EAS as well as the pubococcygeus muscles can sustain voluntary activation for only about 1 min.[16] On voiding, disappearance of all EMG activity in the US precedes detrusor contraction. In the central nervous system disorders, however, detrusor contractions may be associated with increase of sphincter EMG activity.[19,20] Detrusor-sphincter dyssynergia can be easily demonstrated by kinesiological EMG performed as a part of cystometric measurement.[12]

Neurogenic incoordinated sphincter behavior has to be differentiated from voluntary contractions that may occur in poorly compliant patients. The pelvic floor muscle contractions of the so-called non-neurogenic voiding disorder may be a learned abnormal behavior, and can be encountered in some women with dysfunctional voiding.[22]

In health the pubococcygeus in woman reveals similar activity patterns to the USs and the EAS at most detection sites: i.e. continuous activity at rest, some (but not invariable) increase of activity during bladder filling, and reflex increases in activity during any activation maneuver performed by the subject (talking, deep breathing, coughing).

The pubococcygeus also relaxes during voiding.[16] However, in disease, the patterns of activation and the coordination between the two sides may be lost.[23]

Any diagnostic value of kinesiological EMG apart from polygraph cystometric recordings to assess detrusor/sphincter coordination has yet to be established.

The demonstration of voluntary and reflex activation of pelvic floor muscles is indirect proof of the integrity of the respective neural pathways and should also be a part of a CNEMG examination, although the latter is performed primarily to diagnose an LMN lesion (see below). In contrast, kinesiological EMG is used mainly for diagnosis of the central nervous system, i.e. UMN lesions.

Concentric needle electromyography

The aim of CNEMG testing is to differentiate abnormal from normally innervated striated muscle. Although EMG abnormalities are detected as a result of a host of different lesions and diseases, there are in principle only two standard manifestations which can occur: disease of the muscle fibers themselves and changes in their innervation.

The concentric needle electrode consists of a central insulated platinum wire that is inserted through a steel cannula. This type of electrode records activity from muscle tissue up to 2.5 mm from the electrode tip.

For the CNEMG examination, an advanced EMG system, that has the facility for quantitative template-based MUP analysis (multi-MUP) is ideal.[24] The commonly used amplifier filter's setting for CNEMG is 5 Hz to 10 kHz. This must be identical to those set when reference values were compiled, and needs to be checked if MUP parameters are to be measured.

Because of easy access, sufficient muscle bulk, and relative ease of examination, the EAS is the most practical muscle for CNEMG testing of the lower sacral segments.[17,25] To examine the subcutaneous EAS muscle the needle is inserted about 1 cm from the anal orifice, to a depth of a 3–6 mm. For the deeper EAS muscle, 1–3 cm deep insertions are made at the anal orifice, at an angle of about 30° to the anal canal axis.[25] For MUP analysis, both EAS muscles can be sampled and the data pooled.[17] For kinesiological assessment, however, the subcutaneous and the deep muscles must be examined separately.[17]

Both left and right EAS muscles should almost always be examined, by needle insertions into the middle of the anterior and posterior halves. The needle is angled backwards and forwards in a systematic manner (through two insertion sites on each side).[26]

CNEMG examination of the EAS muscle can be divided into observation of insertion activity and of spontaneous denervation activity, and assessment of MUPs and of interference pattern (IP). In addition, it is suggested that the number of continuously active MUPs during relaxation be observed,[18] as well as MUP recruitment on reflex and voluntary activation.[26]

In normal muscle, needle movement elicits a short burst of 'insertion activity,' which is due to mechanical stimulation of excitable membranes. This is recorded at a gain of 50 μV per division, which is also used to record spontaneous denervation activity (sweep speed 5–10 ms/division). Absence of insertion activity with appropriately placed needle electrode[25] usually means complete atrophy of the muscle. Such complete atrophy of all EAS muscles on both sides was found in 9% of men after cauda equina lesions.[27]

Immediately after an acute complete denervation, all MU activity ceases, and (apart from insertion activity) no electrical activity can be recorded. Ten to twenty days later insertion activity becomes more prominent and prolonged and abnormal spontaneous activity appears in the form of short biphasic spikes (fibrillation potentials) and biphasic potentials with prominent positive deflections (positive sharp waves) (Figure 40.3A). This type of activity is referred to as 'spontaneous denervation activity' and originates from denervated single muscle fibers.

In partially denervated muscle, some MUPs remain and mingle eventually with spontaneous denervation activity. As the MUPs in sphincter muscles are also short and mostly bi- or triphasic, as are fibrillation potentials, it takes considerable EMG experience to differentiate one from another. In this situation, examination of the bulbocavernosus muscle is particularly useful because in contrast to sphincter muscles it lacks ongoing activity of low-threshold MU during relaxation (see Figure 40.3A).[26]

In longstanding partially denervated muscles, peculiar abnormal activity called simple or complex repetitive discharges appears, caused by repetitive firing of groups of potentials. This activity may be provoked by needle movement, muscle contraction, etc., or may occur spontaneously, rhythmically. This activity may sometimes be found in USs of patients without any other evidence of neuromuscular disease, and indeed without lower urinary tract problems, although in such cases it is not prominent. A type of repetitive discharge activity called 'decelerating bursts (DB) and complex repetitive discharges (CRD)' can be found in the external US muscles of some young women. The DBs produce the myotonic-like sound similar to underwater recordings of whales. The CRDs, however, sound like a helicopter over the loudspeaker on the EMG system. This activity may be so abundant that it is thought to cause involuntary muscle contraction and urinary retention.[28]

In contrast to limb muscles, where electrical silence is present on relaxation, in sphincter muscles some MUPs are continuously firing. Additional sphincter MUPs can be activated reflexly or voluntarily, and it has been shown that there are two MUP populations with different characteristics: reflexly or voluntarily activated high-threshold MUPs,

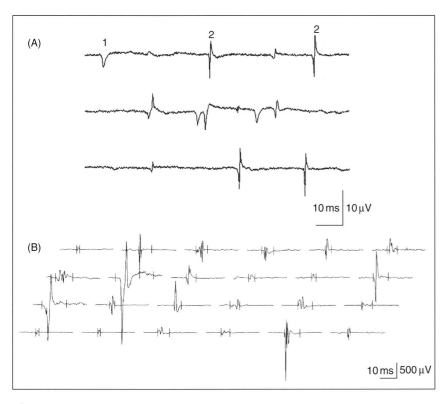

Figure 40.3

Findings of electromyographic (EMG) examination using a standard concentric EMG needle in a 36-year-old man after surgical decompression of the cauda equina due to central herniation of the intervertebral disc L4–L5. The patient had long-term sacral dysfunctions: atonic bladder (emptied by abdominal straining), severe constipation, and severe erectile dysfunction. (A) The EMG activity during relaxation in the left bulbocavernosus muscle 2 months after surgical decompression of the cauda equina. Note the distinct spontaneous denervation activity in the form of biphasic potentials with prominent positive deflections: positive sharp waves (1) and short biphasic spikes (fibrilation potentials (2)): No motor unit potentials (MUPs) could be recruited in that muscle reflexly or voluntarily, which pointed to complete denervation of the muscle. (B) The MUPs sampled (by multi-MUP analysis) from the left subcutaneous external anal sphincter (EAS) muscle during a control uroneurophysiological examination 7 months later. Mean duration was 7.3 ms ($Z = +0.7 -$ SD above the mean), mean area was 808 μVms ($Z = +4.2$), and the mean number of turns was 4.3 ($Z = +1.5$). Good reinnervation of the muscle after (probably) complete denervation, pointed to a combination of neurapraxia (block in nerve transmission) and axonotmesis (degeneration of the nerve fibers with preserved continuity of nerve roots) as opposed to neurotmesis (nerve roots severed) as a mechanism of the cauda equina injury.

which are larger than continuously active low-threshold MUPs. As a consequence, to increase accuracy of MUP analysis, for a template-based multi-MUP analysis, standardization of activity level during sampling at which 3–5 MUPs are sampled on a single muscle site is recommended.[13]

In partially denervated sphincter muscle there is a loss of MUs. To quantify this exactly, use of multi-MUP analysis was proposed.[18] By this approach, apart from the number of remaining MUs after partial denervation (i.e. in cauda equina lesions), the segmental and suprasegmental inputs to motor neurons within the anterior spinal horns as well as the excitation level of the motor neurons can be assessed. This approach was found particularly useful in patients with idiopathic fecal incontinence, but has not been studied in patients with neurogenic bladders.[18]

With axonal reinnervation after complete denervation, nascent MUPs appear first, being short-duration, low-amplitude, bi- and triphasic potentials, soon becoming polyphasic, serrated, and of prolonged duration.

Changes due to collateral reinnervation are reflected by prolongation of the waveform of the MUPs (Figure 40.4), which may have small, late components (satellites). In newly formed axon sprouts endplates, neuromuscular transmission is insecure, resulting in MUPs instability (jitter and blocking of individual components). Over a period of time, provided there is no further denervation, the reinnervating axonal sprouts increase in diameter, so that activation of all parts of the reinnervated MU becomes nearly synchronous, which increases the amplitude and reduces the duration of the MUPs (see Figure 40.4). This phenomenon may be different in sphincter muscles in ongoing

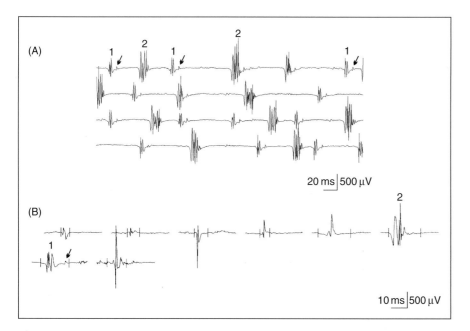

Figure 40.4

Findings of electromyographic (EMG) examination using a standard concentric EMG needle in a 36-year-old man with myelitis of the conus medullaris. The patient had several episodes of urinary and fecal incontinence, impaired sensation of bladder and rectum fullness, and moderate erectile dysfunction, all of which resolved spontaneously after a few months. (A) The EMG activity in the right deeper external anal sphincter (EAS) muscle during voluntary activation 2 months after the beginning of the disease. Note the extremely polyphasic motor unit potentials (MUPs) of increased duration, and late potential (arrows). Consecutive firing of the same MUP slightly changed, which points to MUP instability. No spontaneous denervation activity, and no low threshold MUPs continuously firing during relaxation were present. Reflex recruitment of MUPs was severely reduced but present in the same muscle. All these findings indicated subacute partial (moderately severe) denervation of the muscle. (B) During the same EMG examination only 8 MUPs needed to be sampled (by multi-MUP analysis) from the same muscle to obtain 3 MUPs with values of duration, area, and the number of turns above the upper outlier limit. To declare muscle pathological (neurogenic) using outlier criterion this number (3 out of 20 or less MUPs) is needed. Although at the same time mean values for duration, area, and the number of turns were also all pathological ($Z > 2.0$), they cannot be used in this situation to declare muscle neuropathic, because less than 20 MUPs were sampled. Two MUPs from (A) are also presented below (Nos 1 and 2). Note that averaging used by multi-MUP analysis changed the shape of unstable MUPs (reduced number of phases and turns).

degenerative disorders such as MSA, where long-duration MUPs seem to remain a prominent feature of MUs.[29] Less-pronounced increase in MUP amplitude on reinnervation in sphincter muscles might also be due to a less-efficient fusion of individual muscle fiber potentials in muscles with short spike components of MUPs (also in facial muscles).

Three techniques are available to systematically examine individual MUPs. The first MUP analysis technique follows an algorithm similar to that used by the early electromyographers of Buchthal and his school, who carried out the first quantitative MUP assessments.[30] They measured MUP duration and amplitude from paper records of EMG activity, whereas nowadays the MUPs are automatically analyzed on the screen. Using this modified manual-MUP analysis the highest number of MUPs (up to 10) can be obtained from the muscle site at low levels of activity (at higher levels of activation the baseline becomes unsteady). It takes 2–3 min for each site to be analyzed. This technique is demanding for the operator, because reproducible MUPs have to be identified, the one with the smoothest

baseline chosen, and, in most cases, the duration cursors set manually, which inevitably introduces personal bias.[24]

The introduction of the trigger and delay unit led to its widespread use in analysis of individual MUPs.[31] On applying this technique, during a constant level of EMG activity, the trigger unit is set on a steadily firing MUP. This approach is particularly useful for detection of late MUP components, and then inclusion into MUP duration measurement. The number of MUPs at each site depends on the version of the technique used. In some systems only the highest amplitude MUP can be triggered, which enables sampling of only 1–3 MUPs from each examination site. Single-MUP analysis is time consuming, provides fewer MUPs than the other two described techniques, and is biased towards high amplitude and high threshold MUPs. Furthermore, it is also prone to personal bias.[24]

The recent and sophisticated CNEMG techniques are available only on advanced EMG systems; such is the template operated multi-MUP analysis (Figures 40.3 and 40.4).[32] The needle must be located so that a 'crisp' sounding pattern of EMG activity can be heard over the loudspeaker, indicating that the needle electrode is near to muscle fibers. Then, during an appropriate level of EMG activity, the operator starts the analysis and the computer takes the previous (last) 4.8 s period of the signal. From that signal MUPs are automatically extracted, quantified, and sorted into up to six classes. MUP classes, representing consecutive discharges of a particular MUP, are then averaged and presented (see Figures 40.3 and 40.4). Cursors are set automatically using a computer algorithm that, in addition to certain amplitude deflection, demands the minimum angle of the MUP trace towards the baseline.[32] After acquisition, the operator has to edit the MUPs. Thus, from each examination site up to six different MUPs can be obtained.[24,32,33] Multi-MUP analysis is the fastest and the easiest to apply of the three quantitative MUP analysis techniques mentioned. It can be applied at continuous activity during sphincter muscle relaxation, as well as at slight to moderate levels of activation.[13,24] The multi-MUP technique has (like single-MUP analysis) difficulties with highly unstable and/or polyphasic MUPs. It often fails to sample them, sorts the same MUP to several classes (recognizes it as different MUPs – duplicates), cuts prolonged MUPs into two, or distorts them by averaging. The MUPs with unsteady baseline (unclear beginning or end) need to be recognized and deleted.[29] The multi-MUP technique samples a slightly lower number of MUPs per muscle compared with the manual-MUP technique.[24]

In the small half of the sphincter muscle, collecting 10 different MUPs has been said to be a minimal requirement on using single-MUP analysis. Using manual-MUP and multi-MUP techniques, sampling of 20 MUPs (standard number in limb muscles) from each EAS muscle presents no problem in healthy controls and most patients (see Figures 40.3B).[24] Normative data obtained from the EAS muscle by standardized EMG technique using all these three MUP analyses have been published.[24] Analysis made from the same taped EMG signal, using reference data for mean values and outliers[34] (see Figure 40.4), revealed similar sensitivity of manual-MUP, single-MUP, and multi-MUP analysis for detecting neuropathic changes in the EAS muscle of patients with chronic cauda equina lesions.[24]

A number of MUP parameters are used in the diagnosis of neuromuscular disease (see Figure 40.5). Traditionally, MUP amplitude and duration were measured, and the number of phases was counted.[30] In a study comparing the sensitivity of individual MUP parameters for differentiating normal from neuropathic sphincter muscles of patients with chronic lesion to the cauda equina, area was the most sensitive, followed by the number of turns, and size index. A high correlation between MUP parameters was also shown in the same study, which points to probable redundancy of using all available MUP parameters.[35]

Indeed, a recent study performed in the EAS muscle revealed that probably only the parameters of area, duration,

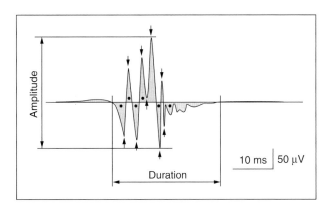

Figure 40.5
The motor unit potential (MUP) parameters. Amplitude is the voltage difference (μV) between the most positive and most negative point of the MUP trace. The MUP duration is the time (ms) between the first deflection and the point when the MUP waveform finally returns to the baseline. The number of MUP phases (small circles) is defined by the number of MUP areas (see below) alternately below and above the baseline, and can be counted as the 'number of baseline crossings plus one'. Turns (arrows) are defined as changes in direction of the MUP trace that are larger than the specified amplitude (100 μV). The MUP area measures the integrated surface of the MUP waveform (shaded).

and the number of turns are needed in MUP analysis. Other MUP parameters (amplitude, the number of phases, duration of the negative peak, thickness, size index) appear to be redundant, and their use might reduce specificity of MUP analysis.[36]

The MUP area is measured as the total surface between the MUP trace and the baseline of the EMG signal (msμV) (see Figure 40.5). It is largely determined by the activity of muscle fibers within a 2.0 mm radius to the recording concentric needle electrode.[37]

The MUP duration is the time (ms) between the first deflection and the point when the MUP waveform finally returns to the baseline (see Figure 40.5). It depends on the number of muscle fibers of a particular MU within 2.5 mm diameter and is little affected by the proximity of the recording electrode to the nearest fiber.[37] The difficulty with the duration measurement is in defining the beginning and end of the MUP. During manual positioning of duration cursors, amplifier gain is crucial: at higher gain, MUPs seem longer.[38] It is unclear whether to include late components (satellite potentials) into MUP duration or not. Late components are defined as the part of MUP starting at least 3 ms after the end of the main spike of the MUP.[38] Although it was agreed not to include them into MUP duration measurement,[38,39] it seems that their exclusion might reduce the sensitivity of MUP analysis, at least in MSA.[40] However, no valid normative data for MUP parameters with inclusion of late components have been published.

A turn is defined as a change in direction of the MUP trace, which is larger than specified amplitude (100 μV) (Figure 40.5). The number of MUP turns cannot distinguish between neuropathic and myopathic muscles, but this is not relevant in the EAS muscle since myopathy confined exclusively to the striated sphincter muscles is unknown.

In addition to continuous firing of low-threshold MUPs in sphincters, additional high-threshold MUPs[13] are recruited voluntarily and reflexly (see Figure 40.4B). By such maneuvers, the amount of recruitable MUs is estimated. Normally, MUPs should intermingle to produce a dense IP on the oscilloscope screen when muscle is contracted well, and during a strong cough.

The IP can be assessed using a number of automatic quantitative analyses, the turn/amplitude analysis being the most popular.[41] However, quantitative IP analysis was shown to be only half as sensitive as the MUP analysis techniques in distinguishing between normal and neuropathic muscles.[24] However, with the needle electrode in focus, qualitative assessment of IP during voluntary or reflex muscle contraction by coughing is recommended.

In summary, template-based multi-MUP analysis is as sensitive as the traditional MUP analysis techniques,[24] fast (5–10 min per muscle), easy to apply, less prone to personal bias, and is a clinically useful technique.[27] In the EAS muscle its use is further facilitated by the availability of common normative data, which are unaffected by age, gender,[42] number and characteristics of vaginal deliveries,[33] mild chronic constipation,[43] or EAS muscle examined (the subcutaneous or the deeper).[17] All these make multi-MUP analysis the technique of choice for quantitative analysis of the EAS reinnervation.

Single fiber electromyography

The aim of single fiber electromyography (SFEMG) testing is similar to CNEMG – to differentiate normal from abnormal striated muscle. The SFEMG electrode has similar external proportions to a concentric needle electrode, but instead of having the recording surface at the tip, a fine insulated platinum or silver wire embedded in epoxy resin is exposed through an aperture on the side 1–5 mm behind the tip. The platinum wire forms the recording surface, and has a diameter of 25 μm. It will pick up activity from within a hemispherical volume of 0.3 mm in diameter. This is very much smaller than the volume of muscle tissue from which a concentric needle electrode records, which has an uptake area of 2.5 mm diameter. Because of the arrangement of muscle fibers in a normal MU, an SFEMG needle will record only 1–3 single muscle fibers from the same MU. When recording with an SFEMG needle, the amplifier filters are set so that low-frequency activity is eliminated (500 Hz to 10 kHz). Thus, the contribution

of each muscle fiber appears as a short biphasic positive–negative action potential.

The SFEMG parameter that reflects MU morphology is the fiber density, which is defined as the mean number of muscle fibers belonging to an individual MU per detection site. To assemble these data, recordings from 20 different intramuscular detection sites are necessary.[44] The normal fiber density for the EAS is below 2.0.[45,46] Changes with age have been reported,[47] showing women to have significantly greater fiber density than men.[46]

The fiber density is increased in reinnervated muscle. The technique has been particularly applied to sphincter muscles in order to correlate increased fiber density findings to incontinence.[48] Due to its technical characteristics, SFEMG electrode is able to record even small changes that occur in MUs due to reinnervation, but is less suitable to detect changes due to denervation itself (i.e. abnormal insertion and spontaneous denervation activity).

The SFEMG electrode is also most suitable to record any instability of MUPs, although this is not routinely assessed in pelvic floor muscles for diagnostic purposes. The instability is revealed as jitter, which is defined as the variability with consecutive discharges of the interpotential interval between two muscle fiber action potentials belonging to the same MU. It may be increased not only in diseases affecting neuromuscular transmission but also by recent reinnervation.

Single fiber electromyography vs concentric needle electromyography

Quantified CNEMG provides the same information on reinnervation changes in muscle as the SFEMG parameter of fiber density,[49,50] but, in addition, CNEMG will reveal spontaneous denervation activity. In muscle after severe partial denervation, the areas of fibrosis are silent to EMG exploration, and the results are based only on the remaining MUP activity. The remaining innervated muscle is easier to establish with CNEMG, which records from a larger volume of tissue. Furthermore, a CNEMG examination can be extended in the same diagnostic session from, for example, lumbar and upper sacral myotomes to the lower sacral myotomes, after a cauda equina lesion. A concentric electrode can also be employed at the same diagnostic session for recording evoked direct and reflex muscle responses. SFEMG electrodes are more sophisticated, and as a consequence much more expensive. In contrast to CNEMG electrodes, no disposable SFEMG electrodes are available.

Use of CNEMG is the method of choice in routine examination of skeletal muscle, and is generally available in clinical neurophysiology laboratories, whereas SFEMG is not so widely used. As a consequence, SFEMG, although an established electrodiagnostic technique, is not recommended for clinical electrophysiological evaluation of patients with neurogenic bladders.

Sacral reflexes

The term sacral reflex refers to electrophysiologically recordable responses of pelvic floor muscles to (electrical) stimulation of sensory fibers in the uro-genito-anal region. In the lower sacral segments there are two common clinically elicited reflexes, the anal and the BCR. Both have the afferent and the efferent limb of their reflex arc in the pudendal nerve, and are centrally integrated at the S2 to S4 cord levels. Electrophysiological correlates of these reflexes have been described.

Measurements of latencies and amplitudes of reflex responses and evoked potentials, including sympathetic skin responses, relate not only to conduction in peripheral and central neural pathways but also to transmission across synapses and within networks of central nervous system interneurons. Therefore, conduction may be influenced by factors that are not apparent from a simplified anatomical model (see Figure 40.1). For example, changes in the threshold, amplitude, and latency of the BCR occur as a consequence of changes in the physiological state of the bladder,[51,52] and differ in pathological conditions (i.e. suprasacral spinal cord lesions).[53]

The aim of electrophysiological testing of sacral reflexes is to assess integrity of the sacral (S2–S4) spinal reflex arc, and to evaluate excitation levels of sacral spinal cord motor neurons.

It is possible to use electrical,[54,55] mechanical,[56,57] or magnetic[58] stimulation. Whereas the latter two modalities have only been applied to the penis and clitoris, electrical stimulation can be applied at various sites: to the dorsal penile/clitoral nerve, perianally, and (using a catheter-mounted ring electrode) at bladder neck/proximal urethra.[59] In clinical practice, electrical and mechanical stimulation of the penis or clitoris can be used (Figure 40.6), so this will be discussed in some detail.

The sacral reflex evoked on the dorsal penile or the clitoral nerve stimulation was shown to be a complex response, often comprising two components (Figure 40.7). The first component, with latency of about 33 ms, is the response that has been most often called the BCR. It is stable, does not habituate, and is based on variability of single motor neuron latency reflex discharges; it is thought to be an oligosynaptic reflex. The second component has a similar latency to the sacral reflexes evoked by stimulation perianally or from the proximal urethra. The variability of single motor neuron reflex responses within this component is much larger, as is typical for a polysynaptic reflex.[10] The second component is not always demonstrable as a discrete response. Double electrical stimuli may be used to facilitate the reflex response when both components cannot be elicited using single electrical pulses.[60]

Sacral reflex responses recorded with needle or wire electrodes can be analyzed separately for each side of the

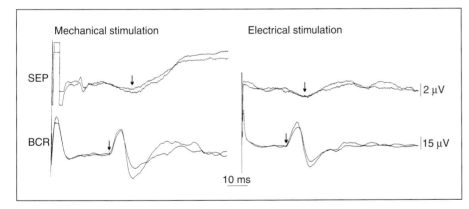

Figure 40.6

Bulbocavernosus reflex (BCR) responses and pudendal somatosensory evoked potentials (SEP) recorded simultaneously in a 9-year-old boy (body height 140 cm), without uroneurological abnormalities. Responses were elicited by consecutive (left) mechanical stimulation (nonpainful squeeze of the penis by the electromechanical hammer) and (right) electrical stimulation (single 20 V stimuli over the dorsal penile nerves). Responses were detected by bifocal montage of the surface electrodes (BCR, active electrode over the external anal sphincter muscle/reference electrode over the bulbocavernosus muscle; SEP, active electrode 2 cm behind Cz/reference electrode on Fz both over the scalp according to the International 10–20 electroencephalography (EEG) System).[68] Measurements were obtained by averaging 100 responses. Latencies to the beginning of the BCR responses (arrows) were 33.4 ms and 25.2 ms; latencies to the first positive peak (P40) (arrowheads) were 47.0 ms and 36.7 ms on mechanical and electrical stimulation, respectively. Peak-to-peak amplitudes of the BCR responses were 69 μV and 63 μV; amplitude of P40 measured 2.0 μV and 1.8 μV on mechanical and electrical stimulation, respectively. Note similar amplitudes but pronounced differences in latency measurements caused by mechanical characteristics of electromechanical hammer used in this study. Latency of the pudendal SEP on electrical stimulation in this child was already within (Z = −1.9) normative limits for adults (41 ± 2.3 ms).[69]

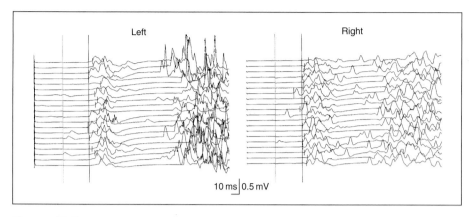

Figure 40.7

Findings of uroneurophysiological examination in a 32-year-old man 2 months after traumatic fracture of pubic bones and urethral rupture. After surgical repair of urethra, the patient continued to leak urine and complained of moderate erectile dysfunction. His bowel function was normal. On concentric needle electromyography (CNEMG) during relaxation some spontaneous denervation activity was detected in the left, but not the right bulbocavernosus muscle. On reflex and voluntary activation, normal motor unit potentials (MUPs) were recruited. In addition, normal bulbocavernosus reflex (BCR) responses were elicited by electrical stimulation (single 80 mA stimuli over dorsal penile nerves), and CNEMG electrode detection in the left and right bulbocavernosus muscles. Left and right latency of the first component of the BCR: 29 ms (marked by solid vertical line). Note also the second component of the BCR. Electrophysiological examination thus confirmed the integrity of the neural structures, and revealed only very slight axonal damage to the left pudendal nerve. Such mild damage could not result in prominent urinary incontinence reported by patient. This was probably due to direct damage to the bladder neck, urethra, or possibly urethral sphincter or its terminal innervation. Similarly, erectile dysfunction was most probably caused by local injury and not by more proximal nervous lesion.

EAS or each bulbocavernosus muscle (see Figure 40.7). Using unilateral dorsal penile nerve blocks, the existence of two unilateral BCR arcs has been demonstrated.[61] Thus, by detection from the left and right bulbocavernosus (and probably also the EAS) muscles, separate testing of both BCR arcs can be performed. Sensitivity of the test can be increased also by use of the inter-side latency difference (normative limits in case of simultaneous bilateral detection: <3 ms).[61] This is important, because in cases of unilateral (sacral plexopathy, pudendal neuropathy) or asymmetrical lesions (cauda equina), which are common, a healthy BCR arc may obscure a pathological one. Similarly, using mechanical stimulation (light touch or pinprick) of the perianal area on each side, with needle detection from the subcutaneous EAS muscles of each side (left and right) during the CNEMG, a separate testing of both reflex arcs can be performed. In the authors' laboratories, testing of BCR on electrical stimulation is performed in conjunction with a CNEMG if no brisk reflex response is present on mechanical stimulation of the perianal/perineal region and recording from the EAS muscle.[26]

Standardization of the technique has been proposed.[1] It was recommended that surface stimulation electrodes be placed on the penis/clitoris, and 10 single, 0.2 ms long stimuli be applied at supramaximal intensity at time intervals of 2 s (=0.5 Hz). Recording is by concentric needle or surface electrodes placed into/over the EAS, or bulbocavernosus

muscle in men, using filters: 10 Hz to 10 kHz; sweep speed, 10 ms/div; and gain, 50–1000 μV/div. Onset latency is the only parameter measured.[1]

Sacral reflex responses on stimulation of the dorsal penile and clitoral nerve have been said to be of value in patients with cauda equina and other LMN lesions, although it is recognized that a reflex with a normal latency does not exclude the possibility of an axonal lesion in its reflex arc (see Figure 40.7). The sensitivity and specificity of sacral reflex responses in patients with conditions associated with neurogenic bladders are not known. In diabetics the nerve conduction studies performed in limbs are more sensitive in revealing peripheral neuropathy than sacral reflex latencies.

Abnormally short latency of BCR has been claimed to suggest either the abnormally low position of conus medullaris in tethered cord syndrome[62] or a suprasacral cord lesion.[63]

Mechanical stimulation has been used to elicit BCR in both sexes[56] and has been found to be a robust technique. Either a standard commercially available reflex hammer or a customized electromechanical hammer can be employed. Such stimulation is painless and can be used in children.[57] The latency of the mechanically elicited BCR is comparable to that elicited electrically. Differences are caused by the somewhat longer pathway for mechanically evoked stimulation (stimulates receptors instead of peripheral nerve) as well as by the variability in the time course of the mechanical stimulation device (see Figure 40.6).[57]

Recently, responses of the bulbocavernosus muscle after mechanical suprapubic stimulation were also described.[64] It was hypothesized that this is a polysynaptic reflex elicited by the stimulation of the bladder wall tensoreceptors, which could be involved in pathogenesis of detrusor-sphincter dyssynergia in some patients with neurogenic bladders.[64]

Sacral reflex testing should be a part of the diagnostic battery of which CNEMG exploration of the pelvic floor muscles is the most important part. Electrophysiological assessment of sacral reflexes is a more quantitative, sensitive, and reproducible way of assessing the S2–S4 reflex arcs than any of the clinical methods.[65] The results, however, should be interpreted with caution, always being mindful of the clinical context.

Pudendal somatosensory evoked potentials

The pudendal SEP is easily recorded following electrical stimulation of the dorsal penile or clitoral nerve.[66,67] This response is, as a rule, of highest amplitudes at the central recording site (Cz – 2 cm: Fz of the International 10–20 electroencephalography (EEG) System)[68] and is highly reproducible (see Figure 40.6). Amplitudes of the P40 measure 0.5–12 μV. The first positive peak at 41 ± 2.3 ms (called P1 or P40) is usually clearly defined in healthy subjects using a stimulus 2–4 times stronger than sensory threshold current strength.[69] Later negative (at around 55 ms) and then further positive waves are interindividually quite variable in amplitude and expression and, furthermore, have little known clinical relevance.

Pudendal SEP recordings on penile/clitoral stimulation are sometimes useful in patients with sensory loss in the lower sacral dermatomes, and brisk BCR on clinical examination such that an UMN lesion is suspected.[26] Pudendal SEPs were recorded in patients with neurogenic bladder dysfunction due to multiple sclerosis but it is now known that in this clinical situation the tibial cerebral SEPs are more often abnormal than the pudendal SEP, and only in exceptional cases is the pudendal SEP abnormal but the tibial normal, suggesting an isolated conus involvement.[70] Pudendal SEP measurements were also measured in patients with neurogenic bladders due to spinal cord lesions and diabetes. Pathological pudendal SEPs seemed to predict poor surgical outcomes after resection of a tight filum terminale.[71]

A study that looked at the value of the pudendal SEP for detecting relevant neurological disease when investigating urogenital symptoms found it to be of lesser value than a clinical examination looking for signs of spinal cord disease in the lower limbs (i.e. lower limb hyper-reflexia and extensor plantar responses).[72] However, there may be circumstances, such as when a patient is complaining of loss of bladder or vaginal sensation, where it is reassuring to be able to record a normal pudendal SEP. The method as such is valid and robust, but its clinical value, particularly in the investigation of incontinence, is minimal.

Uroneurophysiological tests that are not of diagnostic value in individual patients with neurogenic bladders

Neurophysiology of the sacral motor system

Motor nerve conduction studies

Recording of the muscle response (compound motor action potential or M-wave)[39] on electrical stimulation of its motor nerve is the routine method of electrophysiological evaluation of limb nerves. By stimulating the nerve at two levels, motor nerve conduction velocity can be calculated, which distinguishes between lesions of myelin and axons causing motor weakness. For this purpose, however, the technique requires access to the nerve at two well-separated points for stimulation and measurement of the distance between them, a requirement which cannot be easily met in the pelvis. Thus, the only electrophysiological parameter of motor conduction that can be measured also in the pelvic floor is the pudendal nerve terminal motor latency (PNTML).

Latency measures the fastest-conducting fibers, but give little or no information about the loss of biological units generating electrical currents (axons, etc.), which is the determinant of functional importance. However, latencies depend less on irrelevant biological and technical factors, and are therefore more robust measurements than evoked potentials or reflex studies. On the other hand, the amplitude of the compound potential correlates with the number of activated biological units. (A conduction block and pathological dispersion of conduction velocities within a neural pathway also affect amplitudes.) Amplitudes are thus the more relevant physiological parameter, but M-wave amplitudes of the EAS, US, or other pelvic floor muscles on stimulation of the pudendal nerves have unfortunately not yet proved contributory.

PNTML is usually measured by stimulation with a special surface electrode assembly fixed on a gloved index finger – the St Mark's electrode.[73] This consists of a bipolar stimulating electrode fixed to the tip of the gloved finger, with the recording electrode pair placed 8 cm proximally on the base of the finger. The finger is inserted into the rectum. Stimulation of the pudendal nerve is performed close to the ischial spine and the recording is performed from the EAS muscle. Using this stimulator, the PNTML for the anal sphincter MEP is typically around 2 ms.

Prolongation of the PNTML measured by the St Mark's electrode was found in a variety of patient groups, and was taken as a sign of damage to the pudendal nerve. This has led to the term pudendal neuropathy, which is used particularly by coloproctologists. Some workers less familiar with theoretical principles of clinical neurophysiology equate a prolongation of PNTML with pelvic floor denervation. This, however, is mistaken, as prolongation of latency is a poor measure of denervation, as already explained. What type of abnormality this latency prolongation indicates is unclear, as there have not been any relevant morphological studies.

Delays of PNTML in patient groups, even when present, were short – approximately 0.1–0.3 ms – and it is unlikely that these represent a functionally relevant change.

In practice, the PNTML is unhelpful for diagnosis in individual patients with sacral dysfunction.[74–76] Elicitability of a compound motor action potential in pelvic floor muscles (using the perianal stimulation) may be helpful in patients with combined UMN and LMN lesions in whom no MUP activity can be recorded. In this situation the presence of compound motor action potential rules out complete peripheral (axonal) lesion.

Anterior sacral root (cauda equina) stimulation

Transcutaneous stimulation of deeply situated nervous tissue became possible with the development of special electrical and magnetic stimulators. When applied over the spine at the exit from the vertebral canal, spinal roots can be stimulated, and there have been reports of these techniques applied to the sacral roots.[59,77,78]

Electrical or magnetic stimulation depolarizes underlying neural structures in a nonselective fashion, and concomitant activation of several muscles innervated by lumbosacral segments occurs. It has been shown that responses from gluteal muscles may contaminate attempts to record from the sphincters and lead to error.[79] Thus, surface recordings from sphincter muscles are inadvisable.

Recording of MEP with magnetic stimulation has been less successful than with electrical stimulation, at least with standard coils, and there are often large stimulus artifacts. Positioning of the ground electrode between the recording electrodes and the stimulating coil may decrease the artifact.[80]

Demonstrating the presence of a perineal MEP on stimulation over lumbosacral spine and recording with a CNEMG electrode may occasionally be helpful, but an absent response has to be evaluated with caution. The clinical value of the test has yet to be established.

Assessment of central motor pathways

Using the same magnetic or electrical stimulation it has been shown to be possible to stimulate the motor cortex and record a response from the pelvic floor. Magnetic stimulation is not painful and cortical electrical stimulation is nowadays only used for intraoperative monitoring. The aim of these techniques is to assess conduction in the central motor pathways.

By electrical stimulation over the motor cortex of healthy subjects, MEPs in the EAS,[79,80] the US,[81] and the bulbocavernosus[79] muscles were reported. The mean latencies were 30–35 ms if no facilitatory maneuver was used. If, however, stimulation is performed during a period of slight voluntary contraction of the muscle of interest, the latencies of MEPs shortened significantly (for up to 8 ms), as has been shown in limb muscles.

By applying stimulation both over the scalp and in the back (at level L1), and subtracting the latency of the respective MEPs, a central conduction time (i.e. time of conduction in central motor pathways from the motor cortex) could be obtained. Central conduction times of approximately 22 ms without, and about 15 ms with, the facilitation (i.e. slight voluntary contraction) have been reported.[77]

Substantially longer central conduction time in patients with multiple sclerosis and spinal cord lesions as compared to healthy controls have been found,[78] but as all those patients had clinically recognizable cord disease, the diagnostic contribution of the technique remains doubtful.

A well-formed sphincter MEP with a normal latency in a patient with a functional disorder or a medicolegal case may occasionally be helpful, but there is no established clinical use for this type of testing.

Neurophysiology of the sacral sensory system

Electroneurography of the dorsal penile nerve

Electroneurography of the dorsal penile nerve is used to assess sensory nerve conduction of lower sacral segments. Theoretically, normal amplitude sensory nerve action potential (SNAP) of dorsal penile nerves in an insensitive penis distinguishes a lesion of sensory pathways proximal to the dorsal spinal ganglion (central pathways, cauda equina) from a lesion of and distal to ganglion (sacral plexus, pudendal nerves). By placing a pair of stimulating electrodes across the penile glans and a pair of recording electrodes across the base of the penis a SNAP can be recorded (with amplitude of about 10 μV). The sensory conduction velocity of the dorsal penile nerve has been reported as 27 m/s. The method was claimed to be helpful in diagnosing neurogenic erectile dysfunction as a consequence of sensory penile neuropathy,[82] but the problems of measuring the conduction distance pose considerable practical difficulties and the test is rarely used.

More practical seems to be the method of stimulating the pudendal nerve by the St Mark's electrode transrectally, and recording from the penis.[83]

Electroneurography of dorsal sacral roots

SNAPs on stimulation of dorsal penile and clitoral nerves may be recorded intraoperatively when the sacral roots are exposed. This has been found helpful in preserving roots relevant for perineal sensation in spastic children undergoing dorsal rhizotomy and possibly decreasing the incidence of postoperative voiding dysfunction.[84] At the level of lower thoracic and upper lumbar vertebrae a low-amplitude (<1 μV) spinal SEP can be recorded with surface electrodes. It is a monophasic negative potential with a mean peak latency of about 12.5 ms[69] and is probably due to postsynaptic activity in the spinal cord. Responses using surface electrodes are often unrecordable in obese healthy men[77] and in many women.

With epidural electrodes, sacral root potentials on stimulation of the dorsal penile nerve could only be recorded in 13, and cord potentials in 9 out of 22 subjects; latencies of these spinal SEPs were 11.9 ± 1.8 ms,[85] substantiating the results obtained by surface recording.[69]

No use of such recordings out of the operating room has been established.

Cerebral somatosensory evoked potentials on electrical stimulation of urethra, bladder, and anal canal

These responses are claimed to be more relevant to neurogenic bladder dysfunction than the pudendal SEP, as the Aδ sensory afferents from bladder and proximal urethra, which convey impulses from these regions, accompany the autonomic fibers in the pelvic nerves (see above).

Cerebral SEP can be obtained on stimulation of the bladder urothelium. When making such measurements, it is of utmost importance to use bipolar stimulation in the bladder or proximal urethra, because otherwise

somatic afferents are depolarized due to spread of electrical current. These cerebral SEPs have been shown to have maximum amplitude over the midline (Cz – 2 cm: Fz) but even so may be of low amplitude (1 μV and less) and variable configuration, making it difficult to identify the response in some control subjects. The typical latency of the most prominent negative potential (N1) is about 100 ms.[86]

However, clinical usefulness of such recordings has not been established.

Autonomic nervous system tests

All of the neurophysiological methods for evaluation of the neurogenic bladder discussed so far assess the thicker myelinated fibers only, whereas it is the autonomic nervous system, the parasympathetic part in particular, which is the most relevant for bladder function. Although in most instances local involvement of the sacral nervous system (such as due to trauma or compression) will usually involve both somatic and autonomic fibers together, there are some local pathological conditions that cause isolated lesions of the autonomic nervous system, such as mesorectal excision of carcinoma[87] or prostatectomy.[88] In addition, several types of peripheral neuropathy preferentially affect thin autonomic fibers. Methods assessing the parasympathetic and sympathetic systems directly would thus be very helpful. Information on parasympathetic bladder innervation can to some extent be obtained by cystometry, which, however, is a test of overall organ function and usually cannot locate the lesion. Although not strictly an electrophysiological test, thermal sensory testing was found useful in assessment of the thin sensory nerve fibers from sacral segments,[88,89] which are often affected concomitantly with thin autonomic fibers.

Sympathetic skin response

The sympathetic nervous system mediates sweat gland activity in the skin. On stressful stimulation a potential shift can be recorded with surface electrodes from the skin of palms and soles, and has been reported to be a useful parameter in assessment of neuropathy involving unmyelinated nerve fibers. The response, SSR, can also be recorded from perineal skin and from the penis. The SSR is a reflex that consists of myelinated sensory fibers, a complex central integrative mechanism, and a sympathetic efferent limb (with postganglionic nonmyelinated C fibers).[90] The stimulus used in clinical practice is usually an electrical pulse delivered to the upper or lower limb (to mixed nerves), but the genital organs can also be stimulated. The latencies of SSR on the penis following stimulation of a median nerve at the wrist have been reported as between 1.5[91] and 2.3 s[92] and could be obtained in all normal subjects with a large variability. The responses rapidly habituate, and depend on a number of endogenous and exogenous factors, including skin temperature, which should be above 28°C. Only an absent SSR can be taken as abnormal.

There is no consensus on the clinical value of SSR testing in sacral dysfunction.

Corpus cavernosum electromyography

Electrodiagnostic tests of sacral parasympathetic nerve function, as for instance corpus cavernosum EMG, also called spontaneous cavernosal activity,[93] would in principle constitute the most definitive indicator of neurogenic sacral organ involvement. Further research to validate this and other potentially useful methods such as detrusor EMG will clarify their place in both research and diagnostics; currently, these tests cannot be suggested for patient diagnosis.

Patient groups with neurogenic bladders in whom uroneurophysiological tests are of clinical value

Parkinsonism

Neuropathic changes can be recorded in sphincter muscles of patients with multiple system atrophy (MSA).[19,29,50,94–97] Multiple system atrophy is a progressive neurodegenerative disease, which is often (particularly in its early stages) mistaken for Parkinson's disease. Urinary incontinence in both genders, and erectile dysfunction in men are early features of the condition, often present for some years before the onset of typical neurological features.[96] Autonomic failure causing postural hypotension and cerebellar ataxia causing unsteadiness and clumsiness may be additional features. The disease is usually (in 80% of patients) unresponsive to antiparkinsonian treatment. As a part of the neurodegenerative process, loss of motor neurons occurs in Onuf's nucleus, so that partial but progressive denervation of the sphincter and the bulbocavernosus muscles occurs[19] and recorded MUPs show changes of reinnervation.[29,95]

Sphincter EMG has been demonstrated to be of value in distinguishing between idiopathic Parkinson's disease and MSA,[29,95] but may not be sensitive in the early phase of the

disease,[19] and not specific after 5 years of parkinsonism.[97] Prolonged duration of MUPs[29,95] abnormal spontaneous activity,[94] as well as diminished number of continuously active low-threshold MUs and IP abnormalities[98] have been described EMG markers for degeneration of Onuf's nucleus occurring in patients with MSA. The changes of chronic reinnervation may be found in other parkinsonian syndromes such as progressive supranuclear palsy (PSP),[99] in whom neuronal loss in Onuf's nucleus was also demonstrated histologically.[100] Chronic reinnervation changes can also be demonstrated as an increase in fiber density on SFEMG.[50] In contrast to previous reports, a recent study failed to demonstrate significant differences between two small groups of MSA and Parkinson disease patients.[98] This might be a consequence of excluding late components from MUP duration, which was made also in another study that did not find MUP analysis useful.[94] In a small number of patients with MSA or primary autonomic failure, the EAS muscle CNEMG was reported sensitive and specific for men, but nonspecific for women, in supporting a diagnosis of MSA.[101] Kinesiological EMG performed during urodynamics can also be valuable in Parkinson's disease[19] and in MSA[20] patients documenting loss of coordination between detrusor and US muscles (detrusor-sphincter dyssynergia).

CNEMG includes observation of denervation activity[94] and quantitative MUP analysis,[29,95] and is clearly indicated in patients with suspected MSA, particularly in the early stages of the disease.[97] If the test is normal early in the disease, but suspicion of the disease persists, it might be of value to repeat the test at some later date.[19]

Cauda equina and conus medullaris lesions and spinal dysrhaphisms

Lesions to the cauda equina and/or conus medullaris are an important cause of pelvic floor dysfunction. Usually the neural tissue damage is caused by compression within the spinal canal due to disc protrusion, spinal fractures, epidural hematomas, tumors, congenital malformations, etc. Unfortunately, accidental damage to cauda equina may occur during surgical interventions, mainly on lumbar discs.

Patient presentation depends very much on the etiology of the lesion. In cases of disc protrusion, spinal fractures, and epidural hematomas, presentation is often dramatic. Acute severe back pain radiating to legs, associated by numbness and tingling in legs (particularly posterior aspects of thighs), buttocks, and perineal region are noted first. Urinary retention with overflow incontinence and, later, severe constipation follow. When damage is due to disc protrusion, history of previous back pain with sciatica, in spinal fractures the history of trauma, and in epidural hematomas of coagulation disorder, anticoagulation therapy, or recent spinal surgery is usually present. With tumors, the presentation of the cauda equina lesion is much more insidious.

After detailed clinical examination of the perineal region (with particular emphasis on perianal sensation), CNEMG of the EAS muscle (and sometimes bulbocavernosus muscle – see below) and electrophysiological evaluation of BCR (when absent clinically) need to be considered.[26]

Generally stated, detection of pathological spontaneous activity by CNEMG has good sensitivity and specificity to reveal moderate and severe partial denervation, and complete denervation, of pelvic floor muscles 3 weeks or more after injury to the cauda equina and/or conus medullaris (see Figure 40.3A). Traumatic lesions to the lumbosacral spine or particularly to the pelvis are probably the only acquired condition where complete denervation of the perineal muscles can be observed. (Complete denervation of all EAS muscles was present in 9% of men with cauda equina/conus medullaris lesions.)[27] Most other lesions will, by contrast, cause partial denervation. CNEMG of the bulbocavernosus muscles is of particular importance a few weeks after partial denervation in the lower sacral myotomes to detect spontaneous denervation activity.[26]

CNEMG (MUP analysis) can show changes of reinnervation, which appear months after injury.[24] Following a cauda equina lesion, the MUPs are likely to be prolonged and polyphasic,[102] and other MUP parameters are also increased (see Figures 40.3A and 40.4B).[24,27] Similar marked changes are seen in patients with lumbosacral myelomeningocele. EMG was found to contribute to prediction of functional outcome in children with spina bifida.[103]

BCR is useful in evaluation of subjects with cauda equina and/or conus medullaris lesions to assess the integrity of the reflex arc. In patients with a tethered cord syndrome measurement of BCR latency can be of additional value, as a very short reflex latency in this clinical situation supports the possibility of the abnormally low position of the conus medullaris.[62] Although in patients with a normal position of conus medullaris urodynamic studies better predicted occurrence of a tight filum terminale, pathological pudendal SEPs correlated with poor surgical outcomes.[71]

Electrophysiological assessment is useful to determine the sequels of the lesion, and in insidious cases for reaching the diagnosis.

Sacral plexus and pudendal nerve lesions

Neurological lesions located in the sacral plexus and pudendal nerves are less common than lesions of the cauda equina or conus medullaris. They can be caused by pelvic fractures,[104] hip surgery,[104] complicated deliveries,[105] malignant infiltration, local radiotherapy,[106] and by use of

orthopedic traction tables.[107] They are more often unilateral. In principle, one can distinguish between such a lesion and a cauda equina or the conus medullaris lesions by unilateral absence of dorsal penile SNAP, and absent spontaneous denervation activity in the paravertebral muscles. However, both of these tests are difficult to perform (due to difficult unilateral dorsal penile/clitoral nerve stimulation, and absent paravertebral muscles in the lower sacral segments, respectively), so localization of the lesion will usually be made clinically, or in the case of extensive sacral plexus lesions, by examination of the first sacral and lower lumbar segments.

Urinary retention in women

For many years it was said that isolated urinary retention in young women was due either to psychogenic factors or was the first symptom of onset of multiple sclerosis. However, CNEMG in this group has demonstrated that many such patients have profuse complex repetitive discharges (CRDs) and decelerating burst (DB) activity in the US muscle.[108]

Why this activity should occur is not known but in the syndrome described by one of the authors, it was associated with polycystic ovaries.[109] Most commonly, the initial episode of urinary retention is precipitated by a gynecological surgical procedure using general anesthesia, at the mean age of 28, and the condition does not progress to a general neurological disorder.[110] It was shown that this pathological spontaneous activity endures during micturition and may cause interrupted flow.[22] The disorder of sphincter relaxation appears to lead to secondary changes in detrusor function – either instability or failure of contractility.

Because CNEMG will detect both changes of denervation and reinnervation as occur with a cauda equina lesion (see above), as well as this peculiar abnormal spontaneous activity, it can be argued that this test is mandatory in women with urinary retention.[22,108] It should certainly be carried out before stigmatizing a woman as having psychogenic urinary retention.

Patient groups with neurogenic bladders in whom uroneurophysiological tests are of research interest

Uroneurophysiological techniques have been important in research, substantiated hypotheses that a proportion of patients with sacral dysfunction, such as stress urinary and idiopathic fecal incontinence, have involvement of the nervous system,[73,111] established the function of the sacral nervous system in patients with suprasacral spinal cord injury,[112] and revealed the consequences of particular surgeries.[113] However, in individual patients from these groups, uroneurophysiological tests are unlikely to be contributory.

Generalized peripheral neuropathies

Generalized peripheral neuropathies, particularly those that affect thin nerve fibers, can also cause neurogenic bladder. Most important causes of such neuropathies are diabetes mellitus and acute inflammatory demyelinizing polyneuropathy (AIDP or Guillain–Barré syndrome). Most of these neuropathies are length-dependent, with longer fibers first and more severely affected. As a consequence, electrophysiological tests applied on distal lower limb nerves will usually be more sensitive than when applied to nerves that innervate the perineal area/pelvic floor (see above).

Diseases of the central nervous system

Kinesiological tests, performed as a part of cystometric measurements, are often useful in patients with CNS signs having diagnosis of neurogenic bladder. Electrodiagnostic tests of conduction performed in patients with central lesions are only very occasionally indicated. PSEP were found to provide information of diagnostic relevance in the initial diagnostic evaluation of patients with multiple sclerosis, and was also suggested as a screening test for cystometric evaluation in this population.[114] CNEMG is not indicated in central lesions unless segmental spinal cord (conus medullaris) involvement[70] is suspected (see above).[1]

Conclusion

Several electrophysiological tests have been proposed for evaluation of the pelvic floor, the sphincter muscles, and their motor and sensory innervation. Although all tests mentioned in this chapter continue to be of research interest, it is particularly the CNEMG, which is of definite usefulness in everyday routine diagnostic evaluation of selected groups of patients with pelvic floor dysfunction, those with atypical parkinsonism, those with traumatic spinal and pelvic lesions, or young women with urinary retention.

It is expected that new computer-assisted techniques of CNEMG analysis will improve the usefulness of the test as

a diagnostic method to reveal neuropathic pelvic floor muscle involvement.

Further research into and experience with other discussed neurophysiological tests will reveal their contribution to clinical assessment of individual patients, which is presently unknown.

References

1. Fowler CJ, Benson JT, Craggs MD, Vodušek DB, Yang CC, Podnar S. Clinical neurophysiology. In: Abrams P, Cardozo L, Khoury S, Wein A, eds. Incontinence. Plymouth (UK) Health Publication Ltd., 2002; 8b:389–424.

2. Vodušek DB, Fowler CJ. Clinical neurophysiology. In Fowler CJ, ed. Neurology of bladder, bowel and sexual dysfunction. Boston: Butterworth-Heinemann, 1999: 109–143.

3. Fowler CJ, Sakakibara R, Frohman EM, et al, eds. Neurologic bladder, bowel and sexual dysfunction. Amsterdam: Elsevier Science, 2001.

4. Jorge JM, Wexner SD. Etiology and management of fecal incontinence. Dis Colon Rectum 1993; 36:77–97.

5. Agachan F, Chen T, Pfeifer J, et al. A constipation scoring system to simplify evaluation and management of constipated patients. Dis Colon Rectum 1996; 39:681–685.

6. Jackson S, Donovan J, Brookes S, et al. The Bristol Female Lower Urinary Tract Symptoms questionnaire: development and psychometric testing. Br J Urol 1996; 77:805–812.

7. Donovan JL, Peters TJ, Abrams P, et al. Scoring the short form ICSmaleSF questionnaire. International Continence Society. J Urol 2000; 164:1948–1955.

8. Rosen RC, Riley A, Wagner G, et al. An international index of erectile function (IIEF): a multidimensional scale for assessment of erectile dysfunction. Urology 1997; 49:822–830.

9. Quirk FH, Heiman JR, Rosen RC, et al. Development of a sexual function questionnaire for clinical trials of female sexual dysfunction. J Womens Health Gend Based Med 2002; 11:277–289.

10. Vodušek DB, Janko M. The bulbocavernosus reflex. A single motor neuron study. Brain 1990; 113:813–820.

11. Chantraine A, De Leval J, Depireux P. Adult female intra- and peri-urethral sphincter-electromyographic study. Neurourol Urodynam 1990; 9:139–144.

12. Mathers SE, Kempster PA, Swash M, Lees AJ. Constipation and paradoxical puborectalis contractions in anismus and Parkinson's disease; a dystonic phenomenon? J Neurol Neurosurg Psychiatry 1988; 51:1503–1507.

13. Podnar S, Vodušek DB. Standardization of anal sphincter EMG: low and high threshold motor units. Clin Neurophysiol 1999; 110:1488–1491.

14. Chantraine A, Leval J, Onkelinx A. Motor conduction velocity in the internal pudendal nerves. In: Desmedt JE, ed. New developments in electromyography and clinical neurophysiology, Vol. 2. Basel: Karger, 1973:433–438.

15. Jesel M, Isch-Treussard C, Isch F. Electromyography of striated muscle of anal urethral sphincters. In: Desmedt JE, ed. New developments in electromyography and clinical neurophysiology, Vol. 2. Basel: Karger, 1973:406–420.

16. Deindl FM, Vodušek DB, Hesse U, Schussler B. Activity patterns of pubococcygeal muscles in nulliparous continent women. Br J Urol 1993; 72:46–51.

17. Podnar S, Vodušek DB. Standardization of anal sphincter electromyography: uniformity of the muscle. Muscle Nerve 2000; 23:122–125.

18. Podnar S, Mrkaić M, Vodušek DB. Standardization of anal sphincter electromyography: quantification of continuous activity during relaxation. Neurourol Urodyn 2002; 21:540–545.

19. Stocchi F, Carbone A, Inghilleri M, et al. Urodynamic and neurophysiological evaluation in Parkinson's disease and multiple system atrophy. J Neurol Neurosurg Psychiatry 1997; 62:507–511.

20. Sakakibara R, Hattori T, Uchiyama T, et al. Urinary dysfunction and orthostatic hypotension in multiple system atrophy: which is the more common and earlier manifestation? J Neurol Neurosurg Psychiatry 2000; 68:65–69.

21. Chancellor MB, Kaplan SA, Blaivas JG. Detrusor-external sphincter dyssynergia. In: Bock G, Whelan J, eds. Neurobiology of incontinence. Chichester: John Wiley, 1990:195–213.

22. Deindl FM, Vodušek DB, Bischoff C, et al. Dysfunctional voiding in women: which muscles are responsible? Br J Urol 1998; 82:814–819.

23. Deindl FM, Vodušek DB, Hesse U, Schussler B. Pelvic floor activity patterns: comparison of nulliparous continent and parous urinary stress incontinent women. A kinesiological EMG study. Br J Urol 1994; 73:413–417.

24. Podnar S, Vodušek DB, Stålberg E. Comparison of quantitative techniques in anal sphincter electromyography. Muscle Nerve 2002; 25:83–92.

25. Podnar S, Rodi Z, Lukanovič A, Vodušek DB. Standardization of anal sphincter EMG: technique of needle examination. Muscle Nerve 1999; 22:400–403.

26. Podnar S, Vodušek DB. Protocol for clinical neurophysiologic examination of pelvic floor. Neurourol Urodyn 2001; 20:669–682.

27. Podnar S, Oblak C, Vodušek DB. Sexual function in men with cauda equina lesions: a clinical and electromyographic study. J Neurol Neurosurg Psychiatry 2002; 73:715–720.

28. Fowler CJ, Kirby RS, Harrison MJG. Decelerating bursts and complex repetitive discharges in the striated muscle of the urethral sphincter associated with urinary retention in women. J Neurol Neurosurg Psychiatry 1985; 48:1004–1009.

29. Palace J, Chandiramani VA, Fowler CJ. Value of sphincter EMG in the diagnosis of Multiple System Atrophy. Muscle Nerve 1997; 20:1396–1403.

30. Buchthal F. Introduction to electromyography. Copenhagen: Scandinavian University Press, 1957.

31. Czekajewski J, Ekstedt J, Stålberg E. Oscilloscopic recording of muscle fiber action potentials. The window trigger and delay unit. Electroenceph Clin Neurophysiol 1969; 27:536–539.

32. Stålberg E, Falck B, Sonoo M, et al. Multi-MUP EMG analysis – a two year experience in daily clinical work. Electroenceph Clin Neurophysiol 1995; 97:145–154.

33. Podnar S, Lukanovič A, Vodušek DB. Anal sphincter electromyography after vaginal delivery: neuropathic insufficiency or normal wear and tear? Neurourol Urodyn 2000; 19:249–257.

34. Stålberg E, Bischoff C, Falck B. Outliers, a way to detect abnormality in quantitative EMG. Muscle Nerve 1994; 17:392–399.

35. Podnar S, Vodušek DB. Standardization of anal sphincter electromyography: utility of motor unit potential parameters. Muscle Nerve 2001; 24:946–951.

36. Podnar S, Mrkaić M. Predictive power of different motor unit potential parameters in anal sphincter electromyography. Muscle Nerve 2002; 26:389–394.

37. Nandedkar S, Sanders D, Stålberg E, Andreassen S. Simulation of concentric needle EMG motor unit action potentials. Muscle Nerve 1988; 11:151–159.

38. Stålberg E, Andreassen S, Falck B, et al. Quantitative analysis of individual motor unit potentials: a proposition for standardized terminology and criteria for measurement. J Clin Neurophysiol 1986; 3:313–348.

39. Anon. AAEE glossary of terms used in clinical electromyography. Muscle Nerve 1987; 10(8 Suppl):G1–G60.

40. Podnar S, Fowler CJ. Sphincter electromyography in diagnosis of multiple system atrophy: technical issues. Muscle Nerve 2004.

41. Nandedkar SD, Sanders DB, Stålberg EV. Automatic analysis of the electromyographic interference pattern. Part II: Findings in control subjects and in some neuromuscular diseases. Muscle Nerve 1986; 9:491–500.

42. Podnar S, Vodušek DB, Stålberg E. Standardization of anal sphincter electromyography: normative data. Clin Neurophysiol 2000; 111:2200–2207.

43. Podnar S, Vodušek DB. Standardization of anal sphincter electromyography: effect of chronic constipation. Muscle Nerve 2000; 23:1748–1751.

44. Stålberg E, Trontelj JV. Single fiber electromyography: studies in healthy and diseased muscle, 2nd edn. New York: Raven Press, 1994.

45. Neill ME, Swash M. Increased motor unit fiber density in the external anal sphincter muscle in ano-rectal incontinence: a single fiber EMG study. J Neurol Neurosurg Psychiatry 1980; 43:343–347.

46. Jameson JS, Chia YW, Kamm MA, et al. Effect of age, sex and parity on anorectal function. Br J Surg 1994; 81:1689–1692.

47. Laurberg S, Swash M. Effects of aging on the anorectal sphincters and their innervation. Dis Colon Rectum 1989; 32:737–742.

48. Snooks SJ, Badenoch DF, Tiptaft RC, Swash M. Perineal nerve damage in genuine stress incontinence. Br J Urol 1985; 57:422–426.

49. Vodušek DB, Janko M, Lokar J. EMG, single fiber EMG and sacral reflexes in assessment of sacral nervous system lesions. J Neurol Neurosurg Psychiatry 1982; 45:1064–1066.

50. Rodi Z, Vodušek DB, Denišlič M. External anal sphincter electromyography in the differential diagnosis of parkinsonism. J Neurol Neurosurg Psychiatry 1996; 60:460–461.

51. Dyro FM, Yalla SV. Refractoriness of striated sphincter during voiding: studies with afferent pudendal reflex arc stimulation in male subjects. J Urol 1986; 135:732–736.

52. Kaiho Y, Namima T, Uchi K, et al. Electromyographic study of the striated urethral sphincter by using the bulbocavernosus reflex: study on change of sacral reflex activity caused by bladder filling. Nippon Hinyokika Gakkai Zasshi 2000; 91:715–722.

53. Sethi RK, Bauer SB, Dyro FM, Krarup C. Modulation of the bulbocavernosus reflex during voiding: loss of inhibition in upper motor neuron lesions. Muscle Nerve 1989; 12:892–897.

54. Ertekin Ç, Reel F. Bulbocavernosus reflex in normal men and patients with neurogenic bladder and/or impotence. J Neurol Sci 1976; 28:1–15.

55. Vodušek DB, Janko M, Lokar J. Direct and reflex responses in perineal muscles on electrical stimulation. J Neurol Neurosurg Psychiatry 1983; 46:67–71.

56. Dykstra D, Sidi A, Cameron J, et al. The use of mechanical stimulation to obtain the sacral reflex latency: a new technique. J Urol 1987; 137:77–79.

57. Podnar S, Vodušek DB, Tršinar B, Rodi Z. A method of uroneurophysiological investigation in children. Electroenceph Clin Neurophysiol 1997; 104:389–392.

58. Loening-Baucke V, Read NW, Yamada T, Barker AT. Evaluation of the motor and sensory components of the pudendal nerve. Electroenceph Clin Neurophysiol 1994; 93:35–41.

59. Vodušek DB. Evoked potential testing. Urol Clin N Am 1996; 23:427–446.

60. Rodi Z, Vodušek DB. The sacral reflex studies: single versus double pulse stimulation. Neurourol Urodynam 1995; 14:496–497(abs).

61. Amarenco G, Kerdraon J. Clinical value of ipsi- and contralateral sacral reflex latency measurement: a normative data study in man. Neurourol Urodyn 2000; 19:565–576.

62. Hanson P, Rigaux P, Gilliard C, Biset E. Sacral reflex latencies in tethered cord syndrome. Am J Phys Med Rehabil 1993; 72:39–43.

63. Bilkey WJ, Awad EA, Smith AD. Clinical application of sacral reflex latency. J Urol 1983; 129:1187–1189.

64. Amarenco G, Bayle B, Ismael SS, Kerdraon J. Bulbocavernosus muscle responses after suprapubic stimulation: analysis and measurement of suprapubic bulbocavernosus reflex latency. Neurourol Urodyn 2002; 21:210–213.

65. Blaivas JG, Zayed AA, Labib KB. The bulbocavernosus reflex in urology: a prospective study of 299 patients. J Urol 1981; 126:197–199.

66. Haldeman S, Bradley WE, Bhatia N. Evoked responses from the pudendal nerve. J Urol 1982; 128:974–980.

67. Haldeman S, Bradley WE, Bhatia N, et al. Cortical evoked potentials on stimulation of pudendal nerve in women. Urology 1983; 6:590–593.

68. Guérit JM, Opsomer RJ. Bit-mapped images of somatosensory evoked potentials after stimulation of the posterior tibial nerves and dorsal nerve of the penis/clitoris. Electroenceph Clin Neurophysiol (EP) 1991; 80:228–237.

69. Vodušek DB. Pudendal somatosensory evoked potential and bulbocavernosus reflex in women. Electroenceph Clin Neurophysiol 1990; 77:134–136.

70. Rodi Z, Vodušek DB, Denišlič M. Clinical uro-neurophysiological investigation in multiple sclerosis. Eur J Neurol 1996; 3:574–580.

71. Selcuki M, Coskun K. Management of tight filum terminale syndrome with special emphasis on normal level conus medullaris (NLCM). Surg Neurol 1998; 50:318–322.

72. Delodovici ML, Fowler CJ. Clinical value of the pudendal somatosensory evoked potential. Electroenceph Clin Neurophysiol 1995; 96:509–515.

73. Kiff ES, Swash M. Normal proximal and delayed distal conduction in the pudendal nerves of patients with idiopathic (neurogenic) faecal incontinence. J Neurol Neurosurg Psychiatry 1984; 47:820–823.

74. Barnett JL, Hasler WL, Camilleri M. American Gastroenterological Association medical position statement on anorectal testing techniques. American Gastroenterological Association. Gastroenterology 1999; 116:732–760.

75. Osterberg A, Graf W, Edebol Eeg-Olofsson K, et al. Results of neurophysiologic evaluation in fecal incontinence. Dis Colon Rectum 2000; 43:1256–1261.

76. Suilleabhain CB, Horgan AF, McEnroe L, et al. The relationship of pudendal nerve terminal motor latency to squeeze pressure in patients with idiopathic fecal incontinence. Dis Colon Rectum 2001; 44:666–671.

77. Opsomer RJ, Caramia MD, Zarola F, et al. Neurophysiological evaluation of central-peripheral sensory and motor pudendal fibers. Electroenceph Clin Neurophysiol 1989; 74:260–270.

78. Eardley I, Nagendran K, Lecky B, et al. The neurophysiology of the striated urethral sphincter in multiple sclerosis. Br J Urol 1991; 67:81–88.

79. Vodušek DB, Zidar J. Perineal motor evoked responses. Neurourol Urodynam 1988; 7:236–237(abs).

80. Jost WH, Schimrigk K. A new method to determine pudendal nerve motor latency and central motor conduction time to the external anal sphincter. Electroenceph Clin Neurophysiol 1994; 93:237–239.

81. Thiry AJ, Deltenre PF. Neurophysiological assessment of the central motor pathway to the external urethral sphincter in man. Br J Urol 1989; 63:515–519.

82. Bradley WE, Lin JT, Johnson B. Measurement of the conduction velocity of the dorsal nerve of the penis. J Urol 1984; 131:1127–1129.

83. Amarenco G, Kerdraon J. Pudendal nerve terminal sensitive latency: technique and normal values. J Urol 1999; 161:103–106.

84. Deletis V, Vodušek DB, Abbott R, et al. Intraoperative monitoring of dorsal sacral roots: minimizing the risk of iatrogenic micturition disorders. Neurosurgery 1992; 30:72–75.

85. Ertekin Ç, Mungan B. Sacral spinal cord and root potentials evoked by the stimulation of the dorsal nerve of penis and cord conduction delay for the bulbocavernosus reflex. Neurourol Urodynam 1993; 12:9–22.

86. Hansen MV, Ertekin Ç, Larsson LE. Cerebral evoked potentials after stimulation of the posterior urethra in man. Electroenceph Clin Neurophysiol 1990; 77:52–58.

87. Pietrangeli A, Bove L, Innocenti P, et al. Neurophysiological evaluation of sexual dysfunction in patients operated for colorectal cancer. Clin Auton Res 1998; 8:353–357.

88. Lefaucheur JP, Yiou R, Salomon L, et al. Assessment of penile small nerve fiber damage after transurethral resection of the prostate by measurement of penile thermal sensation. J Urol 2000; 164:1416–1419.

89. Lee JC, Yang CC, Kromm BG, Berger RE. Neurophysiologic testing in chronic pelvic pain syndrome: a pilot study. Urology 2001; 58:246–250.

90. Arunodaya GR, Taly AB. Sympathetic skin response: a decade later. J Neurol Sci 1995; 129:81–89.

91. Opsomer RJ, Pesce F, Abi Aad A, et al. Electrophysiologic testing of motor sympathetic pathways: normative data and clinical contribution in neurourological disorders. Neurourol Urodynam 1993; 12:336–338(abs).

92. Daffertshofer M, Linden D, Syren M, et al. Assessment of local sympathetic function in patients with erectile dysfunction. Int J Impotence Res 1994; 6:213–225.

93. Colakoglu Z, Kutluay E, Ertekin Ç. The nature of spontaneous cavernosal activity. BJU Int 1999; 83:449–452.

94. Schwarz J, Kornhuber M, Bischoff C, Straube A. Electromyography of the external anal sphincter in patients with Parkinson's disease and multiple system atrophy: frequency of abnormal spontaneous activity and polyphasic motor unit potentials. Muscle Nerve 1997; 20:1167–1172.

95. Eardley I, Quinn NP, Fowler CJ, et al. The value of urethral sphincter electromyography in the differential diagnosis of parkinsonism. Br J Urol 1989; 64:360–362.

96. Beck RO, Betts CD, Fowler CJ. Genitourinary dysfunction in multiple system atrophy: clinical features and treatment in 62 cases. J Urol 1994; 151:1336–1341.

97. Libelius R, Johansson F. Quantitative electromyography of the external anal sphincter in Parkinson's disease and multiple system atrophy. Muscle Nerve 2000; 23:1250–1256.

98. Giladi N, Simon ES, Korczyn AD, et al. Anal sphincter EMG does not distinguish between multiple system atrophy and Parkinson's disease. Muscle Nerve 2000; 23:731–734.

99. Valldeoriola F, Valls-Sole J, Tolosa ES, Marti MJ. Striated anal sphincter denervation in patients with progressive supranuclear palsy. Mov Disord 1995; 10:550–555.

100. Scaravilli T, Pramstaller PP, Salerno A, et al. Neuronal loss in Onuf's nucleus in three patients with progressive supranuclear palsy. Ann Neurol 2000; 48:97–101.

101. Ravits J, Hallett M, Nilsson J, et al. Electrophysiological tests of autonomic function in patients with idiopathic autonomic failure syndromes. Muscle Nerve 1996; 19:758–763.

102. Fowler CJ, Kirby RS, Harrison MJ, et al. Individual motor unit analysis in the diagnosis of disorders of urethral sphincter innervation. J Neurol Neurosurg Psychiatry 1984; 47:637–641.

103. Tsai PY, Cha RC, Yang TF, et al. Electromyographic evaluation in children with spina bifida. Zhonghua Yi Xue Za Zhi (Taipei) 2001; 64:509–515.

104. Stoehr M. Traumatic and postoperative lesions of the lumbosacral plexus. Arch Neurol 1978; 35:757–760.

105. Feasby TE, Burton SR, Hahn AF. Obstetrical lumbosacral plexus injury. Muscle Nerve 1992; 15:937–940.

106. Vock P, Mattle H, Studer M, Mumenthaler M. Lumbosacral plexus lesions: correlation of clinical signs and computed tomography. J Neurol Neurosurg Psychiatry 1988; 51:72–79.

107. Amarenco G, Ismael SS, Bayle B, et al. Electrophysiological analysis of pudendal neuropathy following traction. Muscle Nerve 2001; 24:116–119.

108. Fowler CJ, Kirby RS. Electromyography of the urethral sphincter in women with urinary retention. Lancet 1986; 1(8496):1455–1457.

109. Fowler CJ, Christmas TJ, Chapple CR, et al. Abnormal electromyographic activity of the urethral sphincter, voiding dysfunction, and polycystic ovaries: a new syndrome? BMJ 1988; 297(6661): 1436–1438.

110. Swinn MJ, Wiseman OJ, Lowe E, Fowler CJ. The cause and natural history of isolated urinary retention in young women. J Urol 2002; 167:151–156.

111. Snooks SJ, Barnes PR, Swash M, Henry MM. Damage to the innervation of the pelvic floor musculature in chronic constipation. Gastroenterology 1985; 89:977–981.

112. Koldewijn EL, Van Kerrebroeck PE, Bemelmans BL, et al. Use of sacral reflex latency measurements in the evaluation of neural function of spinal cord injury patients: a comparison of neuro-urophysiological testing and urodynamic investigations. J Urol 1994; 152:463–467.

113. Liu S, Christmas TJ, Nagendran K, Kirby RS. Sphincter electromyography in patients after radical prostatectomy and cystoprostatectomy. Br J Urol 1992; 69:397–403.

114. Sau G, Siracusano S, Aiello I, et al. The usefulness of the somatosensory evoked potentials of the pudendal nerve in diagnosis of probable multiple sclerosis. Spinal Cord 1999; 37:258–263.

41

Practical guide to diagnosis and follow-up of patients with neurogenic bladder dysfunction

Erik Schick and Jacques Corcos

Introduction

Many traumatic, congenital, tumoral, or degenerative neurological pathologies have direct consequences on vesi-courethral function. Imaging techniques will give information on the anatomical and morphological status of the urinary tract. Endoscopy will provide further information, such as mucosal appearance, small tumors, urethral stenosis, the degree of prostatic enlargement, and urethrovesical mobility in females. Urodynamics is the only diagnostic tool that allows functional evaluation of the urinary tract. It does not replace any of the other diagnostic modalities, but rather complements them. It plays a major role in therapeutic decisions and during follow-up.

Neurogenic bladder dysfunction after trauma

Traumatic injury to the central nervous system (cerebral or spinal) is often followed by the so-called spinal shock phase (see also Chapter 14). The bladder is areflexic during this phase, which may last from 2 weeks up to 8 weeks,[1,2] but sometimes up to 1 year.[3,4] Complete urodynamic evaluation during this period is useless.[5] Intermittent catheterization is the best treatment modality.

In the case of an incomplete spinal cord lesion, the reappearance of bladder sensation will indicate the end of the spinal shock phase. In the case of a complete lesion, the reappearance of osteotendinous reflexes, urine spillage around the urethral catheter if it was left in place, and incontinence episodes between intermittent catheterizations will suggest the presence of some kind of bladder activity. The first urodynamic evaluation is made at this time.

The site of the neurological lesion will give some indication as to the type of neurogenic bladder function to expect. Lesion above T7 results in hyperreflexic bladder, whereas lesion at T11 or below results in areflexic bladder. Lesion between T8 and T10 constitutes the 'gray zone', and can result either in hyperreflexic or areflexic bladder.[4] Vesico-sphincteric dyssynergia is more difficult to predict because only two-thirds of hyperreflexic bladders will be accompanied by dyssynergic voiding.[4]

Neurogenic bladder dysfunction after non-traumatic neurological pathology

Usually, the urologist will see these patients with a well-defined neurological diagnosis when urinary symptoms are already present. In this case, immediate urodynamic evaluation is indicated, together with other diagnostic modalities such as urine culture, ultrasonographic imaging of the upper urinary tract, and free flowmetry, if possible.

Autonomic dysreflexia

Autonomic dysreflexia is an exaggerated sympathetic response to afferent stimulation when spinal cord injury (SCI) is at the level of T6 or above (see also Chapter 13). Acute, life-threatening autonomic dysreflexic episodes can be controlled by chlorpromazine (1 mg) or phentolamine (5 mg), given intravenously.[6] On a long-term basis, chronic α-adrenergic blockade in small doses, such as prazosin (1 mg daily), will be helpful.[7] Our practice is to administer nifedipine (10 mg), a calcium channel blocking agent, sublingually to patients with a potential risk of developing acute autonomic dysreflexia during urological manipulations (e.g. endoscopy, urodynamics), 30 min before these procedures (Figure 41.1).

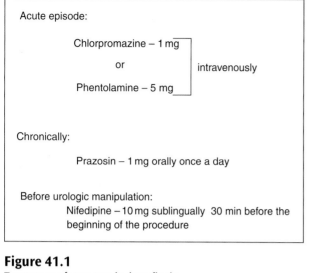

Acute episode:

Chlorpromazine – 1 mg
or   intravenously
Phentolamine – 5 mg

Chronically:

Prazosin – 1 mg orally once a day

Before urologic manipulation:
Nifedipine – 10 mg sublingually 30 min before the beginning of the procedure

Figure 41.1
Treatment of autonomic dysreflexia.

Renal surveillance

In a follow-up study by Donelly et al of paraplegics from World War II, renal disease was the most common cause of death in the first 20 years after the injury, accounting for 40% of all deaths.[8] More recently, in a series of 406 consecutive SCI patients followed for 15 years, Webb et al[9] reported a death-rate of 0.5% (2/406) secondary from renal complications. This highlights the importance of dedicated follow-up to significantly reduce kidney-related mortality in these patients.

Renal ultrasound[10] combined with plain radiography of the abdomen[11] tends to replace intravenous pyelography (IVP) in upper urinary tract evaluation.[12] Color flow Doppler sonography could eventually replace retrograde cystography in the detection of vesicoureteral reflux. In a recent study, Papadaki et al[13] reported that color Doppler ultrasonography diagnosed all grade IV and V, 87.5% of grade III, 83.3% of grade II, and 57.4% of grade I refluxes. There were 6 false-positive and 5 false-negative findings among 187 SCI adults.

In many major SCI centers, radionuclide renograms are used for routine follow-up of renal function, instead of IVP.[6] A study by Phillips et al[14] showed that a decline in effective plasma flow was the best predictor for therapeutic intervention.

It has been our practice to obtain a renal ultrasonogram and a plain abdominal X-ray in all patients with neurogenic bladder dysfunction as part of their initial evaluation, together with urodynamic studies. The results of the latter give information on pressure conditions in the bladder. With a high-pressure system, the upper urinary tract is at high risk for deterioration, and upper tract monitoring

should be more frequent (every 6–12 months). In the case of a low-pressure system, this danger is only relative, and we undertake renal ultrasound study approximately every 3–5 years if no change in clinical symptoms suggests modification of the bladder's pressure status. However, if clinical symptoms change, ultrasonography of the kidneys and urodynamic studies are repeated promptly. Figure 41.2 summarizes, in a schematic way, our initial evaluation and follow-up of patients with neurogenic bladder dysfunction.

Urodynamics

Urodynamics are cornerstones in the diagnosis and management of neurogenic bladder dysfunction. In this respect, the main parameters that require special attention are high detrusor pressure during the filling or storage phase of the bladder (decreased bladder wall compliance and/or sustained detrusor contraction), and detrusor-external sphincter dyssynergia during micturition. (The problem of compliance has been detailed in Chapter 11 and that of detrusor-sphincter dyscoordination in Chapter 12.) Well-conducted, multichannel (video)urodynamic evaluation will highlight these conditions and consequently allow the initiation of appropriate therapeutic measures that should ultimately transform a high-pressure system to a low-pressure system.

Endoscopy

Cystourethroscopy is an essential part of the initial evaluation of all patients with neurogenic bladder dysfunction. It allows visualization of anatomic urethral occlusion, especially in the male. It should be emphasized that there is a fundamental difference between occlusion and obstruction. Urethral occlusion means a more or less pronounced change in urethral caliber, such as a fibrotic stricture. This can be diagnosed endoscopically. In contrast, obstruction is a dynamic concept, which, from the hydrodynamic point of view and simplified to some extent,[15] essentially means a 'high-pressure–low-flow' relationship. This can be diagnosed by urodynamics. Benign prostatic enlargement illustrates the relationship between the two concepts. Endoscopically, one can observe a protrusion of the lateral lobes of the prostate into the urethral lumen, joining each other on the midline. From this picture, however, it is not possible to extrapolate how the detrusor will contract, and how the urethra will relax to allow voiding to take place. In other words, one cannot estimate to what extent this prostatic enlargement will interfere with flow and be responsible for an eventual obstruction.

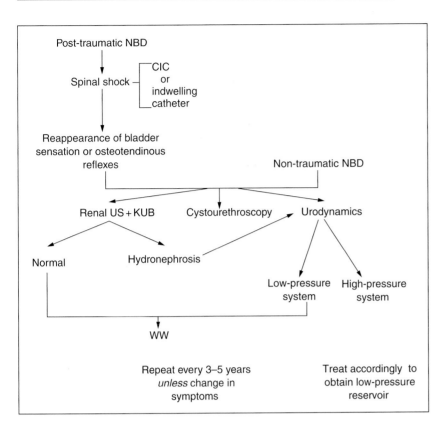

Figure 41.2
Diagnosis and follow-up of patients with neurogenic bladder dysfunction. US, ultrasound; CIC, clean intermittent catheterization; KUB, plain abdominal X-ray; NBD, neurogenic bladder dysfunction; WW, watchful waiting.

In the female, the best chance to visualize stress incontinence is to ask the patient to cough when the bladder has reached its cystometric capacity, at the end of the cystoscopic examination. Also, the best condition to evaluate the bladder neck hypermobility is when the bladder is completely empty.

In both sexes, bladder wall trabeculation suggests an overactive bladder, rather than outlet obstruction (see also Chapter 35).

References

1. Light JK, Faganel J, Beric A. Detrusor areflexia in suprasacral spinal cord injuries. J Urol 1985; 134:295–297.

2. Chancellor MB, Kiilholma P. Urodynamic evaluation of patients following spinal cord injury. Sem Urol 1992; 10:83–94.

3. Wheeler JS Jr, Walter JW. Acute urologic management of the patient with spinal cord injury: initial hospitalisation. Urol Clin N Am 1993; 20:403–411.

4. Perlow DL, Diokno AC. Predicting lower urinary tract dysfunctions in patients with spinal cord injury. Urology 1981; 18:531–535.

5. Chancellor MB. Urodynamic evaluation after spinal cord injury. Phys Med Rehab Clin N Am 1993; 4:273–298.

6. Chancellor MB, Blaivas JG. Spinal cord injury. In: Chancellor MB, Blaivas JG, eds. Practical neurourology. Boston: Butterworth-Heinemann, 1995:99–118.

7. McGuire EJ. Immediate management of the inability to void. In: Parsons FK, Fitzpatrick JM, eds. Practical urology in spinal cord injury. London: Springer Verlag, 1991:5–10.

8. Donelly J, Hackler RH, Bunts RC. Present urologic status of the World War II paraplegic: 25-year follow-up. Comparison with status of the 20-year Korean War paraplegic and the 5-year Vietnam paraplegic. J Urol 1972; 108:558–562.

9. Webb DR, Fitzpatrick JM, O'Flynn JD. A 15-year follow-up of 406 consecutive spinal cord injuries. Br J Urol 1984; 56:614–617.

10. Bodley R. Imaging in chronic spinal cord injury – indications and benefits. Eur J Radiol 2002; 42:135–153.

11. Morcos SK, Thomas DG. A comparison of real-time ultrasonography with intravenous urography in the follow-up of patients with spinal cord injury. Clin Radiol 1988; 39:49–50.

12. Chagnon S, Vallée C, Laissy JP, Blery M. Ultrasonographic evaluation of the urinary tract in patients with spinal cord injuries. Systematic comparison with intravenous urography in 50 cases. J Radiol (Paris) 1985; 66:801–806.

13. Papdaki PJ, Vlychou MK, Zavras GM, et al. Investigation of vesicoureteral reflux with colour Doppler sonography in adult patients with spinal cord injury. Eur Radiol 2002; 12:366–370.

14. Phillips JP, Jadvar H, Sullivan G, et al. Effect of radionuclide renograms on treatment of patients with spinal cord injury. Am J Roentgenol 1997; 169:1045–1047.

15. Kranse R, van Mastrigt R. Relative bladder outlet obstruction. J Urol 2002; 168:565–570.

Part V

Classification

42

Classification of lower urinary tract dysfunction

Anders Mattiasson

Introduction

A system of classification lives only as long as it is generally perceived to correspond to the reality it is intended to describe. The need to revise it is thus present on a continuous basis. The current classification system for disorders and terminology in the lower urinary tract[1–3] needs to be revised.[4] The new approach described herein does not represent any generally accepted system, but rather is a proposal for a new manner in which to view the reality. It is rooted in disorder/illness processes and injuries being described in terms of structure and function and not, as previously (and presently), primarily in terms of consequential effects such as symptoms. Actually, we should be speaking of lower urinary tract disorders. Dysfunction in fact describes only one half of the structure + function pair. We should also be quite aware that a classification that we use as researchers due to, among other things, pedagogical reasons, must ultimately be separated from the one which we in the capacity of caregivers use in contact with, for example, the patients.

In this chapter the general classification of lower urinary tract disorders comprises the subject matter, and thus does not specifically deal with the present system for classification of neurogenic disorders, since this is presented in Parts II and III. A consistent and uniform way of looking at things comprises the basis of a functioning classification system. What one chooses as the basis for the system is in fact of crucial significance. In most of the other fields of medicine, illnesses and injuries are described in pathophysiological terms. So the case ought to be the same on the part of the lower urinary tract. Hence, it is difficult to maintain a system that is based upon a description of the circumstances for the genesis of different forms of urinary incontinence. In certain cases it is the patient's experiences that are the point of departure, such as with urge and so-called overactive bladder, whereas physical exertion or stress is the point of departure in other cases. It is more constructive to describe how the tissues and organs are engaged on different levels in terms of structure and function (S + F) right down to the cell and molecular biology level, and to then describe what the consequences are that give rise to symptoms and difficulties and other conceivable consequential effects.[4] This can be illustrated as in Figure 42.1.

By deciding to use S + F as a basis for a classification system, a decision has been made once and for all as far as it concerns this system precisely. All divisions and categorizations must then, in its continuation, also fit in with each other in the holistic spirit described above. Structure and function are different ways of regarding and expressing the same thing. Complete covariance can be presumed to exist in a well-balanced situation. Structural changes do not occur without altered functionality and vice versa.

This is how the situation appears in a simple system (Figure 42.2). When multiple tissues and multiple organs are connected together, as in the lower urinary tract, new conditions arise, where the different parts come to influence each other. In reality, they are all part of a balanced situation

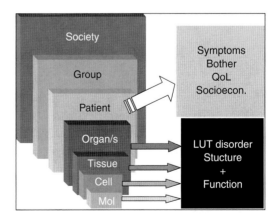

Figure 42.1
Lower urinary tract disorders are best described in pathophysiological terms of structure and function. Symptoms and bother are secondary phenomena, and therefore not as suitable for the primary classification. QoL, quality of life; Socioecon., socioeconomics; Mol, molecule.

intended to fulfill the task of storing and evacuating urine, and an imbalance in one of the parts inexorably comes to have an effect on the other component parts. The lower urinary tract acts as a single functional unit.

All of the different parts of the micturition cycle and the different components of the lower urinary tract cannot, however, be included in a fully comprehensive classification system without them being represented at all levels. This is especially important as the lower urinary tract contains within itself functions that are diametrically opposed in every individual part, i.e. in a part of the micturition cycle optimized for storage and in a different part for emptying. In such a case it is important to capture all these parts as well as the transition forms between them. Hence not only should the bladder, trigone/bladder neck, and urethra be included but also the vagina, prostate, pelvic floor, as well as all the different types of supporting structures. Vessels and nerves have not been mentioned, but are included of course, and strictly speaking the parts of the nervous system involved must also be included in order to form a whole (Figure 42.3).

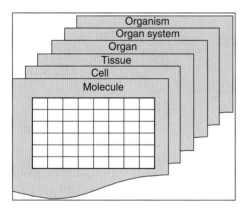

Figure 42.2
All levels and all parts of the lower urinary tract and its innervation can be included in one matrix.

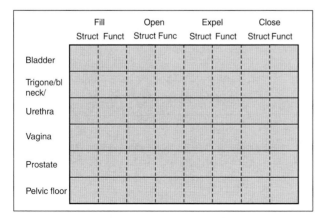

Figure 42.3
When all parts of the lower urinary tract and the whole micturition cycle are characterized regarding both structure and function, the result will be a complete recognition pattern.

The micturition cycle

The classification and thus the description of lower urinary tract disturbances is directly dependent on where one finds oneself in the micturition cycle. Due to the filling and discharge functions being so intimately intertwined, it is often difficult to distinguish which signals are related to what parts of the urinary tract. For example, during filling of the bladder, activity including detrusor contractions can arise too early. This is in fact activity that is characteristic of emptying that appears here during filling. How should this be classified? To do this, the initial point of departure must be fixed. Since the functional status of the lower urinary tract changes in step with the filling and emptying, we must have multiple well-defined points of departure. These actually differ from one another, and collectively represent the entire micturition cycle. The activity that belongs in the different phases can be represented graphically with a simple sketch (Figure 42.4) that depicts the pressure conditions in the bladder and urethra during the different parts of the micturition cycle.

It is logical to make a new division of the micturition cycle in such a manner that the emptying also encompasses the short transitions between storage and evacuation. It is of course precisely at their beginning and ending, respectively, that the storage pattern is broken. The commencement of micturition concerns the direct preparations for emptying, such as the pressure drop in the urethra that takes place during the flow of urine itself. This also applies for the cessation of micturition when the pressure conditions are restored after the flow has ended. The entire storage phase is then governed by a picture that in itself is dynamic, but which in terms of pressure is essentially constant. It is an important and critical point in the micturition cycle when diametrically opposed functions, in contrast to those that have been prevailing, normally for a number of hours, need to be established

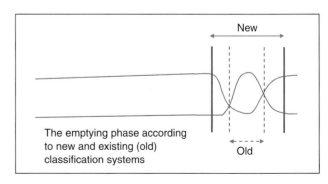

Figure 42.4
When the pressure changes of the bladder and the urethra before and after the expulsion of urine are both included in the emptying phase, this also means that the storage and the emptying phases of the micturition cycle have been redefined.

in order to perform the emptying. The storage-to-emptying turning point is quite important and it has been proposed that it be given an identity of its own, namely the 'SE turn'.

The balance between the lower urinary tract and the nervous system

The lower urinary tract and the parts of the nervous system involved in the micturition cycle balance each other in a purposeful manner independently of the functional phase (Figure 42.5). They are so intimately associated that they can be regarded as the partners in a marriage, i.e. a unit in which both parts are needed to a similar degree. The fact that a large part of the nervous system is situated functionally and anatomically between the lower urinary tract and that part of the nervous system where important coordination and perception are located also makes it easy to view the lower urinary tract as being in a position of dependence. In the classification system that is based upon structure and function, no distinction is drawn between the lower urinary tract and the nervous structures involved.

During the storage phase, an adjustment occurs in the bladder wall for the increasing volume without any appreciable rise in pressure. Nevertheless, the afferent input increases and gradually increasing activity can be read in, for example, the external sphincter in step with the filling of the bladder. Continence is preserved at the bladder neck level, i.e. a low-pressure system for closure. Somatic and adrenergic innervation of striated and smooth musculature are the most influential neuromuscular mechanisms of the closure function. In connection with exertion, activation of the pelvic floor and compression of the urethra become significant factors in the maintenance of continence. Cholinergic innervation via the pelvic nerves is regarded as being inhibited during the bladder's filling phase.

Upon initiation of emptying, a significant change occurs in the nervous and muscular activity. The outflow tract and the urethra must be opened and bladder contraction initiated. Positive feedback must be established and maintained all the way to complete bladder emptying. In order to cause the opening of the intermediate segment and the external sphincter, the stimulation of the smooth and striated muscle contraction that participates in the closure is minimized, i.e. adrenergic and somatic nervous activity is inhibited. At the same time, a contraction probably occurs of certain muscle fibers in order for the funnelling of the outflow tract to be able to take place. In addition, relaxation-mediating substances are released to ensure an open outflow tract and the least possible resistance. The bladder contraction is certainly effectuated primarily under cholinergic influence; however, other substances do seem to be of significance, particularly with functional disorders. We also know that altered activity in C fibers in the bladder is significant in the genesis of increased activation of the entire system for emptying preparedness. This is perhaps also significant for normal functioning, even though the perception has long been that they are normally tacit.

This switching between diametrically different functional states has spawned the 'on-and-off' concept. For individual structures and functions, it works well for describing a course of events. However, the whole is comprised of a number of on-and-off pairs, which do not operate in step with each other; hence, the designation ceases to be appropriate. When one adds that simultaneously exciting and inhibiting influences on nerves and/or muscles seem to be typical for different parts of the lower urinary tract during both filling and emptying, one understands why on-and-off can only be used to describe the occurrence of reciprocity in itself, not the course of events in the lower urinary tract.

A special situation exists in the lower urinary tract in the manner in which mechanisms are activated to guarantee the shutting off of the outflow and urethra, and thus continence, at the same rate as which a preparedness is also built up to be able to open up precisely these structures instantaneously. One cannot rule out the possibility that

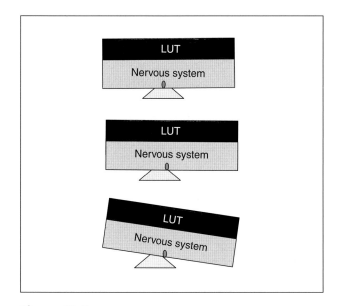

Figure 42.5
The lower urinary tract (LUT) and the nervous system are balancing each other. All parts influence each other. The system becomes more lable with increasing filling of the bladder (triangle). A disturbance can be balanced out, i.e. a disorder can be present without causing any symptoms.

the activation of the continence-preserving external urethral sphincter leads to an activation of afferent pathways which have an inhibitory effect in the spinal cord and on the pelvic nerves. When the contraction in the sphincter is voluntarily released on command from higher centers, inhibitory influence that prevents the activation of the micturition reflex disappears, and activation with accompanying opening of the outflow tract can occur. With such an arrangement, the apparently paradoxical arrangement with the simultaneous building up of activity that promotes both filling and emptying would appear to be both possible and easily explained.

It is possible to say, as shown in Figure 42.5, that the degree of instability in the system increases with an increasing degree of bladder filling. Under normal circumstances the system is of course in balance; however, in the event of illness/injury the main focus is displaced, albeit with retained balance, i.e. without any signs of any disorder. When the process proceeds or when the system is provoked, e.g. through an increasing degree of bladder filling, an imbalance arises, i.e. symptoms appear. It is not always the case that this imbalance is synonymous with symptoms presenting themselves. For example, with a bladder outlet obstruction, reduced detrusor functionality can arise secondarily to the outlet obstruction without the individual experiencing any symptoms. The same applies of course with other types of disruptions.

Classification according to involvement of the nervous system

In principle it can be said that all disruptions that give rise to symptoms have a neurogenic component by definition, since the center for the perception of the illness/injury is located in the same nervous system on a slightly higher level, and there, among other things, it contains the consciousness (Figure 42.6).

If the disorder/injury has its origin purely in the nervous system (1), the disruption can be regarded as primarily neurogenic; however, as soon as the lower urinary tract becomes involved it then contains both a neurogenic as well as a LUT component. The situation is the same with illnesses and injuries that engage the lower urinary tract itself, i.e. most often they are both neurogenic and LUT primarily at the same time (2). However, one can say that they are partly neurogenic and partly LUT. Conditions such as benign prostatic hyperplasia (BPH) without an effect on the lower urinary tract or changes in, for example, ligaments, can probably be said to be non-neurogenic (4). However, this applies only as long as they do not give rise to symptoms; otherwise, they must be classified as secondarily neurogenic (3) (Figure 42.7).

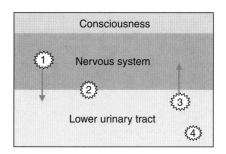

Figure 42.6
Different types of lower urinary tract disorders and their relation to the nervous system (see also Figure 42.7).

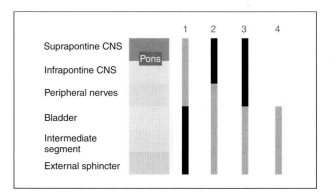

Figure 42.7
Different types of lower urinary tract disorders and their relation to the nervous system (see also Figure 42.6). Light bars refer to primary site of disorder/lesion, dark bars to secondary involvement. 1, primary neurogenic; 2, partly neurogenic, primary; 3, secondarily neurogenic; 4, non-neurogenic, LUT.

Partly neurogenic disorders usually involve a loss – e.g. neuromuscular injuries with female disorders – whereas secondary neurogenic usually means compensation – e.g. with BPH and outlet obstruction. Hence, as a consequence, the treatment is often a nature of supplemental factors with female disorders, whereas the removal of that which is in excess is the solution with, for example, BPH with outlet obstruction.

If we were to turn it all around and proceed from the lower urinary tract, the classification should, from top to bottom, be 'LUT, secondary', 'partly LUT, primary', 'LUT, primary', and LUT instead.

Disorder, consequences, and comorbidity

Primary LUT disorders can thus be partly non-neurogenic, partly secondary, or partly neurogenic. The non-neurogenic conditions, which do not provide symptoms, will not be taken up for further discussion here. Those that are partly neurogenic encompass a pathophysiological process/lesion which probably rarely stops with this, but rather due to the presence of the disease process changes will appear both in it and in the tissues/organ that is affected, in this case the lower urinary tract. This in turn involves changes in structure and innervation in the area that is primarily encompassed, which becomes the object of a process of change. This can in turn naturally lead to symptoms in the same manner as the original disorder or injury.

Precisely because the lower urinary tract is so close-knit functionally and morphologically, processes which injure a part of it will often ultimately also damage the whole. Figure 42.8 shows how different factors can be related in an entire chain, and that an individual symptom can be difficult to connect clinically to a certain factor.

Complicating factors are often logically intertwined with the disorder, even if the link may be latent. With comorbidity, the situation is however slightly different. Many of the changes which are a property of the organism as a whole or of other organ systems can affect the lower urinary tract and either initiate dysfunctional conditions on their own, or in conjunction with other causes, or affect a previously existing illness process (Figure 42.9). An example of a situation where difficulties can exist in reading what contributes to an illness picture is an outflow obstruction with BPH as well as simultaneous metabolic factors, possibly with an influence on the autonomous innervation of the lower urinary tract.

Patterns of recognition

In theory, one can collect information on structure and functionality as measurements of different types in all parts of the lower urinary tract during all parts of the micturition cycle (Figure 42.10).

By illustrating this graphically on a simulated three-dimensional display, different disorder conditions are recognizable by their distinctive features, i.e. as patterns of recognition. Information on completely normal individuals of both genders and at different ages would serve as a reference. An example of a pattern of recognition is shown in Figure 42.10. At present it is not possible to work with such an abundance of detail; however, the largest and most important of the parts must represent the whole. It then is advantageous to seek to attain a degree of representation

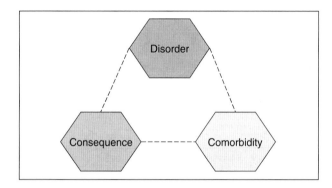

Figure 42.9
The interdependence of the disorder, its consequences, and the influence from other disease processes.

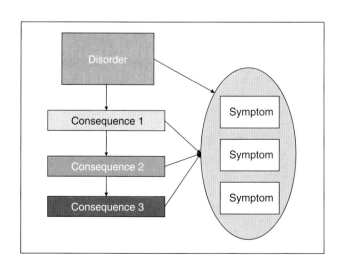

Figure 42.8
In a given clinical situation it is often unclear from what part of the pathophysiological process that symptoms emanate.

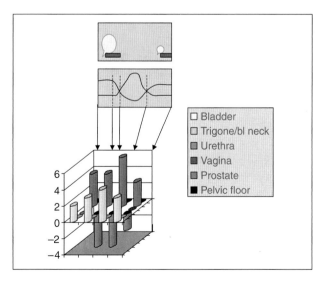

Figure 42.10
A simulated three-dimensional recognition pattern can reflect the influence of the disorder and its consequences, i.e. the impact on the lower urinary tract in different parts of the micturition cycle. Arbitrary scale.

for different levels in the lower urinary tract and its functions. To include the bladder and external sphincter seems quite natural, but so does including the parts that play a central role in the pressure-changing phases, i.e. the trigone, bladder neck, and proximal urethra. Since we do not know precisely the details of the functional contributions of these structures to low-pressure shutting during storage and funnelling as well as pressure decreases during emptying, we can amalgamate them into an intermediate segment with intermediate functionality.

Figure 42.11 illustrates three parts – the external sphincter, the intermediate segment, and the bladder – for a normal man (A) and woman (C) as well as during emptying with the unisex picture A'C'. Figure 42.11B shows how the prostate has a negative influence on the dynamics of the intermediate segment and also how the lumen is restricted by adenomas with a reduced flow of urine as a consequence, whereas Figure 42.11D shows how it can appear with incontinent women, i.e. with a higher flow than normal. Both are examples of what one could call harmonic disorders.

A harmonic micturition cycle?

Lower urinary tract functionality in women with incontinence appears to be characterized by diminished outflow resistance and more efficient emptying than normal, whereas increased resistance and more difficult emptying as well as a changed voiding pattern seem to be typical for men with an outlet obstruction. One could say that it is easier for women to trigger emptying as a consequence of

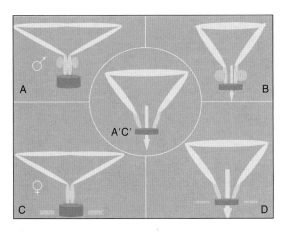

Figure 42.11
A simplified, reduced model of the lower urinary tract, introducing the intermediate segment. Three essential components – the bladder, the intermediate segment, and the external sphincter – of the lower urinary tract in both men and women are in this model. To this can be added the pelvic floor in the female and the prostate in the male. Further explanations are given in the text.

the decline in neuromuscular functionality, whereas for men it is easier to trigger and more difficult to empty due to the appearance of an obstruction. Even if both men and women show altered innervation as an element of these changes, the synchronization between the different component parts is still preserved. With such harmonic disorders the fundamental pattern of the micturition cycle is actually preserved. Even if overactivity, obstructions, or dislocations – via, for example, provocations – occur, the synchronization still continues to be maintained.

However, with disharmonic conditions, this pattern is broken such that simultaneously occurring activities in different parts of the lower urinary tract functionally oppose each other, resulting for example in an unsettled filling phase or more difficult emptying with an obstruction. This is first and foremost characteristic of primarily neurogenic disturbances, and what is especially characteristic are the occurrences of contractions for the purposes of producing a closing of the musculature on the outflow tract simultaneously with the bladder contracting and showing a pressure increase.

With central neurogenic disruptions, the picture is dominated by mass motor behavior, dyssynergy, and overactivity. With peripheral neurogenic and mixed disruptions there is usually a lower degree of activity, synergy more often than not, and both overactivity and underactivity are common occurrences. Disharmonic disruptions can arise without any form of micturition reflex, with pathological reflexes, and range to being with normal reflexes. The activity can thus at times be aberrant, i.e. arise unexpectedly during a part of the micturition cycle where it should normally not occur, such as overactivity. If this is synchronized with other parts so that the result, for example, becomes a premature micturition reflex, then it has a completely different clinical significance than if it were to appear to be unsynchronized and a bladder contraction takes place for a discharge that does not participate in the opening up, or which even actively shuts, as with detrusor-sphincter dyssynergy. Harmonic and disharmonic disruptions can thus be designated as synchronous or asynchronous.

By far the most disruptions that are not primarily neurogenic are characterized by overactivity. Even if sensory overactivity is occurring, it is motor overactivity that is dominating. We prefer to view the bladder during filling and the urethra and discharge during emptying as being passive; then we contrast our perception of the functional condition with the conspicuous activity that they both show during emptying and filling, respectively. This is a way of looking at it that leads to errors in terms of classification. The bladder is characterized, like the discharge and urethra, by both activity and passivity simultaneously during both filling and emptying. To then attribute to solely the more obvious and visible parts of these many different activities the epithet 'active' or 'overactive' does not lead to a firm foundation for classification: that not only excitation and contraction but also an inhibitory nervous influence can be designated to be an activity is in a way easy to comprehend.

Time-related changes

When a disorder process finds a foothold, completely regardless of whether it is spreading itself or not, it leads to changes in other parts of the lower urinary tract by affecting the balance. As time goes on, this imbalance grows if new balancing factors do not counterbalance the changes. Step by step those parts which are situated at the levels above the illness/injury become involved. Usually it is chronic conditions with a time scale spanning decades (Figure 42.12).

Trophic-structural changes are the rule, and are usually most pronounced in individuals who have higher degrees of obstruction and/or overactivity.[5] With women, it primarily involves, simply put, what is being lost; with men, what is being added; and with neurogenic disturbances, what is being reorganized. So, in addition to effects on the dynamics of the intermediate segment, a mechanical effect on the lumen of the urethra, and a certain flow limitation, a changed prostate also has effects on the bladder and therewith the nervous system. If no progress occurs in the primary process, growth in the secondarily arising changes will probably still occur. When remedying a problem in the lower urinary tract it is thus important that one can take hold of the problem by the root: i.e. don't treat problems that are related to the influence of the bladder first of all, but remedy the negative influence of the prostate on the urethra and the intermediate segment as the first priority. Although this is probably self-evident, it nevertheless deserves to be mentioned in this context.

The process that leads to female incontinence, and which probably began with trauma in connection with childbirth, is chronic and progressive in its nature, bringing post-polio syndrome to mind. Functional disturbances in the lower urinary tract are nearly always chronic conditions that cannot always be reversed, just compensated for, and naturally in the best case can even be prevented. Changes conditioned by the age of the organism must also be added to the pathophysiological process. It is therefore important to classify all age groups among both genders.

Bladder outlet obstruction

Bladder outlet obstruction (BOO) usually develops slowly, i.e. over many years.[5,6] It is much more common among men and mainly involves an impediment in the bladder neck and/or prostate.[7] An altered micturition pattern typically occurs, both with regard to the distribution of the instances of micturition during the day as well as to the characteristics of the individual instance of emptying in terms of how quickly and efficiently the emptying is initiated and carried out. We can also see how a pattern in the development of the obstruction picture grows over time as being to a large extent dependent upon the reaction to the impediment and not necessarily involving the impediment itself by looking at the lower urinary tract above the impediment and the nervous system reacting to the occurrence of a downstream impediment to emptying.[8] The impediment may be constant, but the reaction may become variable over time. Using current obstruction classification techniques, a clear discrepancy exists between the symptom picture that the patient reports and the findings of examinations we make with, for example, urodynamics in the form of pressure–flow measurements,[9,10] probably because our formula for obstruction is far too simplified. Factors that are related to an elevated urethral resistance ought to be complemented with a number of additional factors, as set out below.

The development of an obstruction of the lower urinary tract is most often a slow process taking many years. It usually involves successively more difficult emptying. The point in time of establishment is difficult to determine, as is obvious in an illustration of obstruction as a process besides the static condition we use for classification of obstruction today (Figure 42.13). In the typical case, an obstruction is a progressive process, and the development itself of an impediment is part of this process, i.e. a part of the obstruction; therefore, we must also include these circumstances in the new equation in order to describe impediments to evacuation of the bladder.

The obstruction can be characterized in different ways, depending upon where in the development cycle of the reaction to this change one finds oneself (Figure 42.14). An additional argument is that the obstruction concept is composed of and also encompasses all types of impediments to the emptying phase, not only increased urethra resistance as with prostate adenoma or the like but also

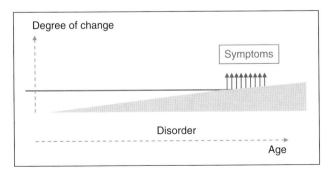

Figure 42.12
Non-malignant disorders of the lower urinary tract often develop slowly over considerable periods of time.

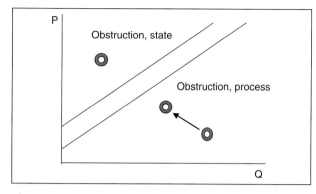

Figure 42.13
Obstruction is presently defined as illustrated in the upper left part of this nomogram from the International Continence Society (ICS). Obstruction can, however, also be a process over time, with a change in the direction of recognized obstruction.

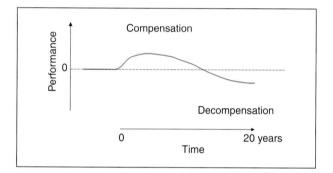

Figure 42.14
Given a certain increased, but over time unchanged, urethral outlet resistance, changes that are induced in the bladder, the nervous system, and in vessels can contribute to compensation with detrusor pressure increase during contraction, etc., in an early phase. One of the consequences of this changed function and the following remodeling of the bladder wall will be a decreased performance at comparable levels later during this process, and thus a decompensation.

changes in the level of the bladder neck, which in such cases can either be isolated or occur together with, for example, BPH (Figure 42.15).

An obstruction below the external sphincter as with, for example, a urethral stricture gives a different clinical picture than the one which appears when the bladder outflow and external sphincter are engaged. With a stricture, features of irritative difficulty such as urges, etc. are seldom seen, whereas this is common with more proximal obstructive processes.

Female incontinence

That the relationships between different female incontinence groups using the currently prevailing classification

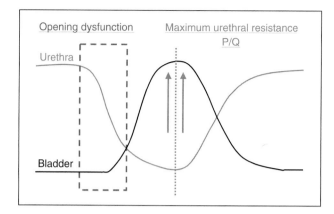

Figure 42.15
The increased detrusor pressure and the decreased urinary flow rate (not shown) used to reflect an outlet obstruction is only representing the moment of maximum performance, which means that an impediment of the opening function might only be caught and classified as an obstruction when we have included any hindrance to the emptying phase (shown as 'New' in Figure 42.4) in our definition of obstruction.

system, which of course builds upon the stress, urge, mixed, and overactivity terminology, have not become clearer over the years is certainly related to an insufficient knowledge of the structure and functionality of the underlying disorder processes, and thus the possibility of making comparisons.[11]

Neuromuscular insufficiency, triggering of normal or pathological reflex activity with or without sensations of urgency, and possible occurrences of incontinence can be described with the simple schedule illustrated in Figure 42.16. More detailed investigations of the different groups, particularly of the urethra and the pelvic floor, have in recent years only managed to move the different incontinence groups closer to each other.[12,13] Changes which they share include a weakness in the musculature of the urethra, pelvic floor, and vaginal wall, which should have a closing effect during stress, and a – possibly of reactive origin – faster establishment of the opening phase and more effective emptying pattern during micturition. A swift activation of emptying seems to be present, which involves a lowering of the pressure in the urethra. This pattern seems to be just as common in incontinent women without urgency, i.e. those that must be classified under stress incontinence using the current terminology.

What could such observations then mean for the classification of disorder(s) eventually leading to female incontinence? One cannot rule out that such opening activity comprises one, and perhaps the foremost, of the least common denominators for different types of female incontinence.[14] Stress incontinence would then not only be

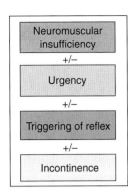

Figure 42.16
A neuromuscular insufficiency in the lower urinary tract might be present in many more women than those being incontinent. Urgency, overactivity, and incontinence might or might not be present. The relation between different types of female incontinence might be better understood.

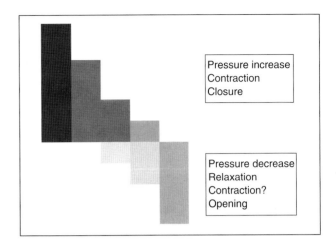

Figure 42.17
The ability to increase the urethral pressure during squeeze seems to also prevent pressure fall and urethral relaxation, whereas incontinent women who often have a reduced ability to increase the intraurethral pressure also present with a urethral relaxation. (Reproduced with permission from Teleman and Mattiasson 2002.)

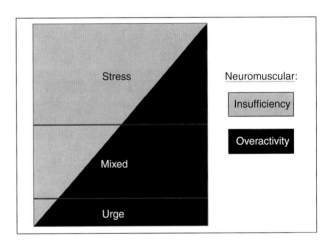

Figure 42.18
A combination of neuromuscular insufficiency and overactive behavior of the lower urinary tract could be a better way than stress, urge, and mixed to describe the condition giving rise to incontinence in women.

comprised of a passive component with insufficient closure due to imperfect contraction during stress but also have an active component in the form of a relaxation, a pressure drop, and opening of the urethra in the same situations. Such easily triggered relaxation activity that is associated with urgency would become classified in our present system as overactive bladder or mixed and urge incontinence, depending upon whether the leakage needs to be triggered with physical exertion and whether urge sensations are present or not. In contrast, using the pathophysiological process for classification would in its functional part instead be characterized by a loss of the functionality in closing abilities of the musculature and instead reveal the penetration of a relaxation-mediating component in a manner that is illustrated by a movement from left to right in Figure 42.17.

To bring together a new model that builds upon the simultaneous occurrence of neuromuscular insufficiency and an increased tendency for activation of emptying-encouraging mechanisms with the traditional stress, mixed, and urge model would give a result that looks like Figure 42.18.

Increased lower urinary tract activity

There are many different types of overactivity.[15] All possible nervous activity and a set of different transmitters or so-called neuromodulators can play important roles in the genesis of overactivity. Solely afferent overactivity with a sensory experience connected to it does exist. Solely efferent overactivity is somewhat more difficult to imagine; however, we certainly all believe that it is possible that purely efferential mechanisms can have an influence on, for example, reflex arches and cause overactivity to arise.

Combinations are common. Afferent overactivity is probably the driver in by far the most cases. A lower urinary tract that is disconnected from a functional context, i.e. without the passage of urine, does not make a nuisance of itself if complicating factors such as infections do not arise.

One often speaks of the significance of neurogenic and myogenic factors. It is important to map out both nerves and muscles; however, without the presence and contribution of both, there will not be much coordinated activity. Isolated myogenic activity with tonus and tension effects on the walls of the lower urinary tract can be found despite this.

Significant trophic changes are often a part of the pathophysiological process, with illnesses and disruptions to the functionality of the lower urinary tract. This is quite natural since structure and functionality go hand-in-hand. At the same time, it is worth noting that the prerequisites for pliability in this case seem particularly large, as nerves and muscles appear to interact: e.g. through the production and influence of nerve-stimulating growth factors.

Since the pattern of overactivity with a pressure drop in the urethra which immediately precedes the rise in bladder pressure is the same as what one sees at the onset of micturition, it appears reasonable to presume that the sequence of events is the same in both situations (Figure 42.19). If such is the case, then one can also characterize the overactivity as LUT instead of detrusor, since all parts of the lower urinary tract seem to be engaged. In addition, it is certainly more precise to call overactivity of this type emptying-related instead of filling-related, as is currently the case with the classification of symptoms related to so-called overactive bladder (Figure 42.20).

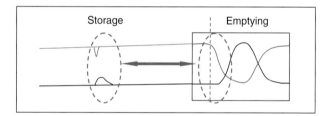

Figure 42.19
The same sequence of events with a urethral pressure fall that precedes the detrusor pressure increase is found in both overactivity and at the start of a normal micturition cycle. It seems reasonable to see this overactivity as emptying-related in nature rather than storage-related.

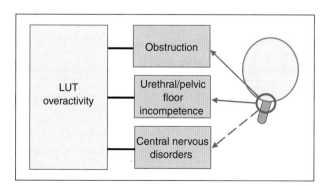

Figure 42.20
The proximal urethra is a probable trigger zone for LUT overactivity in both men and women. Another zone is comprised by the bladder.

A simplified structure and function based classification of lower urinary tract disorders

Since it is not possible to map out all parts of every patient, there is a strong desire to be able to limit one's observations with respect to structure and functionality to a reasonable number. A simplified model that allows this should be able to include observations from the bladder and the outlet/urethra at an early point during bladder filling, at a late point in the filling phase, and with a provocation at the latter or both, as well as also having observations relating to the emptying of the bladder. With this, we must be able to move the focus from the bladder to also encompassing the outlet, urethra, prostate/pelvic floor, as well as including an evaluation of nervous functions as a part of our routine status. In doing so, we will be able to see the pathophysiological process and the disorder or injury as forming a basis for our classification. The symptom picture and other consequences should be added in order to describe manifestations which the patient experiences of the changes that have arisen. In a simplified model we cannot handle anything other than those structures and functions that we regard as being most essential in the micturition cycle. Among these, we count the bladder and the external sphincter, and then we should include the function that is responsible for shutting and opening at the bladder neck level and in the proximal urethra. Along these lines we probably would include the trigone, bladder neck, with men the preprostatic urethra, smooth musculature in the proximal urethra, and the mucous membrane in this area. It is more practical to regard these in their interrelationships and quite simply call them the intermediate segment and the intermediate function (Figure 42.21).

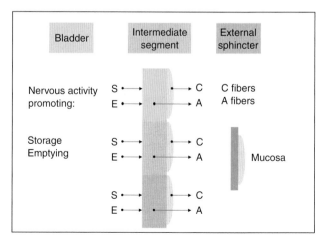

Figure 42.21
A simplified representation of the lower urinary tract and its innervation. S and E denote storage and emptying, respectively, whereas A and C refer to afferent nerve fibers.

For women one can add the pelvic floor to these and, for men, the prostate (Figure 42.22). Activity or morphology concerning efferent nerves that promote filling and emptying can be added, as well as different modalities of afferent innervation, $A\delta$ and C fibers, respectively (Figure 42.23). Figure 42.22 illustrates how BPH can be envisioned to affect both the intermediate segment and the urethra lumen. This is a theoretical model, which, if true, would

explain in a simple manner why a prostate enlargement can be of significance for both the urethra resistance with an established flow as well as for the capability to open the urethra during the initiation of the emptying.

How comprehensive in the sense of how widespread and how intensive a change is and how large an engagement it creates in the surrounding tissues and structures is important to include in a good classification. In addition, one should have a picture of whether afferent and efferent innervation in the three different fundamental parts displays normal characteristics or whether signs of altered innervation/functionality exist. This appears to be knowledge of increasing importance. Placing an extra emphasis on nerves and nervous activity is in line with the fundamental classification model, which proceeds from the neurogenic component in a disruption of the LUT. How this should be carried out and the means by which one should procure this information are of course important questions, but are not covered here. A theoretical model to describe LUT neuromuscular activity might have an appearance similar to that shown in Figure 42.23. After sufficient experience has been built up, one can probably content oneself with a few of the parameters mentioned. A simplified pattern of recognition could then look like Figure 42.24 in its basic structure.

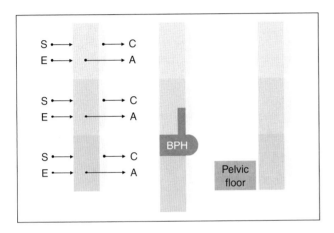

Figure 42.22
Benign prostatic hyperplasia (BPH) might influence not only the urethral lumen but also have a negative impact on the intermediate segment and, for example, bladder neck function. In the female, changes in the pelvic floor might be significant for the whole of the lower urinary tract. S and E denote storage and emptying, respectively, whereas A and C refer to afferent nerve fibers.

Consequences of disorders

The symptoms and the difficulties that an individual feels and experiences are of course completely central for how one should regard the illness/injury. However, they are

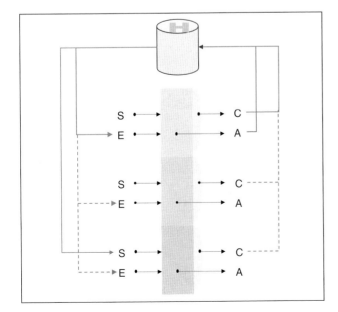

Figure 42.23
Representation of how both A- and C-fiber mediated activity can induce motor events in all parts of the LUT.

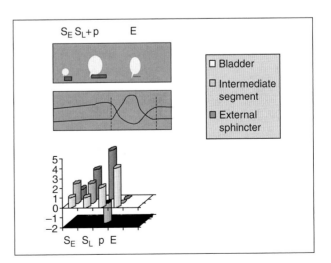

Figure 42.24
A simplified pattern of recognition can be based on a reduced number of observations, and thus provide a framework for clinical use. S_E = storage, early; S_L = storage, late; p = provocation; E = emptying. Arbitrary scale.

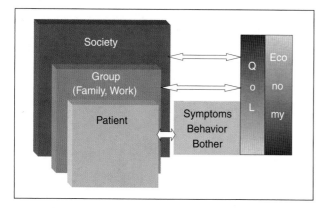

Figure 42.25
Important consequences of the patient's disorder are symptoms, behavior, bother, consequences for quality of life (QoL), and the socioeconomic situation. With increasing consequences, an increased interest should be expected from different groups and from society at large.

consequences of what has been incurred, and thus are secondary to their nature in a classification context (Figure 42.25). That the quality of life is affected to a significant degree by disruptions to the functionality of the lower urinary tract is clear, and likewise that the financial consequences for both the individual and society are most often significant. Their mutual interrelationship can be illustrated by Figure 42.25. A number of different confirming instruments has already been prepared in order to estimate the scope and significance of these consequences, and continued developmental work will provide us with still better measuring instruments.

References

1. Abrams P, Blaivas JG, Stanton SL, Andersen JT. The standardisation of terminology of lower urinary tract function. Scand J Urol Nephrol Suppl 1988; 114(5):5–19.

2. Abrams P, Cardozo L, Fall M, et al. The standardisation of terminology of lower urinary tract function: report from the Standardisation Sub-committee of the International Continence Society. Neurourol Urodyn 2002; 21(2):167–178.

3. Blaivas JG, Appell RA, Fantl JA, et al. Definition and classification of urinary incontinence: recommendations of the Urodynamic Society. Neurourol Urodyn 1997; 16:149–151.

4. Mattiasson A. Characterisation of lower urinary tract disorders: a new view. Neurourol Urodyn 2001; 20:601–621.

5. Hald T, Brading AF, Horn T, et al. Pathophysiology of the urinary bladder in obstruction and ageing. In: Denis, Griffiths, Khoury, et al, eds. Proceedings of the 4th International Consultation on Benign Prostatic Hyperplasia (BPH), 1997:129–178.

6. Patel M, Tewari A, Furman J. Prostatic obstruction and effects on the urinary tract. In: Narayan P, ed. Benign prostatic hyperplasia. Edinburgh: Churchill Livingstone, 2000:139–150.

7. Abrams P, Griffiths D. The assessment of prostatic obstruction from urodynamic measurements and from residual urine. Br J Urol 1979; 51:129–134.

8. Griffiths D, Höfner K, van Mastrigt R, et al. Standardisation of terminology of lower urinary tract function: pressure-flow studies of voiding, urethral resistance, and urethral obstruction. Neurourol Urodyn 1997; 16:1–18.

9. Bates P, Bradley WE, Glen E, et al. Third report on the standardisation of terminology of lower urinary tract function. Procedures related to the evaluation of micturition: pressure flow relationships, residual urine: Br J Urol 1980; 52:348–359; Euro Urol 6:170–171; Acta Urol Jpn 27:1566–1568; Scand J Urol Nephrol 1981; 12:191–193.

10. Bates P, Bradley WE, Glen E, et al. Fourth report on the standardisation of terminology of lower urinary tract function. Terminology related to neuromuscular dysfunction of lower urinary tract. Br J Urol 1981; 52:233–235; Urology 17:618–620; Scand J Urol Nephrol 15:169–171; Acta Urol Jpn 27:1568–1571.

11. Koelbl H, Mostwin J, Boiteeux JP, et al. Pathophysiology. In: Abrams, Cardozo, Khoury, Wein, eds. Proceedings from the 2nd International Consultation on Incontinence, 2001:202–241.

12. Petros PE, Ulmsten UI. An integral theory and its method for the diagnosis and management of female urinary incontinence. Scand J Nephrol Suppl 1993; 153:1–93.

13. Teleman P, Gunnarsson M, Lidfeldt J, et al. Urodynamic characterisation of women with naïve urinary incontinence – a population based study in subjectively incontinent and healthy 53–63 years old women. Eur Urol 2002; 42:583–589.

14. Mattiasson A, Teleman P. A common urethral motor disorder in all types of female incontinence. Submitted to publisher.

15. Fall M, Geirsson G, Lindström S. Toward a new classification of overactive bladders. Neurourol Urodyn 1995; 14:635.

Part VI

Treatment

43

Conservative treatment

Jean-Jacques Wyndaele

Introduction

Conservative treatment is the most applied treatment modality in neurogenic bladder. The reasons for this are clear: most conservative therapeutic methods are cheap, available to the vast majority of patients around the world and, within the limits of proper application, complications are rare.

In this chapter we will give an overview of most techniques used in conservative treatment, including behavioral techniques, physiotherapy, and catheterization.

Behavioral techniques

The philosophy behind behavioral techniques is that one can only have a reasonable chance of acquiring a balanced bladder if daily life adjustments are made to the new situation of the lower urinary tract function caused by the neuropathy. Adjustments can be:

- Scheduled voiding at fixed times during the day when sensation is pathological.
- Voiding several times consecutively in order to lower a residual.
- Increasing the voiding interval to treat frequency. This includes 'bladder drill', aimed at retraining the bladder to hold more urine and inhibit inappropriate detrusor contractions during the filling phase of the micturition cycle.
- Adapting drinking habits, which includes balanced spread of fluid intake and advice on avoiding caffeinated beverages and identifying individual bladder irritants.
- Making the toilet more accessible and improving the patient's mobility.
- Changing drugs intake if these influence diuresis and/or bladder function.
- Treatment of other physical or psychological problems such as constipation and depression.[1]

Hadley divided scheduling regimens into four conceptual categories: bladder training, habit retraining, timed voiding, and prompted voiding.[2]

Keeping a voiding diary can offer information on functional bladder capacity, leakage, and sensation, which are important data for adjusting treatment and for a better understanding by patient and physician. Keeping a voiding diary can also have a therapeutic effect and, by itself, can lead to greater comfort.[3]

Behavioral adaptation and advice is important in all patients.

Physiotherapy

Detrusor overactivity from defective central inhibition or increased detrusor afferent activity can be improved by reinforcing inhibitory pathways. In the storage phase a number of detrusor inhibitory reflexes have been described as emanating from the detrusor via the sympathetic nerves and from the pelvic floor and external urethral sphincter via pudendal afferents.[4] The latter reflex implies that the resting tone in the pelvic floor and external urethral sphincter (supplied by branches of the pudendal nerve: S2–4) has an inhibitory effect on the detrusor. Furthermore, active contraction of these muscle fibers is said to enhance this inhibitory effect. Consequently, pelvic floor training should benefit those patients with weak pelvic musculature. The nerve roots of S2–4 are also involved in some muscles of the lower limb, and there is evidence that activation of S2–4 myotomes may have an inhibitory effect on the detrusor. These muscles include the gluteus maximus, the plantar flexors, and some small muscles of the foot. Hence, one can observe young children activating these myotomes, standing on tiptoes to suppress urgency, and there is no reason why adults cannot use this 'trick'.[5,6]

The sacral dermatomes include the saddle area and the back of the thighs and legs. In particular, the anus, clitoris, and glans penis are well supplied with sensory nerves, and activation of these afferents can inhibit the detrusor.[6]

Centrally, when these afferents are activated by electrical stimulation, they have at least two effects: (1) by provoking the inhibitory sympathetic neurons to the ganglia and the detrusor and (2) by providing central inhibition of the pre-ganglionic bladder motor neurons through a direct route in the sacral cord. Some young girls have been observed to 'curtsy' to control urgency. The pressure of the heel on the perineum presumably activates the sacral dermatomes, in addition to possibly elevating the bladder neck and supporting the proximal urethra. When learning bladder drill for urgency and urge incontinence, patients can be taught to sit down (on a rolled-up towel is best) and press on/squeeze the clitoris/glans penis and so activate the appropriate dermatomes. This reduces urgency, inhibits/reduces unwanted bladder contractions, and helps the patient to defer voiding, aiming to increase the functional bladder capacity. The daily use of transcutaneous electrical nerve stimulation (TENS) over S2–4 dermatomes has also been shown to have a beneficial effect on reducing urgency and urge incontinence. Self-adhesive electrodes delivering 2 Hz stimulation placed bilaterally over S3 in 40 children showed 67.5% response.[7] Sacral stimulation at 10 Hz over S3 in 71 adults with chronic sensory urgency, detrusor instability, or detrusor hyperreflexia during urodynamics showed a significant improvement in cystometric volumes with a concomitant reduction in detrusor pressure compared with pre-stimulation cystometry.[8] TENS applied over the peroneal or posterior tibial nerve is another option for activating sacral afferents.

There is abundant evidence to support the use of maximal electrical stimulation to activate the detrusor inhibitory reflexes from the anal and vaginal regions using electrodes specially designed for this purpose. Optimum electrical parameters include low-frequency (5–10 Hz) alternating rectangular pulses at maximum intensity. This activates the sympathetic inhibitory system to the bladder and the central inhibitory pathway to parasympathetic motor neurons, which have all been shown to operate at low frequencies.[9] In a group of 74 patients with detrusor instability and urge incontinence treated with maximal electrical stimulation, 51 were subjectively cured or significantly improved. Objectively, a significant decrease in frequency and significant increase in bladder volume were demonstrated.[10] A further study by Eriksen et al[11] demonstrated initial clinical and urodynamic cures in 50% of 48 women suffering from idiopathic detrusor instability following seven 20-min treatments of maximal stimulation using a vaginal and an anal electrode simultaneously. In addition, a significant improvement was observed in a further 33%. At 1 year follow-up, a persisting therapeutic effect was found in 77% and no serious side-effects were reported.[11] Also, maximal stimulation on the thigh muscles gave such effect.[12]

Detrusor hypoactivity may also respond to physiotherapy in the form of techniques to facilitate detrusor activity.

Activation of stretch receptors in the bladder wall can instigate a detrusor contraction, and so pressing or tapping over the bladder may set off a detrusor contraction. Likewise, bending forward and straining may help to initiate detrusor activity. However, suprapubic tapping and straining are risky techniques, as described below. Bladder emptying may be further enhanced by ensuring relaxation of the pelvic floor.

Furthermore, using maximal electrical stimulation of the pelvic floor muscles, Plevnik et al[13] treated six patients with spinal cord lesions from C5 to T4, all demonstrating detrusor-sphincter dyssynergia, in whom urinary retention developed. After two to four 20-min treatments over 4 weeks, using vaginal or anal electrodes and monophasic square pulses of 1 ms, frequency of 20 Hz and 50–90 mA, a reduction in maximal urethral pressure was reported. In addition, uninhibited detrusor contractions were reduced in four patients and reflex voiding by tapping was successful in all patients.

Intravesical transurethral bladder stimulation is used to rehabilitate the neurogenic bladder.[14] Its therapeutic goals are to achieve a sensation of bladder filling, to initiate a detrusor contraction, and to achieve conscious urinary control. The procedure combines direct stimulation of the bladder receptors with visual feedback using patient observance of cystometric pressure changes. The effects are technique-dependent.[15]

Several other techniques of pelvic floor physiotherapy can be successfully used in patients with neurogenic bladder: Biofeedback and relaxation can have indications in patients with partly preserved voluntary and/or sensory function.

Intravesical biofeedback has been used successfully in improving the sensation of bladder fullness and control of involuntary contractions.[16]

Triggered reflex voiding is much less applied than a decade ago, but nevertheless it is still used. Bladder reflex triggering comprises various maneuvers performed by the patient in order to elicit reflex detrusor contractions by exteroceptive stimuli.[17] The pathophysiological background is unphysiological in suprasacral lesions for which the technique is mostly used: it comprises C-fiber activation, bladder contraction involuntary and not sustained, detrusor-striated sphincter dyssynergia or detrusor-bladder neck dyssynergia, and autonomic dysreflexia.[18] Only in the minority of patients will triggering lead to balanced voiding. Complications such as infection,[19,20] upper urinary tract alterations/deterioration, and incontinence are frequent. If applied, patients should be encouraged to find the best individual trigger zone and points: suprapubic tapping, thigh scratching, squeezing the glans penis and the scrotal skin, pulling on the crines pubis, as well as anal/rectal manipulation may be effective.[21]

Suprapubic tapping must be stopped in most patients when micturition starts, permitting the fast-reacting striated sphincter to relax, whereas the slowly reacting detrusor may still remain in contraction. As soon as micturition stops, tapping has to be applied again.

Drugs or surgery may be necessary to decrease outflow resistance and to improve reflex incontinence. Videourodynamics are strongly advised to find out if the urodynamic situation is safe. Triggered voiding is contraindicated in cases of:

- inadequate detrusor contraction
- unbalanced voiding
- vesico-uretero-renal reflux
- reflux in the seminal vesicles or in the vas
- uncontrollable AD
- persistence of recurrent urinary tract infections.

Bladder expression comprises various maneuvers aimed at increasing intravesical pressure in order to enable/facilitate bladder emptying. The most commonly used are the Valsalva (abdominal straining) and the Credé (manual compression of the lower abdomen) maneuvers. Bladder expression has been recommended for a long time for patients with so-called lower motor neuron lesions, resulting in a combination of an underactive detrusor with an underactive sphincter or with an incompetent urethral closure mechanism of other origin. Clinical experience has shown that by using Valsalva or Credé maneuvers many patients are able to empty their bladders, albeit mostly incompletely. Urodynamics/videourodynamics have demonstrated that, despite high intravesical pressures during straining, the urinary flow may be very poor due to an inability to open the bladder neck, or to a mechanical obstruction at the level of the striated external sphincter by bending and compression of the urethra. Moreover, Clarke and Thomas[22] showed in flaccid male paraplegics that the major component of urethral resistance is a constant, adrenergically innervated muscular resistance in the external sphincter region.

With increasing time, more than 40% of the patients on straining show influx into the prostate and the seminal vesicles, and complications due to the high pressures such as reflux to the upper urinary tract. Measures to facilitate bladder expression can be the use of α-blockers, but they usually cause or increase urinary stress incontinence.

Contraindications are:

- sphincter hyperreflexia and detrusor-sphincter dyssynergia
- vesico-uretero-renal reflux
- reflux into the male adnexa
- hernias
- hemorrhoids
- urethral pathology
- symptomatic urinary tract infections.

Some patients use the anal sphincter stretch described by Low and Donovan[23] with success.

Intermittent catheterization and intermittent self-catheterization

Intermittent catheterization (IC) and intermittent self-catheterization (ISC) have become widely used in the last 40 years. Many studies show good results and limited complications, leading to a better prognosis and a better quality of life in many patients with neurologic bladder[24–26] (Table 43.1).

IC and ISC are nowadays considered as the methods of choice for the management of neurologic bladder dysfunction.[18]

Results depend on the techniques used, which involves the types of catheters and lubricants, the catheter manipulation and introduction, and the rules needed for a short-term and long-term successful application.

Many types of catheters are used, made of different material. Some are packed in a sheet/bag, others are reusable.[27] Some have a urethral introducer that permits bypassing the colonized 1.5 cm of the distal urethra and which resulted in a significant lower infection rate in hospitalized men with spinal cord injury.[28] Studies comparing materials in a randomized controlled way are scarce. Lundgren et al[29] found, in the rabbit, that a high osmolality is important in hydrophilic catheters with regards to removing friction and urethral trauma. Waller et al[30] had the same experience in men. Wyndaele et al[31] evaluated the use of a hydrophilic catheter in 39 male patients with neurogenic bladder using conventional catheters over a long period. The hydrophilic catheter proved as easy to use but was better tolerated. Satisfaction was better, especially in patients who experienced problems with conventional catheters. Some patients were unsatisfied for reasons of practical use or for economical reasons.

Most catheters require the use of some kind of lubricant, especially in men. Lubricants are applied on the catheter or are instilled into the urethra.[32] In some countries patients use oil or merely water as a lubricant. For patients with preserved urethral sensation, a local anesthetic jelly may be needed. Catheters with a hydrophilic and self-lubricated surface need activation with tap water or sterile water.

For adults, size 10–14 F for males and size 14–16 F for females are mostly used, but a bigger size/lumen may be necessary for those with bladder augmentation or cloudy urine that results from another origin. No studies on IC compared sizes in a randomized way.

Two main techniques have been adopted: a sterile (SIC) and a clean IC (CIC). The sterile non-touch technique advocated by Guttmann and Frankel implicates the use of

Table 43.1 *Outcome of continence study*

Authors	Number of patients	Follow-up	Adjunctive treatment	Result of continence
Iwatsubo et al[118]	60 spinal cord lesions		Overdistention during shock phase	100% continent
Kornhuber and Schultz[120]	197 multiple sclerosis			Continence improved with elimination of residual urine
Kuhn et al[121]	22 spinal cord lesions	5 years	No	Continence did not change
Lindehall et al[122]	26 meningomyeloceles	7.5–12 years		24/26 better
Madersbacher and Weissteiner[116]	12 f	2–4 years		50% dry; other 50% some grade of incontinence
McGuire and Savastano[119]	22 f	2–11 years	Surgery 27%	Continent 73%
Vaidyanathan et al[124]	7 spinal cord lesions	14–30 months	Bladder relaxant drugs intravesically	84% dry, 3 dampness at awakening
Waller et al[123]	30 spinal cord lesions	5–9 years	6 anticholinergics	22 dry, 8 incontinent
Wyndaele et al[117]	30 (18 m, 12 f)	3–30 months	6 anticholinergic, 1 colocystoplasty	73% continent + 13% improvement
Wyndaele and Maes[84]	75 (69 neurogenic)	1.5–12 years	38 anticholinergics	47 dry, 22 seldom wet, 6 wet at least once a day

f = female; m = male.

sterile materials handled with sterile gloves and forceps. In an intensive care unit, some advocate wearing a mask and a sterile gown as well. In some centers, during a bladder training program SIC used to be performed only by a catheter team, which has proven to obtain a very low infection rate.[33] Nowadays, the sterile technique is mostly used only during a restricted period of time and in a hospital setting. In the majority of cases a clean technique is used.

Self-catheterization is done in many different positions: supine, sitting, or standing. Female patients may use a mirror or a specially designed catheter to visualize the meatus. After a while, most women do not need these aids anymore.

The basic principles of urinary catheter introduction are well known: the catheter must be introduced in a noninfecting and atraumatic way. Noninfecting means cleaning hands, using a noninfected catheter and lubricant, and cleaning the meatal region before catheter introduction. Atraumatic requires a proper catheter size, sufficient lubrication, and gentle introduction through the urethra, sphincter area, and bladder neck.[34,35] The catheter has to be introduced until urine flows out. Urine can be drained

directly in the toilet, in a urinal, plastic bag, or other reservoir. The catheter should be kept in place until urine flow stops. Then it should be pulled out slowly, while gentle Valsalva or bladder expression is done in order to completely empty residual urine. When properly done, the residual urine should be maximum 6 ml.[36] However, Jensen et al measured residual urine repeatedly with ultrasonography and found residual urine in 70% of the catheterizations in their group of 12 patients with spinal cord lesion. The residual urine could exceed 50 ml and even 100 ml.[37]

Finally, the end of the catheter should be blocked to prevent backflow of the urine or air into the bladder. Hydrophilic catheters can be left in place for a short time only to prevent suction by the urethral mucosa, which may make removal difficult.

During the rehabilitation phase, clean intermittent self-catheterization (CISC) can be taught very early to patients with good hand function.[38]

When resources are limited, catheters are reused for weeks and months: some are resterilized or cleaned by soaking in an antiseptic solution or boiling water. Microwaving to resterilize rubber catheters has also been described. Reused supplies do not seem to be related to an increased likelihood of urinary tract infection.[39,40]

The frequency of catheterization needed can depend on many factors, such as bladder volume, fluid intake, post-void residual, and urodynamic parameters (bladder compliance, detrusor pressure). Usually it is recommended to catheterize 4–6 times a day during the acute phase after spinal cord lesion. Some patients will need to keep this frequency if IC is the only way of bladder emptying. Other patients will catheterize 1–3 times a day to check and evacuate residual urine after voiding or on a weekly basis during bladder retraining.[41] Use of a portable ultrasound device in IC has been evaluated.[42,43]

Adjunctive therapy to overcome high detrusor pressure is often needed. Anticholinergic drugs or bladder relaxants are often indicated in patients with bladder overactivity. For patients who develop a low-compliance bladder, upper tract deterioration or severe incontinence injection of botulinum toxin in the bladder wall or surgery as bladder augmentation may be necessary.[44,45] Where a too high diuresis is noted during the night due to diurnal variation of anti-diuretic hormone, DDAVP (desmopressin) can be safely and effectively used.[46,47] In cases of catheterization difficulty at the striated sphincter, botulinum toxin injection in the sphincter can help.[48] In individuals with tetraplegia, reconstructive hand surgery can be indicated.[49] For those with poor hand function or difficulty in reaching the meatus, assistive devices might be needed.[50]

Education is very important. Teaching programs have been successful in non-literate persons in developing countries and in quadriplegic patients.[51,52]

It is clear that IC can improve incontinence or can make patients with neurogenic bladder continent. To achieve this, bladder capacity should be sufficient, bladder pressure kept low, urethral resistance high enough, and care taken to balance between fluid intake, residual urine, and frequency of catheterization.

Not all patients starting with IC continue this treatment and several reasons can exist for this (Table 43.2). A main reason to stop is continuing incontinence. Main reasons to continue are continence and autonomy of the patients.[53] Bakke and Malt found that, among those who practiced IC independently, 25.8% were sometimes and 6% were always averse, especially young patients and females. Aversion seemed to be related above all to nonacceptance of their chronic disability.[54] A recent retrospective analysis in spinal cord injury patients showed that, of patients on CIC at discharge, 52% discontinued the method and reverted to an indwelling catheter because of dependence on caregivers, spasticity interfering with catheterization, incontinence despite anticholinergic agents, and lack of availability of external collective devices for female patients.[55]

The introduction of a catheter several times a day can give rise to complications. One of the most frequent complications is infection of the urinary tract (UTI). Prevalence of UTI varies widely in the literature. This is due to the various methods used for evaluation, the different techniques of IC, different frequencies of urine analysis, different criteria for infection and the administration or not of prophylaxis to the group of patients studied, and much more. Some publications give the percentage of sterile urine at between 12 and 88%.[24,56–61] Eleven percent prevalence for asymptomatic UTI and 53% for symptomatic bacteriuria are given in different series.[62,63] Bakke found that in 407 patients, 252 with neurogenic bladder, during an observation period of 1 year, 24.5% of patients had nonclinical UTI, 58.6% had minor symptoms, 14.3% had more

Table 43.2 *Reasons for stopping intermittent self-catheterization*

Authors	Catheter-free	Incontinence	Inconvenience	Infection	Physical status	Choice of patient
Bakke[131]	10%		5%	4%	3%	
Diokno et al[125]	17%	2%	2%		7%	
Hunt et al[132]	10%					
Maynard and Glass[126]	12%					6%
Sutton et al[130]		6%	6%	3%	3%	3%
Timoney and Shaw[129]		36%				
Whitelaw et al[127]	5%		5%		5%	5%
Webb et al[128]	9%		3%		2%	2%

comprehensive or frequent symptoms, while 2.6% claimed major symptoms.[64]

In the acute stage of spinal cord injury (SCI), with proper management, urine can be kept sterile for 15–20 days without antibiotic prophylaxis and for 16–55 days if prophylaxis is given.[65–67] Prieto-Fingerhut et al[68] determined the effect of sterile and nonsterile IC on the incidence of urinary tract infection in 29 patients after SCI in a randomized controlled trial. With urine analysis on a weekly basis they found a 28.6% UTI incidence in the group on sterile IC, whereas a 42.4% incidence was found in the nonsterile catheterization group. The cost of antibiotics for the sterile IC group was only 43% of the cost for those on nonsterile IC. However, the cost of the sterile IC kits was 371% of the cost of the kits used by the nonsterile IC group, bringing the total cost of the sterile program to 277% of the other program. Rhame and Perkash[65] found that in 70 SCI patients in the initial rehabilitation hospitalization treated with sterile catheterization and a neomycin–polymyxin irrigant, 54% of patients developed an infection, at an overall rate of 10.3 infections per 1000 patient-days on IC. Bakke and Volset[69] found that factors that may predict the occurrence of clinical UTI in patients using clean IC were low age and high mean catheterization volume in women, low age, neurogenic bladder dysfunction, and nonself-catheterization in men, in addition to urine leakage in patients with neurogenic dysfunction and the presence of bacteriuria. If antibacterial prophylaxis was used, fewer episodes of bacteriuria were noticed, but significantly more clinical UTIs were seen. Shekelle et al reviewed the risk factors for UTI in adults with spinal cord dysfunction[70] and found increased bladder residual volume to be a risk factor. Patients on IC had fewer infections than those with indwelling catheters.

In order to diagnose UTI, it should be recommended that the urine be obtained by catheterization.[71] The frequency of examining urine samples differs greatly between studies: daily use of a dipslide technique during the acute phase after SCI, once a week during the subacute phase, and monthly or a few times a year in long-term care.[72–74]

If a urine culture reveals more than 10^4 cfu/ml, this indicates significant bacteriuria. Pyuria alone is not considered reliable in patients with neurogenic bladder.[75,76] The bacteria found are mostly *Escherichia coli*, *Proteus*, *Citrobacter*, *Pseudomonas*, *Klebsiella*, *Staphylococcus aureus*, and *Streptococcus faecalis* in short-term cases, while the same bacteria plus *Acinetobacter* are found in the long-term IC patients.[77,78] *E. coli* is considered the dominant species.[64] The detection of *E. coli* on the periurethra corresponds, at a much higher percentage, with bacteriuria than if other bacteria are found.[79] *E. coli* isolates from patients who develop symptomatic UTI may be distinguished from bacteria recovered from patients who remain asymptomatic and possibly from normal fecal *E. coli*.[80]

Urinary sepsis is fortunately rare.[81,82] Previous treatment with an indwelling catheter represents a special risk to develop sepsis.[83] In his thesis Wyndaele[34] found the period of 24 hours to 3 days after changing from indwelling to IC drainage when UTI was present to be dangerous for the development of sepsis.

Wyndaele and Maes[84] found several relationships between IC and UTI. If catheterization is begun by patients with recurrent or chronic UTI and urinary retention, the incidence of infection decreases and patients may become totally free of infection. If symptomatic infections occur, improper practice of IC or misuse can often be found. Chronic infection persists after IC has been started, if the cause of the chronicity remains.

To prevent UTI, a noninfecting technique is needed. But also some additional factors can play a role in infection prevention. Nursing education is important and educational intervention by a clinic nurse is a simple, cost-effective means of decreasing the risk of UTIs in individuals with SCI on IC who are identified as at risk.[85] Anderson[67] found a fivefold incidence when IC was performed 3 times a day compared with 6 times a day. Also, prevention of bladder overdistention is important.[57,70] Crossinfection is less if IC during hospitalization is performed by a catheter team or by the patients themselves. As residual urine plays a role in infection, attention must be made to empty the bladder completely.

Treatment of UTI is necessary if the infection is symptomatic. Waites et al[86] treated men with SCI on IC and saw susceptible organisms disappear from urine in all and significantly reduced in the perineum and urethra. However, they were replaced shortly after by resistant Gram-positive cocci. This shows the importance of reserving antibiotics for symptomatic patients only and of taking into account the data from the antibiogram. The value of nontreatment for chronic nonsymptomatic bacteriuria throughout a hospitalization has been demonstrated.[87]

With antibacterial prophylaxis, several studies have shown a lowered infection rate.[88–94] Cranberry juice has been evaluated recently, but results are unclear.[94] Several studies have considered the risk of developing dangerous resistance against antibiotics when prophylaxis is given either orally or by instillation.[95–97] Galloway et al[98] state that the threat of emergence of resistant organisms, the risk to patients of side-effects of the antibiotics, the expense, and the risk to other patients from crossinfection with resistant organisms are strong arguments against prophylactic antibacterials. Therefore, it would seem logical to use antibacterial prophylaxis only for a short time, such as during the initial stage of IC. It does seem to be less indicated for long-term use, although it can help specific patients to lower the rate of symptomatic infections for which no well-defined cause is found.

Urethritis and epididymo-orchitis have been reported in several case series (Table 43.3). With a long-term

Table 43.3 *Literature data on genitourinary complications in patients on intermittent catheterization*

Author	Total no. of patients	Urethritis	Meatal stricture	Epididymitis	Urethral stricture
Bakke[131]	407 (206 m)	1%		1%	
Hellstrom et al[140]	41 (26 m)			3	
Kuhn et al[121]	22 (11 m)		1		1
Labat et al[138]	68 (48 m)	9 m		3	
Lapides et al[133]	100 (34 m)	2 m	–	–	–
Lapides et al[134]	218 (90 m)	2 m	–	2	
Maynard and Diokno[137]	28 (m?)			4 (1 with infected penile prosthesis)	
Maynard and Glass[139]	34 (m?)			3	2
Orikasa et al[135]	26 (13 m)			1	
Perkash and Giroux[142]	50 m			5	
Perrouin-Verbe et al[53]	159 (113 m)			10% short term, 28% long term	5.3%
Thirumavalan and Ransley[141]				12%	
Waller et al[123]	30 SCI (26 m)			2	4
Webb et al[128]				2%	
Wyndaele et al[136]	30 (18 m)	2 m		2	
Wyndaele and Maes[84]	75 (33 m)		3	6	7

m = male, SCI, spinal cord injury.

indwelling catheter, a larger prevalence is seen.[34] Genital infections can lower fertility in SCI patients.[99] If IC is used to empty the neurogenic bladder, better sperm quality and better pregnancy rates have been found than with indwelling catheterization.[100,101]

Prostatitis can be a cause of recurrent UTI: either acute or chronic, it is difficult to diagnose in patients with neurogenic bladder, and special tests have been developed for this.[102,103] The overall incidence was previously thought to be around 5–18%[71] but 33% may be a more realistic figure.[104]

Urethral bleeding is frequently seen in new patients and occurs regularly in one-third on a long-term basis.[105] Trauma of the urethra, especially in men, can cause false passages, meatal stenosis but the incidence is rare (see Table 43.3). The incidence of urethral strictures increases with a longer follow-up, with most events occurring after 5 years of IC.[53,84] Former treatment with an indwelling catheter causes more complications. Urethral changes were also documented in SCI men on IC for an average of 5 years, using one single reusable silicone catheter for an average of 3 years.[106] IC technique and catheter type

are claimed to be important factors.[30,107,108] Urethral trauma with false passages in neurogenic patients on CIC can be treated successfully with 5 days of antibiotics and 6 weeks of indwelling catheter. The false passage will also disappear on cystoscopy and IC can be safely restarted.[109]

Other complications such as hydronephrosis, vesico-ureteral reflux, and bladder cancer seem to relate rather to infection, bladder trabeculation, detrusor pressure, or neuropathy than to IC itself.[110]

Bladder calculi caused by the introduction of pubic hair,[111,112] loss of the catheter in the bladder,[113] bladder perforation, and bladder necrosis[114] have been case reports on rare complications of IC.

And what if IC or ISC is not possible? There can be several reasons for this: bad hand function and no relative to perform the catheterization, unwillingness of the patient, cost, lack of knowledge from carers, persistent incontinence, general bad condition, or difficulty to reach the meatus. In many cases these problems may be overcome with proper treatment. However, in some cases an indwelling catheter will be used.

Transurethral and suprapubic catheters

Transurethral and suprapubic catheters have been used for a long time. The dangers of the techniques have been well documented and the complications are well known. If they are used, it is very important to stick to good rules of management:

- Catheter size 12–14.
- Place the catheter properly with the balloon in the bladder. It is important to be especially careful in the presence of a spastic sphincter.
- Control the outflow regularly to avoid overdistention.
- Change the catheter regularly several times a week in an acute situation, every 10 days if possible, and every 4–6 weeks in a chronic patient who has few complications.
- Anticholinergic drugs may be important in patients with bladder hyperreflexia.
- Antibacterial drugs should not be used to prevent or to treat an asymptomatic infection of the urine. With an indwelling catheter, the prevalence of infection is 100% if the catheter is used for more than a couple of weeks. In the case of symptomatic infection, treatment is necessary.
- There is no general agreement on clamping of the catheter. In cases of severe incontinence unsuccessfully treated with drugs, a continuous outflow is not the only conservative possibility.
- Complications are frequent. The transurethral catheter can cause acute septic episodes, urethral trauma and bleeding, false passages, strictures, diverticuli and fistuli of the urethra, bladder stones, squamous cell bladder carcinoma, epididymo-orchitis, and prostatitis. With application of good treatment rules, many of these conditions can be largely avoided.
- The presence of an indwelling catheter should be known to all who take care of the patient: OT, PT, and of course the nursing staff.

Appliances (condom catheters, penile clamps)

Their use aims at collecting leaking urine into a device, thus preventing urinary spilling and giving better hygienic control, better control of unpleasant odor and a better quality of life. A condom catheter is indicated in all male patients with urinary incontinence provided that there is no skin/penile lesion, and intravesical pressures during storage and voiding phase are urodynamically proven to be safe.

No absolute contraindications for such appliances seem to exist.

Condom catheters are not invasive and permit us to avoid most of the complications related to indwelling catheters. Old versions were reusable external collecting devices that fitted rather loosely around the penis. They are still preferred by a few paralysed patients who have been accustomed to them for a long time, especially those with a retractile penis.

The actual types are thin conical-shaped sheaths made of different sorts of material. They fit over the shaft of the penis, fixed with some type of glue or occlusive strip. The tips are open and connected with the tube of a urinary collecting device. In recent years special condoms and special devices allowing urethral catheterization without removing the condom have been manufactured.

While the advantages of condom catheters over indwelling catheters and incontinence pads are evident, they are not without problems and complications, sometimes severe:

- Fixation to the skin can be difficult with a smaller and/or retractile penis and/or abundant pubic fat. The problem can be partly overcome by using the proper size and proper fixation glue/strip. A penile prosthesis can be a solution in the case of a retractile small penis.
- Obstruction of urine flow is a rather common problem, due to twisting or kinking of the tip of the condom or the collecting tube. To prevent this, most of the currently available condom catheters are reinforced at the tip.
- Lesions of the penis can be secondary to mechanical damage to the skin from an excessively tight condom worn for a prolonged time. One way of prevention is to discontinue the use of the condom during part of the day or night. Another source of skin lesion is allergy to the material of the condom, usually to latex. Such an allergy is not uncommon, i.e. in myelomeningocele patients. The use a latex-free condom is the solution.
- Urinary tract infection.

Newman and Price[115] found bacteriuria in more than 50% of patients using a condom catheter. One of the few factors correlated with increased risk for UTI was less than daily change of the condom.

Penile clamps are not recommended for patients with neuropathic voiding dysfunction, because of the danger of skin and urethral lesions.[18]

References

1. Wyndaele JJ. Les techniques comportementales. In: Corcos J, Schick E, eds. Les vessies neurogènes de l'adulte. Paris: Masson, 1996: 197–202.

2. Hadley EC. Bladder training and related therapies for urinary incontinence in older people. JAMA 1986; 256:372–379.

3. Dowd T, Kolcaba K, Steiner R. Using cognitive strategies to enhance bladder control and comfort. Holist Nurs Pract 2000; 14:91–103.

4. Mahoney DT, Laferte RO, Blais DJ. Integral storage and voiding reflexes; a neurophysiologic concept of continence and micturition. Urology 1980; 9:95–106.

5. Shafik A. Study of the response of the urinary bladder to stimulation of the cervix uteri and clitoris – "The genitovesical Reflex": an experimental study. Int Urogynecol J 1995; 6:41–46.

6. Laycock J. What can the specialist physiotherapist do? In: Wyndaele JJ, Laycock J, eds. Multidisciplinary conservative treatment for the neurogenic bladder. Wokingham: Incare, 2002:14–18.

7. Hoebeke P, De Paepe H, Renson C, et al. Transcutaneous neuromodulation in non-neuropathic bladder sphincter dysfunction in children: preliminary results. Neurourol Urodyn 1999; 18(4):263–264.

8. Walsh IK, Keane PF, Johnston SR, et al. Non-invasive antidromic sacral neurostimulation to enhance bladder storage. Neurourol Urodyn 1999; 18(4):380.

9. Lindstrom S, Fall M, Carlsson C-A, et al. The neurophysiological basis of bladder inhibition in response to intravaginal electrical stimulation. J Urol 1983; 129:405–410.

10. Fossberg E, Sorensen S, Ruutu M, et al. Maximal electrical stimulation in the treatment of unstable detrusor and urge incontinence. Eur Urol 1990; 18:120–123.

11. Eriksen BC, Bergmann S, Eik-Ness SH. Maximal electrostimulation of the pelvic floor in female idiopathic detrusor instability and urge incontinence. Neurourol Urodyn 1989; 8:219–230.

12. Okada N, Igawa A, Ogawa A, Nishizawa O. Transcutaneous electrical stimulation of thigh muscles in the treatment of detrusor overactivity. Br J Urol 1998; 81:560–564.

13. Plevnik S, Homan G, Vrtacnik P. Short-term maximal electrical stimulation for urinary retention. Urol 1984; 24:521–523.

14. Katona F. Stages of vegetative afferentation in reorganization of bladder control during intravesical electrotherapy. Urol Int 1975; 30:192–203.

15. De Wachter S, Wyndaele JJ. Quest for standardization of electrical sensory testing in the lower urinary tract: the influence of technique related factors on bladder electrical thresholds. Neurourol Urodyn 2002; 21:1–6.

16. Wyndaele JJ, Hoekx L, Vermandel A. Bladder biofeedback for the treatment of refractory sensory urgency in adults. Eur Urol 1997; 32:429–432.

17. Andersen JT, Blaivas JG, Cardozo L, Thuroff J. Lower urinary tract rehabilitation techniques: seventh report on the standardisation of terminology of lower urinary tract function. Neurourol Urodyn 11:593–603.

18. Madersbacher H, Wyndaele JJ, Igawa Y, et al. Conservative management in the neuropathic patient. In: Abrams P, Khoury S, Wein A, eds. Incontinence. Health Publication, 1999:775–812.

19. Stover SL, Lloyd LK, Waites KB, Jackson AB. Neurogenic urinary infection. Neurolog Clin 1991; 9:741–755.

20. Lloyd LK, Kuhlemeier KV, Stover SL. Initial bladder management in spinal cord injury: does it make a difference? J Urol 1986; 135:523–526.

21. Rossier A, Bors E. Detrusor response to perineal and rectal stimulation in patients with spinal cord injuries. Urol Int 1964; 10:181–190.

22. Clarke SJ, Thomas DG. Characteristics of the urethral pressure profile in flaccid male paraplegics. Br J Urol 1981; 53:157–161.

23. Low AI, Donovan WD. The use and mechanism of anal sphincter stretch in the reflex bladder. Br J Urol 1981; 53:430–432.

24. Guttmann L, Frankel H. The value of intermittent catheterization in the early management of traumatic paraplegia and tetraplegia. Paraplegia 1966; 4:63–83.

25. Lapides J, Diokno A, Silber S, Lowe B. Clean intermittent self-catheterization in the treatment of urinary tract disease. J Urol 1972; 107:458–461.

26. Maynard FM, Diokno A. Clean intermittent catheterization for spinal cord injured patients. J Urol 1982; 128:477–480.

27. Wu Y, Hamilton BB, Boyink MA, Nanninga JB. Re-usable catheter for longterm intermittent catheterization. Arch Phys Med Rehab 1981; 62:39–42.

28. Bennett CJ, Young MN, Razi SS, et al. The effect of urethral introducer tip catheters on the incidence of urinary tract infection outcomes in spinal cord injured patients. J Urol 1997; 158:519–521.

29. Lundgren J, Bengtsson O, Israelsson A, et al. The importance of osmolality for intermittent catheterization of the urethra. Spinal Cord 2000; 38:45–50.

30. Waller L, Telander M, Sullivan L. The importance of osmolality in hydrophilic urethral catheters a crossover study. Spinal Cord 1998; 36:368–369.

131. Wyndaele JJ, De Ridder D, Everaert K, et al. Evaluation of the use of Urocath-Gel catheters for intermittent self-catheterization by male patients using conventional catheters for a long time. Spinal Cord 2000; 38:97–99.

32. Hedlund H, Hjelmas K, Jonsson O, et al. Hydrophilic versus non-coated catheters for intermittent catheterization. Scand J Urol Nephrol 2001; 35:49–53.

33. Lindan R, Bellomy V. The use of intermittent catheterization in a bladder training program, preliminary report. J Chron Dis 1971; 24:727–735.

34. Wyndaele JJ. Early urological treatment of patients with an acute spinal cord injury. Thesis Doctor in Biomedical Science, State University of Ghent, 1983.

35. Corcos J. Traitements non médicamenteux des vessies neurogènes. In: Corcos J, Schick E, eds. Les vessies neurogènes de l'adulte. Paris: Masson, 1996:173–187.

36. Stribrna J, Fabian F. The problem of residual urine after catheterization. Acta Univ Carol Med 1961; 7:931–943.

37. Jensen AE, Hjeltnes N, Berstad J, Stanghelle JK. Residual urine following intermittent catheterisation in patients with spinal cord injuries. Paraplegia 1995; 33:693–696.

38. Wyndaele JJ, De Taeye N. Early intermittent selfcatheterization after spinal cord injury. Paraplegia 1990; 28:76–80.

39. Champion VL. Clean technique for intermittent self-catheterization. Nurs Res 1976; 25:13–18.

40. Silbar E, Cicmanec J, Burke B, Bracken RB. Microwave sterilization. Method for home sterilization of urinary catheter. J Urol 1980; 141:88–90.

41. Opitz JL. Bladder retraining: an organized program. Mayo Clin Proc 1976; 51:367–372.

42. Anton HA, Chambers K, Clifton J, Tasaka J. Clinical utility of a portable ultrasound device in intermittent catheterization. Arch Phys Med Rehab 1998; 79:172–175.

43. De Ridder D, Van Poppel H, Baert L, Binard J. From time dependent intermittent selfcatheterisation to volume dependent selfcatheterisation in multiple sclerosis using the PCI 5000 Bladdermanager. Spinal Cord 1997; 35:613–616.

44. Schurch B, Stöhrer M, Kramer G, et al. Botulinum-A toxin for treating detrusor hyperreflexia in spinal cord injured patients: a new alternative to anticholinergic drugs? Preliminary results. J Urol 2000; 164:692–697.

45. Mast P, Hoebeke P, Wyndaele JJ, et al. Experience with augmentation cystoplasty. A review. Paraplegia 1995; 33:560–564.

46. Kilinc S, Akman MN, Levendoglu F, Ozker R. Diurnal variation of antidiuretic hormone and urinary output in spinal cord injury. Spinal Cord 1999; 37:332–335.

47. Chancellor MB, Rivas DA, Staas WE Jr. DDAVP in the urological management of the difficult neurogenic bladder in spinal cord injury: preliminary report. J Am Paraplegia Soc 1994; 17:165–167.

48. Wheeler JS Jr, Walter JS, Chintam RS, Rao S. Botulinum toxin injections for voiding dysfunction following SCI. J Spinal Cord Med 1998; 21:227–229.

49. Kiyono Y, Hashizume C, Ohtsuka K, Igawa Y. Improvement of urological-management abilities in individuals with tetraplegia by reconstructive hand surgery. Spinal Cord 2000; 38:541–545.

50. Bakke A, Vollset SE. Risk factors for bacteriuria and clinical urinary tract infection in patients treated with clean intermittent catheterization. J Urol 1993; 149:527–531.

51. Parmar S, Baltej S, Vaidynanathan S. Teaching the procedure of clean intermittent catheterization. Paraplegia 1993; 31:298–302.

52. Sutton G, Shah S, Hill V. Clean intermittent self-catheterization for quadriplegic patients – a five year follow up. Paraplegia 1991; 29:542–549.

53. Perrouin-Verbe B, Labat JJ, Richard I, et al. Clean intermittent catheterization from the acute period in spinal cord injury patients. Longterm evaluation of urethral and genital tolerance. Paraplegia 1995; 33:619–624.

54. Bakke A, Malt UF. Psychological predictors of symptoms of urinary tract infection and bacteriuria in patients treated with clean intermittent catheterization: a prospective 7 year study. Eur Urol 1998; 34:30–36.

55. Yavuzer G, Gok H, Tuncer S, et al. Compliance with bladder management in spinal cord injury patients. Spinal Cord 2000; 38:762–765.

56. Pearman JW. Prevention of urinary tract infection following spinal cord injury. Paraplegia 1971; 9:95–104.

57. Lapides J, Diokno AC, Lowe BS, Kalish MD. Follow-up on unsterile intermittent self-catheterization. J Urol 1974; 111:184–187.

58. Donovan W, Stolov W, Clowers D, Clowers M. Bacteriuria during intermittent catheterization following spinal cord injury. Arch Phys Med Rehab 1978; 59:351–357.

59. Maynard F, Diokno A. Urinary infection and complications during clean intermittent catheterization following spinal cord injury. J Urol 1984; 132:943–946.

60. Murray K, Lewis P, Blannin J, Shepherd A. Clean intermittent self-catheterization in the management of adult lower urinary tract dysfunction. Br J Urol 1984; 56:379–380.

61. Wyndaele JJ. Clean intermittent self-catheterization in the prevention of lower urinary tract infections. In: Van Kerrebroeck PH, Debruyne F, eds. Dysfunction of the lower urinary tract: present achievements and future perspectives. Bussum: Medicom, 1990:187–195.

62. Sutton G, Shah S, Hill V. Clean intermittent self-catheterization for quadriplegic patients – a five year follow up. Paraplegia 1991; 29:542–549.

63. Whitelaw S, Hamonds J, Tregallas R. Clean intermittent self-catheterization in the elderly. Br J Urol 1987; 60:125–127.

64. Bakke A. Clean intermittent catheterization – physical and psychological complications. Scand J Urol Nephrol Suppl 1993; 150:1–69.

65. Rhame FS, Perkash I. Urinary tract infections occurring in recent spinal cord injury patients on intermittent catheterization. J Urol 1979; 122:669–673.

66. Ott R, Rosier AB. The importance of intermittent catheterization in bladder re-education of acute spinal cord lesions. In: Proc Eighteenth Vet Admin Spinal Cord Injury Conf 1971; 18:139–148.

67. Anderson RU. Prophylaxis of bacteriuria during intermittent catheterization of the acute neurogenic bladder. J Urol 1980; 123:364–366.

68. Prieto-Fingerhut T, Banovac K, Lynne CM. A study comparing sterile and nonsterile urethral catheterization in patients with spinal cord injury. Rehab Nurs 1997; 22:299–302.

69. Bakke A, Vollset SE. Risk factors for bacteriuria and clinical urinary tract infection in patients treated with clean intermittent catheterization. J Urol 1993; 149:527–531.

70. Shekelle PG, Morton SC, Clark KA, et al. Systematic review of risk factors for urinary tract infection in adults, with spinal cord dysfunction. J Spinal Cord Med 1999; 22:258–272.

71. Barnes D, Timoney A, Moulas G, et al. Correlation of bacteriological flora of the urethra, glans and perineum with organisms causing urinary tract infection in the spinal injuries male patient. Paraplegia 1992; 30:851–854.

72. King RB, Carlson CE, Mervine J, et al. Clean and sterile intermittent catheterization methods in hospitalized patients with spinal cord injury. Arch Phys Med Rehab 1992; 73(9):798–802.

73. Darouiche R, Cadle R, Zenon G 3rd, et al. Progression from asymptomatic to symptomatic urinary tract infection in patients with SCI: a preliminary study. J Am Parapleg Soc 1993; 16:219–224.

74. National Institute on Disability and Rehabilitation Research Consensus Statement Jan 27–29, 1992. The prevention and management of urinary tract infections among people with spinal cord injuries. J Am Parapleg Soc 1992; 15:194–204.

75. Gribble MJ, Puterman ML, McCallum NM. Pyuria: its relationship to bacteriuria in spinal cord injured patients on intermittent catheterization. Arch Phys Med Rehab 1989; 70:376–379.

76. Menon EB, Tan ES. Pyuria: index of infection in patients with spinal cord injuries. Br J Urol 1992; 69:141–146.

77. Noll F, Russe O, Kling E, Botel U, Schreiter F. Intermittent catheterisation versus percutaneous suprapubic cystostomy in the early management of traumatic spinal cord lesions. Paraplegia 1988; 26:4–9.

78. Yadav A, Vaidyanathan S, Panigraphi D. Clean intermittent catheterization for the neuropathic bladder. Paraplegia 1993; 31:380.

79. Schlager TA, Hendley JO, Wilson RA, et al. Correlation of periurethral bacterial flora with bacteriuria and urinary tract infection in children with neurogenic bladder receiving intermittent catheterization. Clin Infect Dis 1999; 28:346–350.

80. Hull RA, Rudy DC, Wieser IE, Donovan WH. Virulence factors of *Escherichia coli* isolates from patients with symptomatic and asymptomatic bacteriuria and neuropathic bladders due to spinal cord and brain injuries. J Clin Microbiol 1998; 36:115–117.

81. McGuire EJ, Diddel G, Wagner F Jr. Balanced bladder function in spinal cord injury patients. J Urol 1977; 118:626–628.

82. Sperling KB. Intermittent catheterization to obtain catheter-free bladder in spinal cord injury. Arch Phys Med Rehab 1978; 59:4–8.

83. Barkin M, Dolfin D, Herschorn S, et al. The urological care of the spinal cord injury patient. J Urol 1983; 129:335–339.

84. Wyndaele JJ, Maes D. Clean intermittent self-catheterization: a 12 year follow up. J Urol 1990; 143:906–908.

85. Barber DB, Woodard FL, Rogers SJ, Able AC. The efficacy of nursing education as an intervention in the treatment of recurrent urinary tract infections in individuals with spinal cord injury. SCI Nurs 1999; 16:54–56.

86. Waites KB, Canupp KC, Brookings ES, DeVivo MJ. Effect of oral ciprofloxacin on bacterial flora of perineum, urethra, and lower urinary tract in men with spinal cord injury. J Spinal Cord Med 1999; 22:192–198.

87. Lewis RI, Carrion HM, Lockhart JL, Politano VA. Significance of symptomatic bacteriuria in neurogenic bladder disease. Urology 1984; 23:343–347.

88. Pearman JW. The value of kanamycin-colistin bladder instillations in reducing bacteriuria during intermittent catheterization of patients with acute spinal cord injury. Br J Urol 1979; 51:367–374.

89. Haldorson AM, Keys TF, Maker MD, Opitz JL. Nonvalue of neomycin instillation after intermittent urinary catheterization. Antimicrob Agents Chemother 1978; 14:368–370.

90. Murphy FJ, Zelman S, Mau W. Ascorbic acid as urinary acidifying agent. II: Its adjunctive role in chronic urinary infection. J Urol 1965; 94:300–303.

91. Stover SL, Fleming WC. Recurrent bacteriuria in complete spinal cord injury patients on external condom drainage. Arch Phys Med Rehab 1980; 61:178–181.

92. Johnson HW, Anderson JD, Chambers GK, Arnold WJ, Irwin BJ, Brinton JR. A short-term study of nitrofurantoin prophylaxis in children managed with clean intermittent catheterization. Pediatrics 1994; 93:752–755.

93. Kevorkian CG, Merritt JL, Ilstrup DM. Methenamine mandelate with acidification: an effective urinary antiseptic in patients with neurogenic bladder. Mayo Clin Proc 1984; 59:523–529.

94. Jepson RG, Mihaljevic L, Craig J. Cranberries for preventing urinary tract infections. Cochrane Database Syst Rev 2000; (2):CD001321.

95. Dollfus P, Molé P. The treatment of the paralysed bladder after spinal cord injury in the accident unit of Colmar. Paraplegia 1969; 7:204–205.

96. Vivian JM, Bors E. Experience with intermittent catheterization in the southwest regional system for treatment of spinal injury. Paraplegia 1974; 12:158–166.

97. Pearman JW, Bailey M, Riley LP. Bladder instillations of trisdine compared with catheter introducer for reduction of bacteriuria during intermittent catheterization of patients with acute spinal cord trauma. Br J Urol 1991; 67:483–490.

98. Galloway A, Green HT, Windsor JJ, et al. Serial concentrations of C-reactive protein as an indicator of urinary tract infection in patients with spinal injury. J Clin Pathol 1986; 39:851–855.

99. Allas T, Colleu D, Le Lannon D. Fonction génitale chez l'homme paraplégique. Aspects immunologiques. Presse Med 1986; 29:2119.

100. Ohl DA, Denil J, Fitzgerald-Shelton K, et al. Fertility of spinal cord injured males: effect of genitourinary infection and bladder management on results of electroejaculation. J Am Parapleg Soc 1992; 15:53–59.

101. Rutkowski SB, Middleton JW, Truman G, et al. The influence of bladder management on fertility in spinal cord injured males. Paraplegia 1995; 33:263–266.

102. Kuhlemeier KV, Lloyd LK, Stover SL. Localization of upper and lower urinary tract infections in patients with neurogenic bladders. SCI Dig 1982:336–342.

103. Wyndaele JJ. Chronic prostatitis in spinal cord injury patients. Paraplegia 1985; 23:164–169.

104. Cukier J, Maury M, Vacant J, Mlle Lucet. L'infection de l'appareil urinaire chez le paraplégique adulte. Nouv Presse Med 1976; 24:1531–1532.

105. Webb R, Lawson A, Neal D. Clean intermittent self-catheterization in 172 adults. Br J Urol 1990; 65:20–23.

106. Kovindha A, Na W, Madersbacher H. Radiological abnormalities in spinal cord injured men using clean intermittent catheterization with a re-usable silicone catheter in developing country. Poster 86 presented during the Annual Scientific Meeting of IMSOP, Sydney, 2000:112 [Abstract].

107. Mandal AK, Vaidaynathan S. Management of urethral stricture in patients practising clean intermittent catheterization. Int Urol Nephrol 1993; 25:395–399.

108. Vaidyanathan S, Soni BM, Dundas S, Krishnan KR. Urethral cytology in spinal cord injury patient performing intermittent catheterisation. Paraplegia 1994; 32:493–500.

109. Michielsen D, Wyndaele JJ. Management of false passages in patients practising clean intermittent self catheterisation. Spinal Cord 1999; 37:201–203.

110. Damanski M. Vesico-ureteric reflux in paraplegics. Br J Surg 1965; 52:168–177.

111. Solomon MH, Foff SA, Diokno AC. Bladder calculi complicating intermittent catheterization. J Urol 1980; 124:140–141.

112. Amendola MA, Sonda LP, Diokno AC, Vidyasagar M. Bladder calculi complicating intermittent clean catheterization. Am J Roentgenol 1983; 141:751–753.

113. Morgan JDT, Weston PMT. The disappearing catheter – a complication of intermittent self-catheterization. Br J Urol 1990; 65:113–114.

114. Reisman EM, Preminger GM. Bladder perforation secondary to clean intermittent catheterization. J Urol 1989; 142:1316–1317.

115. Newman E, Price M. External catheters: hazards and benefits of their use by men with spinal cord lesions. Arch Phys Med Rehab 1985; 66:310–313.

116. Madersbacher H, Weissteiner G. Intermittent self-catheterization, an alternative in the treatment of neurogenic urinary incontinence in women. Eur Urol 1977; 3:82–84.

117. Wyndaele JJ, Oosterlinck W, De Sy W. Clean intermittent self-catheterization in the chronical management of the neurogenic bladder. Eur Urol 1980; 6:107–110.

118. Iwatsubo E, Komine S, Yamashita H, et al. Over-distension therapy of the bladder in paraplegic patients using self-catheterisation: a preliminary study. Paraplegia 1984; 22:201–215.

119. McGuire EJ, Savastano J. Comparative urological outcome in women with spinal cord injury. J Urol 1986; 135:730–731.

120. Kornhuber HH, Schutz A. Efficient treatment of neurogenic bladder disorders in multiple sclerosis with initial intermittent catheterization and ultrasound-controlled training. Eur Neurol 1990; 30:260–267.

121. Kuhn W, Rist M, Zach GA. Intermittent urethral self-catheterisation: long term results (bacteriological evolution, continence, acceptance, complications). Paraplegia 1991; 29:222–232.

122. Lindehall B, Moller A, Hjalmas K, Jodal U. Long-term intermittent catheterization: the experience of teenagers and young adults with myelomeningcele. J Urol 1994; 152:187–189.

123. Waller L, Jonsson O, Norlén L, Sullivan L. Clean intermittent catheterization in spinal cord injury patients: long-term followup of a hydrophilic low friction technique. J Urol 1995; 153:345–348.

124. Vaidyanathan S, Soni BM, Brown E, et al. Effect of intermittent urethral catheterization and oxybutynen bladder instillation on urinary continence status and quality of life in a selected group of spinal cord injury patients with neuropathic bladder dysfunction. Spinal Cord 1998; 36:409–414.

125. Diokno AC, Sonda LP, Hollander JB, Lapides J. Fate of patients started on clean intermittent self-catheterization 10 years ago. J Urol 1983; 129:1120–1122.

126. Maynard FM, Glass J. Management of the neuropathic bladder by clean intermittent catheterization: 5 year outcomes. Paraplegia 1987; 25:106–110.

127. Whitelaw S, Hamonds J, Tregallas R. Clean intermittent self-catheterization in the elderly. Br J Urol 1987; 60:125–127.

128. Webb R, Lawson A, Neal D. Clean intermittent self-catheterization in 172 adults. Br J Urol 1990; 65:20–23.

129. Timoney AG, Shaw PJ. Urological outcome in female patients with spinal cord injury: the effectiveness of intermittent catheterization. Paraplegia 1990; 28:556–563.

130. Sutton G, Shah S, Hill V. Clean intermittent self-catheterization for quadriplegic patients – a five year follow up. Paraplegia 1991; 29:542–549.

131. Bakke A. Clean intermittent catheterization – physical and psychological complications. Scand J Urol Nephrol suppl 1993; 150:1–69.

132. Hunt GM, Oakeshott P, Whitacker RH. Intermittent catheterization: simple, safe and effective but underused. BMJ 1996; 312:103–107. [References]

133. Lapides J, Diokno AC, Lowe BS, Kalish MD. Follow-up on unsterile intermittent self-catheterization. J Urol 1974; 111:184–187.

134. Lapides J, Diokno AC, Gould FR, Lowe BS. Further observations on self-catheterization. J Urol 1976; 116:169–172.

135. Orikasa S, Koyanagi T, Motomura M, et al. Experience with non-sterile intermittent selfcatheterization. J Urol 1976; 115:141–142.

136. Wyndaele JJ, Oosterlinck W, De Sy W. Clean intermittent self-catheterization in the chronical management of the neurogenic bladder. Eur Urol 1980; 6:107–110.

137. Maynard FM, Diokno A. Clean intermittent catheterization for spinal cord injured patients. J Urol 1982; 128:477–480.

138. Labat JJ, Perrouin-Verbe B, Lanoiselée JM, et al. L'autosondage intermittent propre dans la rééducation des blesses medullaires et de la queue de cheval II. Ann Réadapt Méd Phys 1985; 28:125–136.

139. Maynard FM, Glass J. Management of the neuropathic bladder by clean intermittent catheterization: 5 year outcomes. Paraplegia 1987; 25:106–110.

140. Hellstrom P, Tammela T, Lukkarinen O, Kontturi M. Efficacy and safety of clean intermittent catheterization in adults. Eur Urol 1991; 20:117–121.

141. Thirumavalan VS, Ransley PG. Epididymitis in children and adolescents on clean intermittent catheterization. Eur Urol 1992; 22:53–56.

142. Perkash I, Giroux J. Clean intermittent catheterization in spinal cord injury patients: a followup study. J Urol 1993; 149:1068–1071.

44

Systemic and intrathecal pharmacological treatment

Shing-Hwa Lu and Michael B Chancellor

Introduction

The principal causes of urinary incontinence in patients with neurogenic bladder are detrusor hyperreflexia (DH) and/or incompetence of urethral closing function. Thus, to improve urinary incontinence the treatment should aim at decreasing detrusor activity, increasing bladder capacity, and/or increasing bladder outlet resistance. Pharmacological therapy has been particularly helpful in patients with relatively mild degrees of neurogenic bladder dysfunction. Patients with more profound neurogenic bladder disturbances may require pharmacological treatment to augment other forms of management such as intermittent catheterization. The two most commonly used classes of agents are anticholinergics and α-adrenergic blockers (Table 44.1). Intravesical pharmacological therapy is discussed in Chapter 45.

Table 44.1 *Systemic drugs for incontinence due to detrusor hyperreflexia and/or low compliant detrusor*

Bladder relaxant drugs:
   Propantheline
   Oxybutynin
   Tolterodine
   Propiverine
   Trospium
   Flavoxate
   Tricyclic antidepressants

Drugs for incontinence due to neurogenic sphincter deficiency:
   Alpha-adrenergic agonists
   Estrogens
   Tricyclic antidepressants

Drugs for facilitating bladder emptying:
   Alpha-adrenergic blockers
   Cholinergics

Drugs for incontinence due to detrusor hyperreflexia and/or low-compliant detrusor

Bladder relaxant drugs

Anticholinergic agents are the commonly used pharmacological agents in the management of neurogenic bladder. Anticholinergic agents are employed to suppress DH. Although there is an abundance of drugs available for the treatment of DH, for many of them, efficacy is estimated based on preliminary open studies rather than on controlled clinical trials.[1] However, drug effects in individual patients may be practically important. In developing countries, most of the bladder relaxant drugs listed below are not available, mainly due to economical reasons, which makes the pharmacological treatment of DH in these countries difficult.

General indications of pharmacological treatment in DH are:

1. to improve or eliminate reflex incontinence
2. to eliminate or prevent a high intravesical pressure situation
3. to enhance the efficacy of intermittent catheterization (IC), triggered voiding, and indwelling catheters.

Spinal DH is mostly associated with a functional outflow obstruction due to detrusor-sphincter dyssynergia (DSD). For the most part, pharmacotherapy is used to suppress reflex detrusor activity completely and facilitate IC. Bladder relaxant drugs decrease detrusor contractility also during voiding. With this situation, residual urine increases and must then be assisted or accomplished by IC.

Propantheline

Propantheline bromide was the classically described oral antimuscarinic drug. Despite its success in uncontrolled case series, no adequate controlled study of this drug for DH is available.[1,2] The usual adult oral dosage is 7.5–30 mg three to four times daily, although higher doses are often necessary.[3]

Oxybutynin

Oxybutynin hydrochloride is a moderately potent antimuscarinic agent with a pronounced muscle relaxant activity and local anesthetic activity as well.[1,3–5]

Several double-blind controlled studies have shown its efficacy for DH.[6–11] The overall rate of good results (more than 50% symptomatic improvement) was 61–86% with 5 mg three times per day. Side-effects were noted in all studies and severity increased with dosage. The overall incidence of possible side-effects was 12.5–68%. Most of them are related to antimuscarinic action, with dry mouth as the most common complaint.

A once-a-day controlled-release formulation of oxybutynin, oxybutynin XL (Ditropan XL®), was recently developed. Parallel-group, randomized, controlled clinical trials comparing the efficacy and safety of controlled-release oxybutynin, oxybutynin XL, with conventional, immediate-release oxybutynin in patients with overactive bladder demonstrated that the urge urinary incontinence episodes declined log-linearly, and no significant difference was observed between the two formulations.[12–14] However, there was a trend toward higher efficacy with oxybutynin XL than with immediate-release oxybutynin at the same dose in one study. Dose–dry mouth analysis showed that the probability of dry mouth with an increasing dose was significantly lower with oxybutynin XL than with immediate-release oxybutynin.[15]

Recent experience with oxybutynin in neurogenic bladder patients

O'Leary et al evaluated the effects and tolerability of extended-release oxybutynin chloride on the voiding and catheterization frequency of a population of multiple sclerosis (MS) patients with neurogenic bladder.[16] This was a 12-week prospective dose titration study of extended-release oxybutynin (oxybutynin XL). Multiple sclerosis patients were recruited for this study from the MS clinic within the university. Entry criteria included a post-void residual (PVR) of <200 ml (in the noncatheterized subjects). Exclusions included those with urine results indicating pyuria in the presence of a positive urine culture. These tests were repeated at 6 and 12 weeks. After a 7-day washout period, patients recorded episodes of voiding or catheterization and incontinence for three consecutive days. Patients received initial doses of 10 mg oxybutynin XL in the first week. Doses were escalated to weekly or biweekly intervals to a maximum of 30 mg/day. Tolerability information was collected at each follow-up visit.

Twenty patients completed the study: the mean age was 46.3 years (range 24–61), and 75% of the patients were women. Subjects reported clinical improvement with decreased urinary frequency and incontinence episodes after dosing was escalated to 30 mg. Seventeen patients chose a final effective dose greater than 10 mg, with 13 patients taking at least 20 mg/day at the end of the study. There were no serious adverse events during the course of the study.

The authors concluded that controlled-release oxybutynin is safe and effective in MS patients with neurogenic bladder. The onset of clinical efficacy occurs within 1 week and daily doses up to 30 mg may be indicated and are well tolerated.

In a similar study, but performed in spinal cord injured (SCI) patients, O'Leary et al evaluated the urodynamic changes with extended-release oxybutynin chloride in SCI patients with defined DH.[17]

This was a 12-week prospective dose titration study of extended-release oxybutynin (oxybutynin XL). SCI subjects with urodynamically defined DH were recruited for this study. After a 7-day washout period, patients were evaluated by videourodynamic study and then treatment at a dose of 10 mg was initiated. Doses were increased in weekly intervals to a maximum of 30 mg/day. Micturition frequency diaries and urodynamics were completed at baseline and repeated at week 12. Tolerability information was collected at each follow-up visit.

Ten patients (mean age 49 years) with complete or incomplete SCI were enrolled. Subjects reported clinical improvement, with decreased urinary frequency and incontinence episodes after dosing was escalated to 30 mg. All patients chose a final effective dose greater than 10 mg with 4 patients taking 30 mg/day. Mean cystometric bladder capacity increased 274 ml to 380 ml ($p = 0.008$). No patient had serious adverse events during the course of the 12-week study.

The authors concluded that oxybutynin XL is safe and effective in SCI patients with detrusor hyperreflexia. The onset of clinical efficacy occurs within 1 week and daily doses up to 30 mg, if indicated, are well tolerated.

Tolterodine

Tolterodine is a new competitive muscarinic receptor antagonist.[18,19] Recently, several randomized, and double-blind controlled studies in patients with overactive bladder have demonstrated its beneficial effect.[20–28] Jonas et al reported on a randomized, double-blind, placebo-controlled study of tolterodine including urodynamic analysis in a total of 242 patients:[20] 2 mg twice daily was significantly more effective than placebo in increasing maximum cystometric bladder capacity and volume at first contraction after 4 weeks' treatment. However, there are no published reports on the specific effect on DH.

The better tolerability profile of tolterodine compared with oxybutynin has been confirmed in another randomized study on detrusor overactivity.[23] Tolterodine (2 mg twice daily) appears to be as effective as oxybutynin (5 mg three times daily), but is much better tolerated, especially in regards to dry mouth. In a meta-analysis of a four-multicenter prospective trial of 1120 patients, moderate to severe dry mouth was reported in 6% of patients receiving the placebo, 4% of patients receiving 1 mg twice daily tolterodine, 17% of patients receiving 2 mg twice daily tolterodine, and 60% of those patients receiving conventional 5 mg three times daily oxybutynin.[21] The other randomized controlled trial of tolterodine by Malone-Lee et al demonstrated superior tolerability than and comparable efficacy to oxybutynin in individuals 50 years old or older with overactive bladder.[26]

Van Kerrebroeck et al reported a comparative study of the efficacy and safety of tolterodine extended release (ER; 4 mg once daily), tolterodine immediate release (IR; 2 mg twice daily), as well as placebo in 1529 adult patients with overactive bladder.[27] The primary efficacy variable was the change in mean number of incontinence episodes per week, which decreased 53% from baseline in the tolterodine ER group, 45% with tolterodine IR, and 28% in the placebo group. Tolterodine ER and IR provided a similar significant reduction in incontinence episodes vs placebo. Post-hoc analysis of the data using median values, based on rational of skewed data distribution, demonstrated improved efficacy of tolterodine ER vs IR. Dry mouth was significantly lower with tolterodine ER than tolterodine IR (23% tolterodine ER, 31% tolterodine IR, and 8% placebo). The incidence of other side-effects was similar to placebo in the tolterodine ER and tolterodine IR groups.

A comparative study between controlled-release oxybutynin (oxybutynin XL) and immediate-release tolterodine (tolterodine IR) was recently published:[28] 378 patients were randomized to receive either oxybutynin XL 10 mg (n = 185) or tolterodine IR 4 mg (2 mg twice daily) (n = 193). The populations were evenly matched with respect to demographics. Oxybutynin XL reduced the number of weekly episodes of urge incontinence from 25.6 to 6.1 instances. Tolterodine IR decreased the number of weekly episodes from 24.1 to 7.8 instances. Oxybutynin XL demonstrated better efficacy (p = 0.03) compared with tolterodine IR. Dry mouth and central nervous system side-effects were similar between oxybutynin XL and tolterodine IR.

Although tolterodine has a documented effect on overactive bladder, further studies on the effect of the drug on DH in the neuropathic population are necessary. Comparative studies of tolterodine ER with propiverine, trospium, or oxybutynin XL, especially with regard to tolerability, could be useful to evaluate its position among other bladder relaxant drugs besides conventional oxybutynin or tolterodine.

Propiverine

Propiverine hydrochloride is a benzylic acid derivative with musculotropic (calcium antagonistic) activity and moderate antimuscarinic effects.[29] Several randomized double-blind, controlled clinical studies of this drug in patients with DH have been reported.[30–32] In a placebo-controlled, double-blind, randomized, prospective, multicenter trial, Stöhrer et al evaluated the efficacy and tolerability of propiverine (15 mg three times daily for 14 days) as compared to placebo in 113 patients suffering from DH caused by spinal cord injury.[30] The majority of patients practiced IC for bladder emptying. The maximum cystometric bladder capacity increased significantly in the propiverine group, on average by 104 ml. Sixty-three percent of the patients expressed a subjective improvement of their symptoms under propiverine in comparison to only 23% of the placebo group.

Takayasu et al conducted a double-blind, placebo-controlled multicenter study in 70 neurogenic patients.[31] During a treatment period of 14 days, 20 mg propiverine once daily or placebo were administered. An increase of maximum bladder capacity, a decrease of maximum detrusor pressure, and an increase of residual urine were also obtained in this Japanese study, all of which were statistically significant compared with placebo. Madersbacher et al, in a placebo-controlled, multicenter study, demonstrated that propiverine is a safe and effective drug in the treatment of DH; it is as effective as oxybutynin, but the incidence of dry mouth and its severity is less with propiverine (15 mg, three times daily) than with oxybutynin (5 mg twice daily).[32]

Trospium

Trospium is a quaternary ammonium derivative with mainly antimuscarinic actions. In a placebo-controlled, double-blind study in 61 patients with spinal DH, significant improvements in maximum cystometric capacity and maximum detrusor pressure were demonstrated with 20 mg of trospium twice daily for 3 weeks compared with placebo.[33] Few side-effects were noted, compared with placebo. Madersbacher et al compared the clinical efficacy and tolerance of trospium (20 mg twice daily) and oxybutynin (5 mg three times daily) in a randomized, double-blind, urodynamically controlled, multicenter trial in 95 patients with spinal cord injuries and DH.[34] They found that the two drugs are equal in their effects on DH (increase of the cystometric bladder capacity by 30% and decrease of the maximum detrusor pressure by 30%), but trospium has fewer severe side-effects (incidence of severe dry mouth 5% with trospium vs 25% with oxybutynin).[34]

Flavoxate

Flavoxate hydrochloride has a direct inhibitory action on detrusor smooth muscle *in vitro*. Early clinical trials with flavoxate have shown favorable effects in patients with DH.[35,36] Several randomized controlled studies have shown that the drug has essentially no effects on detrusor overactivity.[10,37,38]

Tricyclic antidepressants

Many clinicians have found tricyclic antidepressants, particularly imipramine hydrochloride, to be useful agents for facilitating urine storage, both by decreasing bladder contractility and by increasing outlet resistance.[3,39] However, no sufficiently controlled trials of tricyclic antidepressants in terms of DH in neuropathics have been reported. Nevertheless, in some developing countries tricyclic antidepressants are the only bladder relaxant substances that people can afford. The down side with tricyclic antidepressants is the narrow safety profile and side-effects. The potential hazard of serious cardiovascular toxic effect should be taken into consideration.[1] Combination therapy using antimuscarinics and imipramine may have synergistic benefits [*Level 5*].

Drugs for incontinence due to neurogenic sphincter deficiency

Several drugs, including alpha-adrenergic agonists,[40–45] estrogens,[46] beta-adrenergic agonists,[47] and tricyclic antidepressants,[48] have been used to increase outlet resistance [*Level 4*]. No adequately designed controlled studies of any of these drugs for treating neuropathic sphincter deficiency have been published. In certain selected cases of mild to moderate stress incontinence, a beneficial effect may be obtained [Grade D].[1]

Drugs for facilitating bladder emptying

Alpha-adrenergic blockers

Alpha adrenoceptors have been reported to be predominantly present in the bladder base, posterior urethra, and prostate. Alpha-blockers have been reported to be useful in neurogenic bladder by decreasing urethral resistance during voiding. Recently, a multicenter placebo-controlled, double-blind trials of urapidil – an alpha-blocker on neurogenic bladder dysfunction – by means of a pressure–flow study, demonstrated significant improvement of straining and of the sum of urinary symptom scores, which was associated with significant improvement of urodynamic parameters (decreases in the pressure at maximum flow rate and the minimum urethral resistance) over the placebo [*Level 1*].[49,50]

Alpha-adrenergic blockade also helps to prevent excess sweating secondary to spinal cord autonomic dysreflexia. Sweat glands, primarily responsible for thermoregulatory factors, are innervated by postganglionic cholinergic neurons of the sympathetic system. Alpha-receptor blockade inhibits this postsynaptic neuronal uptake of norepinephrine (noradrenaline) and reduces neurologic sweating.[51]

Cholinergics

In general, bethanechol chloride seems to be of limited benefit for detrusor areflexia and for elevated residual urine volume. Elevated residual volume is often due to sphincter dyssynergia. It would be inappropriate to potentially increase detrusor pressure when there is concurrent DSD.[52]

Therapy for sphincter dyssynergia

In patients with sufficient manual dexterity, the most reasonable treatment option is to abolish the involuntary detrusor contractions (to insure continence) and then to institute intermittent self-catheterization (in order to empty the bladder).[53,54] Treatment options include catheterization (either intermittent or continuous) external sphincterotomy, pharmacological therapy, urinary diversion, biofeedback, functional electrical stimulation, and several new minimally invasive alternatives to external sphincterotomy (Table 44.2).

Unfortunately, there is no class of pharmacological agents that will selectively relax the striated musculature of the pelvic floor. Several different drugs have been used to treat detrusor-external sphincter dyssynergia (DESD), including

Table 44.2 *Therapy of detrusor-external sphincter dyssynergia*

Conventional surgery:
  External sphincterotomy

Pharmacological:
  Baclofen (oral or intrathecal)
  Dantrolene
  Benzodiazepine
  Possibly alpha-adrenergic blockade
  Possibly clonidine

Minimally invasive techniques:
  Sphincter stent
  Balloon sphincter dilatation
  Laser sphincterotomy
  Botulinum toxin injection

Circumventing the problem:
  Intermittent catheterization
  Indwelling catheterization (urethral or suprapubic)
  Urinary diversion

the benzodiazepines, dantrolene, baclofen, and alpha-adrenergic blocking agents.[55–58] Baclofen and diazepam exert their actions predominantly within the central nervous system, whereas dantrolene acts directly on skeletal muscle. Although these drugs are capable of providing variable relief of muscle spasticity, their efficacy is far from complete, and troublesome muscle weakness, adverse effects on gait, and a variety of other side-effects minimize their overall usefulness.[55]

Alpha-adrenergic antagonists have been extensively used for DESD. The rationale for their use is their proven efficacy on internal urinary sphincter (bladder neck and prostate) smooth muscle obstruction. Unfortunately, there is no good clinical study to support the use of alpha blockade for DESD.

In addition, there is a report of preliminary success using oral clonidine in 4 of 5 patients with DESD.[59] Continuous intrathecal baclofen infusion has been shown to be effective in diminishing DESD in up to 40% of patients with DESD.[60]

Alpha-adrenergic blockade

Although most researchers would agree that alpha blockers exert their favorable effects on voiding dysfunction primarily by affecting the smooth muscle of the bladder neck and proximal urethra, there are suggestions that they may affect striated sphincter tone as well.[61] Other data suggest that they may exert some effects on the symptoms of voiding dysfunction by decreasing bladder contractility. Alpha antagonists have been shown to be clinically effective in relieving internal sphincter obstruction by their effect on

the bladder neck and prostate.[62,63] Whether the striated external urinary sphincter receives sympathetic innervation remains controversial. Most of the research has been carried out only in laboratory animals, where both the presence and absence of alpha receptors have been reported at the external sphincter level.[64–66] Clinical correlation of the effects of alpha antagonists on the striated external urinary sphincter during micturition is lacking. Most clinical studies have based their conclusions on effects on the passive urethral pressure profile (UPP).[67,68]

The SCI male, with both neurogenic vesical dysfunction and DESD, offers an ideal opportunity to study the interrelationship between the function of the bladder and both the internal and external urinary sphincters.[69] The effect of alpha-adrenergic innervation and its clinical significance on the two sphincters is more readily apparent in such patients.

Mobley treated 37 patients with neurogenic bladder with phenoxybenzamine and noted 78% success.[70] Unfortunately, no objective data – including urodynamic parameters, length of follow-up, or indications of improvement – were specified. Whitfield et al found a significant decrease in the UPP with alpha blockade in 25 patients with neurogenic vesical dysfunction.[71] However, actual voiding pressure was not reported.

Using intravenous phentolamine, Awad et al noted a significant decrease in pressure along the entire length of the urethra in both sexes, including the peak pressure zone.[72] Olsson et al proposed that a constant state of sympathetic tonus to the internal sphincter exists, and that inhibition of this tonus during micturition results in bladder neck opening.[73]

Research providing evidence against a clinically significant effect of a sympathetic antagonist on the external sphincter includes a report by McGuire et al.[74] They reported on 9 patients with neurogenic bladders and severe autonomic dysreflexia who demonstrated dramatic improvement with phenoxybenzamine. The urethral resistance was unassociated with spasticity of the striated muscle and was abolished by administration of phenoxybenzamine. This documents abnormal urethral smooth muscle activity in SCI patients but fails to demonstrate a sympathetic effect on the external sphincter musculature.

Rossier et al used a pudendal block plus phentolamine to study the effect on the external sphincter.[75] The authors concluded that there was no significant sympathetic innervations of striated muscle in humans. Pudendal nerve blocks have demonstrated sphincter dyssynergia to be mediated through the pudendal nerves via spinal reflex arcs. Phentolamine affects on bladder activity suggest that blockade of alpha-adrenergic receptors inhibits primarily the transmission in vesical and/or pelvic parasympathetic ganglia, and acts only secondarily through direct depression of the vesical smooth muscle. Their neuropharmacological results raise strong doubts as to the existence

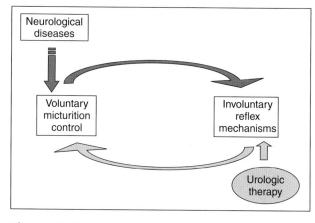

Figure 44.1
Involuntary reflex micturitional mechanisms were developed in the patients with neurological disorders. The aim of urologic therapy including neuropharmacological therapy is to convert the involuntary reflex micturition into more natural voluntary micturition control such as improving detrusor hyperreflexia (DH), and/or disorders of urethral closing function by decreasing detrusor activity, increasing bladder capacity, and/or modulating bladder outlet resistance.

of clinically significant sympathetic innervation of the striated urethral muscle in humans.

Terazosin, a selective alpha$_1$-blocker, was examined in 15 normotensive (SCI) patients.[52] DESD without obstruction of the bladder neck or prostate was documented using videourodynamic evaluation in all patients. Urodynamic testing was performed both before and after treatment was initiated with terazosin (5 mg nightly). Voiding pressure before and during terazosin therapy averaged 92 ± 17 and 88 ± 27 cmH$_2$O, respectively ($p = 0.48$). After subsequent external sphincterotomy or sphincter stent placement, the voiding pressure was reduced to 38 ± 15 cmH$_2$O ($p < 0.001$).

Nine other patients suffered from persistent voiding symptoms after previous sphincterotomy. Each was subsequently treated with oral terazosin. Of 5 patients who improved with this treatment, urodynamic parameters demonstrated obstruction only at the bladder neck, with no evidence of obstruction at the level of the external sphincter. The 4 patients who failed to improve were documented to have an open bladder neck but obstruction at the level of the external sphincter.

This study supports that even though alpha$_1$-sympathetic blockade does not significantly relieve functional obstruction caused by DESD. Also noted was that terazosin is helpful in diagnosing and treating internal sphincter (bladder neck and prostate) obstruction, especially in patients who have persistent voiding symptoms after external sphincterotomy. Other selective alpha$_1$-adrenergic blockade should yield results similar to terazosin.

Patients demonstrating clinical improvement with terazosin therapy, despite no urodynamic verification of improvement in DESD, may be responding to treatment of autonomic dysreflexia symptoms.[76,77] The patients may feel better because of diminished autonomic dysreflexia activity, despite ongoing DESD.[78] Another reason for clinical improvement without resolution of DESD may be an undiagnosed functional obstruction at the level of the urethral smooth musculature, which should improve with alpha$_1$ blockade, rather than true DESD. This is supported by studies by Yalla et al.[79]

Baclofen

Baclofen depresses monosynaptic and polysynaptic excitation of motor neurons and interneurons in the spinal cord and possibly functions as a glycine and gamma-aminobutyric acid (GABA) agonist.[55,56] GABA has been identified as the major inhibitory transmitter in the spinal cord.[80]

Baclofen has been found useful in the treatment of skeletal spasticity attributable to a variety of causes, especially multiple sclerosis and traumatic spinal cord lesions.[55] Hacken and Krucker found intravenous, but not oral, baclofen effective for patients with detrusor-sphincter dyssynergia, with the side-effects of weakness and dizziness common.[58]

Leyson et al studied high-dose oral baclofen in 25 SCI patients.[81] They concluded that baclofen was helpful in decreasing the resting urethral pressure at the level of the sphincter. Residual urine decreased in 73% of their cases. However, only 20% of the patients demonstrated a reduction in intravesical pressure at high doses of between 140 and 160 mg daily. The safety of long-term oral baclofen is also of significant concern. This study verified the very limited role, if any, that baclofen may have in the treatment of DESD.

Florante et al reported that 73% of their patients with voiding dysfunction caused by acute and chronic spinal cord injury had lower striated sphincter responses and decreased residual urine volumes after oral baclofen treatment.[82] However, a very high daily dose of 120 mg was used. The potential side-effects of baclofen include drowsiness, insomnia, rash, pruritus, dizziness, and weakness. The drug may impair the ability to walk or stand, and is not recommended for the management of spasticity resulting from cerebral lesions or disease. Sudden withdrawal has been shown to provoke hallucinations, anxiety, and tachycardia; hallucinations during treatment, which have been responsive to reductions in dosage, have also been reported.[83,84]

Benzodiazepines

Few references are available that provide valuable data on the use of any of the diazepines in the treatment of DESD.

The benzodiazepines potentiate the action of GABA at both presynaptic and postsynaptic sites in the brain and spinal cord.[85,86] We have not found the recommended oral doses of diazepam to be effective in controlling DESD. Anecdotal improvement may simply be attributable to the antianxiety effect of the drug.

Beta-adrenergic agonists

Beta-adrenergic agonists, especially those with prominent beta characteristics, are able to produce relaxation of slow-twitch skeletal muscles.[73] Gosling et al have reported that a portion of the external urethral sphincter comprising the outermost urethral wall consists exclusively of slow-twitch fibers, whereas the striated muscle fibers of the levator ani contain both fast- and slow-twitch fibers.[87] This type of action may account, at least in part, for the decrease in ure-thral profile parameters seen with terbutaline. There is no clinical evidence of successful treatment of DESD with beta-adrenergic agonists.

Dantrolene

Dantrolene sodium exerts its effects by a direct peripheral relaxation action on skeletal muscle.[55,85] Dantrolene has been shown to dissociate excitation–contraction coupling in the sarcoplasmic reticulum of muscle.[56] Hackler et al reported improvement in voiding function in approximately half of their patients with DESD treated with dantrolene.[57]

However, dosages significantly above the recommended daily maximum were required, whereas significant side-effects, especially weakness, were common. Harris and Benson reported that the generalized weakness which dantrolene may induce is often significant enough to compromise its therapeutic effects.[88] Other potential side-effects include euphoria, dizziness, diarrhea, and hepatotoxicity. Fatal hepatitis has been reported in approximately 0.1–0.2% of patients treated with the drug for 60 days or longer, whereas symptomatic hepatitis may occur in 0.5% of patients treated for more than 60 days; chemical abnormalities of liver function are noted in approximately 1%.[89]

Drugs to increase bladder pressure

Modalities that have been tried to increase intravesical pressure to achieve bladder emptying such as suprapubic percussion, Credé's maneuver, and use of bethanechol chloride are not effective and may potentially be detrimental.[68]

Increasing the detrusor pressure without simultaneously relaxing the outlet is associated with upper urinary tract morbidity and can aggravate autonomic dysreflexia.[90]

Intrathecal baclofen pump

The use of an intrathecal baclofen pump has also received some attention in the treatment of DESD.[60] These pumps were implanted for severe spasticity and some of the patients experienced improvement in bladder and sphincter functions. Nanninga et al reported their experience in 7 patients for relief of severe spasticity.[91] Six patients demonstrated an increase in bladder capacity and 4 were able to perform IC and remain dry. A slight decrease in maximum intravesical pressure was seen in all the patients. Talalla et al noted an inconsistent effect of intrathecal baclofen on urethral pressure in 6 SCI patients.[92] Two patients had significant reduction in maximum urethral and maximum detrusor pressures. Side-effects included half of the patients noticing that reflex erections were reduced or abolished for at least 24 hours following intrathecal baclofen. The authors reported that this side-effect has deterred other patients from considering this treatment modality.

There is also a case report of improvement in DESD with intrathecal baclofen in one patient with hereditary spastic paraplegia and voiding dysfunction.[93] However, it is not known if intrathecal baclofen merely reduced pelvic floor spasticity, eliminated lower extremity artifacts, or truly abolished DESD.[94]

At the present time intrathecal baclofen pump implantation for the primary diagnosis of DESD does not seem warranted because of the invasive spinal surgery, cost, and viable alternatives. It may be helpful for DESD in patients who also have lower severe extremities spasticity uncontrolled by oral pharmacological therapy. The intrathecal baclofen pump may also be promising for patients with refractory detrusor hyperreflexia.

Neurogenic bladder drug development

During the past few years, research in neuro-urology has stimulated the development of new therapeutic approaches for incontinence, including the intravesical administration of afferent neurotoxins such as capsaicin and resiniferatoxin. What are the research priorities for the future? It will be important to focus on the development of neuropharmacological agents that can suppress the unique components of abnormal bladder reflex mechanisms and thereby act selectively to decrease symptoms without altering normal voiding function. To end this chapter, we would like to speculate on a few areas of research which we feel may pay off within the next 5 years with new and better treatment of neuropathic urinary incontinence.

Bladder-specific K⁺ channel openers. Can truly bladder smooth muscle or afferent neuron-specific potassium channel openers be developed. This treatment may alleviate the overactive and sensitive bladder without any dry mouth.

Intravesical vanilloid treatment. Can the clinical utility of intravesical resiniferatoxin be perfected so that the preferred therapy for neurogenic bladder is a simple outpatient 30 min instillation of 30 ml resiniferatoxin that will last 3 months without systemic side-effects?

Anticholinergic drugs. Can the pharmaceutical companies develop a truly bladder-specific and effective anticholinergic drug with no dry mouth?

Tachykinin antagonists. These substances are appealing in that they may be effective without increasing residual urine volumes. Can clinically useful and safe NK antagonists be developed?

Stress incontinence drugs. Urethral smooth and/or skeletal muscle specific alpha agonist or 5-HT reuptake inhibitor that may treat stress urinary incontinence. We need an effective drug for stress incontinence.

Advances in neuro-urology. Beyond the horizon of near-term advancement, we predict a brave new paradigm in neuro-urology. What has already started is the evolution of unstoppable forces of change in medicine that include pharmacogenomics, tissue engineering, and gene therapy. These will change how we practice urology and gynecology.

Pharmacogenomics. Medicine will be tailored to the genetic make-up of each individual. Through microarray gene chip technology, we will know how a patient metabolizes medications and the patient's receptor(s) profile and allergy risk. These factors can be screened against a list of medications prior to therapy. A physician will then be able to always prescribe the best drug for each patient without the risk of allergic reaction.

Tissue engineering. Rapid advances are being made feasible in tissue and organ reconstruction using autologous tissue and stem cells. We envisage a day, in the not too distant future, when stress incontinence is cured not with a cadaver ligament and metal screws into the bones but rather a minimally invasive injection of stem cells that will not only bulk up the deficient sphincter but also actually improve the sphincter's contractility and function.

Gene therapy. Diabetic neurogenic bladder and visceral pain may be cured with one or more injections of a gene vector that the physician will inject into the bladder or urethra. Injection of a nerve growth factor via a herpes virus vector into the bladder of a diabetic bladder may restore bladder sensation and innervation. Can the introduction of a virus that expresses the production of endorphin that is site- and nerve-specific help alleviate pelvic visceral pain, regardless of the cause?

References

1. Andersson K-E. Current concepts in treatment of disorders of micturition. Drugs 1988; 35:477.

2. Blaivas JG, Labib KB, Michalik J, Zayed AAH. Cystometric response to propantheline in detrusor hyperreflexia: therapeutic implications. J Urol 1980; 124:259.

3. Wein AJ. Neuromuscular dysfunction of the lower urinary tract and its treatment. In: Walsh, Retik, Vaughan, and Wein AJ, eds. Campbell's urology, 7th edn. 1997:953–1006.

4. Anderson GF, Fredericks CM. Characterization of the oxybutynin antagonism of drug-induced spasms in detrusor. Pharmacology 1972; 15:31.

5. Yarker YE, Goa KL, Fitton A. Oxybutynin. A review of its pharmacodynamic and pharmacokinetic properties, and its therapeutic use in detrusor instability. Drugs Aging 1995; 6(3):243.

6. Thompson IM, Lauvetz R. Oxybutynin in bladder spasm, neurogenic bladder, and enuresis. Urology 1976; 8:452.

7. Hehir M, Fitzpatrick JM. Oxybutynin and prevention of urinary incontinence in spinal bifida. Eur Urol 1985; 11(4):254.

8. Gajewski JB, Awad SA. Oxybutynin versus propantheline in patients with multiple sclerosis and detrusor hyperreflexia. J Urol 1986; 135(5):966.

9. Koyanagi T, Maru A, et al. Clinical evaluation of oxybutynin hydrochloride (KL007 tablets) for the treatment of neurogenic bladder and unstable bladder: a parallel double-blind controlled study with placebo. Nishi Nihon Hinyouki 1986; 48:1050. [in Japanese]

10. Zeegers AGM, Kiesswetter H, Kramer AEJ, Jonas U. Conservative therapy of frequency, urgency and urge incontinence: a double blind clinical trial of flavoxate hydrochloride, oxybutynin chloride, emepronium bromide and placebo. World J Urol 1987; 5:57.

11. Thüroff JW, Bunke B, Ebner A, et al. Ramdomized, double-blind, multicenter trial on treatment of frequency, urgency and urge incontinence related to detrusor hyperactivity: oxybutynin versus propantheline versus placebo. J Urol 1991; 145:813.

12. Anderson RU, Mobley D, Blank B, et al. Once a day controlled versus immediate release oxybutynin chloride for urge incontinence. J Urol 1999; 161:1809.

13. Birns J, Lukkari E, Malone-Lee JG. A randomized controlled trial comparing the efficacy of controlled-release oxybutynin tablets (10 mg once daily) with conventional oxybutynin tablets (5 mg twice daily) in patients whose symptoms were stabilized on 5 mg twice daily of oxybutynin. BJU Int 2000; 85(7):793–798.

14. Versi E, Appell R, Mobley D, et al. Dry mouth with conventional and controlled-release oxybutynin in urinary incontinence. The Ditropan XL Study Group. Obstet Gynecol 2000; 95:718.

15. Gupta SK, Sathyan G, Lindemulder EA, et al. Quantitative characterization of therapeutic index: application of mixed-effects modeling to evaluate oxybutynin dose-efficacy and dose-side effect relationships. Clin Pharmacol Ther 1999; 65:672.

16. O'Leary M, Erickson JR, Smith CP, McDermott C, Horton J, Chancellor MB. Effect of controlled release oxybutynin on neurogenic bladder function in spinal cord injury. J Spinal Cord Med 2003; 26(2):159–162.

17. O'Leary M, Erickson JR, Smith CP, et al. Bladder function in spinal cord injured patients changes in voiding patterns in multiple sclerosis patients with controlled release oxybutynin. Int MS J 2002;

18. Nilvebrant L, Andersson K-E, Gillberg P-G, et al. Tolterodine – a new bladder selective antimuscarinic agent. Eur J Pharmacol 1997; 327:195.

19. Nilvebrant L, Hallen B, Larsson G. Tolterodine – a new bladder selective muscarinic receptor antagonist: preclinical pharmacological and clinical data. Life Sci 1997; 60:1129.

20. Jonas U, Hofner K, Madersbacher H, Holmdahl TH. Efficacy and safety of two doses of tolterodine versus placebo in patients with detrusor overactivity and symptoms of frequency, urge incontinence, and urgency: urodynamic evaluation. The International Study Group. World J Urol 1997; 15:144.

21. Appell RA. Clinical efficacy and safety of tolterodine in the treatment of overactive bladder: a pooled analysis. Urology 1997; 50:90–96.

22. Rentzhog L, Stanton SL, Cardozo L, et al. Efficacy and safety of tolterodine in patients with detrusor instability: a dose-ranging study. Br J Urol 1998; 81:42.

23. Abrams P, Freeman R, Anderstrom C, Mattiasson A. Tolterodine, a new antimuscarinic agent: as effective but better tolerated than oxybutynin in patients with an overactive bladder. Br J Urol 1998; 81:801.

24. Van Kerrebroeck PE, Amarenco G, Thuroff JW, et al. Dose-ranging study of tolterodine in patients with detrusor hyperreflexia. Neurourol Urodyn 1998; 17:499.

25. Goessl C, Sauter T, Michael T, et al. Efficacy and tolerability of tolterodine in children with detrusor hyperreflexia. Urology 2000; 55:414.

26. Malone-Lee J, Shaffu B, Anand C, Powell C. Tolterodine: superior tolerability than and comparable efficacy to oxybutynin in individuals 50 years old or older with overactive bladder: a randomized controlled trial. J Urol 2001; 165:1452.

27. Van Kerrebroeck P, Kreder K, Jonas U, et al. Tolterodine once-daily: superior efficacy and tolerability in the treatment of the overactive bladder. Urology 2001; 57:414.

28. Appell RA, Sand P, Dmochowski R, et al. Prospective randomized controlled trial of extended-release oxybutynin chloride and tolterodine tartrate in the treatment of overactive bladder: results of the OBJECT Study. Mayo Clin Proc 2001; 76:358.

29. Tokuno H, Chowdhury JU, Tomita T. Inhibitory effects of propiverine on rat and guinea-pig urinary bladder muscle. Naunyn-Schmiedeberg's Arch Pharmacol 1993; 348:659.

30. Stöhrer M, Madersbacher H, Richter R, et al. Efficacy and safety of propiverine in SCI-patients suffering from detrusor hyperreflexia – a double-blind, placebo-controlled clinical trial. Spinal Cord 1999; 37:196.

31. Takayasu H, Ueno A, Tuchida S, et al. Clinical effects of propiverine hydrochloride in the treatment of urinary frequency and incontinence associated with detrusor overactivity: a double-blind, parallel, placebo-controlled, multicenter study. Igaku no Ayumi 1990; 153:459. [in Japanese]

32. Madersbacher H, Halaska M, Voigt R, et al. A placebo-controlled, multicentre study comparing the tolerability and efficacy of propiverine and oxybutynin in patients with urgency and urge incontinence. BJU Int 1999; 84:646.

33. Stöhrer M, Bauer P, Giannetti BM, et al. Effects of trospium chloride on urodynamic parameters in patients with detrusor hyperreflexia due to spinal cord injuries. A multicentre placebo-controlled double-blind trial. Urol Int 1991; 47:138.

34. Madersbacher H, Stöhrer M, Richter R, et al. Trospium chloride versus oxybutynin: a randomized, double-blind, multicentre trial in the treatment of detrusor hyperreflexia. Br J Urol 1995; 75:452.

35. Kohler FP, Morales PA. Cystometric evaluation of flavoxate hydrochloride in normal and neurogenic bladder. J Urol 1968; 100:729.

36. Pedersen E, Bjarnason EV, Hansen P-H. The effect of flavoxate on neurogenic bladder dysfunction. Acta Neurol Scand 1972; 48:487.

37. Robinson JM, Brocklehurst JC. Emepronium bromide and flavoxate hydrochloride in the treatment of urinary incontinence associated with detrusor instability in elderly women. Br J Urol 1983; 55:371.

38. Chapple CR, Parkhouse H, Gardener C, Milroy EJ. Double blind, placebo-controlled, crossover study of flavoxate in the treatment of idiopathic detrusor instability. Br J Urol 1990; 66:491.

39. Barrett D, Wein AJ. Voiding dysfunction diagnosis, classification and management. In: Gillenwater JY, Grayhack JT, Howards SS, Duckett JW, eds. Adult and pediatric urology, 2nd edn. St Louis: Mosby-Year Book, 1991:1001–1099.

40. Diokno AC, Taub M. Ephedrine in treatment of urinary incontinence. Urology 1975; 5:624.

41. Raezer DM, Benson GS, Wein AJ, Duckett JW Jr. The functional approach to the management of the pediatric neuropathic bladder: a clinical study. J Urol 1977; 177:649.

42. Awad SA, Downie JW, Kiriluta HG. Alpha-adrenergic agents in urinary disorders of the proximal urethra, part I: sphincteric incontinence. Br J Urol 1978; 50:332.

43. Ek A, Andersson K-E, Gullberg B, Ulmsten K. The effects of long-term treatment with norephedrine on stress incontinence and urethral closure pressure profile. Scand J Urol Nephrol 1978; 12:105.

44. Stewart BH, Banowski LHW, Montague DK. Stress incontinence: conservative therapy with sympathomimetic drugs. J Urol 1976; 115:558.

45. Bauer S. An approach to neurogenic bladder: an overview: Probl Urol 1994; 8:441.

46. Beisland HO, Fossberg E, Sander S. On incompetent urethral closure mechanism: treatment with estriol and phenylpropanolamine. Scand J Urol Nephrol 1981; 60(Suppl): 67.

47. Gleason D, Reilly R, Bottaccini M, Pierce MJ. The urethral continence zone and its relation to stress incontinence. J Urol 1974; 112:81.

48. Gilja I, Radej M, Kovacic M, Parazajders J. Conservative treatment of female stress incontinence with imipramine. J Urol 1984; 132:909–911.

49. Yasuda K, Yamanishi T, Homma Y, et al. The effect of urapidil on neurogenic bladder: a placebo controlled double-blind study. J Urol 1996; 156:1125.

50. Yamanishi T, Yasuda K, Kawabe K, et al. A multicenter placebo-controlled, double-blind trial of urapidil, an α-blocker, on neurogenic bladder dysfunction. Eur Urol 1999; 35: 45.

51. Chancellor MB, Erhard MJ, Hirsch IH, Staas WE. Prospective evaluation of terazosin for the treatment of autonomic dysreflexia. J Urol 1994; 151:111–113.

52. Chancellor MB, Erhard MJ, Rivas DA. Clinical effect of alpha-1 antagonism by terazosin on external and internal urinary sphincter. J Am Parapleg Soc 1993; 16:207–214.

53. Lapides J, Diokno AC, Silber SJ, Lowe BS. Clean intermittent self-catheterization in the treatment of urinary tract disease. J Urol 1972; 107:7458–7461.

54. Maynard FM, Diokno AC. Clean intermittent catheterization for spinal cord injury patients. J Urol 1982; 128:477–480.

55. Cedarbaum JM, Schleifer LS. Drugs for Parkinson's disease, spasticity, and acute muscle spasms. In: Gilman AG, Rail TW, Nies AS, Taylor P, eds. Goodman and Gilman's the pharmacological basis of therapeutics, 8th edn. New York: Pergamon, 1990:463–484.

56. Bianchine J. Drugs for Parkinson's disease: centrally acting muscle relaxants. In: Gilman AG, Goodman LS, Gilman A, eds. The pharmacological basis of therapeutics, New York: MacMillian, 1980;475–495.

57. Hackler RH, Broecker BH, Klein FA, Brady SM. A clinical experience with dantrolene sodium for external urinary sphincter hypertonicity in spinal cord injured patients. J Urol 1980; 124:78–81.

58. Hacken HJ, Krucker V. Clinical and laboratory assessment of the efficacy of baclofen on urethral sphincter spasticity in patients with traumatic paraplegia. Eur Urol 1977; 3:237–240.

59. Herman RM, Wainberg MC. Clonidine inhibits vesico-sphincter reflexes in patients with spinal cord lesions. Arch Phys Med Rehab 1991; 72:539–545.

60. Steers WD, Meythaler JM, Haworth C, et al. Effects of acuter bolus and chronic continuous intrathecal baclofen on genitourinary dysfunction due to spinal cord pathology. J Urol 1992; 148:1849–1855.

61. Hacken HJ. Clinical and urodynamic assessment of alpha adrenolytic therapy in patients with neurogenic bladder function. Paraplegia 1980; 18:229.

62. Caine M. The present role of alpha-adrenergic blockers in the treatment of benign prostatic hypertrophy. J Urol 1986; 136:1.

63. Lepor J, Gup DI, Baumann M, Shapiro E. Laboratory assessment of terazosin and alpha-1 blockade in prostatic hyperplasia. Urology 1988; [Suppl] 32:21.

64. Elbadawi A, Schenk EA. A new theory of the innervation of bladder musculature. Part 4: Innervation of the vesicourethral junction and external urethral sphincter. J Urol 1974; 111:613.

65. Awad SA, Downie JW. Sympathetic dyssynergia in the region of the external sphincter. A possible source of lower urinary tract obstruction. J Urol 1977; 118:636–640.

66. Dixon JS, Gosling JA. Light and electron microscopic observation on noradrenergic nerves and striated muscle cells of the guinea pig urethra. Am J Anat 1977; 149:121.

67. Awad SA, Downie JW. Relative contributions of smooth and striated muscles to canine urethral pressure profile. Br J Urol 1976; 48:347–354.

68. Yalla SV, Rossier AB, Fam B. Dyssynergic vesicourethral responses during bladder rehabilitation in spinal cord injury patients: effects of spurapubic percussion, crede method and bethanechol chloride. J Urol 1976; 115:575.

69. Kaplan SA, Chancellor MB, Blaivas JG. Bladder and sphincter behavior in patients with spinal cord lesions. J Urol 1991; 46:113–117.

70. Mobley DF. Phenoxybenzamine in the management of neurogenic vesical dysfunction. J Urol 1976; 116:737–738.

71. Whitfield HN, Doyle PT, Mayo ME, Poopalasingham N. The effect of adrenergic blocking drugs on outflow resistance. Br J Urol 1976; 47: 823–827.

72. Awad SA, Downie JW, Lywood DW, et al. Sympathetic activity in the proximal urethra in patients with urinary obstruction. J Urol 1976; 115:545–547.

73. Olsson AT, Swanberg E, Svedinger L. Effects of beta adrenoceptor agonists on airway smooth muscle and on slow contracting skeletal muscle: In vitro and in vivo results compared. Acta Pharmacol Toxicol 1979; 44:272.

74. McGuire EJ, Wagner F, Weiss RM. Treatment of autonomic dysreflexia with phenoxybenzamine. J Urol 1976; 115:53–55.

75. Rossier AB, Fam BA, Lee IY, et al. Role of striated and smooth muscle components in the urethral pressure profile in the traumatic neurogenic bladder: a neuropharmacological and urodynamic study. Preliminary report. J Urol 1982; 128:529–535.

76. Sizemore GW, Winternitz WW. Autonomic hyper-reflexia-suppression with alpha-adrenergic blocking agents. N Engl J Med 1970; 282:795.

77. Scott MB, Morrow JW. Phenoxybenzamine in neurogenic bladder dysfunction after spinal cord injury. II. Autonomic dysreflexia. J Urol 1978; 119:483–484.

78. Chancellor MB, Karasick S, Erhard MJ, et al. Intraurethral wire mesh prosthesis placement in the external urinary sphincter of spinal cord injured men. Radiology 1993; 187:551.

79. Yalla SV, Rossier AB, Fam BA, et al. Functional contribution of autonomic innervation to urethral striated sphincter: studies with parasympathomimetic, parasympatholytic and alpha adrenergic blocking agents in spinal cord injury and control male subjects. J Urol 1977; 117:494–499.

80. Bloom FE. Neurohumoral transmission and the central nervous system. In: Gilman AG, Rail TW, Nies AS, Taylor P, eds. Goodman and Gilman's the pharmacological basis of therapeutics, 8th edn. New York: Pergamon, 1990:244–268.

81. Leyson JFJ, Martin BF, Sporer A. Baclofen in the treatment of detrusor-sphincter dyssynergia in spinal cord injury patients. J Urol 1980; 124:82–84.

82. Florante J, Leyson J, Martin F, Sporer A. Baclofen in the treatment of detrusor-sphincter dyssynergia in spinal cord injury patients. J Urol 1980; 124:82–84.

83. Roy CW, Wakefield IR. Baclofen pseudopsychosis: case report. Paraplegia 1986; 24:318.

84. Rivas DA, Chancellor MB, Hill K, Friedman M. Neurologic manifestations of baclofen withdrawal. J Urol 1993; 150:1903–1905.

85. Davidoff RA. Antispasticity drugs: mechanisms of action. Ann Neurol 1985; 17:107.

86. Lader M. Clinical pharmacology of benzodiazepines. Ann Rev Med 1987; 38:19.

87. Gosling JA, Dixon JS, Critchley HOD, et al. A comparative study of the human external sphincter and periurethral levator ani muscles. Br J Urol 1981; 153:35.

88. Harris JD, Benson GS. Effect of dantrolene on canine bladder contractility. Urology 1980; 16:229.

89. Ward A, Chaffman MO, Sorkin EM. Dantrolene. A review of its pharmacodynamic and pharmacokinetic properties and therapeutic use in malignant hyperthermia, the neuroleptic syndrome and an update of its use in muscle spasticity. Drugs 1986; 32:130.

90. McGuire EJ, Woodside JR, Borden TA, Weiss RM. The prognostic significance of urodynamic testing in myelodysplastic patients. J Urol 1981; 126:205–209.

91. Nanninga JB, Frost F, Penn R. Effect of intrathecal baclofen on bladder and sphincter function. J Urol 1989; 142:101–105.

92. Talalla A, Grundy D, Macdonell R. The effect of intrathecal baclofen on the lower urinary tract in paraplegia. Paraplegia 1990; 8:420–427.

93. Bushman W, Steers WD, Meythaler JM. Voiding dysfunction in patients with spastic paraplegia: urodynamic evaluation and response to continuous intrathecal baclofen. Neurourol Urodynam 1993; 12:163–170.

94. Kums JJ, Delhaas EM. Intrathecal baclofen infusion in patients with spasticity and neurogenic bladder disease. World J Urol 1991; 9:153–156.

45

Intravesical pharmacological treatment

Carlos Silva and Francisco Cruz

Introduction

The increasing interest around intravesical pharmacological therapy for neurogenic bladder overactivity is essentially due to the fact that it circumvents systemic administration of active compounds. This offers two potential advantages. First, intravesical therapy is an easy way to provide high concentrations of pharmacological agents in the bladder tissue without causing unsuitable levels in other organs. Secondly, the action of effective drugs inappropriate for systemic administration can be restricted to the bladder. Although extremely attractive, it must, however, be kept in mind that intravesical pharmacological therapy should be introduced as a second-line treatment in patients refractory to conventional oral anticholinergic therapy or patients who do not tolerate its systemic side-effects.

Drugs susceptible to decreasing or abolishing detrusor contractions by the intravesical route block either the sensory input or the parasympathetic outflow to the detrusor muscle. Drugs that block the sensory input include capsaicin and resiniferatoxin, two compounds of the vanilloid family. Drugs that block the parasympathetic outflow include botulinum A toxin and anticholinergic compounds.

Vanilloid substances

Common vanilloids, VR1 receptor, and desensitization

Capsaicin, which is extracted from hot chilli peppers, and resiniferatoxin (RTX), which is extracted from *Euphorbia resinifera*, a cactus-like plant abundant in northern Africa, are the most well-studied compounds of this family. The name vanilloid derived from the presence of a homovanillyl ring in capsaicin and RTX molecules (Figure 45.1). However, such a designation became a misnomer, as new compounds with properties similar to those of capsaicin or

RTX were identified which do not possess a homovanillyl ring in their structure. Examples of such compounds include polygodial, scutigeral, and olvanil.[1]

Vanilloid substances bind to a receptor – named vanilloid receptor type 1 or VR1 – that occurs in the membrane of type C, unmyelinated sensory fibers.[2,3] VR1 is a nonselective ion channel that belongs to the transient resting potential family of ion channels, being for that reason also denominated TRPV1 in more recent publications.[4] Once activated, VR1 allows a massive Ca^{2+} and Na^+ inflow into the neuron. This causes a brief excitation, followed by a prolonged desensitization, during which the neuron is

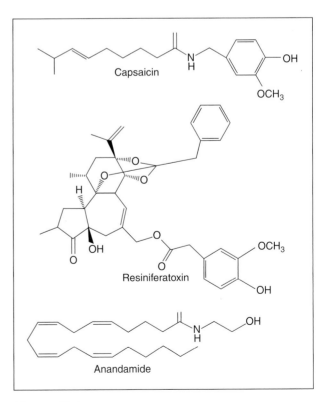

Figure 45.1
Molecular structures of capsaicin, resiniferatoxin, and anandamide.

unresponsive to natural stimuli.[1] Only desensitization has therapeutic implications. It is, however, a poorly understood phenomenon. It depends on Ca^{2+} inflow, since desensitization does not occur in sensory neurons kept in culture mediums lacking the calcium ion. It is believed that high intracellular Ca^{2+} levels arrest the voltage-sensitive Ca^{2+} conductance, disrupt metabolic critical pathways, and release neuropeptides such as substance P (SP) or calcitonin gene-related peptide (CGRP).[1] In addition, desensitization may also induce prolonged neuromessenger modifications in sensory fibers, such as a down-regulation of SP[5] and an up-regulation of galanin synthesis.[6] The latter peptide is usually not expressed by sensory neurons.[6]

It is intriguing that an endogenous vanilloid-like substance binding to VR1 has not yet been identified. At present, the endogenous substance closest to capsaicin or RTX is anandamide, a lipid synthesized in brain tissue, vascular endothelium, and macrophages.[7] Anandamide, although lacking a homovanillyl ring, has a long chain similar to that occurring in typical vanilloids (see Figure 45.1). Interestingly, anandamide also evokes Ca^{2+} inflow through VR1 receptors.[3,8]

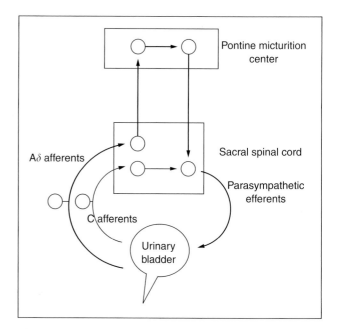

Figure 45.2
Neuronal pathways controlling micturition.

Rationale for intravesical vanilloid application

Capsaicin does not interfere with reflex detrusor contractions in intact animals but suppresses them in chronic spinal animals.[9] This finding by de Groat et al was subsequently explained by the existence of two micturition reflex pathways fed by distinct sensory input (Figure 45.2).[9] One pathway, a supraspinal loop passing through the pontine micturition center, was triggered by Aδ-fiber sensory input. The other pathway, a neuronal pathway totally lodged in the sacral spinal cord, was dependent upon C-fiber sensory input. Interestingly, the former pathway controlled micturition in intact animals, whereas the latter was active only in spinal transected animals. These experimental findings pushed Fowler et al to instill capsaicin into overactive bladders of patients with spinal cord lesions.[10] As intravesical capsaicin suppressed detrusor activity, that study indirectly confirmed the existence of a C-fiber-mediated spinal micturition reflex in man.[10]

Clinical experience with intravesical capsaicin

More than 100 patients with bladder overactivity of spinal origin received intravesical capsaicin in six non-controlled[11–16] and one controlled[17] clinical trial (Tables 45.1 and 45.2). In general, treatments followed the methodology initially suggested by Fowler et al in 1992.[10] Capsaicin was dissolved in 30% alcohol and 100–125 ml (or half of the bladder capacity if lower than that volume) of 1–2 mmol/l solutions were instilled into the bladder and left in contact with the mucosa for 30 min.

Best clinical results were found among patients with incomplete spinal cord lesions caused by multiple sclerosis, trauma, or infectious diseases who maintained some degree of bladder sensation and emptied the bladder by micturition. Success rates, defined as complete continence or satisfactory improvement, reached 70–90% (see Table 45.1).[11,15,16] In addition, capsaicin also decreased urinary frequency and attenuated urge to urinate.[11,15,16] In patients with complete spinal cord lesions the success rate was much lower. Geirsson et al[12] obtained full continence in only 20% and partial improvement in another 20% of patients with cervical cord lesions (see Table 45.1). The effect of capsaicin on micturition symptoms was long-lasting, exceeding 6 or even 9 months in some cases.[11,15,16] Upon reinstillation, capsaicin maintained the efficacy found at the first administration.[11,15,16]

Urodynamic improvement occurred in 70–90% of the patients (see Table 45.1). In particular, a 47–156% increase of bladder capacity was observed. The effect of capsaicin on maximal detrusor pressure is less clear. Although three studies have reported a 20–30 cmH$_2$O decrease in maximal detrusor pressure,[11,16,17] another study was unable to demonstrate any significant decrease.[12]

One randomized controlled study that compared capsaicin against 30% ethanol, the vehicle solution, should be mentioned (see Table 45.2).[17] Twenty cases were

Table 45.1 *Open clinical studies with intravesical capsaicin*

Study	Dose/patients	Frequency		FDC (ml)		MCC (ml)		DP (cmH$_2$O)		Clinical and urodynamic improvement
		Before	After	Before	After	Before	After	Before	After	
Fowler et al[11]	1 or 2 mmol/l 12 patients					124	274	58	40	Clinical improvement 75% Full continence 40%
Geirsson et al[12]	2 mmol/l 10 patients					195	293	82	90	Clinical improvement 40% Full continence 20% Urodynamic improvement 90%
Das et al[13]	0.1–2 mmol/l 5 patients					124	231			Clinical improvement 60%
Igawa et al[14]	1–2 mmol/l 5 patients					72	185			Clinical improvement 100%
Cruz et al[15]	1 mmol/l 10 patients	15	8	97	173	151	288			Clinical improvement 90% Full continence 80% Urodynamic improvement 70%
De Ridder et al[16]	1–2 mmol/l 49 patients					194	247	58	28	Clinical improvement 82%
Fowler (in De Ridder et al[16])	1–2 mmol/l 18 patients	12.7	6.4			169	320	68	49	Clinical improvement 78% Full continence 61%

FDC, volume to first detrusor contraction; MCC, maximum cystometric capacity; DP, maximum detrusor voiding pressure.

Table 45.2 *Comparative study between intravesical capsaicin and vehicle solution (30% ethanol)*

Study	Dose/ patients	Incontinence		Frequency		MCC (ml)		DP (cmH$_2$O)		Subjective improvement
		Before	After	Before	After	Before	After	Before	After	
De Séze et al[17]	1 mmol/l capsaicin 10 patients	3.9	0.6*	9.3	6.1*	169	299*	77	53*	100%
	Placebo 10 patients	5.1	4	11.1	12.2	157	182	64	69	10%

MCC, maximum cystometric capacity; DP, maximum detrusor voiding pressure; * indicates a statistically significant change.

randomized to receive capsaicin (10 cases) or 30% ethanol (10 cases). All patients that received capsaicin found significant regression of incontinence and urge sensation, whereas only one ethanol-treated patient had amelioration.

Clinical experience with intravesical resiniferatoxin

The first non-controlled trials with this vanilloid included 34 patients, most of them with incomplete spinal cord lesions (Table 45.3).[18–21] Different RTX concentrations, 10 nmol/l, 50 nmol/l, 100 nmol/l, and 10 μmol/l, were tested. RTX brought an immediate improvement or disappearance of urinary incontinence in 67–85% of the patients and a 30% decrease in their daily urinary frequency. The effect was long-lasting, up to 12 months, only in patients receiving 50 nmol/l or higher doses of RTX.[18,21] In patients treated with doses as high as 10 μmol/l, a transient urinary retention due to detrusor hypoactivity occurred.[20]

Urodynamic improvement was observed in most of the treated patients. For example, the volume to first detrusor contraction increased 40% after 50–100 nmol/l RTX. Maximal bladder capacity increased 25% after 10 nmol/l,[19] 80% after 50–100 nmol/l,[18,21] and 120% after 10 μmol/l solutions.[20] Maximal detrusor pressure was decreased only after 10 μmol/l RTX.

RTX was compared against the vehicle solution (10% ethanol in saline) in a recent randomized ongoing study (Table 45.4).[22] The discomfort was similarly low in both arms. A significant improvement of urinary frequency and incontinence was found only in the RTX arm. In addition, only patients receiving RTX had an increase of the volume to first detrusor contraction and of maximal bladder capacity, 35% and 80% above the pre-treatment values, respectively. Another three studies compared 50–100 nmol/l RTX against 1–2 mmol/l capsaicin (Table 45.5).[23–25] RTX was better tolerated and its effects on continence and urodynamic parameters were equivalent[25] or superior[24] to those induced by capsaicin.

Safety of intravesical vanilloids

The most frequent problem seen with capsaicin instillation is suprapubic burning pain felt by patients with preserved bladder sensation. It starts immediately after the beginning of the treatment and may require vigorous analgesic medication and prompt capsaicin evacuation. Preliminary bladder anesthesia with lidocaine (lignocaine) may provide partial relief.[11,15,26] In addition, a transient worsening of the urinary symptoms may occur during the first 1–2 weeks after instillation which should not be interpreted as a treatment failure.[11,15,26] Another side-effect of capsaicin needs to be stressed. In patients with high, complete spinal cord lesions, capsaicin can trigger severe episodes of autonomic dysreflexia.[12,15] In contrast, these side-effects did not occur with RTX instillation.[18,21,22]

Human contact with capsaicin and RTX was not initiated with intravesical application of these vanilloids. Capsaicin is consumed in the daily diet of millions of people and historical reports indicate that RTX has been used for medicinal purposes over many centuries, mainly as analgesic unguent.[27] Nevertheless, the contact of vanilloid compounds with the bladder mucosa represents a new challenge, the consequences of which have not yet been fully evaluated. In agreement with these concerns, bladder biopsies were obtained from patients repeatedly instilled with capsaicin[28] or RTX.[29] Examinations under the conventional and electronic microscopes were unable to detect any significant change in the transitional mucosa of those patients.

The ideal patient, the ideal vanilloid, and how to apply it

Patients with small contracted bladders or bedridden due to severe neurological disorders responded very poorly to capsaicin or RTX instillation.[11,30] In addition, in patients

Table 45.3 Open clinical studies with intravesical resiniferatoxin

Study	Dose/patients	Incontinence		Frequency		FDC (ml)		MCC (ml)		DP (cmH$_2$O)		Clinical improvement
		Before	After	Before	After	Before	After	Before	After	Before	After	
Cruz et al[18]	50 or 100 nmol/l	3.6	1.5	14	10	134	184	182	330	80	70	80% at 3 months
Silva et al[21]	7 + 14 patients											
Lazzeri et al[19]	10 nmol/l							175	216	69	61	67% at 2 weeks
	6 patients											33% at 4 weeks
Lazzeri et al[20]	10 μmol/l							190	421	75	21	85% at 4 weeks
	7 patients											

FDC, volume to first detrusor contraction; MCC, maximum cystometric capacity; DP, maximum detrusor voiding pressure.

Table 45.4 *Comparative study between intravesical RTX and vehicle solution (10% ethanol)*

Study	Dose/patients	Incontinence		Frequency		FDC (ml)		MCC (ml)	
		Before	After	Before	After	Before	After	Before	After
Cruz et al[22]	50 nmol/l RTX 12 patients	3	1.3*	9.2	7.3*	139	185*	185	326*
	Placebo 11 patients	1.8	1	10	9.6	109	110	180	189

FDC, volume to first detrusor contraction; MCC, maximum cystometric capacity; * indicates a statistically significant change.

Table 45.5 *Comparative studies between intravesical capsaicin and resiniferatoxin*

Study	Dose/patients	Incontinence		Frequency		FDC (ml)		MCC (ml)		DP (cmH$_2$O)		Subjective improvement
		Before	After	Before	After	Before	After	Before	After	Before	After	
Giannatoni et al[24]	Capasaicin 2 mmol/l 12 patients	3	2.3	5.8	5.6	165	195	183	219	76	69	33%
	RTX 100 nmol/l 12 patients	4.2	1.9*	6.6	4.8*	176	275*	196	357*	71	68	92%
de Sèze et al[25]	Capsaicin 1 mmol/l 19 patients	6	2.6*	11.1	6.4*			174	300*	75	75	67%
	RTX 50 nmol/l 21 patients	6.9	4.3	9.5	9.4			195	320*	75	71	56%
Park et al[23]	Capsaicin 2 mmol/l 7 patients							108	156*	75	60	57%
	RTX 10 nmol/l 6 patients							115	222*	58	53	83%

FDC, volume to first detrusor contraction; MCC, maximum cystometric capacity; DP, maximum detrusor voiding pressure; * indicates a statistically significant change.

with complete spinal cord transection 50–100 nmol/l RTX solutions, although increasing bladder capacity, usually do not render bladders fully arreflexic.[12] These patients might benefit from higher RTX concentrations,[20] but this aspect requires further investigation.

At present, RTX seems preferable to capsaicin, because of its reduced pungency. RTX is available only as a dry powder. A 10 μmol/l stock solution in pure ethanol (1 mg RTX dissolved in 159 ml of ethanol) must be prepared and kept at 4°C in a glass container,[18,21,22] because of RTX instability in plastic containers.[31] Solutions for instillation are then prepared immediately before treatment.[18,21,22] For example,

to prepare 100 ml of 50 nmol/l solution in 10% ethanol in saline, 0.5 ml of the stock solution should be added to 9.5 ml of pure ethanol and 90 ml of saline. Due to their low pungency, the instillation of 50–100 nmol/l RTX solutions can be carried out as an outpatient procedure without any form of preliminary bladder anesthesia.[18,21,22] A three-way urethral catheter is inserted, the urine is emptied, and the RTX solution is instilled for 30 min. Phasic detrusor contractions can occur during instillation, although they become more spaced towards the end of the treatment. Leakage of RTX solution can, however, be prevented by maintaining the urethral catheter gently pulled against the bladder neck. At the end of the treatment, the bladder is evacuated and rinsed with saline and the patients are discharged home. Urinary tract infections should be prevented by a judicious use of prophylactic antibiotics.

If capsaicin is the chosen vanilloid, 1 mmol/l solutions can be obtained by dissolving 0.3 g of capsaicin in 1000 ml of 30% ethanol in saline.[10] Instillation is carried out as described for RTX. However, in patients with some bladder sensation remaining, strong analgesic treatment is usually required to alleviate bladder pain.[11,15,16] Furthermore, patients with spinal cord transection at high levels should be carefully monitored due to their susceptibility to severe episodes of autonomic dysreflexia.[12,15] Adequate treatment must be readily accessible for immediate administration.

Botulinum A toxin

Botulinum A toxin is a neurotoxin produced by *Clostridium botulinum*, a facultative anaerobe. It causes muscular paralysis by preventing the release of acetylcholine from cholinergic nerve endings at the neuromuscular junction.[32] This property was shown to relax the external urethral sphincter and improve bladder emptying in patients with detrusor-sphincter dyssynergia.[33,34] More recently, botulinum A toxin was also shown to relax the detrusor smooth muscle and reduce bladder overactivity in spinal patients.[35] This treatment requires multiple bladder injections. Therefore, although being reviewed in this chapter, it should be realized that it implicates more than a simple bladder instillation.

Clinical experience with botulinum A toxin

Schurch et al[35] were the first to use botulinum A toxin in the treatment of bladder overactivity resistant to anticholinergic drugs. In a nonrandomized study, 17 patients with complete and 4 patients with incomplete traumatic spinal cord injuries who emptied the bladder by intermittent self-catheterization underwent botulinum A toxin detrusor injections (Table 45.6). Botulinum A toxin (Botox®) was diluted in normal saline in order to obtain a concentration of 10 units/ml. Under visual control through a cystoscope, 30 injections of 1 ml (10 units of botulinum A toxin) were performed in 30 different locations above the trigone. A flexible 6F injection needle was used to deliver the toxin in the detrusor smooth muscle. In general, detrusor paralysis started 2 weeks later. At 6 weeks, urodynamic evaluation revealed a significant increase of bladder capacity and a significant decrease in maximum

detrusor voiding pressure that was still present at 36 weeks (see Table 45.6). Seventeen patients became completely continent, 7 patients without any additional anticholinergic medication and 10 patients requiring a lower daily dose. Interestingly, in susceptible patients, episodes of autonomic dysreflexia disappeared.

The initial experience with botulinum A toxin injections was recently confirmed in a multicenter nonrandomized clinical trial conducted in Europe and involving 184 patients (see Table 45.6).[36] Detrusor relaxation and continence was achieved in all cases but two-thirds of the patients still had to maintain a daily dose of anticholinergics.[36] The long-lasting effect of the first treatment, up to 1 year, appears to be maintained in subsequent injections.

Botulinum A toxin has been recently assayed in children with myelomeningocele (see Table 45.6).[37,38] As in adults, the toxin also increased bladder capacity and decreased maximal detrusor pressure. For the moment, the success rate in terms of continence and cessation of anticholinergic medication seems inferior to that observed in adults (see Table 45.6). In children, botulinum A toxin dose (Botox®) has to be calculated according to body weight. Schulte-Baukloh et al[37] suggested a dose of 12 units/kg of weight up to a maximum dose of 300 units, whereas Corcos et al[38] used 4 units/kg. The duration of detrusor paralysis is still unknown.

Side-effects of botulinum A toxin injections in the bladder appear to be minimal: the most feared one, paralysis of the striated musculature due to circulatory leakage of the toxin, was never reported. Currently, it is not known whether the prolonged deficit of parasympathetic tonus induces detrusor muscle atrophy. Furthermore, repeated injections of botulinum A toxin may lose efficacy due to the appearance of antibodies against the toxin.

Ideal patient for botulinum A toxin treatment

Patients should understand that following botulinum A toxin injection urinary retention will occur due to detrusor paralysis. Therefore, currently, ideal patients for botulinum A toxin treatment are those performing intermittent catheterization who maintain significant incontinence or high intravesical pressures in spite of a correct anticholinergic medication.

Botulinum A toxin is available under the tradenames of Botox® and Dysport®. The two varieties have been compared in some controlled studies. Available information indicates that Botox® is roughly three times more potent than Dysport®.[39] Therefore, if the latter variety is chosen, it may be necessary to triplicate the doses indicated for Botox®. Whatever the type of botulinum A toxin used,

Table 45.6 Experience with botulinum A toxin bladder injections

Study	Patients	Dose/protocol	Follow-up	FDC (ml)		MCC (ml)		DP (cmH₂O)		RV (ml)		Compliance (ml/cmH₂O)		Improvement
				Before	After	Before	After	Before	After	Before	After	Before	After	
Schurch et al[35]	19 adults	200–300 IU 20–30 sites 10 U/ml/site Trigone spared	6 weeks	215.8	415.7	296.3	480.5	65.6	35	261.8	490.5	32.6	62.1	Urodynamic improvement 100% Full continence 89%
Reitz et al[36]	184 adults	200–300 IU 20–30 sites 10 U/ml/site Trigone spared	12 weeks			272	420	61	30	236	387	32	72	Subjective improvement 100%
			36 weeks			272	352	61	44	236	291	32	51	Subjective improvement 100%
Corcos et al[38]	16 children (8–20 years)	4 IU/kg 20–30 sites	3 months			221	307	33.7	12.3					Subjective improvement 80% Full continence 68%
Schulte-Baukloh et al[37]	17 children (mean age 10.8 years)	85–300 IU 30–40 sites	2–4 weeks	95	201	137	215	59	40			20	45	40% overall decrease in incontinence score

Open clinical trials. FDC, volume to first detrusor contraction; MCC, maximum cystometric capacity; DP, maximum detrusor voiding pressure; RV, residual urine volume.

a common drawback of this treatment is its cost. A dose of 300 units of botulinum A toxin might exceed US$1500, and to which one must add the cost of a cystoscopy. Moreover, a substantial number of patients will still require permanent anticholinergic medication.

Anticholinergic drugs

Oxybutynin is the anticholinergic drug most frequently used by the intravesical route. Intravesical oxybutynin has been offered mainly to patients in whom oral administration has no effect or evokes severe side-effects, with a 55–90% success rate.[40–45] Treatment can be maintained over long periods of time without any form of bladder toxicity.[46,47] The reason why oxybutynin is better tolerated by the intravesical rather than the oral route is still incompletely understood. As a matter of fact, plasma concentrations of oxybutynin after intravesical or oral administration were shown to be similar.[43] A plausible explanation may, therefore, rest on the level of N-desethyloxybutynin, an active metabolite of oxybutynin, which is in general lower after intravesical than after oral administration. However, it should be kept in mind that drug absorption through the bladder may still evoke anticholinergic systemic side-effects, leading to treatment discontinuity in a significant number of cases.[48]

At the present time, there are no oxybutynin formulations ready for intravesical application. Thus, for adult patients, a 5 mg oxybutynin tablet must be crushed and dissolved in 30 ml of distilled water or saline and instilled twice or three times daily. The solution should not be evacuated until the next voiding, since maximum effect may take 3–4 hours to occur.[49] For children, it is advisable to start with 1.25 mg (one-quarter of a 5 mg oxybutynin tablet in 5 ml of sterile water) three times daily and adjust the dose according to the response.[48] The inconvenience of crushing oxybutynin tablets before every instillation can be avoided if purified oxybutynin preparations are available, usually as 5 ml vials containing 5 mg of oxybutynin.[50]

However, the need for 2–3 daily instillations restricts intravesical oxybutynin to patients on intermittent catheterization. To obviate this inconvenience long-acting intravesical oxybutynin formulations are being investigated. Hydroxypropylcellulose that adheres to the bladder mucosa or small reservoirs that can be placed in the bladder cavity may be used in the future to induce intravesically a slow and sustained release of oxybutynin.[51,52]

Electromotive drug administration (EMDA), which uses an electrical field to enhance the migration of ionized molecules (iontophoresis) through a particular tissue, has also been suggested as an alternative to increase absorption of intravesical oxybutynin.[53,54] A Foley catheter containing a silver positive electrode is introduced and the bladder is evacuated and rinsed with distilled water to remove urinary solutes that might be dragged by the electric current. The bladder is then filled with an oxybutynin solution. Negative electrode pads are placed on the paraumbilical area.[55] Riedl et al administered, by EMDA, 15–50 mg of oxybutynin to 14 patients with detrusor hyperreflexia by applying a 15 mA electric current for 20 min. Clinical and urodynamic improvement lasting several weeks occurred in half of the patients.[55] Di Stasi et al[56] also found significant clinical and urodynamic improvement in 10 patients refractory to standard anticholinergic therapy after EMDA of 5 mg oxybutynin (5 mA electric current for 30 min). Although attractive, it is still unclear why the therapeutic effect of intravesical oxybutynin given by EMDA lasts longer than after passive instillation. Moreover, it is intriguing why oxybutynin-induced systemic side-effects are less intense after EMDA than after passive intravesical administration in spite of the fact that high doses of the drug are dragged into the bladder tissue by EMDA. Future studies are, therefore, strongly recommended before a widespread use of intravesical EMDA.

Other drugs, such as trospium chloride, verapamil, tolterodine, atropine, diltiazem, and imipramine, have been used sporadically by intravesical route to decrease bladder overactivity but their effects remain to be compared with oxybutynin.[45,57]

References

1. Szallasi A, Blumberg PM. Vanilloid (capsaicin) receptors and mechanisms. Pharmacol Rev 1999; 51:159–211.

2. Caterina MJ, Schumacher MA, Tominaga M, et al. The capsaicin receptor: a heat-activated ion channel in the pain pathway. Nature 1997; 389:816–824.

3. Hayes P, Meadows J, Gunthorpe MJ, et al. Cloning and functional expression of a human orthologue of rat vanilloid receptor-1. Pain 2000; 88:205–215.

4. Gunthorpe MJ, Benham CD, Randall A, Davies JB. The diversity in the vanilloid (TRPV) receptor family of ion channels. Trends Pharmacol Sci 2002; 23:183–191.

5. Szallasi A, Farkas-Szallasi T, Tucker JB, et al. Effects of systemic resiniferatoxin on substance P mRNA in rat dorsal root ganglia and substance P receptor mRNA in the spinal cord. Brain Res 1999; 815:177–184.

6. Avelino A, Cruz C, Cruz F. Nerve growth factor regulates galanin and c-jun overexpression occurring in dorsal root ganglion cells after intravesical resiniferatoxin application. Brain Res 2002; 951:264–269.

7. Di Marzo V, De Petrocellis L, Sepe N, et al. Biosynthesis of anandamide and related acylethanolamides in mouse J774 macrophages and N18 neuroblastoma cells. Biochem J 1996; 316:977–984.

8. Zygmunt PM, Peterson J, Andersson DA, et al. Vanilloid receptors on sensory nerves mediate the vasodilator action of anandamide. Nature 1999; 400:452–457.

9. de Groat WC, Kawatani M, Hisamitsu T, et al. Mechanisms underlying the recovery of urinary bladder function following spinal cord injury. J Auton Nerv Syst 1990; 30(suppl):S71–S77.

10. Fowler CJ, Jewkes D, McDonald WI, et al. Intravesical capsaicin for neurogenic bladder dysfunction. Lancet 1992; 339:1239.

11. Fowler CJ, Beck RO, Gerrard S, et al. Intravesical capsaicin for the treatment of detrusor hyperreflexia. J Neurol Neurosurg Psychiatry 1994; 57:169–173.

12. Geirsson G, Fall M, Sullivan L. Clinical and urodynamic effects of intravesical capsaicin treatment in patients with chronic traumatic spinal detrusor hyperreflexia. J Urol 1995; 154:1825–1829.

13. Das A, Chancellor MB, Watanabe T, et al. Intravesical capsaicin in neurogenic impaired patients with detrusor hyperreflexia. J Spinal Cord Med 1996; 19:190–193.

14. Igawa Y, Komiyama I, Nishizawa O, Ogawa A. Intravesical capsaicin inhibits autonomic dysreflexia in patients with spinal cord injury. Neurourol Urodyn 1996; 15:374–375. [Abstract]

15. Cruz F, Guimarães M, Silva C, et al. Desensitization of bladder sensory fibers by intravesical capsaicin has long lasting clinical and urodynamic effects in patients with hyperactive or hypersensitive bladder dysfunction. J Urol 1997; 157:585–589.

16. De Ridder D, Chandiramani V, Dasgupta P, et al. Intravesical capsaicin as a treatment for refractory detrusor hyperreflexia: a dual center study with long-term followup. J Urol 1997; 158:2087–2092.

17. de Séze M, Wiart L, Joseph PA, et al. Capsaicin and neurogenic detrusor hyperreflexia. A double blind placebo controlled study in 20 patients with spinal cord lesions. Neurourol Urodyn 1998; 17:513–523.

18. Cruz F, Guimarães M, Silva C, Reis M. Suppression of bladder hyperreflexia by intravesical resiniferatoxin. Lancet 1997; 350:640–641.

19. Lazzeri M, Beneforti P, Turini D. Urodynamic effects of intravesical resiniferatoxin in humans: preliminary results in stable and unstable detrusor. J Urol 1997; 158:2093–2096.

20. Lazzeri M, Spinelli M, Beneforti P, et al. Intravesical resiniferatoxin for the treatment of detrusor hyperreflexia refractory to capsaicin in patients with chronic spinal cord diseases. Scand J Urol Nephrol 1998; 32:331–334.

21. Silva C, Rio ME, Cruz F. Desensitization of bladder sensory fibers by intravesical resiniferatoxin, a capsaicin analog: long-term results for the treatment of detrusor hyperreflexia. Eur Urol 2000; 38:444–452.

22. Cruz F, Silva C, Ribeiro M, Avelino A. The effect of intravesical resiniferatoxin in neurogenic forms of bladder overactivity. Preliminary results of a randomised placebo controlled clinical trial. Neurourol Urodyn 2002; 21:426–427. [Abstract]

23. Park WH, Kim HG, Park BJ, et al. Comparison of the effects of intravesical capsaicin and resiniferatoxin for treatment of detrusor hyperreflexia in patients with spinal cord injury. Neurourol Urodyn 1999; 18:402. [Abstract]

24. Giannantoni A, Di Stasi SM, Stephen RL, et al. Intravesical capsaicin versus resiniferatoxin in patients with detrusor hyperreflexia: a prospective randomized study. J Urol 2002; 167:1710–1714.

25. de Sèze M, Wiart L, de Sèze M, et al. Efficacy and tolerance of intravesical instillation of capsaicin and resiniferatoxin for the treatment of detrusor hyperreflexia in spinal cord injured patients. A double-blind controlled study: preliminary results. Neurourol Urodyn 2002; 21:41–42. [Abstract]

26. Chandiramani V, Peterson T, Duthie GS, Fowler CJ. Urodynamic changes during therapeutic intravesical instillations of capsaicin. Br J Urol 1996; 77:792–797.

27. Appendino G, Szallasi A. Euphorbium: modern research on its active principle, resiniferatoxin, revives an ancient medicine. Life Sci 1997; 60:681–696.

28. Dasgupta P, Chandiramani V, Parkinson MC, et al. Treating the human bladder with capsaicin: is it safe? Eur Urol 1998; 33:28–31.

29. Silva C, Avelino A, Souto-Moura C, Cruz F. A light and electron microscope histopathological study of the human bladder mucosa after intravesical resiniferatoxin application. BJU Int 2001; 88:355–360.

30. Cruz F. Desensitization of bladder sensory fibers by intravesical capsaicin or capsaicin analogs. A new strategy for treatment of urge incontinence in patients with spinal detrusor hyperreflexia or bladder hypersensitivity disorders. Int Urogynecol J 1998; 9:214–220.

31. Szallasi A, Fowler CJ. After a decade of intravesical vanilloid therapy: still more questions than answers. Lancet Neurology 2002; 1:167–172.

32. Jankovic J, Brin MF. Botulinum toxin: historical perspective and potential new indications. Muscle Nerve 1997; 6(suppl):129–145.

33. Dykstra DD, Sidi AA. Treatment of detrusor-sphincter dyssynergia with botulinum A toxin: a double-blind study. Arch Phys Med Rehab 1990; 71:24–26.

34. Schurch B, Hauri D, Rodic B, et al. Botulinum-A toxin as a treatment of detrusor-sphincter dyssynergia: a prospective study in 24 spinal cord injury patients. J Urol 1996; 155:1023–1029.

35. Schurch B, Schmid DM, Stohrer M. Treatment of neurogenic incontinence with botulinum toxin A. N Engl J Med 2000; 342:665.

36. Reitz A, von Tobel J, Stohrer M, et al. European experience of 184 cases treated with botulinum-A toxin injections into the detrusor muscle for neurogenic incontinence. Neurourol Urodyn 2002; 21:427–428. [Abstract]

37. Schulte-Baukloh H, Michael T, Schobert J, et al. Efficacy of botulinum-A toxin in children with detrusor hyperreflexia due to myelomeningocele: preliminary results. Urology 2002; 59:325–328.

38. Corcos J, Al-Taweel W, Pippi Salle J, et al. The treatment of detrusor hyperreflexia using botulinum A toxin in myelomeningocele patients unresponsive to anticholinergic. Neurourol Urodyn 2002; 21:332–333. [Abstract]

39. Odergen T, Hjaltason H, Kaakkola, S, et al. A double blind, randomised, parallel group study to investigate the dose equivalence of Dysport® and Botox® in the treatment of cervical dystonia. J Neurol Neurosurg Psychiatry 1998; 64:6–12.

40. Brendler BCH, Radebaugh LC, Mohler JL. Topical oxybutynin chloride for relaxation of dysfunctional bladders. J Urol 1989; 141:1350–1352.

41. Madersbacher H, Jilg G. Control of detrusor hyperreflexia by the intravesical instillation of oxybutynin hydrochloride. Paraplegia 1991; 29:84–90.

42. Greenfield SP, Fera M. The use of intravesical oxybutynin chloride in children with neurogenic bladder. J Urol 1991; 146:532–534.

43. Massada CA, Kogan BA, Trigo-Rocha FE. The pharmacokinetics of intravesical and oral oxybutynin chloride. J Urol 1992; 148:595–597.

44. Weese DL, Roskamp DA, Leach GE, Zimmern PE. Intravesical oxybutynin chloride: experience with 42 patients. Urology 1993; 41:527–530.

45. Frohlich G, Burmeister S, Wiedeman A, Bulitta M. Intravesical instillation of trospium chloride, oxybutynin and verapamil for relaxation of the bladder detrusor muscle. A placebo controlled, randomized clinical test. Arzneimittelforschung 1998; 48:486–491.

46. Prasad KV, Vaidyanathan S. Intravesical oxybutynin chloride and clean intermittent catheterisation in patients with neurogenic vesical dysfunction and decreased bladder capacity. Br J Urol 1993; 72:519–522.

47. Mizunaga M, Miyata M, Kaneko S, et al. Intravesical instillation of oxybutynin hydrochloride therapy for patients with a neurogenic bladder. Paraplegia 1994; 32:25–29.

48. Palmer LS, Zebold K, Firlit CF, Kaplan WE. Complications of intravesical oxybutynin chloride therapy in the pediatric myelomeningocele population. J Urol 1997; 157:638–640.

49. Lose G, Norgaad JP. Intravesical oxybutynin for treating incontinence resulting from an overactive detrusor. BJU Int 2001; 87:767–771.

50. Buyse G, Verpoorten C, Vereecken R, Casaer P. Treatment of neurogenic bladder dysfunction in infants and children with neurospinal dysraphism with clean intermittent (self)-catheterisation and optimized intravesical oxybutynin hydrochloride therapy. Eur J Pediatr Surg 1995; 5(suppl 1):31–34.

51. Saito M, Tabuchi F, Otsubo K, Miyagawa I. Treatment of overactive bladder with modified intravesical oxybutynin chloride. Neurourol Urodyn 2000; 19:683–688.

52. Dmochowski RR A, Appell RA. Advancements in pharmacologic management of the overactive bladder. Urology 2000; 1(suppl):41–49.

53. Gurpinar T, Truong LD, Wong HY, Griffith DP. Electromotive drug administration to the urinary bladder: an animal model and preliminary results. J Urol 1996; 156:1496–1501.

54. Di Satsi SM, Giannantoni A, Massoud R, et al. Electromotive administration of oxybutynin into the human bladder wall. J Urol 1997; 158:228–233.

55. Riedl CR, Knoll M, Plas E, Pfluger H. Intravesical electromotive administration technique: preliminary results and side effects. J Urol 1998; 159:1851–1856.

56. Di Stasi SM, Giannantoni A, Vespasiani G, et al. Intravesical electromotive administration of oxybutynin in patients with detrusor hyperreflexia unresponsive to standard anticholinergics regimens. J Urol 2001; 165:491–498.

57. Mattiasson A, Ekstrom B, Andersson KE. Effects of intravesical instillation of verapamil in patients with detrusor hyperactivity. J Urol 1989; 141:174–177.

46

Transdermal oxybutynin administration

G Willy Davila

Introduction

Overactive bladder (OAB) is a chronic condition characterized by symptoms of urinary urgency, frequency, and nocturia, with or without urge incontinence, caused by involuntary contractions of the detrusor smooth muscle during bladder filling. It it estimated to affect approximately 34 million individuals in the United States, mostly women, and can have a markedly negative impact on quality of life. Long-term therapy for OAB is generally required to maintain symptomatic relief. Bladder training and other nonpharmacologic interventions may be effective in many cases, but lack of patient motivation and poor compliance restrict the long-term effectiveness of these approaches.[1,2] The mainstay of treatment for OAB is therefore pharmacologic therapy with antimuscarinic drugs. Unfortunately, they are limited in their clinical utility because of their propensity to induce dose-limiting side-effects, such as dry mouth, constipation, and sedation, thereby reducing patient compliance.

Oxybutynin, the primary antimuscarinic drug used to treat the symptoms of OAB, has been available for oral administration for more than 25 years. Although other drugs have now reached the market, oxybutynin remains a favorable treatment option.

The mechanism of action of oxybutynin, a cholinergic muscarinic receptor antagonist, is to competitively inhibit the binding of acetylcholine at postganglionic cholinergic receptor sites in the bladder smooth muscle. Oxybutynin also independently relaxes bladder smooth muscle and has local anesthetic properties.[3] Following oral administration, oxybutynin is extensively metabolized to the active compound N-desethyloxybutynin (N-DEO). N-DEO plasma levels have been associated with anticholinergic side-effects. With the development of a controlled-release oral formulation, and now with transdermal delivery, metabolism is reduced, efficacy is maintained, and side-effects are decreased. The contributions of the parent compound to efficacy and the metabolite to anticholinergic side-effects are becoming increasingly clear as more clinical experience is gained with improved delivery systems. The therapeutic effectiveness of oxybutynin is dose-related and occurs in conjunction with improvement in urodynamic parameters. Oxybutynin reduces the number of impulses reaching the detrusor muscle, thereby delaying the initial desire to void and increasing bladder capacity.[4]

As higher oral doses of oxybutynin are administered to achieve efficacy, dry mouth becomes more pronounced; therefore, alternative routes of administration have been tried. Intravesical therapy was found to alter the pharmacokinetic properties – a significantly lower concentration of the primary metabolite, N-DEO, reaches the systemic circulation, resulting in fewer anticholinergic side-effects.[5] Instillation of oxybutynin directly into the bladder is clinically effective and in most cases causes minimal or no dry mouth.[6] Because this route of administration is impractical, it is currently used only in special clinical circumstances.[7]

Recently, an oxybutynin transdermal delivery system (Oxytrol™, Watson Pharmaceuticals, Inc., Salt Lake City, Utah)[8] has been shown to provide continuous delivery of oxybutynin over 96 h, by way of a matrix-type delivery system applied to the patient's skin. This route of administration alters the pharmacokinetic profile of oxybutynin, thereby minimizing anticholinergic side-effects without compromising clinical efficacy.[9]

Transdermal drug delivery

Background

Transdermal drug administration for the pharmacologic treatment of systemic conditions has the known advantage of avoidance of presystemic gastrointestinal and hepatic 'first-pass' metabolism, which allows administration of lower doses to achieve similar plasma concentrations. Other advantages include avoidance of gastrointestinal interactions, consistent drug release over a prolonged period of time, ease of patient compliance, and utility when oral or parenteral drug administration is not ideal.

Transdermal application systems are currently in use for the treatment of angina pectoris, chronic pain syndromes, and motion sickness; to provide hormone replacement therapy and contraception; and for assistance with smoking cessation.

Transdermal systems (TDSs) vary in the technology used for delivering drugs across the stratum corneum (first layer of skin) and in their dosing frequencies. For example, the first marketed transdermal delivery system employed both a drug reservoir and rate-controlling semipermeable membrane and required daily dosing. Subsequently, hormone replacement therapy with estradiol has been administered for 3½ to 7 days using a matrix-type TDS to women with symptoms associated with menopause.

Transdermal drug therapy for the overactive bladder

The currently available oxybutynin TDS is a matrix-type system requiring twice-weekly dosing. It is composed of three layers (Figure 46.1), as follows:

- The first layer is a backing film that provides the occlusion required for drug absorption.
- The second layer is the basis of the matrix technology and contains:

    a thin film of acrylic adhesive, which enables the system to attach to the skin
    oxybutynin dissolved in an acrylic adhesive
    glycerol triacetate (triacetin, USP), a nonalcoholic permeation enhancer that improves the ability of the drug to penetrate the skin.

- The third layer is a release liner that is peeled off for application.

The design of the matrix-type delivery system allows a controlled rate of drug absorption by means of a chemical method of enhancing skin permeation. Flux enhancers, or chemical penetration enhancers, improve permeation of the drug through the dermal layer, thereby allowing for diffusion into the systemic circulation.[10]

Pharmacokinetic advantage

The oxybutynin TDS has a significant pharmacokinetic advantage over oral oxybutynin, as it avoids presystemic metabolism of the parent compound. Presystemic metabolism refers to the metabolism of the parent compound, prior to entering the systemic circulation, by the CYP450 enzyme system in the gastrointestinal tract and liver following oral administration. With transdermal oxybutynin administration, the avoidance of presystemic metabolism lowers the extent to which the primary metabolite, N-DEO, becomes available to the systemic circulation, thus resulting in fewer anticholinergic side-effects, such as dry mouth, constipation, and drowsiness.

Steady and predictable diffusion of oxybutynin across the stratum corneum has been demonstrated.[9] In studies of human subjects, it has been shown that a 39 cm^2 TDS containing 36 mg of drug will deliver an average dose of 3.9 mg/day and result in average plasma concentrations of oxybutynin of about 4 ng/ml during twice-weekly application (Figure 46.2). In human subjects, the application of oxybutynin TDS to three distinct skin sites – the buttock, hip, and abdomen – showed the same absorption profile.[11]

Bioavailability studies in human subjects showed that after the application of the first oxybutynin TDS, the parent compound becomes available to target tissues within 2 h, peaks at about 24 h, and is sustained at a steady

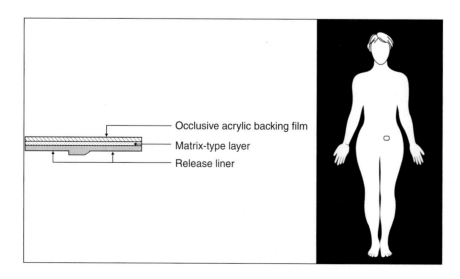

Occlusive acrylic backing film
Matrix-type layer
Release liner

Figure 46.1
A cross section of the matrix-type oxybutynin TDS (transdermal system). Placement of the oxybutynin TDS on the lower abdominal skin region.

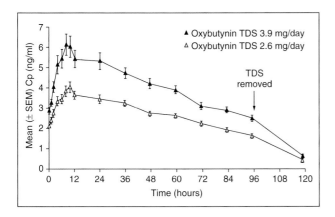

Figure 46.2
Plasma concentrations (Cp) were measured (SEM = standard error of the mean) following the subject's third application. The oxybutynin TDS (transdermal system) was removed after 96 hours.

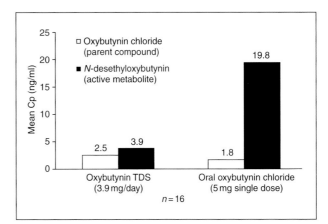

Figure 46.3
Mean plasma concentrations (Cp) were measured after a single 96-hour application of oxybutynin TDS 3.9 mg/day and a single 5 mg oral dose of oxybutynin chloride in 16 healthy subjects.

level for over 96 h. Steady-state concentrations are reached with the second application.[9]

In patients with OAB, plasma concentrations showed a linear relationship between the dose of oxybutynin TDS and plasma concentrations of both the parent compound, oxybutynin, and the active metabolite, N-DEO. This occurred from the lower (1.3 mg/day) to the upper (5.2 mg/day) dose studied.[12]

To show the alteration in first-pass hepatic and gastrointestinal metabolism of the parent oxybutynin compound during transdermal delivery, 16 human subjects participated in a study in which the plasma concentrations of the active metabolite and parent compound were measured following both oral and transdermal drug administration.[13] In the oral oxybutynin group, the average plasma concentration for N-DEO was 19.8 ng/ml and for the parent compound was 1.8 ng/ml, a ratio of approximately 10:1. In the oxybutynin TDS group, average plasma concentrations for N-DEO, the active metabolite, and the parent compound were 3.9 and 2.5 ng/ml, respectively, a ratio of approximately 1.2:1, showing the contrast of transdermally to orally administered oxybutynin in pharmacokinetic properties (Figure 46.3).

Clinical efficacy in the overactive bladder

The efficacy of oxybutynin TDS in the treatment of OAB was demonstrated in two clinical trials. The pivotal trial enrolled 520 patients and consisted of a 12-week, double-blind, placebo-controlled initial phase in which three doses of oxybutynin TDS (1.3, 2.6, and 3.9 mg/day) were compared with placebo. For patients receiving oxybutynin

TDS 3.9 mg/day, the median number of episodes of urinary incontinence decreased from 31 per week at baseline to 12 per week at end point (Figure 46.4), showing significance ($p = 0.017$) in the end-point change from baseline comparison to placebo (-19 vs -14.5, respectively). A supportive efficacy end point, the mean daily urinary frequency, decreased by 2.3 urinations per day from a baseline of 12 and was significant ($p = 0.046$) in comparison to placebo (-2.3 vs -1.7, respectively). In addition, the measured urinary voided volume increased significantly and quality of life scores improved in the group receiving oxybutynin TDS 3.9 mg/day.[14] Patients in all TDS treatment groups then entered a 12-week, open-label, dose-titration period and again experienced reductions in the number of urinary incontinence episodes per week.

In an earlier 6-week, dose-identification trial, 76 patients who had previously responded to treatment with oral oxybutynin were randomized to active treatment with either TDS or oral immediate-release oxybutynin. Dosages were titrated for each group, according to anticholinergic side-effects at weeks 2 and 4. Mean daily incontinence episodes were reduced from washout to end of treatment by approximately 5 in both groups ($p < 0.0001$), with no significant difference between transdermal and oral therapy (Figure 46.5). After 6 weeks of treatment, daily incontinence episodes were reduced to 2.4 ± 2.4 in the transdermal group and 2.6 ± 3.3 in the oral group.[12] A total of 8 patients in the TDS group and 10 patients in the oral group were continent on completion of the study.

Cystometry was performed before and at the end of treatment (Figure 46.6). Bladder volume (mean $\pm$ SD) at first detrusor contraction increased by 66 ± 126 ml for the transdermal group ($p = 0.005$) and 45 ± 163 ml in the oral group ($p = 0.1428$). Maximum bladder capacity

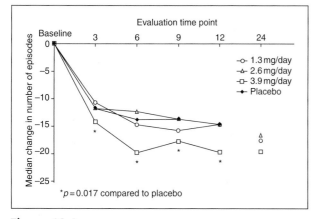

Figure 46.4
Patients taking oxybutynin TDS 3.9 mg/day had a significant decrease in the number of urinary incontinence episodes per week from baseline (BL) to end point.

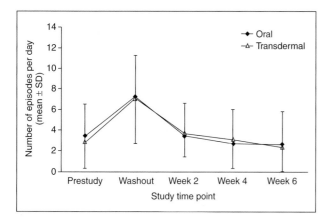

Figure 46.5
Incontinence episodes (mean ± SD) in 72 patients receiving titrated doses of both oral and transdermal oxybutynin during 6 weeks of treatment.

(mean ± SD) increased 53 ± 8 and 51 ± 138 ml in the transdermal (*p* = 0.0011) and the oral (*p* = 0.0538) groups, respectively.[12]

Side-effect profile

The improved anticholinergic side-effect profile of oxybutynin TDS over oral oxybutynin is the most important clinical consequence of this novel route of oxybutynin administration.

In the pivotal trial of 520 patients who received either TDS oxybutynin in doses of 1.3 mg/day, 2.6 mg/day, or 3.9 mg/day, or placebo, the overall frequency of dry mouth was 7.0% for the oxybutynin TDS group and 8.3% for

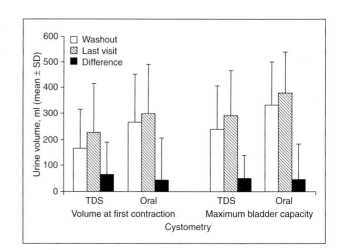

Figure 46.6
Bladder volume at first contraction and maximum bladder capacity in patients receiving TDS (*n* = 33) and oral (*n* = 30) oxybutynin in patients at washout and after 6 weeks of treatment. Patients received titrated doses of oxybutynin between time points.

placebo. Constipation, which can be especially troublesome in older patients, occurred in only 3% of subjects receiving either TDS oxybutynin or placebo. The incidence of dizziness and somnolence was similar to that of the placebo group.[14] The most common adverse event of TDS oxybutynin is a skin reaction at the application site – generally pruritus (16.8%) or erythema (5.6%). In all clinical trials for patients treated with the largest available patch, 3.9 mg/day of TDS oxybutynin (*n* = 331), application site reaction occurred in 14.8% of patients and was mostly mild or moderate in severity and completely reversible.[14]

A review of published clinical trial reports, such as the OBJECT study, shows the incidence of anticholinergic side-effects for oral oxybutynin formulations to be higher than reported in the TDS oxybutynin pivotal clinical trial (Table 46.1).

Dose escalation and occurrence of dry mouth

The first clinical trial of oxybutynin TDS (*n* = 76) was designed to determine the dose limitation in patients with OAB, based on tolerability of anticholinergic side-effects in two parallel groups taking either oral or TDS oxybutynin. Patients entered the trial based on their pre-study dose of oral oxybutynin at one of three TDS dose levels – 2.6, 3.9, or 5.2 mg/day – and had their dose increased every 2 weeks to the maximum of 5.2 mg/day, according to their tolerance of dry mouth. At the 6-week study visit, 68% of the patients receiving oxybutynin TDS had titrated to the maximal dose of 5.2 mg/day compared with 32% of

Table 46.1 *Incidence of dry mouth for orally administered anticholinergic drugs*

Published clinical trials	OXY (%)	OXY er (%)	TOL (%)	OXY TDS (%)	PLA (%)
Appell et al:[15] 　OXY er, 10 mg/d 　TOL, 2 mg bid		28.1	33.2		
Davila et al:[12] 　OXY TDS, 2.6–5.2 mg od 　OXY, 10–20 mg od	94[b]			38[b]	
Dmochowski et al:[14] 　OXY TDS, 3.9 mg od 　PLA				9.6	8.3
Tapp et al:[16] 　OXY, 5 mg qid 　PLA	29				10
Thuroff et al:[17] 　OXY, 5 mg tid 　PLA	48				12
Birns et al:[18] 　OXY, 5 mg bid 　OXY er, 10 mg od	16.7	22.6			
Versi et al:[19] 　OXY, 5–20 mg[a] 　OXY er, 5–20 mg[a]	7 (5 mg) 26 (10 mg) 39 (15 mg) 45 (20 mg)	4 (5 mg) 9 (10 mg) 19 (15 mg) 40 (20 mg)			
Anderson et al:[20] 　OXY, 5 mg od-qid[a] 　OXY er, 5–30 mg, od[a]	87	68			
Burgio et al:[21] 　OXY, 2.5 mg od to 5 mg tid[a]	96.9				

[a] Titrated doses.
[b] At maximum tolerated dose.

OXY, oxybutynin; TOL, tolterodine; TDS, transdermal system; PLA, placebo; er, extended-release formulation; od, daily; bid, twice daily; tid, three times daily; qid, four times daily.

patients taking oral oxybutynin.[12] No patient using the oxybutynin TDS had intolerable dry mouth; 62% did not report any dry mouth; and only 11% had moderate, tolerable dry mouth at the final visit.[12] This low incidence of dry mouth, the major anticholinergic side-effect of oxybutynin, contrasts with incidences of 9% intolerable and 59% moderate but tolerable incidence for oral oxybutynin.

Convenience and quality of life

Patients may exercise, shower, or bathe with the TDS in place. The translucent nature of the oxybutynin TDS improves aesthetic acceptability to the patient. The quality of life (QoL) Incontinence Impact Questionnaire showed a significant improvement ($p < 0.05$) compared with that of placebo (Figure 46.7).

Discussion

Transdermal delivery is a novel approach for the administration of oxybutynin to patients with OAB. Although oxybutynin has a long-established history of efficacy in reducing the number of episodes of urge incontinence, a large percentage of patients discontinue oral oxybutynin because of intolerable anticholinergic side-effects, dry mouth in particular. Because side-effects are dose-related, it has not been possible for most patients to tolerate higher,

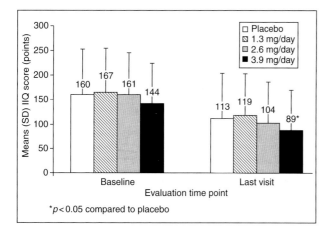

Figure 46.7
Patients with oxybutynin TDS reported improved quality of life on the Incontinence Impact Questionnaire (IIQ) during the double-blind treatment period. Numerical values are in inverse relation to quality of life.

more therapeutically effective doses. The TDS was developed to minimize anticholinergic side-effects by modifying the metabolism and plasma concentration profile of oxybutynin.

By avoiding presystemic gastrointestinal and hepatic metabolism, transdermal delivery of oxybutynin reduces the incidence of anticholinergic side-effects, specifically dry mouth, while maintaining its efficacy in controlling the symptoms of OAB. The incidence of dry mouth is dose-related and reported to be 7.0% overall for oxybutynin TDS and similar to placebo (8.3%).

In conclusion, the pharmacokinetic changes that result from transdermal administration of oxybutynin make it possible to achieve higher plasma levels of oxybutynin with much lower dosing compared to oral administration. Dosing of oxybutynin can thus be optimized without intolerable anticholinergic side-effects. The TDS offers a convenient, efficacious, and well-tolerated route of administering oxybutynin to patients with symptoms of OAB.

References

1. Frewen W. Role of bladder training in the treatment of the unstable bladder in the female. Urol Clin N Am 1979; 6:273–277.

2. Oldenburg B, Millard RJ. Predictors of long term outcome following a bladder re-training programme. J Psychosom Res 1986; 30:691–698.

3. Rovner ES, Wein AJ. Modern pharmacotherapy of urge urinary incontinence in the USA: tolterodine and oxybutynin. BJU Int 2000; 86:44–54.

4. United States Pharmacopeial Convention. Oxybutynin: systemic. In: United States Pharmacopeial Convention, ed. Drug information for the health care professional. Englewood, CO: Micromedex, 2001:2300–2302.

5. Buyse G, Waldeck K, Verpoorten C, et al. Intravesical oxybutynin for neurogenic bladder dysfunction: less systemic side effects due to reduced first pass metabolism. J Urol 1998; 160:892–896.

6. Dmochowski RR, Appell RA. Advancements in pharmacologic management of the overactive bladder. Urology 2000; 56:41–49.

7. Madersbacher H, Jilg G. Control of detrusor hyperreflexia by the intravesical instillation of oxybutynin hydrochloride. Paraplegia 1991; 29:84–90.

8. Watson Pharmaceuticals I. Data on File, Oxytrol™ NDA 21-351. 2001.

9. Zobrist RH, Thomas H, Sanders SW. Pharmacokinetics and metabolism of transdermally administered oxybutynin. Clin Pharmacol Ther 2002:P94. [Abstract]

10. Ranade VV. Drug delivery systems: 6. Transdermal drug delivery. J Clin Pharmacol 1991; 31:401–418.

11. Sanders SW, Thomas H, Zobrist RH. Population pharmacokinetics of transdermally administered oxybutynin. Clin Pharmacol Ther 2002:P34. [Abstract]

12. Davila GW, Daugherty CA, Sanders SW. A short-term, multicenter, randomized double-blind dose titration study of the efficacy and anticholinergic side effects of transdermal compared to immediate release oral oxybutynin treatment of patients with urge urinary incontinence. J Urol 2001; 166:140–145.

13. Zobrist RH, Schmid B, Feick A, et al. Pharmacokinetics of the R- and S-enantiomers of oxybutynin and N-desethyloxybutynin following oral and transdermal administration of the racemate in health volunteers. Pharm Res 2001; 18:1029–1034.

14. Dmochowski RR, Davila GW, Zinner NR, et al. Efficacy and safety of transdermal oxybutynin in patients with urge and mixed urinary incontinence. J Urol 2002; 168:580–586.

15. Appell RA, Sand P, Dmochowski R, et al. Prospective randomized controlled trial of extended-release oxybutynin chloride and tolterodine tartrate in the treatment of overactive bladder: results of the OBJECT Study. Mayo Clin Proc 2001; 76:358–363.

16. Tapp AJ, Cardozo LD, Versi E, Cooper D. The treatment of detrusor instability in post-menopausal women with oxybutynin chloride: a double blind placebo controlled study. Br J Obstet Gynaecol 1990; 97:521–526.

17. Thuroff JW, Bunke B, Ebner A, et al. Randomized, double-blind, multicenter trial on treatment of frequency, urgency and incontinence related to detrusor hyperactivity: oxybutynin versus propantheline versus placebo. J Urol 1991; 145:813–816.

18. Birns J, Lukkari E, Malone-Lee JG. A randomized controlled trial comparing the efficacy of controlled-release oxybutynin tablets (10 mg once daily) with conventional oxybutynin tablets (5 mg twice daily) in patients whose symptoms were stabilized on 5 mg twice daily of oxybutynin. BJU Int 2000; 85:793–798.

19. Versi E, Appell R, Mobley D, et al. Dry mouth with conventional and controlled-release oxybutynin in urinary incontinence. Obstet Gynecol 2000; 95:718–721.

20. Anderson RU, Mobley D, Blank B, et al. Once daily controlled versus immediate release oxybutynin chloride for urge urinary incontinence. J Urol 1999; 161:1809–1812.

21. Burgio KL, Locher JL, Goode PS, et al. Behavioral vs drug treatment for urge urinary incontinence in older women: a randomized controlled trial. JAMA 1998; 280:1995–2000.

47

Management of autonomic dysreflexia

Waleed Altaweel and Jacques Corcos

Autonomic dysreflexia (AD) is a life-threatening condition, and is considered a medical emergency. It is important for physicians dealing with spinal cord injury (SCI) patients to recognize and to be aware of the signs and symptoms of this syndrome. However, the signs and symptoms of AD might be minimal or absent, despite elevated blood pressure. SCI patients might have difficulty disclosing their symptoms when AD presents due to cognitive and verbal communication impairments. The key to successful management is prevention, through patient and family education, proper bladder, bowel, and skin care, and identification and avoidance of noxious stimuli. Health care providers should be aware of the potential causes of AD or treat it when it occurs.

Acute treatment

Normally, patients with SCI at T6 or above have normal systolic blood pressure of 90–110 mmHg. A sudden 20–40 mmHg increase of both systolic and diastolic blood pressure over baseline that is frequently associated with bradycardia may be a sign of AD.

If blood pressure is elevated, the patient needs to be placed upright in the sitting position. This maneuver pools blood in the lower limbs and might reduce the blood pressure.[1,2]

Tight clothing or any constrictive devices should be loosened to allow the blood to pool in the abdomen and lower extremities.[1,2]

SCI patients usually suffer impaired autonomic regulations. During AD, the blood pressure has the potential to fluctuate; therefore it should be monitored frequently (every 5 min) until the patient has stabilized.[1–6]

Triggering factors should be removed; the most common cause of AD is **bladder distention**:

- If an indwelling catheter is not in place, catheterize the patient.[3,7–10] Since catheterization can exacerbate AD, use intraurethral lidocaine (lignocaine) jelly and wait for 2 min to decrease sensory input and to relax the sphincter (Table 47.1).

- If the patient has a Foley catheter, check for obstruction or kinks.
- If the catheter is blocked, try to irrigate with 10–15 ml of warm saline; the use of a large volume or of a cold solution can exacerbate the autonomic dysreflexia. Avoid bladder distention and suprapubic percussion because it can worsen the condition. If this fails to decompress the bladder, change the catheter with lidocaine jelly.
- During bladder decompression, monitor the patient's blood pressure because sudden decompression will normalize it. However, hypotension might occur, especially if the patient has been given antihypertensive medication.
- If blood pressure elevation persists, then suspect **fecal impaction**. It is the second most common cause of AD.[3,7]
- Appropriate precaution should be taken before disimpaction, since additional stimulation could further aggravate AD.[11–13] Use intrarectal lidocaine jelly and wait 2 min before checking for the presence of stool.
- If present, gently disimpact it. If AD worsens, stop the manual evacuation and recheck after 20 min. However, if blood pressure is above 150 mmHg, consider **pharmacological management** before disimpaction:

1. Nifedipine or nitrates are the most commonly used medications during acute attack.[14–16] Nifedipine 10 mg, bitten and swallowed in the immediate-release form, is the preferred method of administration; treatment can be repeated in 30 min. Extreme caution should be exercised in the elderly or in patients with coronary artery disease, as it has been reported that nifedipine can cause hypotension and reflex tachycardia in individuals without SCI.[17]

2. Phenoxybenzamine, 10 mg orally, an alpha-receptor blocker, can be given to treat acute AD. It has been shown that phenoxybenzamine causes relaxation of the internal sphincter and controls the symptoms.[18,19]

3. Glyceryl trinitrate 300–600 μg S/L can be administered in appropriately monitored settings for rapid blood pressure control. It can be repeated

Table 47.1 *Practical acute management of AD*

1.	If an indwelling urinary catheter is not in place, catheterize the patient
2.	If an indwelling urinary catheter is already in place, check the system along its entire length for position, kinks, folds, constrictions, or obstructions
3.	If the catheter appears to be blocked, gently irrigate the bladder with a small amount of fluid, such as normal saline, at body temperature. Avoid manually compressing or tapping on the bladder
4.	If the catheter is draining and the blood pressure remains elevated, suspect fecal impaction; check the rectum for stool, using intrarectal lidocaine jelly as lubricant
5.	If the situation is not corrected, administer an antihypertensive agent with rapid onset and short duration while the causes of AD are being investigated: • nifedipine 10 mg to be repeated every 30 min if necessary. It should be in the immediate-release form; bite-and-swallow is the preferred method, *not* sublingual treatment • nitrates (e.g. glyceryl trinitrate). To be avoided the patient took sildenafil in the past 24 hours • phenoxybenzamine 10 mg orally • captopril 25 mg orally
6.	Use antihypertensives with extreme caution in older persons or people with coronary artery disease
7.	Monitor the individual's symptoms and blood pressure for at least 2 hours after resolution of the AD episode to ensure that blood pressure elevation does not reoccur. AD may resolve because of medication, not because of resolution of the underlying cause
8.	If the response to treatment is poor and/or if the cause of the AD has not been identified, admit the patient for close monitoring, maintenance of pharmacological blood pressure control, and investigation of other possible causes

after 10 min. Sildenafil is being increasingly used to treat erectile dysfunction in SCI patients. Nitrates are contraindicated in patients taking sildenafil. The resulting blood pressure decrease may be huge and dangerous. If sildenafil is used within the last 24 h, another short-acting antihypertensive medication should be given.

4. Captopril 25 mg is an alternative for the management of hypertensive emergencies in AD. It acts within 30 min, achieves levels within 1–3 h and, has a half-life of 2–4 h. A pilot study has shown that it is safe and effective in treating patients with hypertension from AD.[20]

• Blood pressure should be monitored for symptomatic hypotension. If present, the patient should lie down and elevate his legs. If not controlled, then consider intravenous fluids and adrenergic agonist. If the precipitating cause has still not been determined, check for the least-frequent cause.

capable of preventing an AD attack if given shortly before stimulation (Table 47.2).[21] In patients with recurrent attacks, terazosin results in complete suppression of dysreflexic symptoms; a nightly dose of 5 mg reduces the severity, but does not eliminate the need for careful monitoring during provocative procedures.[22]

Anesthetic techniques for controlling AD include topical application for cystoscopy, general anesthesia, and spinal and epidural anesthesia. Lidocaine jelly decreases the sensation and relaxes the sphincter during cystoscopy, but bladder distention may trigger an AD episode despite local anesthesia. In one case report AD occurred despite general anesthesia.[23] Studies have shown that halothane anesthesia is more effective than other agents.[24–26] Spinal anesthesia has been reported to give excellent control,[9] and has been recommended to manage acute AD refractory to medical management.[27] Preoperative evaluation should include determination of the level of injury and history of dysreflexic episodes. Intraoperative and postoperative cardiac monitoring is recommended.[28–30]

Prophylactic treatment of autonomic dysreflexia and anesthetic considerations

Surgical, cystoscopic, urodynamic, and radiological procedures might precipitate acute AD. Nifedipine 10 mg is

Autonomic dysreflexia treatment during pregnancy and labor

Spinal cord injury patients should be monitored for urinary tract infections, fecal impaction, and blood

Table 47.2 *Preventive measures against autonomic dysreflexia*

- Frequent pressure relief in bed/chair

- Avoidance of sunburn/scalds

- Maintenance of regular bowel program

- A well-balanced diet and adequate fluid intake

- Compliance with medications

- For patients with an indwelling catheter:
  - keep the tubing free of kinks
  - keep the drainage bags empty
  - check daily for deposits inside the catheter

- If patients are on an intermittent catheterization program, they should catheterize themselves as often as necessary to prevent overfilling

- If patients void spontaneously, make sure that they have an adequate output

- Patients should carry an intermittent catheter kit when they are away from home

- In all cases: perform routine skin assessments

- Inform the health care staff if you tend to develop AD

- Carry Adalat (nifedipine) 10 mg; give 10 mg orally 30 min before stimulation

pressure during both gestation and labor. AD during pregnancy has the same pathophysiology and management. In addition, before vaginal examinations, urinary catheterizations, or rectal manipulation, use an anesthetic jelly to reduce stimulation. Bladder catheter drainage should be initiated and monitored frequently to avoid obstruction during labor.[31] It has also been proposed that monitoring during labor and delivery should ideally include:

1. an intra-arterial catheter for continuous blood pressure reading
2. telemetry for cardiac rhythm monitoring continuously
3. constant electronic fetal monitoring to identify fetal distress.[32]

A complete anesthesia consultation should be undertaken prior to labor. Epidural anesthesia with a combination of morphine, with bupivacaine,[33] or meperidine alone[34] has been reported in cases of successful deliveries in women with spinal cord lesions. Oral nifedipine, intravenous hydralazine, or trimethaphan has been recommended to control extremely high blood pressures in this population during labor.[33] Intravenous nitroprusside is not recommended because of elevated fetal cyanide levels.[35] Ganglionic-blocking agents with a short duration of action, such as a 0.1% solution of trimethaphan in 5% dextrose by intravenous drip, can be administered in refractory AD cases during labor that are not adequately controlled by regional anesthesia.[35]

Autonomic dysreflexia is a common complication of pregnancy SCI or patients. Prevention remains the most important factor in AD management to avoid morbidity and mortality in patients or their fetus. Patient and health worker should understand the pathophysiology, and causes and management of this syndrome to avoid serious complications.

Conclusion

Autonomic dysreflexia is an emergency often secondary to urological or gynecological problems or manipulations. Its management starts primarily with its prevention. Easy measures can avoid this highly risky event. Facing such events, physicians must be aware of simple procedures and the possible cascade of treatment that could be administered. Pregnancy and anesthesia have to be considered as precipitating factors supporting preventive and aggressive management.

References

1. Cole TM, Kotte FJ, Olsen M, et al. Alterations of cardiovascular control in high spinal myelomalacia. Arch Phys Med Rehab 1967; 48:359–368.

2. Guttman L, Frankel HL, Paeslack V. Cardiac irregularies during labor in paraplegic women. Paraplegia 1965; 66:144.

3. Colachis SC. Autonomic hyperreflexia in spinal cord injury. J Am Parapleg 1992; 15:171.

4. Erickson RP. Autonomic hyperreflexia, pathophysiology and medical management. Arch Phys Med Rehab 1980; 61:431.

5. Kewalramani LS. Autonomic dysreflexia in traumatic myelopathy. Am J Phys Med 1980; 59:1.

6. Kuric J, Hixon AK. Clinical practice guideline: autonomic dysreflexia. Jackson Height, NY: Eastern Paralyzed Veterans Association, 1996.

7. Lee BY, Karmakar MG, Herz BL, et al. Autonomic dysreflexia revisited. J Spinal Cord Med 1995; 18:75. [Review]

8. Lindun R, Joiner E, Frechafer AA, et al. Incidence and clinical features of autonomic dysreflexia in patients with spinal cord injury. Paraplegia 1980; 18:285.

9. Trop CS, Bennett CJ. Autonomic dysreflexia and its urological implications. J Urol 1992; 146:1461. [Review]

10. Wurster RD, Randall WC. Cardiovascular response to bladder distension in patients with spinal transection. Am J Physiol 1975; 228:1288.

11. O'Donnell WF. Urological management in the patient with acute spinal cord injury. Crit Care Clin 1987; 3:599.

12. Silver JR. Vascular reflexes in spinal shock. Paraplegia 1971; 8:231.

13. Muzumdar AS. The mass reflex; an emergency in the quadriplegic patient. Can Med Ass J 1982; 126:376.

14. Braddom RL, Rocco JF. Autonomic dysreflexia: a survey of current treatment. Am J Phys Med Rehab 1991; 70:234.

15. Dyskstra DD, Sidi AA, Anderson LC. The effect of nifedipine on cystoscopy induced autonomic dysreflexia in patients with high spinal cord injuries. J Urol 1987; 138:1115.

16. Thyberg M, Ertzgaard PE, Gylling M, et al. Effect of nifedipine on cystometry, induced elevation of bladder pressure in patients with reflex urinary bladder after a high level spinal cord injury. Paraplegia 1994; 32:308.

17. Grossman E, Messerli FH, Grodzicki T, Kowey P. Should a moratorium be placed on sublingual nifedipine capsules given for hypertensive emergencies and pseudo-emergencies?. JAMA 1996; 276:1328–1331.

18. Scott MB, Marrow JW. Phenoxybenzamine in neurogenic bladder dysfunction after spinal cord injury. Autonomic dysreflexia. J Urol 1978; 119:483.

19. McGuire J, Wagner FM, Weiss RM. Treatment of autonomic dysreflexia with phenoxybenzamine. J Urol 1976; 115:53.

20. Esmail Z, Shalansky K, Sunderji R, et al. Evaluation of captopril for the management of hypertension in autonomic dysreflexia. Pilot study. Arch Phys Med Rehab 2002; 38:604.

21. Lindan R, Lettler EJ, Kedia KR. A comparison of the efficacy of alpha adrenergic blocker and slow calcium channel blocker in autonomic dysreflexia. Paraplegia 1985; 23:34.

22. Viadyanathan S, Soni BM, Sett P, et al. Pathophysiology of autonomic dysreflexia: long-term treatment with terazosin in adult and pediatric spinal cord injury patients manifesting recurrent dysreflexic episodes. Spinal Cord 1998; 36:761.

23. Raeder JC, Gisvold SE. Perioperative autonomic hyperreflexia in high spinal cord lesions: a case report. Case report. Acta Anast Scand 1986; 30:672–673.

24. Ciliberti BJ, Goldfein J, Rovenstine EA. Hypertension during anesthesia in patients with spinal cord injures. Anesthesiology 1954; 15:273–279.

25. Alderson JD, Thomas DG. The use of halothane anesthesia to control autonomic hyperreflexia during transurethral surgery in spinal cord injury patient. Paraplegia 1975; 13:183.

26. Drinker AS, Helrich M. Halothane anesthesia in paraplegic patients. Anesthesiology 1963; 24:399.

27. Nieder RM, O'Higgins JW, Aldrete JA. Autonomic hyperreflexia in urologic surgery. JAMA 1970; 213:867–869.

28. Deasmon J. Paraplegia: problem confronting the anaesthesiologist. Cnad Anesth Soc J 1970; 17:435.

29. Schonwald G, Fish K, Perkash I. Cardiovascular complications during anesthesia in chronic spinal cord injured patients. Anesthesiology 1981; 55:550–558.

30. Fraser A, Edmonds-Seal J. Spinal cord injuries. A review of the problems facing the anesthetist. Anesthesia 1982; 37:1084–1098.

31. Greenspoon JS, Paul RH. Paraplegia and quadriplegia. Special consideration during pregnancy and labor and delivery. Am J Obstet Gynecol 1986; 155:738–741.

32. Gross LL, et al. Pregnancy, labour, delivery and post spinal cord injury. Paraplegia 1992; 30:890.

33. Crosby E, St. Jean B, Reid D, Elliott RD. Obstetrical anesthesia and analgesia in achronic spinal cord-injured women. Can J Anasth 1992; 36:487–494.

34. Baraka A. Epidural meperidine for control of autonomic hyperreflexia in a paraplegic paturient. Anesthesiology 1985; 62:688–690.

35. Tabsh K, Crinkman C, Reff R. Autonomic dysreflexia in pregnancy. Obstet Gynecol 1982; 60:119.

48

Peripheral electrical stimulation

Magnus Fall and Sivert Lindström

General background

Important prerequisites for continence are intactness of the vesicourethral supportive structures and of the smooth and the striated muscles of the urethra, the latter being composed of the intramural striated sphincter and the paraurethral components of the pelvic floor muscles. Most striated muscles of the body are composed of three motor unit types, one with slowly contracting muscle fibers and two with fast contraction properties.[1] The intramural urethral sphincter is special in being composed of slow fibers only, whereas the paraurethral striated muscles have varying numbers of all three types. The three motor unit types differ with respect to their maximal force development, fusion frequency – that is the activation frequency for a smooth sustained contraction – and resistance to fatigue. The slow units develop little force but are resistant to fatigue. Their fusion frequency is about 10 Hz. The fastest units can produce 10–20 times more contraction force but fatigue rapidly. Their fusion frequency is around 40–50 Hz. The intermediate fast units are somewhat weaker but considerably more fatigue-resistant. It follows that the intramural striated sphincter can generate a well-sustained but rather limited increase in urethral pressure. The main function of this muscle seems to be to accomplish urethral closure during bladder filling at rest, when there is little physical stress. In more provocative situations, when the intra-abdominal pressure suddenly increases, e.g. lifting, coughing, and running (when most women with stress urinary incontinence leak), the fast motor units of the paraurethral pelvic floor muscles provide a rapidly induced, strong closing force upon the urethra. This contraction is in fact governed by the central motor program during self-generated increases of the intra-abdominal pressure, thereby allowing these muscles to contract in advance of the pressure rise. They are also promptly reflexly engaged by pressure increases from the outside caused by a sudden push towards the abdominal wall, but in this situation the contraction lags behind the pressure increase. The pressures generated by the pelvic floor muscles upon the urethra clearly exceed the maximal detrusor or

intra-abdominal pressures in intact subjects. Thus, there is normally a reliable safety margin.

Bladder filling is detected by mechanoreceptors in the bladder wall. These receptors respond both to passive distention and to active contraction of the detrusor.[2] The afferent signals are transmitted, mainly via the pelvic nerves, to the spinal cord, and ascend bilaterally in the dorsolateral white matter. The information eventually reaches the cerebral cortex in the medial region of its somatosensory area[3,4] and gives rise to the sensation of bladder filling and urgency. The afferent signal also influences neurons in Barrington's micturition center in the upper pons.[5] When appropriately activated, descending neurons in this center drive preganglionic bladder pelvic neurons in the sacral cord, and thereby induce a micturition contraction. Once initiated, the micturition reflex is self-sustained by a positive feedback mechanism. The reflex detrusor contraction generates an increased bladder pressure and an enhanced activation of bladder mechanoreceptors. This afference, in turn, reinforces the activation of the pontine micturition center and the pelvic motor output to the bladder, resulting in a further increase in bladder pressure and mechanoreceptor afference. When urine enters the urethra, the reflex is further enhanced by activation of urethral receptors.[6] Normally, this positive feedback mechanism ascertains a complete emptying of the bladder during micturition. As long as there is any fluid left in the lumen, the intravesical pressure will be maintained above the threshold for the mechanoreceptors, which will provide a continuous drive for the detrusor.

A drawback with this arrangement is that the reflex system may easily become unstable. Any stimulus that elicits a small burst of impulses in mechanoreceptor afferents may trigger a micturition reflex. To prevent this from happening during the filling phase, the micturition reflex pathway is controlled by several inhibitory mechanisms at spinal and supraspinal levels.[7] The micturition reflex has normally an all-or-nothing character. The pelvic efferents to the bladder are silent during the filling phase but, due to the positive feedback system, they fire maximally during micturition contractions.

Activation of continence reflexes by electrical stimulation

Penile,[8] clitoris,[9] and vaginal electrical stimulation[10,11] activates the motor fibers to the pelvic floor and the intramural urethral sphincter, either directly or by reflex mechanisms, or both.[10–13] At these sites of stimulation, further reflexes are evoked with the afferent limb in the pudendal nerve and with three concomitant central actions: activation of hypogastic inhibitory fibers to the bladder; central inhibition of the pelvic outflow to the bladder; and central inhibition of the ascending afferent pathway from the bladder.[4,12,14] This reflex is silent at rest and seems to be designed to prevent bladder contractions during coitus. Anal stimulation[15,16] inhibits the bladder in a similar fashion by a reflex with its afferent limb in pelvic nerve branches to the anal region,[17] a reflex designed to inhibit the bladder during defecation. Thus, perineal methods for electrical stimulation utilize natural reflexes that are silent during normal, everyday life but capable of sustained bladder inhibition when evoked by continuous or intermittent electrical stimulation.

It is generally believed that in the normal situation, bladder inhibition follows pelvic floor contraction and that bladder inhibition elicited by electrical stimulation would result from pelvic floor activation.[14] However, in animal experimental studies it has been demonstrated that there is rather activation of specific inhibitory pudendal afferents. Lindström et al[12] showed that complete relaxation of the pelvic floor by succinylcholine did not abolish the inhibitory effect of stimulation. Subsequently, it has been demonstrated that there are separate systems for bladder and urethral sphincter activation. In patients with so-called uninhibited overactive bladder there was a dissociation of the ability to exhibit bladder inhibition and sphincter activation, respectively, in 21% of patients.[18] In experiments in cats, Blok and Holstege[19] described separate centers for micturition (M-region pontine center) and storage (L-region pontine center). The M region excites bladder muscle through projections to its motoneurons and inhibits the urethral sphincter through γ-aminobutyric acid (GABA) interneurons, which inhibits the sphincter. The L region acts independently and excites the sphincter motoneurons.

The therapeutic effects of functional electrical stimulation (FES), on the bladder as well as the sphincter mechanism, depends on artificial activation of nerves. The first requirement for an effect is that the stimulation intensity is high enough to evoke an activity in the relevant nerves. The threshold intensity varies inversely with the fiber diameter, distance between the nerves and the stimulating electrodes, and the pulse configuration. Large myelinated fibers, like efferents to the pelvic floor, have the lowest threshold. Anogenital cutaneous afferents involved in bladder inhibition and pelvic floor muscle reflexes (bulbocavernosus reflex) have intermediate values, whereas afferents responsible for pain sensation have the highest. In practice the distance between electrode and nerve fiber is more important. Thus, all external electrodes induce skin or mucosal sensations at much lower intensities than pelvic floor contractions by direct stimulation of the motor fibers. For the same reason, the difference between the detection threshold and the pain effects is quite narrow, with the maximal tolerance level reached at intensities about 1.5–2 times the detection threshold.[20] From experimental studies it is clear that the tolerance level is well below that required for maximal bladder inhibition or pelvic floor contraction. It follows that proper electrode design that permits positioning of the electrodes close to the relevant nerves is mandatory to achieve good clinical effects.

Any pulse configuration would do for nerve activation, provided the stimulators can generate high enough intensities (in mA or V). Short square-wave pulses (0.2–0.5 ms) are most effective, however, in terms of charge transfer for a given biological effect.[28,29] To minimize electrochemical reactions at the electrode–mucosa interphase, it is preferable to use biphasic or polarity alternating pulses.

Stimulation frequency is another crucial factor. Due to the contractile properties of the fast and slow motor units, a high stimulation frequency, 50–100 Hz is required for maximal urethral closure. The bladder inhibitory reflex systems operate at much lower frequencies. Maximal inhibition via the sympathetic route is obtained at about 5 Hz, and 5–10 Hz is also the best frequency for central inhibition of the pelvic outflow to the bladder. Since the lower frequency may be unpleasant, 10 Hz stimulation has been recommended as a practical compromise. In clinical experiments in women with detrusor overactivity, cystometric registrations and isobaric volume recordings were performed to document effects during intravaginal electrical stimulation.[21] With these procedures it was easy to demonstrate an abolishment of phasic detrusor contractions and an increase in bladder volume during stimulation, an effect most evident at low-frequency stimulation (10 Hz). Vereecken et al[22] and Vodusek et al[23] observed similar effects but did not see any difference in the degree of bladder inhibition at stimulation frequencies between 5 and 20 Hz. All frequencies in that range do elicit bladder inhibition and it is quite plausible that different clinical conditions, like idiopathic phasic detrusor overactivity vs detrusor overactivity in spinal cord injury, may require somewhat different technique for an optimal response. Detrusor inhibition has likewise been demonstrated by anal[16] or penile surface[8] electrodes. The frequency characteristics are similar for reflexes elicited from anal or genital stimulation. Engagement of larger pudendal nerve branches or selective stimulation of clitoris or penile nerve branches has been found to optimize the effect. It has been suggested that the effect on the bladder can be further improved if the pudendal nerve stimulation is calibrated by electrophysiological monitoring of the 'maximal motor response'.[24]

In trials without drugs, adequate urethral closure was obtained at 20–50 Hz, the lower frequency being a good compromise for patients with mixed stress and urge incontinence. Muscle fatigue is an important problem. When using FES for incontinence, intermittent trains of impulses have been found to reduce this problem.[25,26] Another factor to consider is the long-term effect of chronic stimulation on the pelvic floor muscles. As one effect, it has been proposed that chronic stimulation increases the relative number of slow-twitch fibers in the paraurethral muscles,[27] since it has previously been found for leg muscles that long-lasting slow stimulation may transform intermediate fast motor units to such with mainly slow properties.[28] Slow and intermediate motor units are also recruited first in reflex activation of the motor pool. Intermittent high-frequency stimulation would, if anything, be expected to have the opposite effect, though. To improve urethral closure at sudden increases of the intra-abdominal pressure, stronger fast-twitch fibers would be desirable, not the opposite.

A clinically most significant result of peripheral electrical stimulation is the carry-over or re-education effect: in some patients there is long-term remission of symptoms after repeated electrical stimulation,[10,29–31] sometimes lasting for years.[32] The physiological basis of this seemingly curative effect of stimulation is not yet fully explained but no doubt involves modulation of central nervous activity. A change of peripheral receptor activity after chronic stimulation has been suggested, too,[33,34] which may contribute to a normalization of micturition pattern. Recently, Jiang,[35] during anogenital electrical stimulation in the rat, demonstrated that 5 min stimulation at 10 Hz induced a prolonged increase in the micturition threshold volume, which was maintained for 40 min, presumably involving modulation of synaptic transmission in the central micturition pathway. When intravesical electrical stimulation (IVES) was used, the opposite result was achieved: i.e. prolonged enhancement of the micturition reflex. In further experiments, the specific antagonist CPPene was used to block central glutaminergic receptors of the NMDA type. The IVES-induced decrease in micturition threshold was blocked by prior administration of CPPene. This finding indicates that the IVES-induced modulation of the micturition reflex is due to an enhanced excitatory synaptic transmission in the central micturition reflex pathway.[36] Similar modulation of the inhibitory, central mechanisms during electrical stimulation at relevant sites seems quite likely. A further plausible mechanism is that continence reflexes, once upgraded by artificial electrical stimulation, will be maintained when micturition is normalized, providing the chance of daily voiding and withholding training sessions.

Table 48.1 *Requirements of a stimulator for clinical use*
Adequate electrode design
Sufficient and adjustable stimulation intensity
Short pulse width (range 0.2–0.5 ms)
Biphasic pulses
Variability of stimulation frequency (range 10–50 Hz), depending on clinical demands
Continuous or intermittent stimulation, depending on clinical demands

A further possibility is that chronic stimulation can improve the central motor programs for activation of the relevant striated muscles, in analogy with the stimulation-induced re-education in urge incontinence. Stimulation may also improve the reinervation of partly denervated muscle fibers by enhancing sprouting of surviving motor axons. Activation in animal experiments has been observed to promote the development of large motor units with many muscle fibers.[37] In line with these observations, Smith et al[38] and Fall, Hjälmås, and Lindehall (unpublished work) observed an improvement of stress incontinence in children and youngsters with myelomeningocele and partly denervated pelvic floor.

It is worth noting that electrical pelvic floor stimulation involves the coordinated bladder and urethral function. When treating bladder overactivity, an effect on the sphincter mechanism may be as significant for the patient. It is not an unusual observation that, during ongoing treatment, the patients may still experience urgency and frequency of urination but have regained control of the sphincter. They can thereby postpone voiding – an effect of utmost importance for their ability to resume normal activities of daily life.

Clinical techniques of electrical stimulation

There are two main options for clinical treatment. *Long-term stimulation* implies chronic stimulation at low intensity and requires several hours of treatment per day during several months. This modality was first used by Caldwell et al,[29] who implanted electrodes into the pelvic floor muscles and connected them to a radiolinked stimulator activated from an outside antenna. It was subsequently found that external electrodes yielded similar good results. Different shapes of vaginal and anal electrodes have been tried on a long-term basis. Advantages of long-term external stimulation are that hospital attention is not required and treatment is cheap and self-controlled by the patient.

A disadvantage is that the procedure demands patient persistence. Many patients also find the different devices uncomfortable to wear for a prolonged period of time. Most patients using this treatment prefer to use the device during sleep at night. Today, because of the slow progress of treatment, most of the devices for long-term treatment have gone out of the market.

A different approach was presented by Godec et al.[39] Using anal plug electrodes and needle electrodes inserted into the levator ani muscle, they applied a 15–20 min continuous train of pulses at high intensity, so-called *acute maximal stimulation*. The applications were repeated up to 10 times in the outpatient clinic. Plevnik and Janez[40] and Kralj[41] used a modified technique with only surface electrodes and obtained a successful result in more than 50% of patients. Acute maximal stimulation may be preferable as treatment in urge incontinence owing to an overactive bladder. High-amplitude stimulation induces a more pronounced bladder inhibition and fewer stimulation sessions are required for a curative effect.[12,24] A limiting factor for maximal stimulation by means of external electrodes is that the effective range up to the maximum tolerable level is rather narrow.[20] A stronger effect may be obtained in selected cases by direct stimulation of the pudendal nerve trunk by means of needle electrodes.[42] A combined approach of clinical and home high-intensity stimulation by means of a personal stimulator (*home maximal stimulation*) now seems to be the most popular alternative.[43]

Up to half of the patients regain permanent control (re-education) of the bladder and/or the urethral sphincters after a period of long-term or a sequence of maximal electrical stimulation.[16,32,40–45] In some patients only a temporary improvement may be achieved, and recurrence of symptoms is encountered after a few weeks or months. In these cases, repeated sessions of treatment usually restore control. However, very frequent periods of treatment or daily stimulation is demanding and not readily accepted by all patients. In such a situation, implantation of a sacral root or pudendal nerve stimulator may be a better solution (see Chapter 50).

The problem of randomized controlled trials and functional electrical stimulation

One problem with FES is the relative lack of randomized controlled studies (RCTs). In clinical practice today no treatment is fully accepted if active treatment is not superior to placebo. FES requires the sensation of stimulation to be effective. It has still not been possible to design a study with a genuine placebo equivalent, i.e. electrical stimulation producing the sensation of stimulation with no other effect in the control arm. A nonfunctioning stimulator as control is too easy for the patient to reveal and thus is not an ideal placebo. In an early trial, this method was tested, but the study was not completed because of dropouts in the group having nonfunctioning stimulation devices.[46] Recently, trials have been presented using this principle,[47,48] and a statistically significant effect on stress urinary incontinence was found during active home maximal stimulation compared to the group wearing a device without stimulation. Yamanishi et al[49] treated patients with detrusor overactivity with 15 min stimulation twice daily for 4 weeks, which is comparably a low quantity of stimulation. Still, subjective improvement in the active arm compared with inactive treatment was accomplished, as well as increase of cystometric capacity. Other reports have been contradictory, such as the one by Luber and Wolde-Tsadik[50] treating patients with genuine stress incontinence twice daily for 3 months with no difference between active and control groups.

Control studies are important to determine the 'real' efficacy of varying FES modalities for different diagnoses. They are also desirable to get acceptance of the methods by health insurance authorities. In the recent report of the International Consultation on Incontinence, electrical stimulation was claimed to have an insufficient evidence base depending on the limited number of positive RCTs. Too much emphasis on RCTs, disregarding extensive experience presented in open studies, may lead to a shortsighted abandonment of further experimentation and development of techniques and includes the risk that a useful and harmless option for treatment of stress incontinence and detrusor overactivity is disregarded. Studies of electrical stimulation also entail other risks and problems. If treatment is applied with suboptimal techique, an effect may be overlooked and researchers may be disencouraged to continue further trials.

Electrical stimulation in various neurogenic lower urinary tract dysfunctions

Established indications are **stress urinary incontinence** caused by pelvic floor insufficiency, the efficacy of FES being similar to that of pelvic floor exercises. It has been demonstrated that female stress incontinence depends not only on a defect of the urethral supporting structures but also on partial damage of the innervation to the pelvic floor muscle complex caused by delivery or other traumatic insults.[51] Up to 75% of patients referred for surgery of their stress incontinence may be sufficiently improved by FES so that an operation becomes unnecessary.[16,32,41] Some patients using pelvic floor exercises have defective perception and cannot recognize the relevant muscles, making training impossible. By means of intravaginal stimulation, muscle identification may be possible, and a combined treatment may reinforce their training. In stress incontinence, long-term stimulation at 20–50 Hz is recommended.

The standard therapy of an **overactive bladder** is anticholinergic drug treatment, however limited in usefulness because of more or less pronounced side-effects owing to general effects on the receptor systems. Functional electrical stimulation circumvents this problem by acting directly on the micturition reflex mechanism. Urge incontinence due to detrusor overactivity (DO) is an ideal indication for electrical stimulation.[40,42,44,45,52] Detrusor overactivity is a typical feature of suprasacral spinal cord lesion as well as supraspinal neuropathy. There is an ongoing debate on the etiology and pathogenesis of detrusor overactivity in patients with so-called idiopathic DO. When making a thorough examination, however, subtle neurologic signs may frequently be revealed, mainly affecting the lower extremities,[53] which indicate that we are dealing with a neurogenic bladder disorder. Another feature of DO relevant for the application of electrical stimulation, is that different functional subtypes may be identified. The **uninhibited overactive bladder** subtype[54] responds fairly well to maximal stimulation at 10 Hz, few other methods being applicable. The results are even better in subjects with **phasic detrusor instability**,[54] many of which attain the unique re-education effect, too. In mixed incontinence, an individual assessment is mandatory. If stress urinary incontinence dominates, surgery is usually preferred, but electrical stimulation at 10–20 Hz may be contemplated as an alternative. When DO dominates, electrical stimulation is the therapy of choice, either as repeated maximal stimulation or as self-administered home-maximal stimulation at 10 Hz.

Detrusor overactivity may be a severe symptomatic distress in spinal cord injury with **spinal detrusor hyperreflexia**. In cases refractory to anticholinergic drugs, penile electrical stimulation has been demonstrated to reduce hyperreflexic contractions and urinary leaks.[22,23] Recently, Shah[55] utilized penile electrical stimulation in a physiological study to modulate DO in a homogeneous series of subjects with spinal cord injury. Optimal inhibition of detrusor contraction required currents at least twice the pudendo-anal reflex, irrespective of pulse width, and was achieved with stimulation frequencies between 15 and 20 Hz. Repetitive stimulation resulted in increasing filling volumes before contraction with slow poststimulation return to the baseline volume, indicating not only acute but also prolonged modulation of detrusor inhibitory mechanisms. No doubt, this option of treatment warrants further exploration in this group of patients.

In patients refractory to noninvasive procedures, other techniques are justified, e.g. perineally inserted or implanted electrodes for direct stimulation of the pudendal main nerve trunk.[42,56] Another option is percutaneous stimulation of the sacral nerves, a successful test being followed by implantation of a stimulator for chronic use.

Acknowledgment

The authors acknowledge the support of the Swedish Medical Research Council (Project Nos. 009902-02 and 04767) and the Medical Faculty, Göteborg University.

References

1. Burke RE, Levine DN, Tsairis P, Zajac FE 3rd. Physiological types and histochemical profiles in motor units of the cat gastrocnemius. J Physiol 1973; 234(3):723–748.

2. Iggo A. Tension receptors in the stomach and the urinary bladder. J Physiol 1955; 128:593–607.

3. Badr G, Fall M, Carlsson C-A, et al. Cortical evoked potentials obtained after stimulation of the lower urinary tract. J Urol 1984; 131:306–309.

4. Jiang C-H, Lindström S, Mazières L. Segmental inhibitory control of ascending sensory information from bladder mechanoreceptors in cat. Neurourol Urodyn 1991; 10:286–288.

5. Barrington FJF. The relation of the hind-brain to micturition. Brain 1921; 44:23–53.

6. Barrington FJF. The nervous mechanism of micturition. Q J Exp Physiol 1914; 8:33–71.

7. Lindström S, Fall M, Carlsson C-A, Erlandson B-E. Rhythmic activity in pelvic afferents to the bladder: an experimental study in the cat with reference to the clinical condition "unstable bladder". Urol Int 1984; 39:272–279.

8. Nakamura M, Sakurai T. Bladder inhibition by penile electrical stimulation. Br J Urol 1984; 56:413–415.

9. Madersbacher H, Kiss G, Mair D. Transcutaneous electrostimulation of the pudendal nerve for treatment of detrusor overactivity. Neurourol Urodynam 1995; 14:501–502.

10. Alexander S, Rowan D, Millar W, Scott R. Treatment of urinary incontinence by electric pessary. A report of 18 patients. Br J Urol 1970; 42:184–190.

11. Fall M, Erlandson B-E, Carlsson C-A, Lindström S. The effect of intravaginal electrical stimulation of the feline urethra and urinary bladder. Neuronal mechanisms. Scand J Urol Nephrol 1978; Suppl 44:19.

12. Lindström S, Fall M, Carlsson C-A, Erlandson B-E. The neurophysiological basis of bladder inhibition in response to intravaginal electrical stimulation. J Urol 1983; 129:40.

13. Trontelj TV, Janko M, Godec C, et al. Electrical stimulation for urinary incontinence: a neurophysiological study. Urol Int 1974; 29:213.

14. Teague CT, Merrill DC. Electric pelvic floor stimulation. Mechanism of action. Invest Urol 1977; 15:65–69.

15. Glen E. Effective and safe control of incontinence by the intra-anal plug electrode. Br J Surg 1967; 54:802.

16. Eriksen BC, Bergmann S, Mjolnerod OK. Effect of anal electrostimulation with the 'Incontan' device in women with urinary incontinence. Br J Obstet Gynaecol 1987; 94:147–156.

17. Lindström S, Sudsuang R. Functionally specific bladder reflexes from pelvic and pudendal nerve branches: an experimental study in the cat. Neurourol Urodyn 1989; 8:392–393.

18. Geirsson G, Fall M, Lindström S. Cystometric classification of bladder overactivity: assessment of a new system in 501 patients. Int Urogyn J 1993; 4:186–193.

19. Blok BF, Holstege G. Two pontine micturition centers in the cat are not interconnected directly: implications for the central organisation of micturition. J Comp Neurol 1999; 403:209–218.

20. Ohlsson BL. Effects of some different pulse parameters on the perception of intravaginal and intraanal electrical stimulation. Med Biol Eng Comput 1988; 26:503–505.

21. Fall M, Erlandson B-E, Sundin T, Waagstein F. Intravaginal electrical stimulation. Clinical experiments on bladder inhibition. Scand J Urol Nephrol 1978; (suppl) 44:41–47.

22. Vereecken RL, Das J, Grisar P. Electrical sphincter stimulation in the treatment of detrusor hyperreflexia of paraplegics. Neurourol Urodyn 1984; 3:145–154.

23. Vodusek DB, Light JK, Libby JM. Detrusor inhibition induced by stimulation of pudendal nerve afferents. Neurourol Urodyn 1986; 5:381–389.

24. Vodusek DB, Plevnik S, Vrtacnik P, et al. Detrusor inhibition on selective pudendal nerve stimulation in the perineum. Neurourol Urodyn 1988; 6:389–393.

25. Collins CD. Intermittent electrical stimulation. Urol Int 1974; 29:221.

26. Rottembourg JL, Ghoneim MA, Fretin J, Susset JG. Study on the efficiency of electric stimulation of the pelvic floor. Invest Urol 1976; 13:354–358.

27. Bazeed MA, Thuroff JW, Schmidt RA, et al. Effect of chronic electrostimulation of the sacral roots on the striated urethral sphincter. J Urol 1982; 128:1357–1362.

28. Ridge RM, Betz WJ. The effect of selective, chronic stimulation on motor unit size in developing rat muscle. J Neurosci 1984; 4:2614–2620.

29. Caldwell KP, Cook PJ, Flack FC, James ED. Stress incontinence in females: report on 31 cases treated by electrical implant. J Obstet Gynaecol Br Commonw 1968; 75:777–780.

30. Eriksen BC, Erik-Nes SH. Long-term electrostimulation of the pelvic floor: primary therapy in female stress incontinence? Urol Int 1989; 44:90–95.

31. Fall M, Erlandson B-E, Nilson AE, Sundin T. Long-term intravaginal electrical stimulation in urge and stress incontinence. Scand J Urol Nephrol 1978; (suppl) 44:55–63.

32. Fall M. Does electrostimulation cure urinary incontinence? J Urol 1984; 131:664–667.

33. Janez J, Plevnik F, Korosec L, et al. Changes in detrusor receptor activity after electric pelvic floor stimulation. In: Proceedings of International Continence Society's XIth Meeting, Lund, Sweden; 1981:22.

34. Ishigooka M, Hashimoto T, Sasagawa I, Nakada T. Reduction in norepinephrine content of the rabbit urinary bladder by alpha-2 adrenergic antagonist after electrical pelvic floor stimulation. J Urol 1994; 151:774–775.

35. Jiang CH. Prolonged modulation of the micturition reflex by electrical stimulation. Thesis, Linköping University Medical Dissertations No. 582. Faculty of Health Sciences, Linköping University, Sweden, 1999.

36. Jiang C-H. Modulation of the micturition reflex pathway by intravesical electrical stimulation: an experimental study in the rat. Neurourol Urodyn 1998; 17:543–553.

37. Salmons S, Vrbova G. The influence of activity on some contractile characteristics of mammalian fast and slow muscles. J Physiol 1969; 201:535–549.

38. Schmidt RA, Kogan BA, Tanagho EA. Neuroprostheses in the managment of incontinence in myelomeningocele patients. J Urol 1990; 143:779–782.

39. Godec C, Cass AS, Ayala GF. Bladder inhibition with functional electrical stimulation. Urology 1975; 6:663–666.

40. Plevnik S, Janez J. Maximal electrical stimulation for urinary incontinence: report of 98 cases. Urology 1979; 14:638–645.

41. Kralj B. Treatment of female urinary incontinence by stimulators of the pelvic floor muscles. Artif Org 1981; (suppl)5:609–612.

42. Ohlsson BL, Fall M, Frankenberg-Sommar S. Effects of external and direct pudendal nerve maximal electrical stimulation in the treatment of the uninhibited overactive bladder. Br J Urol 1989; 64:374–380.

43. Plevnik S, Janez J, Vrtacnik P, et al. Short-term electrical stimulation: home treatment for urinary incontinence. World J Urol 1986; 4:24–26.

44. Eriksen BC, Bergmann S, Erik-Nes SH. Maximal electrostimulation of the pelvic floor in female idiopathic detrusor instability and urge incontinence. Neurourol Urodyn 1989; 8:219.

45. Primus G, Kramer G. Maximal external electrical stimulation for treatment of neurogenic or non-neurogenic urgency and/or urge incontinence. Neurourol Urodyn 1996; 15:187–194.

46. Shepherd AM, Blannin JP, Winder A. The English experience of intravaginal electrical stimulation in urinary incontinence – a double blind trial. Proc International Continence Society's 15th Annual Meeting, London, 1985:224–225.

47. Sand PK, Richardson DA, Staskin DR, et al. Pelvic floor electrical stimulation in the treatment of genuine stress incontinence: a multicenter, placebo-controlled trial. Am J Obstet Gynecol 1995; 173:72–79.

48. Yamanishi T, Yasuda K, Hattori T, et al. Pelvic floor electrical stimulation in the treatment of stress incontinence: a placebo-controlled double-blind trial. Neurourol Urodyn 1996; 15:397.

49. Yamanishi T, Yasuda K, Sakakibara R, et al. Randomized, double-blind study of electrical stimulation for urinary incontinence due to detrusor overactivity. Urology 2000; 55:353–357.

50. Luber KM, Wolde-Tsadik G. Efficacy of functional electrical stimulation in treating genuine stress incontinence: a randomized clinical trial. Neurourol Urodyn 1997; 16:543–551.

51. Allen RE, Hosker GL, Smith AR, Warrell DW. Pelvic floor damage and childbirth: a neurophysiological study. Br J Obstet Gynaecol 1990; 97:770–779.

52. Abel I, Ottesen B, Fischer-Rasmussen W, Lose G. Maximal electrical stimulation of the pelvic floor in the treatment of urge incontinence: a placebo controlled study. Neurourol Urodyn 1996; 15:283–284.

53. Ahlberg J, Edlund C, Wikkelsö C, Rosengren L, Fall M. Neurological signs are common in patients with urodynamically verified "idiopathic" bladder overactivity. Neurourol Urodyn 2002; 21:65–70.

54. Fall M, Geirsson G, Lindström S. Toward a new classification of overactive bladders. Neurourol Urodyn 1995; 14:635–646.

55. Shah N. Thesis, University College London Medical School, London, 2002.

56. Janez J, Plevnik S, Vrtacnik P. Maximal electrical stimulation in patients with lower motor neuron lesion. Proc International Continence Society's XIIth Annual Meeting, Leiden, The Netherlands, 1982:115–118.

49

Emptying the neurogenic bladder by electrical stimulation

Graham H Creasey

Principles

Electrical stimulation has been investigated for many years for the purpose of restoring function to the neurogenic bladder, whose functions of micturition and continence may be impaired by either paralysis or hyperreflexia of the detrusor and/or sphincter mechanisms. Ideally, the functions of both emptying and storage should be restored. This would require coordinated contraction of the detrusor and relaxation of the sphincter mechanism for voiding, alternating with relaxation of the detrusor and adequate contraction of the sphincters for continence.

Electrical stimulation is usually thought of as producing muscle contraction, but there are also ways of using it to prevent contraction or produce relaxation. Reflex contraction or relaxation of muscle may be produced by stimulating sensory nerves. When stimulation is applied in this way, modifying activity in the central nervous system, it is sometimes called neuromodulation; this is discussed in other chapters in this book. When stimulation is applied directly to efferent nerves to improve function by producing contraction of muscles it is sometimes called functional neuromuscular stimulation or functional electrical stimulation. This chapter describes such stimulation of sacral efferent nerves to produce emptying of the neurogenic bladder. This process clearly requires that efferent nerves to the bladder be intact, specifically the preganglionic parasympathetic efferents from the sacral segments of the cord which run via the sacral anterior nerve roots, sacral nerves, and pelvic plexus. It is therefore applicable to patients with lesions of the spinal cord above the sacral segments, who can now derive considerable clinical benefit from electrical stimulation to produce safe and effective bladder emptying. Restoration of continence to the neurogenic bladder by electrical stimulation is still under investigation, and chemical or surgical methods are still needed in many cases.

Location of stimulation

A variety of sites of stimulation have been used in patients with suprasacral spinal cord injury or disease, with electrodes on the bladder wall, the pelvic splanchnic nerves, the conus medullaris, the sacral anterior roots, or the mixed sacral nerves. In practice only the latter two sites have reached clinical significance (Figure 49.1).

Electrodes on the bladder wall produced poor results, probably for several reasons including breakage of electrodes with bladder movement, the difficulty of recruiting enough of the detrusor muscle, and the stimulation of afferents producing unwanted reflexes.[1,2] If these problems

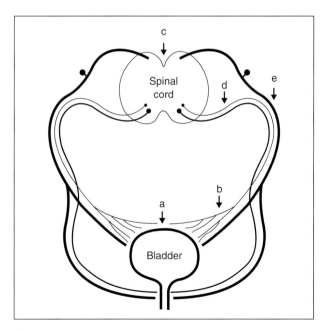

Figure 49.1
Potential sites of stimulation: (a) bladder wall; (b) pelvic nerves; (c) conus medullaris; (d) sacral anterior roots intradurally; and (e) sacral nerves extradurally.

could be solved it might be useful to stimulate postganglionic parasympathetic neurons in the bladder wall for patients whose preganglionic neurons have been damaged by injuries to the sacral segments of the spinal cord or the cauda equina; such patients do not gain bladder function from electrical stimulation at present.

The pelvic splanchnic nerves appear to be a theoretically desirable site but surgical access is difficult and it may be difficult to avoid stimulating sympathetic fibers to the bladder neck and afferent fibers. Good results were claimed in a few patients but little has been published on this route.[3,4]

Stimulation of the conus medullaris was developed by Nashold et al.[5] A laminectomy from T12 to L2 was performed and a pair of electrodes inserted into the gray matter of the conus medullaris at the spinal level giving the highest bladder pressures on electrical stimulation of the dorsal surface of the conus. Nashold reported a good result in 16 of 27 patients followed for 3–10 years; however, the technique has not gained wide acceptance, perhaps because of the difficulty of identifying a location in the cord which could produce coordinated micturition.

Stimulation of the sacral anterior roots was developed by Brindley.[6,7] This site has the advantage that these roots do not usually contain sensory neurons, so direct activation of reflexes rarely occurs. The sacral anterior roots do, however, contain efferent neurons to both detrusor and external urethral sphincter. The lower motor neurons to the sphincter have a lower threshold for electrical activation than the parasympathetic efferent neurons to the detrusor, so it is possible to activate the sphincter without the bladder but not usually the bladder without the sphincter. It used to be thought that attempts to produce voiding would therefore be ineffective and possibly dangerous, by causing co-contraction of detrusor and sphincter. However, Brindley made use of the fact that the smooth muscle of the detrusor contracts and relaxes much more slowly than the striated muscle of the external urethral sphincter. Stimulation in bursts of a few seconds, separated by longer gaps, allows a sustained pressure to be built up in the bladder while allowing the external sphincter to relax rapidly between the bursts, allowing urine to flow during these gaps.[8] Careful long-term clinical follow-up has shown that the brief co-contraction of the sphincter during the bursts does not cause bladder trabeculation or upper tract damage, and effective emptying of the bladder can be produced.

Sensory nerves in the end organs can nevertheless respond to muscle activity, and this may produce reflex contraction, or failure to relax, at the sphincter, even during the gaps between stimulation, a condition resembling detrusor-sphincter dyssynergia, which can hinder the flow of urine in some patients.[9] Sauerwein developed the addition of posterior sacral rhizotomy to this stimulation, carrying out both procedures simultaneously at the level of the cauda equina.[10] This has the great advantage of reducing not only reflex contraction of the sphincter but also reflex contraction

of the bladder, protecting the upper tracts from back pressure and abolishing reflex incontinence. It also abolishes autonomic dysreflexia triggered from contraction of the bladder or lower bowel. It does, however, have other disadvantages, which are discussed below.

If posterior sacral rhizotomy is performed, similar function can be obtained by applying bursts of stimulation to the mixed sacral nerves whose afferent connections to the cord have been divided. Electrodes and cables can thus be implanted extradurally in the sacral spinal canal. The rhizotomy is still best performed intradurally where it is easier to separate sensory from motor roots. It is easiest to separate these where they diverge to enter the conus medullaris and the sensory roots can be divided with little handling of the motor roots. The combination of extradural electrodes and intradural rhizotomy at the conus was developed by Sarrias et al. and is sometimes called the Barcelona technique.[11] However, this involves a second laminectomy at the level of the conus. If there has been a previous spinal fracture or internal fixation at the thoracolumbar junction it is probably safer not to risk destabilizing the spine at this level and to carry out the rhizotomy in the cauda equina. This can be done conveniently at the lower end of the dural sac through the same laminectomy used for implanting extradural electrodes (Figure 49.2).

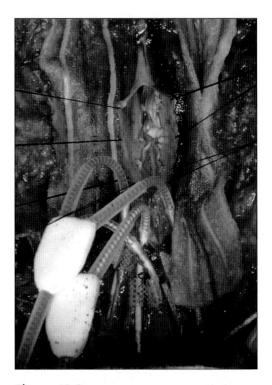

Figure 49.2
Alternative site of posterior rhizotomy with extradural electrodes. The lower end of the dural sac is shown held open with stay sutures to display the divided posterior roots; the electrodes have been attached to the sacral nerves caudal to the end of the dural sac.

Methods

Surgery

General anesthesia should be carried out without anticholinergic medication, which could reduce bladder contraction, and preferably without long-acting skeletal muscle relaxants, so that lower limb muscle responses can be used to assist in identifying nerves. Laminectomy is carried out according to the technique selected from Table 49.1. After opening the dura, sensory roots are distinguished from motor roots by intraoperative stimulation using hook electrodes while recording bladder pressure via a urethral catheter. Under general anesthesia sensory roots do not produce bladder contraction though they may produce reflex contraction of the lower limbs and reflex rises in blood pressure that can be rapid. It is therefore advisable to monitor blood pressure intra-arterially. After division of posterior roots, usually S2–5, electrodes are implanted on the nerves or roots that produce bladder pressure on stimulation, usually S3–4. Electrodes may also be implanted on S2, even if these roots do not produce bladder pressure, for the purpose of producing penile erection. The cables from the electrodes are passed subcutaneously through a cannula, usually to a temporary pocket in the flank. After repositioning the patient, they can be passed subcutaneously to the front of the body, where they are attached to a stimulator implanted in a subcutaneous pocket over the lower chest or abdomen. Detailed instructions are given in Brindley's *Notes for Surgeons and Physicians*, available from the manufacturer.[12]

Equipment

Equipment includes implanted components, external components, and equipment used during surgery. Implantable intradural and extradural electrodes are shown in Figure 49.3. Cables from the electrodes are connected via plugs and sockets to an implantable receiver (Figure 49.4). A 3-channel receiver is typically used if S2–4 are to be stimulated individually with intradural electrodes, whereas a 2-channel receiver can be used if S3 and S4 are stimulated by the same channel, as is often done with extradural electrodes.

The implantable components contain no batteries but are powered and controlled by radio transmission from an external controller programmed by the clinician and operated by the user. Analog and digital versions of the controller are available; their batteries can be charged weekly.

During surgery, hook electrodes connected to a battery-powered nerve stimulator are used for identification of nerves. Medical adhesive is used to seal the connections between plugs and sockets.

The equipment is approved by the US Food and Drug Administration (FDA) as a Humanitarian Use Device and in Europe is CE Marked under the requirements of the Active Implantable Medical Device Directive 90/385/EEC.

Preoperative investigation

It is essential to know that the parasympathetic efferent fibers from the sacral cord to the bladder are capable of producing bladder contraction. This may be tested by cystometry in which it is desirable to see a reflex bladder contraction of at least 35 cmH$_2$O in a woman and 50 cmH$_2$O in a man.[12] Anticholinergics may need to be stopped several days before this procedure, in which case it may be necessary to prepare the patient for increased incontinence and autonomic dysreflexia. The presence of other sacral reflexes such as the anocutaneous reflex, bulbocavernosus reflex, or ankle tendon reflexes and a history of reflex erection help to confirm sacral function.

It is also desirable to confirm adequate bladder capacity and exclude severe fibrosis of the bladder wall. This can usually be determined from the patient's history, particularly when using anticholinergics, but in case of doubt can be confirmed by repeating cystometry under spinal anesthesia.

It is of course desirable to document urinary tract function thoroughly, as well as penile erection and bowel

Table 49.1 *Potential sites of surgery; criteria for selecting a site are given under Discussion*			
Technique	Electrodes	Posterior rhizotomy	Laminectomies
Classical technique	Intradural	Mid cauda equina	L3–5
Barcelona technique	Extradural	Conus medullaris	S1–3 and T12–L1
Alternative technique	Extradural	Low cauda equina	S1–3

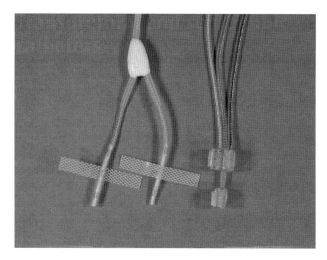

Figure 49.3
Electrodes. On the right is shown an array of intradural electrodes, with three cables corresponding to S2, S3, and S4. On the left is shown a pair of extradural electrodes, for application to left and right sacral nerves at a given segmental level, with a common lead. Three pairs of extradural electrodes may be implanted for S2–4, but more commonly the S3 and S4 nerves are stimulated together, allowing two pairs to be used.

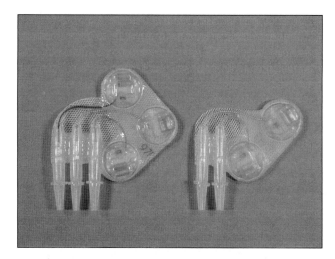

Figure 49.4
Receivers. On the left is shown a 3-channel receiver and on the right a 2-channel receiver. During implantation, cables from the electrodes are attached to the receivers using plugs and sockets located within the vertical tubular structures.

function. The appearance of the bladder neck on video-cystometry probably has prognostic value for stress incontinence, as described below.[13] Bladder diverticula are not necessarily a contraindication but may result in some persistence of urinary tract infection. Ureteric reflux or hydronephrosis are not necessarily a contraindication and may be a strong indication for posterior rhizotomy. If a subject has a suprapubic catheter it is probably preferable to revert to urethral catheterization before surgery to allow adequate closure of the stoma before generating bladder pressure with the stimulator. Prior bladder augmentation, if successful, abolishes the ability of the bladder to generate pressure and therefore renders the patient unsuitable.

Imaging of the lumbosacral spine can be used to exclude structural abnormalities. Separation of the spinal roots intradurally can be complicated by adhesions due to previous subarachnoid hemorrhage (such as from a bullet or stab wound) or spinal meningitis or myelography with an oily contrast medium,[12] and magnetic resonance imaging (particularly with gadolinium enhancement) may aid in the preoperative detection of these adhesions[14] as well as confirming the position of the conus medullaris.

Postoperative management

Extradural electrodes may be tested and brought into use on the first postoperative day. Cystometry and clinical examination should show that rhizotomy is effective; on the rare occasion that bladder reflexes persist, it is easier to return to surgery and complete the rhizotomy before the wound is healed. It is wise to check residual volumes after stimulator-driven voiding for the first few days and adjust the stimulator if necessary with urodynamic monitoring of voiding pressure and flow rate. Many patients may have a high fluid output initially as a result of intravenous fluids or the habit of a high fluid intake, so it may be necessary to void frequently until this is adjusted. Overdistention of the bladder can result in poor contractility and the need to revert to catherization until the bladder recovers.

Some surgeons prefer to postpone the use of intradural electrodes for a few days after surgery to reduce the risk of leakage of cerebrospinal fluid along the cables, but the implant should be tested within 3–4 days; reduced responses at 1 week, particularly of somatic muscles, may indicate nerve damage due to handling at operation. However, the patient can be reassured that the motor responses seen in the first week are likely to return.[12]

Delay in the use of the stimulator can contribute to postoperative constipation, but thereafter regular use of the stimulator usually improves bowel function, though patients may take a few weeks to adjust to a new bowel habit. Initial follow-up by telephone is helpful and thereafter follow-up is recommended at 3 months and annually.

Results

This technique has now been used in several thousand patients, primarily in Europe, where the intradural technique has been predominant, with others in

North America, the Far East, New Zealand, and Australia. Reports have been published from many single-center studies,[10,13,15–22] as well as multi-center studies[23–26] and surveys.[27,28] The stimulator was the subject of conferences at Le Mans, France in 1989,[29] Halifax, Nova Scotia in 1992,[30] Innsbruck, Austria in 1996, and Sydney, Australia in 2000.

Micturition

The majority of subjects with the stimulator use it routinely for producing micturition at home 4–6 times per day. Of the 184 patients reported by van Kerrebroeck et al, 157 (85%) used the stimulator alone; a further four required a subsequent sphincterotomy in order to use it, and a further eight combined its use with intermittent catheterization; 7.6% did not use it for various reasons.[27] Residual volume in the bladder following implant-driven micturition was reduced in 151 patients (89% of users) to less than 30 ml, and in 95% of users to less than 60 ml. No user had a residual greater than 200 ml.

Urine infection

A substantial decrease in urinary tract infection is one of the main benefits of the technique, and has been reported by many groups following the use of the implant.[15,17,23,27,29,31] The reduction in residual volume is probably the main reason, together with greatly reduced use of intermittent or indwelling catheterization. As a result, antibiotic use is also greatly reduced.

Continence of urine

Reflex incontinence due to spinal reflexes is abolished by posterior sacral rhizotomy from S2–5. Some female patients have reported that incontinence can return temporarily if they have a urinary tract infection; this is probably a local reflex as a result of inflammation of the bladder wall, as it always improves following eradication of the infection.

Stress incontinence may persist following surgery in 10–15% of patients, particularly in those who have had previous sphincterotomy or bladder neck resection. McDonagh et al. reported that the state of the bladder neck on videourodynamics prior to sacral rhizotomy appeared to have a bearing on subsequent continence. All patients in their series with a closed bladder neck preoperatively became continent, except one patient who had had two previous sphincterotomies; another patient with previous sphincterotomy but a closed bladder neck prior to rhizotomy became continent. However, three out of four patients with an open bladder neck preoperatively had some degree of incontinence. Pre- or postoperative sphincterotomy appeared to be less of a risk to continence than bladder neck resection.[13] Of 41 early users followed up for 5–13 years, 35 reported continence day and night; of the six who were not continent, four had had previous bladder neck resections.[32] Stress incontinence may also occur *de novo* in a few patients; this is probably in those with an open bladder neck whose continence has been maintained preoperatively by hyperreflexia of the external urethral sphincter; abolition of this hyperreflexia may then result in stress incontinence.

Most paraplegic patients dispense with urine collection devices, but some tetraplegic patients wear a condom and leg bag because of their limited hand function.

Urodynamics

Bladder capacity

Posterior rhizotomy dramatically increases bladder capacity by abolishing detrusor hyperreflexia; urodynamic filling of the areflexic bladder is best limited to under 400 ml to avoid stretching of the detrusor. McDonagh et al showed that functional bladder capacity increased by at least 140 ml, and an average of 404 ml (range 140–680), in all patients who had posterior rhizotomy, an increase that was statistically significant at the level of $p < 0.00001$.[13] Van Kerrebroeck et al, who took particular care not to overdistend the bladder postoperatively, found an average increase in cystometric capacity of 332 ml ($p < 0.001$) in patients who had undergone posterior rhizotomy.[33]

Bladder compliance

Since compliance is volume-dependent, it is desirable to compare it at the same volumes pre- and postoperatively; Van Kerrebroeck used the maximal preoperative cystometric capacity of each patient as this volume, and found that patients who had undergone posterior rhizotomy had a statistically significant increase in compliance from 8 to 53 ml/cmH$_2$O. The postoperative compliance, at 500 ml, was over 50 ml/cmH$_2$O in 12 of 13 patients.[33]

Detrusor pressure

Detrusor pressure can be controlled by programming the external controller, and fluctuates with bursts of stimulation. Pressures in the bladder during electrically activated micturition have been reported by several authors. Cardozo et al reported that the maximum voiding pressure was on average 55 cmH$_2$O with a range of 22–82 cmH$_2$O.[34]

Arnold et al recorded a mean peak pressure of 88 cmH$_2$O and mean trough pressure of 40 cmH$_2$O and concluded that this did not appear to be harmful.[15] Madersbacher et al reported a mean peak pressure of 71 cmH$_2$O (range 55–90) and noted that post-stimulus voiding did not appear to induce detrusor hypertrophy.[17] In the first 50 patients to receive the implant, bladder trabeculation was reported to have decreased in 13 patients when followed up at 1–9 years, and no patient in this group showed evidence of increased trabeculation.[32] Van Kerrebroeck recorded a mean peak voiding pressure of 89 cmH$_2$O.[33] It is likely that voiding pressure is less significant for the upper tracts than storage pressure, which is usually reduced by posterior rhizotomy.

Upper tracts

The improvement in bladder capacity and compliance which follow posterior rhizotomy reduce the risk of upper tract damage and can result in improvement in pre-existing ureteric reflux or hydronephrosis.[10] In a multi-center review of 184 patients, reflux was present in nine patients before the operation: after implantation it was improved or abolished in seven of these and persisted in two. No patient in this group developed reflux with the use of the stimulator.[27] Eight of the 184 subjects showed upper tract dilatation preoperatively: of these, the dilatation improved in seven and deteriorated in one. No patient in this series developed upper tract dilatation *de novo* after implantation of the stimulator.[27]

Pain

Stimulation is never painful in patients with complete spinal cord injury and almost never in patients who undergo posterior rhizotomy. Intradural stimulation of anterior roots would usually be expected to be painless, even without rhizotomy, since these roots are usually purely motor. However, among the first 50 patients, implanted over 20 years ago, all of whom had intradural implants but not all of whom had rhizotomy, three were unable to use the implant because of pain on stimulation, and four others found use of the stimulator to some extent painful. All these patients had preserved pain sensitivity in the sacral dermatomes preoperatively.[35] It may be that current can sometimes spread from the intradural electrodes to activate nearby sensory roots, but a few patients have continued to experience pain on stimulation in spite of a thorough sacral posterior rhizotomy. This led to the belief that some anterior roots can contain sensory fibers, which has been confirmed experimentally.[36] A modified implant with a larger number of channels has been developed for use in such patients, to allow more selective stimulation of individual roots.[12] Extradural stimulation of mixed sacral nerves would be unacceptably painful if pain sensitivity was present in the sacral dermatomes and rhizotomy was not performed.

Autonomic dysreflexia

The symptoms of autonomic dysreflexia associated with contraction of the bladder or lower bowel are greatly reduced by posterior rhizotomy. Slight rises in blood pressure may occur with stimulation in rhizotomized patients, perhaps as a result of somatic muscle contraction in the sacral segments, or the presence of afferent nerves in anterior roots, but these are not sufficient to prevent use of the device.[37] If rhizotomy were not performed, extradural stimulation of mixed sacral nerves would be likely to cause significant blood pressure rises, at least in patients with cervical and upper thoracic lesions.

Nerve damage

Accidental damage to motor nerve fibers at the time of operation is less likely to occur with extradural electrodes than intradural, because of the greater surgical handling of anterior roots in the latter procedure and the lack of supporting fibrous tissue intradurally. It is dependent on surgical care and experience. It can be most sensitively detected by testing for any loss of skeletal muscle responses to the use of the stimulator during the first postoperative week, and may also become evident as a temporary loss of bladder response. It usually takes the form of neuropraxia or axonotmesis and is therefore temporary, but bladder responses may take from 2 to 6 months to return as the axons regrow, thus delaying the use of the implant for micturition.

Some patients have now been using the stimulator for 20 years or more without apparent deterioration in nerve function. The histological appearance of stimulated nerves was reported as normal in the case of two patients who died (one by suicide and one from myocardial infarction) after using the implant for 3 and 5 years, respectively.[31]

Leakage of cerebrospinal fluid

Early intradural implants sometimes had leakage of cerebrospinal fluid along the cables passing through the dura. The implant has since been modified by the addition of a grommet to seal the cables to the dura, and the incidence of this complication appears to have been greatly reduced.

It is rarely a problem with extradural electrodes, even though the dura may have been opened in the vicinity of the cables to perform rhizotomy.

Implant infection

Infection of the implants has been rare, particularly since a technique of coating them with antibiotics was introduced in 1982. Rushton et al reported in 1989 that one out of 104 coated implants had become infected, and in this case infection appeared to have been introduced at a subsequent operation to close a leak of cerebrospinal fluid.[38] Brindley reported a 1% infection rate for the first 500 implants.[28] The infection rate for a variety of similar implants has been shown to be significantly reduced by antibiotic coating, but not by systemic perioperative antibiotics.[38] Nevertheless, many surgeons use systemic perioperative antibiotic prophylaxis aimed at both Gram-positive and Gram-negative organisms.

If the receiver becomes infected, and this is detected promptly before infection has spread along the cables, it is sometimes possible to divide the cables at a sterile location in the flank and remove the receiver, leaving the electrodes in place. If the infection has spread along the cables to the electrodes, it is necessary to remove all the implanted components. In either case, vigorous treatment with antibiotics followed by a waiting period of at least 6 months is advisable before reimplanting a stimulator.

Implant reliability

The implanted components have proved to be remarkably reliable. A survey of the first 500 implants showed that faults occurred on average once every 19.2 implant-years.[39] The commonest site for faults has been in cables, which are sometimes mechanically damaged by movement. Repair or replacement of the device is usually possible, often with minor surgery, and special equipment is available from the manufacturer to facilitate repairs.[12]

Failures in the external transmitter have been more common and have primarily been due to breaks in the antenna lead, but do not require reoperation.

Penile erection

In about 60% of patients, sustained full erection sufficient for coitus can be produced by stimulation of S2, although not all of these patients use it for coitus.[23] In many of the remaining 40% of patients, a partial erection is produced and this may be useful when attaching a condom for urine

drainage. Some centers have reported less success with erection when using extradural electrodes; these require higher levels of stimulation to pass equivalent current through the epineurium.

Bowel function

Stimulation, primarily of S3, produces contraction of the lower bowel as far proximal as the splenic flexure, and increases the frequency of defecation, probably by enhancing colonic motility.[40–43] By careful adjustment of the Finetech stimulator, MacDonagh et al were able to produce defecation routinely with the stimulator alone in 6 of 12 patients, and to reduce the time spent each week in bowel emptying from 2.5 h to half an hour.[44]

Costs

A prospective three-center study in the Netherlands collected the actual costs of hospital care, self-care, and travel expenses associated with bladder function of 52 patients before and after the procedure and through 2 years of follow-up. A model of the long-term costs indicated a break-even point of approximately 8 years, after which the procedure resulted in reduced costs.[25] In the USA a retrospective study of costs of bladder and bowel care using structured interviews in 12 patients indicated a break-even point of 5 years; the lower figure may be related to a shorter length of postoperative hospitalization in the North American patients.[45]

Discussion
Selection of patients

Patients with complete spinal cord injury above the conus medullaris and inefficient reflex micturition may be considered at any time after the first few months of injury, particularly if they have complications such as frequent or chronic urine infection, reflex incontinence resistant to medication, or autonomic dysreflexia triggered by bladder or bowel.

In patients with incomplete injuries:

1. it is wise to wait until 2 years after injury to allow any recovery to occur
2. it is necessary to determine whether the implant is likely to be painful
3. it is particularly important to weigh the advantages of posterior rhizotomy against any loss of function which it may cause.

Some patients with multiple sclerosis are suitable, subject to the reservations above. A few adult patients with suprasacral meningomyelocele may also be suitable, but the growth of young children might displace the electrodes if implanted in them. Betz has investigated the use of extensible leads, and has implanted stimulators in patients as young as 14 after evaluation of their skeletal maturity.[46,47] Children with spinal cord injury have a significant risk of developing scoliosis during adolescence, so it may be worth waiting until this is unlikely, or combining implantation with spinal instrumentation if that is needed.

In assigning priorities the following generalizations may be of use:

- Patients with complete spinal cord lesions are more straightforward to investigate and treat by this technique than patients with incomplete lesions.
- Women with reflex incontinence have more to gain than men, because of the lack of satisfactory urine-collecting devices for females, and have less to lose from posterior rhizotomy.
- Patients with recurrent infection have more to gain than those without. Those with persistently high reflex bladder pressures endangering renal function or with autonomic dysreflexia triggered by bladder or bowel are likely to benefit from posterior rhizotomy; this operation provides the opportunity to implant a stimulator, which may then provide them with a preferable alternative to intermittent catheterization.
- Men with poor or absent reflex erection have more to gain and less to lose than those whose reflex erections already suffice for coitus.
- Paraplegic men are more likely to benefit from continence, whereas some tetraplegic men may continue to wear a condom and leg bag at least during the day because of the difficulty in handling urine bottles and clothing.

Selection of surgical technique

Each of the techniques described above can produce excellent results in the hands of a careful surgeon who performs the operation sufficiently often to maintain skill.

The classical technique, implanting electrodes and performing the rhizotomy at the level of the cauda, has the advantage of a single laminectomy. There is a slight risk of cerebrospinal fluid leakage along the cables, and if the cables later break at the site of exit through the dura they are difficult to repair at this site; extradural electrodes can be added to restore function. If the rhizotomy at the cauda later proves to be incomplete it can be revised at the conus.

The Barcelona technique, implanting extradural electrodes and performing intradural rhizotomy at the conus, has the advantage that it is easier to distinguish sensory from motor roots at the conus and little handling of the motor roots is necessary; in addition, the sacral nerves extradurally have a fibrous covering continuous with the dura and are more robust than the intradural anterior roots. It is therefore probably less likely that the motor neurons will be damaged by intraoperative handling, at least in the hands of a new operator. Extradural electrodes may be the only type possible if there is severe intradural arachnoiditis. If the rhizotomy at the conus proves to be incomplete, it can be revised within a few days at the same site or later at the cauda, provided that intrathecal bleeding has not led to arachnoiditis.

The alternative technique, implanting extradural electrodes and performing rhizotomy at the lower end of the cauda, combines the advantages of a single laminectomy with those of the Barcelona technique, and avoids any risk of destabilizing the spine at the thoracolumbar junction if there has been a previous fracture or internal fixation at that level. It is slightly more difficult to identify all the posterior roots in the cauda than at the conus, so there may be a slightly higher incidence of incomplete rhizotomy.

Extradural separation of sensory and motor fibers is difficult and may damage the nerves, and is rarely performed.[48]

Detrusor-sphincter dyssynergia

Many of the complications of the neurogenic bladder are due to co-contraction of the external urethral sphincter or its failure to relax, and many forms of electrical stimulation produce contraction of the sphincter in addition to the detrusor. Several approaches to reducing sphincter contraction during electrical stimulation have been investigated. Tanagho et al used a variety of surgical procedures such as pudendal neurotomy, levatorotomy, pudendal nerve stimulation, and increasingly extensive posterior rhizotomy,[49] but effective voiding was only produced in about one-third of subjects.

Brindley and Craggs suggested the use of anodal block to prevent propagation of action potentials in the large somatic axons to the external sphincter while allowing propagation in the small parasympathetic fibers to the detrusor.[50] They demonstrated the principle experimentally and early models of the Brindley stimulator included the option of a triangular waveform for this purpose. This option was later omitted when clinical follow-up showed that post-stimulus voiding was safe and effective for voiding, at least when combined with posterior rhizotomy.

In our laboratory we showed in chronically spinalized dogs that anodal block could be used to produce contraction of the bladder with little contraction of the external urethral sphincter. However, voiding was still hindered by reflex activation of urethral muscle unless posterior rhizotomy was performed.[51,52]

High-frequency stimulation can also be applied selectively to large axons to produce either fatigue or block, while allowing smaller axons and their muscles to be activated. This has been applied by implants in chronically spinalized dogs in Montreal.[53] Although voiding pressures were not significantly different with selective stimulation, the urethral pressures were much lower and voiding was produced with low residual volumes without evidence of reflux over a 6-month period in these animals.

The role of posterior rhizotomy

Division of all the posterior roots from S2 to S5 can produce substantial benefits to a patient with a neurogenic bladder; it can also have some significant disadvantages and has therefore been a subject of some debate.

During the early 1980s sacral anterior root implants, using intradural electrodes to stimulate motor nerves, were often done without deliberate rhizotomy, though posterior roots may have been damaged accidentally in some cases.[35] Most of these patients had useful function, though some may have had persisting autonomic dysreflexia and some needed subsequent sphincterotomy.

Tanagho et al reported extradural implants on 22 patients, most of whom had other procedures to reduce outlet resistance; with increasing experience, they commented that 'more extensive dorsal rhizotomy is essential to achieve good voiding'.[49]

Talalla et al placed electrodes extradurally in seven patients without posterior rhizotomy or pudendal neurectomy and, although initial results were promising,[54] Talalla and Bloom subsequently concluded that this combination was not effective.[9]

Kirkham et al recently implanted extradural electrodes without rhizotomy in five patients with spinal cord injury. Reflex bladder contraction was preserved and could be inhibited by using the electrodes to stimulate only afferent neurons in the sacral nerves, but voiding was hindered in several patients, probably by reflex contraction of the sphincter.[55]

The major advantages of posterior rhizotomy are:

1. A great increase in bladder compliance and capacity (except in the few cases where poor compliance is due to fibrosis), thereby protecting the upper tracts from ureteric reflux and hydronephrosis.
2. The abolition of uninhibited reflex bladder contractions, thereby reducing reflex incontinence and the need for anticholinergic medication and its side-effects.
3. The abolition of reflex contraction of the sphincter, thereby reducing detrusor-sphincter dyssynergia.

4. The abolition of autonomic dysreflexia triggered from the bladder or rectum.

The disadvantages of posterior rhizotomy include:

1. The loss of perineal sensation if present.
2. The loss of reflex erection and reflex ejaculation if present, although these are not always functional after spinal cord injury. Some patients are capable of a modified form of orgasm by stimulating the sacral dermatomes after spinal cord injury and this too would be abolished by sacral rhizotomy. Erection is commonly produced by the implant and even more effectively by injection of papaverine or prostaglandins into the corpora cavernosa. Seminal emission can now be produced from a high proportion of spinal cord injured men by rectal probe electrostimulation, even after rhizotomy, and the procedure does not damage the implant.
3. The loss of reflex micturition and reflex defecation. The micturition produced by the implant is usually much more effective than reflex micturition, but if the implant is not used for any reason a patient will have to resort to intermittent or indwelling catheterization. Similarly, a patient with rhizotomy who uses the implant will generally become less constipated, but will be more constipated if the implant is not used.

A decision about posterior rhizotomy should therefore be made in each case. Brindley suggests the following policy:

- In women with complete lesions – who have less to lose and much to gain from continence – complete posterior rhizotomy is usually advised.
- In men with complete lesions and without useful reflex erection or ejaculation, the same policy may be followed, but if useful reflexes or sensation are present, the advantages and disadvantages of rhizotomy should be weighed with the patient.

The advantages of the combined procedure are such that implantation of the stimulator is now rarely performed without posterior rhizotomy, and this practice is likely to continue until a suitable alternative to surgical rhizotomy is found.

References

1. Bradley W, Timm G, Chou S. A decade of experience with electronic simulation of the micturition reflex. Urol Int 1971; 26:283–303.

2. Halverstadt D, Parry W. Electronic stimulation of the human bladder: nine years later. J Urol 1975; 113:341–344.

3. Burghele T. Electrostimulation of the neurogenic urinary bladder. In: Lutzmeyer Wea, ed. Urodynamics. Upper and lower urinary tract. Berlin: Springer-Verlag, 1973:319–322.

4. Kaeckenbeeck B. [Electrostimulation of the bladder in paraplegia. Method of Burghele–Ichim–Demetrescu.] Acta Urol Belg 1979; 47:139–140.

5. Nashold BS Jr, Friedman H, Grimes J. Electrical stimulation of the conus medullaris to control the bladder in the paraplegic patient. A 10-year review. Appl Neurophysiol 1981; 44:225–232.

6. Brindley GS. An implant to empty the bladder or close the urethra. J Neurol Neurosurg Psychiatry 1977; 40:358–369.

7. Brindley GS, Polkey CE, Rushton DN. Sacral anterior root stimulators for bladder control in paraplegia. Paraplegia 1982; 20:365–381.

8. Brindley GS. Emptying the bladder by stimulating sacral ventral roots. J Physiol 1974; 237:15P–16P.

9. Talalla A, Bloom J. Sacral electrical stimulation for bladder control. In: Illis LS, ed. Functional stimulation (spinal cord dysfunction, III). Oxford: Oxford University Press, 1992:206–218.

10. Sauerwein D. [Surgical treatment of spastic bladder paralysis in paraplegic patients. Sacral deafferentation with implantation of a sacral anterior root stimulator.] Urologe A 1990; 29:196–203.

11. Sarrias M, Sarrias F, Borau A. The "Barcelona" technique. Neurourol Urodyn 1993; 12:495–496.

12. Brindley G. The Finetech–Brindley Bladder Controller: Notes for surgeons and physicians. Welwyn Garden City, Herts, England: Finetech Medical Ltd., 1998.

13. MacDonagh RP, Forster DMC, Thomas DG. Urinary continence in spinal injury patients following complete sacral posterior rhizotomy. Br J Urol 1990; 66:618–622.

14. Delamarter RB, Ross JS, Masaryk TJ, et al. Diagnosis of lumbar arachnoiditis by magnetic resonance imaging. Spine 1990; 15:304–310.

15. Arnold E, Gowland S, MacFarlane M, et al. Sacral anterior root stimulation of the bladder in paraplegics. Aust NZ J Surg 1986; 56:319–324.

16. Herlant M, Colombel P. Electrostimulation intra-durale des racines sacrees anterieures chez les paraplegiques. Historique, reultats, indications. Annales de Réadaptation et de Médecine physique 1986; 29:405–411.

17. Madersbacher H, Fischer J, Ebner A. Anterior sacral root stimulator (Brindley): experiences especially in women with neurogenic urinary incontinence. Neurourol Urodyn 1988; 7:593–601.

18. Robinson L, Grant A, Weston P, et al. Experience with the Brindley anterior sacral root stimulator. Br J Urol 1988; 62:553–557.

19. Nordling J, Hald T, Kristensen JK, et al. [An implantable radio-controlled sacral nerve root stimulator for control of urination.] Ugeskr Laeger 1988; 150:978–980.

20. Borau A, Vidal J, Sarrias F, et al. Electro-estimulación de las raices sacras anteriores para el control esfinteriano en el lesionado medular. Médula Espinal 1995; 1:128–133.

21. Schurch B, Rodic B, Jeanmonod D. Posterior sacral rhizotomy and intradural anterior sacral root stimulation for treatment of the spastic bladder in spinal cord injured patients. J Urol 1997; 157:610–614.

22. van der Aa HE, Alleman E, Nene A, Snoek G. Sacral anterior root stimulation for bladder control: clinical results. Arch Physiol Biochem 1999; 107:248–256.

23. Egon G, Barat M, Colombel P, et al. Implantation of anterior sacral root stimulators combined with posterior sacral rhizotomy in spinal injury patients. World J Urol 1998; 16:342–349.

24. Van Kerrebroeck PEV, van der Aa HE, Bosch JLHR, et al. Sacral rhizotomies and electrical bladder stimulation in spinal cord injury: clinical and urodynamic analysis. Eur Urol 1997; 31:263–271.

25. Wielink G, Essink-Bot ML, Van Kerrebroeck PEV, Rutten FFH. Sacral rhizotomies and electrical bladder stimulation in spinal cord injury: cost-effectiveness and quality of life analysis. Eur Urol 1997; 31:441–446.

26. Creasey G, Grill J, Korsten M, et al. An implantable neuroprosthesis for restoring bladder and bowel control to patients with spinal cord injuries: a multi-center trial. Arch Phys Med Rehab 2001; 82:1512–1519.

27. Van Kerrebroeck P, Koldewijn E, Debruyne F. Worldwide experience with the Finetech-Brindley sacral anterior root stimulator. Neurourol Urodyn 1993; 12:497–503.

28. Brindley GS. The first 500 patients with sacral anterior root stimulator implants: general description. Paraplegia 1994; 32:795–805.

29. Colombel P, Egon G. [Electrostimulation of the anterior sacral nerve roots. An International Congress – Le Mans – 24–25 November 1989.] Ann Urol Paris 1991; 25:48–52.

30. Brindley GS. History of the sacral anterior root stimulator, 1969–1982. Neurourol Urodyn 1993; 12:481–483.

31. Brindley GS, Rushton DN. Long-term follow-up of patients with sacral anterior root stimulator implants. Paraplegia 1990; 28:469–475.

32. Brindley GS. Sacral anterior root stimulators for bladder control in paraplegia: the first 50 cases. J Neurol Neurosurg Psychiatry 1986; 49:1104–1114.

33. Van Kerrebroeck P, Koldewijn E, Wijkstra H, Debruyne F. Urodynamic evaluation before and after intradural posterior rhizotomies and implantation of the Finetech-Brindley anterior sacral root stimulator. Urodinamica 1992; 1:7–16.

34. Cardozo L, Krishnan KR, Polkey CE, et al. Urodynamic observations on patients with sacral anterior root stimulators. Paraplegia 1984; 22:201–209.

35. Brindley G, Polkey C, Rushton D, Cardozo L. Sacral anterior root stimulators for bladder control in paraplegia: the first 50 cases. J Neurol Neurosurg Psychiatry 1986; 49:1104–1114.

36. Schalow G. Efferent and afferent fibres in human sacral ventral nerve roots: basic research and clinical implications. Electromyogr Clin Neurophysiol 1989; 29:33–53.

37. Schurch B, Knapp PA, Jeanmonod D, et al. Does sacral posterior rhizotomy suppress autonomic hyper-reflexia in patients with spinal cord injury? Br J Urol 1998; 81:73–82.

38. Rushton DN, Brindley GS, Polkey CE, Browning GV. Implant infections and antibiotic-impregnated silicone rubber coating. J Neurol Neurosurg Psychiatry 1989; 52:223–229.

39. Brindley GS. The first 500 sacral anterior root stimulators: implant failures and their repair. Paraplegia 1995; 33:5–9.

40. Varma JS, Binnie N, Smith AN, et al. Differential effects of sacral anterior root stimulation on anal sphincter and colorectal motility in spinally injured man. Br J Surg 1986; 73:478–482.

41. Binnie N, Smith A, Creasey G, Edmond P. Motility effects of electrical anterior sacral nerve root stimulation of the parasympathetic supply of the left colon and anorectum in paraplegic subjects. J Gastrointest Mot 1990; 2:12–17.

42. Binnie N, Smith A, Creasey G, Edmond P. The effects of electrical anterior sacral nerve root stimulation on pelvic floor function in paraplegic subjects. J Gastrointest Mot 1991; 3:39–45.

43. Binnie NR, Smith AN, Creasey GH, Edmond P. Constipation associated with chronic spinal cord injury: the effect of pelvic parasympathetic stimulation by the Brindley stimulator. Paraplegia 1991; 29:463–469.

44. MacDonagh RP, Sun WM, Smallwood R, et al. Control of defecation in patients with spinal injuries by stimulation of sacral anterior nerve roots. Br Med J 1990; 300:1494–1497.

45. Creasey GH, Dahlberg JE. Economic consequences of an implanted neuralprosthesis for bladder and bowel management. Arch Phys Med Rehab 2001; 82:1520–1525.

46. Akers JM, Smith BT, Betz RR. Implantable electrode lead in a growing limb. IEEE Trans Rehab Eng 1999; 7:35–45.

47. Merenda LA, Spoltore TA, Betz RR. Progressive treatment options for children with spinal cord injury. SCI Nurs 2000; 17:102–109.

48. Sauerwein D, Ingunza W, Fischer J, et al. Extradural implantation of sacral anterior root stimulators. J Neurol Neurosurg Psychiatry 1990; 50:681–684.

49. Tanagho EA, Schmidt RA, Orvis BR. Neural stimulation for control of voiding dysfunction: a preliminary report in 22 patients with serious neuropathic voiding disorders. J Urol 1989; 142:340–345.

50. Brindley GS, Craggs MD. A technique for anodally blocking large nerve fibres through chronically implanted electrodes. J Neurol Neurosurg Psychiatry 1980; 43:1083–1090.

51. Grunewald V, Bhadra N, Creasey GH, Mortimer JT. Functional conditions of micturition induced by selective sacral anterior root stimulation: experimental results in a canine animal model. World J Urol 1998; 16:329–336.

52. Bhadra N, Grunewald V, Creasey G, Mortimer JT. Selective suppression of sphincter activation during sacral anterior nerve root stimulation. Neurourol Urodyn 2002; 21:55–64.

53. Abdel-Gawad M, Boyer S, Sawan M, Elhilali MM. Reduction of bladder outlet resistance by selective stimulation of the ventral sacral root using high frequency blockade: a chronic study in spinal cord transected dogs. J Urol 2001; 166:728–733.

54. Talalla A, Bloom JW, Nguyen Q. Successful intraspinal extradural sacral nerve stimulation for bladder emptying in a victim of traumatic spinal cord transection. Neurosurgery 1986; 19:955–961.

55. Kirkham AP, Knight SL, Craggs MD, et al. Neuromodulation through sacral nerve roots 2 to 4 with a Finetech-Brindley sacral posterior and anterior root stimulator. Spinal Cord 2002; 40:272–281.

50

Central neuromodulation

Philip EV Van Kerrebroeck

Introduction

A multitude of neurological disorders can affect the bladder and although the incidence of lower urinary tract dysfunction is different among the various neurological entities, an important percentage of patients develop voiding dysfunction.[1] Incontinence and poor evacuation of urine with residual urine and recurrent urinary tract infections can cause important morbidity. In patients with spinal cord injury the lack of ability to control the storing and evacuation function of the bladder is one of the most prominent aspects of their handicap.

Besides these bladder problems with a proven neurological basis, a vast group of patients suffers from lower urinary tract dysfunction without an evident neurological cause. These are patients with different forms of so-called idiopathic dysfunctional voiding.

Therapeutic modalities are pharmacological treatment, eventually in combination with clean intermittent catheterization. Lifelong continuation of this therapy, however, is a major issue mainly because of side-effects. Furthermore, in most patients, especially in females, incontinence remains a problem even with maximal pharmacological treatment. The failure of pharmacological manipulation has led to the development of surgical approaches such as augmentation cystoplasty, sphincteric incisions, and artificial sphincter implantation. However, a considerable number of patients with neurogenic bladder dysfunction continue to have significant urological problems although maximal classical therapy is applied. Therefore the use of electrical stimulation to control storage and evacuation of urine has become an important tool in the urological treatment of voiding dysfunction.

The aim of electrical stimulation for voiding dysfunction is to treat incontinence due to a lack of activity in the striated muscles of the urethral closure mechanism by improvement of the contraction of the sphincter mechanism or to overcome incontinence due to detrusor hyperactivity by reduction of detrusor contractions. Furthermore, electrical stimulation can be used to permit evacuation of a paraplegic bladder by provocation of detrusor contractions or to control micturition in the hyperreflex bladder by a combination of dampening of spontaneous reflex excitability and controlled activation of the detrusor.

These aims can be fulfilled by stimulation of the efferent nerves to the lower urinary tract or by modulation of reflex activity as a consequence of stimulation of afferent nerves. Different modalities to apply electrical current to the lower urinary tract are available. Surface electrodes can be used as nonimplantable devices.[2] Insertable plugs in the anal canal or the vagina are applied to treat incontinence.[3–5] Intravesical electrostimulation is performed in children with meningomyelocele.[6–8] Implantable prostheses are available to induce bladder contraction in order to evacuate urine in paraplegic bladders or to control detrusor contraction in hyperreflexic bladders.[9–11] Another type of prosthesis permits the modulation of symptomatic voiding dysfunction such as urge incontinence, urgency/frequency syndrome, and retention.[12,13]

Electrical stimulation for chronic lower urinary tract dysfunction

Chronic lower urinary tract dysfunction, such as urge incontinence, urgency/frequency syndrome, and bladder evacuation problems, presents a challenge. Most patients are initially treated conservatively with bladder retraining, pelvic floor exercises, and biofeedback. In the majority, this regimen will be supplemented with drugs. However, about 40% of patients with these forms of lower urinary tract dysfunction do not achieve an acceptable condition with these forms of treatment and remain a therapeutic problem. Alternative procedures with variable success rates such as bladder transection, transvesical phenol injection of the pelvic plexus, augmentation cystoplasty, and even urinary diversion are being advocated.

During recent decades, functional electrical stimulation has gained interest in the treatment of this type of lower urinary tract dysfunction. Different stimulation sites, such as the vagina or the anus, have been reported to be successful. Since the 1960s, transcutaneous neurostimulation applied to the third or fourth sacral foramen has been tried as a method of controlling functional lower urinary tract disorders.[14] Unilateral sacral segmental stimulation with a permanent electrode at the level of the sacral foramen S3 or S4 (sacral neuromodulation) can offer an alternative nondestructive mode of treatment for patients presenting with voiding dysfunction and chronic pelvic pain refractory to conservative measures. Since 1981 a clinical trial has been underway to evaluate the effectiveness of this method. Since that time, experience has been gathered in the evaluation, surgery, and follow-up of patients presenting with voiding dysfunction and pelvic pain who have been treated with sacral foramen electrode implants.[15] The goal of such treatment is to relieve the symptoms by rebalancing micturition control.

The mode of action of this so-called sacral neuromodulation is still unclear but it has been hypothesized that the electrical current modulates reflex pathways involved in the filling and evacuation phase of the micturition cycle.[16] Stimulation of Aδ myelinated fibers of the sacral roots S3 and S4 decreases the spastic behavior of the pelvic floor and enhances the tone of the urethral sphincter. The threshold for the somatic component of the spinal nerve that innervates the pelvic floor is lower than that for the autonomic component to the bladder. Therefore, simultaneous bladder contraction is avoided during stimulation. In many subjects the primary voiding dysfunction appears to begin with unstable urethral activity, which activates the voiding reflexes, leading to detrusor instability and the associated urgency, frequency, and incontinence. The inhibitory effect of the enhanced urethral sphincter tone suppresses detrusor instability and stabilizes detrusor activity.

Ideal candidates for neuromodulation are patients presenting with urge incontinence, urinary urgency/frequency, and evacuation problems. Patients who have failed numerous other therapies should not be excluded from neuromodulation as they often show an excellent response to this technique.

Sacral neuromodulation is planned as a long-term treatment, but patients are first tested by means of a temporary trial stimulation for 3–7 days. This trial stimulation consists of two steps. The first phase is the acute testing, followed by the so-called subchronic phase. During an outpatient procedure and under local anesthesia, one of the sacral foramina, preferably the third one, is punctured with a 20-gauge hollow needle. The proximal and distal tip of the needle is not isolated and allows electrical stimulation.

Typical responses to stimulation of each nerve level are seen at both the local (perineum) and distant (foot and toe) sites. S3 stimulation produces a contraction of the levator muscles (bellows-like contraction) as well as detrusor and urethral sphincter contraction. Signs of S3 stimulation in the lower extremities include plantar flexion of the great toe. Subjectively, patients report a pulling sensation in the rectum during S3 stimulation, with variable sensations being perceived in the scrotum and the tip of the penis by men or the labia and vagina in women. S4 stimulation results in a contraction of the levator ani muscle (bellows-like contraction), with no activity being noted in the foot or leg. The sacral root at either site with the best clinical (subjective) or urodynamic response is selected and the intensity of the current adapted to the sensation of stimulation.

Through the needle a temporary electrode is placed and the needle is removed. This electrode remains in the vicinity of the sacral root selected and passes through the sacral foramen, subcutaneous tissue, and the skin. When the acute motoric responses with stimulation are confirmed, the electrode is connected to an external stimulator. Then starts the subchronic phase of the trial stimulation. Patients will check the effect for 3–7 days based on voiding diaries. Urodynamic examination is a possible other control of the effect.

Patients with a good clinical and preferably urodynamic result can be candidates for a permanent implant. This implant consists of a surgically implanted electrode with four contact points (Pisces quad lead Model 3886, Medtronic Inc., Minneapolis, Minnesota, USA) connected to a pacemaker (Interstim stimulator, Medtronic Interstim, Tolchenau, Switzerland).

Implantation is performed under general anesthesia. After a midline incision over the sacrum, the fascia overlying the foramina at one side of the sacrum is opened, giving access to the foramen selected. Acute stimulation with a needle will be repeated in order to confirm the motoric responses. The permanent electrode is positioned in the foramen with the four contact points in the neighborhood of the sacral nerve. The electrode is fixed to the posterior wall of the sacral with nonresorbable sutures and passed subcutaneously to an incision in one of the flanks. After closure of the wounds, the patient is placed in a lateral position. A subcutaneous pocket is created lateral of the umbilicus. The flank wound is opened and the electrode is connected with the pulse generator using a connection cable that is passed subcutaneously to an abdominal pocket. The pacemaker is fixed to the rectus fascia. Recently an alternative technique has been presented in which a gluteal pocket is created to receive the pulse generator. This method has the advantage that the surgery can be performed in one position. Furthermore, morbidity, especially pain at the implant side, seems to be reduced.

Generally, low amplitudes (1.5 to 5.5 V, 210 μs pulse duration at 10 to 15 cycles/s) are sufficient for stimulation of the somatic nerve fibers. With these parameters, no dyssynergia of the bladder and striated urethral musculature is induced even when voiding is initiated with the stimulator on.

Previous reports indicate an overall success rate of 60–75% at initial trial stimulation.[15] Of the patients selected after subchronic trial stimulation who underwent permanent implantation, up to 83% have derived major benefit from the definitive procedure.[17] This effect appears to be durable, as evidenced by the late results. However, about 20% of patients who respond well on trial stimulation fail to reproduce the same result after chronic stimulation. Based on clinical parameters it appears that patients with detrusor overactivity and urethral instability have the best result.[18]

Recently, the results of a multinational, multicenter clinical trial of this method were presented.[19] In a group of 155 patients with therapy-resistant urge incontinence, 98 (63%) reacted sufficiently on the temporary trial stimulation. Of these, 38 were followed for 1 year with a successful outcome in 30 (79%).

Similar multicenter, multinational studies in patients with urgency/frequency and chronic voiding problems have been published with similar results.[20,21] Also, with long-term follow-up, results seem to be persistent over time.[22] However after permanent implantation about 20% of patients with initially favorable PNE test results fail to respond for yet unknown reasons. Further research to indicate additional parameters that may be used as reliable predictors of success is necessary.

Neuromodulation seems to be an effective treatment modality in patients with various forms of lower urinary tract dysfunction. This technique is a valuable addition to our treatment options when conservative measures fail.

References

1. Wein AJ, Raezer DM, Benson GS. Management of neurogenic bladder dysfunction in the adult. Urology 1976; 8:432–443.

2. Bradley WE, Timm GW, Chou SN. A decade of experience with electronic stimulation of the micturition reflex. Urol Int 1971; 26:283–302.

3. Godec C, Cass AS, Ayala GF. Electrical stimulation for incontinence. Technique, selection and results. Urology 1976; 7:388–397.

4. Merrill DC. The treatment of detrusor incontinence by electrical stimulation. J Urol 1979; 122:515–517.

5. Fall M. Does electrostimulation cure urinary incontinence? J Urol 1984; 131:664–667.

6. Katona F. Stages of vegetative afferentiation in reorganization of bladder control during intravesical electrotherapy. Urol Int 1975; 30:192–203.

7. Seiferth J, Heising J, Larkamp H. Experiences and critical comments on the temporary intravesical electrostimulation of neurogenic bladder in spina bifida children. Urol Int 1978; 33:279–284.

8. Madersbacher H, Pauer W, Reiner E. Rehabilitation of micturition by transurethral electrostimulation of the bladder in patients with incomplete spinal cord lesions. Paraplegia 1982; 20:191–195.

9. Caldwell KP, Flack FC, Broad AF. Urinary incontinence following spinal injury treated by electronic implant. Lancet 1965; 39:846–847.

10. Brindley GS, Polkey CE, Rushton DN, Cardozo L. Sacral anterior root stimulators for bladder control in paraplegia: the first 50 cases. J Neurol Neurosurg Psychiatry 1986; 49:1104–1114.

11. Tanagho EA, Schmidt RA, Orvis BR. Neural stimulation for control of voiding dysfunction: a preliminary report in 22 patients with serious neuropathic voiding disorders. J Urol 1989; 142:340–345.

12. Markland C, Merrill D, Chou S, Bradley W. Sacral nerve root stimulation: a clinical test of detrusor innervation. J Urol 1972; 107:772–776.

13. Schmidt RA. Advances in genitourinary neurostimulation. Neurosurgery 1986; 18:1041–1044.

14. Habib HN. Experiences and recent contributions in sacral nerve stimulation for both human and animal. Br J Urol 1967; 39:73–83.

15. Schmidt RA. Applications of neurostimulation in urology. Neurourol Urodyn 1988; 7:585.

16. Thon WF, Baskin LS, Jonas U, et al. Neuromodulation of voiding dysfunction and pelvic pain. World J Urol 1991; 9:38.

17. Bosch JLHR, Groen J. Sacral (S_3) segmental nerve stimulation as a treatment for urge incontinence in patients with detrusor instability: results of chronic electrical stimulation using an implantable neural prosthesis. J Urol 1995; 154:504–507.

18. Koldewijn EL, Rosier PF, Meuleman EJ, Koster AM, Debruyne FM, Van Kerrebroeck PE et al. Predictors of success with neuromodulation in lower urinary tract dysfunction: results of trial stimulation in 100 patients. J Urol 1994; 152:2071–2075.

19. Janknegt RA, Van Kerrebroeck PhEV, Lycklama à Nijeholt AA, et al. Sacral nervemodulation for urge incontinence: a multinational, multicenter randomized study. J Urol 1997; 157, 4:1237.

20. Hassouna MM, Siegel SW, Nyeholt AA, et al. Sacral neuromodulation in the treatment of urgency-frequency symptoms: a multicenter study on efficacy and safety. J Urol 2000; 163(6):1849–1854.

21. Jonas U, Fowler CJ, Chancellor MB, et al. Efficacy of sacral nerve stimulation for urinary retention: results 18 months after implantation. J Urol 2001; 165:15–19.

22. Bosch JL, Groen J. Sacral nerve neuromodulation in the treatment of patients with refractory motor urge incontinence: long-term results of a prospective longitudinal study. J Urol 2000; 163(4):1219–1222.

51

Intravesical electrical stimulation of the bladder

Helmut G Madersbacher

Background

Already in 1887 the Danish surgeon Saxtorph[1] described intravesical electrical stimulation (IVES) for the 'atonic bladder' by inserting a transurethral catheter with a metal stylet in it and with a neutral electrode on the lower abdomen. In 1899 two Viennese surgeons, Frankl-Hochwart and Zuckerkandl,[2] stated that intravesical electrotherapy was more effective in inducing detrusor contractions than external faradization. In 1975 Katona[3] introduced this method for the treatment of neurogenic bladder dysfunction. Ebner et al[4] demonstrated in cat experiments that intravesical electrostimulation activates the mechanoreceptors within the bladder wall.

Further basic research was undertaken by Jiang et al,[5] who demonstrated that IVES at low frequencies ($\geqslant 20$ Hz) had a better modulatory effect than at higher frequencies. Jiang[6] proved in the animal experiment that IVES induced modulation of the micturition reflex due to an enhanced excitatory synaptic transmission in the central micturition reflex pathway. The observed modulation may account for the clinical benefit of IVES treatment.

The afferent stimuli induced by IVES travel along afferent pathways from the lower urinary tract to the corresponding cerebral structures. This 'vegetative afferention'[3] results in the sensation of bladder filling/urge to void, with subsequent enhancement of active contractions and possibly also voluntary control over the detrusor (Figure 51.1).

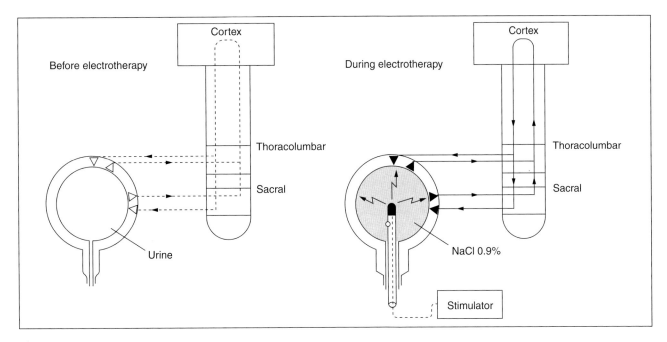

Figure 51.1
Intravesical electrostimulation activates the mechanoreceptors within the bladder wall, thus increasing the efferent input from the bladder and consequently the efferent output to the bladder. (Reproduced with permission from Ebner et al.[4])

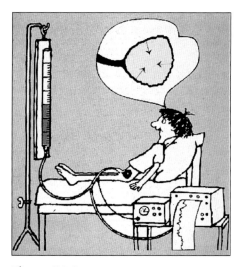

Figure 51.2
With intravesical electrostimulation a feedback training is mediated by enabling the patient to observe the change of the detrusor pressure on a water manometer: the patient is able to realize when a detrusor contraction takes place.

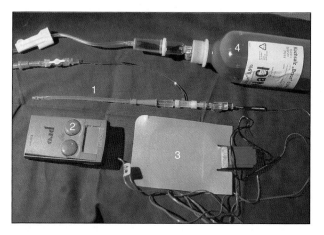

Figure 51.3
IVES armamentarium: 1, Disposable catheter with the electrode in it; 2, battery-operated stimulator; 3, neutral electrode; 4, saline (0.9%).

Colombo et al[7] demonstrated that intravesical electrostimulation also induces electrical changes on higher micturition centers, measured by electroencephalography (EEG). The evaluation of viscerosensory cortical evoked potentials after transurethral electrical stimulation has been proved to be useful in determining whether a patient is suitable for IVES or not.[8]

A feedback training is mediated by enabling the patient to observe the change of the detrusor pressure on a water manometer; thus the patient is able to realize when a detrusor contraction takes place. This also facilitates voluntary control (Figure 51.2).

Various synonyms were used in the literature for intravesical electrical stimulation, such as bladder stimulation, intravesical bladder stimulation, transurethral electrostimulation of the bladder, and intravesical, transurethral bladder stimulation.

Technique

The technique involves a catheter, with a stimulation electrode (cathode) in it, being introduced into the bladder and connected to a stimulator. Saline (0.9%) is used as the current leading medium within the bladder. The anode (neutral) electrode (14 × 9 cm) is attached to the skin in an area with preserved sensation, usually in the lower abdomen (Figure 51.3). According to Ebner et al[4] the following stimulation parameters have proved to be most effective in the animal experiment: pulse width, 2 ms; frequency, 20 Hz; and current, 1–10 mA. Some researchers use square unipolar pulses for continuous stimulation,[9]

whereas others use intermittent stimulation with bursts and gaps that can be varied (1–10 s) along with the rise time and the time of the plateau within the burst. With intermittent electrostimulation, each therapy session takes 60–90 min, with continuous stimulation 20 min, on a daily basis, 5 days a week, until the maximum response is reached. For patients who have never experienced the urge to void – e.g. children with myelomeningocele or children who have lost this ability – IVES is combined with a biofeedback training: on a water manometer attached to the system the patient is able to observe the change in the detrusor pressure. This way he is able to realize that the sensation experienced is caused by a bladder contraction. This external feedback also facilitates achievement of voluntary control.

Results

The results presented are based on 31 studies: 6 are basic research papers (animal experiments and clinical research), one is a randomized controlled trial, there are 2 reviews within an editorial, one pro and one contra IVES, and the others are case series.

Intravesical electrical stimulation of the bladder is still a controversial therapy for patients with neurogenic detrusor dysfunction, although basic research during the last decade has evidenced the mechanism of its action and its efficacy.[4,6] At least, in animal experiments, optimal parameters have been determined.[4,10]

The controversy about the value of IVES for detrusor (re-)habilitation is also reflected in an editorial recently published, in which Kaplan[11] reported favorable results in 288 children who received at least one series (20 outpatient sessions, 90 min long): 87% of patients have control and void or catheterize with sensation or have improved bladder compliance. Eighteen percent have gained full control, they void synergistically and are continent, whereas before they were either voiding poorly and incontinent or used clean intermittent catherization and were more or less dry. Forty-four percent void with sensation and are in biofeedback to try and gain control. Finally, in 13% the treatment failed, but the patients maintained their condition. Moreover, the results seen in an 'early' group were followed up 10 years later. As long as no intervening neurosurgical insult occurred, less than 3% of cases needed to return for a tune-up to maintain their 'healthy bladder'. The average number of daily sessions to achieve these results was 47.

In contrast, the results reported by Decter[12] were less favorable. In 25 patients during a 5-year period with, all together, 938 sessions of stimulation, bladder capacity increased greater than 20% in regards to the age-adjusted and end-filling bladder pressure and showed clinically significant decreases in 28% of patients. In response to a questionnaire, 56% of parents noted a subjective improvement in their childrens' bladder function. However, the urodynamic improvements achieved after IVES did not significantly alter the daily voiding routine in these children.[13]

The only randomized controlled prospective clinical trial[14] could not find differences between active and sham treatment; however, only 15 sessions were performed at first and another 15 sessions of IVES were applied after a 3-month hiatus. Moreover, the inclusion criteria were not defined.

Other studies are either individual case-controlled studies (*Level of evidence 3B*) or case series (*Level of evidence 4*). They cannot be compared due to different or non-defined inclusion criteria, different technique details (different time of electrostimulation, varying follow-ups), and some with only a small number of patients included.[15–31] Recently, Gladh[9] presented the results of 44 children (mean age 10.5 years), 20 of them with neurogenic bladder dysfunction: with a mean follow-up of 2.5 years, 64% had their bladder emptying normalized, 11 of 15 children on clean intermittent catheterization (CIC) have terminated catheterization, 8 of them with neurogenic bladder dysfunction; 7 children had no remaining benefit of the treatment.

Prerequisites for successful intravesical electrical stimulation

None of the research really focused on the inclusion criteria. According to the basic research, only those with some intact afferent fibers from the bladder to the cortex and those with spinal cord lesions with the presence of pain sensation in the sacral dermatomes S3 and S4 can benefit from IVES. According to Nathan and Smith,[32] the pathways of the bladder proprioception and for pain lie close together. The value of viscerosensoric cortical evoked potentials from the bladder neck was demonstrated by Kiss et al.[8] A precise indication seems to be one prerequisite for a good result. Regarding children with myelomeningocele, one must also take into account that myelomeningocele bladders at birth may have a threefold increase in connective tissue compared to normal controls.[33] According to clinical experience, significant decrease of receptors tempers the enthusiasm for intravesical electrical stimulation in this particular group of patients.

Implications for practice

Basically, intravesical electrotherapy is able to improve neurogenic bladder dysfunction, primarily by stimulating $A\delta$ mechanoafferents inducing bladder sensation and the urge to void and consequently increasing the efferent output with improvement of micturition and conscious control. Therefore, IVES is the only available option to induce/improve bladder sensation and to enhance the micturition reflex in incomplete central or peripheral nerve damage. However, proper indication is crucial and this type of therapy should only be applied in those with intact afferent fibers between the bladder and the cortex if possible, proved by the evaluation of viscerosensoric cortical evoked potentials. *If these premises are respected, IVES is effective.*

Intravesical electrical stimulation is *safe*; no side-effects have been reported, beyond an occasional urinary infection. The question of cost-effectiveness was raised by Kaplan,[11] who stated that the most commonly used alternative for these patients is bladder augmentation, which is 'miles apart in terms of cost, discomfort and short- and long-term complications'.

One benefit of IVES was noted by most of the authors: improved sensation documents satisfactory long-term results. The patients with successful IVES get great satisfaction from knowing when their bladder is full and when it is time to catheterize or to void. Moreover, even without direct bowel stimulation, patients noted significant improvement in the warning of bowel fullness and gained greater control for their bowel movements.

IVES can only be effective with certain prerequisites, the most important being that at least some afferent fibers between the bladder and the CNS are intact and the detrusor is able to contract. The method is safe, and no real complications have been reported.

Conclusions

- Basic research during the last decade has proved the underlying working concept.
- The results reported in the literature are controversial, mainly because of different inclusion and exclusion criteria.
- In the only sham-controlled study the treatment period is too short and the inclusion and exclusion criteria are not really defined.
- The alternative may be either life long intermittent catheterization or bladder augmentation. In this regards, IVES is *cost-effective*.
- It is worthwhile to apply intravesical electrostimulation, bearing in mind inclusion and exclusion criteria, especially when trying to verify functioning afferent fibers between the bladder and the cortex.

Recommendations

- Intravesical electrotherapy is able to improve neurogenic bladder dysfunction, primarily by stimulating Aδ mechanoreceptor afferents inducing bladder sensation and the urge to void and consequently increasing the efferent output with improvement of micturition and conscious control.
- IVES is the only available option to induce/improve bladder sensation and to enhance the micturition reflex in patients with incomplete central or peripheral nerve damage.
- Indication is crucial and IVES should only be applied if afferent fibers between the bladder and the cortex are still intact and if the detrusor muscle is still able to contract.
- *If these premises are respected, IVES is effective.*
- The ideal indication is the neuropathic underactive – hyposensitive and hypocontracile – detrusor.

Further research

There is definitely a need for placebo-(sham-)controlled prospective studies with clear inclusion and exclusion criteria and clear definitions of the aims. Recently De Wachter and Wyndaele[34] demonstrated in animal experiments and models that the position of the stimulating electrode, as well as the amount of saline within the bladder, may be crucial for the effect. Additional research is needed to clarify these aspects of IVES.

References

1. Saxtorph MH. Stricture urethrae – fistula perinee – retentio urinae. Clinisk Chirurgi. Copenhagen: Gyldendalske Fortlag 1878:265–280.

2. Frankel vL, Zuckerkandl O. In: Hrsg. H Senator, Die erkrankungen der blase. Wien: Alfred Höbler Verlag, 1899:101.

3. Katona F. Stages of vegetative afferentiation in reorganization of bladder control during electrotherapy. Urol Int 1975; 30:192–203.

4. Ebner A, Jiang CH, Lindström S. Intravesical electrical stimulation – an experimental analysis of the mechanism of action. J Urol 1992; 148:920–924.

5. Jiang CH, Lindström S, Mazières L. Segmental inhibitory control of ascending sensory information from bladder mechanoreceptors in cat. Neurourol Urodyn 1991; 10:286–288.

6. Jiang CH. Modulation of the micturition reflex pathway by intravesical electrical stimulation: an experimental study in the rat. Neurourol Urodyn 1998; 17(5):543–553.

7. Colombo T, Wieselmann G, Pichler-Zalaudek K, et al. Central nervous system control of micturition in patients with bladder dysfunctions in comparison with healthy control probands. An electrophysiological study. Urologe A 2000; 39(2):160–165.

8. Kiss G, Madersbacher H, Poewe W. Cortical evoked potentials of the vesicourethral junction – a predictor for the outcome of intravesical electrostimulation in patients with sensory and motor detrusor dysfunction. World J Urol 1998; 16(5):308–312.

9. Gladh G. Intravesical electrical stimulation in children with micturition dysfunction. Proc ICS 2002, Heidelberg, 2002: 22. [Abstract]

10. Buyle S, Wyndaele JJ, D'Hauwers K, et al. Optimal parameters for transurethral intravesical electrostimulation determined in an experiment in the rat. Eur Urol 1998; 33(5):507–510.

11. Kaplan WE. Intravesical electrical stimulation of the bladder: Pro. Editorial. Urology 2000; 56(1):2–4.

12. Decter RM. Intravesical electrical stimulation of the bladder: Contra. Editorial. Urology 2000; 56(1):2–4.

13. Decter RM, Snyder P, Laudermilch C. Transurethral electrical bladder stimulation: a follow-up report. J Urol 1994; 152:812–814.

14. Boone TB, Roehrborn CG, Hurt G. Transurethral intravesical electrotherapy for neurogenic bladder dysfunction in children with myelodysplasia: a prospective, randomized clinical trial. J Urol 1992; 148:550–554.

15. Eckstein HG, Katona F. Treatment of neuropathic bladder by transurethral electrical stimulation. Lancet 1974; 1:780–781.

16. Nicholas JL, Eckstein HB. Endovesical electrotherapy in treatment of urinary incontinence in spina bifida patients. Lancet 1975; 2:1276–1277.

17. Denes J, Leb J. Electrostimulation of the neuropathic bladder. J Pediatr Surg 1975; 10(2):245–247.

18. Janneck C. Electric stimulation of the bladder and the anal sphincter – a new way to treat the neurogenic bladder. Prog Pediatr Surg 1976; 9:119–139.

19. Seiferth J, Heising J, Larkamp H. Intravesical electrostimulation of the neurogenic bladder in spina bifida children. Urol Int 1978; 33(5):279–284.

20. Seiferth J, Larkamp H, Heising J. Experiences with temporary intravesical electro-stimulation of the neurogenic bladder in spina bifida children. Urologe A 1978; 17(5):353–354.

21. Schwock G, Tischer W. The influence of intravesical electrostimulation on the urinary bladder in animals. Z Kinderchir 1981; 32(2): 161–166.

22. Madersbacher H, Pauer W, Reiner E, et al. Rehabilitation of micturition in patients with incomplete spinal cord lesions by transurethral electrostimulation of the bladder. Eur Urol 1982; 8:111–116.

23. Kaplan WE, Richards I. Intravesical bladder stimulation in myelodysplasia. J Urol 1988; 140:1282–1284.

24. Madersbacher H. Intravesical electrical stimulation for the rehabilitation of the neuropathic bladder. Paraplegia 1990; 28:349–352.

25. Lyne CJ, Bellinger MF. Early experience with transurethral electrical bladder stimulation. J Urol 1993; 150:697–699.

26. Kölle D, Madersbacher H, Kiss G, Mair D. Intravesical electrostimulation for treatment of bladder dysfunction. Initial experience after gynecological operations. Gynakol Geburtshilfliche Rundsch 1995; 35(4):221–225.

27. Cheng EY, Richards I, Kaplan WE. Use of bladder stimulation in high risk patients. J Urol 1996; 156:479–752.

28. Cheng EY, Richards I, Balcom A, et al. Bladder stimulation therapy improves bladder compliance: results from a multi-institutional trial. J Urol 1996; 156:761–764.

29. Primus G, Trummer H. Intravesical electrostimulation in detrusor hypocontractility. Wien Klin Wochensch 1993; 105(19):556–557.

30. Kroll P, Jankowski A, Martynski M. Electrostimulation in treatment of neurogenic and non-neurogenic voiding dysfunction. Wiad Lek 1998; 51(Suppl 3):92–97.

31. Pugach JL, Salvin L, Steinhardt GF. Intravesical electrostimulation in pediatric patients with spinal cord defects. J Urol 2000; 164:965–968.

32. Nathan PW, Smith MC. The centripetal pathway from the bladder and urethra within the spinal cord. J Neurol Neurosurg Psychiatry 1951; 14:262–280.

33. Shapiro E, Becich MJ, Perlman E, Lepor H. Bladder wall abnormalities in myelodysplastic bladders: a computer assisted morphometric analysis. J Urol 1991; 145(5):1024–1029.

34. De Wachter S, Wyndaele JJ. Personal Communication, 2001.

52

Surgery to improve reservoir function

Manfred Stöhrer

Introduction

Compensated bladder storage is a function that is decisive for the quality of life and life expectancy of patients with neurogenic lower urinary tract dysfunction. It is characterized by low-pressure storage with physiological storage pressure as the maximum value. Storage pressure does not increase significantly before filling volume reaches 300 ml. The volume at which this pressure increase occurs is defined as the reflex volume.[1] Continence is better and the pressure load on the upper urinary tract is lower when the reflex volume is higher. When this condition cannot be achieved by medical treatment, a number of surgical interventions are available. Electrical stimulation and intestinal replacement are described elsewhere. The surgical procedures outlined here are effective for the majority of patients and are minimally invasive.

Two prerequisites are fundamental: intact detrusor musculature (no fibrosis) and satisfactory management of bladder emptying, preferably by intermittent catheterization. Should detrusor elasticity be impaired by morphologic conditions, (partial) bladder replacement is the only option. These changes, caused by tissue scarring, are the result of 'mismanagement' over several years. When the patient is treated correctly, this pathology will seldom occur.

In principle, to normalize the detrusor muscle its nervous supply can be altered by chemical receptor blockers, such as botulinum A toxin, which is the simplest and most promising method of ensuring compensated storage.[2,3]

For non-responders or when the effect is unsatisfactory, detrusor myectomy (partial auto-augmentation) is a possible alternative.[4,5] Some authors have expanded this simple intervention, with the use of omentum or gastrointestinal components to cover the mucosa at the site of the muscular defect after surgery.[6–9]

Should these procedures fail, clam cystoplasty offers a compromise before embarking on extensive enterocystoplasty.[10] All three methods can help patients with both complete or incomplete lesions.

Available for high and complete lesions, deafferentation by transection of the S2–S4 vertebral roots is an additional procedure to completely block detrusor overactivity.[11] In these cases, alternative emptying (preferably by intermittent catheterization) is necessary too, unless sacral root electrostimulation is applied.[12,13]

Table 52.1 presents an overview of the surgical options that could improve storage function in patients with neurogenic detrusor overactivity.

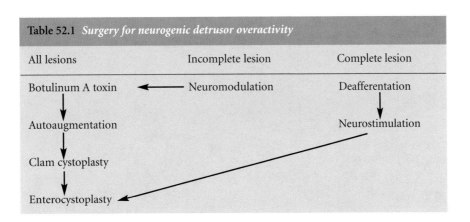

Table 52.1 *Surgery for neurogenic detrusor overactivity*

All lesions	Incomplete lesion	Complete lesion
Botulinum A toxin	← Neuromodulation	Deafferentation
Autoaugmentation		Neurostimulation
Clam cystoplasty		
Enterocystoplasty		

Botulinum A toxin injections in the detrusor

Botulinum A toxin has been known for many years to be not only one of the most potent venoms but also a very effective drug for the suppression of chronic muscular spasticity. It has been applied since 1980 to spastic striated muscles in many neurologic and orthopedic domains.[14,15] Aesthetic plastic surgeons use it much more extensively.[16] In urology, it was injected initially in the external sphincter to treat detrusor-sphincter dyssynergia.[17] In 1998, detrusor injections were given to patients with neurogenic lower urinary tract dysfunction in Germany and Switzerland. The first results were published in 1999.[2,3]

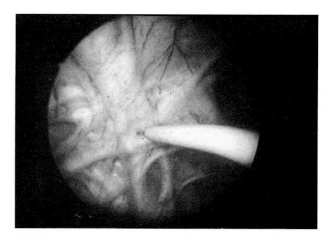

Figure 52.1
Botulinum A toxin injection in detrusor trabecule.

Mode of action

Botulinum toxin has several subtypes. Subtype A is the most effective, and the only one that is available commercially: a product of *Clostridium botulinum*, it is a strong natural venom. The molecule is composed of light and heavy nucleic acid chains connected by a disulfide ring. It blocks presynaptic nerve endings at the cholinergic neuron and prevents acetylcholine secretion, leading to temporary chemical denervation and loss of nerve activity in the target organ. The process is reversible by nerve regeneration, as new nerve endings will sprout from the neuron and reconstitute connections to the target organ. The time course of this process is dependent on the target organ type and is individually variable; it takes roughly between 3 and 4 months in the urethral sphincter, and 6–14 months in the detrusor. The average efficacy period in patients studied after detrusor injection is 10–12 months. Maximal efficacy is observed after about 2 weeks, remains pronounced until about 3 months after the injection, and then subsides slowly and continually.

Two varieties of botulinum A toxin are available: Botox® and Dysport®. The efficacy ratio between these two products is about 1:3. Dysport demonstrates greater dispersion. It thus appears rational to use a lower dilution to avoid its dispersion into the circulation. This mechanism may explain the isolated cases of generalized muscle weakness described in the literature.[18] We have not observed this effect in our patients who have been treated with Botox®.

Indication

Botulinum A toxin injections into the detrusor are indicated when anticholinergic medication is not effective or not tolerated. As this procedure is the least invasive of all available options in these cases, it should be the method of first choice when conservative treatment fails.

Its fundamental prerequisite is an effective bladder emptying after the treatment. Our experience shows that aseptic intermittent catheterization is preferred. When the detrusor overactivity is enhanced by acute urinary tract infection, the action of the toxin is insufficient to suppress it, and episodes of reflex incontinence may occur.

Method of application

Botox 300 IU (or Dysport 750–1000 IU) are given for the treatment of neurogenic detrusor overactivity. The agent is dissolved in 15 ml saline and injected in 0.5 ml aliquots through a standard endoscopic needle (30 injection sites) over the entire muscle. For children, the dosage is reduced in relation to body weight. The injections are administered preferably in visible muscular structures (trabecules) (Figure 52.1). The trigone and ureteric orifices are spared to prevent possible reflux. Thus, 10 IU Botox are injected at each site. An indwelling catheter is placed for 24 h. Antibiotic prophylaxis is started preoperatively and continued for 1 week. After removal of the indwelling catheter the patient practices intermittent catheterization – most patients adopt this routine before treatment. Peroperative anticholinergic treatment is continued during the first postoperative week and then discontinued completely.

Results

In our center, 141 patients were treated from early 1998 until October 2002: 222 treatment sessions were performed, including multiple treatments. The underlying condition was traumatic spinal cord lesion in the majority of patients, with small groups suffering from multiple sclerosis or myelomeningocele. Patients with low bladder compliance caused by structural changes in the detrusor wall (fibrosis) secondary to neurological disease were excluded from this treatment. Patients at risk from autonomic dysreflexia or who preserved their bladder sensation were treated under local or general anesthesia.

The condition of these patients and of those who were evaluated in cooperation with the center in Zurich was checked by videourodynamics preoperatively and at 12 and 36 weeks postoperatively. The parameters studied were reflex volume, maximal voiding detrusor pressure, cystometric bladder capacity, detrusor compliance, and continence status (Figures 52.2–52.5). Patient satisfaction and the post-treatment dosage of anticholinergics were also recorded. Significant improvement of all parameters was achieved in nearly all patients (95%). Reflex volume and cystometric capacity showed considerable amelioration after 6 weeks and most responders (>90%) were continent, unless urinary tract infection was present. Spontaneous voiding was eliminated, and thus the residual

was equal to the capacity. Treatment was successful, even in children. The condition of many patients with pre-existing autonomic dysreflexia improved significantly. It was not known why 5% of patients did not respond to botulinum A toxin injections, although immunity caused against the toxin by the presence of antibodies after earlier contact with it might be one reason.

Blocked nerve endings regenerate slowly – after 36 weeks, the condition of patients had deteriorated in comparison to that at 6 weeks, but was still significantly better than preoperatively. The mean efficacy period in our patients was 10–12 months. These results have been confirmed in a European multicenter study comprising over 200 patients.

Repeated botulinum A treatment sessions did not result in any loss of efficacy. In our patients, 51 had two injection sessions, 21 had three, 6 had four, and 3 had five, and increased toxin tolerance was not found.

Botox or Dysport application led to essentially similar outcomes, but generalized muscle weakness was observed in three patients after Dysport application. As discussed above, dispersion and dilution could have been determining

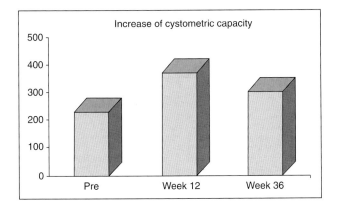

Figure 52.2
Increase of cystometric capacity at 12 and 36 weeks after botulinum treatment.

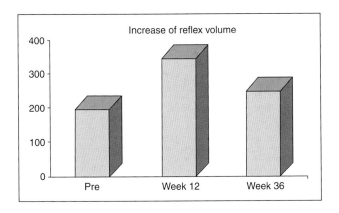

Figure 52.3
Increase of reflex volume at 12 and 36 weeks after botulinum treatment.

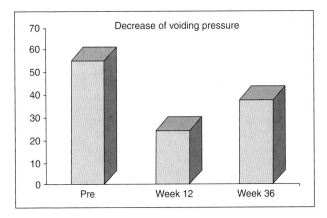

Figure 52.4
Decrease of voiding pressure at 12 and 36 weeks after botulinum treatment.

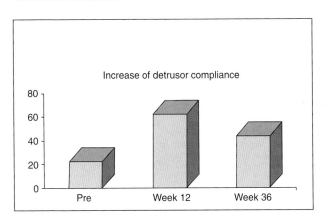

Figure 52.5
Increase of detrusor compliance at 12 and 36 weeks after botulinum treatment.

factors here; thus, we decided to reduce the dilution volume to 7.5 ml when using Dysport. Whether this will diminish or prevent the occurrence of these generalized adverse effects is still an open question.

In summary, detrusor injections of botulinum A toxin represent an effective treatment for neurogenic detrusor overactivity. Because this therapy has not been approved by the medical authorities in most countries, its use should be considered only with the appropriate precautions and documentation.

Recent literature

This procedure[2,3] has raised much interest since its introduction, but, apart from conference reports, the number of publications in the literature is still sparse. Its mechanism of action has been studied in rats[19] and preliminary trials have confirmed its efficacy also in myelomeningocele children.[20]

Partial detrusor myectomy (autoaugmentation)

The basis of this therapy is partial removal of the overactive detrusor without compromising the underlying mucosa. It decreases storage pressure and increases bladder capacity. The essential advantage of the procedure is its low invasivity and abstinence from covering the defect with intestinal tissue sections. This option remains available when later, more invasive procedures might become necessary.

Indication

Aggressive detrusor overactivity that is refractory to conservative treatment and that also does not respond to botulinum A toxin can be corrected by autoaugmentation. After this treatment, intermittent catheterization is compulsory. The functional transformation caused by the procedure needs time to be expressed. This period is at least 1 year, and the procedure is contraindicated if enough time is not available due to the patient's condition. Degenerative changes in the detrusor musculature, causing a reduction of anesthetic bladder capacity, are also a contraindication.

Method

The bladder anterior wall and dome are approached, and the peritoneum is freed from the bladder until about halfway down the bladder posterior wall. The bladder is filled to about 200 ml, and a circular section of the detrusor muscle with a radius of about 4 cm around the urachus is resected. The mucosa is left intact (Figures 52.6 and 52.7). The diverticulum created in this way will reduce storage pressure and improve bladder capacity after a period of 1–2 years. An indwelling catheter is left for 2 days when the mucosa has not been perforated during the procedure. When mucosal perforation has occurred, the indwelling catheter is placed for a maximum of 2 weeks and is clamped intermittently for 3–4 days, putting a low-grade load on the diverticulum.[5,21] In a few patients, ancillary injection with botulinum A toxin to accelerate the process of functional transformation has recently shown partial success.

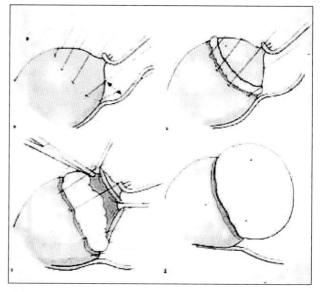

Figure 52.6
The autoaugmentation procedure (side view).

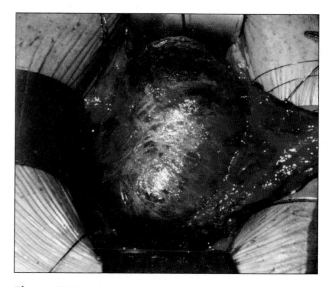

Figure 52.7
Surgical view during autoaugmentation procedure.

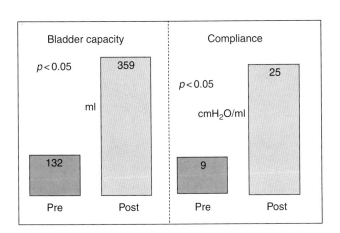

Figure 52.8
Bladder capacity and detrusor compliance after autoaugmentation.

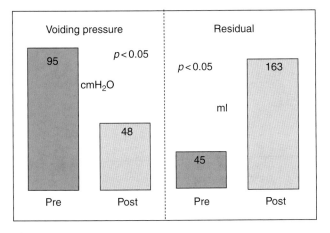

Figure 52.9
Voiding pressure and residual after autoaugmentation.

In 1989, Cartwright and Snow published a paper on a similar procedure in dogs and in a child.[4] Also in 1989, we performed this for the first time in a man with an incomplete spinal cord lesion. Cartwright and Snow attached the bladder to the iliopsoas, whereas we only do the simple resection. This simpler approach produces good results. The peritoneum remains closed, and covering of the defect is unnecessary.[5,21]

Results

From 1989 to October 2002 we treated 93 patients by this method. After the introduction of botulinum A toxin injections for the same indication, the number of autoaugmentations declined considerably, but nonresponders to botulinum A toxin are good candidates for autoaugmentation. The efficacy of this procedure has been documented by videourodynamics, preoperatively, 6–12 weeks and 1 year postoperatively, and at 1–2 year intervals thereafter. Its outcome parameters are improvement of incontinence, bladder compliance, maximum detrusor pressure during voiding, cystometric capacity, residual urine, reduced use of anticholinergics, and patient satisfaction. All parameters are significantly ameliorated after a mean follow-up period of over $6^{1}/_{2}$ years in about two-thirds of patients (Figures 52.8 and 52.9). Patients who have been lost to follow-up are rated as nonresponders. The patient population consists mainly of complete and incomplete spinal cord lesions, plus multiple sclerosis and myelomeningocele. The interval between surgery and a satisfactorily improved functional condition was 3 months to 2 years (Figures 52.10 and 52.11). One woman who

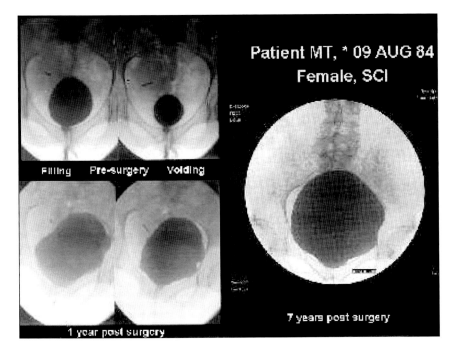

Figure 52.10
X-ray views of female patient pre, and 1 and 7 years post autoaugmentation.

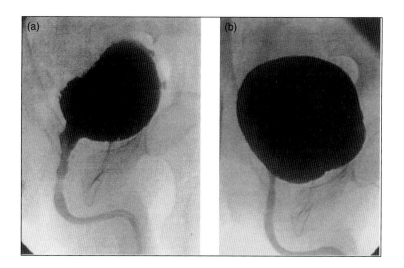

Figure 52.11
X-ray views of male patient pre (a)
and 5 months after (b) autoaugmentation.

received an artificial sphincter after autoaugmentation and thus lost the opportunity for overflow incontinence suffered a bladder rupture at 600 ml capacity. Her condition was resolved by surgery without any sequelae. Four patients submitted to further procedures with intestinal replacement.

It is of the utmost importance to realize that functional improvement does not occur immediately after treatment, but may take a long time. One of our patients had already elected for intestinal augmentation but after 2 years a positive result was obtained. Published modifications of the method, including covering the defect with omentum or intestinal sections, have not produced better outcomes. One major advantage of this uncomplicated procedure is that the peritoneum is not opened. Based on my 13 years of experience, I thus see no need to change it.

Recent literature

In a review comparing enterocystoplasty and detrusor myectomy,[22] it is stated that: 'For most clinical indications detrusor myectomy has offered comparable success or significant improvement in bladder function without incurring the significant complication rate of enterocystoplasty.' Another review[23] attests that: 'The principle of urothelial preservation, introduced by autoaugmentation, is very promising in the effort to create a compliant urinary reservoir without metabolic disturbance and without the risk of cancer.' In a review comparing Ingelman–Sundberg bladder denervation, detrusor myectomy, and augmentation cystoplasty,[24] it is argued that augmentation cystoplasty has the highest success rate but a 'much higher likelihood of early and late post-operative complications' and, thus, the less invasive methods should be favored if feasible. Two long-term follow-up studies on children[25,26] underscore the contraindication of hypertonic/poorly compliant bladders.

In this author's view, the use of backing tissue to cover the detrusor defect[26–28] does not contribute to improvement of the clinical result. The procedure, as presented in this chapter, offers fast repair of – nearly inevitable – mucosal perforations. This is probably the reason why a laparoscopic access for this surgery has not become established.[29,30]

Clam cystoplasty

This relatively simple bladder augmentation with only slight per-operative risks inserts an intestinal segment in the bladder defect that is made by incision of the posterior bladder wall.[10] The results so far are good,[31,32] but the procedure is far more invasive than autoaugmentation and might induce late complications from bowel use.

S2–S4 Deafferentation

Another option to achieve a low-pressure bladder without intestinal patches is the transection of the S2–S4 roots on both sides. Unlike the methods described above, this procedure is indicated only in patients with complete spinal cord lesions. The transection causes complete detrusor acontractility – the bladder must be emptied by intermittent catheterization. As many of these patients have high-level lesions, the required dexterity is often unavailable. In those cases, combination with sacral electrostimulation (e.g. Brindley stimulator) is feasible, as the stimulator can be operated quite easily.[12] Improvement of the technique might enhance the quality of stimulated voiding.[33] Deafferentation is also an option for patients with pronounced spasticity who are able to handle intermittent catheterization. Patients must be informed about the adverse effects on their sexual functions (demise of lubrification, loss of reflex erection).

Conclusion

The procedures described in this chapter are sufficient to achieve compensated storage in the vast majority of patients. More complicated interventions, necessary for nonresponders, are described in other chapters of this book.

References

1. Stöhrer M, Goepel M, Kondo A, et al. The standardization of terminology in neurogenic lower urinary tract dysfunction with suggestions for diagnostic procedures. Neurourol Urodyn 1999; 18:139–158.

2. Stöhrer M, Schurch B, Kramer G, et al. Botulinum-A toxin in the treatment of detrusor hyperreflexia in spinal cord injury: a new alternative to medical and surgical procedures? Neurourol Urodyn 1999; 18:401–402.

3. Schurch B, Stöhrer M, Kramer G, et al. Botulinum A-toxin for treating detrusor hyperreflexia in spinal cord injured patients: a new alternative to anticholinergic drugs? Preliminary results. J Urol 2000; 164:692–697.

4. Cartwright PC, Snow BW. Bladder auto-augmentation: early clinical experience. J Urol 1989; 142:505–508.

5. Stöhrer M, Kramer G, Goepel M, et al. Bladder autoaugmentation in adult patients with neurogenic voiding dysfunction. Spinal Cord 1997; 35:456–462.

6. Dewan PA, Stefanek W. Autoaugmentation gastrocystoplasty: early clinical results. Br J Urol 1994, 74:460–464.

7. Nguyen DH, Mitchell ME, Horowitz M, et al. Demucosalized augmentation gastrocystoplasty with bladder autoaugmentation in pediatric patients. J Urol 1996; 156:206–209.

8. Carr MC, Docimo SG, Mitchell ME. Bladder augmentation with urothelial preservation. J Urol 1999; 162:1133–1136.

9. Perovic SV, Djordjevic ML, Kekic ZK, Vukadinovic VM. Bladder autoaugmentation with rectus muscle backing. J Urol 2002; 168:1877–1880.

10. Mast P, Hoebeke P, Wyndaele JJ, et al. Experience with augmentation cystoplasty. A review. Paraplegia 1995; 33:560–564.

11. Diokno AC, Vinson RK, McGillicuddy J. Treatment of the severe uninhibited neurogenic bladder by selective sacral rhizotomy. J Urol 1977; 118:299–301.

12. Sauerwein HD. The use of nerve deafferentation and stimulation in the paraplegic female patient. In: Raz S, ed. Female urology. Philadelphia: WB Saunders, 1996: 656–664.

13. Van Kerrebroeck PE, Koldewijn EL, Debruyne FM. Worldwide experience with the Finetech–Brindley sacral anterior root stimulator. Neurourol Urodyn 1993; 12:497–503.

14. National Institutes of Health. Clinical use of botulinum toxin. National Institutes of Health Consensus Development Conference Statement, Nov. 12–14, 1990. Arch Neurol 1991; 48:1294–1298.

15. Jankovic J, Schwartz KS. Longitudinal experience with botulinum toxin injections for treatment of blepharospasm and cervical dystonia. Neurology 1993; 43:834–836.

16. Bulstrode NW, Grobbelaar AO. Long-term prospective follow-up of botulinum toxin treatment for facial rhytides. Aesthetic Plast Surg 2002; 26:356–359.

17. Schurch B, Hauri D, Rodic B, et al. Botulinum-A toxin as a treatment of detrusor-sphincter dyssynergia: a prospective study in 24 spinal cord injury patients. J Urol 1996; 155:1023–1029.

18. Wyndaele JJ, Van Dromme SA. Muscular weakness as side effect of botulinum toxin injection for neurogenic detrusor overactivity. Spinal Cord 2002; 40:599–600.

19. Smith CP, Somogyi GT, Chancellor AM. Emerging role of botulinum toxin in the treatment of neurogenic and non-neurogenic voiding dysfunction. Curr Urol Rep 2002; 3:382–387.

20. Schulte-Baukloh H, Michael T, Schobert J, et al. Efficacy of botulinum-A toxin in children with detrusor hyperreflexia due to myelomeningocele: preliminary results. Urology 2002; 59: 325–327.

21. Stöhrer M, Kramer A, Goepel M, et al. Bladder auto-augmentation – an alternative for enterocystoplasty: preliminary results. Neurourol Urodyn 1995; 14:11–23.

22. Leng WW, Blalock HJ, Fredriksson WH, et al. Enterocystoplasty or detrusor myectomy? Comparison of indications and outcomes for bladder augmentation. J Urol 1999; 161:758–763.

23. Cranidis A, Nestoridis G. Bladder augmentation. Int Urogynecol J Pelvic Floor Dysfunct 2000; 11:33–40.

24. Westney OL, McGuire EJ. Surgical procedures for the treatment of urge incontinence. Tech Urol 2001; 7:126–132.

25. Marte A, Di Meglio D, Cotrufo AM, et al. A long-term follow-up of autoaugmentation in myelodysplastic children. BJU Int 2002; 89:928–931.

26. Carr MC, Docimo SG, Mitchell ME. Bladder augmentation with urothelial preservation. J Urol 1999; 162:1133–1136.

27. Oge O, Tekgul S, Ergen A, Kendi S. Urothelium-preserving augmentation cystoplasty covered with a peritoneal flap. BJU Int 2000; 85:802–805.

28. Perovic SV, Djordjevic ML, Kekic ZK, Vukadinovic VM. Bladder autoaugmentation with rectus muscle backing. J Urol 2002; 168:1877–1880.

29. McDougall EM, Clayman RV, Figenshau RS, Pearle MS. Laparoscopic retropubic auto-augmentation of the bladder. J Urol 1995; 153:123–126.

30. Siracusano S, Trombetta C, Liguori G, et al. Laparoscopic bladder auto-augmentation in an incomplete traumatic spinal cord injury. Spinal Cord 2000; 38:59–61.

31. Chartier-Kastler EJ, Mongiat-Artus P, Bitker MO, et al. Long-term results of augmentation cystoplasty in spinal cord injured patients. Spinal Cord 2000; 38:490–494.

32. Arikan N, Turkolmez K, Budak M, Gogus O. Outcome of augmentation sigmoidoplasty in children with neurogenic bladder. Urol Int 2000; 64:82–85.

33. Schumacher S, Bross S, Scheepe JR, et al. Restoration of bladder function in spastic neuropathic bladder using sacral deafferentation and different techniques of neurostimulation. Adv Exp Med Biol 1999; 462:303–309.

53

Surgery to improve bladder outlet function

Gina Defreitas and Philippe Zimmern

Introduction

The bladder outlet in patients with neurogenic voiding dysfunction is subject to two main abnormalities: outlet underactivity, leading to urine leakage with increased intra-abdominal pressure; nonrelaxing urethral sphincter obstruction, resulting in reduced urine flow at the time of bladder emptying.[1] This chapter is therefore divided into two sections: surgical treatment of the underactive or incompetent bladder outlet and surgical treatment of the nonrelaxing or hyperactive bladder outlet (detrusor-sphincter dyssynergia or DSD). Procedures currently used to alleviate sphincteric deficiency in the neurogenic bladder population are injection of urethral bulking agents, slings, artificial urethral sphincters, bladder neck reconstruction procedures, and bladder neck closure. The surgical options currently available for the treatment of intractable DSD are sphincterotomy, insertion of a temporary or permanent urethral stent, balloon dilatation of the external sphincter, and use of a chronic indwelling catheter. The choice of surgical treatment depends on a number of factors, the most important of which are sex of the patient, the patient's comorbidities and functional status, the severity of urine leakage, whether or not the patient has had previous anti-incontinence procedures, patient and caregiver preferences, and, last but not least, the experience and expertise of the surgeon.

This chapter will focus on indications, surgical techniques, results, and complications of the various treatment options currently employed to treat bladder outlet pathology in the neurogenic bladder population. Literature dealing with the use of these surgical procedures in patients with non-neurogenic voiding dysfunction will not be discussed. Definitions and urodynamic terminology will conform to the recommendations published in the most recent report of the standardization sub-committee of the International Continence Society.[1]

Surgical management of the incompetent bladder outlet

Urethral bulking agents

Introduction

The first use of an injectable substance to treat urinary incontinence dates back to 1938 when Murless instilled sodium murrhate into the anterior vaginal wall.[1] Since then, a number of advancements have been made in agent composition, patient selection, and injection technique. Agents that have been employed for urethral injection include autologous fat, polytetrafluoroethylene (polytef, Teflon), bovine collagen (Contigen), and pyrolytic carbon-coated zirconium oxide beads (Durasphere). In 1984, Lewis et al performed periurethral Teflon injections in female patients with neurogenic bladder on intermittent catheterization and noted a favorable result on continence.[2] Subsequently, several investigators have published data on the use of urethral bulking agents to treat urinary incontinence in patients with neurogenic voiding dysfunction. Although the bulk of the literature deals with children, adults with neuropathic bladder have been addressed in a few case series. Since the majority of experience has been accrued with glutaraldehyde cross-linked bovine collagen, and it is currently the most widely used bulking agent for the treatment of urinary incontinence, this section will focus on the results obtained with this substance. The Food and Drug Administration (FDA), secondary to problems with granuloma formation and particle migration, has not approved Teflon for the treatment of urinary incontinence.[3] To date there have not been any studies published dealing with the use of autologous fat or Durasphere in patients with neurogenic bladder dysfunction.

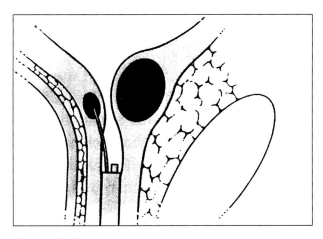

Figure 53.1
Correct placement of periurethral collagen. Injection should be at the proximal urethra in the submucosal plane. (Reproduced with permission from Functional reconstruction of the urinary tract and gynaeco-urology, 1st edn, 2002, Fig. 9.79 c and d.)

The use of bulking agents to treat incontinence has several advantages. Delivery is minimally invasive, relatively easy to learn, and entails low morbidity. Furthermore, treatment with injectable substances does not jeopardize the performance and efficacy of other anti-incontinence procedures later on. The liabilities of this technology stem from a lack of durability and poorer effectiveness when compared to other, albeit more invasive, treatment modalities. This disadvantage often leads to repeat injections, which can elevate the cost of a procedure already known to be expensive.[4]

Collagen biocompatibility, durability, and allergenicity

The collagen used for urethral injection is harvested from bovine corium, which is treated to decrease its antigenicity, and then cross-linked with glutaraldehyde to improve its durability and resistance to degradation by host collagenase.[5] Comprised of 95% type I collagen and 5% type III collagen, it is marketed under the trade names Contigen, Zyderm, and Zyplast (Bard Corp., Atlanta, GA and Collagen Corp., Palo Alto, CA). Bovine collagen has weak antigenicity in humans with 1–3% of patients having a positive skin test.[5] Concerns over developing an autoimmune response to human collagen after injection with bovine collagen appear to be unfounded, since no direct relation between collagen injection and autoimmune disease has been demonstrated in clinical practice.[6] The product is not latex-free, and for this reason, the manufacturer package insert states that a positive skin test may be more prevalent in myelomeningocele patients; however, no literature or experimental data exist to substantiate this finding.

Bovine collagen was approved by the FDA for treatment of intrinsic sphincter deficiency in 1993. Since then, no reports of local or distant migration in animals or humans have surfaced. The host inflammatory response is mild and little granuloma formation occurs. The substance is supposed to undergo gradual degradation over the course of 3–19 months and becomes a matrix for host collagen deposition and neo-vascularization.[7] Three-dimensional ultrasonographic imaging of the urethra, however, has found persistence of bovine collagen in the tissues up to 4 years post-injection,[8] indicating that resorption of this substance may be slower and more variable than was previously proposed.

Mechanism of action

In the neuropathic urethra, sphincteric deficiency is caused by denervation of the musculature of the bladder neck, proximal urethra, external sphincter, and pelvic floor.[9]

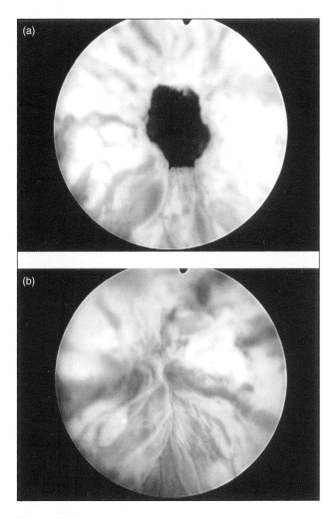

Figure 53.2
(a) Intraoperative cystoscopic view of open proximal urethra before collagen injection. (b) Intraoperative cystoscopic view of properly coapted proximal urethra after collagen injection.

Collagen and other injectable agents theoretically work by increasing the length of bladder neck and proximal urethral mucosa apposition, thereby improving the efficiency of compression of the sphincter mechanism in response to increases in intra-abdominal pressure.[9,10] McGuire et al have determined that injectable agents exert their mechanism of action by increasing the Valsalva leak point pressure (VLPP) but not the detrusor leak point pressure (DLPP) or voiding pressure.[11] This finding has been substantiated by several other authors including Bomalaski et al, who found that in neurogenic bladder patients who experience clinical improvement with collagen injections, the VLPP increased an average of 26 cmH_2O, compared with an increase of only 8 cmH_2O in patients who were not helped by the treatment.[4]

Urethral bulking agents are not thought to increase bladder outlet resistance and, therefore, the pressure at which the bladder empties. For this reason, they are postulated to have an advantage in the treatment of neurogenic incontinence over slings and artificial sphincters, which may cause elevated detrusor pressures and upper tract deterioration.[12,13] So far, there have been no reports of renal compromise related to the use of injectable agents. Chernoff et al, however, have reported significant postoperative urodynamic changes in 3 children with neurogenic bladder who were treated with transurethral collagen injections with decreased compliance and appearance of a DLPP where none had previously existed. These investigators warn of possible bladder decompensation in patients with small-capacity, low-compliance bladders who undergo injection of urethral bulking agents.[14]

Delivery methods

There are three methods for the injection of bulking agents in the treatment of stress urinary incontinence: periurethral, transurethral, and antegrade.[15] Before the use of collagen, 0.1 ml of skin test collagen must be injected subcutaneously into the volar surface of the forearm and observed for 4 weeks to rule out sensitivity. If the test is negative, then collagen injections can proceed. The skin test must be readministered prior to any repeat collagen treatments. Prior to injection, all patients should have a negative urine culture and receive perioperative antibiotics to prevent urosepsis post-procedure. This is especially important for the neurogenic bladder population, in whom urinary tract infections (UTIs) and bacteriuria are common. Children require a general anesthetic, but most adults, especially if they are insensate below the waist secondary to neurologic pathology, can tolerate the injection under local anesthetic or intravenous sedation. Some urologists prefer to inject all patients under general anesthetic in order to have better control over placement of the submucosal blebs. The patient is placed in the dorsal lithotomy position no matter which method of injection is used.

Periurethral technique. This method is often used in women. The urethra is injected with 2% lidocaine (lignocaine) jelly, and 1% lidocaine is injected periurethrally at 3 and 9 o'clock. A 20-gauge spinal needle is inserted at the 3 o'clock position and advanced under cystoscopic vision within the submucosal space toward the urethral lumen just distal to the bladder neck and proximal urethra. The bulking agent is slowly injected with the needle bevel facing the lumen until a mucosal bleb is raised. This process is repeated on the opposite side at 9 o'clock until the cystoscopic appearance of the lumen resembles that of lateral prostatic lobes meeting in the midline.

Transurethral technique. Although preferred for males, this method is often used in females as well. It requires a 21–24F cystoscope that can accommodate a 5F working element. A zero, 12, or 30 degree lens can be used.[16] The cystoscope is placed in the urethral lumen just proximal to the external sphincter and a needle delivery system (often 20-gauge) is placed through the working port of the cystoscope. The submucosal space is entered at 3 or 9 o'clock with the needle bevel pointing towards the urethral lumen. The bulking material is slowly injected until a sufficient bleb is raised. The process is repeated on the opposite side or anywhere else necessary to achieve good coaptation. Care should be taken to avoid more than one puncture at any single injection site in order to minimize extrusion. As with the periurethral technique, the cystoscope should not be advanced past the injection sites, because this can result in compression or extrusion of material and loss of the mucosal bleb.

Antegrade technique. This approach was developed in an attempt to achieve better closure of the bladder neck in males with scarred, noncompliant urethras postprostatectomy. It can also be used in children or adults with previous bladder neck reconstruction in whom the urethral passage may not be wide enough or compliant enough to accommodate a cystoscope of the caliber needed to employ the needle delivery system. It can be done under general anesthetic, intravenous sedation, or spinal anesthesia. The bladder is distended with irrigation fluid and a suprapubic cystotomy is performed under cystoscopic guidance, then dilated to allow placement of a sheath large enough to accommodate the cystoscope. Antegrade cystoscopy is performed and the material is injected submucosally around the bladder neck until coaptation occurs. A suprapubic tube is left in postoperatively for 24–72 hours.

Postoperative care

Patients are discharged once they are able to void. If they go into retention, they can be taught intermittent catheterization with a small-caliber catheter. Some investigators place narrow-lumen urethral catheters for 24–72 hours post-procedure.[17] If the patient was performing intermittent catheterization preoperatively, he can usually resume catheterization with an 8–12F tube the same day of the procedure with little fear of significant molding of the material.[9,12]

Indications and patient selection

The role of injectable agents for the treatment of urinary incontinence in the neurogenic bladder population remains hard to define. Perhaps this is because there are no randomized controlled trials comparing one treatment modality with another in this subset of patients, and the literature mainly consists of case series comprised of small numbers and short follow-up. In examining these data, however, a few patterns emerge.

It is often said that the ideal candidate for urethral collagen injection has a stable, compliant, good capacity bladder with low VLPP.[12,14] Many investigators believe that detrusor overactivity or decreased compliance should be treated with anticholinergics and/or augmentation cystoplasty before attempting to treat an incompetent outlet with bulking agents.[12,18] Perez et al, however, in their series of 32 patients with neurogenic bladder, found that the presence of detrusor overactivity and decreased compliance did not adversely affect the clinical outcome.[19]

In addition to its role in leakage prevention, injection of collagen into the bladder neck and proximal urethra has also been used to provide outlet resistance in order to increase the bladder capacity of children with exstrophy-epispadias complex prior to bladder neck reconstruction.[20] Although this technique has been successful in a small number of patients, not every author has found this to be the case.[14]

Many investigators regard urethral bulking agents as adjuncts to other forms of treatment, but do not believe them capable of providing a durable cure for incontinence in the majority of patients with neurogenic voiding dysfunction when used as the sole source of intervention.[13,17,21] This is particularly true in the subset of children with exstrophy-epispadias complex who have undergone bladder neck reconstruction yet remain incontinent. Many of these patients were rendered dry or experienced substantial improvement after collagen injection.[12,17,19,20] Bomalaski et al, in their study of 40 children with neurogenic bladder, found statistically greater improvement in continence and postoperative satisfaction in the exstrophy-epispadias group than in the myelomeningocele group.[4]

Groups of investigators in Canada have determined that preoperative urodynamic data could not predict the clinical result of collagen injection.[12,18] Chernoff et al, however, in their series of 11 children, found that a preoperative VLLP of greater than 45 cmH$_2$O was predictive of injection failure.[14] A patulous bladder neck was thought to be a positive predictor of success by Kim et al, whose series of patients undergoing collagen injection contained 8 children with neurogenic bladder, 4 of whom had this finding on examination and were dry post-injection. These authors speculated that this cystoscopic feature, although indicative of a severely incompetent bladder outlet, may be a sign of more pliable, less-scarred tissue which would allow for optimal injection and, therefore, improved long-term treatment success.[22]

Contraindications to the use of injectable collagen for the treatment of urinary incontinence are known collagen sensitivity (a positive skin test), untreated detrusor over-activity, and untreated urinary tract infection. Scarring secondary to previous surgery or radiation treatment may decrease retention of collagen in tissue, thus contributing to its relatively poor efficacy.[9,17]

Results

Analysis of the studies published in the last 10 years on treatment of urinary incontinence with collagen injection reveals that the benefits derived from this agent by patients with neuropathic voiding dysfunction are comparable to those seen in the non-neurogenic incontinence population (Table 53.1). The proportion of patients rendered dry ranges from 20 to 50% in the majority of studies, although cure rates as low as 5% have been reported. The improvement rate, which is often the only outcome stated, ranges anywhere from 15 to 76%. The data are difficult to interpret and compare, since there is no standard definition of cure and improvement, and these terms are not always clearly delineated within the methodology of each study.

Most patients received between 1 and 4 injections, with the majority of responders having had only 1 or 2 treatments before assessment of clinical efficacy was made. The total volume of collagen injected ranged from 0.4 to 55 ml, with a total of less than 10 ml typically administered by most authors. In our experience, continence is rarely attained if a trial of 1 or 2 injections fails to achieve any improvement. We have recently begun to employ three-dimensional ultrasound of the urethra as an objective outcome measure to aid in the decision as to whether or not to offer repeat collagen injection to patients who have failed to experience clinical improvement.[8] The administration of further collagen may be costly and delay more effective treatment, particularly if postoperative three-dimensional ultrasound imaging demonstrates either poor or good retention of collagen, and the patient's incontinence persists.

Although most studies reported moderate treatment efficacy with follow-up of 1–6.3 years, some investigators found collagen to be disappointing in terms of treatment outcome. In 20 children with neurogenic stress incontinence, Sundaram et al reported only 30% improvement in leakage status post-collagen injection, while the rest

Table 53.1 Results of glutaraldehyde cross-linked collagen in patients with neurogenic incontinence

Investigator	Year and patient population	Number of patients	Mean follow-up (months)	Mean amount collagen (ml)	Results	Complications	Comments
Capozza et al[20]	1995 pediatric	25 – 9 NB, 16 EE	Range 9–36; no mean given	3 range 2.1–4.5	76% improved 9/9 NB, 10/16 EE	None	EEC patients had prior NB reconstruction
Bennett et al[9]	1995 adult	11 – 5 MMC, 5 SCI, 1 SC tumor	24 range 12–32	Females – 55 Males – 56	28% cured 36% improved	1 transient difficulty catheterizing	Series contained 9 men, 2 women
Ben-Chaim et al[17]	1995 3 adults, 16 children	19 – all EE	26 range 9–84	4 range 0.4–12	53% improved	1 UTI/epididymo-orchitis, 1 bladder perforation	15 patients had prior NB reconstruction
Perez et al[14]	1996 pediatric	32 – 24 MMC, 7 EE, 1 sacral teratoma	10 range 3–19	10 MMC, 7.5 EE range 3.5–17	MMC – 20% dry, 28% improved EEC – 43% dry, 14% improved	1 urosepsis, 2 transient worsening of incontinence	3/7 EEC patients had undergone previous NB reconstruction
Bomalaski et al[14]	1996 pediatric	40 – 25 MMC, 12 EE, rest non-neurogenic	25.2 range 3–75.6	10.2 range 2.5–22.5	22% cure, 54% improved Statistically significant decrease in pad use, dry interval, incontinence grade	None	8 patients followed for 4.5 years had overall cure/improvement of 86% Greater success with EE than with MMC
Leonard et al[12]	1996 pediatric	18 – 10 MMC, 6 EE	15 range 5–21	5 range 2.4–13	MMC – 3/6 cured, 2 improved EE – 2 cured, 2 improved	None	4 patients had ileocysto-plasty, 7 had NB reconstruction, 4 had epispadias repair
Chernoff et al[14]	1997 pediatric	11 – 7 MMC, 1 SCI, 2 EE, 1 uro-genital sinus defect	14.4 range 4–20	Maximum injected 15 ml	36% dry, 18% improved	None	4 patients had previous ileocystoplasty, 3 had NB reconstruction
Sundaram et al[21]	1997 pediatric	20 – 12 MMC, 4 EE, 4 other neurogenic bladder causes	15.2 range 9–23	7.3 range 3–18	5% dry, 25% improved, 10 had transient improvement	None	2 patients had prior NB reconstruction
Kassouf et al[18]	2001 pediatric	20 – all MMC	50.4	6.3 range 2–13	10% dry, 15% improved, 14 had transient improvement	None	80% on CIC, all had stable bladder preoperation

CIC, clean intermittent catheterization; EEC, exstrophy-epispadias complex; SCI, spinal cord injury; NB, neurogenic bladder.

experienced transient improvement lasting an average of 52 days.[21] In children with myelomeningocele on intermittent catheterization, Kassouf et al found that only one-quarter of patients had a durable treatment response, with the rest failing at 3 months.[18] Suboptimal outcomes have been attributed in part to disruption of the collagen blebs by catheterization shortly after injection, but Sundaram et al did not find any difference in the outcome between patients on intermittent catheterization and those who voided spontaneously.[21]

Complications have been few and minor, consisting of UTI, urosepsis, epididymo-orchitis, transient difficulty with catheterization, and temporary worsening of urinary incontinence.[9,17,19] One patient sustained a bladder perforation requiring laparotomy and operative repair 3 days after injection which was felt by the investigators to be secondary to overfilling at the time of the procedure and subsequent difficulty emptying the bladder completely.[17]

Conclusion

In summary, treatment of stress urinary incontinence with glutaraldehyde cross-linked bovine collagen in the neurogenic bladder population has been demonstrated to be safe and variably successful, with follow-up extending past 5 years. Almost all the literature, however, deals with children, and very little data exist for adults with spinal cord injury or other acquired forms of neuropathic voiding dysfunction. Children with exstrophy-epispadias who have had previous bladder neck reconstruction have been found to be suitable candidates for collagen injection, as have patients with myelomeningocele. The relative efficacy of

injectable agents, coupled with their minimally invasive nature and ease of administration, has continued to fuel the search for novel substances. Animal and human studies examining the feasibility of submucosal injection of autologous ear chondrocytes and autologous muscle-derived cells are currently underway in an attempt to find more durable, more biocompatible, and less allergenic alternatives to bovine collagen.[23,24] The ideal injectable agent has not yet been devised.

Bladder neck slings and wraps

Introduction

The fascial sling and the artificial urethral sphincter (AUS) are the two most commonly employed surgical treatments for patients with urinary incontinence secondary to neurogenic outlet incompetence. The pros and cons of bladder neck sling and artificial urethral sphincter are listed in Table 53.2. The issue of how much tension to place on the fascial sling is not as problematic in the neurogenic bladder population as it is in patients with stress urinary incontinence (SUI), since retention in a patient with neurogenic bladder who already performs intermittent catheterization (IC) is usually a treatment goal rather than a complication. Furthermore, the incidence of tension-induced erosion is low when autologous fascia is utilized as the sling material. Unfortunately, long-term experience with the bladder neck sling in the neurogenic bladder population is seldom reported, with most case series documenting mean follow-up times of less than 4 years. It is thus unknown whether

Table 53.2 *Advantages and disadvantages of fascial bladder neck sling and artificial urethral sphincter (AUS)*		
Surgical option	Advantages	Disadvantages
Bladder neck sling	1. No foreign body insertion 2. 'Pop-off' valve – allows leakage to occur at high intravesical pressure, protecting upper tracts 3. No concern with contamination of surgical field and infection seeding when performing a concomitant bladder augment	1. Majority of patients must catheterize to empty bladder 2. Less efficacious in males than females
AUS	1. Highly effective even for severe outlet incompetence 2. No 'pop-off' valve – may lead to upper tract deterioration in patients with poor preoperative compliance and high intravesical pressures 3. Allows some patients to void spontaneously without need for catheterization	1. Risk of revision for mechanical failure 2. Risk of infection and erosion

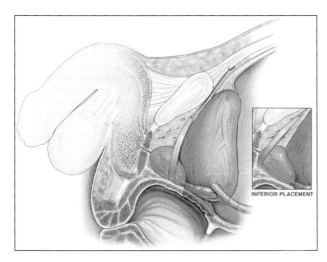

INFERIOR PLACEMENT

Figure 53.3
Placement of rectus fascia sling in a male patient. Sling is placed at the bladder neck posterior to the seminal vesicles.

or not the fascial sling in young women with myelomeningocele may be disrupted by pregnancy and childbirth.[25]

Indications and patient selection

The ideal candidate for this procedure is a female patient with bladder outlet incompetence, preserved urethral length, and a well-managed bladder on IC.

Whether or not to perform enterocystoplasty in addition to a procedure to occlude the bladder outlet is a complex decision based on preoperative urodynamic and radiographic assessment. Bladder augmentation alone may be sufficient to cure incontinence in some neurogenic bladder patients despite low outlet resistance,[26] particularly in male children who have the potential for increased outlet competence with pubertal prostate growth. Conversely, supporting the bladder neck with a sling may be enough to abolish leakage if the preoperative urodynamic assessment, performed with some form of bladder outlet occlusion, shows a stable bladder with sufficient capacity and normal compliance.[27] Whether or not to perform both procedures together, or to do one before the other, is somewhat controversial. In general, a cystogram showing a wide open bladder neck and a VLPP less than 30 cmH$_2$O are indications of intrinsic sphincter deficiency, in which case a procedure to improve bladder outlet competence is recommended. Adherence to these guidelines, however, cannot always predict the patient's postoperative status. As Kreder and Webster demonstrated, a bladder neck sling may cause de-novo detrusor overactivity (DO) or decreased bladder capacity and compliance if performed without enterocystoplasty, despite a preoperative urodynamic work-up documenting normal detrusor parameters.[27] To avoid

subjecting the patient to a second operation, some investigators have advocated the routine performance of concomitant enterocystoplasty and rectus fascial sling in all patients with neurogenic incontinence.[28,29] One such proponent of this practice, Decter, found that the rate of postoperative leakage was higher in patients who did not undergo bladder augmentation along with bladder neck sling compared with patients who had both procedures.[29] The downside of this systematic approach, however, is that even though it saves some patients the morbidity of a second surgery, it may needlessly subject some others to the risks of enterocystoplasty.

Surgical techniques

Prior to undergoing a bladder neck sling, patients must have a negative urine culture. Perioperative broad-spectrum antibiotics are administered and, if a bladder augmentation is performed, they are continued postoperatively for a few days.

A bowel preparation should be considered in all patients undergoing concomitant enterocystoplasty. When performing both a sling and a bladder augment, the fascial harvest and bladder neck dissection are usually performed prior to the augmentation. Once the augment is completed, the fascial sling is positioned and secured in place.

A midline incision provides the best exposure if an enterocystoplasty is also to be done, but a Pfannenstiel incision can be employed, staying extraperitoneal, if only a sling is required.[30] The bladder neck dissection is often done via the abdominal incision, but a transvaginal or combined transabdominal–transvaginal approach can be employed in adult women, and has even been accomplished in adolescent girls with the help of a mediolateral episiotomy.[31] In the transabdominal dissection, the endopelvic fascia is incised bilaterally, the bladder neck and proximal urethra are freed circumferentially, and a Penrose drain is placed around the bladder neck. A finger in the vagina, or the rectum in males, can aid in the posterior dissection.[30] Some surgeons prefer just to clear a tunnel beneath the bladder neck rather than mobilizing around it completely.[28] In males, the dissection is identical to that performed for AUS bladder neck cuff placement, in that a plane is entered posterior to the bladder neck but anterior to the seminal vesicles.[32] The transvaginal dissection, if employed, is approached via a vertical midline or inverted U incision in the anterior vaginal wall. The incision should extend from 1.5 cm proximal to the urethral meatus to 1 cm proximal to the bladder neck, which is identified with the aid of the balloon of a urethral Foley catheter. The vaginal mucosa is dissected off the underlying periurethral fascia to expose the urethrovesical junction. After perforating the endopelvic fascia, the retropubic space is entered on either side of the bladder neck using a combination of sharp and

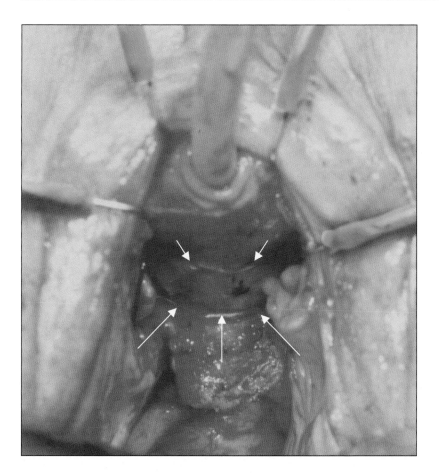

Figure 53.4
Correct placement of rectus fascia sling at the proximal urethra in a female patient (arrows indicate superior and inferior edges of the rectus sling).

blunt dissection. This dissection allows a ligature carrier to be passed safely from the suprapubic region to the vaginal area under fingertip guidance.

A strip of autologous rectus fascia 1.5–2 cm in width and 6–10 cm in length is usually employed, although fascia lata may also be used. Marlex slings have also been placed, but the likelihood of infection and erosion is increased compared to autologous fascia.[32] The rectus fascia can be harvested transversely or longitudinally as a free graft, or one end of the fascial strip may be left attached to the anterior abdominal wall as a pedicle and secured to the opposite rectus sheath. In males, the sling is usually placed around the bladder neck and superior aspect of the prostate, although some surgeons place it around the distal prostatic urethra, where coaptation may be easier to achieve.[33] In females, the fascial strip is positioned around the bladder neck and proximal urethra. The sling is often sutured to the lateral edges of the bladder neck with absorbable suture to prevent rolling and displacement that may cause excessive urethral angulation or compression. If employing a free fascial graft, a zero or number one polypropylene stitch is passed through each end of the graft before the sling is positioned around the bladder neck. When the operation is done transvaginally, the sutures are brought out through the lower anterior abdominal wall using a ligature carrier

passed through the retropubic space into the vaginal incision under fingertip guidance. The sutures are then tied down suprapubically at the end of the procedure. Some investigators have used Gortex bolsters or pledgets to prevent suture pull-through,[25,31] but this is not essential. Alternatively, the edges of fascia can be secured to Cooper's ligament[4] or the symphysis pubis.[29]

Several techniques have been recommended to optimize sling tension. In patients with neurogenic bladder on IC there is little concern with causing retention, but one should avoid tying the sutures too tightly to prevent urethral erosion and atrophy.[34] Elder describes filling the bladder with saline via a suprapubic tube and increasing tension on the sling until urethral leakage no longer occurs with manual bladder compression.[25] Other authors have tied the sutures so that no further movement of a Foley balloon at the bladder neck occurs, or so that 1 or 2 fingers can be placed between the knots and the fascia.[31] The sling sutures can also be tightened under cystoscopic control until the bladder neck appears closed.[29,30] Decter has suggested that because of the prostate bulk, more tension needs to be applied to the sutures in males than in females to achieve adequate urethral elevation and compression.[29] The surgeon should ensure that catheterization can be performed before finalizing sling tension.[28]

Some surgeons leave a suprapubic tube and urethral Foley catheter in postoperatively, remove the Foley catheter within 1–2 weeks, and then the suprapubic tube once catheterization can be performed with no difficulties. Others leave just a suprapubic tube, which is removed after 1–3 weeks, depending on whether or not an enterocystoplasty was also performed.

Wrap procedures in which a pedicle of bladder detrusor, a strip of rectus fascia, or a distally based rectus/pyramidalis myofascial flap is used to encircle the bladder neck completely, have been employed by various authors in order to provide circumferential compression, tapering, and suspension of the bladder outlet.[33,35,36] In some cases, one end of the wrap is secured to the anterior abdominal wall fascia in order to elevate the bladder neck.[35] It has been theorized that catheterization may be easier with the bladder neck wrap than with the sling, since the suspending force is evenly distributed around the bladder neck, thereby avoiding urethral kinking.[33,36]

Some investigators, in addition to placing a sling support beneath the bladder neck, have tapered it to improve urethral coaptation and reduce sling tension, in an attempt to decrease the likelihood of erosion.[32] Techniques which have been described include excising a full-thickness diamond of tissue along the anterior aspect of the bladder neck and reapproximating the edges of mucosa and detrusor muscle with absorbable sutures, or, alternatively, excising full-thickness wedges of anterior bladder neck and prostate from the edges of a vertical midline incision extending to the level of the verumontanum, and tapering it over a 16F catheter.[30,32]

Results and complications

The literature on bladder neck slings to treat neurogenic urinary incontinence consists largely of case series, made up of pediatric or a mixture of pediatric and adult patients (Table 53.3). Mean follow-up ranges from 9 months to 4.5 years. Published success rates depend on the definition of dryness used by the author. Continence has been described as no leakage occurring in between intermittent catheterization intervals of 3–4 hours or more, wearing less than 1 pad per day, or dry during the daytime only, with no consideration given to nocturnal incontinence. Most investigators report overall continence rates greater than 70%, with women faring better (85%) than men (69%) in some studies.[28,29,31–33] Kurzrock et al suggest that this discrepancy in sling effectiveness between the sexes may be because the prostate makes it more difficult to close and elevate the proximal urethra.[33] Fascial bladder neck wraps have not been found to be any more effective at preventing urinary leakage than slings.[33,35,36]

Complications specific to the rectus fascia sling are relatively rare and include sling breakdown resulting in postoperative leakage as a result of fascial breakage or suture pullout and urethral erosion.[29,30] The urethra may become angulated, resulting in difficulty with catheterization or retraction of the meatus into the vaginal introitus.[30] Care needs to be taken when passing a cystoscope via the urethra post-sling insertion. Elder[25] and Barthold et al[35] have described cases in which patients who were initially dry after surgery became incontinent after the performance of transurethral instrumentation. Bladder perforation may occur in patients with augmented bladders and bladder neck slings who are not compliant with IC, or in whom catheterization has become difficult.[28,35,37] Other reported complications are incisional hernia, de-novo DO, retroperitoneal hematoma, and bladder neck contracture when the outlet is tapered along with sling insertion.[30,32]

Conclusion

The rectus fascia bladder neck sling has been shown to be a versatile and valuable addition to the armamentarium of the reconstructive surgeon. Despite its lower rate of success in males with neurogenic incontinence, the lack of requirement for foreign materials and relative ease of implantation make it an attractive option for treatment of the incompetent reservoir outlet in a wide variety of patients. The long-term durability of the bladder neck sling, however, is still unknown. This is an important consideration, particularly for children, in whom the procedure may have to last decades. Many authors speculate that with growth the sling should maintain its functional obstruction of the bladder outlet, but longer follow-up is required.

Artificial urinary sphincters

Introduction

Ever since the first published clinical report in 1973 by Scott, the AUS has been used extensively to treat sphincteric incontinence.[38] High rates of efficacy and patient satisfaction, but also substantial revision rates secondary to mechanical failure as well as problems with infection and erosion resulting in sphincter removal have been reported. The high initial cost of the device, compounded with the cost of replacing components when they malfunction or wear out, makes it an expensive treatment option. Despite its availability since the 1970s, concerns have also been raised regarding silicone shedding, particularly in children, since the long-term sequelae of silicone migration is unknown.[39] There have been relatively few large series of AUS use in neurogenic patients, and there are no controlled trials comparing its efficacy to that of fascial slings or bladder neck reconstruction.

Table 53.3 Results of fascial slings and wraps in patients with neurogenic bladder outlet incompetence

Study	Year and patient population	Number and type of patients	Mean follow-up (months)	Surgical technique	Results	Other surgical procedures
Elder[25]	1990 adult and pediatric M and F	**14:** 10 F, 4 M all MMC	12 range 7–27	Periurethral or peri-prostatic RF sling, tied on abdominal wall	85.7% dry 1 nocturnal enuresis only	12 concomitant bladder augmentation
Herschorn and Radomski[32]	1992 adult M	**13:** 10 MMC, 3 SCI	34.3 range 5.5–49	2 Marlex, 11 RF pedicle sutured to opposite rectus sheath, BN tapering	69.2% dry	All had concomitant augmentation
Decter[29]	1993 adult and pediatric M and F	**10:** 6 F, 4 M 8 MMC, 2 SA	26.4	RF sling in 5, fascia lata in 5, symphyseal fixation	67% with augment dry, 25% without augment dry	6 concomitant bladder augmentations
Chancellor et al[113]	1993 adult F	**14:** neurogenic, patulous urethras	24 range 6–60	RF pedicle sling sutured to opposite abdominal wall	100% dry	5 concomitant augmentations, 5 cutaneous urostomy
Gormley et al[31]	1994 F adolescents	**15:** 8 MMC, 2 SA, 1 imperforate anus, 3 BN trauma	54 range 6–102	RF sling, combined abdominal and vaginal dissection, tied over abdominal wall	84.6% dry (2 redos using larger piece of RF) 1 using 1 pad/day	2 concomitant augmentations, 5 prior bladder outlet procedures
Walker et al[30]	1995 adult and pediatric M and F	**17:** 9 F, 8 M 10 MMC, 3 sacral lipoma, 4 other	16.2	RF sling, some with bladder neck tapering	94.1% dry 1 has some SUI	11 concomitant augmentations, 9 prior BN procedures
Kakizaki et al[34]	1995 adult and pediatric mostly M	**13:** 10 M, 3 F 8 MMC, 2 pelvic surgery, 1 SCI, 2 non-neurogenic patients	36 range 4–63	Sling of RF in 8, fascia lata in 5; BN placement in 11, bulbous urethra in 2; tied over abdominal wall	69.2% dry 23% improved	9 concomitant bladder augmentations

Reference	Year/population	Patients	Procedure	Follow-up (months)	Results	Comments
Kurzrock et al[33]	1996 pediatric M and F	24: 9 F, 15 M all MMC	Bladder wall pedicle wrap suspended to pubic symphysis	Range 9–14	100% F dry 66.7% M dry	6 prior augmentations, 1 prior RF sling
Fontaine et al[28]	1997 adult F	21: 9 MMC, 8 SCI, 3 SA, 1 sacral lipoma	RF sling done transabdominally, sutured to Cooper's	28.6 range 6–60	85.7% dry day and night 95.2% dry day only	All had concomitant bladder augmentation
Barthold et al[35]	1999 pediatric mostly F	27: 20 F, 7 M 21 MMC, 2 SA, 4 other	10 RF slings, 18 RF wraps, both secured to anterior abdominal wall	Wrap 43.2 sling 25.2	Wrap 28% dry, sling 50% dry ($p > 0.05$) 14.3% M dry, 50% F dry ($p = 0.02$)	19 concomitant, 1 prior, 2 subsequent augmentations, 17 Mitrofanoffs
Austin et al[37]	2001 pediatric M and F	18: 10 M, 8 F 16 MMC, 2 SCI	RF sling tied over anterior abdominal wall	21.2 range 6–57	78% dry, 2 dry with repeat sling	4 concomitant, 2 prior augmentations
Mingin et al[36]	2002 pediatric and adult M and F	37: 14 M, 23F 36 neurogenic, 1 traumatic	Distally based rectus/pyramidalis myofascial flap wrapped around BN and sewn to contralateral RF	48 range 6–120	92% (34) dry 2 M failures, 1 F failure	33 concomitant augmentations, 9 Mitrofanoff stomas, 5 reimplantations

MMC, myelomeningocele; SCI, spinal cord injury; SA, sacral agenesis; M, male; F, female; RF, rectus fascia; BN, bladder neck; SUI, stress urinary incontinence.

History and design evolution

The AUS 800 represents the culmination of a number of design modifications which have occurred since 1975 when the patent for the original device, the AMS 721, was issued to American Medical Systems (Minnetonka, Minnesota). This early model operated on the hydraulic principle still employed by the modern AUS, but there was no way to control the occlusive force applied to the urethra and the large number of components made it difficult to implant.[40] In 1980, the AMS 721 was altered to overcome these problems by streamlining the design and incorporating a pressure-regulating balloon reservoir, which was then marketed as the AMS 761. The AMS 742, 791, and 792 represented further design simplifications and introduced the concept of delayed activation in order to allow for tissue healing. With these devices, a second surgical procedure was needed to activate the pump.[40]

In 1982, the AMS 800 was introduced and is the only AUS currently available on the market.[41] Like its predecessors, it consists of three components: a cuff which fits around the urethra or bladder neck; a balloon fluid reservoir which is implanted in the abdomen; and a pump which is implanted in the scrotum or labia to control activation. The cuff is composed of an outer layer of Dacron (polyethylene terephthalate) monofilament backing an inner silicone shell, and is available in sizes ranging from 4 to 11 cm with 0.5 cm increments. Three different balloon reservoirs are available with plateau pressures of 51–60 cmH$_2$O, 61–70 cmH$_2$O and 71–80 cmH$_2$O. The pump and reservoir are also made of silicone and are connected to each other and the pump by kink-resistant color-coded tubing. The sphincter is implanted fully primed with isotonic radiopaque fluid or normal saline in its deactivated state.

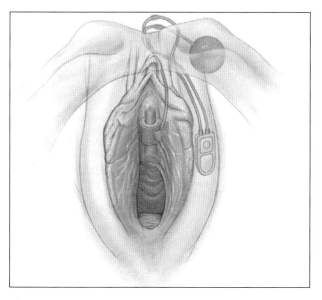

Figure 53.5
Placement of the AMS-800 in a female patient. (Reproduced with permission from The urinary sphincter, Chapter 34, Fig. 5.)

The device is activated a few weeks later by sharply squeezing the bulb of the pump. This maneuver allows fluid to exit the reservoir and enter the hollow cuff, thereby occluding the urethra or bladder neck lumen. When the patient wishes to void, he pumps the bulb to direct fluid out of the cuff and back into the reservoir. Fluid moves back into the cuff, closing it automatically within 3–5 min. Should urethral or bladder instrumentation be necessary, the unit can be locked or deactivated by pressing a button on the pump.

In 1988, a cuff with Dacron backing that was narrower than the silicone surface facing the urethra (narrow-backed cuff) was incorporated into the AMS 800 design along with alterations in the manufacturing process used to make the reservoir. These modifications improved durability and decreased urethral pressure atrophy.[42] There have been no further changes to the AMS 800 design.

Indications and patient selection

All patients in whom an AUS is being considered should undergo preoperative urodynamic testing to document the severity and mechanism of incontinence and to assess bladder function. Determination of detrusor parameters may require bladder neck occlusion with a Foley catheter balloon during the filling phase.[43] As for the fascial sling, the ideal candidate for an AUS should have a stable bladder with good compliance and capacity as well as a good emptying. Elevated detrusor pressures can lead to upper tract deterioration once the outlet is occluded by the sphincter cuff. De Badiola et al compared the preoperative and postoperative urodynamic parameters of 23 pediatric patients who received an AUS for neurogenic sphincteric incompetence. Patients with filling pressures of less than 50 cmH$_2$O with preoperative bladder capacities greater than or equal to 60% of that expected for age and/or a preoperative compliance greater than 2 ml/cmH$_2$O, were less likely to require subsequent augmentation for persistent incontinence and upper tract changes.[44] The average time to cystoplasty in patients who developed high intravesical pressures after AUS implantation was 14 months.[44]

Many authors advocate an AUS as primary treatment for patients who can void spontaneously.[45] Patients, however, should be informed that IC may have to be performed in the future, particularly if they receive a bladder augment or, in men, if prostatic growth later in life produces outlet obstruction. The AUS has also been employed as secondary treatment for patients who have failed other forms of bladder outlet surgery. Aliabadi and Gonzalez described 15 patients who had failed multiple urethral and bladder neck surgeries and were salvaged with an AUS, resulting in an overall continence rate of 73%.[46]

The optimal timing for US insertion in the pediatric population with neurogenic incontinence is controversial.

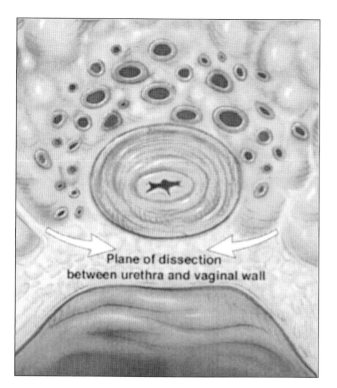

Figure 53.6
Transvaginal view of urethra and anterior vaginal wall to show dissection plane between the vagina and urethra/bladder neck.

Kryger et al found no difference in the number of AUS removals, continence rate, revision rate, augmentation rate, or number of complications in patients who received an AUS before age 11 compared to those placed later in life. AUS insertion, in fact, may be easier in prepubertal patients secondary to the shallower pelvis and lesser degree of periurethral venous plexus engorgement. Revisions for retraction of the pump in the scrotum were uncommon, occurring only in 1 of their 25 patients.[45] Levesque et al also found no increase in the rate of AUS revision post-puberty, with a follow-up of 12.1 years.[47]

Although Fulford et al[41] have reported a cuff erosion rate of 44% in females, and Levesque et al[47] found a higher rate of erosion in girls who had previous bladder neck surgery, other investigators have not. Salisz et al described successful AUS insertion in women despite intraoperative injuries to the vagina, bladder, or urethra. Their technique involved closing the injury primarily, placing the cuff within a different plane of dissection around the bladder neck, and delaying sphincter activation for a minimum of 6 weeks.[48]

Surgical technique

AUS insertion can be performed under general or spinal anesthesia. The cuff is usually placed around the bladder neck in women and children and around the bulbar urethra in males. The dorsal lithotomy position is favored in order to access the perineum for bulbar urethral placement, or to place a finger in the vagina to aid in transabdominal dissection of the bladder neck. The urine should be sterile before surgery and the skin should be free of dermatitis or candidiasis. Broad-spectrum perioperative intravenous antibiotics are administered. Strict sterile precautions are followed in the operating room and many surgeons prepare the patient with a 10–15 min antiseptic soap scrub before painting the abdomen and perineum with an antiseptic solution. Once the patient has been draped, a Foley catheter is inserted into the bladder.

Dissection of the bladder neck proceeds in much the same fashion as for placement of a fascial sling (see earlier). A 2-cm wide window behind the bladder neck is adequate for cuff placement, and a right-angled clamp is used to pass the measuring device around the bladder neck. Bladder neck cuff sizes range from 6 to 11 cm in diameter. Limited injuries to the bladder or vagina can be repaired primarily, but rectal injuries require abortion of the procedure. Once the appropriate-sized cuff is placed around the bladder neck, the cuff tubing is brought out through the rectus fascia via a separate stab incision superior to the pubis. The reservoir is placed in the retropubic space with its tubing penetrating the rectus fascia near the cuff tubing. A 71–80 cmH$_2$O balloon is often used for bladder neck occlusion. The reservoir can also be inserted into the peritoneal cavity, a location preferred by some to permit better balloon expansion.[40]

The anterior rectus sheath is closed and the balloon reservoir is filled with 22 ml of normal saline or an iso-osmotic contrast solution for postoperative X-ray imaging of the AUS. The pump mechanism is placed subcutaneously in the most dependent part of the scrotum or the labia. This space is created by passing a long curved Kelly clamp or sponge forceps from the lower edge of the suprapubic incision into the hemiscrotum or labium. The site of pump placement depends on whether the patient is left- or right-handed. A Babcock clamp can be placed around the pump tubing to prevent it from riding up while the components are being assembled. All tubing must be cleared of bubbles and blood clots before being connected. Straight or right-angled connectors can be used and secured with the quick-connect system or hand-tied with 2–0 or 3–0 polypropylene sutures in revision cases. The device should be cycled intraoperatively to make sure the cuff inflates and deflates properly. Some surgeons perform this maneuver while visualizing the cuff directly with flexible cystoscopy. Others perform perfusion sphincterometry to confirm proper sphincter function, to exclude unsuspected urethral injury, and to determine the refill time of the device.[49] All AUS components and incisions are irrigated copiously with antibiotic solution throughout the procedure. Before closing the incision, the AUS is deactivated by squeezing the button on the pump before it refills completely.

Placement of the cuff around the bulbar urethra begins by making a vertical incision in the perineum with its midpoint at the lower edge of the ischeal tuberosities. A Lonestar or Turner–Warwick retractor is recommended for better exposure. After incising the bulbocavernosus muscle along its midline, the bulbar urethra is mobilized circumferentially for a distance of 2–3 cm. If the urethra is injured, then the procedure should be terminated and the Foley catheter left indwelling after the injury is repaired with fine absorbable suture. A measuring device is passed around the urethra and the appropriate-sized cuff is placed. Most adult male patients will be fitted a 4.5 cm cuff, but sizes of 4 and 5 cm are also available. The cuff tubing and tab are withoriented laterally so that neither one abuts the base of the penis, which can be uncomfortable postoperatively. The reservoir is placed in the retropubic space through a separate abdominal incision. The operation proceeds as described above.

To circumvent retention secondary to edema, a catheter is usually left in the bladder overnight and removed the next morning. Patients are discharged on oral antibiotics for 10–14 days after completing 24–48 hours of intravenous therapy. Patients should avoid heavy lifting, straining, and intercourse for 4–6 weeks. The AUS is activated in the clinic 4–6 weeks after its insertion and the patient is instructed in its use. Patients should inform medical personnel that they have an AUS when entering the hospital for surgery or any other procedure that may involve bladder catheterization, since the cuff should be deactivated beforehand to avoid damage to the device and the urethra. Patients should also carry the AUS information card provided by the manufacturer and obtain a Medicalert bracelet in case of accident or injury.

Results and complications

In patients with neurogenic sphincteric incontinence, the AUS has been reported to result in continence rates from 59–92%, revision rates of 27–57%, and removal rates of 19–41% (Table 53.4).[45,47,50–55] Perioperative and immediate postoperative complications include bladder neck, urethral and rectal perforations, UTIs, wound infections, and scrotal hematomas.[50,51] In the long term, mechanical problems are the most common reason for revision surgery and include tubing kinks, fluid loss secondary to pump, reservoir or cuff leaks, pump migration, pump dysfunction, and connector separation.[42,52,53,55] Non-mechanical complications consist of urethral atrophy, infection, erosion, and elevated bladder storage pressures which can result in reflux, hydronephrosis, and renal insufficiency.[42,47,50] In the Mayo Clinic series of 323 AUS patients, 26 of whom had myelomeningocele, both types of complications were shown to decrease after 1988 with incorporation of the narrow-backed cuff and improved manufacturing

process: the rate of mechanical failure fell from 21 to 7.5% and the non-mechanical failure rate dropped from 17 to 9%.[42]

Infection, one of the most dreaded complications, results in sphincter removal, and accounts for 4–5% of most series.[40] Proposed mechanisms include contamination during the procedure, exposure of the AUS to chronically infected urine, and hematogenous spread of bacteria with seeding of the device.[56] The presence of an infection is often indicated by skin erythema, induration at the pump or reservoir site, erosion of the cuff through the urethra, or erosion of the pump through the scrotal or labial skin. Microorganisms recovered from infected AUS include *Staphylococcus epidermidis*, β-streptococcus, *Bacteroides fragilis*, *Escherichia coli*, *Pseudomonas*, and diphtheroid species.[56–58] A pseudocapsule made of myofibroblasts surrounds the silicone parts of the AUS and may confer protection against bacteria, which can be liberated into the bloodstream at the time of cystoplasty or with systemic infections.[57] The infection rate does not appear to increase in patients who catheterize compared to those who void spontaneously or who empty their bladders using the Credé maneuver.[57] Some investigators have found a definite increase in the occurrence of infection when cystoplasty is performed concomitantly with AUS insertion.[47,51] Holmes et al found an increased incidence of infection to be associated with prior bladder neck surgery in the neurogenic bladder population and recommended performing the AUS insertion before doing the augmentation in patients who have this risk factor.[56] Miller et al performed simultaneous bladder augmentation and AUS insertion using a variety of different bowel segments and found a 6.9% infection rate (2/29 patients). They suggested performing gastrocystoplasty along with AUS insertion since there were no infections associated with the use of stomach in their series.[58]

Erosion rates range from 6 to 31% in contemporary neurogenic bladder series and are the major cause of sphincter removal. Erosion can occur secondary to infection, ischemia from high cuff pressures, devascularization from prior surgery or radiation, and traumatic catheterization.[41,50,56] Factors which increase the likelihood of erosion include prior bladder neck surgery, placement of the cuff around the bulbar urethra in children, and placement of the cuff around the bowel used to form a neobladder.[41,50,55] Guralnick et al recently described AUS cuff placement through a dissection plane deep to the tunica albuginea of the corporal bodies in 31 men who experienced erosion or atrophy at the original cuff site. They were able to salvage continence in 84% of cases, but there was the potential for postoperative deterioration of erectile function.[59]

Patients who receive an AUS must undergo long-term urologic follow-up with urodynamic bladder monitoring and serial upper tract imaging to detect the onset of upper tract deterioration. High intravesical pressure requires the institution of anticholinergic medications, or, if this fails,

Table 53.4 *Results of artificial urinary sphincter insertion for the treatment of incontinence in patients with neurogenic bladder*

Study	Year	Patient population	Type and location of sphincter	Mean follow up time	Results	Complications
Bellioli et al[53]	1992	Adolescents 37: 35 male, 2 female 33 MMC, 3 SA, 1 pelvic surgery	2 AMS 792, 35 AMS 800 33 BN, 4 BU	4.5 years range 1–8.5	59% dry day and night 90% dry day only	2 upper tract deteriorations 38% reoperation rate for mechanical problems 1 infection, 1 BN perforation, 1 scrotal hematoma
Gonzalez et al[52]	1995	Pediatric 19 males all neurogenic	11 AMS 800 8 AMS 721 or 792 all BN placement	8 years	84.2% continent 73.8% catheterizing	36.8% postoperative augmentation rate 1 renal loss 10% new hydro
Levesque et al[47]	1996	Adult and pediatric Most with MMC 36: 22 male, 14 female before 1985 After 1985 18 children	Before 1985: 6 AMS 792, 18 AMS 292, 12 AMS 800 After 1985: all AMS 800 All BN placement	13.7 years	Mean survival time 12.1 years 82% dry 64% catheterizing 59% continent	6 developed renal failure 42% required postoperative augmentation
Singh and Thomas[51]	1996	Mostly adult 90: 75 male, 15 female 65 MMC, 19 SCI, 5 SA, 1 sacral angioma	82 AMS 800 8 AMS 792 BU and BN	4 years range 1–10	92% continent 79% with detrusor overactivity required augmentation 78% catheterizing	28% reoperation rate 6 infections, 7 erosions, 8 system failures, 2 pump failures, 1 cut tube, 1 rectal perforation, 1 bladder perforation
Simeoni et al[50]	1996	Pediatric 107: 74 male, 33 female 92 MMC	AMS 800 98 BN, 9 BU	61 months minimum of 12	41% continent with no revisions 21% augmentation rate	Immediate: 4 UTI, 2 wound infection, 3 scrotal hematoma, 3 urinary fistula, 2 retention 25% removal rate 59% revision rate 13% erosion rate

Table 53.4 Continued

Table 53.4 *Continued*

Study	Year	Patient population	Type and location of sphincter	Mean follow up time	Results	Complications
Fulford et al[41]	1997	Adult and pediatric 61: 43 male, 18 female 34 neurogenic, 15 post-radiation prostatectomy, 12 other	Combination of AMS 791, 792, and 800 BU and BN placement	10–15 years	75% functioning	49 with 1 or more revision 13% continent with original AUS *in situ* 31% erosion rate, 2/3 in 1st year after placement
Elliot and Barrett[42]	1998	Adult 323: 313 male, 10 female 70 neurogenic	All AMS 800 139 without narrow cuff backing 184 with narrow cuff backing 272 BU, 51 BN	68.8 months range 18–153	Males 27% reoperation rate, females: 60% reoperation rate 90.4% functioning at 5 years, 72% no reoperation at 5 years	Mechanical failure: 21% pre-cuff, 7.6% post-cuff Non-mechanical failure: 17% pre-cuff, 9% post-cuff
Kryger et al[45]	2001	Pediatric 32: 25 male, 7 female Group 1 – insertion before age 11 (21) Group 2 – insertion after age 11 (11)	AMS 800 – 21 Pre-AMS 800 – 11	1 year 15.4 years	Group 1 – 54% intact, all dry Group 2 – 64% intact, 86% dry No statistical significant difference between groups	56% revision rate Group 1 – 43% removed: 4 infection, 5 erosion Group 2 – 36% removed: 1 infection, 3 erosions
Castera et al[55]	2001	Pediatric 49: 39 male, 10 female 38 MMC, 7 exstrophy, 4 trauma	All AMS 800 29 BN 20 BU	7.5 years range 2–11	67% dry: 86% dry with no prior surgery, 37.5% dry with prior BN surgery	20% erosion, 4% infection, 12% mechanical failure
Spiess et al[54]	2002	Pediatric 30 males with MMC	All AMS 800	6.5 years	63% dry, 20% slightly wet	Only 8.3% lasted >100 months, mean lifetime 4.9 years

MMC, myelomeningocele; SA, sacral agenesis; SCI, spinal cord injury; BN, bladder neck; BU, bulbar urethra; UTI, urinary tract infection.

augmentation. Hydronephrosis or reflux is usually refractory to medical management and indicates a need for cystoplasty. The proportion of AUS recipients with neurogenic bladder who ultimately require augmentation cystoplasty ranges from 4 to 42%.[46,50,52,55] Patients who are noncompliant with surveillance protocols may develop upper tract damage. A number of authors have described the occurrence of chronic renal failure in patients with incontinence of neurologic etiology who received an AUS and were then lost to follow-up for long periods of time.[42,46,53]

Conclusions

When it was first marketed in the early 1970s, the AUS represented a major advancement in the treatment of patients with severe incontinence secondary to sphincteric deficiency. The device has undergone many design modifications since its first inception, all of which have served to increase its efficacy and lower its complication rate. Erosion and infection rates are low in well-selected patients. The possibility of requiring repeat surgery for mechanical failure is high, as is the cost of these revisions, but the AUS will, no doubt, continue to be utilized in the treatment of urinary incontinence.

Bladder neck reconstruction

Introduction

In 1908, Young described a technique for increasing bladder outlet resistance by narrowing the urethra and bladder neck lumen to the size of a silver probe.[60] Since this first description of bladder neck reconstruction was published, there have been many modifications to the surgical procedure. At first, reconfiguring the bladder outlet to increase its resistance was thought to be contraindicated in the neurogenic bladder population because of the subsequent necessity for IC.[61] Many investigators, however, have found this technique to be a viable alternative to bladder neck sling, AUS, or urinary diversion in patients with neurologic lesions who require treatment for severe sphincteric incompetence provided that the patient and/or caregiver is capable of performing IC and is compliant with this routine. These procedures are technically challenging and a successful outcome is highly dependent on the operative experience of the surgeon.

The main types of bladder neck reconstruction that have been utilized in the neurogenic bladder population are the Kropp anterior bladder wall flap valve and the Salle anterior bladder wall flip-flap. The Young–Dees–Leadbetter posterior bladder wall flap is primarily used for the treatment of bladder exstrophy, but has been reported

in patients with neurogenic sphincteric deficiency. The Tanagho and Smith bladder neck reconstruction, which is mostly of historic interest, has been described in patients with post-prostatectomy incontinence and will not be covered in this section.[61,62] The majority of the literature deals with the pediatric population, since it is in this age group that urologic intervention is first sought. The Kropp and Salle procedures work on the flap valve principle popularized by Mitrofanoff. As the bladder fills with urine, increases in intravesical pressure are transmitted to the valve constructed from anterior bladder wall, thereby increasing leak point threshold and preventing incontinence.[63] The Young–Dees–Leadbetter reconstruction prevents urine leakage by increasing bladder neck and urethral length and decreasing their caliber, two maneuvers which result in an increase in outlet resistance.[60]

Young–Dees–Leadbetter procedure

The Young–Dees–Leadbetter bladder neck reconstruction, as it was first described by Leadbetter in 1964, involves lengthening the urethra and creating a new bladder neck using a flap of posterior bladder wall which incorporates the trigone. The ureters are reimplanted 3–4 cm superiorly so that the trigonal muscle can be utilized. The posterior bladder wall is not mobilized in order to keep the blood and nervous supply intact, thereby helping to prevent slough and denervation of the bladder wall flap. The vertical midline cystotomy which was made to reimplant the ureters is carried into the urethra, and longitudinal lateral incisions are made on either side of the urethra and bladder neck. These incisions begin at the apex of the midline urethral incision and extend along the bladder base through the old ureteric orifice sites and 1–2 cm beyond them on the posterior bladder wall.

The resulting lateral bladder flaps are denuded of mucosa to leave a posterior strip of bladder 1.5 cm wide and 3 cm long.[64] These flaps are then folded over on each other using an 8–10F urethral catheter as a guide to caliber and closed in two layers. The mucosal layer is closed with interrupted fine absorbable suture and the muscle layer is opposed in an overlapping fashion using a fine running suture of absorbable material. The bladder neck closure is completed in layers: mucosa, muscle, and serosa. The end result is a urethra which is lengthened by 4–5 cm. The dog ears of bladder that remain are incorporated into the bladder wall closure, since resection of these segments can result in a substantial decrease in bladder capacity.[60] A urethral catheter and suprapubic tube are often placed, although some surgeons prefer to forgo urethral stenting. If employed, the urethral Foley catheter is removed within 3–4 weeks and the suprapubic tube is discontinued once the patient is able to empty the bladder by voiding or intermittent catheterization.

Placement of a silicone sheath around the bladder neck reconstruction to facilitate the insertion of an artificial urethral sphincter cuff later on if required was advocated by Mitchell et al in 1985. These authors, however, later abandoned this practice upon experiencing a 67% erosion rate at a mean of 4 years after operation.[65] Ransley's group, however, has reported a lower erosion rate of 14% after decreasing the thickness of the silicone sheath and interposing omentum between the sheath and the bladder neck.[65,66]

Kropp bladder neck reconstruction

The Kropp procedure was first described by Kropp and Aangwafo in 1986. It lengthens the urethra by attaching it to a tube of bladder muscle which is implanted into the posterior bladder wall through a submucosal tunnel to create a one-way flap valve that allows a catheter to be passed but prevents urine from leaking out. A rectangular flap 5–7 cm × 2–2.5 cm is outlined on the anterior bladder wall with stay sutures. This flap is left attached to the bladder neck and the bladder is separated completely from the bladder neck. The anterior wall flap is rolled into a tube over a 10–12F Foley catheter and sutured together with 4–0 chromic catgut. A submucosal tunnel is developed between the ureteric orifices, and the tube is pulled through this tunnel. The bladder is drawn back down to the bladder neck and sutured with absorbable sutures. The ostia of the new urethra is sutured to the posterior bladder wall. This method can also be accomplished using a posterior strip of bladder, which is tunneled into the anterior bladder wall.[67]

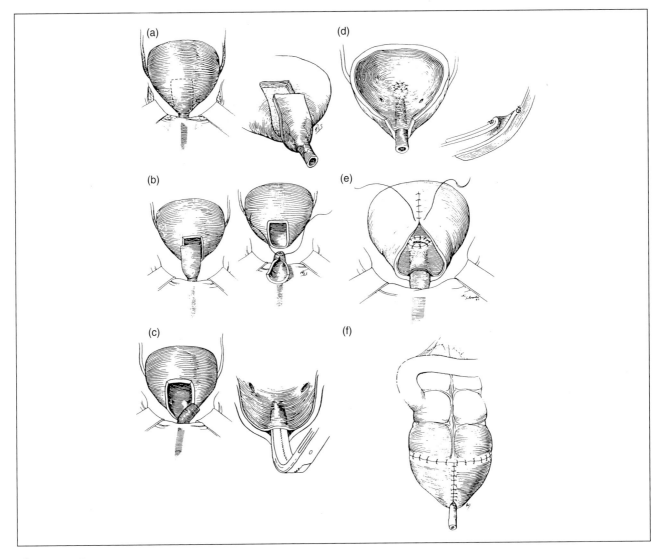

Figure 53.7
Kropp anterior flap-valve bladder neck reconstruction. (Reproduced with permission from Kropp and Angwolfo, J Urol 1986; 135:533–536.)

Two modifications to the Kropp bladder neck reconstruction were described by Belman and Kaplan and subsequently adopted widely by other surgeons, including the originator of the Kropp procedure.[68] These alterations involve leaving the bladder neck attached to the bladder and making a groove in the posterior bladder wall into which the tube is laid, then suturing the epithelium over the tube rather than creating a submucosal tunnel.[69] Mollard et al demuscularized the bladder tube, leaving only mucosa to tunnel in some cases, and reimplanted one of the ureters cephalad to make more room to tunnel the tube in the posterior bladder wall.[63]

Pippi Salle bladder neck reconstruction

In 1994, Pippi Salle described his own version of the anterior wall flap valve in 15 dogs and 6 children with myelomeningocele. The Salle bladder neck reconstruction is a modification of the Kropp design in which the urethra is lengthened with an anterior bladder wall flap 4–5 cm × 1–1.7 cm, which is sutured to the posterior wall in an onlay fashion. In the original description, the ureters are reimplanted superiorly using the Cohen cross-trigonal technique. A border of mucosa 0.1 cm wide is removed from the flap to obtain separate non-overlapping suture lines. The edges of the posterior bladder wall are then sewn over the lengthened urethra to create a flap valve. A urethral catheter is left in for 2–3 weeks.[70] In 1997 Salle and colleagues described a number of modifications to the original technique. The first involved making two longitudinal incisions in the trigonal mucosa to better expose the muscle for suturing to the exposed muscle edges of the anterior wall flap, then suturing the lateral edges of posterior wall mucosa over the flap to help prevent leakage of urine and fistula formation. The second modification was to widen the base of the flap to improve its blood supply but to leave the distal tip narrow to attain the correct lumen size when fashioning the neourethra. In some cases, a superior extension of mucosa was taken with the anterior wall flap and folded back over the intravesical urethra to cover it and prevent fistula formation. Lastly, the authors described the creation of a lateral anterior wall flap in 4 patients who had a midline scar in the anterior bladder wall from previous surgery. Ureteric reimplantations were not performed routinely in this later series.[71]

Indications and patient selection

All patients being considered for bladder neck reconstruction should undergo urodynamic assessment and

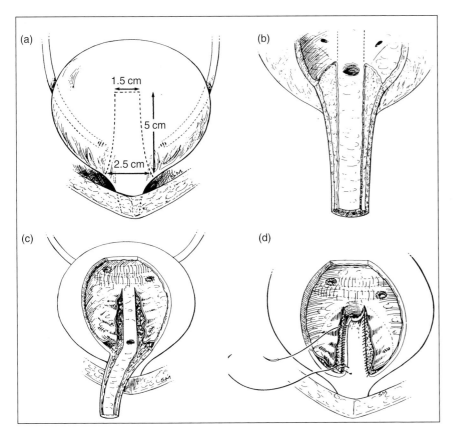

Figure 53.8
Pippi Salle flip-flap bladder reconstruction. (Reproduced with permission from Pippi-Salle, J Urol 1994; 152:803–806.)

voiding cystourethrogram to document the mechanism of incontinence and the degree of urethral incompetence. The filling phase should be carried out with a Foley balloon occluding the bladder outlet to determine bladder capacity, stability, and compliance.[43] Cystoscopy may aid in assessing the characteristics of the bladder wall and outlet before surgery. The urodynamic prerequisites for bladder neck reconstruction are similar to those for the AUS or bladder neck sling: a stable, adequate capacity bladder (see above). The majority of authors recommend the concomitant performance of bladder augmentation, since increasing outlet resistance will often lead to elevated storage pressures and the use of bladder wall to reconstruct the outlet can significantly decrease bladder capacity.[72,73]

Although bladder neck reconstruction can be performed as a salvage procedure for patients who have failed bladder neck sling or AUS insertion,[74] many authors advocate considering it as a primary option in patients who have total incontinence secondary to a patulous, wide-open bladder neck, since compromised blood supply from previous surgery will decrease the success of the operation.[69] Bladder neck reconstruction in general is not suitable for the correction of mild stress urinary incontinence, since it has a significant complication rate.

The Young–Dees–Leadbetter bladder neck reconstruction is mainly employed in the treatment of anatomic bladder outlet defects encountered in the exstrophy-epispadias complex; there have been few reports of its use in patients with neurogenic bladder. Continence rates are not as high in patients with neuropathic outlet incompetence as they are in the exstrophy population, and some investigators have documented better results in females than in males.[75]

The Kropp procedure was specifically designed for the treatment of neurogenic incontinence and functions on the assumption that all patients will need to catheterize to empty the bladder. It is often performed as a last resort to achieve continence before AUS insertion. Mollard et al[63] and Snodgrass[73] prefer to use the Kropp procedure as first-line bladder outlet management in females and reserve the AUS for males, with the rationale that lengthening the urethra in boys may make it more difficult for them to perform IC. Waters et al, however, in a review of catheterization problems in patients who had had Kropp reconstruction, found that the problem was experienced by equal numbers of boys and girls.[68] The Salle technique has been employed with equal success in patients with incontinence secondary to neurogenic bladder and exstrophy-epispadias complex.[70,71,76,77]

Results and complications

The Young–Dees–Leadbetter procedure and its numerous modifications have produced continence rates up to 60–80% when performed in the exstrophy population.[78,79] Published series employing this technique in neurogenic bladder patients are small, but success has been reported to be lower, with continence rates of 50–60% over a follow-up period of greater than 5 years.[75,80,81] Complications have included UTIs, de-novo vesicoureteral reflux (VUR), urethral and bladder neck fistulas, SUI, difficulty catheterizing, and bladder neck strictures, particularly in patients who have had previous bladder neck surgery.[75,79]

The Kropp bladder neck reconstruction has enjoyed continence rates of 80–94%, but this has been tempered by difficult catheterization rates of 10–44% (Table 53.5).[63,67–69,72,73] This problem is thought to occur secondary to the tube being compressed as it passes through the submucosal tunnel, or the suture line running along the back wall of the tube causing formation of an elevated scar.[67,70] An overdistended bladder resulting from delay in catheterization can also compress the valve, making it difficult to pass a drainage tube.[72] In later series, investigators have noted a decrease in the occurrence of catheterization problems when the urethral catheter was left in 4–5 weeks after bladder neck reconstruction.[69] In most cases, this situation is alleviated by passing a catheter under cystoscopic guidance and leaving it in for a few weeks, then having the patient resume catheterization.[68] Other patients who have trouble passing a catheter require bladder neck dilatation or endoscopic resection of the roof of the neourethra. Occasionally, open revision of the flap valve is required.[67,72] Snodgrass has described the performance of an appendicovesicostomy concomitant to the Kropp procedure as a means of providing an alternative route of bladder drainage should the patient be unable to catheterize via the reconstructed bladder outlet.[73]

Other complications encountered with the Kropp technique include pyelonephritis, peritonitis secondary to bladder perforation, de-novo VUR, and fistula formation between the valve and the bladder resulting in incontinence. The Kropp procedure is highly effective at increasing bladder neck resistance and can result in the attainment of a VLPP of greater than 60 cmH$_2$O in many patients.[69] This high level of continence, coupled with the possibility of difficult catheterization in a patient who may also have an enterocystoplasty, can result in perforation of the augmented portion of the bladder, with subsequent peritonitis, cases of which have culminated in death.[72] New-onset VUR is thought to be a consequence of elevated intravesical pressures as a result of increased outlet resistance, disruption of the trigonal musculature when tunneling the tube, or VUR which was present preoperatively but was not observed on cystourethrogram.[71,73] A small proportion of patients who develop de-novo VUR fail to resolve it spontaneously and require ureteric reimplantation. Fistulas can occur at areas of devascularization along suture lines or as a consequence of traumatic

Table 53.5 *Results of Kropp bladder neck reconstruction in patients with neurogenic incontinence*

Procedure	Study	Year	Patients	Follow-up time	Concomitant surgeries	Results	Complications
Kropp	Kropp and Angwafo[67]	1986	Pediatric 7 male, 6 female 13 MMC	8–36 months	6 augments, 2 reimplants, 2 undiversions	92% dry	4/6 IC problems 4 de-novo VUR
Kropp	Belman and Kaplan[69]	1989	Pediatric 18: 16 MMC, 2 SA, 10 male	Not stated	14 augments	78% dry, 4 hours	44% IC problems 4 de-novo VUR, 1 pyelonephritis
Kropp	Nill et al[72]	1990	Pediatric and adult 24: MMC and MS 14 female	1.5–7 years	19 reoperations to perform bladder augmentation	83% dry	46% IC problems 1 vesicocutaneous fistula, 5 reoperations on valve, 9 peritonitis, 8 bladder stones, 10 de-novo VUR
Kropp	Mollard et al[63]	1990	Pediatric 16 girls 15 MMC, 1 other	Not stated	6 augments, 7 reimplants	81% dry	12.5% IC problems 2 valve failures
Kropp (Belman and Kaplan modifications)	Snodgrass[73]	1997	Pediatric 23: 13 male all MMC	Mean 27 months range 3–72	20 augments	91% dry	17% IC problems all in males, 2 valve fistulas, 50% de-novo VUR

MMC, myelomeningocele; SA, sacral agenesis; IC, intermittent catheterization; VUR, vesicoureteric reflux.

Table 53.6 *Results of Salle and Young–Dees–Leadbetter bladder neck reconstruction in patients with neurogenic incontinence*

Procedure	Study	Year	Patients	Follow-up time	Concomitant surgery	Results	Complications
Salle	Pippi Salle et al[70]	1994	Pediatric 6: 3 males All with MMC	Mean 16.8 months range 7–24	Not stated	4/6 (67%) dry	1 flap fistula, 1 re-operation to narrow flap, 1 de-novo VUR, 1 pyelo
Salle	Rink et al[77]	1994	Pediatric 3 MMC females	12–15 months	Cohen reimplants 2 augments	2/3 dry, 1 noctural leakage	None
Salle	Mouriquard et al[76]	1995	Pediatric 8 girls: 7 MMC, 1 other	Mean 6.7 months range 2–18	6 augments	38% dry day and night 88% dry during day	1 flap fistula, 1 bladder calculi
Salle	Pippi Salle et al[71]	1997	Pediatric 17: 13 neurogenic, 4 EE	Mean 25.6 months range 9–49	Not stated	70% dry 9/13 neurogenic dry, 3/4 EE dry	2 flap fistulas, 2 IC problems (all in EEC), 12% de-novo VUR
Young–Dees–Leadbetter vs AUS	Sidi et al[80]	1987	Pediatric 11 BN reconstruction: 9 female 16 AUS: all male 17 MMC, 6 SA, 4 other	BNR Mean 3.2 years range 1–5 AUS Mean 5.7 years range 1–12	BNR: 64% dry AUS: 69% dry	BNR reoperation rate 0.8/patient AUS reoperation rate 1.5/patient	BNR: 9 augments AUS: 2 augments
Young–Dees–Leadbetter	Donnahoo et al[75]	1999	Pediatric 38: 25 female 32 MMC, 3 SA, 13 other	Mean 9 years range 1–17	8 silicone sheath placements, 36 reimplants, 22 augments	50% dry 12.5% partially dry 63% girls vs 25% boys dry with primary bladder neck reconstruction	10.5% IC problems 62.5% silicone sheath erosion, 14% perforation of augmented bladder

MMC, myelomeningocele; SA, sacral agenesis; EE, exstrophy-epispadias; IC, intermittent catheterization; VUR, vesicoureteric reflux; AUS, artificial urethral sphincter; BNR, bladder neck reconstruction instrumentation or catheterization and usually require open revision of the flap valve in order to achieve continence.

The Salle anterior bladder wall flap has continence rates which are slightly lower than the Kropp procedure, but does not have the high incidence of catheterization difficulty which has plagued the other technique. The occurrence of fistulas between the flap valve and bladder is a problem particularly noted with the Salle procedure and catheterization problems were experienced by some of the exstrophy patients in the later series published by Pippi Salle et al (Table 53.6).[70,71]

Conclusion

In summary, bladder neck reconstruction is one of the earliest surgical treatments devised for treating urinary incontinence secondary to an incompetent bladder neck and proximal urethra. All these procedures, while they have the advantage of utilizing the patient's own tissue, are technically challenging and are associated with a number of complications, some of which may require numerous surgical revisions. Bladder neck reconstruction should not be performed in patients who have mild degrees of urinary incontinence that may be cured by urethral collagen injections or a fascial sling. Bladder neck reconstruction should be reserved for patients with severe outlet incompetence and should only be performed by an experienced surgeon. Despite the availability of the AUS and popularity of the fascial sling, bladder neck reconstruction in its many forms continues to have a role in the treatment of patients with neurogenic bladder and exstrophy-epispadias complex who suffer from total urinary incontinence.

Bladder neck closure

Introduction

Bladder neck closure is considered a last-resort procedure.[82] It is indicated in patients with outlet incompetence who have failed multiple anti-incontinence procedures, patients who are poor surgical candidates and cannot tolerate lengthy, complex reconstructive procedures, and in patients with destroyed urethras which cannot be rebuilt.[83] Closure of the bladder neck can be combined with a catheterizable cutaneous stoma or a chronic indwelling suprapubic tube depending on the constitutional and functional status of the patient.

In female spinal cord injury patients who have been managed with a chronic indwelling Foley catheter, bladder neck closure and suprapubic tube insertion can improve quality of life by eliminating leakage of urine alongside the tube, which can cause chronic skin breakdown, and facilitate return to sexual activity by eliminating the urethral catheter.[84,85]

The disadvantages of bladder neck closure are its irreversibility; its abolishment of the pop-off valve, which necessitates long-term monitoring of the upper tracts to prevent occult renal deterioration;[86] and unpredictable effects on potency and ejaculation when performed in young males.[82] Patients who are managed with bladder neck closure and a chronic suprapubic tube must undergo surveillance cystoscopy in order to monitor for the formation of bladder calculi and squamous neoplasia.[83] There is also a persistent risk of infection secondary to the indwelling catheter.[84]

Transposition of the female urethra to the suprapubic area to form a continent catheterizable stoma has been described, but it is not suitable for obese patients or patients with a significant amount of periurethral scarring secondary to previous surgical procedures or years of chronic indwelling urethral Foley management.[83,84,86] Reconstruction using vaginal wall or bowel has also been attempted in females with destroyed urethras but the success rate with these procedures is low.[87] Alternatively, a tight fascial sling can be used to achieve a functional bladder neck closure, provided that the patient has a urethral length of at least 1.5–2 cm.[88]

Surgical technique

Bladder neck closure can be performed via the transabdominal or transvaginal route. In the transabdominal approach, a transverse suprapubic incision or vertical midline incision is made and the bladder neck is mobilized. In males, the bladder is transected just cranial to the prostate after ligating the superficial dorsal venous complex and dissecting the neurovascular bundles away. The prostate is usually left intact in order to preserve fertility and antegrade ejaculation. In cases of urethral stricture or prostatorectal fistula which compromise drainage of prostatic secretions and act as a nidus of infection, the prostate is removed to avoid abscess formation. In females the bladder is transected at the vesicourethral junction once the deep dorsal vein has been ligated. Intravenous indigo carmine or ureteric catheters are used to help identify the ureteric orifices. The bladder is mobilized posteriorly to the level of the ureteric orifices. A sponge stick in the vagina can aid in identifying the correct plane of dissection.

Once the posterior and inferior aspects of the bladder have been mobilized out of its dependent position in the pelvis, the bladder neck opening is closed ventrally in two layers: mucosa and muscle with serosa. A suprapubic tube is placed and brought out through a separate stab incision before closing the bladder neck completely, and if the bladder closure is to be combined with a continent catheterizable stoma it is constructed and attached to the bladder at this stage. The urethral stump is closed dorsally in two layers and an omental flap is mobilized and placed between the closed urethral stump and the bladder neck closure to prevent fistula formation.[82,84] A drain is usually left in the space of Retzius. Postoperatively, anticholinergics are administered to prevent bladder spasms. Reid et al have described a different technique of bladder neck closure which involved denuding the bladder neck mucosa through a midline cystotomy, excising a cuff of bladder neck, then closing the denuded muscle with a purse string suture.[89]

The transvaginal approach is typically employed in females with urethral destruction secondary to chronic indwelling Foley catheter drainage who are to be managed with bladder neck closure and suprapubic tube placement. The patient is placed in the dorsal lithotomy position and a suprapubic tube is placed using a Lowsley retractor. This technique is employed to circumvent the difficulty inherent in distending a small contracted bladder with an incompetent outlet.

The patient is placed in the Trendelenburg position to displace the bowels cephalad and the curved Lowsley retractor is inserted into the urethra and pointed towards the anterior abdominal wall 1–2 cm above the pubic symphysis. A small fascial incision is made over the tip of the retractor, which is pushed out through the skin incision.

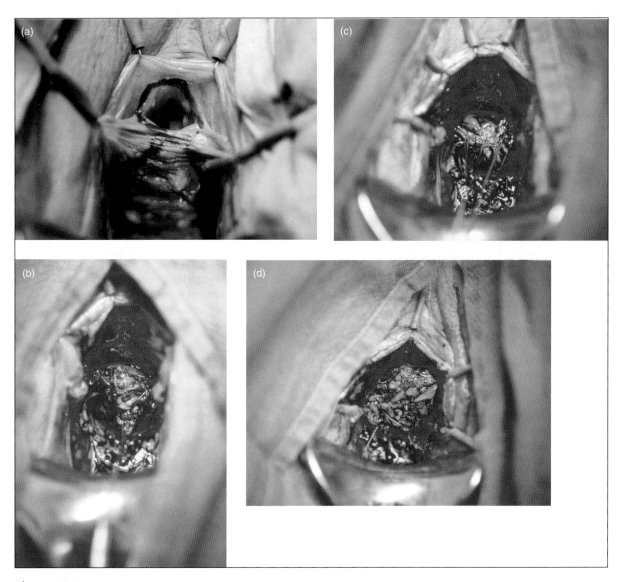

Figure 53.9
Transvaginal bladder neck closure. (a) Creation of anterior vaginal wall flap. Destroyed urethra is circumscribed. (b) Bladder neck is mobilized and urethral reminant excised. First tension-free layer of bladder neck closure. (c) Transversal second layer closure to protect against a secondary vesicovaginal fistula. (d) Placement of Martius flap tunneled beneath labia minora. (Reproduced with permission from Glenn's Urologic Surgery, 5th edn, 1998, Chapter 49, Figs 49.1–49.4.)

The tip of a large-bore Foley catheter is grasped in its jaws and pulled back into the bladder. Intravesical placement of the catheter can be confirmed by irrigation of the tube or cystoscopic inspection.[90]

An incision circumscribing the urethral opening is extended into an inverted U incision on the anterior vaginal wall. The endopelvic fascia is pierced on either side of the bladder neck in order to free it up completely from the pubic bone and the pubourethral ligaments are transected. Intravenous indigo carmine is given to visualize the ureteric orifices. The scarred urethra, if present, is excised and the bladder neck closed in two layers: first in the vertical, and then in the horizontal direction. The second suture line should contain tissue from the bladder neck to the anterior wall located behind the symphysis to transfer the closed bladder neck to the retropubic space and remove it from a dependent position. The integrity of the closure is checked by filling the bladder through the suprapubic tube. A Martius flap is interposed between the bladder neck and anterior vaginal wall to help prevent vesicovaginal fistula formation and the vaginal wall flap is closed over the Martius flap as a third layer. A vaginal pack containing antibiotic solution is left in for 24 hours,[83] and anticholinergics are administered to prevent bladder spasms.

Bladder neck closure is highly effective at treating incontinence secondary to an incompetent bladder outlet. Continence rates of 75–100% have been reported in the literature, with mean follow-up times ranging from 1.5 to 3 years.[82–87,91,92] The main technical complication is bladder neck fistulization with continued leakage of urine, which has been reported to occur in 6–25% of cases.[84,89–92] The rate of fistulization is low in series which adhere to the following surgical principles: mobilization of the bladder from its dependent position in the pelvis, closure of the bladder neck and urethral stump in multiple layers without tension, and interposition of well-vascularized tissue such as omentum or a labial fat pad between the urethra and bladder neck. No adverse effect on potency or ejaculation was noted by Hoebeke et al, who performed the procedure in nine young males.

Surgical treatment of the hyperactive bladder outlet

Introduction

For several years it has been recognized that detrusor-external sphincter dyssynergia (DESD), a common condition in patients with suprasacral spinal cord lesions, is associated with elevated intravesical pressure, which can result in substantial morbidity and mortality. DESD is defined as a detrusor contraction concurrent with an involuntary contraction of the urethral and/or peri-urethral striated muscle during voiding.[93] During urodynamic assessment, DESD is denoted by an increase in electromyographic activity of the sphincter or pelvic muscles associated with an involuntary detrusor contraction. On voiding cystourethrogram or videourodynamic assessment, dilation of the bladder neck due to a contracted external sphincter is observed during bladder emptying.[94] The condition leads to a complication rate in excess of 50%, resulting in urosepsis, hydronephrosis, nephrolithiasis, and vesicoureteric reflux, all of which can terminate in renal insufficiency and, eventually, dialysis.[95,96] DESD is also associated with autonomic dysreflexia, particularly in patients with injuries above the T5 spinal cord level. Since its description by Emmett et al in 1948, sphincterotomy has been recommended to treat DESD in a subset of spinal cord injured males who are at risk for renal damage.[97] By incising the external sphincter to render it incompetent, one can transform intermittent incontinence into continous incontinence, which can be managed with a condom catheter drainage device.[98] Sphincterotomy is irreversible and has been associated with intraoperative bleeding and erectile dysfunction. A reduction in long-term efficacy has also been observed which may require repeat external sphincter or bladder neck incision.[99] Long-term use of a condom catheter can lead to skin ulceration, urethrocutaneous fistula, and penile retraction.[98] Despite these drawbacks, sphicterotomy is still considered the gold standard to which other treatments for DESD are compared.

A urethral stent was first used by Milroy et al in 1988 to treat stricture disease.[100] Subsequently, it has been employed in benign prostatic hyperplasia (BPH) therapy and as an alternative to sphincterotomy in patients with DESD. Most of the experience with external sphincter stenting has been with the Urolume prosthesis (American Medical Systems, Minnetonka, Minnesota), a nonmagnetic superalloy woven into a mesh cylinder which is inserted endoscopically across the external sphincter to hold it open. The geometry and elasticity of the stent material exerts a radial force which maintains its position within the urethral lumen until epithelialization occurs.[101] Other urethral stents which have been used to circumvent DESD include the Ultraflex (Boston Scientific Corp., Boston, MA), which is made of a single elastalloy wire, and the Memokath (Engineers and Doctors A/S, Homback, Denmark), a coil made of thermosensitive titanium/nickel alloy. Sphincteric stenting has several advantages over sphincterotomy. It is an easier and quicker procedure that is associated with shorter hospital stay and cost.[101] Unlike sphincterotomy, stent insertion is potentially reversible, a characteristic which appeals to spinal cord injured patients still hoping for a cure.[94] Furthermore, sphincteric stents are

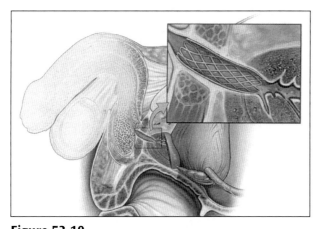

Figure 53.10
Sagittal view of male pelvis to show placement of urethral stent across external sphincter.

not associated with diminished erectile ability or significant blood loss.[94] Despite these advantages, insertion of a stent across the external sphincter raises some legitimate concerns. The stent is a foreign body which is placed in contact with urine, resulting in encrustation.[94] Difficult removal of the Urolume stent occasionally resulting in urethral injury has also been reported.[102,103]

Another minimally invasive treatment for the dyssynergic external sphincter, balloon dilatation, has also recently been described.[104] More experience is needed to determine its long-term merit.

Indications and patient selection

Both sphincterotomy and urethral stents are employed in the treatment of DESD in male spinal cord injured patients with DO refractory to anticholinergics and IC, or in those unable or unwilling to carry out this conservative treatment.[99] Sphincteric stents have been used not only as primary treatment for DESD but also for patients who have failed previous sphincterotomy.[94,105] Relative contraindications to stenting include patients who are known to be recurrent stone formers, patients who have had previous bladder neck (BN) incisions or TURP (transurethral rejection of the prostate), and patients who have an artificial urinary sphincter.[94,105,106] Chancellor et al, in the North American Multicenter Urolume Trial, found that a wide-open bladder neck secondary to previous bladder neck or prostatic surgery predisposed patients to stent migration.[94] McInerney and colleagues placed stents in 3 men with spinal cord injuries and DESD who had artificial urinary sphincters.[105] The voiding parameters of these men were not improved, and, due

to perineal discomfort, one stent was eventually removed with great difficulty.

The Memokath stent has been found to be easier to remove than the Urolume device and has been advocated as a short-term treatment option for DESD. This stent may be used as an alternative to an indwelling catheter in recent spinal cord injured patients who are likely to regain enough upper extremity function to be able to perform self-catheterization, or for patients who would like to try condom catheter drainage before committing themselves to Urolume or sphincterotomy.[107] Men who are undergoing electroejaculation may also benefit from the Memokath, since the device can be easily removed and replaced later on.[107]

Sphincterotomy or sphincteric stenting with condom catheter drainage is preferable to a chronic indwelling Foley catheter, which is still often used as the management of last resort in quadriplegic patients who do not have the manual dexterity or caregiver support to perform IC or change a condom catheter. Chronic indwelling catheters are associated with recurrent urosepsis, bladder calculi, and squamous cell carcinoma in this patient population.[108]

Sphincterotomy techniques

Before proceeding with incision of the external sphincter, the patient should have a negative urine culture. The patient is placed in the dorsal lithotomy position and perioperative intravenous antibiotic prophylaxis is administered. The type of anesthesia required depends on the amount of sensation and severity of autonomic dysreflexia experienced by the individual. Intravenous sedation with or without calcium channel or alpha-antagonist prophylaxis for hypertensive crisis may be all that is needed.

Sphincterotomy is usually performed under endoscopic video control with a 24F resectoscope and Collins knife or loop electrocautery attachment. A cut is made anteriorly at the 12 o'clock or 11 o'clock position away from the neurovascular bundles to minimize the risk of bleeding and erectile dysfunction. The incision is taken from the prostatic urethra just proximal to the verumontanum to the proximal bulbar urethra. The cut must extend through the muscle fibers of the sphincter to the level of the corpus spongiosum tissue of the proximal bulb.[109] Hemostasis is attained with the electrocautery, and a 22F three-way Foley catheter is placed in the bladder. Continuous bladder irrigation is run for 24–48 hours to prevent clot retention and the patient is discharged once the urine is clear. The catheter is removed 4–7 days after the procedure and a condom catheter is applied to the penis for bladder drainage.

Sphincterotomy performed with the Nd:YAG contact laser has been described as an alternative to electrocautery.[110,111] A chisel or round-tip probe is deployed through the instrument port of a 21 or 23F cystoscope with a 30 degree lens. The sphincterotomy is performed anteriorly, as with electrocautery, with the probe tip in contact with the tissue to be vaporized. Repeated passes are made over the area until the required depth is attained. Cutting tissue requires settings of 25–50 W and hemostasis is achieved with lower energy settings of 15–25 W. Laser sphincterotomy may take a longer time than conventional electrocautery, especially if there is a large amount of scarring from previous surgery.[111]

Whether or not to perform bladder neck incision concomitant with sphincterotomy to optimize bladder emptying is somewhat controversial. Some investigators state that the bladder neck should not be incised immediately, as there is often delayed relaxation of the bladder outlet after sphincterotomy, and performing a bladder neck incision will result in complete incontinence with continuous urine leakage.[99] Other surgeons cut the bladder neck in addition to the external sphincter when preoperative urodynamics demonstrate bladder neck obstruction.[109,110] In their series of laser sphincterotomies, Perkash[110] performed concomitant laser bladder neck incisions at 3 and 9 o'clock, whereas Rivas et al[111] cut the bladder neck in the midline at 6 o'clock.

Results and complications of sphincterotomy

The results of some contemporary series of spinal cord patients treated with sphincterotomy are listed in Table 53.7. Incising the external sphincter results in statistically significant decreases in maximum detrusor pressure, post-void residual, and the occurrence of autonomic dysreflexia. Bladder capacity is usually maintained. Complications include bleeding, clot retention, urosepsis, erectile dysfunction, and sphincterotomy failure secondary to urethral scarring. Making the incision anteriorly at 12 or 11 o'clock, rather than posterolaterally, has lowered the likelihood of damage to the urethral blood supply and cavernous body innervation, resulting in decreased rates of clot retention and erectile dysfunction compared with older series.[109,111] The need for repeat sphincterotomy secondary to scarring and stenosis of the external sphincter is usually evident within 12 months of having the procedure, but can occur years later.[99] Repeat sphincterotomy rates range from 9%, when the laser is employed, to 31%, with the use of conventional electrocautery.[109,110] Other complications said to be decreased with laser sphincterotomy compared to electrocautery are severe bleeding and erectile dysfunction. In the absence of a prospective randomized trial, there is no conclusive

proof of the superiority of laser to electrocautery. The post-void residual often persists after incising the external sphincter, but many authors do not consider this finding an indication of treatment failure unless the patient continues to have recurrent UTIs due to urinary stasis.[98,109] Treatment failure despite a technically perfect sphincterotomy occurs in 10–50% of men treated for DESD. Reasons for failure include problems fitting the condom catheter as well as detrusor areflexia, which can result in poor bladder emptying despite an incompetent bladder outlet.[98,109,112]

Sphincteric stenting techniques

As with sphincterotomy, the patient is placed in the dorsal lithotomy position and is given perioperative antibiotic coverage. The Urolume device is packaged in a preloaded 24F cystoscopic insertion tool that accommodates a zero degree urethroscope. The Urolume comes in lengths of 2, 2.5, and 3 cm. The Ultraflex device comes in 2–5 cm lengths with 0.5 cm increments. The 3 cm length is usually adequate for two-thirds of patients being treated for DESD,[113] and, with the 5 cm Ultraflex prosthesis, only 10% of patients were found to need placement of a second stent.[114] If required, however, more than one device can be placed in order to span the entire external sphincter. Temporary suprapubic drainage is established intraoperatively to ensure good visibility and postoperative bladder drainage. Under direct vision, the insertion tool is introduced into the urethra and advanced to the level of the verumontanum, then released. The stent usually retracts 1–2 mm after deployment, and this should be accounted for when deciding on the position to release the device.[110,111] The stent should cover the caudal half of the verumontanum, leaving the ejaculatory ducts unblocked. The distal end should extend at least 5 mm into the bulbar urethra, well beyond the distal aspect of the external sphincter. If placement is incorrect, the Urolume can be moved or removed with endoscopic forceps. The Ultraflex can be pulled back using a suture located on its distal end which is removed after confirmation of proper placement.[114] When needed, a second stent should be placed overlapping the first by approximately 5 mm to completely bridge the sphincteric area.[115]

The Memokath stent is also inserted under direct vision mounted on a flexible or rigid cystoscope. Intraoperative fluoroscopy is used after filling the bladder with 200 ml of dilute contrast to monitor for distal movement that may occur with removal of the scope after stent deployment.[112] Once the stent is positioned correctly within the urethral lumen, saline warmed to 50°C is instilled into the device to cause expansion. Irrigation of the stent with cold saline (<10°C) renders it soft for easy removal with alligator forceps.[116]

Table 53.7 *Contemporary results of sphincterotomy in the treatment of detrusor–external sphincter dyssynergia*

Study	Year	Number and type of patients	Type of sphincterotomy	Mean follow-up (months)	Previous surgery	Results	Complications
Rivas et al[111]	1994	22 SCI males 14 quads 8 paras	Nd:YAG contact laser (round probe)	14 range 3–20	7% previous electrocautery sphincterotomy	18 successful Decreased voiding pressure and PVR ($p < 0.01$)	13.6% repeat sphincterotomy 1 skin ulceration, 1 urethrocutaneous fistula
Vapneck et al[109]	1994	16 SCI males 13 quads 3 paras	14 electrocautery 1 open 1 cold knife	39 range 3–96		50% success 8/16 still used condom drainage	5 repeat sphincterotomy, 1 spinal headache, 1 urosepsis/ADR Long term: 3 recurrent UTIs, 2 penile skin problems, 2 ADR, 1 combo of above
Perkash[110]	1996	76 SCI males 32% – bladder neck stenosis or BPH 32% bulbar strictures 54% quads 46% paras	Nd:YAG contact laser (chisel tip probe) Sphincterotomy ± bladder neck/ prostatic incisions	27 range 16–41	56% previous electrocautery sphincterotomy	Decreased voiding pressure ($p < 0.0003$), decreased ADR	Overall 11.8% 7 repeat sphincterotomy 2 blood loss >100 ml
Fontaine et al[98]	1996	92 SCI males 47 quads 45 paras	Electrocautery	20.6		Objective improvement in 83.7% Subjectively improved in 73%, ADR resolution in 93.2%, decreased PVR ($p < 0.001$)	Overall 10.6% 8.1% repeat sphincterotomy 4 hematurias 1 transfusion 4 de-novo ADR 2 bacteremia

SCI, spinal cord injury; ADR, autonomic dysreflexia; PVR, post-void residual; quad, quadraplegic; para, paraplegic; BPH, benign prostatic hyperplasia.

Postoperative oral antibiotics are usually continued for 10–14 days.[94,111] A condom catheter is used to drain the bladder postoperatively. The patient can be discharged within 24 hours. A pelvic X-ray is recommended to confirm proper position of the prosthesis before discharge. The suprapubic tube can be removed a few days later once adequate bladder emptying via the condom catheter is documented. Urethral catheterization should be avoided for at least 3 months to avoid displacement of the stent before epithelialization occurs.

Stent removal can be accomplished under intravenous sedation or general anesthesia. The resectoscope on low cutting current is used to remove all epithelium overlying the stent. The prosthesis is then grasped with alligator forceps and pulled through the scope or pushed into the bladder and removed through the scope obturator.[103,113] The stent may unravel into individual wires and may need to be removed piece-by-piece. When the stent begins to separate, more than one procedure may be required in order to remove the prosthesis completely.[115] Fluoroscopy or a pelvic X-ray should be obtained to ensure complete stent removal.

Results and complications of sphincteric stenting

Several series examining the performance of urethral stents in the treatment of DESD have found statistically significant decreases in voiding pressure, post-void residual, and autonomic dysreflexia with no change in bladder capacity (see Table 53.8).[94,102,114] In a prospective nonrandomized trial comparing sphincterotomy to the Urolume stent, Rivas et al found no statistically significant differences in treatment outcomes between these two modalities.[101] The stent, however, was associated with a significantly shorter operative time, decreased length of hospital stay, and less blood loss when compared to sphincterotomy. Long-term complications that have been found to occur with the Urolume include epithelial hyperplasia, stent encrustation, stent migration, urethral obstruction, secondary bladder neck obstruction, and difficult stent removal.[94,100,103,106] The Memokath device is associated with a high rate of migration, recurrent UTIs, and calcification, making it more suitable for the short-term treatment of DESD.[102,112]

Urothelial hyperplasia first occurs during growth of urethral mucosa over the stent, and usually resolves by the time the stent is completely covered, a process which can take anywhere from 3 months to 1 year.[94] Incorporation of the device into the urethral wall lowers the likelihood of stone formation, infection, and migration.[100,114] Epithelial hyperplasia can lead to stent obstruction in 5% of cases, which can be remedied with endoscopic resection.[94] Calcific encrustation may occur at the ends of the

Urolume device, which are the last areas to become epithelialized.[102]

Stent migration is the most common reason for stent removal and can usually be diagnosed by cystoscopy or a pelvic X-ray. The most recent report of the North American Multicenter Urolume Trial found a 28.7% rate of stent migration, with approximately 40% of cases occurring within the first 3 months after insertion.[94] Reasons for stent migration include previous bladder neck or prostatic surgery, previous sphincterotomy, urethral catheterization before epithelialization took place, and dislodgement during stool disimpaction or patient transfers.[94,103] Wilson et al, in a recent review of stent failures, discovered urethral obstruction in one patient who had had tandem stents placed, secondary to one stent telescoping on the other more proximal stent.[103] The long-term rate of secondary bladder neck obstruction is 26.3% with the Urolume endoprosthesis,[94] and is thought to be a result of bladder neck dyssynergia masked by the presence of DESD.[106] If conservative management with alpha-blockade fails, then bladder neck incision or resection can be performed.

Despite several large series detailing the ease with which the Urolume can be removed even when completely epithelialized, many investigators have reported cases of stent explantation which were difficult and tedious.[102,103] Despite following the manufacturer's directions for prosthesis removal, the stent has been known to disintegrate and unravel, requiring piecemeal removal of each individual wire in a time-consuming process. Wilson et al described two cases of challenging stent removal, one of which required making a perineal incision, and the other resulting in avulsion of the urethral mucosa.[103]

Balloon dilatation of the external urethral sphincter

The concept of dilating the urethra with a balloon in order to treat high intravesical pressure was first described by Bloom et al, who employed this technique to lower the leak point pressures of 18 children with myelomeningocele.[117] Since then, Chancellor et al have compared the short-term results of balloon dilatation of the external sphincter to sphincterotomy and stent insertion in the treatment of spinal cord injured men with DESD. All three modalities were found to be equivalent in terms of decreasing voiding pressure, post-void residual, and autonomic dysreflexia at a mean follow-up time of 15 months. Complications occurring in 20 cases of balloon dilatation were blood transfusion (1), recurrent sphincteric obstruction (3), and bulbar urethral stricture (1).[104]

Table 53.8 *Results of urethral stents for the treatment of detrusor-external sphincter dyssynergia*

Study	Year	Number and type of patients	Type of stent	Mean follow-up (months)	Previous surgery	Results	Complications
Rivas et al[101]	1994	26 had stent, 20 sphincterotomy	Urolume vs sphincterotomy Patients selected treatment	Range 6–20		Shorter OR time, hospitalization time, lower blood loss, no difference in decrease in PVR, voiding pressure, or capacity	Stents – 15.4% migration, 2 BNO Sphincterotomy – 2 transfusions, 2 repeat ORs, 1 erectile dysfunction
Sauerwein et al[115]	1995	51 SCI males	Urolume (see above)	Range 12–36	All had sphincterotomy, 22 BNI, 18 TURBN	All had lowered ADR and voiding pressures, increased compliance	25.5% initial ADR, 9.8% migration, 5.9% explantation, 1 poor emptying
McFarlane et al[106]	1996	11 SCI males	Wallstent (American Medical Systems, UK) now Urolume	69.6 range 36–89		36.4% success – decreased PVR, maximum detrusor pressure	1 urosepsis at insertion, 5 BNO, 2 explantations, 1 recurrent UTI, 1 encrustation
Shaw et al[107]	1997	14 SCI males	Memokath (see above)	Maximum 24		50% success – decreased PVR, hydro, ADR	42.9% migration 1 mucosal hyperplasia, 1 recurrent UTI
Low and McRae[112]	1998	24 SCI males	Memokath (Engineers and Doctors A/S, Hornback, Denmark)	16 range 2–24	13 had 1 or more sphincterotomies 4 TURP, 4 other	29.1% success – decreased PVR, ADR, and UTIs	20.8% migration 25% recurrent UTIs, 12.5% de-novo ADR, 16.7% poor emptying, 4.1% encrustation
Chancellor et al[116]	1999	160 males 100 SCIs, 8 MS, 1 spinal vascular accident, 1 SC tumor	Urolume (American Medical Systems, Minnetonka, Minnesota)	60	46 had 1 or more sphincterotomies 11 TURP, 11 TURBN, 4 BNI	Significantly decreased voiding pressure, PVR, ADR, hydro, UTIs	15% explanted 28.7% migration 33% hematuria 26.3% BNO 2 urosepsis
Chartier-Kestler et al[114]	2000	40 males 30 SCI, 6 MS, 4 other	Ultraflex (Boston Scientific Corp., Boston, MA)	16.9	5 – 1 or more sphincterotomies 4 TUIP, 2 TURP, 3 VIU	Decreased PVR, decreased ADR in 63.1%	1 explantation for UTIs, 2 BNOs\ transient hematuria

SCI, spinal cord injury; PVR, post-void residual; ADR, autonomic dysreflexia; BNO, bladder neck obstruction; UTI, urinary tract infection; BPH, benign prostatic hyperplasia; TURP transurethral resection of the prostate; BNI, bladder neck incision; TURBN, transurethral resection of bladder neck contracture.

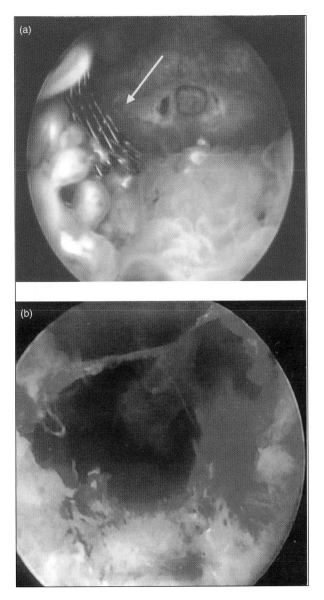

Figure 53.11
Urethral avulsion (a) stent exposed on right side (arrow); (b) after stent removal.

Conclusion

In summary, treatment of the male neurogenic bladder patient with refractory DESD continues to be challenging. Sphincterotomy and urethral stents will undoubtedly continue to be used in the management of these difficult cases. While there are now several different surgical options to choose from in addition to sphincterotomy, none of these treatment modalities has been shown to be superior to another with respect to efficacy, and each is fraught with its own unique liabilities and complications. Hopefully, future technical advances in the construction and composition of urethral stents will decrease their rate of migration and improve the ease of explantation. The results of balloon

dilatation are still too preliminary to speculate as to whether this technique will become a viable option for the treatment of DESD.

Conclusions

The surgeon endeavoring to treat a patient with urinary incontinence secondary to neuropathic bladder outlet incompetence has a number of surgical options at his disposal. Injectable agents are often employed in female patients with mild degrees of incontinence, patients who leak small amounts post-bladder neck sling or reconstruction, and patients who are not operative candidates or who are reluctant to undergo open surgery. The sling and AUS are commonly used when a more durable, long-term solution for incontinence is required. Because slings may be more successful in females than in males, some surgeons prefer to use slings as their first-line treatment in females and AUS as their primary treatment in males with neurogenic sphincteric incompetence. Reluctance to utilize the AUS in females stems from concerns of cuff erosion. The fascial sling may be preferable to the AUS in patients who do not wish to have a foreign body implanted or who, because of their comorbidities or surgical history, are at high risk for cuff erosion or infection of the device. Bladder neck reconstruction techniques are still performed at some specialized centers with experience in treating myelomeningocele and exstrophy-epispadias patients, but their popularity is waning secondary to high complication rates, especially in patients who have already undergone bladder neck surgery. Bladder neck closure is a suitable option for select patients who have failed multiple surgical attempts to increase outlet resistance or who have poor functional and constitutional status.

Sphincterotomy and urethral stents have both been shown to be effective at treating DESD. As some recent reports have illustrated, however, the currently available urethral stents many not be as easily removed or as complication-free as was once thought. Choice of treatment option is often guided by what the patient perceives as the irreversibility of sphincterotomy compared to urethral stenting.

References

1. Murless BC. The injection treatment of stress incontinence. J Obstet Gynaecol 1938; 45:67–73.

2. Lewis RI, Lockhart JL, Politano VA. Periurethral polytetrafluoroethylene injections in incontinent female subjects. J Urol 1984; 131:459–462.

3. Malizia AA Jr, Reiman HM, Myers RP, et al. Migration and granulomatous reaction after periurethral injection of Polytef (Teflon). JAMA 1984; 251:3277–3281.

4. Bomalaski MD, Bloom DA, McGuire EJ, Panzi A. Glutaraldehyde cross-linked collagen in the treatment of urinary incontinence in children. J Urol 1996; 155:699–702.

5. Kryger JV, Gonzalez R, Barthold JS. Surgical management of urinary incontinence in children with neurogenic sphincteric incompetence. J Urol 2000; 163:256–263.

6. Cooperman L, Micheli D. The immunogenicity of injectable collagen II. A retrospective review of 72 tested and treated patients. J Am Acad Dermatol 1984; 10:647–651.

7. Leonard MP, Carring DA, Epstein JI. Local tissue reaction to the suburethral injection of glutaraldehyde cross-linked bovine collagen in humans. J Urol 1990; 143:1209.

8. Defreitas GA, Wilson TS, Zimmern PE, Forte TB. Three dimensional ultrasonography: an objective outcome tool to assess collagen distribution in women with stress urinary incontinence. Urology 2003; 62(2):232–236.

9. Bennett JK, Green BG, Foote JE, Gray M. Collagen injections for intrinsic sphincter deficiency in the neuropathic urethra. Paraplegia 1995; 33:697–700.

10. Wan J, McGuire EJ, Bloom DA, Ritchey ML. The treatment of urinary incontinence in children using glutaraldehyde cross-linked collagen. J Urol 1992; 148:127–130.

11. McGuire EJ, Fitzpatrick CC, Wan J, et al. Clinical assessment of urethral sphincteric function. J Urol 1993; 150:1452–1454.

12. Leonard MP, Decter A, Mix LW, et al. Treatment of urinary incontinence in children by endoscopically directed bladder neck injection of collagen. J Urol 1996; 156:637–641.

13. McGuire EJ, Apell RA. Transurethral collagen injection for urinary incontinence. Urology 1994; 43:413–415.

14. Chernoff A, Horowitz M, Combs A, et al. Periurethral collagen injection for the treatment of urinary incontinence in children. J Urol 1997; 157:2303–2305.

15. Kershen RT, Atala A. New advances in injectable therapies for the treatment of incontinence and vesicoureteral reflux. Urol Clin N Am 1999; 26:81–94.

16. Nataluk EA, Assimos DG, Kroov RL. Collagen injections for treatment of urinary incontinence secondary to intrinsic sphincter deficiency. J Endourol 1995; 9:403–406.

17. Ben-Chaim J, Jeffs RD, Peppas DS, Gearhart JP. Submucosal bladder neck injections of glutaraldehyde cross-linked bovine collagen for the treatment of urinary incontinence in patients with the exstrophy/epispadias complex. J Urol 1995; 154:862–864.

18. Kasouff W, Capolicchio G, Berardinucci G, Corcos J. Collagen injection for treatment of urinary incontinence in children. J Urol 2001; 165:1666–1668.

19. Perez LM, Smith EA, Parrot TS, et al. Submucosal bladder neck injection of bovine dermal collagen for stress urinary incontinence in the pediatric population. J Urol 1996; 156:633–636.

20. Capozza N, Caione P, De Gennaro M, et al. Endoscopic treatment of vesico-ureteric reflux and urinary incontinence: technical problems in the pediatric patient. Br J Urol 1995; 75:538–542.

21. Sundaram CP, Reinberg Y, Aliabadi HA. Failure to obtain durable results with collagen implantation in children with urinary incontinence. J Urol 1997; 157:2306–2307.

22. Kim YH, Kattan MW, Boone TB. Correlation of urodynamic results and urethral coaptation with success after transurethral collagen injection. Urology 1997; 50:941–948.

23. Bent AE, Tutrone RT, McLennan MT, et al. Treatment of intrinsic sphincter deficiency using autologous ear chondrocytes as a bulking agent. Neurourol Urodyn 2001; 20:157–165.

24. Yokoyama T, Yoshimura N, Dhir R, et al. Persistence and survival of autologous muscle derived cells versus bovine collagen as potential treatment of stress urinary incontinence. J Urol 2001; 165:271–276.

25. Elder JS. Periurethral and puboprostatic sling repair for incontinence in patients with myelodysplasia. J Urol 1990; 144:434–437.

26. Raz S, McGuire EJ, Ehrlich RM, et al. Fascial sling to correct male neurogenic sphincter incompetence: the McGuire/Raz approach. J Urol 1988; 139:528–531.

27. Kreder KJ, Webster G. Management of the bladder outlet in patients requiring enterocystoplasty. J Urol 1992; 147:38–41.

28. Fontaine E, Bendaya S, Desert JF, et al. Combined modified rectus fascial sling and augmentation ileocystoplasty for neurogenic incontinence in women. J Urol 1997; 157:109–112.

29. Decter RM. Use of the fascial sling for neurogenic incontinence: lessons learned. J Urol 1993; 150:683–686.

30. Walker RD, Flack CE, Hawkins-Lee B, et al. Rectus fascial wrap: early results of a modification of the rectus fascial sling. J Urol 1995; 154:771–774.

31. Gormley EA, Bloom DA, McGuire EJ, Ritchey ML. Pubovaginal slings for the management of urinary incontinence in female adolescents. J Urol 1994; 152:822–825.

32. Herschorn S, Radomski SB. Fascial slings and bladder neck tapering in the treatment of male neurogenic incontinence. J Urol 1992; 147:1073–1075.

33. Kurzrock EA, Lowe P, Hardy BE. Bladder wall pedicle wraparound sling for neurogenic urinary incontinence in children. J Urol 1996; 155:305–308.

34. Kakizaki H, Shibata T, Shinno Y, et al. Fascial sling for the management of urinary incontinence due to sphincter incompetence. J Urol 1995; 153:644–647.

35. Barthold JS, Rodriguez E, Freedman AL, et al. Results of the rectus fascial sling and wrap procedures for the treatment of neurogenic sphincteric incontinence. J Urol 1999; 161:272–274.

36. Mingin GC, Youngren K, Stock JA, Hanna MK. The rectus myofascial wrap in the management of urethral sphincter incompetence. BJU Int 2002; 90:550–553.

37. Austin PF, Westney L, Leng WW, et al. Advantages of rectus fascial slings for urinary incontinence in children with neuropathic bladders. J Urol 2001; 165:2369–2372.

38. Scott FB, Bradley WE, Timm GW. Treatment of urinary incontinence by an implantable prosthetic device. Urology 1973; 1:252–259.

39. Reinberg Y, Manivel JC, Gonzalez R. Silicone shedding from artificial urinary sphincter in children. J Urol 1993; 150:694–696.

40. Hajivassiliou CA. The development and evolution of artificial urethral sphincters. J Med Eng Technol 1998; 22:154–159.

41. Fulford SCV, Sutton C, Bales G, et al. The fate of the 'modern' artificial urinary sphincter with a follow-up of more than 10 years. Br J Urol 1997; 79:713–716.

42. Elliot DS, Barrett DM. Mayo Clinic long-term analysis of the functional durability of the AMS 800 artificial sphincter: a review of 323 cases. J Urol 1998; 159:1206–1208.

43. Woodside JR, McGuire EJ. Technique for detection of detrusor hypertonia in the presence of urethral sphincteric incompetence. J Urol 1982; 127:740–743.

44. De Badiola FIP, Castro-Diaz D, Hart-Austin C, Gonzalez R. Influence of preoperative bladder capacity and compliance on the outcome of artificial sphincter implantation in patients with neurogenic sphincter incompetence. J Urol 1992; 148:1483–1495.

45. Kryger JV, Lerverson G, Gonzalez R. Long-term results of artificial urinary sphincters in children are independent of age at implantation. J Urol 2001; 165:2377–2379.

46. Aliabadi H, Gonzalez R. Success of the artificial sphincter after failed surgery for incontinence. J Urol 1990; 143:987–990.

47. Levesque PE, Bauer SB, Atala A, et al. Ten year experience with the artificial urinary sphincter in children. J Urol 1996; 156:625–628.

48. Salisz JA, Diokno AC. The management of injuries to the urethra, bladder or vagina encountered during the difficult placement of the artificial urinary sphincter in the female patient. J Urol 1992; 148:1528–1530.

49. Leach GE, Raz S. Perfusion sphincterometry. Method of intraoperative evaluation of artificial urethral sphincter function. Urology 1983; 21:312–314.

50. Simeoni J, Guys JM, Mollard P, et al. Artificial urinary sphincter implantation for neurogenic bladder: a multi-institutional study in 107 children. Br J Urol 1996; 78:287–293.

51. Singh G, Thomas DG. Artificial urinary sphincter in patients with neurogenic bladder dysfunction. Br J Urol 1996; 77:252–255.

52. Gonzalez R, Merino FG, Vaughn M. Long-term results of the artificial urinary sphincter in male patients with neurogenic bladder. J Urol 1995; 154:769–770.

53. Bellioli G, Campobasso P, Mercurella A. Neuropathic urinary incontinence in pediatric patients: management with artificial sphincter. J Ped Surg 1992; 27:1461–1464.

54. Spiess PE, Capolicchio JP, Kiruluta G, et al. Is an artificial sphincter the best choice for incontinent boys with spina bifida? Review of our long term experience with the AS-800 artificial sphincter. Can J Urol 2002; 9:1486–1491.

55. Castera R, Podesta ML, Ruarte A, et al. 10-year experience with artificial urinary sphincter in children and adolescents. J Urol 2001; 165:2373–2376.

56. Holmes NM, Kogan BA, Baskin LS. Placement of artificial urinary sphincter in children and simultaneous gastrocystoplasty. J Urol 2001; 165:2366–2368.

57. Light K, Lapin S, Vohra S. Combined use of bowel and the artificial urinary sphincter in reconstruction of the lower urinary tract: infectious complications. J Urol 1995; 153:331–333.

58. Miller EA, Mayo M, Kwan D, Mitchell M. Simultaneous augmentation cystoplasty and artificial urinary sphincter placement: infection rates and voiding mechanisms. J Urol 1998; 160:750–753.

59. Guralnick ML, Miller E, Toh KL, Webster GD. Transcorporal artificial urinary sphincter cuff placement in cases requiring revision for erosion and urethral atrophy. J Urol 2002; 167:2075–2079.

60. Leadbetter GW. Surgical correction of total urinary incontinence. J Urol 1964; 91:261–266.

61. Tanagho EA. Bladder neck reconstruction for total urinary incontinence: 10 years experience. J Urol 1981; 125:321–326.

62. Tanagho EA, Smith DA, Meyers FH, Fisher R. Mechanism of urinary continence II. Technique for surgical correction of incontinence. J Urol 1969; 101:305–313.

63. Mollard P, Mouriquand P, Joubert P. Urethral lengthening for neurogenic urinary incontinence (Kropp's procedure): results of 16 cases. J Urol 1990; 143:95–97.

64. Ferrer FA, Tadros YE, Gearhart J. Modified Young–Dees–Leadbetter bladder neck reconstruction: new concepts about old ideas. Urology 2001; 58:791–796.

65. Kropp BP, Rink RC, Adams MC, et al. Bladder outlet reconstruction: fate of the silicone sheath. J Urol 1993; 150:703–706.

66. Hollowell JG, Ransley PG. Surgical management of incontinence in bladder extrophy. Br J Urol 1991; 68:543–548.

67. Kropp KA, Angwafo FF. Urethral lengthening and reimplantation for neurogenic incontinence in children. J Urol 1986; 135:533–536.

68. Waters PR, Chehade NC, Kropp KA. Urethral lengthening and reimplantation: incidence and management of catheterization problems. J Urol 1997; 158:1053–1056.

69. Belman AB, Kaplan GW. Experience with the Kropp anti-incontinence procedure. J Urol 1989; 141:1160–1162.

70. Pippi Salle JL, Fraga JCS, Amarante A, et al. Urethral lengthening with anterior bladder wall flap for urinary incontinence: a new approach. J Urol 1994; 152:803–806.

71. Pippi Salle JL, McLorie GA, Bagli DJ, Khoury AE. Urethral lengthening with anterior bladder wall flap (Pippi Salle procedure): modifications and extended indications of the technique. J Urol 1997; 158:585–590.

72. Nill TG, Peller PA, Kropp KA. Management of urinary incontinence by bladder tube urethral lengthening and submucosal reimplantation. J Urol 1990; 144:559–563.

73. Snodgrass W. A simplified Kropp procedure for incontinence. J Urol 1997; 158:1049–1052.

74. Gearhart JP, Canning DA, Jeffs RD. Failed bladder neck preconstruction: options for management. J Urol 1991; 146:1082–1084.

75. Donnahoo KK, Rink RC, Cain MP, Casale AJ. The Young–Dees–Leadbetter bladder neck repair for neurogenic incontinence. J Urol 1999; 161:1946–1949.

76. Mouriquand PDE, Phillips SN, White J, et al. The Kropp-onlay procedure (Pippi Salle procedure): a simplification of the technique of urethral lengthening. Preliminary results in eight patients. Br J Urol 1995; 75:656–662.

77. Rink RC, Adams MC, Keating MA. The flip-flap technique to lengthen the urethra (Salle procedure) for treatment of neurogenic urinary incontinence. J Urol 1994; 152:799–802.

78. Lepor H, Jeffs RD. Primary bladder closure and bladder neck reconstruction in classical bladder extrophy. J Urol 1983; 130:1142–1145.

79. Leadbetter GW. Surgical reconstruction for complete urinary incontinence: a 10 to 22-year followup. J Urol 1985; 133:205–206.

80. Sidi AM, Reinberg Y, Gonzalez R. Comparison of artificial sphincter implantation and bladder neck reconstruction in patients with neurogenic urinary incontinence. J Urol 1987; 138:1120–1122.

81. Rink RC, Mitchell M. Bladder neck reconstruction in the incontinent child: bladder neck/urethral reconstruction in the neuropathic bladder. Dial Ped Urol 1987; 10:5.

82. Hoebeke P, De Kuyper P, Goeminne H, et al. Bladder neck closure for treating pediatric incontinence. Eur Urol 2000; 38:453–456.

83. Zimmern PE, Hadley HR, Leach GE, Raz S. Transvaginal closure of the bladder neck and placement of a suprapubic catheter for destroyed urethra after long-term indwelling catheterization. J Urol 1985; 134:554–557.

84. Syme RRA. Bladder neck closure for neurogenic incontinence. Aust NZ J Surg 1981; 2:197–200.

85. Chancellor MB, Erhard MJ, Kilholma PJ, et al. Functional urethral closure with pubovaginal sling for destroyed female urethra after long-term urethral catheterization. Urology 1994; 43:499–505.

86. Das S, Amar AD. Abdominal transposition of the female urethra. J Urol 1986; 135:373–375.

87. Litweller SE, Zimmern PE. Closure of bladder neck in the male and female. In: Graham SD, Glen JF, eds. Glenn's Urologic surgery, 5th edn. Wolters Kluwer, 1998: 407–414.

88. Chancellor MB, Erhard JM, Kilholma PJ, et al. Functional urethral closure with pubovaginal sling for destroyed female urethra after long-term urethral catheterization. Urology 1994; 43:499–505.

89. Reid R, Schneider K, Fruchtman B. Closure of the bladder neck in patients undergoing continent vesicostomy for urinary incontinence. J Urol 1978; 120:40–42.

90. Zeidman EJ, Chiang H, Alarcon A, Raz S. Suprapubic cystotomy using the Lowsley retractor. Urology 1988; 32:54.

91. Hensle TW, Kirsch AJ, Kennedy WA, Reiley EA. Bladder neck closure in association with continent urinary diversion. J Urol 1995; 154:883–885.

92. Jayanathi VR, Churchill BM, McLorie GA, Khoury AE. Concomitant bladder neck closure and Mitrofanoff diversion for the management of intractable urinary incontinence. J Urol 1995; 154:886–888.

93. Abrams P, Cardozo L, Fall M, et al. The standardization of terminology of lower urinary tract function: report from the standardization sub-committee of the International Continence Society. Neurourol Urodyn 2002; 21:167–178.

94. Chancellor MB, Gajewski J, Ackman CF. Long-term followup of the North American Multicenter Urolume Trial for the treatment of external detrusor-sphincter dyssynergia. J Urol 1999; 161:1545–1550.

95. Kaplan SA, Chancellor MB, Blaivas JG. Bladder and sphincter behavior in patients with spinal cord lesions. J Urol 1991; 146:113.

96. McGuire EJ, Brady S. Detrusor-sphincter dyssynergia. J Urol 1979; 121:774.

97. Emmett J, Paut R, Dunn J. Role of the external urethral sphincter in the normal bladder and cord bladder. J Urol 1948; 59:439–454.

98. Fontaine E, Hajari M, Rhein F, et al. Reappraisal of endoscopic sphincterotomy for post-traumatic neurogenic bladder: a prospective study. J Urol 1996: 155:277–280.

99. Noll F, Sauerwein D, Stohrer M. Transurethral sphincterotomy in quadraplegic patients: long term follow up. Neurourol Urodyn 1995; 14:351–358.

100. Milroy EJG, Chapple CR, Cooper JE, et al. A new treatment for urethral strictures. Lancet 1988; 1(8600):1424–1427.

101. Rivas DA, Chancellor MB, Bagley D. Prospective comparison of external sphincter prosthesis placement and external sphincterotomy in men with spinal cord injury. J Endourol 1994; 8:89–93.

102. Shaw PJR, Milroy EJG, Timoney AG, et al. Permanent external striated sphincter stents in patients with spinal injuries. Br J Urol 1990; 66:297–302.

103. Wilson TS, Lemack GE, Dmochowski RR. Urolume stents: lessons learned. J Urol 2002; 167:2477–2480.

104. Chancellor MB, Rivas DA, Abdill CK, et al. Prospective comparison of external sphincter balloon dilatation and prosthesis placement with external sphincterotomy in spinal cord injured men. Arch Phys Med Rehab 1994; 75:297–305.

105. McInerney PD, Vanner TF, Harris SAB, Stephenson TP. Permanent urethral stents for detrusor sphincter dyssynergia. Br J Urol 1991; 67:291–294.

106. McFarlane JP, Foley SJ, Shah PJR. Long-term outcome of permanent urethral stents in the treatment of detrusor-sphincter dyssynergia. Br J Urol 1996; 78:729–732.

107. Shah NC, Foley SJ, Edhem I, Shah PJR. Use of Memokath temporary urethral stent in treatment of detrusor-sphincter dyssynergia. J Endourol 1997; 11:485–488.

108. Watanabe T, Rivas DA, Smith R, et al. The effect of urinary tract reconstruction on neurologically impaired women previously treated with an indwelling urethral catheter. J Urol 1996; 156:1926–1928.

109. Vapnek JM, Couillard DR, Stone AR. Is sphincterotomy the best management of the spinal cord injured bladder? J Urol 1994; 151:961–964.

110. Perkash I. Contact laser sphincterotomy: further experience and longer follow-up. Spinal Cord 1996; 34:227–233.

111. Rivas DA, Chancellor MB, Staas WE, Gomella LG. Contact neodymium:yttrium-aluminum-garnet laser ablation of the external sphincter in spinal cord injured men with detrusor sphincter dyssynergia. Urology 1995; 45:1028–1031.

112. Low AI, McRae PJ. Use of the Memokath for detrusor-sphincter dyssynergia after spinal cord injury – a cautionary tale. Spinal Cord 1998; 36:39–44.

113. Chancellor MB, Karusick S, Erhard MJ, et al. Placement of a wire mesh prosthesis in the external urinary sphincter of men with spinal cord injuries. Radiology 1993; 187:551–555.

114. Chartier-Kastler EJ, Bussel TB, Chancellor MB, Denys P. A urethral stent for the treatment of detrusor-striated sphincter dyssynergia. BJU Int 2000; 86:52–57.

115. Sauerwein D, Gross AJ, Kutzenberger J, Ringert RH. Wallstents in patients with detrusor-sphincter dyssynergia. J Urol 1995; 154:495–497.

116. Chancellor MB, Rivas DA, Linsenmeyer T, et al. Multicenter trial in North America of Urolume urinary sphincter prosthesis. J Urol 1994; 152:924–930.

117. Bloom DA, Knechtel JM, McGuire EJ. Urethral dilation improves bladder compliance in children with myelomeningocele and high leak point pressures. J Urol 1990; 144:430–433.

54

Urinary diversion

Greg G Bailly and Sender Herschorn

Introduction

The goals of urologic management of neurogenic bladder dysfunction are to achieve and maintain low-pressure urinary storage and voiding, with preservation of the upper urinary tract and achievement of urinary continence. Long-term management has been facilitated by the widespread acceptance of clean self-intermittent catheterization (CIC).[1] The introduction of new medications over the past few years has also contributed to management. The vast majority of patients with neurogenic bladder dysfunction can be managed without resorting to urinary diversion. However, there continues to be patients who are unwilling or unable to perform self-catheterization or to be intermittently catheterized. There are others who despite appropriate management are unable to maintain low-pressure urinary storage and voiding and/or continence. It is these patients who may benefit from lower urinary tract reconstruction and urinary diversion rather than resort to indwelling Foley catheters.

Patients with neurogenic bladder dysfunction are followed regularly with clinical evaluation, laboratory testing with serum creatinine and urine cultures, upper tract imaging (usually ultrasound), and urodynamic studies. The storage and voiding problems are usually addressed with a combination of CIC and various medications. Males with spinal cord injuries are frequently managed with condom drainage with or without CIC. However, outlet-relaxing procedures, such as transurethral sphincterotomy[2] or Urolume stent,[3] are occasionally needed in suprasacral cord injury patients with high detrusor pressures and sphincter dyssynergia. Neurogenic bladders in women may be harder to manage. Urethral CIC may be difficult for wheelchair-bound women and incontinence between CICs may also be more difficult to contain.

The aim of long-term follow-up of patients with neurogenic bladder disease is to prevent any changes that may lead to upper tract compromise. The complications of high intravesical pressures are well described and include upper tract dilatation, reflux, stones, pyelonephritis, and renal failure.[4,5] In addition, the patients may present with clinical symptoms. Changes in overall health can often be the first sign that the bladder may not be functioning satisfactorily. Worsening of incontinence, recurrent urinary tract infections, autonomic dysreflexia, suprapubic or back pain, as well as changes in the neurologic status of some patients, often indicate an alteration in lower urinary tract. These important clues can direct the urologist toward the appropriate investigations.

An outline of management of neurogenic bladder in relation to urinary diversion is shown in Figure 54.1. Urinary diversion, although frequently employed in the past for the treatment of neurogenic bladder dysfunction, is now only required in special circumstances. The commonly accepted indications include hydronephrosis that may be accompanied by progressive renal deterioration secondary to ureteral obstruction from a thick-walled bladder or intractable ureterovesical reflux, recurrent episodes of urosepsis, and persistent storage or emptying failure when CIC is impossible.[6] If, in the opinion of the urologist, the upper tract deterioration and/or storage problem cannot be managed with bladder augmentation surgery alone then urinary diversion may be indicated. Another reason for diversion is when urethral CIC is not feasible.

Unmanageable incontinence, while not life-threatening, may lead to skin breakdown, persistent infection, social isolation, and negative psychological impact on patients. When procedures such as bulking agents, slings, artificial sphincters, and augmentation cystoplasty are unsuccessful or contraindicated, and/or urethral CIC is not possible, urinary diversion may be considered. Often the diversion is as an alternative to an indwelling catheter. Although there have been no randomized prospective long-term trials, patients with indwelling catheters have more morbidity, such as infectious complications, calculi, and radiographic abnormalities, than those managed with CIC.[7,8] Although a long-term Foley catheter may be convenient, safe, and effective for some patients, urinary diversion may be a reasonable option. The various types of diversions will be discussed in this chapter.

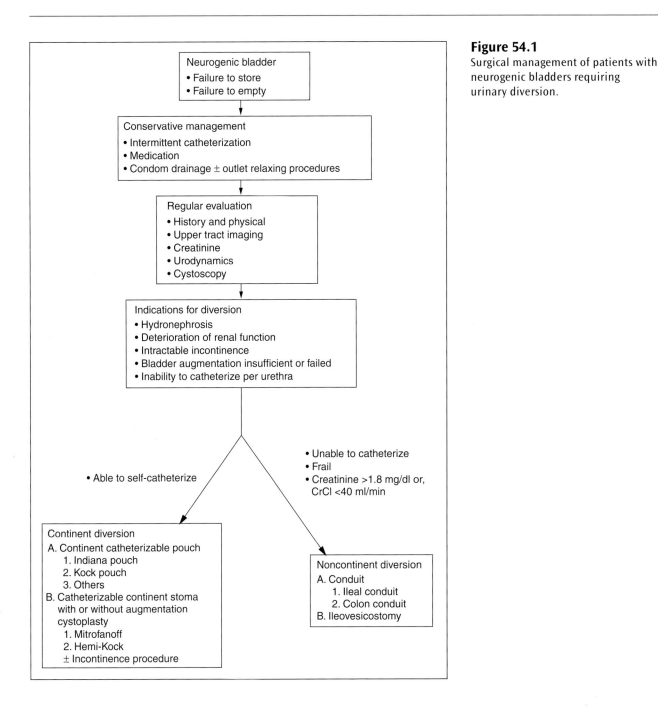

Figure 54.1
Surgical management of patients with neurogenic bladders requiring urinary diversion.

The choice of urinary diversion: patient considerations

The selection of a urinary diversion procedure is largely based on the surgeon's opinion and experience. Several important patient characteristics are considered when choosing an appropriate form of diversion (see Figure 54.1). The patient's ability to self-catheterize must be evaluated as it significantly impacts on whether to construct a noncontinent or continent form of urinary diversion. Patients who cannot perform self-catheterization of an abdominal stoma

because of underlying neurologic disease or poor manual dexterity are not well suited for continent diversions. Other medical conditions may also exclude a patient from undergoing a continent diversion. Elderly, debilitated patients with other significant medical co-morbidities are generally not good candidates for continent diversion. In addition to poor outcomes, these patients have higher perioperative risks. Continent diversions often take longer to perform and have increased potential for complications compared with noncontinent diversion, and therefore proper patient selection is paramount to successful outcome.

Renal insufficiency is a relative contraindication to continent forms of diversion.[9,10] Continent diversion allows longer exposure time of urine to the intestinal mucosa, thereby increasing the risk of electrolyte disturbances, particularly in the patient with renal insufficiency. As a general rule, it has been recommended that patients with a preoperative creatinine of greater than 1.8 mg/dl (180 μmol/l) should undergo a noncontinent form of diversion.[10] A patient with borderline renal function should have a creatinine clearance calculated. A minimal creatinine clearance of 40 ml/min should be documented before the patient is deemed an appropriate candidate for a continent diversion.[11] Hepatic function should also be evaluated. Significant hepatic dysfunction increases the risk of developing hyperammonemia if the liver is unable to adequately process the ammonium chloride that may be produced by bacterial growth in retained urine of a pouch.[9]

Once the patient has been assessed it is important that the surgeon work with the patient and family/caregivers, without forcing the patient into one direction or another. The patient's willingness, ability, and motivation to comply with self-care and follow-up are other crucial considerations. Speaking to other patients with various forms of diversion often helps the patient better understand the surgery. The Internet may also provide valuable information on different forms of diversion. The surgeon should inform the patient of all potential risks and benefits of each type of diversion. The surgeon's experience, opinion, and review of the literature are important in protecting the patient from inappropriate or unrealistic expectations. Ultimately the decision is made on an individual basis by the patient and family with physician input.

General principles of surgery
Preoperative preparation

History and physical examination are required to ascertain any risk factors that may affect bowel segment selection. These include previous surgery, regional enteritis, ulcerative colitis, diverticulitis, intraperitoneal malignancy, and prior bowel resection. The patient should be seen preoperatively by the enterostomal therapist to have appropriate marking of the stoma site. The site is selected by patient anatomy and preference. A bag should stay on or the patient (or caregiver) should be able to catheterize comfortably. Usually the site is marked with the patient in the sitting position. The appropriate site will vary depending on the patient's body habitus, spinal column stability, and ability to see and access various abdominal locations. Rather than the traditional right lower quadrant site, other locations such as the left side, umbilicus, or supraumbilical regions may have to be considered. The site should be indicated with ink and then the skin etched with a needle after the patient is anesthetized at the time of surgery.

Bowel preparation

The patient usually receives mechanical bowel preparation prior to surgery, in an attempt to reduce the amount of feces in the colon. An antibiotic bowel preparation may be used to reduce the bacterial count. Bowel preparation has been shown to decrease the rates of wound infection, intraperitoneal abscesses, and anastomotic dehiscence rate.[12,13]

Although the true benefit of mechanical bowel preparation is poorly defined in the literature, most urologic, colon, and rectal surgeons in North America routinely prescribe mechanical bowel preparations.[14,15] The type of preparation varies from center to center, but usually includes Fleet Phospho-soda (sodium phosphate), polyethylene glycol electrolyte (PEG) solution (GoLYTELY or NuLYTELY, Braintree Laboratories, Braintree, Massachusetts), or magnesium citrate. PEG solution requires administration of approximately 4 liters of fluid but is safe in most cases since there is virtually no net absorption of ions or water in the gut.

Oral sodium phosphate, i.e. Fleet Phospho-soda (C.B. Fleet Co., Lynchburg, Virginia), has replaced PEG at many centers, because it appears to be better tolerated by patients.[15] This compound acts as an osmotic cathartic, causing large volumes of water to be translocated into the bowel, which results in diarrhea and bowel cleansing. Two 45 ml doses are usually ingested 4 hours apart on the night before surgery.[16] At least three 8-ounce glasses of water should be consumed after each dose, with as much clear liquid as possible until midnight. When compared with PEG, Phospho-soda has been shown to be better tolerated and equally effective, with similar wound infection rates.[17] Patients appear to prefer Phospho-soda to PEG.[18,19] It is, however, contraindicated in patients with renal insufficiency, symptomatic congestive heart failure, or liver failure with ascites.[14] Most clinical studies have also excluded patients with creatinines greater than 2 mg/dl.[17,18]

Antibiotic coverage

Preoperative antibiotic coverage for elective bowel surgery continues to be controversial. Urologists tend to use prophylactic antibiotics based on information extrapolated from the colorectal surgery literature. However, the literature is not clear on what to give and how to give it, and there are no clear consistent recommendations. In an extensive review of the use of antibiotic and mechanical preparations in urologic diversion surgery, Ferguson and colleagues recommended 1 g of oral-based neomycin and 1 g metronidazole at 5 and 11 p.m. on the night before surgery.[14]

The use of antibiotics administered intravenously within an hour prior to making the skin incision is less controversial.

The Centers for Disease Control and Prevention (CDC) recommends a second-generation cephalosporin, such as cefoxitin or cefotetan, over a first-generation cephalosporin, such as cefazolin, for surgery of the rectum or colon.[20] Additional doses may be required during the surgery based on the half-life of the antibiotic, or if blood loss exceeds 1 liter, and the duration of the surgery. The benefit of continued prophylactic antibiotics during the postoperative period is unproven. The CDC also recommended that prophylactic antibiotics not be continued more than 24 hours.[21]

Surgical principles
Intestinal anastomosis

Since urinary diversion is dependent on reconstructing various segments of bowel, it is important to understand certain basic principles of intestinal surgery. Much of the morbidity and mortality associated with urinary diversion in the immediate postoperative period relates to intestinal complications.[22] The fundamental principles of intestinal anastomoses include adequate mobilization, maintenance of blood supply, apposition of serosa to serosa of the two bowel segments, and creation of a watertight and tensionless anastomotic line. The various methods of performing the enteroenterostomy are well described.[23] Sutures or staples can be used with similar efficacy and complication rates.[23]

Ureterointestinal anastomoses

Many different types of ureterointestinal anastomoses have been used in urinary diversion surgery, but all should follow basic surgical principles. Only as much ureter as necessary should be mobilized to create a tensionless anastomosis. Periadventitial tissue should remain to ensure adequate blood supply. The anastomosis with the intestine should be performed with fine (4-0 or 5-0) delayed absorbable sutures, with the creation of a watertight mucosa-to-mucosa apposition. At our center, we frequently retroperitonealize the anastomoses for further protection.

The issue of antirefluxing ureteric anastomoses is controversial. While some experimental literature indicates a benefit, the results of clinical studies of colonic conduits with antirefluxing anastomoses are equivocal. Deterioration of the upper tracts for ileal and colon conduits has been reported in 10–60% of patients.[23] In one widely quoted historic series, 49% of the upper tracts showed changes after conduit diversion, 16% of which had a blood urea nitrogen increase of 10 mg/dl or

more.[24] Deterioration of the upper tracts is usually a consequence of either infection or stones, or less commonly obstruction at the ureteral intestinal anastomosis.[23] In a prospective randomized comparison of ileal and colonic conduits into which one ureter was implanted with and the other without an antireflux technique, renal scarring was more prominent on the refluxing side.[25] However, split renal function tests showed no difference after 10 years.[26] These findings and those of others do not support the use of nonrefluxing ureterointestinal anstomoses for conduits. The final decision often rests with the surgeon's preference. At our center, we use refluxing anastomoses (Bricker or Wallace technique) for ileal conduits (Figures 54.2 and 54.3).

The ureterointestinal anastomoses of continent reservoirs may be refluxing or nonrefluxing.[27] Depending upon which continent reservoir is chosen, the nonrefluxing mechanism can be constructed from intussuscepted bowel, by tunneled implantation of the ureters, or by providing a long proximal loop or other techniques such as the split-nipple or LeDuc mucosal groove.[27]

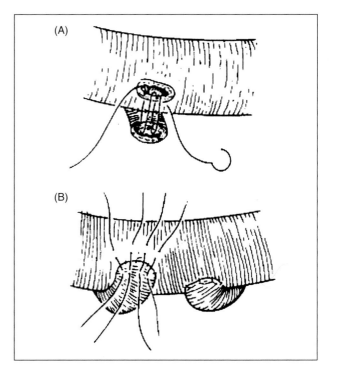

Figure 54.2
Bricker ureterointestinal anastomosis. (A) A full-thickness serosa and mucosal plug is removed from the bowel. Interrupted 5-0 delayed absorbable suture approximates the ureter to the full thickness of the bowel mucosa and serosa. (B) A supportive suture layer can be added from the adventitia of the ureter to the serosa of the bowel. (Reproduced with permission from McDougal.)[23]

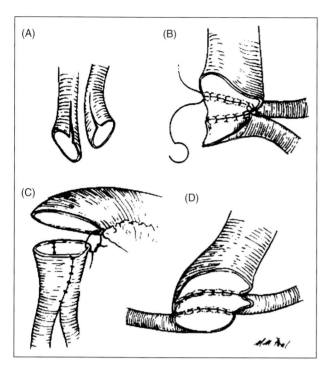

Figure 54.3
Wallace ureterointestinal anastomosis. (A) Both ureters are spatulated and are laid adjacent to each other. (B) The apex of one ureter is sutured to the apex of the other ureter. The medial walls of both ureters are then sutured together with interrupted or running 5-0 delayed absorbable suture. The lateral walls are then sutured to the bowel. (C) A 'Y-type' variant of above. (D) The 'head-to-tail' variant. (Reproduced with permission from McDougal.)[23]

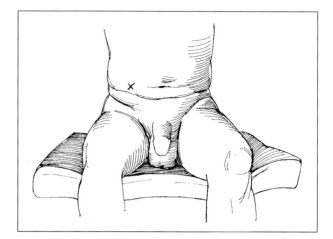

Figure 54.4
The stoma site is selected and marked on the surface of the abdomen where the skin is not rolled into folds while the patient is either sitting or standing. (Reproduced with permission from Hinman.)[27]

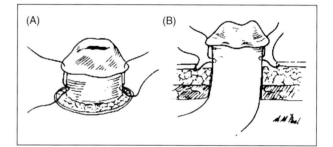

Figure 54.5
Rosebud stoma: 5–6 cm of intestine is brought through the abdominal wall. The open bowel is sutured to the skin with four quadrant sutures of 3-0 delayed absorbable sutures that pass through the skin edge, then catch the adventitia of the bowel well below the level of the skin, and finally go through the mucosal edge, thus everting the stoma. Additional sutures are placed through the skin and bowel edge between the quadrant sutures to close the gap. (Reproduced with permission from McDougal.)[23]

The stoma

The stoma is a very important aspect of the surgery. Much of the success of a stoma can be dependent on appropriate selection of the stomal site, as outlined above. A noncontinent stomal site should accommodate a collection device that does not leak, while maintaining patient comfort when wearing clothes. It should meet these requirements in the standing, sitting, and supine position (Figure 54.4). A commonly used stoma for an incontinent conduit is the nipple, or 'rosebud', described by Brooke in 1954[28] (Figure 54.5). It is usually created as the last step in the conduit construction.

The catheterizing stoma of the continent diversions is often placed in the lower quadrant of the abdomen through the rectus muscle and below the 'bikini line', or at the umbilicus. The umbilicus, or even higher, is the preferred location for someone in a wheelchair, because of easier access.

Diversions
Noncontinent urinary diversion

The first attempt at using isolated segment of bowel for urinary diversion was reported in 1908 by Verhoogen, who described a technique to divert urine into an isolated segment of ileum and ascending colon.[29] Construction of the ileal loop conduit was first reported by Seiffert in 1935.[30] Unfortunately, his procedure lacked effective means to collect and store urine. It was not until Bricker reported his technique that the ileal conduit became an acceptable method of urinary diversion.[31] Noncontinent diversions generally are ileal conduits, although various forms of conduits can be constructed from colon or jejunum. An alternative form of noncontinent diversion to the conduit is an ileovesicostomy.

Ileal conduit

Background. Since 1950, the Bricker ileal conduit has been the standard for noncontinent urinary diversion.[31] Still, today, the ileal conduit remains the most popular form of urinary diversion.[32] It is the most straightforward of the diversionary procedures to construct, with overall fewer potential complications than continent diversions.[32] It is the most appropriate urinary diversion in elderly, debilitated patients and in those who lack the hand–eye coordination or manual dexterity for self-catheterization, or the motivation to care for a continent pouch.

Technique. Little has changed since Bricker described his technique of the ileal conduit in 1950.[32] Blood supply is based on the superior mesenteric artery (SMA). The jejunal and ileal branches of the SMA anastomose to form arcades of vessels, which can be easily transilluminated through the mesentery during the operation for preservation of the blood supply to the conduit.

A lower vertical midline incision is made from the symphysis pubis to the umbilicus or beyond. The ureters are identified and transected approximately 3–4 cm above the bladder. The left ureter is brought under the sigmoid colon through the sigmoid mesentery to the right side, taking care to avoid damage to both the sigmoid and ureteral blood supply. The ileum is inspected to ensure healthy disease-free tissue. About 15–20 cm from the ileocecal valve, a 15–20 cm segment of ileum is selected, a length that will extend from the sacral promontory to the abdominal wall without tension. Two windows are constructed in the mesentery, with care taken to keep the base of the mesentery as wide as possible to prevent ischemia of the segment. The distal window usually measures 10–15 cm, and the proximal window can be much shorter at 3–5 cm. The bowel is transected, and the disconnected ileal segment is placed inferior to the remaining bowel segments. The bowel is reanastomosed using staplers or a standard two-layer closure. The mesenteric trap is closed. The ureteroileal anastomoses are performed either separately, as with the Bricker technique, or the ureters are joined together, as in the Wallace technique, at the proximal end of the loop.[33] The final step is the creation of the stoma (Figure 54.6).

Colon conduit

Background. A colon conduit may be chosen when there are functional or anatomical factors that preclude the use

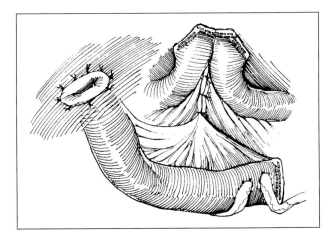

Figure 54.6
The ileal conduit at completion. (Reproduced with permission from Hinman.)[27]

of ileum. It has a larger diameter than ileum and can usually be easily mobilized into any portion of the abdomen or pelvis. The three types of colon conduits are transverse, sigmoid, and ileocecal, each having specific indications with advantages and disadvantages. The transverse colon is used in individuals who have received extensive pelvic irradiation. It is also an excellent segment when an intestinal pyelostomy needs to be performed. The sigmoid conduit is a good choice in patients undergoing a pelvic exenteration who will have a colostomy. An ileocecal conduit has an advantage of providing a long segment of ileum if a distal segment of ureter needs replacement. Because of the large lumen of the colon, stomal stenosis is rare. It is also used in situations in which reflux of urine from the conduit to the upper tracts is thought to be undesirable, as antireflux ureteral anastomoses are relatively easy to perform due to the thick wall. Contraindications to the use of transverse, sigmoid, and ileocecal conduits include the presence of inflammatory large bowel disease and severe chronic diarrhea.[23]

Ileal vesicostomy

The concept of ileal vesicostomy arose from the successful management of pediatric neurogenic bladders by creation of a vesicostomy. It is an alternative to an ileal conduit in some patients. It avoids the complications of ureterointestinal anastomosis, while maintaining the native ureteral antireflux mechanism. The small segment of ileum from the bladder to the abdominal acts to maintain low pressure in the bladder. The ileal segment is often referred to as a 'chimney', the distal end of which is brought up to the abdominal wall and a 'rosebud' stoma fashioned. It is important to use as short a segment of ileum as possible and to avoid a circular anastomosis between the ileum and the bladder. Redundancy of bowel may inhibit urinary flow and lead to electrolyte disturbances, which will be discussed below.[34] Theoretically, this results in a low-pressure reservoir that, if indicated at a later date, can be converted back to normal anatomy.

Technique. With the patient in the supine position, a lower midline incision is usually adequate. A 10–15 cm ileal segment is isolated, depending on what length is required to bridge the gap between the abdominal wall and bladder dome, leaving approximately 20 cm of terminal ileum and the ileocecal valve intact. The bowel anastomosis is performed as described previously. The bladder is mobilized from the pelvic wall by dividing its lateral attachments, and the bladder dome is generously opened transversely. The proximal ileal segment is spatulated approximately 4–6 cm along its antimesenteric border, and anastomosed to the open bladder with 2-0 absorbable sutures. The distal tubularized segment is brought out to the abdominal wall at a predetermined site and a stoma is created, as in the ileal conduit (Figure 54.7). A Foley catheter is left indwelling and exits through the stoma. An ileovesicostomy cystogram is performed 3 weeks postoperatively to ensure adequate healing of the suture line, and if there is no leak, the catheter is removed.[34]

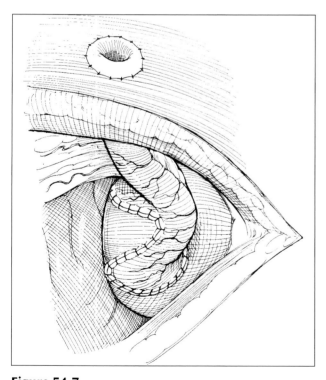

Figure 54.7
The ileovesicostomy. (Reproduced with permission from Hinman.)[27]

Continent urinary diversion
Background

Continent urinary diversion includes any reservoir subserved by a catheterizable efferent mechanism other than the native urethra and bladder neck.[35] Continent urinary diversion is often performed in patients with malignancy who require cystectomy and/or urinary diversion. It may also be used for appropriate patients with neurogenic bladder dysfunction who require diversion and wish to remain continent. In this setting, we generally try to preserve the bladder while adding capacity with an augmentation, thus maintaining the native ureteral antireflux mechanism. When this cannot be achieved due to significant bladder disease, a supravesical continent catheterizable pouch may be a better option. In the next section we will review the continent supravesical reservoirs and the continent bladder stoma.

The continent supravesical reservoir
Continence mechanisms

Although various forms of continent diversions were attempted in the past, it was not until 1982 when Kock et al reported the successful construction of an ileal reservoir that renewed interest in continent diversion was generated.[36] Its use in the neurogenic bladder population requires careful evaluation of physical and mental capabilities to ensure proper patient selection.

Continent catheterizable pouches are more complex to construct than conduits. Perhaps the single most demanding technical aspect of a catheterizable pouch is the creation of the continence mechanism. Four techniques are well described in the literature. The first involves using the appendix or a pseudoappendiceal tube fashioned from ileum or right colon and is sometimes performed for right colon pouches.[10]

The second type of continence mechanism used in right colon pouches is the tapered and/or imbricated terminal ileum and ileocecal valve. It involves imbrication or plication of the ileocecal valve region along with tapering of the more proximal ileum in the fashion of a neourethra.[37–40] This technique has been criticized by some because of the loss of the ileocecal valve and the potential consequence of more frequent bowel movements in some patients.

The third type of continence mechanism is an intussuscepted nipple valve, or more recently, the flap valve. The creation of the nipple valve may be technically demanding, and is associated with the highest complication and reoperation rate.[37] A significant learning curve is required, and thus this technique is not meant for the surgeon who performs the occasional continent pouch. Many modifications have been made to the original Kock pouch description, because of the long-term instability of the nipple valve in some patients. Despite the modifications, nipple valve failure can be observed in 10–15% of cases with the most experienced surgeons.[37] Failure may result from eversion and effacement of the intussusception and ischemic atrophy requiring a new nipple to be constructed. As well, stone formation on eroded or exposed staples can present a problem. Recently, a group from the University of Southern California has developed a new procedure, the T pouch, which uses a simpler and possibly more reliable procedure to create a flap valve, which results in both a continence and antireflux mechanism.[41]

The fourth procedure involves the construction of a hydraulic valve, as in the Benchekroun nipple.[42] This procedure has been largely abandoned because of nipple destabilization and stomal stenosis and will not be discussed.

Types of continent supravesical reservoirs

Indiana pouch

The Indiana pouch was first reported by Rowland and colleagues from the University of Indiana in 1985, and has since become one of the most popular forms of continent urinary diversion.[38] It uses the right colon as a reservoir while using reinforcement of the ileocecal valve for continence and tunneled tenial ureteral implantation for antireflux (Figure 54.8). The remaining ileal limb acts as the 'neourethra', which can be tapered and brought out through the abdominal wall as a stoma (Figure 54.9). Several variations of the Indiana pouch exist, including the Florida (Tampa) pouch[39] and the University of Miami pouch.[40]

Kock pouch (continent ileal reservoir)

Unlike the Indiana pouch, the Kock pouch involves the use of only small bowel to create a low-pressure reservoir.[36] Continence of urine and prevention of reflux to the upper tracts is achieved by constructing 'nipple valves' (Figure 54.10). It has been criticized for being technically difficult and associated with a high complication rate. As such, many urologists have abandoned it. However, the Kock limb (nipple valve) remains an important procedure for constructing a continent catheterizable stoma, such as with the hemi-Kock augmentation cystoplasty.

Other types of pouches that have been reported include the Mainz pouch, the UCLA pouch, the T pouch, and the Penn pouch.[37]

Continent bladder stoma

At our center, we aim to preserve the patient's native bladder if possible, thereby performing an augmentation cystoplasty and incorporating a continent bladder stoma.

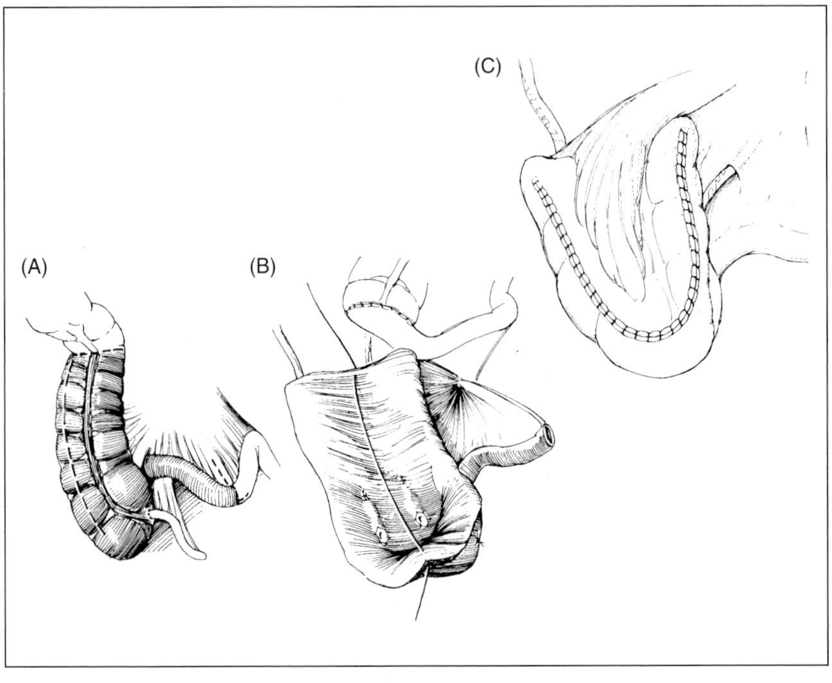

Figure 54.8
Indiana pouch. (A) A 25–30 cm segment of cecum, ascending colon, and hepatic flexure, in addition to an 8–10 cm of terminal ileum, is selected. The ascending colon is split down the antimesenteric border to within 2 cm of the caudal tip. (B) An ileocolostomy is performed using a suture technique or by a stapled method. The ureters are inserted by a submucosal technique. (C) A Malecot catheter is placed through the wall of the lowest part of the complex, in a position to allow direct exit through the abdominal wall. The U-shaped defect is closed by folding the distal portion of the colon into the proximal end and sutured into place with a running 3-0 absorbable suture. A serosal Lembert stitch with occasional lock stitches is added. The ileum is left to form the cutaneous conduit with tapering, as shown in Figure 54.9. (Reproduced with permission from Hinman.)[27]

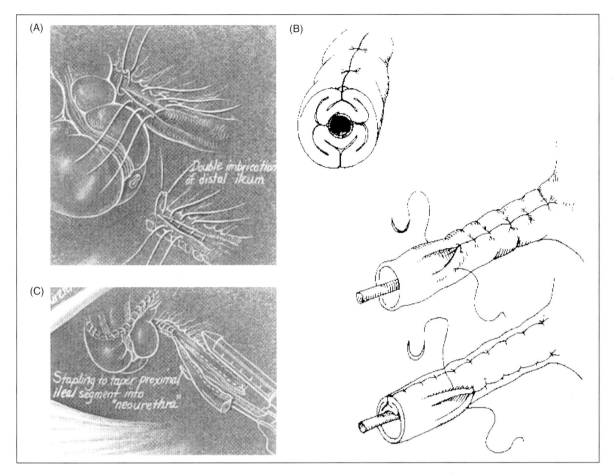

Figure 54.9
Tapering of ileal cutaneous conduit for Indiana pouch. Apposing Lembert sutures are applied on each side of the terminal ileum. Excess ileum can also be tapered by a stapling technique. (Reproduced with permission from Benson and Olsson.)[37]

Preserving the bladder and avoiding the ureterointestinal anstomoses should lead to fewer complications. Two popular methods of achieving a continent catheterizable bladder stoma are the Mitrofanoff procedure and the hemi-Kock (nipple valve) with or without formal augmentation cystoplasty. Urethral continence may be addressed simultaneously if necessary. Depending on the severity, it may involve a pubourethral sling, insertion of an artificial urinary sphincter, or closure of the bladder neck.[43]

The Mitrofanoff principle

In 1980, Mitrofanoff described a procedure in which the isolated appendix was anastomosed to the bladder at one end and the other end brought out to the skin.[44,45] The appendix is mobilized on its mesenteric pedicle and implanted on the bladder dome (Figure 54.11–54.13). The proximal lumen is tunneled under the bladder mucosa as an antireflux mechanism. As the reservoir fills, the rise in intravesical pressure is transmitted through the epithelium and to the implanted conduit, coapting its lumen. This mucosal tunneling technique is key to achieving continence.

The appendix has many advantages over methods for creating a continent catheterizable stoma.[46] The intraluminal pressure can rise nearly threefold that of the reservoir itself.[47] Perhaps the most important aspect of the flap-valve mechanism is the tunnel length to lumen ratio. Urodynamic evaluation has shown that a minimal tunnel length of 2 cm is required to achieve continence.[48] The Mitrofanoff principle can be used in native bladder, enterocystoplasty, or in a continent urinary reservoir. Because it is so reliable in preventing incontinence, it may place the patient at risk for upper tract deterioration or spontaneous rupture of the bladder or reservoir if regular catheterization is not performed. The appendix is particularly well suited for children because it is relatively longer and the abdominal wall is thinner. It also circumvents many of the secondary complications associated with using the ileocecal valve or other bowel segments.

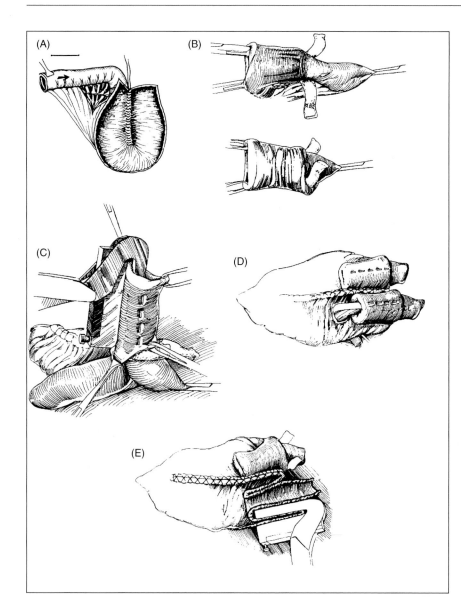

Figure 54.10
Construction of a nipple valve for the Kock pouch. (A) A 15 cm segment of terminal ileum is isolated and opened along its antimesenteric wall. The proximal 10 cm serves as the continent intussusception and the distal 5–10 cm as the patch. The size of the patch varies according to the size of the excised segment. (B) A Babcock clamp is advanced into the terminal ileum, the full thickness of the intussuscipiens is grasped, and it is prolapsed into the pouch. (C) Three rows of 4.8 mm staples are applied to the intussuscepted nipple valve using the TA55 stapler. (D) A small buttonhole is made in the back wall of the ileal plate to allow the anvil of the TA55 stapler to be passed through and advanced into the nipple valve. A fourth row of staples is applied. The figure shows two valve mechanisms. In this instance, there would be only one. (E) The anvil of the stapler can be directed between the two leaves of the intussuscipiens and the fourth row of staples applied in this manner. The figure shows two valve mechanisms. In this instance, there would be only one. (Reproduced with permission: (A) from Ghoneim MA, Kock NG, Lycke G, El-Din AB. An appliance-free, sphincter-controlled bladder substitute. J Urol 1987; 138:1150–1154; (B–E) from Hinman[27] and Benson and Ollson.)[37]

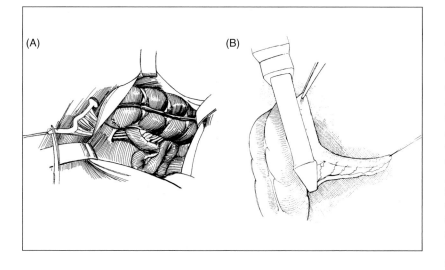

Figure 54.11
Mitrofanoff (appendicovesicostomy). (A) Stay sutures are placed at the base of the appendix, and the wall of the cecum is incised circumferentially to take a small cuff of cecum with the appendix. The appendiceal mesentery is separated a short distance from that of the cecum, preserving all of the appendiceal blood supply. The cecal defect is closed. The appendix is extraperitonealized behind the ileocecal junction. For umbilical placement of the stoma, it is not necessary to extraperitonealize the appendix. (B) For a short appendix or an obese patient, the appendix can be made longer by incorporating some of the cecal wall. (Reproduced with permission from Hinman.)[27]

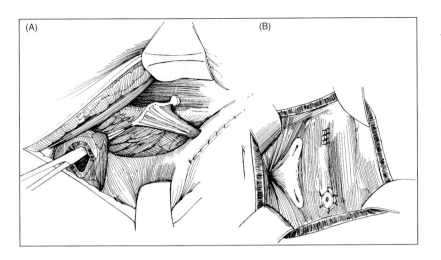

Figure 54.12
Through a cystotomy, a submucosal tunnel is made in the posterolateral wall of the bladder, beginning well above the right ureteral orifice. The appendix tip is implanted. A bladder augmentation is usually done next. (Reproduced with permission from Hinman.)[27]

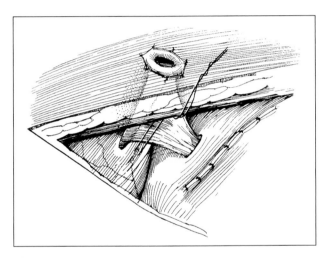

Figure 54.13
The appendiceal base is passed through an opening in the abdominal wall muscles large enough to accommodate a finger. The appendiceal opening is sutured to the skin (sometimes at the umbilicus). The bladder should be hitched to the anterior abdominal wall, and a catheter left in the appendix. (Reproduced with permission from Hinman.)[27]

Hemi-Kock augmentation enterocystoplasty

As an alternative to the Mitrofanoff procedure, patients may undergo a hemi-Kock ileocystoplasty with continent stoma permitting abdominal catheterization into the bladder. At our center, we have performed this procedure on various patients: wheelchair-dependent patients when urethral catheterization is difficult or impossible due to physical disability; patients who are unable to perform intermittent urethral catheterization; or patients who had a urethra that could not be rehabilitated due to trauma or surgery.[49] This procedure can be performed in conjunction with an incontinence procedure, including closure of the bladder neck in select cases.

Through a lower midline incision, the bladder is accessed and, in the case of an augmentation, the bladder is bivalved (clammed) in an anteroposterior direction in the midline from the bladder neck to 1 cm above the trigone. The ileal segment is measured from a point 25–30 cm proximal to the ileocecal valve. The next 15 cm proximal to this segment are for the nipple valve and the efferent limb. Up to another 45 cm is isolated on a mesenteric pedicle if an augmentation is performed. The intussuscepted nipple valve is constructed with three lines of TA55 staples, including one line that attaches the nipple to the segment. If no augmentation is performed, the bowel segment with the nipple is approximated to the bladder incision, and the third TA55 staple line fastens the nipple directly to the bladder wall. The catheterizing limb is brought out through the lower abdominal wall, usually on the right side, although other sites, including the umbilicus, can be used (Figure 54.14).

In a review of 47 patients who had construction of a hemi-Kock nipple valve as a catheterizable bladder stoma, Herschorn reported that 36 were dry or had mild leakage, and 44 (94%) patients considered their surgery to be successful compared with their preoperative management at a mean follow-up of 56 months.[50] Six patients required valve revision and/or stomal hernia surgery within the first 2 years. After the technique was modified by tapering the efferent limb, there was a significant decrease in revision rate. Kreder and colleagues have also reported success with using the hemi-Kock as a catheterizable bladder stoma.[51]

Complications of urinary diversion

The complications of urinary diversion can be categorized as either technical–surgical, metabolic, or neuromechanical.[23] Surgical complications are related to the reconstruction

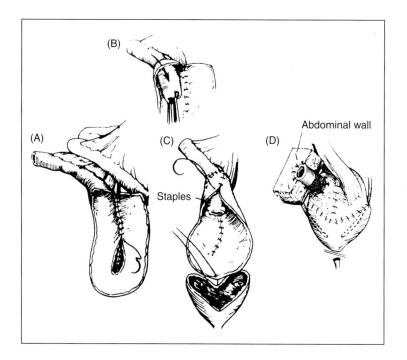

Figure 54.14
Hemi-Kock augmentation cystoplasty. (A) The distal segment of 15 cm for the efferent limb remains tubularized while the 45 cm for the augmentation has been detubularized. (B) Construction of the valve for continence. (C) Anastomosis of the augmentation to the 'clammed' bladder. (D) The efferent limb has been brought through the abdominal wall as a stoma. (A urethral continence procedure or urethral closure may be done for continence.) (Adapted from Kreder et al.)[51]

of the bowel and diversionary unit. Metabolic complications are the result of how the reabsorption of solutes is altered by the contact of urine with the bowel. The neuromechanical aspects involve the configuration of the reconstructed urinary reservoir and conduits and how this impacts on storage of urine.

Surgical complications

The complications associated with intestinal urinary diversion are displayed in Table 54.1. Postoperative surgical complications can also be classified as early or late. Nurmi and co-workers[71] reported on 144 patients with ileal conduits and found that the most common early postoperative complication was wound infection, followed by ureteroileal leakage, intestinal obstruction, intestinal fistulas, and acute pyelonephritis. Long-term complications were related to the delayed sequelae of intestinal surgery: stomal stenosis; ureteroileal stenosis; elongation of the loop; subsequent failure of the loop to propel urine adequately; and deterioration of the upper urinary tract.

The complications that can occur with ureterointestinal anastomosis include leakage, stenosis, reflux in antireflux anastomoses, and pyelonephritis. Urine leakage usually presents within the first 7–10 days postoperatively with an incidence of 3–9%.[72,73] The use of soft ureteral stents has reduced the incidence. Fortunately, most leaks resolve with time and proper drainage, but they have been associated with periureteral fibrosis and scarring, leading to stricture formation.[23] The incidence of ureteric stenosis is approximately 1–14%.[23] Stricture formation can be asymptomatic

and occur at any time in the life of the patient; hence the importance of yearly or biennial upper tract imaging. Strictures can be anywhere along the ureter, as well as at the anastomosis. A common location is where the left ureter crosses over the aorta beneath the inferior mesenteric artery. When a stricture is detected it is usually treated first by endourologic or percutaneous means using balloon dilatation or incision. Although these methods offer less morbidity to the patient, the long-term success rate is lower than open repair (90% vs 50%).[74,75]

Stomal complications are the single most common problem encountered in the postoperative period after diversion.[23] Early problems include bowel necrosis, bleeding, dermatitis, parastomal hernia, prolapse, obstruction, stomal retraction, and stomal stenosis. The incidence of stomal stenosis has been reported in 20–24% of patients with ileal conduits and 10–20% of those with colon conduits.[23] Stomal problems can frequently be improved or prevented with proper stomal care and better-fitting appliances.

Metabolic complications

Electrolyte abnormalities

Electrolyte abnormalities may result from absorption and excretion of water and solutes from the bowel surface. They are dependent on the segment of bowel used, the surface area of the bowel, the amount of time the urine is exposed to the bowel, the concentration of the solutes in the urine, renal function, and pH. Jejunal conduits are rarely performed because of their potential

Table 54.1 *Complications of urinary intestinal diversion*

Complications	Type of diversion	Patients (complications/no.)	Incidence (%)
Bowel obstruction	Ileal conduit	124/1289	10
	Colon conduit	9/230	5
	Gastric conduit	2/21	10
	Continent diversion	2/250	4
Ureteral intestinal obstruction	Ileal conduit	90/1142	8
	Antireflux colon conduit	25/122	20
	Colon conduit	8/92	9
	Continent diversion	16/461	4
Urine leak	Ileal conduit	23/886	3
	Colon conduit	6/130	5
	Continent diversion	104/629	17
	Ileum colon	5/123	4
Stomal stenosis or hernia	Ileal conduit	196/806	24
	Colon conduit	45/227	20
	Continent diversion	28/310	9
Renal calculi	Ileal conduit	70/964	7
	Antireflux colon conduit	5/94	5
Pouch calculi	Continent diversion	42/317	13
Acidosis requiring treatment	Ileal conduit	46/296	16
	Antireflux colon conduit	5/94	5
	Gastric conduit	0/21	0
	Continent diversion		
	Ileum	21/263	8
	Colon or colon-ileum	17/63	27
Pyelonephritis	Ileal conduit	132/1142	12
	Antireflux colon conduit	13/96	13
	Continent diversion	15/296	5
Renal deterioration	Ileal conduit	146/808	18
	Antireflux colon conduit	15/103	15

Source: from McDougal.[23]

[a] Composite from the literature. Follow-up averages 5 years for ileal conduits, 3 years for colon conduits, 2 years for gastric conduits, and 2 years for continent diversions.

[b] Data from references 52–70

metabolic complications. They can cause hyponatremia, hypochloremia, hyperkalemia, and metabolic acidosis, leading to lethargy, nausea, vomiting, dehydration, weakness, and hyperthermia. This syndrome is more profound if the proximal jejunum is used. Ileum and colon diversions may result in similar abnormalities: hyperchloremic metabolic acidosis. Abnormalities may be worse with continent diversions than conduits because of the exposure time of the bowel to urine. However, normal kidneys can usually correct the abnormalities. Clinical symptoms can include easy fatigability, anorexia, weight loss, polydipsia, and lethargy. Regardless of the type of diversion, patients require regular screening of their electrolytes.[23]

Magnesium deficiency, drug intoxication, or abnormalities in ammonia metabolism

These factors are uncommon, but may lead to alteration of the sensorium. Each should be identified and treated accordingly. Drugs more likely to be a problem are those that are absorbed by the gastrointestinal tract and excreted unchanged by the kidneys, e.g. phenytoin.[76] Methotrexate toxicity has been documented in a patient with an ileal conduit.[77] The problems with chemotherapeutic agents, in particular the antimetabolites, are relatively rare, but caution should be given to patients with continent diversions receiving chemotherapy. In this case, it is recommended that a pouch be drained during the time the toxic drugs are being administered.

Osteomalacia

Osteomalacia is loss of mineralized bone while the osteoid component increases. It may occur in patients with urinary diversion secondary to a combination of persistent acidosis, vitamin D resistance, and excessive calcium loss by the kidney.[23] The degree to which each of these factors contributes to the syndrome varies from patient to patient. With this syndrome comes lethargy, joint pain, especially on the weightbearing joints, and proximal myopathy. Serum calcium may be low or normal, and the alkaline phosphatase is usually elevated. Treatment involves correcting the acidosis and providing dietary supplements of calcium and rarely vitamin D. It is especially important to prevent acidosis in patients who are at risk of developing osteoporosis with aging to spare them the possibility of severe bone disease.

Bacteriuria and clinical infection

Bacteriuria and clinical infection are reported in most series of patients with bowel incorporated into the urinary tract, and the theoretical basis is well described.[78] Urine in the bowel may have a higher pH than normal and is less bacteriostatic. Distended bowel may become ischemic, and the disrupted mucosal barrier may allow translocation of bacteria into the systemic circulation. Intestinal mucus may also act as a template for formation of bacterial biofilms and perpetuate the bacteriuria.[79]

Bacteriuria, bacteremia, and sepsis occur with greater frequency when patients have intestinal diversions, especially in those with conduits. About three-quarters of those with conduits have bacteriuria at any time, yet many of them are asymptomatic and do not require treatment for their colonization. The main indication to treat asymptomatic bacteriuria is the presence of cultures dominant for *Proteus* or *Pseudomonas* spp. It has been suggested that these organisms may contribute to upper tract damage.[23]

The majority of patients with catheterized pouches will have chronic bacteriuria. Most urologists do not suggest treating asymptomatic bacteriuria.[80] Patients are usually well protected from pyelonephritis from their nonrefluxing ureterointestinal anastomosis. With a symptomatic pouch infection or pyelonephritis, antibiotic treatment should be administered. True pouch infections may require long courses of antibiotics, and, if frequently recurrent, we occasionally employ regular pouch instillation with antibiotics. A condition known as 'pouchitis' is manifested by pain in the region of the pouch along with increased pouch contractility.[23] The patient may experience sudden explosive

discharge of urine from the continent stoma in this setting. This type of scenario usually responds to longer courses of antibiotics.

Because of the devastating consequences with infection and possibly perforation, these patients and caregivers must be well informed regarding urinary retention. It may occur from simply not catheterizing the stoma or occasionally when the stoma, particularly with the nipple valve, obstructs or does not allow entrance of a catheter. This is considered a true emergency and the patient is instructed to seek attention from experienced medical personnel. It is recommended that various sizes and types of catheters are used, including the coude tip catheter. Sometimes, flexible cystoscopy is necessary. When significant manipulation of the stoma/pouch is required, we recommend leaving a catheter in for a short period due to edema.

Other metabolic complications

There is substantial evidence that urinary intestinal diversion has a negative impact on bone growth and development.[81] These effects are most prominent in children who have diversions performed prior to puberty.

Most *stones* formed in intestinal urinary diversions are composed of calcium, magnesium, and ammonium phosphate. Patients with hyperchloremic metabolic acidosis, pre-existing pyelonephritis, and urinary tract infection with urea-splitting organisms are at the greatest risk of developing stones.[82] A major cause of calculus formation in conduits and pouches is the presence of a foreign body, such as staples or nonabsorbable sutures.

The exact risk of developing *cancer* in a segment of bowel that has been incorporated into the urinary tract is unknown. After bladder augmentation for benign disease, there have been at least 14 cases of malignancy reported in the literature.[83,84] In a series of 2000 patients with a maximum follow-up of 22 years, only 1 case of malignancy was reported.[85]

Neuromechanical complications

Perforation of a cutaneous continent diversion or augmentation cystoplasty with catheterizable stoma occurs infrequently. In the former, the incidence of perforation/rupture is in the range of 1–2%.[86] In a survey of 1700 patients in Scandinavia, 20 episodes of perforation occurred in 18 patients.[87] Rupture may occur from reservoir catheterization, endoscopic examination, a fall, or spontaneously. The signs and symptoms may be vague, especially in patients with neurological disease, who may not sense fullness. This possible complication should be kept in mind when these patients present with pain, and consideration should be given to performing enterocystography or a CT scan. Since the perforation may cause peritonitis, prompt recognition and possible surgical exploration may be necessary.

Quality of life

In addition to maintaining low-pressure urinary storage and protecting the upper tracts, urinary diversion in the patient with a neurogenic bladder aims to improve the patient's quality of life (QoL). Often this translates into providing a reliable state of urinary continence, which positively impacts on the patients' lives. QoL issues in neurogenic bladder patients who have undergone urinary diversion are infrequently described in the literature. Much of what we know is extrapolated from cancer patients, who, in many ways, are a different patient population. Whether one procedure is better than another is very much based on what factors were considered when choosing which type of diversion. Newer or more complicated methods do not always result in a better QoL.[88] Herschorn and Hewitt,[89] in their series of 59 augmentation cystoplasties in neurogenic bladder patients, 35 of whom had a continent bladder stoma, reported the results of a patient questionnaire. Forty-one patients were 'delighted', 12 were 'pleased', and 6 were 'mostly satisfied' with their urinary tract management. This was despite one-third having some degree of incontinence. Most of the patients had been managed with indwelling catheters preoperatively.

Another important issue regarding continent vs noncontinent forms of diversion is the effect on the body image and sexuality of the patient. In a series of 18 neurologically impaired women treated with indwelling catheters, Watanabe and co-workers[90] reported the effect of urinary tract reconstruction on self-esteem and sexual function. On a scale of 0 (worst) to 5 (best), mean scores for self-esteem improved from 1 preoperatively to 4 postoperatively, self-image from 1 to 4, sexual desire from 2 to 4, and ability to cope with disability from 1 to 4, respectively. In 4 of the 15 women who were sexually active preoperatively, the frequency of sexual intercourse doubled from a mean of 3 to 6 times per month, respectively, and all 4 women reported improved sexual satisfaction. All 13 patients with pelvic pain and 5 with symptoms of autonomic dysreflexia noticed significant improvement if not complete resolution of the symptoms.

These reports confirm the positive effect that improvement in urinary tract management has on patients' QoL. It also underscores the need for evaluating patients' QoL in response to treatment and for further studies.

Conclusion

Considerable progress has been made in the surgical management of neurogenic bladder disease. Prior to 1950 the only diversion available was ureterosigmoidostomy, but infections, electrolyte problems, and long-term development of carcinomas discouraged its use. The ileal conduit then became the standard for urinary diversion and has essentially remained so, especially for patients with bladder cancer who need cystectomies. The procedure is standardized and the long-term risks and benefits are well known.

In the last 15 years continent diversions have become established as a reasonable alternative to an ileal conduit. In addition, procedures, such as continent bladder stomas, which address continence and catheterization difficulties with an intact bladder, have emerged as another option. The risks, benefits, and long-term outcomes are becoming more widely known. The availability of these procedures has improved the management and QoL for patients in whom conservative therapy has failed.

References

1. Barkin M, Dolfin D, Herschorn S. The urologic care of the spinal cord injured patient. J Urol 1983; 129:335–339.

2. Madersbacher H, Scott FB. Twelve o'clock sphincterotomy. Urol Int 1975; 30:75–81.

3. Chancellor M, Gajewski J, Ackman CFD, et al. Long-term follow-up of the North American Multicenter Urolume Trial for the treatment of external detrusor-sphincter dyssynergia. J Urol 1999; 161:1545–1550.

4. Rivas D, Karasick S, Chancellor M. Cutaneous ileocystostomy (a bladder chimney) for the treatment of severe neurogenic vesical dysfunction. Paraplegia 1995; 33:530–535.

5. Madersbacher H, et al. Conservative management in the neuropathic patient (Committee 19). In: Abrams P, Khoury S, Wein A, eds. Incontinence. London: Health Publication Ltd, 1999:755–812.

6. Wein AJ. Neuromuscular dysfunction of the lower urinary tract and its management. In: Walsh PC, Wein AJ, Vaughan ED Jr, Retik AB, eds. Campbell's urology, 8th edn. Philadelphia: WB Saunders, 2002:931–1026.

7. Weld KJ, Dmochowski RR. Association of level of injury and bladder behavior in patients with post traumatic spinal cord injury. Urology 2000; 55:490–494.

8. Jamil F, Williamson M, Ahmed YS, et al. Natural fill urodynamics in chronically catheterized patients with spinal cord injury. BJU Int 1999; 83:396–399.

9. Mills RD, Studer UE. Metabolic consequences of continent urinary diversion. J Urol 1999; 161:1057–1066.

10. Benson MC, Olsson CA. Continent urinary diversion. Urol Clin N Am 1999; 26(1):125–147, ix.

11. Kristjansson A, Davidsson T, Mansson W. Metabolic alterations at different levels of renal function following continent urinary diversion through colonic segments. J Urol 1997; 157:2099–2103.

12. Irvin TT, Goligher JC. Aetiology of disruption of intestinal anastomosis. Br J Surg 1973; 60:461.

13. Dion YM, Richards GK, Prentis JJ, Hinchey EJ. The influence of oral versus parenteral preoperative metronidazole on sepsis following colon surgery. Ann Surg 1980; 192:221–226.

14. Ferguson KH, McNeil JJ, Morey AF. Mechanical and antibiotic bowel preparation for urinary diversion surgery. J Urol 2002; 167:2352–2356.

15. Nichols RL, Smith JW, Garcia RY, et al. Current practices of preoperative bowel preparation among North American colorectal surgeons. Clin Infect Dis 1997; 24:609–611.

16. Henderson JM, Barnett JL, Turgeon DK, et al. Single-day, divided-dose oral sodium phosphate laxative versus intestinal lavage as preparation for colonoscopy: efficacy and patient tolerance. Gastrointest Endosc 1995; 42:238–240.

17. Oliveira L, Wexner SD, Daniel N, et al. Mechanical bowel preparation for elective colorectal surgery. A prospective, randomized, surgeon blinded trial comparing sodium phosphate and polyethylene glycol-based oral lavage solutions. Dis Col Rectum 1997; 40:585–587.

18. Thomson A, Naidoo P, Crotty B. Bowel preparation for colonoscopy: a randomized prospective trial comparing sodium phosphate and polyethylene glycol in a predominantly elderly population. J Gastroenterol Hepatol 1996; 11:103–106.

19. Heymann TD, Chopra K, Nunn E, et al. Bowel preparation at home: prospective study of adverse effects in elderly people. BMJ 1996; 313:727–730.

20. Mangram AJ, Horan TC, Pearson ML, et al. Guideline for prevention of surgical site infection, 1999. Centers for Disease Control and Prevention (CDC) Hospital Infection Control Practices Advisory Committee. Am J Infect Control 1999; 27:97–103.

21. Rowe-Jones DC, Peel AL, Kingston RD, et al. Single dose cefotaxime plus metronidazole versus three dose cefuroxime plus metronidazole as prophylaxis against wound infection in colorectal surgery: multicentre prospective randomised study. BMJ 1990; 300:18–22.

22. Mansson W, Colleen S, Stigsson L. Four methods of uretero-intestinal anastomoses in urinary conduit diversion. Scand J Urol Nephrol 1979; 13:191–199.

23. McDougal WS. Use of intestinal segments and urinary diversion. In: Walsh PC, Retik AB, Vaughan ED, et al, eds. Campbell's urology, 8th edn. Philadelphia: WB Saunders, 2002:3745–3788.

24. Schwarz GR, Jeffs RD. Ileal conduit urinary diversion in children: computer analysis of follow-up from 2 to 16 years. J Urol 1975; 114:285–288.

25. Kristjansson A, Wallin L, Månsson W. Renal function up to 16 years after conduit (refluxing or anti-reflux anastomosis) or continent urinary diversion. I. Glomerular filtration rate and patency of uretero-intestinal anastomosis. Br J Urol 1995; 76:539–545.

26. Kristjansson A, Bajc M, Wallin L, et al. Renal function up to 16 years after conduit (refluxing or anti-reflux anastomosis) or continent urinary diversion. II. Renal scarring and location of bacteriuria. Br J Urol 1995; 76:546–550.

27. Hinman F. Atlas of urologic surgery, 2nd edn. Philidelphia: WB Saunders, 1998:682.

28. Brooke BN. Ulcerative colitis and its surgical management, 1st edn. Edinburgh: Churchill Livingstone, 1954:92.

29. Verhoogen J. Neostomie uretero-caecale: formation d'une nouvelle poche vesicale et d'ub nouvel eretre. Assoc Franc Urol 1908; 12:362.

30. Seiffert L. Die Darm-"Siphonblase." Arch Klin Chir 1935; 183:569.

31. Bricker EM. Bladder substitution after pelvic evisceration. Surg Clin N Am 1950; 30:1511.

32. Williams O, Vereb MJ, Libertino JA. Non-continent urinary diversion. Urol Clin N Am 1997; 24(4):735–744.

33. Wallace DM. Uretero-ilestomy. Br J Urol 1970; 42:529–534.

34. Atan A, Konety BR, Nangia A, Chancellor MB. Advantages and risks of ileovesicostomy for the management of neuropathic bladder. Urology 1999; 54:636–640.

35. Kaefer M, Retik AB. The Mitrofanoff principle in continent urinary reconstruction. Urol Clin N Am 1997; 24(4):795–811.

36. Kock NG, Nilson AE, Nilsson LO, et al. Urinary diversion via a continent ileal reservoir: clinical results in 12 patients. J Urol 1982; 128:469.

37. Benson MC, Olsson CA. Cutaneous continent urinary diversion. In: Walsh PC, Retik AB, Vaughan ED, et al, eds. Campbell's urology, 8th edn. Philadelphia: WB Saunders, 2002:3789–3834.

38. Rowland RG, Mitchell ME, Bihrle R. The cecoileal continent urinary reservoir. World J Urol 1985; 3:185–190.

39. Lockhart JL. Remodeled right colon: an alternative urinary reservoir. J Urol 1987; 138:730–734.

40. Bejany DE, Politano VA. Stapled and nonstapled tapered distal ileum for construction of a continent colonic urinary reservoir. J Urol 1988; 140:491–494.

41. Stein JP, Lieskovsky G, Ginsberg DA, et al. The T pouch: an orthotopic ileal neobladder incorporating a serosal lined ileal antireflux technique. J Urol 1998; 159:1836–1842.

42. Benchekroun A. Hydraulic valve for continence and antireflux: a 17 year experience of 210 cases. Scand J Urol Nephrol Suppl 1992; 142:70–72.

43. Leng WW, McGuire EJ. Reconstructive surgery for urinary incontinence. Urol Clin N Am 1999; 26(1):61–80, viii.

44. Mitrofanoff P. Cystostomie continente trans-appendiculaire dans le traitement des vessies neurologiques. Chir Pediatr 1980; 21:297–305.

45. Keating MA, Rink RC, Adams MC. Appendicovesicostomy: a useful adjunct to continent reconstruction of the bladder. J Urol 1993; 149:1091.

46. Hinman F Jr. Functional classification of conduits for continent diversion. J Urol 1990; 144:27.

47. Malone RR, D'Cruz VT, Worth PHL, Woodhouse RJ. Why are continent diversions continent? J Urol 1989; 141:303A.

48. Watson HS, Baur SB, Peters CA, et al. Comparative urodynamics of appendiceal and ureteral Mitrofanoff conduits in children. J Urol 1995; 154:878.

49. Herschorn S, Thijssen AJ, Radomski SB. Experience with the hemi-Kock ileocystoplasty with a continent catheterizable stoma. J Urol 1993; 149:998–1001.

50. Herschorn S. Durability of the hemi-Kock continent bladder stoma. J Urol 2001; 165(5):suppl 88. [Abstract]

51. Kreder K, Anurag KD, Webster GD. The hemi-Kock ileocystoplasty: a versatile procedure in reconstructive urology. J Urol 1992; 147:1248–1251.

52. Adams MC, Mitchell ME, Rink RC. Gastrocystoplasty: an alternative solution to the problem of urological reconstruction in the severely compromised patient. J Urol 1988; 140:1152–1156.

53. Althausen AF, Hagen-Cook K, Hendren WH III. Nonrefluxing colon conduit: experience with 70 cases. J Urol 1978; 120:35–39.

54. Beckley S, Wajsman Z, Pontes JE, Murphy G. Transverse colon conduit: a method of urinary diversion after pelvic irradiation. J Urol 1982; 128:464–468.

55. Boyd SD, Schiff WM, Skinner DG, et al. Prospective study of metabolic abnormalities in patients with continent Kock pouch urinary diversion. Urology 1989; 33:85–88.

56. Castro JE, Ram MD. Electrolyte imbalance following ileal urinary diversion. Br J Urol 1970; 42:29–32.

57. Elder DD, Moisey CU, Rees RWM. A long-term follow-up of the colonic conduit operation in children. Br J Urol 1979; 51:462–465.

58. Flanigan RC, Kursh ED, Persky L. Thirteen year experience with ileal loop diversion in children with myelodysplasia. Am J Surg 1975; 130:535–538.

59. Hagen-Cook K, Althausen AF. Early observations on 31 adults with nonrefluxing colon conduits. J Urol 1979; 121:13–16.

60. Jaffe BM, Bricker EM, Butcher HR Jr. Surgical complications of ileal segment urinary diversion. Ann Surg 1968; 167:367–376.

61. Loening SA, Navarre RJ, Narayana AS, Culp DA. Transverse colon conduit urinary diversion. J Urol 1982; 127:37–39.

62. Malek RS, Burke EC, DeWeerd JH. Ileal conduit urinary diversion in children. J Urol 1971; 105:892–900.

63. Middleton AW Jr, Hendren WH. Ileal conduits in children at the Massachusetts General Hospital from 1955 to 1970. J Urol 1976; 115:591–595.

64. Pitts WR Jr, Muecke EC. A 20-year experience with ileal conduits: the fate of the kidneys. J Urol 1979; 122:154–157.

65. Richie JP. Intestinal loop urinary diversion in children. J Urol 1974; 111:687–689.

66. Schmidt JD, Hawtrey CE, Flocks RH, Culp DA. Complications, results, and problems of ileal conduit diversions. J Urol 1973; 109:210–216.

67. Schwarz GR, Jeffs RD. Ileal conduit urinary diversion in children: computer analysis of follow-up from 2 to 16 years. J Urol 1975; 114:285–288.

68. Shapiro SR, Lebowitz R, Colodny AH. Fate of 90 children with ileal conduit urinary diversions a decade later: analysis of complications, pyelography, renal function, and bacteriology. J Urol 1975; 114:289–295.

69. Smith ED. Follow-up studies on 150 ileal conduits in children. J Pediatr Surg 1972; 7:1–10.

70. Sullivan JW, Grabstald H, Whitmore WF Jr. Complications of ureteroileal conduit with radical cystectomy: review of 336 cases. J Urol 1980; 124:797–801.

71. Nurmi M, Puntala P, Alanen A. Evaluation of 144 cases of ileal conduits in adults. Eur Urol 1988; 15:89–92.

72. Beckley S, Wajsman Z, Pontes JE, Murphy G. Transverse colon conduit: a method of urinary diversion after pelvic irradiation. J Urol 1982; 128:464–468.

73. Loening SA, Navarre RJ, Narayana AS, Culp DA. Transverse colon conduit urinary diversion. J Urol 1982; 127:37–39.

74. Kramolowsky EV, Clayman RV, Weyman PJ. Endourological management of ureteroileal anastomotic strictures: is it effective? J Urol 1987; 137:390–394.

75. Kramolowsky EV, Clayman RV, Weyman PJ. Management of ureterointestinal anastomotic strictures: comparison of open surgical and endourological repair. J Urol 1988; 139:1195–1198.

76. Savarirayan F, Dixey GM. Syncope following ureterosigmoidostomy. J Urol 1969; 101:844–845.

77. Bowyer GW, Davies TW. Methotrexate toxicity associated with an ileal conduit. Br J Urol 1986; 60:592.

78. McDougal WS. Metabolic complications of urinary intestinal diversion. J Urol 1992; 147:1199–1208.

79. Blyth B, Ewalt DH, Duckett JW, et al. Lithogenic properties of enterocystoplasty. J Urol 1992; 148:575–577.

80. Skinner DG, Lieskovsky G, Skinner E, Boyd S. Urinary diversion. Curr Probl Surg 1987; 24:401–471.

81. Kock MO, McDougal WS, Hall MC, et al. Long-term effects of urinary diversion: a comparison of myelomeningocele patients managed by clean, intermittent catheterization and urinary diversion. J Urol 1992; 147:1343–1347.

82. Dretler SP. The pathogenesis of urinary tract calculi occurring after conduit diversion: I. clinical study; II. conduit study; III. prevention. J Urol 1973; 109:204–209.

83. Treiger BFG, Marshall FF. Carcinogenesis and the use of intestinal segments in the urinary tract. Urol Clin N Am 1991; 18:737–742.

84. Carr LK, Herschorn S. Early development of adenocarcinoma in a young woman following augmentation cystoplasty for undiversion. J Urol 1997; 157:2255–2256.

85. Rowland RG, Regan JS. The risk of secondary malignancies in urinary reservoirs. In: Hohenfellner R, Wammack R, eds. Continent urinary diversion. London: Churchill Livingstone, 1992:299–308.

86. Studer UE, Stenzl A, Mansson W, Mills R. Bladder replacement and urinary diversion. Eur Urol 2000; 38(6):1–11.

87. Mansson W, Bakke A, Bergman B, et al. Perforations of continent urinary reservoirs. Scand J Urol Nephrol 1997; 31:529–532.

88. Mansson A, Mansson W. When the bladder is gone: quality of life following different types of urinary diversion. World J Urol 1999; 17:211–218.

89. Herschorn S, Hewitt R. The patient perspective of long-term outcome of augmentation cystoplasty in the management of neurogenic bladders. Urology 1998; 52:672–678.

90. Watanabe T, Rivas DA, Smith R, et al. The effect of urinary tract reconstruction on neurologically impaired women previously treated with an indwelling urethral catheter. J Urol 1996; 156(6):1926–1928.

Tissue engineering applications for patients with neurogenic bladder

Anthony Atala

Introduction

Regenerative medicine, a recently defined field, involves the diverse areas of tissue engineering, stem cells, and cloning towards the common goals of developing biological substitutes which would restore and maintain normal tissue and organ function.

Tissue engineering follows the principles of cell transplantation, materials science, and engineering towards the development of biological substitutes which would restore and maintain normal function. Tissue engineering may involve matrices alone, wherein the body's natural ability to regenerate is used to orient or direct new tissue growth, or the use of matrices with cells.

When cells are used for tissue engineering, donor tissue is dissociated into individual cells, which are either implanted directly into the host, or expanded in culture, attached to a support matrix, and reimplanted after expansion. The implanted tissue can be either heterologous, allogeneic, or autologous. Ideally, this approach might allow lost tissue function to be restored or replaced *in toto* and with limited complications.[2] The use of autologous cells would avoid rejection, wherein a biopsy of tissue is obtained from the host, the cells are dissociated and expanded *in vitro*, reattached to a matrix, and implanted into the same host.

One of the initial limitations of applying cell-based tissue engineering techniques to urologic organs had been the previously encountered inherent difficulty of growing genitourinary associated cells in large quantities. In the past, it was believed that urothelial cells had a natural senescence that was hard to overcome. Normal urothelial cells could be grown in the laboratory setting, but with limited expansion. Several protocols were developed over the last two decades which improved urothelial growth and expansion.[3–6] Using these methods of cell culture, it is possible to expand a urothelial strain from a single specimen that initially covers a surface area of 1 cm^2 to one covering a surface area of 4202 m^2 (the equivalent area of one football field) within 8 weeks.[3]

Biomaterials in genitourinary tissue engineering may function as an artificial extracellular matrix (ECM), and elicit biological and mechanical functions of native ECM found in tissues of the body. The design and selection of the biomaterial is critical in the development of engineered genitourinary tissues. The biomaterial must be capable of controlling the structure and function of the engineered tissue in a predesigned manner by interacting with transplanted cells and/or the host cells. Generally, the ideal biomaterial should be biocompatible, promote cellular interaction and tissue development, and possess proper mechanical and physical properties.

Generally, three classes of biomaterials have been utilized for engineering genitourinary tissues: naturally derived materials, e.g. collagen and alginate; acellular tissue matrices, e.g. bladder submucosa and small intestinal submucosa; and synthetic polymers, e.g. polyglycolic acid (PGA), polylactic acid (PLA), and poly(lactic-co-glycolic acid) (PLGA). These classes of biomaterials have been tested in respect to their biocompatibility with primary human urothelial and bladder muscle cells.[7,8] Naturally derived materials and acellular tissue matrices have the potential advantage of biological recognition. Synthetic polymers can be produced reproducibly on a large scale with controlled properties of their strength, degradation rate, and microstructure.

Tissue engineering of the urethra

Various strategies have been proposed over the years for the regeneration of urethral tissue. Woven meshes of PGA have been used to reconstruct urethras in animals.[9,10] PGA has been also used as a cell transplantation vehicle to engineer tubular urothelium *in vivo*.[11] When using cells for transplantation, it has been shown that cells from an abnormal environment, if genetically stable, are able to be engineered into normal tissues.[12] A homologous free graft of acellular urethral matrix was used in a rabbit model.[13] All tissue components were seen in the grafted matrix after 3 months, with further improvement over time; however, the smooth muscle in the matrix was less than in normal rabbit urethra and was not well oriented.

Acellular collagen matrices obtained from donor bladder submucosa have proven to be suitable grafts for repairing urethral defects both experimentally and clinically at our institution. Rabbit neourethras reconstructed with acellular matrices demonstrated a normal urothelial luminal lining and organized muscle bundles, without any signs of strictures or complications.[14] These results were confirmed clinically in a series of patients with a history of failed hypospadias reconstruction wherein the urethral defects were repaired with human bladder acellular collagen matrices in an onlay fashion, with the size of the created neourethras ranging from 5 to 15 cm (Figure 55.1).[15] The same technique was used to repair urethral strictures on over 40 adult patients.[16] One of the advantages over nongenital tissue grafts used for urethroplasty is that the collagen-based acellular material is 'off the shelf'. This eliminates the necessity of additional surgical procedures for graft harvesting, which may decrease operative time, as well as the potential morbidity due to the harvest procedure.

It has also been noted that although acellular collagen-based grafts may be suitable for partial onlay urethral replacement, they are not effective for the replacement of tubularized segments, as this results in the collapse of the grafts, with subsequent stricture formation.[17] Tubularized urethral repairs require the application of collagen-based grafts seeded with both urothelial and muscle cells.[17] Total urethral replacement is possible with the use of tissue-engineered constructs composed of urothelial and muscle cell seeded matrices.

Tissue engineering of the bladder

Currently, gastrointestinal segments are commonly used as tissues for bladder replacement or repair. However, gastrointestinal tissues are designed to absorb specific solutes, whereas bladder tissue is designed for the excretion of solutes. When gastrointestinal tissue is in contact with the urinary tract, multiple complications may ensue, such as infection, metabolic disturbances, urolithiasis, perforation, increased mucus production, and malignancy.[18] Due to the problems encountered with the use of gastrointestinal segments, numerous investigators have attempted

alternative methods, materials, and tissues for bladder replacement or repair.

Seromuscular grafts and de-epithelialized bowel segments, either alone or over a native urothelium, have been attempted.[19–26] The concept of demucosalizing organs is not new to urologists. Over four decades ago, in 1961, Blandy proposed the removal of submucosa from intestinal segments used for augmentation cystoplasty to insure that mucosal regrowth would not occur.[19] Hypothetically, this would avoid the complications associated with using bowel in continuity with the urinary tract.[20,21] Since Blandy's initial report, over 25 years transpired before there was a renewed interest in demucosalizing intestinal segments for urinary reconstruction.[22] Since 1988, several other investigators have pursued this line of research.[23–26] These investigative efforts have emphasized the complexity of both the anatomic and cellular interactions present when combining tissues with different functional parameters. The complexity of these interactions is emphasized by the observation that the use of demucosalized intestinal segments for augmentation cystoplasty is limited by either mucosal regrowth or contraction of the intestinal patch.[23,24] It has been noted that removal of only the mucosa may lead to mucosal regrowth, whereas removal of the mucosa and submucosa may lead to retraction of the intestinal patch.[27,28]

Some researchers have combined the techniques of autoaugmentation and enterocystoplasty. An autoaugmentation is performed and the diverticulum is covered with a demucosalized gastric or intestinal segment. In a series of autoaugmentation[25] enterocystoplasty, patients with a neurogenic bladder had either incorporation of stomach or colon. In both groups of patients the mucosa of the enteric segment was dissected away from the underlying muscle, and the resulting mucosa-free graft was used to cover a newly created bladder diverticulum. A satisfactory increase in bladder capacity and compliance was achieved in most patients. In another series of patients who underwent seromuscular colocystoplasty, the bladder capacity increased an average of 2.4-fold in 14 patients.[26] Ten patients had a postoperative bladder biopsy: 7 patients demonstrated urothelium covering the augmented portion of the bladder, 2 patients had regrowth of colonic mucosa, and 1 patient showed a mixture of colonic mucosa and urothelium. Although colonic mucosal regrowth is seen, there is a subset of patients, that may benefit from these procedures, wherein mucous secretion may be reduced or eliminated.[26]

Bladder grafts, initially used experimentally in 1961, have been used recently by various investigators.[29–32] The allogenic acellular bladder matrix has served as a scaffold for the ingrowth of host bladder wall components. The matrix is prepared by mechanically and/or chemically removing the cellular components.

Allogenic bladder submucosa was utilized as a biomaterial for bladder augmentation in dogs.[31] Biomaterials preloaded with cells prior to their implantation showed better tissue regeneration, compared with biomaterials implanted with no cells in which the tissue regeneration depended on the ingrowth of the surrounding tissue. The bladders showed a significant increase in capacity of 100% when augmented with scaffolds seeded with cells, compared with a capacity of 30% for scaffolds without cells (Figure 55.2).

Small-intestinal submucosa (SIS), derived from pig small intestine, has been used for augmentation cystoplasty in dogs.[33] Preoperative mean bladder capacity was 51 ml compared with a postoperative mean capacity of 55 ml. Histologically, the muscle layer was not fully developed. A large amount of collagen was interspersed between a smaller number of muscle bundles. A computerized assisted image analysis demonstrated a decreased muscle-to-collagen ratio, with a loss of the normal architecture in the SIS regenerated bladders. *In-vitro* contractility studies performed on the SIS regenerated dog bladders showed a decrease in maximal contractile response by 50% from those of normal bladder tissues. Cholinergic and purinergic innervation was present.[34]

In multiple studies using different materials as an acellular graft for cystoplasty, the urothelial layer was able to regenerate normally, but the muscle layer, although present, was not fully developed.[30–33] Engineering tissue using selective cell transplantation may provide a means of creating functional new bladder segments.[11] The success of using cell transplantation strategies for bladder reconstruction depends on the ability to use donor tissue efficiently and to provide the right conditions for long-term survival, differentiation, and growth.

Urothelial and muscle cells can be expanded *in vitro*, seeded onto the polymer scaffold, and allowed to attach and form sheets of cells. The cell–polymer scaffold can then be implanted *in vivo*. A series of *in-vivo* urologic associated cell–polymer experiments were performed in mice, rabbits, and dogs.[3,11,31,35]

To better address the functional parameters of tissue-engineered bladders, an animal model was designed that required a subtotal cystectomy with subsequent replacement with a tissue-engineered organ.[36] Dogs underwent a trigone-sparing cystectomy. The animals were randomly assigned to one of three groups. Animals underwent closure of the trigone without a reconstructive procedure, reconstruction with a cell-free bladder-shaped biodegradable matrix, or reconstruction using a bladder-shaped biodegradable matrix that delivered autologous urothelial and smooth muscle cells. The cell populations had been separately expanded from a previously harvested autologous bladder biopsy. Preoperative and postoperative urodynamic, radiographic, gross, histological, and immunocytochemical analyses were performed serially at 1, 2, 3, 4, 6, and 11 months, postoperatively.[36]

The cystectomy-only controls and polymer-only grafts maintained average capacities of 22% and 46% of preoperative values, respectively. An average bladder capacity of 95% of the original pre-cystectomy volume was achieved in the tissue-engineered bladder replacements. These findings were confirmed radiographically. The subtotal cystectomy reservoirs, which were not reconstructed, and polymer-only reconstructed bladders showed a marked decrease in bladder compliance (10% and 42%, respectively). The compliance of the tissue-engineered bladders showed almost no difference from preoperative values that were measured when the native bladder was present (106%). Histologically, the polymer-only bladders presented a pattern of normal urothelial cells with a thickened fibrotic submucosa and a thin layer of muscle fibers. The retrieved tissue-engineered bladders showed a normal cellular organization, consisting of a trilayer of urothelium, submucosa, and muscle (Figure 55.3). Immunocytochemical analyses for desmin, α-actin, cytokeratin 7, pancytokeratins AE1/AE3, and uroplakin III confirmed the muscle and urothelial phenotype. S-100 staining indicated the presence of neural structures. The results from this study showed that it is possible to tissue engineer bladders which are anatomically and functionally normal.[36] Human bladders have been created using the same techniques.

Clinically, cells used for tissue engineering may be harvested from abnormal bladders. We investigated the contractility of tissue-engineered bladder smooth muscle derived from patients with functionally normal bladders and functionally abnormal neuropathic and exstrophic bladders.[12] The tissue-engineered cells showed similar expression of smooth muscle marker proteins (α-actin and myosin) regardless of their origin. All scaffolds showed similar muscle formation and were α-actin positive. At retrieval, the muscle cell-seeded scaffolds exhibited contractile activity to electrical field stimulation and carbachol. There was no statistical difference between the three different types of muscle cells seeded (normal, neurogenic, and exstrophic). The results of this study were also consistent with prior findings that, in diseased bladders, a large portion of the pathologic effects seen are due to increased fibrosis, whereas the cells retain their genetic stability.

Injectable therapies using tissue engineering techniques

Both urinary incontinence and vesicoureteral reflux are common conditions affecting the genitourinary system, wherein injectable bulking agents can be used for treatment. The goal of several investigators has been to find alternative implant materials that would be safe for human use.[37] Long-term studies were conducted to determine the effect of injectable chondrocytes *in vivo*.[38] It was initially determined that alginate, a liquid solution of gluronic and mannuronic acid, embedded with chondrocytes, could serve as a synthetic substrate for the injectable delivery and maintenance of cartilage architecture *in vivo*. A biopsy of the ear could be easily and quickly performed, followed by chondrocyte processing and endoscopic injection of the autologous chondrocyte suspension for therapy.

Chondrocytes can be readily grown and expanded in culture. Neocartilage formation can be achieved *in vitro* and *in vivo* using chondrocytes cultured on synthetic biodegradable polymers.[38] This system was adapted for the treatment of vesicoureteral reflux in a porcine model.[39] Chondrocytes were harvested from the left auricular surface of surgically created refluxing mini-swine and expanded. The animals underwent endoscopic repair of reflux with the injectable autologous chondrocyte solution on the right side only. Serial cystograms showed no evidence of reflux on the treated side and persistent reflux in the uncorrected control ureter in all animals. The harvested ears had evidence of cartilage regrowth within 1 month of chondrocyte retrieval.

At the time of sacrifice, gross examination of the bladder injection site showed a well-defined rubbery to hard cartilage structure in the subureteral region. Histologic examination of these specimens showed evidence of normal cartilage formation. The polymer gels were progressively replaced by cartilage over time. Aldehyde fuschin-alcian blue staining suggested the presence of chondroitin sulfate.

Using the same line of reasoning as with the chondrocyte technology, the possibility of using autologous muscle cells was also investigated.[40] *In-vivo* experiments were conducted in mini-pigs and reflux was successfully corrected. In addition to its use for the endoscopic treatment of reflux and urinary incontinence, the system of injectable autologous cells may also be applicable for the treatment of other medical conditions, such as rectal incontinence, dysphonia, plastic reconstruction, and wherever an injectable permanent biocompatible material is needed.

Recently, the first human application of cell-based tissue engineering technology for urologic applications has occurred with the injection of chondrocytes for the correction of vesicoureteral reflux in children (Figure 55.4) and for urinary incontinence in adults. The clinical trials are currently ongoing.[37,41–43]

The potential use of injectable, cultured myoblasts for the treatment of stress urinary incontinence has recently been investigated in preliminary experiments.[44] Primary myoblasts obtained from mouse skeletal muscle were transduced *in vitro* to carry the β-galactosidase reporter gene and were then incubated with fluorescent microspheres which would serve as markers for the original cell population. Cells were then directly injected into the proximal urethra and lateral bladder walls of nude mice with a microsyringe in an open surgical procedure. Tissue was harvested up to 35 days post-injection, analyzed histologically, and assayed for β-galactosidase expression. Myoblasts expressing β-galactosidase and containing fluorescent microspheres were found at each of the retrieved time points. In addition, regenerative myofibers expressing β-galactosidase were identified within the bladder wall. By 35 days post-injection, some of the injected cells expressed the contractile filament a-smooth muscle actin, suggesting the possibility of myoblastic differentiation into smooth muscle. The authors reported that a significant portion of the injected myoblast population persisted *in vivo*. The fact that myoblasts can be transfected, survive after injection, and begin the process of myogenic differentiation further supports the feasibility of using cultured cells of muscular origin as an injectable bioimplant.

Gene therapy and tissue engineering

Genetically engineered cells

Cells can be engineered to secrete growth factors for various applications, such as for promoting angiogenesis for tissue regeneration.[45] Angiogenesis, the process of new blood vessel formation, is regulated by different growth factors. These growth factors stimulate endothelial cells, which are already present in the patient's body, to migrate to the implanted area of need, where they proliferate and differentiate into blood vessels.[46] One of the major molecules which promotes and regulates angiogenesis is vascular endothelial growth factor (VEGF).[47] Several methods have been used experimentally to deliver VEGF *in vivo*. The growth factor protein can be directly injected into tissues.[48] However, the rapid clearance of VEGF proteins from the vascular system limits its effect to only minutes. The *VEGF* gene could be delivered to tissues using various techniques; however, the transfection efficiency is low, the onset of action is delayed for up to 48–72 h after the *VEGF* cDNA is incorporated, and the effect is transient, lasting only several days.[48,49]

An approach which has been pursued in our laboratory to increase and stimulate rapid vascularization *in vivo* was to engineer a cell line to secrete high levels of VEGF proteins by gene transfecting the cells with the *VEGF* cDNA. The VEGF-secreting cells were encapsulated in polymeric microspheres. The microspheres allowed nutrients to reach the cells, whereas the VEGF proteins secreted from the cells diffused into the surrounding tissues. The microspheres protected the coated cells from the host immune environment. This novel system of neovascularization was tested *in vitro* and *in vivo* in an animal model. The degree of VEGF secretion and the period of delivery can be regulated by modulating the number of engineered cells encapsulated per microsphere, as well as the number of microspheres injected. A similar strategy has also been pursued for the genetic engineering of antiangiogenic factor secreting cells.[50] These strategies could be useful for antitumor therapy in urology.

Gene therapy for tissue engineered constructs

Based on the feasibility of tissue engineering techniques in which cells seeded on biodegradable polymer scaffolds form tissue when implanted *in vivo*, the possibility was explored of developing a neo-organ system for *in-vivo* gene therapy.[51] In a series of studies conducted in our laboratory, human urothelial cells were harvested, expanded *in vitro*, and seeded on biodegradable polymer scaffolds. The cell–polymer complex was then transfected with *PGL3-luc*, *pCMV-luc*, and *pCMVß-gal* promoter–reporter gene constructs. The transfected cell–polymer scaffolds were then implanted *in vivo* and the engineered tissues were retrieved at different time points after implantation. Results indicate that successful gene transfer may be achieved using biodegradable polymer scaffolds as a urothelial cell delivery vehicle. The transfected cell–polymer scaffold formed organ-like structures with functional expression of the transfected genes.[51] This technology is applicable throughout the spectrum of diseases which may be manageable with tissue engineering. For example, one can envision the use of effecting *in-vivo* gene delivery through the *ex-vivo* transfection of tissue-engineered cell–polymer scaffolds for the genetic modification of diseased corporal smooth muscle cells harvested from impotent patients. Theoretically, the *in-vitro* genetic modification of corporal smooth muscle cells harvested from an impotent patient, resulting in either a reduction in the expression of the *TGF-1* gene or the overexpression of genes responsible for PGE1 production, could lead to the resumption of erectile functionality once these cells were used to repopulate the diseased corporal bodies.

Stem cells for tissue engineering

Most current strategies for engineering urologic tissues involve harvesting of autologous cells from the host diseased organ. However, in situations where extensive end-stage organ failure is present, a tissue biopsy may not yield enough normal cells for expansion. Under these circumstances, the availability of pluripotent stem cells may be beneficial. Pluripotent embryonic stem cells are known to form teratomas *in vivo*, which are composed of a variety of differentiated cells. However, these cells may be

immunocompetent, and may require immunosuppression if used clinically.

The possibility of deriving pluripotent cells from postnatal mesenchymal tissue from the same host, and inducing their differentiation *in vitro* and *in vivo*, was investigated. Pluripotent cells were isolated from human foreskin-derived fibroblasts. Adipogenic, myogenic, and osteoblastic lineages were obtained from these progenitor cells. The cells were grown, expanded, seeded onto biodegradable scaffolds, and implanted *in vivo*, where they formed mature tissue structures. This was the first demonstration that stem cells can be derived from postnatal connective tissue and can be used for engineering tissues *in vivo ex situ*.[52]

Therapeutic cloning for tissue engineering

Recent advances with the cloning of embryos and newborn animals have expanded the possibilities of this technology for tissue engineering and organ transplantation. There are many ethical concerns with cloning in terms of creating humans for the sole purpose of obtaining organs. However, the potential for retrieving cells from early-stage cloned embryos for subsequent regeneration is being proposed as an ethically viable benefit of therapeutic cloning (Figure 55.5). The feasibility of engineering syngeneic tissues *in vivo* using cloned cells was investigated.

Unfertilized donor bovine eggs were retrieved and the nuclear material was removed. Bovine fibroblasts from the skin of a steer were obtained. The nuclear material was removed from the fibroblast and microinjected into the donor egg shell (nuclear transfer). A short burst of energy was delivered, initiating neoembryogenesis. These techniques replicate what was performed to clone the first mammal, Dolly the sheep. However, instead of implanting the embryo into a uterus, the goal would be to harvest stem cells from the embryo, which was created, not from the union of a sperm and an egg, but rather from a skin cell and an egg shell, devoid of any genetic material. To achieve a proof of principle, bypassing the *in-vitro* differentiation, the embryos were placed in the same steer uterus from which the fibroblasts had been obtained. The cloned embryo, with identical genetic material as the steer, was retrieved for tissue harvest. Various cell types were harvested, expanded *in vitro*, and seeded on biodegradable scaffolds. The cell–polymer scaffolds were implanted into the back of the same steer from which the cells were cloned. The implants were retrieved at various time points for analyses. Renal tissue, and cardiac and skeletal muscle were engineered successfully using therapeutic cloning.

These studies demonstrated that cells obtained through nuclear transfer can be successfully harvested, expanded in culture, and transplanted *in vivo* with biodegradable scaffolds where the single suspended cells form and organize into tissue structures, which are the same genetically as the host. These studies were the first demonstration of the use of therapeutic cloning for the regeneration of tissues *in vivo*.[53] One could envision taking one skin cell from a patient, and having the ability to generate most types of tissues for replacement or transplantation, which would be genetically identical and fully biocompatible. Thus, each patient could conceivably have a ready-made supply of their own tissues available on demand.

Conclusion

Tissue engineering efforts are currently being undertaken for every type of tissue and organ within the urinary system. Primary autologous cells, stem cells, and therapeutic cloning are being applied for the creation of tissues and organs. Tissue engineering techniques require expertise in growth factor biology, a cell culture facility designed for human application, and personnel who have mastered the techniques of cell harvest, culture, and expansion. Polymer scaffold design and manufacturing resources are essential for the successful application of this technology.

The first human application of cell-based tissue engineering for urologic applications occurred at our institution with the injection of autologous cells for the correction of vesicoureteral reflux in children. The same technology has been recently expanded to treat adult patients with urinary incontinence. Trials involving urethral tissue replacement using processed collagen matrices are in progress at our center for both hypospadias and stricture repair. Bladder replacement using tissue engineering techniques is being explored. Recent progress suggests that engineered urologic tissues may have a wider clinical applicability in regenerative medicine.

References

1. Murray JE, Merrill JP, Harrison JH. Renal homotransplantation in identical twins. J Am Soc Nephrol 2001; 12(1):201–204.

2. Atala A. Tissue engineering in the genitourinary system. In: Atala A, Mooney D, eds. Tissue engineering. Boston: Birkhauser Press, 1997:149.

3. Cilento BG, Freeman MR, Schneck FX, et al. Phenotypic and cytogenetic characterization of human bladder urothelia expanded in vitro. J Urol 1994;152:655.

4. Scriven SD, Booth C, Thomas DF, et al. Reconstitution of human urothelium from monolayer cultures. J Urol 1997; 158(3 Pt 2): 1147–1152.

5. Liebert M, Wedemeyer G, Abruzzo LV, et al. Stimulated urothelial cells produce cytokines and express an activated cell surface antigenic phenotype. Semin Urol 1991; 9(2):124–130.

6. Puthenveettil JA, Burger MS, Reznikoff CA. Replicative senescence in human uroepithelial cells. Adv Exp Med Biol 1999; 462:83–91.

7. Pariente JL, Kim BS, Atala A. In vitro biocompatibility assessment of naturally-derived and synthetic biomaterials using normal human urothelial cells. J Biomed Mat Res 2001; 55:33–39.

8. Pariente JL, Kim BS, Atala A. In vitro biocompatibility evaluation of naturally derived and synthetic biomaterials using normal human bladder smooth muscle cells. J Urol 2002; 167:1867–1871.

9. Bazeed MA, Thüroff JW, Schmidt RA, Tanagho EA. New treatment for urethral strictures. Urology 1983; 21:53–57.

10. Olsen L, Bowald S, Busch C, et al. Urethral reconstruction with a new synthetic absorbable device. Scand J Urol Nephrol 1992; 26:323–326.

11. Atala A, Vacanti JP, Peters CA, et al. Formation of urothelial structures in vivo from dissociated cells attached to biodegradable polymer scaffolds in vitro. J Urol 1992; 148:658.

12. Lai JY, Yoon CY, Yoo JJ, et al. Phenotypic and functional characterization of in vivo tissue engineered smooth muscle from normal and pathological bladders. J Urol 2002; 168:1853–1858.

13. Sievert KD, Bakircioglu ME, Nunes L, et al. Homologous acellular matrix graft for urethral reconstruction in the rabbit: histological and functional evaluation. J Urol 2000; 163(6):1958–1965.

14. Chen F, Yoo JJ, Atala A. Acellular collagen matrix as a possible "off the shelf" biomaterial for urethral repair. Urology 1999; 54:407–410.

15. Atala A, Guzman L, Retik A. A novel inert collagen matrix for hypospadias repair. J Urol 1999; 162:1148–1151.

16. Kassaby EA, Yoo J, Retik A, Atala A. A novel inert collagen matrix for urethral stricture repair. J Urol 2000;163(supp 4):70.

17. DeFilippo RE, Yoo JY, Chen F, Atala A. Urethral replacement using cell-seeded tubularized collagen matrices. J Urol 2002; 168:1789–1793.

18. McDougal WS. Metabolic complications of urinary intestinal diversion. J Urol 1992; 147:1199.

19. Blandy JP. Neal pouch with transitional epithelium and anal sphincter as a continent urinary reservoir. J Urol 1961; 86:749.

20. Blandy JP. The feasibility of preparing an ideal substitute for the urinary bladder. Ann Roy Coll Surg 1964; 35:287.

21. Harada N, Yano H, Ohkawa T, et al. New surgical treatment of bladder tumors: mucosal denudation of the bladder. Br J Urol 1965; 37:545.

22. Oesch I. Neourothelium in bladder augmentation. An experimental study in rats. Eur Urol 1988; 14:328.

23. Salle J, Fraga C, Lucib A, et al. Seromuscular enterocystoplasty in dogs. J Urol 1990; 144:454.

24. Cheng E, Rento R, Grayhack TJ, et al. Reversed seromuscular flaps in the urinary tract in dogs. J Urol 1994; 152:2252.

25. Dewan PA. Autoaugmentation demucosalized enterocystoplasty. World J Urol 1998; 16:255–261.

26. Gonzalez R, Buson H, Reid C, Reinberg Y. Seromuscular colocystoplasty lined with urothelium (SCLU). Experimental in 16 patients. Urology 1995; 45:124.

27. Atala A. Commentary on the replacement of urologic associated mucosa. J Urol 1995; 156:338.

28. Atala A. Autologous cell transplantation for urologic reconstruction. J Urol 1998; 159:2.

29. Tsuji I, Ishida H, Fujieda J. Experimental cystoplasty using preserved bladder graft. J Urol 1961; 85:42.

30. Probst M, Dahiya R, Carrier S, Tanagho EA. Reproduction of functional smooth muscle tissue and partial bladder replacement. Br J Urol 1997; 79:505–515.

31. Yoo JJ, Meng J, Oberpenning F, Atala A. Bladder augmentation using allogenic bladder submucosa seeded with cells. Urology 1998; 51:221.

32. Sutherland RS, Baskin LS, Hayward SW, Cunha GR. Regeneration of bladder urothelium, smooth muscle, blood vessels, and nerves into an acellular tissue matrix. J Urol 1996; 156:571–577.

33. Kropp BP, Rippy MK, Badylak SF, et al. Small intestinal submucosa: urodynamic and histopathologic evaluation in long term canine bladder augmentations. J Urol 1996; 155:2098–2104.

34. Vaught JD, Kroop BP, Sawyer BD, et al. Detrusor regeneration in the rat using porcine small intestine submucosal grafts: functional innervation and receptor expression. J Urol 1996; 155:374–378.

35. Atala A, Freeman MR, Vacanti JP, et al. Implantation in vivo and retrieval of artificial structures consisting of rabbit and human urothelium and human bladder muscle. J Urol 1993; 150:608.

36. Oberpenning FO, Meng J, Yoo J, Atala A. De novo reconstitution of a functional urinary bladder by tissue engineering. Nat Biotechnol 1999; 17:2.

37. Kershen RT, Atala A. Advances in injectable therapies for the treatment of incontinence and vesicoureteral reflux. Urol Clin 1999; 26:81–94.

38. Atala A, Cima LG, Kim W, et al. Injectable alginate seeded with chondrocytes as a potential treatment for vesicoureteral reflux. J Urol 1993; 150:745.

39. Atala A, Kim W, Paige KT, et al. Endoscopic treatment of vesicoureteral reflux with chondrocyte-alginate suspension. J Urol 1994; 152:641.

40. Cilento BG, Atala A. Treatment of reflux and incontinence with autologous chondrocytes and bladder muscle cells. Dial Pediatr Urol 1995; 18:11.

41. Diamond DA, Caldamone AA. Endoscopic correction of vesicoureteral reflux in children using autologous chondrocytes: preliminary results. J Urol 1999; 162:1185.

42. Caldamone AA, Diamond DA. Long-term results of the endoscopic correction of vesicoureteral reflux in children using autologous chondrocytes. J Urol 2001; 165(6 Pt 2):2224–2227.

43. Bent AE, Tutrone RT, McLennan MT, et al. Treatment of intrinsic sphincter deficiency using autologous ear chondrocytes as a bulking agent. Neurourol Urodyn 2001; 20(2):157–165.

44. Yokoyama T, Chancellor MB, Watanabe T, et al. Primary myoblasts injection into the urethra and bladder as a potential treatment of stress urinary incontinence and impaired detrusor contractility; long term survival without significant cytotoxicity. J Urol 1999; 161:307.

45. Machlouf M, Orsola A, Atala A. Controlled release of therapeutic agents: slow delivery and cell encapsulation. World J Urol 2000; 18:80–83.

46. Polverini PJ. The pathophysiology of angiogenesis. Crit Rev Oral Biol Med 1996; 6:230.

47. Klagsbrun M, D'Amore PA. Regulation of angiogenesis. Ann Rev Physiol 1991; 53:217.

48. Bauters C, Asahara T, Zheng LP, et al. Physiological assessment of augmented vascularity induced by VEGF in ischemic rabbit hindlimb. Am J Physiol 1994; 267:263.

49. Takeshita S, Tsurumi Y, Couffinahl T, et al. Gene transfer of naked DNA encoding for three isoforms of vascular endothelial growth factor stimulates collateral development in vivo. Lab Invest 1996; 75:487.

50. Joki T, Machluf M, Atala A, et al. Continuous release of endostatin from microencapsulated engineered cells for tumor therapy. Nat Biotechnol 2001; 19(1):35–39.

51. Yoo JJ, Atala A. A novel gene delivery system using urothelial tissue engineered neo-organs. J Urol 1997; 158:1066–1070.

52. Bartsch GC, Yoo JJ, De Coppi P, et al. Dermal stem cells for pelvic and bladder reconstruction. J Urol 2002; 167:59a.

53. Lanza RP, Chung HY, Yoo JJ, et al. Generation of histocompatible tissues using nuclear transplantation. Nat Biotechnol 2002;20: 689–696.

56

Restoration of complete bladder function by neurostimulation

Michael Craggs

Introduction

During the past 20 years two key developments using implantable neuroprostheses have had a significant impact on treating and managing patients with a neurogenic bladder. The first of these was the Brindley sacral anterior root stimulator[1] used principally for bladder emptying in (see Chapter 49). The second was the sacral nerve stimulator originally developed by Tanagho and Schmidt for neuromodulating[2,3] a variety of bladder dysfunctions, including the overactive bladder and urinary retention (see Chapter 50). It is timely to consider how these two techniques, among others, may in the future be combined using emerging technologies to restore more complete control of the dysfunctional bladder in people with a suprasacral spinal cord injury (SCI).

Suprasacral lesions to the spinal cord nearly always lead to serious disruption of lower urinary tract function: impairment of voluntary sphincter control and sensation of bladder, fullness, aberrant reflexes of the bladder, and an uncoordinated urinary sphincter[4] (see Chapter 29). As a consequence, bladder emptying is impaired and the result

is reflex incontinence. Reflex incontinence is primarily caused by detrusor hyperreflexia, an aberrant reflex that emerges after a period of spinal shock following SCI (Figure 56.1). It is often associated with dyssynergic contractions of the striated sphincter muscle of the urethra, preventing efficient emptying of the bladder. Persons with SCI frequently develop large residual volumes and urinary tract infections, and are prone to upper urinary tract damage and subsequent renal failure if managed incorrectly.

Medical treatment is usually by a combination of drugs for suppressing detrusor hyperreflexia and intermittent catheterization for emptying the bladder. However, the antimuscarinic drugs used to treat incontinence often have debilitating side-effects, such as constipation, dry mouth, and visual disturbance.

Emptying the bladder can also be very troublesome, especially in women for whom no reliable collection device exists (other than indwelling catheters and bags or ungainly pads), and intermittent catheterization can often introduce bladder infections. Other more radical approaches such as surgery for augmenting the bladder, sphincterotomies, cutting posterior sacral roots to suppress

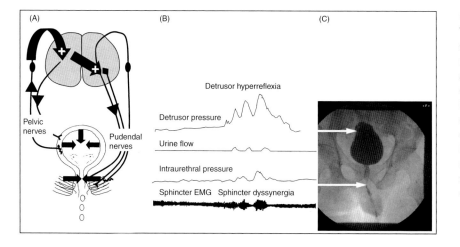

Figure 56.1
The neurogenic bladder in suprasacral spinal cord injury. (A) Aberrant pelvic reflexes causing detrusor hyperreflexia and detrusor-external sphincter dyssynergia. (B) Traces showing the high bladder pressures generated, dyssynergia of the sphincter, associated electromyography (EMG) and urine leakage during videourodynamics. (C) X-ray image shows the bladder and sphincter at the exact time of dyssynergia.

hyperreflexia, or repeated injections of toxins such as Botulinum toxin to paralyse the sphincter and bladder may all have destructive effects which could preclude the use of future developments, including more novel implantable neurostimulating devices.

This chapter briefly reviews some future possibilities for combining existing and emerging science and technologies[5,6] to develop an implantable neuroprosthesis capable of restoring complete control to the bladder and sphincters in SCI. Six areas of development will be addressed:

- sacral anterior root stimulation for emptying the paralysed bladder
- sacral nerve stimulation for suppressing detrusor hyperreflexia
- conditional neuromodulation for automatic control of reflex incontinence
- the sacral posterior and anterior root stimulator implant (SPARSI)
- selective stimulation of sacral roots to prevent detrusor-sphincter dyssynergia
- prospects for complete restoration of bladder control by neuroprosthesis.

Sacral anterior root stimulation for emptying the paralysed bladder

In the 1970s, Brindley and his colleagues developed an implantable device to empty the bladder and control the sphincters[7] (see Chapter 49). The prosthesis uses sacral anterior root stimulation (Finetech–Brindley SARS, Finetech Medical Limited, Welwyn Garden City, UK) to activate bladder motor pathways and produce clinically effective voiding (Figure 56.2). For reflex incontinence and sphincter dyssynergia to be overcome in these patients, the sacral sensory nerve roots from S2 to S4 have to be cut (sacral deafferentation or posterior rhizotomy).

The Finetech–Brindley device has been successfully used in many countries throughout the world.[8] The implant when combined with sacral deafferentation has been shown to be very effective in increasing bladder volume, promoting complete emptying of the bladder, reducing bladder infections, and significantly improving the quality of life for many patients.[9] However, the need for sacral deafferentation (posterior rhizotomy), with the consequent

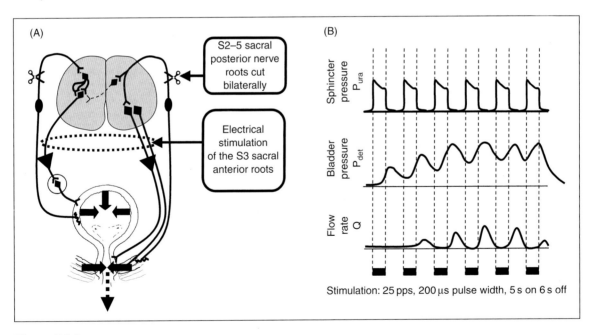

Figure 56.2

Sacral anterior root stimulation (SARS) with sacral deafferention for bladder control. (A) The Finetech–Brindley SARS implantable stimulator uses bilaterally placed intrathecal or extradural electrodes on the S2–S4 sacral roots to activate the preganglionic parasympathetic pathway to produce efficient bladder emptying. A rhizotomy of the corresponding posterior roots (sensory) prevents detrusor hyperreflexia, dyssynergia of the sphincter, and incontinence. (B) Bursts of stimulation activate simultaneously the striated sphincter muscle and detrusor smooth muscle. During the intervals between the bursts the sphincter relaxes rapidly to leave a low urethral resistance whilst the detrusor is still contracting slowly to a higher pressure so as to enable efficient voiding.

loss of reflex erections, reflex ejaculation, bowel problems, and potential pelvic floor weakness can deter many very suitable young male patients from accepting SARS. Furthermore, the hope by some patients of a 'cure' for SCI in the future using neural regeneration and repair techniques is a further obstacle to acceptance. Patients having already suffered accidental damage to their spinal cord are understandably reluctant to then accept deliberate damage. Realistically, a cure for restoring autonomic functions controlling bladder and bowel may take many years to perfect and, meanwhile, management has to try to give the patient the best quality of life. With good medical management of the neurogenic bladder in SCI most patients can now expect a near normal life span and SARS can definitely help many patients, but clearly it would be much more acceptable if it did not involve further destruction of potentially useful reflexes. There may be an alternative solution to sacral deafferentation which involves stimulation of these same afferent pathways rather than cutting them to suppress reflex incontinence.

Sacral root stimulation for suppressing detrusor hyperreflexia

During the 1980s Tanagho and Schmidt developed the use of electrical stimulation of sacral nerves to treat a variety of lower urinary tract problems, including those of the neurogenic bladder[10] (see Chapter 50). Subsequently, a neuroprosthesis was developed (Interstim, Medtronic, Inc., Minneapolis, USA) which comprised an implanted pulse generator attached to a multipole electrode surgically inserted into the S3 sacral foramina for stimulating the

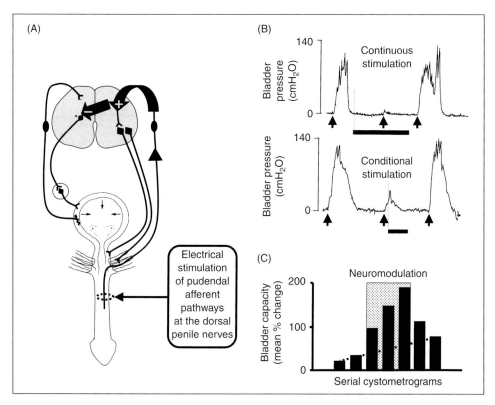

Figure 56.3

Controlling detrusor hyperreflexia by noninvasive neuromodulation through pudendal afferent pathways. (A) By stimulating the dorsal penile (or clitoral) nerves with electrical pulses between 10 and 20 per second and above twice the threshold for the pudendo-anal reflex, it is possible to profoundly suppress detrusor hyperreflexia. (B) The upper trace shows the effect of continuous stimulation of the dorsal penile nerves on the bladder pressure rise associated with a detrusor hyperreflexia contraction provoked at the middle arrow. Control hyperreflexic contractions provoked at the other arrows can be seen before and after stimulation. The lower trace shows the effect of applying neuromodulation conditionally (that is only when detrusor hyperreflexia just appears) in response to provocation at the middle arrow. Again, this response is flanked by control provocations. (C) Repeated cystometrograms with continuous neuromodulation (shaded area), demonstrating significant increases in bladder volume when compared to control fills. Following stimulation the bladder takes some time to restore to its smaller capacity, probably as a result of stretching of the bladder wall during the period of neuromodulation.

mixed sacral nerves.[11] Such stimulation, commonly known as *neuromodulation*, has also been successfully used to increase bladder capacity in patients with an SCI.[12]

Studies using noninvasive multipulse magnetic stimulation over the sacrum to stimulate the mixed extradural sacral roots (S2–4) have demonstrated that the increase in bladder capacity is brought about by suppression of detrusor hyperreflexia in patients with SCI.[13] The mechanism for this 'neuromodulatory' action has yet to be determined in man, but one theory, based on experimental work in animals,[14] suggests that neuromodulation involves inhibitory action by pudendal afferent (sensory) nerve stimulation on pelvic nerve motor pathways to the bladder through spinal cord circuits.[15] Pudendal afferents course through S2–4 posterior (sensory) roots to the spinal cord. Evidence in support of the theory was obtained by electrically stimulating purely pudendal afferent pathways at the level of the dorsal penile[16,17] (or dorsal clitoral) nerves in patients.

Dorsal penile nerve (DPN) stimulation through surface electrodes in patients with SCI produces a profound and repeatable suppression of provoked detrusor hyperreflexia when applied either continuously (pre-emptively) or conditionally (i.e. when bladder pressure just begins to increase)[18,19] (Figure 56.3). Furthermore, in addition to suppressing hyperreflexia, DPN stimulation can produce significant increases in bladder volume, as demonstrated in serial cystometrograms.[20] These effects depend essentially on stimulation, and diminish when stimulation is switched off. Interestingly, intermittent stimulation also appears to produce good results, although the ideal interval between bursts has yet to be determined, balancing the need to suppress every hyperreflexic contraction reliably against preserving the battery life of the stimulator.[21]

In a recent pilot study the same benefit has been shown using a Finetech–Brindley implantable device to stimulate extradural or intradural sacral roots but without

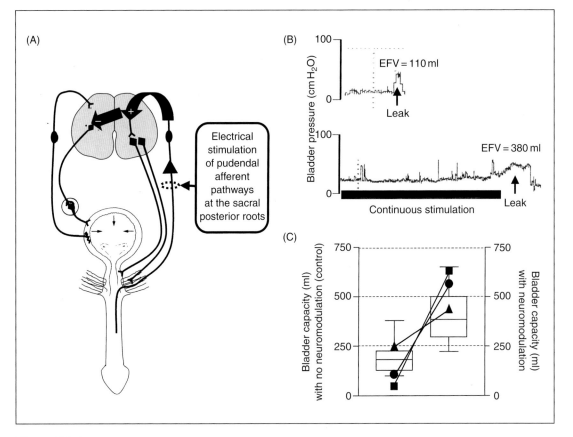

Figure 56.4

Controlling detrusor hyperreflexia and increasing bladder capacity by sacral posterior root stimulation. (A) A Finetech–Brindley implanted stimulator (without deafferentation) is used to apply neuromodulation bilaterally through the S3–S4 sacral roots. (B) Continuous stimulation at about 15 pulses per second (240 μs pulse width) with a current level set to suppress detrusor hyperreflexia significantly increased bladder capacity over control tests (EFV = end-fill volume). (C) The graph shows box and whisker results from a group of 11 patients with SCI tested using continuous neuromodulation through the dorsal penile nerves (DPN) compared with the effect of applying neuromodulation through the posterior roots in 3 patients (solid lines with symbols) from this same group. It can be seen that bladder capacity is markedly increased with stimulation of the roots and compares favorably with the significant group result using DPN stimulation. DPN stimulation may be a good predictor for success with a sacral nerve stimulator.

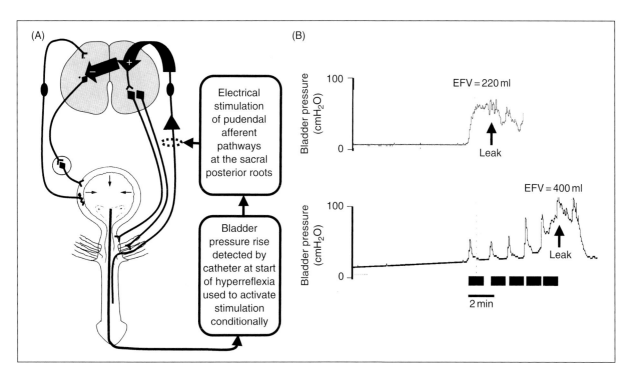

Figure 56.5
Using bladder pressure to automatically control detrusor hyperreflexia with conditional neuromodulation. (A) By measuring bladder pressure with a catheter it is possible to detect exactly when a detrusor hyperreflexic contraction begins and this can be used to activate stimulation of the sacral posterior roots to suppress the contraction automatically. The cystometrograms in this figure were obtained from a patient with an incomplete upper thoracic spinal lesion, but similar results have also been shown in patients with complete lesions. (B) The upper trace shows a cystometrogram without stimulation and a relatively low bladder capacity. The lower trace shows that when a pressure rise is detected, the applied stimulation immediately reduces the pressure, and by automatically repeating this suppression on successive detrusor hyperreflexic contractions a much larger bladder capacity can be achieved. A point is reached at this new maximum capacity when suppression is no longer possible. EFV = end-fill volume.

deafferentation.[22] In a small group of patients with a suprasacral spinal injury, electrodes were placed bilaterally on either the mixed extradural sacral (S2–4) roots or separated anterior and posterior sacral roots (S3) intrathecally. Each patient was assessed preoperatively with DPN stimulation, as described above, to demonstrate the efficacy of neuromodulation. Preliminary results indicated that patients were able to achieve both good suppression of detrusor hyperreflexia and clinically useful increases in bladder volume (Figure 56.4).

Conditional neuromodulation for automatic control of reflex incontinence

In the implant studies described above it was also demonstrated that conditional stimulation, applied only at the onset of hyperreflexic contractions, was at least as good as continuous stimulation at increasing bladder capacity and was sometimes better. Bladder contractions were sensed by measuring intravesical pressure with a standard catheter

and the pudendal afferents stimulated either at the level of the penile dorsal nerve or sacral roots to inhibit bladder contractions (Figure 56.5).[20,22]

A conditional system that detects the onset of unstable bladder contractions and then suppresses them has a number of theoretical advantages. Although continuous neuromodulation is an effective and simple way to increase bladder capacity in spinally injured patients, in many situations it is not ideal. The need for constant current delivery would shorten both battery and electrode life in a completely implanted device, and continuous stimulation of the sacral afferents may have undesirable long-term reflex effects on the anal and urethral sphincters, perhaps exacerbating any residual dyssynergia.

Hence, a device that could stimulate the sacral nerves for neuromodulation only when necessary might have considerable benefits and would have the added advantage that it could provide feedback about bladder fullness to the patient. That is, stimulating pulses associated with the conditional neuromodulation could also be applied to sensate parts of the body to warn of detrusor hyperreflexia at bladder capacity.

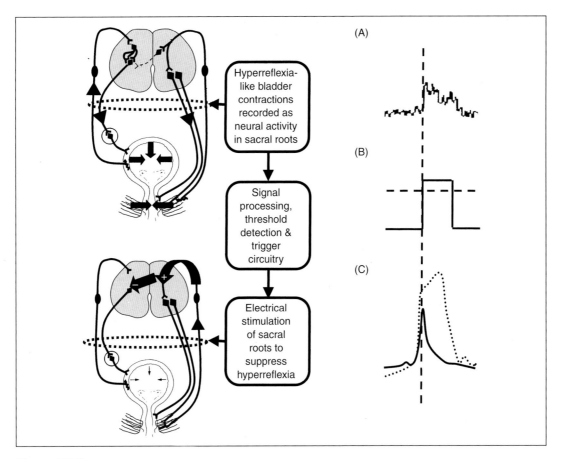

Figure 56.6
Sacral nerve activity as feedback control for conditional neuromodulation. (A) A miniature electrical signal (<0.5 μV) from the sacral nerves associated with a hyperreflexia-like contraction in an experimental animal. (B) Using special signal processing techniques it is possible to detect the changes and then activate stimulation of the sacral posterior roots for conditional neuromodulation. (C) The hyperreflexia-like contraction (dotted line) without neuromodulation is very effectively suppressed (solid line) when stimulation is applied.

What sort of reliable detection system for conditional neuromodulation could be incorporated into an implant? Brindley was the first to suggest that it might be possible to monitor bladder pressure by implant and use the information to control electrical stimulation of the pudendal nerves to inhibit unstable bladder contractions. Subsequently, an implanted applanation tonometer was developed which could be sutured onto the bladder wall to record pressure. However, tests to assess its long-term performance in experimental animals were not very successful, as the device eroded or became dislodged from the bladder.[23] Further obstacles, such as infection and encrustation, preclude the immediate development and implementation of such vesical devices.

Recently it has been shown in experimental animals that it is possible to detect very small electroneurographic signals at fractional microvolt levels, using sophisticated recording techniques, from the afferents in the mixed sacral nerve roots during hyperreflexia-like bladder contractions.[24] The recorded signals could then be used to trigger stimulation of the pudendal or sacral posterior nerves to inhibit conditionally in a feedback loop those same contractions (Figure 56.6).

Some preliminary work in patients with SCI during implantation of sacral anterior root stimulators indicates that detecting bladder contractions from the sacral sensory nerves may also be possible.[25,26] However, although an implanted conditional neuromodulation device may be feasible in people with a spinal cord injury it is likely to be considerably more complex than present devices tried in animals and will have to be very reliable. Implantable microcircuits for detecting minute neural signals in humans which could be used to activate conditional neuromodulation are now being developed for this purpose.[27]

Whether detrusor hyperreflexia is to be controlled by automatic conditional stimulation or simply by continuous neuromodulation the interesting possibility now exists for combining the benefits of bladder emptying with control of reflex incontinence in one implantable sacral root stimulator.

The sacral posterior and anterior root stimulator implant

This new concept is being developed using a single implant (Finetech–Brindley) to combine bladder emptying through sacral anterior root stimulation with posterior sacral root stimulation to prevent reflex incontinence.[28] If successful, the major advantage of SPARSI would be restoration of bladder function without the need for sacral deafferentation.

In a recent study, five patients with a suprasacral spinal injury have been implanted with a standard bilateral extradural Finetech–Brindley device, but without sacral deafferentation, to test the concept of SPARSI. These patients were part of the neuromodulation study described above.[22] A significant finding in this study, reported first in 2001,[29] demonstrated that the benefits of neuromodulation by a SPARSI implant at home were comparable to the effects of oxybutynin in improving functional bladder capacity in the same patient (Figure 56.7). Furthermore, the improvement also compared favorably with the benefits of sacral deafferentation. Another interesting finding, which agrees with other studies of sacral neuromodulation for the overactive bladder (e.g. using the Medtronic sacral nerve stimulator), showed that the effects do not necessarily diminish appreciably with time, but that when stimulation is stopped symptoms such as incontinence return. With SPARSI, bladder capacity always returned to much smaller values in less than 24 h when stimulation was stopped.

Unfortunately in this small group of patients bladder emptying was not always very efficient despite the generation of adequate bladder pressures. The concept of SPARSI using extradural electrodes will only be successful when good bladder emptying (as in the original SARS with posterior rhizotomy) is also achieved. SARS uses post-stimulus voiding to empty the bladder efficiently so that during the intervals between bursts of stimulation, urethral pressure is much lower than bladder pressure, allowing unimpeded urine flow. In SPARSI, where both striated sphincter and bladder reflex pathways are intact, there can be residual increases in urethral pressure as the slow bladder pressure develops in the post-stimulation gap (Figure 56.8). This is reflex detrusor-sphincter dyssynergia, and leads to urinary outflow obstruction, making emptying much less reliable (compare with Figure 56.2).

As Brindley suggested,[9] bladder emptying is improved by posterior rhizotomy, and so implantation of a Finetech–Brindley device for bladder emptying without a rhizotomy in patients with severe detrusor-external sphincter dyssynergia would not currently be advised. Interestingly, Brindley's early patients often did not have a rhizotomy, and most achieved good emptying, but the devices were intrathecal and there was almost certainly posterior root damage in many cases.[30]

The SPARSI concept could achieve its original objective once the problems of bladder emptying are overcome. A number of possible solutions to control detrusor-external sphincter dyssynergia are available – including pharmacotherapy (e.g. Botulinum toxin), stenting, and surgery (sphincterotomy) – but ideally we should find a neurophysiological solution which could be applied through the same stimulating implant.

Selective stimulation of sacral roots to prevent detrusor-sphincter dyssynergia

Sacral anterior roots contain, among other pathways, both the large somatic nerves to the urethral striated sphincter and the small preganglionic parasympathetic nerves to the bladder detrusor smooth muscle. Consequently, during anterior root stimulation, bladder emptying is impaired by coactivation of these two groups of nerve fibers (see Figure 56.2). This is the reason for adopting the post-stimulus voiding technique,[31] which takes advantage of the rapid relaxation of the sphincter and slow contraction of the detrusor to achieve good bladder emptying. This type of voiding is not particularly physiological, but it is efficient. However, in the presence of intact sacral reflexes (i.e. no rhizotomy), the dyssynergia persists in the gap between the bursts of stimulation to prevent efficient emptying, as described above. For this problem to be overcome, tests are now being done using a variety of techniques, including sphincter fatiguing methods and selective nerve blocking ('anode block') of sphincter motor pathways.

The principle of selective electrical stimulation relies on blocking the large nerve fibers to the striated muscles by anodal hyperpolarization to prevent the passage of action potentials down the nerve, while permitting the flow of action potentials along the small motor nerves to the bladder muscle (Figure 56.9). To prevent 'anode-break' excitation when the individual stimulating pulses in the train switch off, they must be switched off slowly.

This method of stimulation was originally shown by Brindley and Craggs to be effective in experimental animals using a specially designed chronically implanted tripolar electrode and triangular-shaped electrical pulses to stimulate the sacral anterior roots selectively.[32] The range of stimulating currents where sphincter motor potentials were blocked while bladder pressure increased was relatively small but effective. However, Brindley and Craggs did not demonstrate bladder emptying in their experiments.

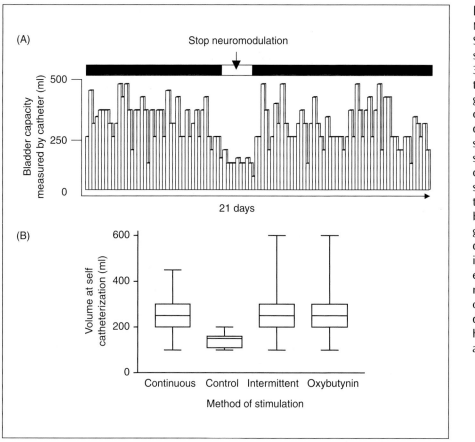

Figure 56.7
Neuromodulation through SPARSI at home. (A) A continuous set of data showing that over a 3-week period neuromodulation through the implant maintained good bladder capacity when compared to a short period during which stimulation was stopped. (B) Continuous stimulation was shown to be comparable to intermittent stimulation given on a 50 s 'on' to 50 s 'off' cycle and both gave bladder volumes statistically greater than no stimulation during a control period. An interesting finding was the near equivalence of benefit with neuromodulation alone or oxybutynin (an anticholinergic drug to block detrusor hyperreflexic contractions) alone.

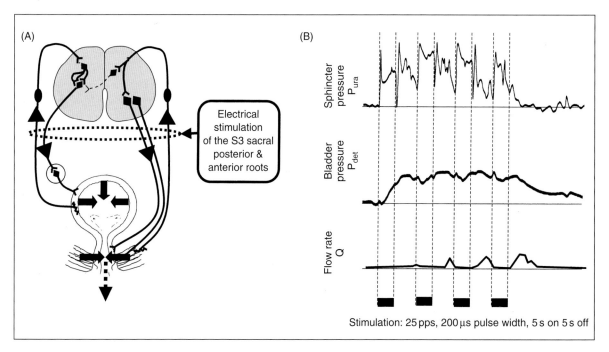

Figure 56.8
Bladder contraction through SPARSI. (A) Stimulation of the mixed sacral roots through extradural electrodes or separated roots through intrathecal electrodes activates both efferent (motor) and afferent (sensory) pathways either directly or reflexly. (B) Good bladder pressures are generated by bursts of stimulation, but voiding is very inefficient in the gaps as a result of reflex contractions of the sphincter, elevating urethral pressure above the bladder pressure (compare with the traces shown in Figure 56.2).

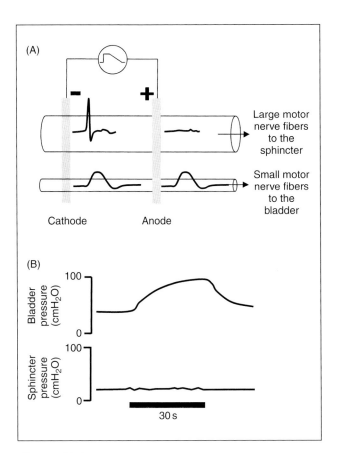

Figure 56.9

Selective blockade of the motor nerves to the sphincter.
(A) Applying triangular or quasitrapezoidal electrical pulses to groups of different diameter nerve fibers in the sacral roots it is possible to find a range of stimulating currents that block the large motor nerves to the striated sphincter at the anode electrode (anode block), while still permitting conduction down the small motor nerves to the bladder detrusor muscle.
(B) Selective anode blockade of the sphincter successfully applied while a good bladder contraction is elicited during stimulation with a train of triangular pulses at 30 pulses per second.

Interestingly, a similar type of tripolar electrode is used in the standard intrathecal Finetech–Brindley SARS implant, so theoretically it should be possible to investigate the possibility of using this technique for actual bladder emptying in patients. However, to prevent reflex effects on all of the motor fibers to the sphincter it may be necessary to apply anode blockade to all of the sacral anterior roots simultaneously.

It has been shown that during implantation of a Finetech–Brindley SARS it is possible to demonstrate intraoperatively that an anode-blocking technique with long rectangular pulses can be used to get selective stimulation in anesthetised patients,[33] but again efficient bladder emptying was not demonstrated. Recently, it has been claimed that physiological micturition (i.e. natural voiding

where the sphincter relaxes during contraction of the bladder to produce a good stream of urine and complete bladder emptying) is possible using a modified Finetech–Brindley intrathecal electrode to activate the bladder in the dog.[34] Unfortunately, this study did not present data to substantiate the claim but did demonstrate a significant lowering of sphincter pressure simultaneous with good bladder pressures during sacral stimulation with quasitrapezoidal pulses.[35]

So, it remains to be seen whether such selective stimulation techniques can produce efficient voiding; the evidence from animal studies is promising[36] but awaits a successful resolution in patients in whom we may wish to preserve all sacral reflexes. When resolved, the concept of SPARSI described above is more likely to become a realistic possibility.

Prospects for complete restoration of bladder control by neuroprosthesis

In this chapter we have considered some old, new, and emerging developments and technologies using sacral root stimulation which together may in the future provide full restoration of bladder control to the neurogenic bladder (Figure 56.10).

In recent times our understanding of the neurophysiology of the lower urinary tract has advanced in ways that may lead to even more sophisticated ways of controlling the neurogenic bladder, bowel, and sexual dysfunction. Of these emerging techniques currently being developed in experimental animal models is the exciting possibility of actually stimulating and recording from the nuclei of origin of the sacral motor pathways in the spinal cord. Intraspinal microstimulation, as it has become known, involves inserting fine wire electrodes into the tracts in these structures.[37–40] Interestingly, as with sacral root stimulation, the problem of controlling the dyssynergia of the urethral sphincter presents as the most difficult problem to be overcome in these experimental studies. Neurophysiological studies have shown that spinal interneurons are very much involved in the segmental coordination of the bladder and sphincters and therefore it may become possible to activate these interneuronal pathways by stimulation to get the synergic control necessary to empty the bladder efficiently.[41] It seems that considerable technical advances will be needed to apply microstimulation, not least the problem of keeping fine microelectrodes in close contact with the appropriate neural substrates while at the same time preventing tethering of the spinal cord, which in itself could cause significant damage.

Whichever future development provides the best and safest solution for controlled neurostimulation it still

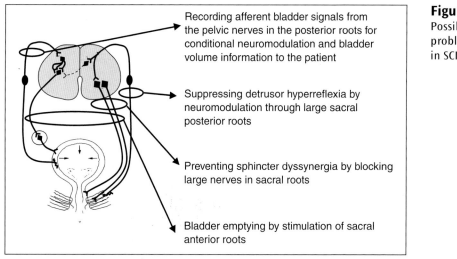

Recording afferent bladder signals from the pelvic nerves in the posterior roots for conditional neuromodulation and bladder volume information to the patient

Suppressing detrusor hyperreflexia by neuromodulation through large sacral posterior roots

Preventing sphincter dyssynergia by blocking large nerves in sacral roots

Bladder emptying by stimulation of sacral anterior roots

Figure 56.10
Possible techniques to overcome problems of the neurogenic bladder in SCI.

remains that for a significant number of patients, with lower motor neuron problems, such as corda equina lesions, the possibilities for restoration of pelvic functions is problematic. For this important group of patients, coordination of the bladder and sphincter is less important than impaired contraction, but problems of incontinence and the inability to void remain impediments to good management and quality of life. Perhaps the new surgical techniques for neural repair and regeneration of the motor pathways may offer some prospect for helping these patients.[42] There may even be a place to assist or combine this neuronal repair with neurostimulation.[43] Although recovery of central afferent pathways is less likely in these repairs, any sacral reflexes that are restored may be more aberrant than in suprasacral injuries and therefore present with new and more difficult challenges to be overcome.

Finally, some of the ideas presented here might be limited by current technology but this is very likely to become realizable in the near future. Such technological advances might include more appropriately designed and stable electrode–nerve interfaces (especially important if the electrodes are to be implanted inside the spinal cord or brain), new implantable integrated electronics capable of processing tiny signals and delivering patterned stimuli, and improved systems for transferring or using power efficiently in implants. A new range of intelligent sensor technology for detecting physiological changes in the body is likely to emerge. The future may also see the increased use of telemetries for computerized control of implants, including the transfer of data to and from these devices to improve function.

Summary

Ultimately, it is hoped that by combining conditional neuromodulation for reflex incontinence with selective neurostimulation for bladder emptying we can completely control the neurogenic bladder without cutting any sacral sensory nerves. The big challenge will probably be to overcome the detrusor-sphincter dyssynergia resulting from the emergence of aberrant reflexes following spinal injury. By preserving all pelvic reflexes, including those for erection, ejaculation, and bowel control, as well as those essential to guard against stress incontinence, we will help to reassure people with a spinal cord injury that this technology will improve their quality of life until the time comes when neural repair becomes a realistic possibility for them.

References

1. Brindley GS, Polkey CE, Rushton DN. Sacral anterior root stimulators for bladder control in paraplegia. Paraplegia 1982; 20:365–381.

2. Schmidt RA. Treatment of the unstable bladder. Urology 1991; 37:28–32.

3. Tanagho EA. Concepts of neuromodulation. Neurourol Urodyn 1993; 12:487–488.

4. Selzman AA, Hampel N. Urologic complications of spinal cord injury. Urol Clin N Am 1993; 20:453–464.

5. Grill WM, Craggs MD, Foreman RD, et al. Emerging clinical applications of electrical stimulation: opportunities for restoration of function. J Rehab Res Dev 2001; 38:641–653.

6. Jezernik S, Craggs M, Grill WM, et al. Electrical stimulation for the treatment of bladder dysfunction: current status and future possibilities. Neurol Res 2002; 24:413–430.

7. Brindley GS. An implant to empty the bladder or close the urethra. J Neurol Neurosurg Psychiatry 1977; 43:1083–1090.

8. van Kerrebroeck PEV. Worldwide experience with the Finetech–Brindley Sacral Anterior Root Stimulator. Neurourol Urodyn 1993; 12:497–503.

9. Brindley GS. The first 500 patients with sacral anterior root stimulator implants: general description. Paraplegia 1994; 32:795–805.

10. Tanagho EA, Schmidt RA. Electrical stimulation in the clinical management of the neurogenic bladder. J Urol 1988; 140:1331–1339.

11. Schmidt RA, Jonas U, Oleson KA, et al. for the Sacral Nerve Stimulation Study Group. Sacral nerve stimulation for the treatment of refractory urinary urge incontinence. J Urol 1999; 162:352–357.

12. Chartier-Kastler EJ, Bosch RJL, Perrigot M, et al. Long-term results of sacral nerve stimulation (S3) for the treatment of neurogenic refractory urge incontinence related to detrusor hyperreflexia. J Urol 2000; 164:1476–1480.

13. Sheriff MKM, Shah PJR, Fowler C, et al. Neuromodulation of detrusor hyperreflexia by functional magnetic stimulation of the sacral roots. Br J Urol 1996; 78:39–46.

14. Lindström S, Fall M, Carlsson CA, Erlandson BE. The neurophysiological basis of bladder inhibition in response to intravaginal electrical stimulation. J Urol 1983; 129:405–410.

15. Craggs MD, McFarlane JP. Neuromodulation of the lower urinary tract. Exp Physiol 1999; 84:149–160.

16. Nakamura M, Sakurai T. Bladder inhibition by penile electrical stimulation. Br J Urol 1984; 56:413–415.

17. Wheeler JS, Walter JS, Zaszczurynski PJ. Bladder inhibition by penile nerve stimulation in spinal cord injury patients. J Urol 1992; 147:100–103.

18. Shah N, Edhem I, Knight SL, Craggs MD. Acute suppression of provoked detrusor hyperreflexia with detrusor sphincter dyssynergia by electrical stimulation of the dorsal penile nerves in patients with a spinal injury. Eur Urol 1998; 33(suppl): 60.

19. Kirkham A, Knight S, Casey A, et al. Conditional neuromodulation of end-fill hyperreflexia to increase bladder capacity in spinally injured patients. Neurourol Urodyn 2000; 19:515–516.

20. Kirkham APS, Shah NC, Knight SL, et al. The acute effects of continuous and conditional neuromodulation on the bladder in spinal cord injury. Spinal Cord 2001; 39:420–428.

21. Zafirakis H, Knight SL, Shah PJR, et al. Intermittent versus continuous electrical stimulation of the dorsal penile nerve on bladder capacity in spinal cord injury. Neurourol Urodyn 2002; 21:400.

22. Kirkham APS, Knight SL, Casey ATM, et al. Neuromodulation of sacral nerve roots 2 to 4 with a Fintech–Brindley sacral posterior and anterior root stimulator. Spinal Cord 2002; 40:272–281.

23. Koldewijn EL, van Kerrebroeck PE, Schaafsma E, et al. Bladder pressure sensors in an animal model. J Urol 1994; 151:1376–1384.

24. Jezernik S, Grill WM, Sinkjaer T. Detection and inhibition of hyperreflexia-like bladder contractions in the cat by sacral nerve root recording and electrical stimulation. Neurourol Urodyn 2001; 20:215–230.

25. Sinkjaer T, Rijkhoff N, Haugland M, et al. Electroneurographic (ENG) signals from intradural S3 dorsal sacral nerve roots in a patient with a suprasacral spinal cord injury. Proc 5th Int Functional Electrical Stimulation Soc Conf, Aalborg, Denmark, 2000:361–364.

26. Grill WM, Creasey GH, Wu K, Takaoka Y. Detection of hyperreflexia-like increases in bladder pressure by recording of sensory nerve activity in human spinal cord injury. Abstract in Proc 5th Int Functional Electrical Stimulation Soc Conf, Aalborg, Denmark, 2000:234.

27. Donaldson N de N, Zhou L, Haugland M, Sinkjaer T. An implantable telemeter for long-term electroneurographic recordings in animals and humans. Proc 5th Int Functional Electrical Stimulation Soc Conf, Aalborg, Denmark, 2000:378–381.

28. Craggs MD, Casey A, Shah PJR, et al. SPARSI: an implant to empty the bladder and control incontinence with posterior rhizotomy in spinal cord injury. Br J Urol Int 2000; 85(suppl 5): 2.

29. Kirkham APS, Knight SL, Casey ATM, et al. Acute and chronic use of a sacral posterior and anterior nerve root stimulator to increase bladder capacity in spinal cord injury. Proc 6th Int Functional Electrical Stimulation Soc Conf, Cleveland, Ohio, USA, 2001:172–174.

30. Brindley GS, Polkey CE, Rushton DN, Cardozo L. Sacral anterior root stimulators for bladder control in paraplegia: the first 50 cases. J Neurol Neurosurg Psychiatry 1986; 49:1104–1114.

31. Jonas U, Tanagho EA. Studies on the feasibility of urinary bladder evacuation by direct spinal cord stimulation. II. Poststimulus voiding: a way to overcome outflow resistance. Invest Urol 1975; 13:151–153.

32. Brindley GS, Craggs MD. A technique of anodally blocking large nerve fibres through chronically implanted electrodes. J Neurol Neurosurg Psychiatry 1980; 43:1083–1090.

33. Rijkhoff NJM, Wijkstra H, van Kerrebroeck PEV, Debruyne FMJ. Selective detrusor activation by electrical sacral nerve root stimulation in spinal cord injury. J Urol 1997; 157:1504–1508.

34. Seif Ch, Braun PM, Bross J, et al. Selective block of urethral sphincter contraction using a modified Brindley electrode in sacral anterior root stimulation of the dog. Neurourol Urodyn 2002; 21:502–510.

35. Fang ZP, Mortimer JT. Selective activation of small motor axons by quasitrapezoidal current pulses. IEEE Trans Biomed Engng 1991; 38:168–174.

36. Grünewald V, Bhadra N, Creasey GH, Mortimer JT. Functional conditions of micturition induced by selective sacral anterior root stimulation. World J Urol 1998; 16:329–336.

37. Carter RR, McCreery DB, Woodford BJ, et al. Micturition control by microstimulation of the sacral spinal cord of the cat: acute studies. IEEE Trans Rehab Engng 1995; 3:206–214.

38. Grill WM, Bhadra N, Wang B. Bladder and urethral pressures evoked by microstimulation of the sacral spinal cord in cats. Brain Res 1999; 836:19–30.

39. Tai C, Booth AM, de Groat WC, Roppolo JR. Colon and anal sphincter contractions evoked by microstimulation of the sacral spinal cord in cats. Brain Res 2001; 889:38–48.

40. Tai C, Booth AM, de Groat WC, Roppolo JR. Penile erection produced by microstimulation of the sacral spinal cord of the cat. IEEE Trans Rehab Engng 1998; 6:374–381.

41. Grill WM. Electrical activation of spinal neural circuits: application to motor system neural prostheses. Neuromodulation 2000; 3:97–106.

42. Carlstedt T. Approaches permitting and enhancing motoneuron regeneration after spinal cord, ventral root, plexus and peripheral nerve injuries. Curr Opin Neurol 2000; 13:683–686.

43. Grill WM, McDonald JW, Peckham PH, et al. At the interface: convergence of neural regeneration and neural prostheses for restoration of function. J Rehab Res Dev 2001; 38:633–639.

57

Neuroprotection and repair after spinal cord injury

W Dalton Dietrich

Introduction

Injury to the spinal cord initiates a cascade of events that ultimately leads to cell death and neurological dysfunction. Various biochemical and molecular pathways are activated after spinal cord injury (SCI) in both the acute and subacute injury setting that may be targeted for therapeutic intervention. Clarification of what dominant injury mechanisms may be attenuated by pharmacological and hypothermic therapies is an active area of investigation. Also, there is much excitement in the area of transplantation and repair therapy in chronic SCI. New strategies are being used to alter the local environment to make it more permissive for axonal regeneration. The replacement of lost cell populations by using transplantation strategies as well as the delivery of genes or proteins to enhance axonal regeneration is another exciting research direction. In this chapter, we review various neuroprotective strategies as well as several transplantation strategies directed toward a cure of paralysis following SCI.

Neuroprotection following spinal cord injury

In acutely injured SCI patients, especially those having incomplete lesions, neuroprotective strategies have the potential of limiting secondary injury mechanisms. Although methylprednisolone (MP) treatment has been reported to benefit a subpopulation of SCI patients,[1] recent publications have questioned the benefits of MP as the standard therapy for acute SCI.[3–5] Thus, new therapies need to be developed and tested. Glutamate, the major endogenous excitatory neurotransmitter in the central nervous system (CNS), has been shown to mediate pathological processes in many injury models, including SCI. With the use of intracerebral microdialysis, sampling of the extracellular space has shown massive release of glutamate as well as other neurotransmitters during and following SCI.[5]

In recent studies, Wrathall and colleagues[6] have reported that treatment with NBQX, a highly selective antagonist of the non-N-methyl-D-aspartate excitatory amino acid receptor, reduces histopathological and functional deficits following traumatic SCI. Likewise, convincing support for the importance of free radicals and lipid peroxidation in SCI models has been derived from studies reporting that oxygen radical scavengers or the use of inhibitors of lipid peroxidation can limit neuronal damage and improve outcome.[7,8] In a model of traumatic brain injury (TBI), the novel inhibitor of lipid peroxidation, LY341122, was reported to improve histopathological outcome only when the agent was given in the early post-injury period.[9] Thus, when evaluating the potential use of agents that block excitotoxic or free radical-mediated damage, questions regarding the therapeutic window for these strategies must be addressed. Obviously, if the window of opportunity has passed prior to the patient's arrival in the emergency room, these pathomechanisms may not be appropriate targets for therapeutic strategies.

A fundamental question regarding pathophysiology of SCI is the nature of cell death: is it necrosis or apoptosis?[10] Necrosis is characterized by the early compromise of cell membrane integrity, leading to a loss of ionic homeostasis and prominent cell swelling. Apoptosis reflects the activation of intrinsic genetic programs, leading to the endonuclease cleavage of DNA and eventual death of the cell.[11] While the death of neurons induced by ischemia or trauma has been classically considered to be necrosis, growing evidence is suggestive that some cells undergo apoptosis following SCI.[11,12] Indeed, recent experimental and clinical data have suggested that the death of oligodendrocytes following traumatic SCI involves activation of apoptotic pathways.[12,13] This research direction is particularly important because the potential for developing antiapoptotic strategies to target late occurring cell death after SCI is a real possibility.[14–16] For example, the antiapoptotic gene *Bcl-2* has been reported to inhibit neuronal death induced by glutamate. The potential use of gene therapy to introduce protective genes into the host to enhance cellular neuroprotective mechanisms or antagonize cytotoxic products associated with apoptosis is an exciting research direction.

An emerging strategy for the treatment of CNS injury is directed toward inflammatory events.[17] Experimental studies have indicated roles of several inflammatory molecules in the pathophysiology, including tumor necrosis factor α (TNFα) and interleukin-β (IL-β), as well as various chemokines.[18,19] In this regard, recent experimental data have demonstrated that the administration of the potent anti-inflammatory cytokine IL-10 improves both histopathological and locomotive function following traumatic SCI in rats.[18] In that study, IL-10 treatment significantly decreased overall contusion volume, preserved the white matter tracts, and improved behavioral recovery as assessed by the Basso, Bresnahan, and Beattie (BBB) open-field test. In terms of therapeutic windows for anti-inflammatory strategies, current investigations are determining how long after SCI IL-10 can be given to promote improved outcome. Interestingly, IL-10 in combination with MP has been reported to reduce tissue injury after SCI.[20] Thus, combination therapy may also be advantageous in specific clinical conditions.

Mild-to-moderate hypothermia has been shown to be neuroprotective in many experimental models of CNS injury.[21,22] Local as well as systemic hypothermia has been used by various laboratories to prevent energy failure, reduce histopathological damage, diminish free radical activity, and elevated levels of glutamate following injury. Recent studies have evaluated the relationship between systemic and epidural temperature after SCI and the effects of moderate systemic hypothermia following traumatic SCI in rats. In one study, post-traumatic hypothermia (32–33°C) initiated 30 min after injury for a 4-hour period significantly protected against locomotive deficits and reduced the area of tissue damage.[23] Experimental findings also indicate that post-traumatic hypothermia following SCI reduces polymorphonuclear leukocyte (PMNL) accumulation.[24] In a recent study, post-traumatic hypothermia significantly reduced myeloperoxidase (MPO) activity (an enzyme for neutrophil infusion) compared with normothermic animals. Thus, a potential mechanism by which hypothermia improves outcome following SCI is by attenuating post-traumatic inflammation. Whether mild systemic or local hypothermia can be used clinically to inhibit the detrimental effects of post-injury hyperthermia and/or protect the spinal cord from secondary injury merits further investigation.

Nitric oxide (NO) has been shown to play an important role in the pathophysiology of SCI.[25,26] Importantly, NO has been reported to be both neurodestructive and neuroprotective, depending on the location and time of release.[27]

In a recent study, the effects of inhibiting inducible NO synthase (iNOS) by aminoguanidine treatment were investigated.[26] Treated rats demonstrated improved hind limb function and decreased histopathological injury compared with nontreated traumatized rats. Immunostaining for iNOS indicated that a significant cellular source of iNOS protein appeared to be invading PMNLs. Thus, in the acute injury state, therapeutic interventions including hypothermia and aminoguanidine may be protective by attenuating the release of NO-induced cytotoxic products from PMNLs. Additional research in the area of neuroprotection is required to clarify what injury mechanisms may be targeted for therapeutic intervention.

Cellular transplantation following spinal cord injury

There is an unprecedented sense of enthusiasm within the scientific community that one day therapeutic strategies will be developed to treat paralysis following SCI. The replacement of lost cell populations by cell transplantation strategies as well as utilizing helper cells to deliver genes or proteins to enhance axonal regeneration is currently being investigated in many laboratories throughout the world.[28] Indeed, several types of intraspinal transplants have effectively treated experimental models of human diseases. The peripheral nervous system provides an appropriate environment for axonal regeneration. David and Aguayo[29] first demonstrated that segments of sciatic nerve could be used as bridges between the medulla and lower cervical or thoracic spinal cord. In that study, evidence was presented that axons from nerve cells in the injured spinal cord and brainstem could elongate for long distances when the glial environment of the CNS was replaced by peripheral nerve. Axonal elongation is thought to be due to the presence of Schwann cells (SCs) that produce neurotrophic factors and synthesize and secrete elements of extracellular matrix, including laminin and cell adhesion molecules. Indeed, the use of guidance channels lined with SCs has been successfully utilized to support axonal regeneration following transection of the adult spinal cord.[30]

Most recently, the axonal growth-promoting properties of adult olfactory ensheathing glia (OEG) and SC-filled guidance channels have been utilized to bridge spinal cord stumps and to enhance regeneration into the host spinal cord.[31] Supraspinal serotinergic axons were reported to cross the transection gap through the bridges and elongate in white and periaqueductal gray. Long-distance regeneration (at least 2.5 cm) of injured ascending propriospinal axons was also observed in the rostral spinal cord. In another study, spinal implantation of OEG was performed in adult rats after rhizotomy to promote axonal regeneration and bladder function.[32] Immediately after rhizotomy,

OEG cells were injected into the vicinity of the sacral parasympathetic nucleus and several roots reattached to the cord with fibrin glue. Importantly, both anatomical regeneration of bladder wall primary afferents as well as recovered bladder function were observed. Taken together, this study and others indicate that EG appear to provide injured spinal axons with factors for long-distance regeneration. Successful regeneration may, therefore, be attained eventually by using a combination of 'helper cell' transplantation strategies following adult CNS injury.

The infusion of various neurotrophins to enhance axonal regeneration following SCI has also been utilized in various experimental models. Grill et al[33] determined the effects of transgenic cellular delivery of neurotrophin-3 (NT-3) on the morphological and functional disturbances following SCI in rats. In that study, experimental subjects received grafts of fibroblasts genetically modified to produce NT-3. Importantly, the local cellular delivery of NT-3 in this model of SCI led to regrowth of corticospinal tracts and improved functional recovery at 1 and 3 months postinjury. In a study of SCs, Tuszynski et al[34] reported robust growth of host neurotrophin-responsive axons after grafting with genetically modified SC, producing high levels of human nerve growth factor (NGF). Thus, the use of genetically engineered cells to locally deliver various neurotrophins represents an important approach to enhancing axonal regeneration.

Neuronal progenitors isolated from the adult CNS may one day be used to replace populations of neurons and oligodendrocytes destroyed following injury. Recently, the consequences of transplanting embryonic stem cells into the injured rat spinal cord on recovery of function has been assessed. McDonald et al[35] transplanted neuro-differentiated mouse embryonic stem cells into the injured spinal cord to determine the fate of these cells as well as to determine whether the transplant procedure led to behavioral recovery. Histological analysis demonstrated that the transplanted cells survived and differentiated into astrocytes, oligodendrocytes, and neurons. Importantly, gait analysis showed improved hind limb function, weight support, and coordination in rats transplanted with stem cells, compared with controls. Ongoing research continues to investigate novel sources of stem cells that one day may be isolated from SCI subjects prior to transplantation procedures.

Although inflammatory processes have been implicated in the pathophysiology of neuronal cell injury following SCI,[18] recent data indicate that activated macrophages may also enhance functional recovery.[36,37] Rapalino et al[37] have reported that bloodborne macrophages stimulated with segments of rat peripheral sciatic nerve and transplanted into the lesion site lead to improved electrophysiological, morphological, and behavioral outcome after SC transection, compared with non-treated animals. Based on these findings, it appears that therapeutic strategies to attenuate inflammatory responses after SCI may have to target early but not later occurring inflammatory processes. Indeed, the inflammatory cascade appears to be extremely complicated, and more experimental work is required to assess what specific inflammatory processes need to be attenuated or promoted after SCI.

Future directions

In terms of both acute neuroprotection and cellular transplantation strategies for the treatment of spinal cord dysfunction, great progress has been made in the last several years. In the area of neuroprotection, future investigations will target combination therapy where multiple strategies may be used to promote more complete protection and recovery of function following SCI. One exciting direction involves the use of mild hypothermia plus pharmacotherapy. Indeed, recent studies in cerebral ischemia found that mild hypothermia plus IL-10 protected the brain better than either therapy alone.[22] Also, following SCI, a synergistic effect of basic fibroblast growth factor (bFGF) and MP on neurological function was reported.[38] In addition, better therapies must be developed to target white matter pathology, which plays an extremely important role in the functional consequences of SCI.

Recent breakthroughs in the cell biology of CNS injury have demonstrated the regenerative capacity of the adult spinal cord to recover function under the right circumstances. Many laboratories throughout the world have reported novel strategies that appear to be successful in converting nonpermissive environments for regeneration into permissive ones. Future studies will continue to investigate combination therapies to target axonal regeneration that may also include neuroprotective strategies to protect cellular transplants and enhance growth. It is conceivable that the use of multiple helper cells in addition to the administration of neuroprotective agents, neurotrophic factors, and antibodies that target inhibitory proteins will all be necessary to one day successfully regenerate the spinal cord. For example, while several recent publications have reported significant degrees of axonal regeneration using peripheral nerve or SC grafts,[39,40] unsuccessful re-entry into the dorsal cord has been a major limitation of this repair procedure.

Recent studies suggest that the formation of an astroglial scar and/or an inhibitory molecular barrier may inhibit fibers from exiting the grafts.[41,42] Thus, strategies including the use of neutralizing antibodies against growth inhibitors or enzyme treatments have been investigated in some regeneration studies.[43–45] In a recent investigation, the effects of degrading chondroitin sulfate proteoglycan with chrondroitinase ABC on sensory and motor projections were studied.[45] Importantly, treatment up-regulated a regeneration-associated protein and promoted regeneration of both ascending sensory and descending corticospinal tract axons. Combination therapies, including bridging strategies, cellular transplantation, growth factor administration, and the blockage of inhibitory factors, may have therapeutic potential for the treatment of human SCI. These reparative strategies, combined with rehabilitative procedures to relearn motor tasks, are critical in the overall cure strategy.[46] As new circuits are formed, remaining as well as new neural pathways must become functional to execute stepping and standing. Thus, the use of robotically based assistive devices may be necessary to promote circuit function and motor recovery as well as improved cardiovascular, pulmonary, and skeletal systems.[46] The correct combination of treatments in both the acute and chronic injury setting continues to be an exciting area of investigation in the field of SCI.

Acknowledgments

I would like to thank The Miami Project faculty and fellows for helpful discussions and Charlaine Rowlette for editorial assistance and manuscript preparation.

References

1. Bracken MB, Shepard M, Holford TR, et al. Administration of methylprednisolone for 24 or 48 hours or tirilazad mesylate for 48 hours in the treatment of acute spinal cord. JAMA 1997; 277:1597–1604.

2. Hulbert RJ. Methylprednisolone for acute spinal cord injury: an inappropriate standard of care. J Neurosurg 2000; 93:1–7.

3. Rabchevsky AG, Fugaccia I, Sullivan PG, et al. Efficacy of methylprednisolone therapy for the injured rat spinal cord. J Neurosci Res 2002; 68:7–18.

4. Short DJ, El Masry WS, Jones PW. High dose methylprednisolone in the management of acute spinal cord injury – a systematic review from a clinical perspective. Spinal Cord 2000; 38:273–286.

5. Painter SC, Wum SW, Faden AI. Alteration in extracellular amino acids after traumatic spinal cord injury. Ann Neurol 1990; 27:96–99.

6. Wrathall JR, Teng YD, Marriott R. Delayed antagonism of AMPA/kainate receptors reduces long-term functional deficits resulting from spinal cord trauma. Exp Neurol 1997; 145:565–573.

7. Behrmann DL, Bresnahan JC, Beattie MS. Modeling of acute spinal cord injury in the rat: neuroprotection and enhanced recovery with methylprednisolone, U-74006F and YM-14673. Exp Neurol 1994; 126:61–75.

8. Liu D, Liu J, Wen J. Elevation of hydrogen peroxide after spinal cord injury detected by using the fenton reaction. Free Rad Biol Med 1999; 27(3/4):478–482.

9. Wada K, Alonso OF, Busto R, et al. Early treatment with a novel inhibitor of lipid peroxidation (LY341122) improves histopathological outcome after moderate fluid percussion brain injury in rats. Neurosurgery 1999; 45:601–608.

10. Keane RW, Kraydieh S, Lotocki G, et al. Apoptotic and anti-apoptotic mechanisms following spinal cord injury. J Neuropathol Exp Neurol 2001; 60:422–429.

11. Kato H, Kanellopoulos GK, Matsuo S, et al. Neuronal apoptosis and necrosis following spinal cord ischemia in the rat. Exp Neurol 1997; 148:464–474.

12. Crowe MJ, Bresnahan JC, Shuman SL, et al. Apoptosis and delayed degeneration after spinal cord injury in rats and monkeys. Nature Med 1997; 3:73–76.

13. Emery E, Aldana M, Bunge M, et al. Apoptosis after traumatic human spinal cord injury. J Neurosurg 1998; 89:911–920.

14. Osawa H, Keane RW, Marcillo AE, et al. Therapeutic strategies targeting caspase inhibition following spinal cord injury in rats. Exp Neurol 2002; 177:306–313.

15. Li M, Ona VO, Chen M, et al. Functional role and therapeutic implications of neuronal caspase-1 -3 in a mouse model of traumatic spinal cord injury. Neuroscience 2000; 99:333–342.

16. Springer JE, Azbil D, Knapp PE. Activation of the caspase-3 apoptosis cascade in traumatic spinal cord injury. Nature Med 1999; 5:943–946.

17. del Zoppo G, Ginis I, Hallenbeck JM, et al. Inflammation and stroke: putative role for cytokines, adhesion molecules and iNOS in brain response to ischemia. Brain Pathol 2000; 10:95–112.

18. Bethea JR, Nagashima H, Acosta MC, et al. Systemically administered interleukin-10 reduces tumor necrosis factor-alpha production and significantly improves functional recovery following traumatic spinal cord injury in rats. J Neurotrauma 1999; 16:851–863.

19. Kinoshita K, Chatzipanteli K, Vitarbo E, et al. Interleukin-1β messenger ribonucleic acid and protein levels after fluid percussion brain injury in rats: the importance of injury severity and brain temperature. Neurosurgery 2002; 51:195–203.

20. Takami T, Oudega M, Bethea JR, et al. Methylprednisolone and interleukin-10 reduce gray matter damage in the contused Fischer rat thoracic spinal cord but do not improve functional outcome. J Neurotrauma 2002; 19(5):653–666.

21. Dietrich WD. Therapeutic hypothermia in experimental models of traumatic brain injury. In: Hayashi N, ed. Brain hypothermia: pathology, pharmacology and treatment of severe brain injury. Tokyo: Springer-Verlag, 2000:39–46.

22. Dietrich WD, Busto R, Bethea JR. Postischemic hypothermia and IL-10 treatment provide long-lasting neuroprotection of CA1 hippocampus following transient global ischemia in rats. Exp Neurol 1999; 158:444–450.

23. Yu CG, Jimenez O, Marcillo AE, et al. Beneficial effects of modest systemic hypothermia on locomotor function and histopathological damage following contusion-induced spinal cord injury in rats. J Neurosurg 2000; 93:85–93.

24. Chatzipanteli K, Yanagawa Y, Marcillo A, et al. Posttraumatic hypothermia reduces polymorphonuclear leukocyte accumulation following spinal cord injury in rats. J Neurotrauma 2000; 17:321–332.

25. Callsen-Cencic P, Hoheisel U, Kask EA, et al. The controversy about spinal neuronal nitric oxide synthase: under which conditions is it up- or down-regulated? Cell Tissue Res 1999; 295:183–194.

26. Chatzipanteli K, Garcia R, Marcillo AE, et al. Temporal and segmental distribution of constitutive and inducible nitric oxide synthases following traumatic spinal cord injury: effect of aminoguanidine treatment. J Neurotrauma 2002; 19:639–651.

27. Sinz EH, Kochanek PM, Dixon CE, et al. Inducible nitric oxide synthase is an endogenous neuroprotectant after traumatic brain injury in rats and mice. J Clin Invest 1999; 104:647–656.

28. Sagen J, Bunge MB, Kleitman N. Transplantation strategies for treatment of spinal cord dysfunction and injury. In: Lanza RP, Langer R, Vacanti JP, eds. Principles of tissue engineering, 2nd edn. New York: Academic Press, 2000:799–820.

29. David S, Aguayo AJ. Axonal elongation into peripheral nervous system "bridges" after central nervous system injury in adult rats. Science 1981; 214:931–933.

30. Xu XM, Guénard V, Kleitman N, Bunge MB. Axonal regeneration into Schwann cell-seeded guidance channels grafted into transected adult rat spinal cord. J Comp Neurol 1995; 351:145–160.

31. Ramón-Cueto A, Plant GW, Avila J, Bunge MB. Long-distance axonal regeneration in the transected adult rat spinal cord is promoted by olfactory ensheathing glia transplants. J Neurosci 1998; 18:3803–3815.

32. Pascual JI, Gudiño-Cabrera G, Insausti R, Nieto-Sampedro M. Spinal implants of olfactory ensheathing cells promote axon regeneration and bladder activity after bilateral lumbosacral dorsal rhizotomy in the adult rat. J Urol 2002; 167:1522–1526.

33. Grill R, Murai K, Blesch A, et al. Cellular delivery of neurotrophin-3 promotes corticospinal axonal growth and partial functional recovery after spinal cord injury. J Neurosci 1997; 17:5560–5575.

34. Tuszynski MH, Weidner N, McCormack M, et al. Grafts of genetically modified Schwann cells to the spinal cord: survival, axon growth and myelination. Cell Trans 1998; 7(2):187–196.

35. McDonald JW, Liu X-Z, Qu Y, et al. Transplanted embryonic stem cells survive, differentiate and promote recovery in injured rat spinal cord. Nature Med 1999; 5:1410–1412.

36. Bethea JR, Dietrich WD. Targeting the host inflammatory response in traumatic spinal cord injury. Curr Opin Neurol 2002; 15:355–360.

37. Rapalino O, Lazarov-Spiegler O, Agranov E, et al. Implantation of stimulated homologous macrophages results in partial recovery of paraplegic rats. Nature Med 1998; 4:814–821.

38. Baffour R, Achanta K, Kaufman J, et al. Synergistic effect of basic fibroblast growth factor and methylprednisolone on neurological function after experimental spinal cord injury. J Neurosurg 1995; 83:105–110.

39. Guest JD, Rao A, Olson L, et al. The ability of human Schwann cell grafts to promote regeneration in the transected nude rat spinal cord. Exp Neurol 1997; 148:502–522.

40. Levi ADO, Dancausse H, Li X, et al. Peripheral nerve grafts promoting central nervous system regeneration after spinal cord injury in the primate. J Neurosurg 2002; (suppl 2) 96:107–205.

41. Snow DM, Lemmon V, Carrino DA, et al. Sulfated proteoglycans in astroglial barriers inhibit neurite outgrowth *in vivo*. Exp Neurol 1990; 109:111–130.

42. Schwab ME, Kapfhammer JP, Bandtlow CE. Inhibitors of neurite growth. Ann Rev Neurosci 1993; 16:565–595.

43. Oudega M, Rosano C, Sadi D, et al. Neutralizing antibodies against neurite growth inhibitor NI-35-250 do not promote regeneration of sensory axons in the adult rat spinal cord. Neuroscience 2000; 100(4):873–883.

44. Bregman BS, Kunkel-Bagden E, Schnell L, et al. Recovery from spinal cord injury mediated by antibodies to neurite growth inhibitors. Nature 1995; 378:498–501.

45. Bradbury EJ, Moon LD, Popat RJ, et al. Chondroitinase ABC promotes functional recovery after spinal cord injury. Nature 2002; 416:636–640.

46. Edgerton VR, deLeon RD, Harkema SJ, et al. Topical review. Retaining the injured spinal cord. J Physiol 2001; 533:15–22.

Part VII

Synthesis of treatment

58

Treatment alternatives for different types of neurogenic bladder dysfunction in adults

Erik Schick and Jacques Corcos

Introduction

Vesicourethral dysfunction secondary to degenerative processes, traumas, or neoplasias of the central or peripheral nervous system will most certainly have a deleterious effect on the patient's quality of life.

For centuries, the prognosis of these pathologies on patient survival was bad. We know from the Edwin Smith papyrus that as far back as 1600 BC the ancient Egyptians were aware of the relationship between the nervous system and urinary bladder function.[1] They considered spinal cord trauma as a 'disease not to treat'.[2]

Statistics on spinal cord trauma are available since World War I. The mortality rate was extremely high in those days – more than 90% – mainly due to urinary complications such as urosepsis and renal insufficiency. Dramatic improvements in prognosis came during World War II when Sir Ludwig Guttmann, in England, established specialized units to take care of these patients, and introduced the method of intermittent catheterization.[3] During the 1970s the use of urodynamics became more widespread, allowing a better understanding of the physiology and pathophysiology of the lower urinary tract. Translation of these new notions has significantly improved the prognosis of these patients.

The main goals in treating patients with neurogenic bladder dysfunction are threefold:

1. to preserve upper urinary tract integrity
2. to insure adequate continence
3. to minimize stone formation and urinary infection.

All these therapeutic goals aim to improve the patient's quality of life and prolong life expectancy.

In the ideal situation, these objectives should be attainable without the necessity of having to rely on a foreign body (i.e. a catheter) permanently installed in the urinary tract.

Therapeutic classification of vesicourethral dysfunction

Several classifications of vesicourethral dysfunction have been proposed in the literature. The latest, and probably the most original, is developed elsewhere in this book by A Matthiasson (see Chapter 42). Based mainly on Krane and Siroky's work, we have elaborated a simple and practical classification that is derived from observations obtained from urodynamic studies, and which focuses on therapeutic goals.[4]

The bladder, as a reservoir, can exhibit only three types of dysfunction:

1. hypo- or areflexia
2. hyperreflexia (including those with decreased contractility)
3. small capacity bladder with or without decreased compliance.

The urethra, the outlet, can be obstructive owing to an anatomical cause (e.g. stenosis, or benign prostatic hyperplasia), functional alterations (e.g. vesicosphincteric dyssynergia), or it can be hypotonic (e.g. incontinence). In clinical practice, most often, both structures function abnormally to varying degrees (Table 58.1).

Urodynamics investigation is the cornerstone of any treatment strategy in neurogenic bladder dysfunction. It allows us to separately evaluate the reservoir function and outlet function, as well as the coordination of these structures during micturition. A well-conducted urodynamics study should answer at least the following questions:

- During the filling phase, is the bladder hyper-, hypo-, or areflexic?
- What is the bladder wall compliance?
- At what bladder volume does the first desire to void appear?
- What is the post-void residual volume and the cystometric capacity?

Table 58.1 *Urodynamic classification of neurogenic bladder dysfunction*

Bladder function	Urethral function
Normal	Hypotonic
Normal	Hypertonic
Hyperreflexic[a]	Normal
Hyperreflexic[a]	Hypotonic
Hyperreflexic[a]	Hypertonic
Hypo- or areflexic	Normal
Hypo- or areflexic	Hypotonic
Hypo- or areflexic	Hypertonic

[a] With or without decreased compliance; with or without impaired contractility.

- Does the bladder represent a high-pressure or a low-pressure system?
- During micturition, is there any kind of infravesical obstruction?
- What is the detrusor contractility, and what is its power?
- As far as the urethra is concerned, what is its 'tonicity' (hypo- or hypertonic) at rest?
- How is increased abdominal pressure transmitted to the urethra in females?
- Is micturition synergic or dyssynergic?

In any kind of neurological pathology associated with vesicourethral dysfunction, even complex situations can be logically analyzed by urodynamics evaluation, which estimates the component of the lower urinary tract that is dysfunctional and to what extent. This allows us to elaborate a logical therapeutic plan that is adapted or personalized to each patient's condition.

Altered reservoir function

As mentioned above, neurological pathology can modify bladder function with three possible end results.

The hypo- or areflexic bladder

In this situation, the bladder cannot empty itself, or can do so only partially, leaving a high post-void residual volume behind. Complete bladder emptying can be promoted by the following techniques.

Clean intermittent catheterization

Whenever the clinical situation permits, clean intermittent catheterization is one of the major approaches taken to ensure adequate bladder emptying. The credit goes to Lapides, who demonstrated that self-catheterization does not need to be sterile and is safe and harmless if the catheter is simply clean.[5–7] His observations, which revolutionized the management of patient bladder evacuation problems, are based on the premise that one of the mechanisms the bladder has to resist bacterial colonization is its periodic and complete emptying.

Transurethral electrical stimulation of the detrusor

Katona et al,[8] who stimulated the bladder wall with a monopolar electrode placed in the bladder *per urethram*, proposed direct stimulation of the detrusor muscle itself. Continuous 60–100 mA current stimulates the mechanoreceptors of the bladder, provoking reflex detrusor contraction.[9] The sacral reflex arc must be intact and the patient must feel the desire to void during the sessions to successfully apply this technique. Daily stimulation sessions of 60–90 min for up to 80 days are necessary. This approach differs significantly from neurostimulation of the sacral roots, since the aim here is to rehabilitate the bladder to regain voluntary control of micturition. The 75% success rate claimed by the original investigators has been confirmed by others[10–13] (see Chapter 51).

Myoplasty of the detrusor

To decrease a large, decompensated bladder, Klarskov et al[14] suggested a partial cystectomy. It has been postulated that this will not only decrease bladder volume but also might increase the contractile efficiency of the detrusor. Hanna,[15] on the other hand, proposed 'remodeling' of the bladder, whereby a part of the bladder wall, stripped of its mucosa, covers the remaining bladder wall, much like a double-breast closure of the abdominal cavity. This would double the thickness of the detrusor, increasing its overall contractility. He operated on 11 patients (9 adults and 2 children): 10 of them have been improved.

Bladder wall strengthening by striated muscle flap

More recently, the group of Tanagho[16] demonstrated in the dog that use of the skeletal muscle, which can be stimulated, may serve to facilitate bladder emptying. Stenzl et al[17] proposed detrusor myoplasty in humans, which consists of transposing a part of the latissimus dorsi muscle around the bladder in such a way that 75% of the bladder wall will be covered by this striated muscle. Of the 11 patients operated on, all were able to void volitionally, and 8 of them no longer required catheterization throughout the follow-up period of 12–46 months.

Pharmacological therapy

Because motor innervation of the detrusor is mainly cholinergic, it seems logical to use this type of medication to enhance bladder emptying. Despite the theoretical advantages of this approach, very little success has been achieved in clinical practice. Awad et al[18] pointed out the importance of the agent's route of administration. They succeeded in obtaining spontaneous voiding and decreasing post-void residual by injecting the medication subcutaneously. Comparable results were not obtained with oral administration. However, it should be noted that side-effects increased with prolonged subcutaneous treatment.

Decreasing urethral resistance

Obviously, decreasing or eliminating urethral resistance should improve bladder emptying. This will be discussed in more detail below.

Summary

The hypo- or areflexic bladder is best managed, whenever possible, by clean intermittent catheterization. Electrostimulation becomes an increasingly valuable alternative, but is still expensive. Direct electrical stimulation of the bladder wall should be attempted when the sacral reflex arc

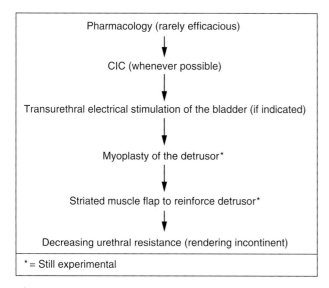

Pharmacology (rarely efficacious)

↓

CIC (whenever possible)

↓

Transurethral electrical stimulation of the bladder (if indicated)

↓

Myoplasty of the detrusor*

↓

Striated muscle flap to reinforce detrusor*

↓

Decreasing urethral resistance (rendering incontinent)

*= Still experimental

Figure 58.1
Algorithm for the treatment of hypo- or areflexic bladder. CIC, clean intermittent catheterization.

is preserved. The time-consuming nature of this approach and the relatively limited indications might prevent its widespread use, in spite of the favorable results reported in the literature. Striated muscle flap is still in its experimental phase. Long-term results in a substantial number of patients are not yet available.

Pharmacological manipulation in this group of patients has limited success and, at the present, has no real indication (Figure 58.1).

The hyperreflexic bladder

The physiopathological consequences of bladder hyperreflexia are threefold:

1. urinary incontinence can be provoked when the amplitude of bladder contractions exceeds urethral closure pressure
2. a low-pressure system can become a high-pressure system if the uninhibited contractions are frequent, with an amplitude over 40 cmH_2O, and/or bladder compliance decreases as a result of progressive bladder wall fibrosis
3. vesicoureteral reflux can develop as a result of hyperreflexia.

Hyperreflexia can be controlled by pharmacological and/or surgical means.

Pharmacological manipulation

Oral administration. In the last decade, a large number of pharmacological substances have been developed to control bladder hyperreflexia. All of these substances have antimuscarinic properties, interfering with M_3 type receptors. Their overall efficacy in neurogenic hyperreflexia is about 50%.[19] No published randomized clinical trials have been performed on the newly developed anticholinergics – Ditropan XL (oxybutynin), tolterodine, Darifenacine, etc. – in the neurogenic bladder patient population. However, 15–30 mg daily doses of Ditropan XL have been found to be very effective in the hyperreflexic bladder in clinical practice.[20,21]

Transcutaneous administration. James et al[22] in a pilot study used nitroglycerin dermal patches to control bladder instability. They observed a reduction in diurnal and nocturnal frequency as well as a decrease in incontinence episodes per 24 hours. More recently, Davila et al[23] reported the results of a multicenter trial with transcutaneous oxybutynin. Compared with oral administration, the transdermal route had equal efficacy and a significantly improved side-effect profile in adults with urge urinary incontinence. This subject is examined in more detail in Chapter 46.

Intravesical treatment. Bladder hyperreflexia involves an intact sacral reflex arc. Intravesically administered substances can act on the efferent or on the afferent branches of this reflex arc.

Anticholinergics block the efferent part of the reflex. Brendler et al[24] used 5 mg of oxybutynin chloride in 20–30 ml of water in 10 incontinent patients. All of them became continent. Madersbacher et al[25] studied oxybutynin in 13 hyperreflexic bladder patients: in 10 of them who presented incontinence between clean intermittent catheterizations, 9 became continent. Even if the oxybutynin serum level was higher after intravesical administration than orally, the side-effects of anticholinergics were totally absent in the intravesical group. In patients with enterocystoplasty, the side-effects were identical to the oral group. This observation led Massad et al[26] to conclude that a hepatic metabolite of oxybutynin is probably responsible for the side-effects. In a recent study of 12 patients with hyperreflexic bladder, Di Stasi et al[27] found that oral oxybutynin had no effect. When administered intravesically, passive diffusion of oxybutynin significantly reduced urinary leakage, but with electromotive diffusion it caused significantly greater post-void residual urine volume and fewer episodes of urinary leakage, together with measurable changes in urodynamic parameters: decreased duration and amplitude of uninhibited contractions as well as increased bladder wall compliance.

Multisite botulinum A toxin injection in the bladder (up to a total of 300 units) has been proposed to control hyperreflexia. Schurch et al[28] reported their experience recently in 31 spinal cord injury (SCI) patients. Bladder capacity and mean reflex volume increased significantly, mean maximum voiding pressure decreased, and post-void residual volume rose. The duration of bladder paresis was at least 9 months, when repeated injections were required.

Among substances interfering with the afferent branch of the reflex arc, one should mention capsaicin, resiniferatoxin and Marcain (bupivacaine). Capsaicin and resiniferatoxin, both vanilloids, block neurotransmission via small demyelinized C fibers, which come into function only after spinal disruption when myelinized Aδ fibers cannot transmit information to the central nervous system. In idiopathic detrusor instability and in suprapontine pathology, where the C-fiber-mediated reflex does not emerge, these substances seem not to be effective.[29] A controlled trial by de Sèze et al[30] showed that capsaicin was significantly more effective than placebo for continence, frequency, urgency, and patient satisfaction. In a meta-analysis by this same group,[31] 84% of patients (97 out of 115) with detrusor hyperreflexia presented some improvement in their symptoms when treated with intravesical capsaicin. Worldwide experience suggests that 60–100% of patients might respond favourably to this kind of therapy by decreasing or eliminating incontinence episodes between clean intermittent catheterizations for 1–9 months without systemic toxicity.[21]

At 1000-fold more potent than capsicin, resiniferatoxin is mainly interesting for the reduced local reaction that it provokes in the bladder.[32] Resiniferatoxin trials were recently summarized by De Ridder and Baert.[33] The results on vanilloids are updated in Chapter 45.

Local anesthetics block axonal conduction in unmyelinated nerve fibers. The clinical response is of very short duration, and no protocol has been proposed using this approach to control detrusor hyperreflexia. An extensive review on the intravesical administration of drugs in patients with bladder hyperreflexia has been published by Ekström.[34]

Intrathecal administration. According to the experience of Steers et al,[35] intrathecal infusion of baclofen, a γ-aminobutric acid (GABA) agonist, proved to be successful in patients with severe spasticity and hyperreflexia. In all of them, hyperreflexia disappeared, bladder capacity increased by 72%, and bladder compliance improved in 16%. Kums et al[36] made similar observations in 9 quadriplegics. In the last decade, however, no report on this approach to treat detrusor hyperreflexia has been found in the literature.

Neurostimulation

Neurostimulation is the term used when electrical stimulation is applied directly to a nerve fiber to achieve a desired function (sphincter contraction or detrusor relaxation). Neuromodulation is the term used when electrical stimulation is applied to indirectly modify sensory and/or motor functions of the lower urinary tract.

Neurostimulation is applied mainly in patients with complete SCI and preserved detrusor function. (It excludes patients with areflexic bladder.) Introduced by Tanagho[37] and Brindley,[38] this technique is most often associated with bilateral sacral posterior rhizotomy to reduce hyperreflexia and autonomic dysreflexia. The success rate is high for bladder function, but less for rectal function.[39–41]

Surgery

Two main surgical procedures have been proposed in the literature to decrease detrusor hyperreflexia and/or to manage low-compliant bladders: partial detrusorectomy (autoaugmentation) and enterocystoplasty. The ultimate goal with each procedure is to increase reservoir capacity and reduce the amplitude of detrusor contractions.

Enterocystoplasty is contemplated in patients with bladder capacity less than 300 ml under anesthesia. Most commonly, a detubularized segment of the distal ileum is used for this purpose, but a detubularized colic segment or part of the gastric wall can also be used.

Excellent long-term results were reported in about 75% of patients, with improvement in another 20%. The most frequent complications were stone formation in the reservoir (20%) and reoperation (15%) to reaugment the bladder.[42]

The main advantages of autoaugmentation over enterocystoplasty are its lower morbidity (the peritoneal cavity is not opened, the gastrointestinal tract is not violated) and, in case of failure, further intestinal substitution is not precluded. We reserve partial detrusorectomy for patients with bladder capacity over 300 ml under general anesthesia. Detrusor myomectomy and enterocystoplasty offer comparable success or improvement.[43]

Summary

The first step in the management of the hyperreflexic bladder should be a pharmacological one. The oral route of administration is used most frequently. Among transdermal anticholinergic patches, oxybutynin is the only one which underwent clinical trials. It showed equal efficacy and a better side-effect profile than the traditional oral route. Intravesical capsaicin will probably be replaced by the better-tolerated resiniferatoxin, but clinical trails have been recently suspended by the sponsoring pharmaceutical companies.[30] Botulinum A toxin injections in the detrusor are promising, but must be repeated, probably on an annual basis or so. No long-term results exist. Intrathecal baclofen is not indicated at present for the treatment of hyperreflexic bladder, but one should remember that if a baclofen infusion pump is installed for other reasons (e.g. uncontrollable skeletal muscle spasticity), the patient might have some benefit from the urological point of view as well. Neurostimulation constitutes the less-invasive surgical alternative. The still very expensive nature of this treatment modality limits its widespread use. More invasive surgical procedures include bladder autoaugmentation or enterocystoplasty, with equally good long-term results and an acceptable complication rate (Figure 58.2).

Altered outlet function
Infravesical obstruction

From the functional point of view, distinction should be made between occlusion and obstruction. Occlusion is a static phenomenon, as it can be observed: e.g., during a cystoscopic examination. Viewing the lateral lobes of the prostate from the verumontanum, one is looking at a static image. It is impossible to extrapolate from this observation how the proximal urethra will relax in response to detrusor contraction and to what degree urethral funneling will allow the normal passage of urine. In contrast, obstruction

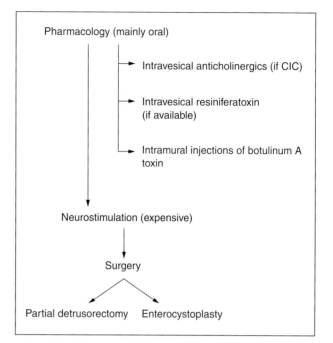

Figure 58.2
Algorithm for the treatment of hyperreflexic bladder. CIC, clean intermittent catheterization.

is a dynamic phenomenon which, in hydrodynamics, means high pressure associated with decreased flow. This can only be objectively demonstrated by urodynamics. Infravesical urethral obstruction can be anatomical (e.g. urethral stenosis) or functional (e.g. vesicosphincteric dyssynergia). We will concentrate on functional obstructions.

The pharmacological approach

From the theoretical point of view, alpha-blocking agents and those that might relax the striated sphincter (together with the pelvic floor) should decrease urethral resistance during micturition. This approach can be beneficial in the neurologically intact patient, but their use in the neurological patient is not very effective. It should be noted, however, that no randomized, double-blind study has demonstrated the role of these substances in the neurological bladder.

Dykstra and Sidi[44] injected botulinum A toxin locally in the striated sphincter once a week for 3 consecutive weeks in 5 patients with proven vesicourethral dyssynergia. Electromyographic (EMG) activity in the striated sphincter has been abolished after injections, while maximum urethral closure pressure, voiding pressure, and post-void residual all decreased. Follow-up of these patients was not provided.

Fowler et al[45] also injected botulinum A toxin in the external sphincter of 6 non-neurological women who exhibited chronic urinary retention. None of the women improved, a failure that might be explained by the fact that these patients were neurologically normal.

Phelan et al[46] recently reported on the efficacy of botulinum toxin injection in the urethral sphincter of men and women with acontractile bladder. All but 1 of the 21 patients treated voided without catheterization, post-void residual decreased by 71%, and voiding pressure by 38%. Transient incontinence was sometimes observed.[47]

In the previously quoted study by Steers et al,[35] intrathecal infusion of baclofen not only abolished bladder hyperreflexia in all patients but also eliminated vesicosphincteric dyssynergia in 40% of them.

Reversible surgical procedures

Intraurethral stents. Growing experience suggests that intraurethral stents are effective in eliminating vesicosphincteric dyssynergia. According to the North American experience, 13% of the prosthesis were withdrawn during the 24-month observation period.[48] The result was 11% in a European study, with a global complication rate of 38%.[49] An excellent in-depth review of the subject, including sphincterotomy, and comparison between the two treatment modalities, have been presented recently by Rivas and Chancellor.[50]

Transurethral balloon dilatation. Chancellor et al[51] proposed hydraulic dilatation of the striated urethral sphincter. Their study, of 17 male patients with vesicourethral dyssynergia, demonstrated interesting results 1 year later: micturition pressure decreased significantly (83 ± 35 cmH$_2$O vs 37 ± 15 cmH$_2$O), as well as post-void residual (163 ± 162 vs 68 ± 59 cmH$_2$O). One year postoperatively, 82% of the patients voided adequately. Even autonomic dysreflexia, when present, was improved. No long-term follow-up was provided.

Overdistention of the female urethra. Overdistention should be very generous to rupture the helicoidal fibers of the urethra. If the bladder neck is competent, stress incontinence

should not result from this approach.[52] Transurethral resection of the bladder neck in females should be avoided, as stress incontinence will most likely be its consequence.

Credé's maneuver. This maneuver is more efficacious, especially in females, when the pelvic floor muscles are paralyzed. The increased abdominal pressure is dissipated in part by the flaccid pelvic floor, and lesser pressure will be exerted simultaneously on the proximal urethra. Bladder evacuation, however, is never complete with this technique.

Irreversible surgical procedures

Transurethral bladder neck/prostate incision/resection. If the patient is able to void during urodynamic testing, distinction can be made between constrictive and compressive obstruction.[53] If the obstruction is constrictive in nature and there is no anatomical stenosis at the level of the anterior urethral, we prefer transurethral incision of the bladder neck, as described a number of years ago by Turner-Warwick.[54] Our incision, however, is not limited strictly to the bladder neck, but goes down to the level of the verumontanum, including the lateral lobes of the prostate as well. We observed less restenosis after incision than after resection of the bladder neck, which is contrary to the experience of others.[52]

Sphincterotomy. In the absence of videourodynamics, it is not always easy to decide when to perform sphincterotomy alone and when to combine it with bladder neck incision. Gardner et al[55] combined cystography and static urethral pressure measurements: their algorithm is illustrated on Figure 58.3. In our experience, X-ray studies are recommended, but not absolutely mandatory. When pressure–flow assessment demonstrates obstruction and maximum urethral closure pressure (MUCP) is high, transurethral surgery can include sphincterotomy as well. If MUCP is low, sphincterotomy is probably not useful.

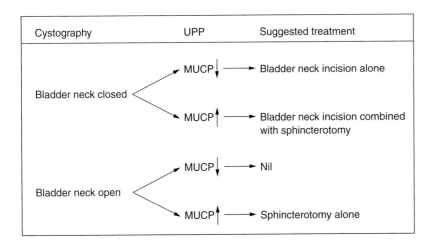

Figure 58.3
Algorithm to decrease urethral resistance. UPP, static urethral pressure profile; MUCP, maximum urethral closure pressure. (Reproduced with permission from Gardner et al.)[55]

Summary

Increased urethral resistance can be weakened by pharmacological means, which, in the form of oral medication, is less efficacious than in the non-neurologic patient. However, it should be the first-line treatment. In case of failure, transurethral injection of botulinum A toxin can be offered. Clinical experience with this form of treatment is limited, and the toxin is not readily available worldwide. Intraurethral stents are effective, but not exempt from causing morbidity and their removal after a prolonged time period can be quite challenging. Balloon dilatation has never gained wide acceptance, despite the fact that it is easy to perform, relatively inexpensive, produces limited complications, and gives good results. Unfortunately, no long-term results are available with this form of therapy. Overdilation of the female urethra should not result in stress urinary incontinence. Sphincterotomy with or without bladder/prostate incision/resection, although the most invasive alternative, remains the gold standard in the management of the obstructive male urethra (Figure 58.4).

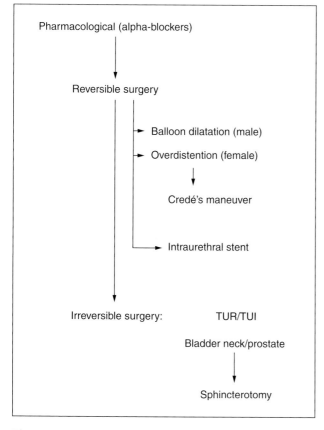

Figure 58.4
Algorithm for the treatment of functional bladder outlet obstruction. TUR, transurethral resection; TUI, transurethral incision.

The hypotonic outlet – incontinence

Urinary incontinence can result from an alteration in reservoir function (hyperreflexia, decreased compliance, small capacity) or a sphincteric failure at the level of the urethra. How to obviate alterations in reservoir function has been discussed previously. In the following sections we will summarize the possibilities of increasing urethral resistance. It should be pointed out that the prerequisite to augmented resistance is a low-pressure bladder reservoir.

Urethropexy

When intrinsic sphincter deficiency and abdominourethral pressure transmission failure are demonstrated in patients with neurogenic bladder, urethropexy can be performed. A detailed description of the multiple techniques proposed in the literature to achieve this is beyond the scope of our chapter. At the moment, Burch urethropexy[56] is the gold standard, as modified by Tanagho.[57] After having been used mainly for the failure of previous urethropexy, and the treatment of stress urinary incontinence without bladder neck hypermobility, sling operations became more popular during the last decade, and indications have been enlarged. However, no randomized study has yet been published to compare retropubic open urethropexy with sling operations. Different sling materials have been used, such as autologous fascia, cadaveric fascia, and a variety of artificial materials. Among the commercially available materials, the tension-free vaginal tape (TVT) technique has gained much popularity, and has the potential to replace the traditional retropubic approach.[58] The precise indications for TVT use are not yet clearly defined in the literature.

Periurethral injections

Berg was the first to report on periurethral injection of Teflon paste in the submucosa of the vesical neck to increase urethral resistance.[59] Because microparticles of this paste have been recovered from the lymphatic ganglia, liver, spleen, brain, and kidney, alternative substances have been proposed.[60] Collagen has been the most widely used substance,[61] followed by autologous fat tissue[62] and silicone microspheres (Genisphere).[63] Pineda and Hadley recently published an extensive review on the subject.[64] The overall success rate in the reported series in females is between 54% and 83% for collagen and 43% and 86% for fat. In men, the overall success rate is between 36% and 100% for collagen. No series were found with fat injection in males. This treatment modality has not been studied in detail in the neurogenic population. Only a few reports reflect the experience in patients with neurogenic bladder dysfunction.[65]

Neurostimulation

Neurostimulation has been summarized previously.

Artificial urinary sphincter

Artificial urinary sphincter remains the gold standard, especially in males, for the treatment of urinary incontinence secondary to sphincter weakness. Fulford et al[66] reported on 68 patients, all of them followed for more than 10 years: 75% of them had satisfactory continence, but only 13% still retained their original device. This suggests that the lifetime of the artificial sphincter is around 10–15 years, which has been confirmed recently by Spiess et al,[67] who studied 30 meningomyelocele children in whom an artificial sphincter was implanted at the bladder neck or the bulbar urethra. Survival analysis of the sphincter device revealed a sharp drop after 100 months, with only 8.3% of the sphincters still functioning beyond this point.

Urethra replacement

When the urethra is judged nonsalvageable from the functional point of view, it can be replaced by a muscular tube obtained from the detrusor. Two main surgical techniques have been described. The Young–Dees–Leadbetter technique creates a muscular tube from the trigone. This necessitates reimplantation of both ureters in an extratrigonal site. Long-term results showed perfect continence in 57% of adults and 70% of children.[68] Tanagho[69] proposed creation of the tube from the anterior bladder wall. This leaves the ureterovesical junction undisturbed. Good to excellent results were obtained in 71.5% of the 56 patients operated on.

Supraurethral derivation

When the clinical situation is such that neither the Young–Dees–Leadbetter operation nor the Tanagho technique is feasible, supraurethral derivation might become necessary. This creates an abdominal stoma which can be continent or incontinent. It frequently implies, especially in females, the simultaneous closure of the bladder neck.

Summary

Failure of the sphincter mechanism in males is best treated by the implantation of an artificial sphincter, which might even be the first line of treatment. Pharmacological substances are rarely effective enough in ensuring continence, and periurethral injections do not resist time. In females suburethral

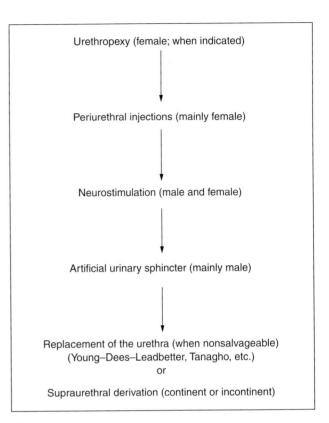

Urethropexy (female; when indicated)

↓

Periurethral injections (mainly female)

↓

Neurostimulation (male and female)

↓

Artificial urinary sphincter (mainly male)

↓

Replacement of the urethra (when nonsalvageable)
(Young–Dees–Leadbetter, Tanagho, etc.)
or
Supraurethral derivation (continent or incontinent)

Figure 58.5
Algorithm for the hypotonic outlet: incontinence.

slings are an interesting option, especially if the patient is on a clean intermittent catheterization regimen. In this case, the sling might even be overstretched to some extent to allow continence, bladder emptying being secured by catheterization. When complete replacement of a nonsalvageable urethra is indicated, both posterior (trigonal) and anterior bladder wall tubes give almost the same good results. It should be kept in mind, however, that these are complex surgical procedures with some degree of associated morbidity. Supraurethral derivation (continent or incontinent) should be considered as a last resort treatment (Figure 58.5).

References

1. Küss R, Grégoire W. Histoire illustrée de l'urologie de l'Antiquité à nos jours. Paris (France): R. Dacosta, 1988.

2. Gutierrez PA, Young RR, Vulpe M. Spinal cord injury – an overview. Urol Cl N Am 1993; 20:373–382. [Quote]

3. Guttman L, Frankel H. The value of intermittent catheterization in the early management of traumatic paraplegia and tetraplegia. Paraplegia 1966; 4:63–84.

4. Schick E. Synthèse thérapeutique: traitement des grands types de vessies neurogènes. In: Corcos J, Schick E, eds. Les vessies neurogènes de l'adulte. Paris (France): Masson et Cie, 1996:203–226.

5. Lapides J, Diokno AC, Silber SJ, Lowe BS. Clean, intermittent self-catheterization in the treatment of urinary tract disease. J Urol 1972; 107:458–461.

6. Lapides J, Diokno AC, Lowe BS, Kalish MD. Follow-up on unsterile, intermittent self catheterization. J Urol 1974; 111:184–187.

7. Diokno AC, Sonda P, Hollander JB, Lapides J. Fate of patients started on clean intermittent self-cathaterization therapy 10 years ago. J Urol 1983; 129:1120–1122.

8. Katona F, Berényi M. Intravesical transurethral electrotherapy in meningomyelocele patients. Acta Paediatr Acad Sci Hung 1975; 16:363–374.

9. Ebner A, Jiang C, Lindström S. Intravesical electrical stimulation – an experimental analysis of the mechanism of action. J Urol 1992; 148:920–924.

10. Madersbacher H, Hetzel H, Gottinger F, Ebner A. Rehabilitation of micturition in adults with incomplete spinal cord lesions by intravesical electrotherapy. Neurourol Urodyn 1987; 6:230–232. [Abstract]

11. Kaplan WE, Richards I. Intravesical transurethral electrotherapy for the neurogenic bladder. J Urol 1986; 136:243–246.

12. Decter RM, Snyder P, Rosvanis TK. Transurethral electrical bladder stimulation: initial results. J Urol 1992; 148:651–653.

13. Lyne CJ, Bellinger MF. Early experience with transurethral electrical bladder stimulation. J Urol 1993; 150:697–699.

14. Klarskov P, Holm-Bentzen M, Larsen S, et al. Partial cystectomy for the myogenous decompensated bladder with excessive residual urine. Urodynamics, histology and 2–13 years follow-up. Scand J Urol Nephrol 1988; 22:251–256.

15. Hanna MK. New concept in bladder remodeling. Urology 1982; 19:6–12.

16. von Heyden B, Anthony JP, Kaula M, et al. The latissimus dorsi muscle for detrusor assistance: functional recovery after nerve division and repair. J Urol 1994; 151:1081–1087.

17. Stenzl A, Strasser H, Klima G, et al. Reconstruction of the lower urinary tract using autologous muscle transfer and cell seeding: current status and future perspectives. World J Urol 2000; 18:44–50.

18. Awad SA, McGinnis RH, Downie JW. The effectiveness of bethanechol chloride in lower motor neuron lesions: the importance of mode of administration. Neurourol Urodyn 1984; 3:173–178.

19. Barrett DM, Wein AJ, Parulkar BG. Surgery for neuropathic bladder. AUA Update Series 1990; 9:298–303.

20. Appell RA. Treatment of overactive bladder with once-daily extended release tolterodine or oxybutynin: the antimuscarinic clinical effectiveness trial (ACET). Curr Urol Rep 2002; 3:343–344.

21. Elliott DS, Barrett DM. Surgical and medical management of the neurogenic bladder. AUA Update Series 2002; 21:138–143.

22. James MJ, Iacovon JW. The use of GNT patches in detrusor instability: a pilot study. Neurourol Urodyn 1993; 12:399–400. [Abstract]

23. Davila GW, Daugherty CA, Sanders SW. Transdermal Oxybutynin Study Group. A short-term, multicenter, randomized double-blind dose titration study of the efficacy and anticholinergic side effects of transdermal compared to immediate release oxybutynin treatment of patients with urge urinary incontinence. J Urol 2001; 166:140–145.

24. Brandler CB, Radebaugh LC, Mohler JL. Topical oxybutynin chloride for relaxation of dysfunctional bladders. J Urol 1989; 141:1350–1352.

25. Madersbacher H, Jilg G. Control of detrusor hyperreflexia by the intravesical installation of oxybutynin chloride. Paraplegia 1991; 29:84–90.

26. Massad CA, Kogan BA, Trigo-Rocha FE. Pharmacokinetics of intravesical and oral oxybutynin chloride. J Urol 1992: 595–597.

27. Di Stasi SM, Giannantoni A, Navarra P, et al. Intravesical oxybutynin: mode of action assessed by passive diffusion and electromotive administration with pharmacokinetics of oxybutynin and N-desethyl-oxybutynin. J Urol 2001; 166:2232–2236.

28. Schurch B, Stöhrer M, Kramer G, et al. Botulinum-A toxin for treating detrusor hyperreflexia in spinal cord-injured parients: a new alternative to anticholinergic drugs? Preliminary results. J Urol 2000; 164:692–697.

29. Fowler CJ. Bladder afferents and their role in overactive bladder. Urology 2002; 59(suppl 5A):37–42.

30. de Sèze M, Wiart L, Joseph PA, et al. Capsaicin and neurogenic detrusor hyperreflexia: a double-blind placebo-controlled study in 20 patients with spinal cord lesions. Neurourol Urodyn 1998; 17:513–523.

31. de Sèze M, Wiart L, Ferrière JM, et al. Intravesical installation of capsaicin in urology: a review of the literature. Eur Urol 1999; 36:267–277.

32. Maggi CA, Patacchini R, Tramontana M, et al. Similarities and differences in the action of resiniferatoxin and capsaicin on central and peripheral endings of primary sensory neurons. Neuroscience 1990; 37:531–539.

33. De Ridder D, Baert L. Vanilloids and the overactive bladder. BJU Int 2000; 86:172–180.

34. Ekström B. Intravesical instillation of drugs in patients with detrusor hyperactivity. Scand J Urol Nephrol 1992; 149(suppl):1–67.

35. Steers WD, Meythaller JM, Haworth C, et al. Effects of acute bolus and chronic continuous intrathecal Baclofen on genito-urinary dysfunction due to spinal cord pathology. J Urol 1992; 148:1849–1855.

36. Kums JJM, Delhaas EM. Intrathecal Baclofen infusion in patients with spasticity and neurogenic bladder disease. Preliminary results. World J Urol 1991; 9:99–104.

37. Tanagho EA, Schmidt RA. Electrical stimulation in the clinical management of the neurogenic bladder. J Urol 1988; 140:1331–1339.

38. Brindley GS, Pulkey CE, Rushton DN, Cardozo L. Sacral anterior root stimulators for bladder control in paraplegia: the first 50 cases. J Neurol Neurosurg Psychiatry 1986; 49:1104–1114.

39. Chartier-Katler EJ, Denys P, Chancellor MB, et al. Urodynamic monitoring during percutaneous sacral nerve neurostimulation in patients with neurogenic detrusor hyperreflexia. Neurourol Urodyn 2001; 20:61–71.

40. Van Kerrebroeck PE, Koldewijn EL, Debruyne FM. Worldwide experience with the Finetech-Brindley sacral anterior root stimulator. Neurourol Urodyn 1993; 12:497–503.

41. Van Kerrebrock PE. Neurostimulation. In: Corcos J, Schick E, eds. The urinary sphincter. New York: Marcel Dekker, 2001:553–563.

42. Flood HD, Malhotra SJ, O'Connell HE, et al. Long-term results and complications using augmentation cystoplasty in reconstructive urology. Neurourol Urodyn 1995; 14:297–309.

43. Leng WW, Blalock HJ, Frederiksson WH, et al. Enterocystoplasty or myomectomy? Comparison of indications and outcomes for bladder augmentation. J Urol 1999; 161:758–763.

44. Dykstra DD, Sidi AA. Treatment of detrusor-sphincter dyssynergia with Botulinum A toxin: a double-blind study. Arch Phys Med Rehab 1990: 71:24–26.

45. Fowler CJ, Betts CD, Christmas TJ, et al. Botulinum toxin in the treatment of chronic urinary retention in women. Br J Urol 1992; 70:387–389.

46. Phelan MW, Franks M, Somogyi GT, et al. Botulinum toxin urethral sphincter injection to restore bladder emptying in men and women with voiding dysfunction. J Urol 2001; 164:1107–1110.

47. Boyd RN, Britton TC, Robinson RO, Borzyskowski M. Transient urinary incontinence after Botulinum A toxin. Lancet 1996; 348(9025):481–482. [Letter]

48. Oesterling JE, Kaplan SA, Epstein HB, et al., and The North American Urolume Study Group. The North American experience with the Urolume endoprosthesis as a treatment for benign prostatic hyperplasia. Long term results. Urology 1994; 44:353–362.

49. Guazzone G, Montorsi F, Coulange Ch, et al. A modified prostatic wallstent for healthy patients with symptomatic benign prostatic hyperplasia: a European multicenter experience. Urology 1994; 44:364–370.

50. Rivas DA, Chancellor MB. Sphincterotomy and sphincter stent prosthesis placement. In: Corcos J, Schick E, eds. The urinary sphincter. New York: Marcel Dekker, 2001:565–582.

51. Chancellor MB, Karasick S, Strup S, et al. Transurethral balloon dilation of the external urinary sphincter: effectiveness in spinal cord-injured men with detrusor-sphincter dyssynergia. Radiology 1993; 187:557–560.

52. Parsons KF. Difficulty with voiding or acute urinary retention having previously voided satisfactorily. In: Parsons KF, Fitzpatrick JM, eds. Practical urology in spinal cord injury. London: Springer-Verlag, 1991:27–42.

53. Schäfer W. Principles and clinical application of advanced urodynamic analysis of voiding function. Urol Cl N Am 1990; 17:553–566.

54. Turner-Warwick R. Clinical problems associated with urodynamic abnormalities with spacial reference to the value of synchronous cine-pressure-flow cystography and the clinical importance of detrusor function studies. In: Lutzeyer W, Melchior H, eds. Urodynamics – upper and lower urinary tract. Berlin: Springer-Verlag, 1970:237–263.

55. Gardner BP, Parsons KF, Machin DG, et al. The urological management of spinal cord damaged patients: a clinical algorithm. Paraplegia 1986; 24:138–147.

56. Burch JC. Cooper's ligament urethrovesical suspension for stress incontinence. Nine year's experience – results, complications, technique. Am J Obstet Gynecol 1968; 100:764–774.

57. Tanagho EA. Colpocystourethropexy: the way we do it. J Urol 1976; 116:751–753.

58. Ulmsten U, Falconer C, Johnson P, et al. A multicenter study of tension-free vaginal tape (TVT) for surgical treatment of stress urinary incontinence. Int Urogynec J Pelvic Floor Dysfunc 1998; 9:210–213.

59. Berg S. Polytef augmentation urethroplasty. Arch Surg 1973; 107:379–381.

60. Malizia AA, Reiman HM, Myers RP, et al. Migration and granulomatous reaction after periurethral injection of polytef (Teflon). JAMA 1984; 251:3277–3281.

61. Corcos J, Fournier C. Periurethral collagen injection for the treatment of female stress urinary incontinence: 4-year follow-up results. Urology 1999; 54:815–818.

62. Santarosa RP, Blaivas JG. Periurethral injection of autologous fat for the treatment of sphincteric incontinence. J Urol 1994; 151:607–611.

63. Barrett DM, Ghoniem G, Bruskewitz R, et al. The Genisphere: a new percutaneously placed anti-incontinence device. J Urol 1990; 141:224A. [Abstract # 141]

64. Pineda EB, Hadley HR. Urethral injection treatment for stress urinary incontinence. In: Corcos J, Schick E, eds. The urinary sphincter. New York: Marcel Dekker, 2001:497–515.

65. Kassouf W, Capolechio J, Bernardinucci G, Corcos J. Collagen injection for treatment of urinary incontinence in children. J Urol 2001; 165:1666–1668.

66. Fulford SC, Sutton C, Bales G, et al. The fate of the 'modern' artificial urinary sphincter with a follow-up of more than 15 years. Br J Urol 1997; 79:713–716.

67. Spiess PE, Capolicchio JP, Kiruluta G, Salle JP, Berardinucci G, Corcos J. Is an artificial sphincter the best choice for incontinent boys with spina bifida? Review of our long term experience with the AS-800 artificial sphincter. Can J Urol 2002; 9:1486:91.

68. Leadbetter GW Jr. Surgical reconstruction for complete urinary incontinence: a 10 to 22 year follow-up. J Urol 1985; 113:205–206.

69. Tanagho EA. Bladder neck reconstruction for total urinary incontinence: 10 years of experience. J Urol 1981; 125:321–326.

59

Treatment alternatives for different types of neurogenic bladder dysfunction in children

Roman Jednak and Joao Luiz Pippi Salle

Introduction

Congenitally acquired lesions of spinal cord development collectively referred to as neurospinal dysraphisms are the most common cause of neurogenic bladder dysfunction in children. Abnormal bladder innervation is found in the overwhelming majority of patients with myelodysplasia, and, consequently, impaired drainage of the lower and upper urinary tract, if not managed appropriately, can be a significant cause of morbidity.

Management goals include establishing satisfactory bladder emptying, maintaining safe bladder storage pressures to prevent upper urinary tract deterioration, avoiding urinary tract infections, and, in the long term, achieving urinary continence. Fortunately, significant advances in the treatment of children with myelodysplasia have resulted in an impressive decrease in the incidence of upper urinary tract deterioration and marked improvements in the achievement of urinary continence. Naturally, this has translated into decreased morbidity and notable improvements in the quality of life for affected children.

Renal damage, nevertheless, remains a real risk and patients require careful evaluation and follow-up. It should also be emphasized that in the myelodysplastic child, the neurologic lesion and bladder dynamics can change with time. Regular urodynamic testing should be performed both in order to identify worsening parameters before upper urinary tract deterioration occurs and to appropriately select management strategies when trying to establish urinary continence.

Here we outline some of the medical and surgical alternatives available when managing the child with neurogenic bladder. The reported outcomes of various surgical techniques in the pediatric population are reviewed.

Management of the bladder

Anticholinergic medications and clean intermittent catheterization

Bladder management is tailored according to the results of urodynamic evaluation.[1–4] Management goals are the maintenance of a compliant low-pressure reservoir that can be regularly emptied in order to both protect the upper urinary tract from deterioration and achieve urinary continence.

Not all children require early clean intermittent catheterization and/or anticholinergic medications.[2,5] Children who empty the bladder effectively in association with synergic or incompetent sphincter function can be observed closely. Clean intermittent catheterization should be started in those patients with a flaccid bladder that empties poorly.[6–8] Latex catheters should be avoided in order to minimize the risk of developing a latex allergy.[9–12] Antibiotic prophylaxis need not be routinely administered in all children but should be considered in those with documented vesicoureteral reflux.[13–15]

Catheterization is ideally performed at intervals of every 3–4 hours. Clean intermittent catheterization used in combination with an anticholinergic medication is indicated in patients with a poorly compliant or hyperreflexic bladder or in those with detrusor-sphincter dyssynergia.[16–24] Detrusor contraction is primarily mediated by the action of acetylcholine.[25,26]

Anticholinergic agents effectively increase the bladder capacity achieved prior to the onset of an uninhibited contraction, decrease the magnitude of uninhibited contractions, and produce an increase in total bladder capacity. Oxybutynin is the most commonly used anticholinergic and in children can be introduced 2–3 times

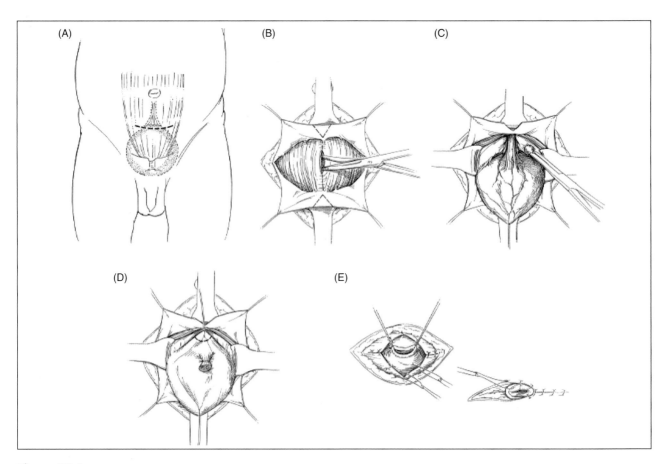

Figure 59.1

Cutaneous vesicostomy. (A) Transverse incision made midway between the umbilicus and symphysis pubis. (B) Modified Pfannenstiel approach. Fascial flaps are raised and the rectus muscles separated in the midline. (C) Urachal remnant, dome, and posterior bladder gradually accessed by progressively retracting the bladder inferiorly and sweeping away the peritoneum. (D) Site for cystostomy selected behind the ligated urachus. (E) Detrusor circumferentially anastomosed to the fascia below the cystostomy. The musosa is matured to the skin with interrupted sutures. (From Keating MA: Incontinent urinary diversion. In Marshall FF (ed): Textbook of Operative Urology. Philadelphia, WB Saunders, 1996, with permission Dr FF Marshall.)

per day at a dose of 0.1–0.2 mg/kg. The medication can be safely used, even in the neonatal period. The most common anticholinergic side-effects encountered in children are dry mouth, constipation, flushing of the skin, blurred vision, and hyperactivity.[27] A newer extended-release formulation that can be administered once daily and may produce fewer adverse effects is also available. Alternatively, intravesical instillation can also be performed. It should be remembered, however, that intravesical instillation is also associated with a similar spectrum of side-effects.[27–33]

Cutaneous vesicostomy

Occasionally, despite maximal efforts, clean intermittent catheterization and anticholinergics are unsuccessful in managing high-risk bladders, controlling reflux, avoiding infections, or preventing upper urinary tract deterioration. In addition, clean intermittent catheterization may not be reliably instituted because of social or anatomic factors. In these cases, cutaneous vesicostomy is a useful and reliable form of temporary urinary diversion in neonates and infants.[34–36] The procedure involves creating a communication between the bladder and the skin of the lower abdominal wall, which allows for free and unobstructed drainage of urine (Figure 59.1).[37] Complications include prolapse, stomal stenosis, stomal eversion, stones, and peristomal dermatitis.[38,39] Anterior bladder wall stomas can allow for posterior bladder wall prolapse. The incidence of prolapse can therefore best be minimized by using a posterior portion of the bladder wall cephalad to the urachus for the vesicostomy.

Bladder augmentation

The objective of bladder augmentation is to create a low-pressure storage reservoir of sufficient capacity to preserve upper urinary tract function and maintain or establish urinary continence when maximal medical therapy is unsuccessful. Advances in surgical techniques have enabled the attainment of these goals with a high degree of reliability, and the experience with bladder enlargement has been extended to a variety of materials and techniques.[40] Most commonly, intestinal segments are selected for bladder augmentation.[41] More recent developments have focused on techniques attempting to preserve the bladder urothelium and thereby avoiding the introduction of intestinal mucosa into the urinary tract.[42–45] Irrespective of the technique used, bladder emptying is usually impaired to some degree and, consequently, most children require clean intermittent catheterization postoperatively. All patients should additionally be made aware of the risk of bladder perforation, a potentially life-threatening complication that may occur following any form of bladder augmentation.[46]

Techniques which do not preserve the urothelium

Ileo- and colocystoplasty. Bladder augmentation using ileum or colon has proven to be a reliable means of increasing bladder capacity and reducing bladder pressures.[47–52] The incorporation of these intestinal segments into the urinary tract, however, is associated with a number of long-term complications.[41] Because of the young patient population typically being treated, this long-term exposure to these complications is of significant concern. Complications most commonly observed include mucus production, bacterial colonization, electrolyte imbalances, metabolic acidosis, somatic growth retardation, and vitamin B_{12} deficiency.[53–57] Other concerns are the risk of calculus formation and the development of malignancy (Table 59.1).[58–66]

Gastrocystoplasty. Stomach first gained popularity as an alternative to colon or ileum in children with chronic renal failure and azotemia as a direct result of its natural acid-secreting ability, which does not worsen the metabolic acidosis.[67,68] The technique is also useful when bowel resection is not an option, as is the case with short-bowel syndrome. Mucus production is less problematic and the acidic urine may also reduce bacterial colonization and the incidence of urinary tract infections. Specific complications include intermittent hematuria, metabolic alkalosis, and the hematuria–dysuria syndrome, which is characterized by bladder or urethral pain and hematuria in

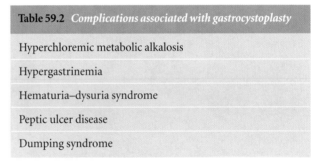

Table 59.1 *Long-term complications associated with ileo- and colocystoplasty*

	Ileum	Colon
Medical		
Hyperchloremic metabolic acidosis	+	+
Vitamin B_{12} deficiency	+	−
Bile salt malabsorption	+	−
Somatic growth retardation	+	−
Osteomalacia/rickets	+	+
Alterations in drug metabolism	+	+
Mucus production	+	+
Bacterial colonization	+	+
Malignancy	+	+
Surgical		
Calculus formation	+	+
Bladder perforation	+	+
Bowel obstruction	+	+

Table 59.2 *Complications associated with gastrocystoplasty*

Hyperchloremic metabolic alkalosis
Hypergastrinemia
Hematuria–dysuria syndrome
Peptic ulcer disease
Dumping syndrome

the absence of infection (Table 59.2).[69,70] Children with incontinence or renal insufficiency/oliguria tend to experience more problems with the hematuria–dysuria syndrome. Since the hematuria–dysuria syndrome does not always respond well to histamine antagonists, this may pose a significant problem in children with normal bladder and urethral sensation.

Techniques which preserve the urothelium

Ureterocystoplasty. The dilated ureter serving a non-functioning kidney can occasionally be used for bladder augmentation (Figure 59.2).[71,72] Success with ureterocystoplasty has been excellent and, since the urothelium is preserved, acid–base disturbances and mucus production are not a problem.[73] In addition, the procedure can be performed using an exclusively extraperitoneal approach.[74] Since the procedure requires a severely dilated ureter and

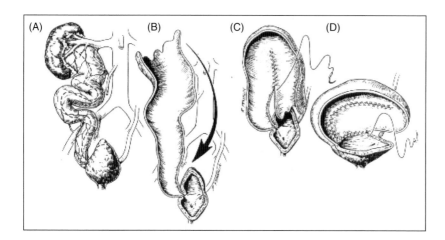

Figure 59.2
Operative stages of ureteral bladder augmentation. (A) Normal blood supply to ureter. (B) Ureteral detubularization following mobilization. (C) Reconfiguration of ureter into U-shaped patch. (D) Anastomosing ureteral patch to native bivalved bladder. (From Churchill BM, et al. Ureteral bladder augmentation. J Urol 1993; 150:716–720.)

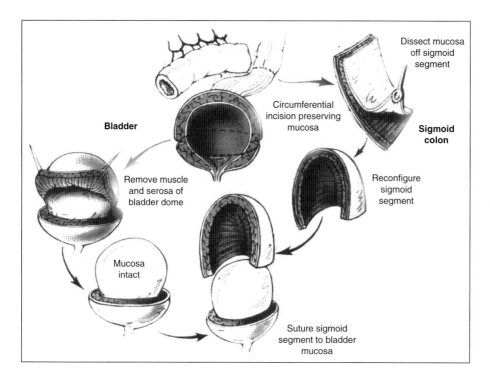

Figure 59.3
Operative technique of seromuscular colocystoplasty lined with urothelium. (Reprinted with modification from Urology 44, Buson et al, Seromuscular colocystoplasty lined with urothelium: experimental study, pp. 743–748, Copyright 1994, with permission from Elsevier Science.)

nonfunctioning kidney, however, its usefulness is limited to specific clinical situations.

Autoaugmentation. Excision or incision of the diseased detrusor with preservation of the urothelium creates a urothelium diverticulum that serves to augment the bladder.[75,76] The benefits of preserving the urothelium are maintained but the reported urodynamic outcomes have varied. Some reports have described only slight improvements in bladder capacity, whereas others have noted improvements in capacity with persistently high bladder pressures.[77–79] One series has reported lower success rates in patients with neurogenic bladder dysfunction.[80]

Seromuscular enterocystoplasty. The complications associated with enterocystoplasty are attributable to the presence of intestinal mucosa within the urinary tract.[41,53–57] Seromuscular enterocystoplasty makes use of demucosalized segments of ileum, colon, or stomach to augment the bladder and thereby avoid the potential disadvantages of urine contact with intestinal mucosa.[43–45] The procedure can be performed with or without preservation of the urothelium. When the urothelium is preserved the detrusor is excised, leaving a urothelial diverticulum over which the seromuscular patch is then placed (Figure 59.3).[81–86] When no attempt is made to preserve the urothelium, a standard clam enterocystoplasty technique is used and the seromuscular patch is used to augment the bladder using the standard enterocystoplasty technique.[87–89]

The importance of postoperative bladder distention has consistently been stressed as essential to achieving an optimal result in all reports describing the technique.[83,86–88,90] This can be achieved by one of two methods. When the urothelium is preserved and the seromuscular patch is positioned over the exposed urothelial bubble, a Foley catheter can be left to straight drainage and positioned 20–30 cm above the level of the symphysis pubis for a period of 4–5 days.[81–83,86,90] A competent bladder outlet is important to optimize bladder distention in this case, and a concomitant bladder outlet procedure is recommended in patients with poor outlet resistance. In addition, since urothelial integrity is critical to minimizing postoperative leaks, performing concomitant procedures that violate the urothelium should be avoided.[83,86,90]

An alternative method makes use of an intravesical silicone mold that maintains the seromuscular patch in a distended state for a period of 10–14 days.[87,88] This technique can be used both when the urothelium is and is not preserved. Short-term results to date have been encouraging, with postoperative urodynamic parameters and continence rates paralleling those of standard augmentation techniques. Mucus production and electrolyte abnormalities do not appear to be a problem.

Management of the bladder outlet

Medications to increase outlet resistance

Adrenergic nerves innervate the muscular fibers of the bladder base. Alpha agonists (ephedrine, pseudoephedrine) produce an increase in bladder outlet resistance and on occasion may improve urine storage.[91–93] The results with these agents, however, are often less than satisfactory, but improvements in continence can occasionally be obtained in children with mild degrees of wetting due to sphincteric incompetence. In addition, side-effects, including hypertension, anxiety, headaches, and insomnia, may be problematic, so that the use of these agents in managing the incompetent bladder outlet remains limited.

Periurethral injection of bulking agents

Bulking agents such as collagen, Teflon, and, more recently, dextranomer/hyaluronic acid copolymer can be injected submucosally at the bladder neck to facilitate mucosal coaptation and achieve continence.[93–103] Continence rates are difficult to interpret since variable criteria have been reported to define success. In addition, some authors have failed to show a durable response with long-term follow-up.[101] When

defined as a dry interval of 4 hours, continence rates are in the range of 5–63%. Success is often dependent on more than one injection, and as a result cost may become an important issue. Predictors of response to the injection of bulking agents are inconsistent but at least one group has noted improved outcomes in patients with detrusor areflexia and low-pressure bladders.[100] Attempts at defining urodynamic characteristics that may serve as predictors of long-term success have been unsuccessful.[104] Importantly, collagen injection has not been found to interfere with bladder neck surgery if this is subsequently required.

Bladder neck suspension and fascial sling procedures

The use of bladder neck suspension techniques for the treatment of the pediatric neurogenic bladder has not gained widespread use. Reported continence rates achieved in girls in association with bladder augmentation have been at least 80%, with the longest period of follow-up being 30 months.

Fascial slings improve outlet resistance by compression and elevation of the urethra. Reported continence rates have varied from 40 to 100% over a follow-up period of at most 4.5 years.[109–118] The majority of patients have been girls. Attempts at improving outlet resistance have led to a number of modifications, including concomitant bladder neck tapering or circumferentially wrapping the bladder neck with rectus fascia, a rectus myofascial flap, or a strip of anterior bladder wall.[119–125] Bladder augmentation is often necessary to improve continence rates and intermittent catheterization is frequently required. Success using the procedure in boys has been reported in several series.[110,113,115–119,121,122,124,125]

Urethral lengthening procedures

The Kropp and Pippi Salle procedures create a fixed increase in bladder outlet resistance by using a portion of the anterior bladder wall to construct a one-way valve. The Kropp procedure consists of performing urethral lengthening with a tubularized segment of anterior bladder wall, which is reimplanted in the posterior intertrigonal area, creating a one-way valve mechanism similar to the antireflux mechanism procedures used for correction of vesicoureteral reflux (Figure 59.4).[126] Increases in intravesical pressures are transmitted to the submucosal urethral tube, thereby increasing closure pressure and preventing incontinence.

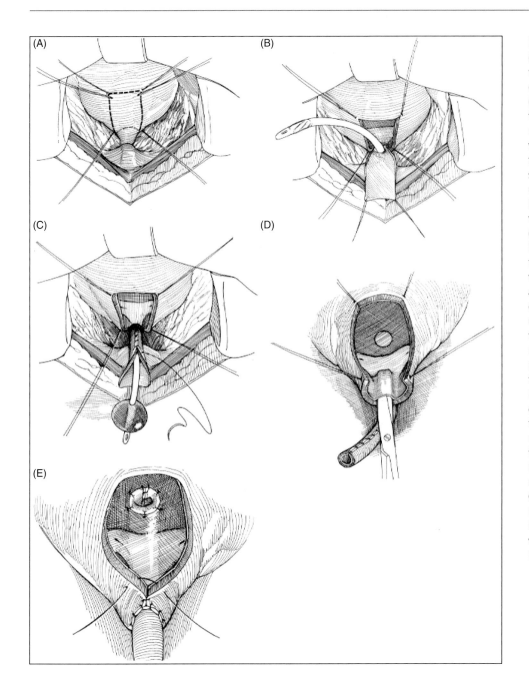

(A)
(B)
(C)
(D)
(E)

Figure 59.4
(A) An anterior bladder wall flap (5 to 7 cm x 2.5 cm wide) is outlined. (B) The junction of the trigone and the bladder neck is identified from within and the mucosa of the bladder neck separated from the urethra. (C) The anterior bladder flap is tubularized with a one-layer suture (interrupted suture in the last 2 cm). (D) A posterior trigonal tunnel (6 x 3 cm wide) is created beginning at the bladder neck and carried upward beyond the ureteral orifices. (E) The tubularized flap is reimplanted in the posterior submucosal tunnel and the anterior bladder wall is sutured over the bladder neck at the base of the neourethra. (Reprinted from Pippi Salle JL: Urethral lengthening for urinary incontinence. In Gearhart, Mouriquand, Rink (eds): Pediatric Urology, Copyright 2001, with permission from Elsevier Science.)

The procedure is technically demanding and, consequently, revisions have been proposed to facilitate creation of the submucosal tube. Mollard and colleagues described resection of the muscular layer of the distal 50% of the tube to make it more pliable and facilitate submucosal tunneling.[127] Snodgrass made use of a longitudinal bladder incision starting from the bladder neck and extending up between the ureteral orifices into which the detrusor tube was laid. Lateral mucosal flaps are then secured to either side of the tube.[128] The Pippi Salle procedure consists of fashioning an anterior bladder wall flap, which is then sutured to the posterior bladder wall in an onlay fashion. The neourethra is then covered with bladder wall and lateral mucosal flaps to fashion a submucosal tunnel (Figure 59.5).[129–131]

Both these techniques commit the patient to intermittent catheterization, which at times may be difficult.[126,128,130,132–134] Overall, more catheterization difficulties seem to be encountered with the Kropp procedure. As a result, thought should be given to performing a concomitant continent catheterizable channel to facilitate intermittent catheterization postoperatively.[135] Because bladder wall is sacrificed to lengthen the urethra, the postoperative development of low bladder capacity and poor compliance is a risk and, consequently, concomitant bladder augmentation is often required with both techniques.[128,130–133,135–137]

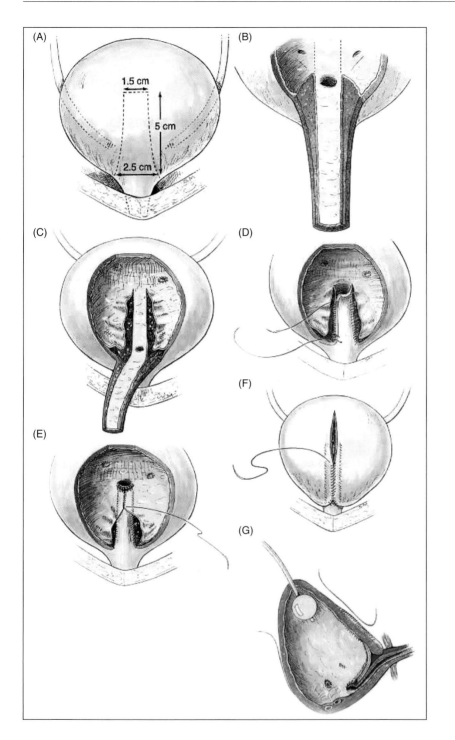

Figure 59.5
(A) Anterior bladder wall flap with a wide base to improve vascular supply. (B) The flap mucosal edges are excised from the muscle to achieve a narrow rectangular mucosal strip with a rich blood supply. This allows a non-overlapping two-layer anastomosis. (C) Parallel incisions are made in the posterior trigonal mucosa. If reimplantation is necessary, both ureters are disconnected and reimplanted superiorly in a cross-trigonal fashion. (D) The anterior flap is dropped onto the incised posterior mucosa and sutured in two layers (mucosa–mucosal and muscle–muscular) to the posterior wall in an onlay fashion. (E) The posterior mucosa lateral to either side of the trigonal incision is mobilized from the detrusor and used to cover the neourethra. (F) The anterior bladder wall is closed in front of the intravesical urethra in a tension-free manner. Tension over the neourethra can cause impairment of the flap vascular supply. (G) Schematic lateral view of the neourethra demonstrating its intravesical position and the flap-valve mechanism when the bladder fills. (From Pippi Salle JL, et al. Modifications of and extended applications for the Pippi Salle procedure. World J Urol 1998; 16: 279–284, Spinger-Verlag publishers, with permission.)

As a result of the potential risk for upper tract deterioration should bladder storage characteristics worsen, careful radiologic and urodynamic follow-up is essential.

Reported continence rates are in the range of 77–91% for the Kropp[126–128,132,133] procedure, whereas those rates for the Pippi Salle[128,130–133,135–137] procedure are in the range of 64–94%. Outcome with the Pippi Salle procedure tends to be more favorable in girls.[136–138]

The artificial urinary sphincter

The artificial urinary sphincter was first introduced in 1974 and has since undergone a number of improvements in design. Continence is achieved by compression of the bladder neck or urethra by an inflatable cuff that can be intermittently deflated to allow for catheterization or voiding. The preferred site of placement in children is around the bladder neck. Patients that empty their bladder without the need for catheterization prior to surgery may continue to do so following sphincter placement[142–150] but, if necessary, intermittent catheterization can be instituted safely.[151,152] It is essential that bladder capacity and compliance be evaluated prior to placing an artificial sphincter, but admittedly this may be difficult in the presence of an incompetent bladder neck.

Some centers have found that preoperative urodynamics may not accurately predict which patient will go on to require bladder augmentation[154] but, nevertheless, failure to recognize a clearly noncompliant bladder preoperatively may put the upper urinary tracts at an unnecessary and significant risk when outlet resistance is increased. In cases where bladder augmentation is required, this can be performed concomitantly without increasing the risk of complications.[155,156]

Despite having favorable preoperative bladder dynamics some patients may develop deterioration in bladder compliance and, therefore, postoperative urodynamic studies and careful radiological and urodynamic follow-up are essential.[143,145–149,157,158] The most common complications include mechanical failure, erosion, and infection. Both erosion and infection result in permanent failure. Revision of the device has been high in most published series, but more recent reports have noted a considerable improvement in the revision rate. Given that the artificial sphincter is a mechanical device with a finite life span, however, it can be expected that most patients will at some time require surgery for revision. Overall, continence rates from 61% to over 95% have been reported in those children having a functional artificial urinary sphincter still in place.[143,144,146–149,159–161]

Conclusions

The treatment of neurogenic bladder dysfunction in children has been a major driving force behind a myriad of innovative surgical solutions: unfortunately, we must accept that none of these are perfect. It also needs to be kept in mind that the successful management of any given patient is defined by a multitude of variables and is not simply a good surgical outcome. Management goals are consistent from patient to patient, but the management strategies are not simply defined by urodynamic studies and urinary tract imaging. Often, the patient's physical limitations as well as their emotional and social needs play a critical role in determining a rational therapeutic strategy.

Before any surgical reconstruction is entertained, available medical management options should be exhausted. Bladder augmentation remains a reliable and highly successful means of dealing with the small capacity, poorly compliant, or hyperreflexic bladder. Far more controversy surrounds the management of the incompetent bladder

neck and the inherent difficulty of dealing with bladder neck incompetence underlies the variety of reconstructive techniques that has been described over the years. The most favorable management approach in a specific clinical situation is therefore often defined by surgeon preference against the background of clearly defined patient expectations. Urodynamic studies performed with a balloon catheter to occlude the bladder neck may facilitate the process.

References

1. McGuire EJ, Woodside JR, Borden TA, Weiss RM. Prognostic value of urodynamic testing in myelodysplastic patients. J Urol 1981; 126:205–209.

2. Bauer SB, Hallett M, Khoshbin S, et al. Predictive value of urodynamic evaluation in newborns with myelodysplasia. JAMA 1984; 252:650–652.

3. Sidi AA, Peng W, Gonzalez R. The value of urodynamic testing in the management of newborns with myelodysplasia: a prospective study. J Urol 1986; 135:90–93.

4. Wang SC, McGuire EJ, Bloom DA. A bladder pressure management system for myelodysplasia – clinical outcome. J Urol 1988; 140:1499–1502.

5. Fernandes ET, Reinberg Y, Vernier R, Gonzalez R. Neurogenic bladder dysfunction in children: review of pathophysiology and current management. J Pediatr 1994; 124:1–7.

6. Lapides J, Diokno AC, Silber S, Lowe BS. Clean, intermittent self-catheterization in the treatment of urinary tract disease. J Urol 1972; 107:458–461.

7. Lapides J, Diokno AC, Lowe BS, Kalish M. Followup on unsterile, intermittent self-catheterization. J Urol 1974; 111:184–187.

8. Lapides J, Diokno AC, Gould FR, Lowe BS. Further observations on self-catheterization. J Urol 1976; 116:169–171.

9. Slater JE, Mostello LA, Shaer C. Rubber-specific IgE in children with spina bifida. J Urol 1991; 146:578–579.

10. Ellsworth PI, Merguerian PA, Klein RB, Rozycki AA. Evaluation and risk factors of latex allergy in spina bifida patients: is it preventable? J Urol 1993; 150:691–693.

11. Pasquariello CA, Lowe DA, Schwartz RE. Intraoperative anaphylaxis to latex. Pediatrics 1993; 91:983–986.

12. Nguyen DH, Burns MW, Shapiro GG, et al. Intraoperative cardiovascular collapse secondary to latex allergy. J Urol 1991; 146:571–574.

13. Kass EJ, Koff SA, Diokno AC, Lapides J. The significance of bacilluria in children on long-term intermittent catheterization. J Urol 1981; 126:223–225.

14. Ottolini MC, Shaer CM, Rushton HG, et al. Relationship of asymptomatic bacteriuria and renal scarring in children with neuropathic bladders who are practicing clean intermittent catheterization. J Pediatr 1995; 127:368–372.

15. Schlager TA, Anderson S, Trudell J, Hendley JO. Nitrofurantoin prophylaxis for bacteriuria and urinary tract infection in children with neurogenic bladder on intermittent catheterization. J Pediatr 1998; 132:704–708.

16. Diokno AC, Kass E, Lapides J. New approach to myelodysplasia. J Urol 1976; 116:771–772.

17. Crooks KK, Enrile BG, Wise HA. The results of clean intermittent catheterization on the abnormal upper urinary tracts of children with myelomeningocele. Ohio State Med J 1981; 77:377–379.

18. Perez-Marrero R, Dimmock W, Churchill BM, Hardy BE. Clean intermittent catheterization in myelomeningocele children less than 3 years old. J Urol 1982; 128:779–781.

19. Geraniotis E, Koff SA, Enrile B. The prophylactic use of clean intermittent catheterization in the treatment of infants and young children with myelomeningocele and neurogenic bladder dysfunction. J Urol 1988; 139:85–86.

20. Joseph DB, Bauer SB, Colodny AH, et al. Clean, intermittent catheterization of infants with neurogenic bladder. Pediatrics 1989; 84:78–82.

21. Klose AG, Sackett CK, Mesrobian H-GJ. Management of children with myelodysplasia: urological alternatives. J Urol 1990; 144:1446–1449.

22. Baskin LS, Kogan BA, Benard F. Treatment of infants with neurogenic bladder dysfunction using anticholinergic drugs and intermittent catheterisation. Br J Urol 1990; 66:532–534.

23. Kasabian NG, Bauer SB, Dyro FM, et al. The prophylactic value of clean intermittent catheterization and anticholinergic medication in newborns and infants with myelomeningocele at risk of developing urinary tract deterioration. Am J Dis Child 1992; 146:840–843.

24. Edelstein RA, Bauer SB, Kelly MD, et al. The long-term urological response of neonates with myelodysplasia treated proactively with intermittent catheterization and anticholinergic therapy. J Urol 1995; 154:1500–1504.

25. de Groat WC, Yoshimura N. Pharmacology of the lower urinary tract. Ann Rev Pharmacol Toxicol 2001; 41:691–721.

26. Yamanishi T, Chapple CR, Chess-Williams R. Which muscarinic receptor is important in the bladder? World J Urol 2001; 19:299–306.

27. Andersson KE, Chapple CR. Oxybutynin and the overactive bladder. World J Urol 2001; 19:319–323.

28. Greenfield SP, Fera M. The use of intravesical oxybutynin chloride in children with neurogenic bladder. J Urol 1991; 146:532–534.

29. Kasabian NG, Vlachiotis JD, Lais A, et al. The use of intravesical oxybutynin chloride in patients with detrusor hypertonicity and detrusor hyperreflexia. J Urol 1994; 151:944–945.

30. Kaplinsky R, Greenfield S, Wan J, Fera M. Expanded followup of intravesical oxybutynin chloride use in children with neurogenic bladder. J Urol 1996; 156:753–756.

31. Painter KA, Vates TS, Bukowski TP, et al. Long-term intravesical oxybutynin chloride therapy in children with myelodysplasia. J Urol 1996; 156:1459–1462.

32. Palmer LS, Zebold K, Firlit CF, Kaplan WE. Complications of intravesical oxybutynin chloride therapy in the pediatric myelomeningocele population. J Urol 1997; 157:638–640.

33. Ferrara P, D'Aleo CM, Tarquini E, et al. Side-effects of oral or intravesical oxybutynin chloride in children with spina bifida. BJU Int 2001; 87:674–677.

34. Cohen JS, Harbach LB, Kaplan GW. Cutaneous vesicostomy for temporary urinary diversion in infants with neurogenic bladder dysfunction. J Urol 1978; 119:120–121.

35. Mandell J, Bauer SB, Colodny AH, Retik AB. Cutaneous vesicostomy in infancy. J Urol 1981; 126:92–93.

36. Snyder HM III, Kalichman MA, Charney E, Duckett JW. Vesicostomy for neurogenic bladder with spina bifida: followup. J Urol 1983; 130:724–726.

37. Duckett JW Jr. Cutaneous vesicostomy in childhood: the Blocksom technique. Urol Clin N Am 1974; 1:485–495.

38. Hurwitz RS, Ehrlich RM. Complications of cutaneous vesicostomy. Urol Clin N Am 1974; 10:503–508.

39. Duckett JW, Ziylan O. Uses and abuses of vesicostomy. AUA Update Series 1995; 14:130–135.

40. Duel BP, Gonzalez R, Barthold JS. Alternative techniques for augmentation cystoplasty. J Urol 1999; 159:998–1005.

41. Gough DCS. Enterocystoplasty. BJU Int 2001; 88:739–743.

42. Ureterocystolasty: the latest developments. BJU Int 2001; 88:744–751.

43. Jednak R, Schmike CM, Ludwikowski B, González R. Seromuscular colocystoplasty. BJU Int 2001; 88:752–756.

44. Close CE. Autoaugmentation gastrocystoplasty. BJU Int 2001; 88:757–761.

45. Lima SVC, Araújo LAP, Vilar FO, et al. Experience with demucosalized ileum for bladder augmentation. BJU Int 2001; 88:762–764.

46. Shekarriz B, Upadhyay J, Demirbilek S, et al. Surgical complications of bladder augmentation: comparison between various enterocystoplasties in 133 patients. Urology 2000; 55:123–128.

47. Hendren WH, Hendren RB. Bladder augmentation: experience with 129 children and young adults. J Urol 1990; 144:445–453.

48. Mitchell ME, Kulb TB, Backes DJ. Intestinocystoplasty in combination with clean intermittent catheterization in the management of vesical dysfunction. J Urol 1986; 136:288–291.

49. Decter RM, Bauer SB, Mandell J, et al. Small bowel augmentation in children with neurogenic bladder: an initial report of urodynamic findings. J Urol 1987; 138:1014–1016.

50. Mitchell ME, Piser JA. Intestinocystoplasty and total bladder replacement in children and young adults: followup in 129 cases. J Urol 1987; 138:579–584.

51. Krishna A, Gough DCS, Fishwick J, Bruce J. Ileocystoplasty in children: assessing safety and success. Eur Urol 1995; 27:62–66.

52. Wang K, Yamataka A, Morioka A, et al. Complications after sigmoidocolocystoplasty: review of 100 cases at one institution. J Pediatr Surg 1999; 34:1672–1677.

53. McDougal WS. Metabolic complications of urinary intestinal diversion. J Urol 1992; 147:1199–1208.

54. Stampfer DS, McDougal WS, McGovern FJ. Metabolic and nutritional complications. Urol Clin N Am 1997; 24:715–722.

55. Nurse DE, Mundy AR. Metabolic complications of cystoplasty. Br J Urol 1989; 63:165–170.

56. Wagstaff KE, Woodhouse CRJ, Duffy PG, Ransley PG. Delayed linear growth in children with enterocystoplasties. Br J Urol 1992; 69:314–317.

57. Mundy AR, Nurse DE. Calcium balance, growth and skeletal mineralisation in patients with cystoplasties. Br J Urol 1992; 69:257–259.

58. Blyth B, Ewalt DH, Duckett JW, Snyder HM. Lithogenic properties of enterocystoplasty. J Urol 1992; 148:575–577.

59. Palmer LS, Franco I, Kogan SJ, et al. Urolithiasis in children following augmentation cystoplasty. J Urol 1993; 150:726–729.

60. Nurse DE, McInerney PD, Thomas PJ, Mundy AR. Stones in enterocystoplasties. Br J Urol 1996; 77:684–687.

61. Khoury AE, Salomon M, Doche R, et al. Stone formation following augmentation cystoplasty: the role of intestinal mucus. J Urol 1997; 158:1133–1137.

62. Kronner KM, Casale AJ, Cain MP, et al. Bladder calculi in the pediatric augmented bladder. J Urol 1998; 160:1096–1098.

63. Mathoera RB, Kok DJ, Nijman RJM. Bladder calculi in augmentation cystoplasty in children. Urology 2000; 56:482–487.

64. Filmer RB, Spencer JR. Malignancies in bladder augmentations and intestinal conduits. J Urol 1990; 143:671–678.

65. Trieger BFG, Marshall FF. Carcinogenesis and the use of intestinal segments in the urinary tract. Urol Clin N Am 1991; 18:737–742.

66. Malone MJ, Izes JK, Hurley LJ. Carcinogenesis. The fate of intestinal segments used in urinary reconstruction. Urol Clin N Am 1997; 24:723–728.

67. Adams MC, Mitchell ME, Rink RC. Gastrocystoplasty: an alternative solution to the problem of urological reconstruction in the severely compromised patient. J Urol 1988; 140:1152–1156.

68. Sheldon CA, Gilbert A, Wacksman J, Lewis AG. Gastrocystoplasty: technical and metabolic characteristics of the most versatile childhood bladder augmentation modality. J Pediatr Surg 1995; 30:283–287.

69. Nguyen DH, Bain MA, Salmonson KL, et al. The syndrome of dysuria and hematuria in pediatric urinary reconstruction with stomach. J Urol 1993; 150:707–709.

70. Kinahan TJ, Khoury AE, McLorie GA, Churchill BM. Omeprazole in post-gastrocystoplasty metabolic alkalosis and aciduria. J Urol 1992; 147:435–437.

71. Bellinger MF. Ureterocystoplasty: a unique method for vesical augmentation in children. J Urol 1993; 149:811–813.

72. Churchill BM, Aliabadi H, Landau EH, et al. Ureteral bladder augmentation. J Urol 1993; 150:716–720.

73. Landau EH, Jayanthi VR, Khoury AE, et al. Bladder augmentation: ureterocystoplasty versus ileocystoplasty. J Urol 1994; 152:716–719.

74. Dewan PA, Nicholls EA, Goh DW. Ureterocystoplasty: an extraperitoneal urothelial bladder augmentation technique. Eur Urol 1994; 26:85–89.

75. Cartwright PC, Snow BW. Bladder autoaugmentation: partial detrusor excision to augment the bladder without use of bowel. J Urol 1989; 142:1050–1053.

76. Cartwright PC, Snow BW. Bladder autoaugmentation: early clinical experience. J Urol 1989; 142:505–508.

77. Reid C, Moorehead JD, Hadley HR. Experience with detrusorectomy procedures. J Urol 1990; 143:331A.

78. Stothers L, Johnson H, Arnold W, et al. Bladder autoaugmentation by vesicomyotomy in the pediatric neurogenic bladder. Urology 1994; 44:110–113.

79. Skobejko-Wlodarska L, Strulak K, Nachulewicz P, Szymkiewicz C. Bladder autoaugmentation in myelodysplastic children. Br J Urol 1998; 81(Suppl 3):114–116.

80. Swami KS, Feneley RCL, Hammonds JC, Abrams P. Detrusor myectomy for detrusor overactivity: a minimum 1-year follow-up. Br J Urol 1998; 81:68–72.

81. Dewan PA, Stefanek W. Autoaugmentation colocystoplasty. Pediatr Surg Int 1994; 9:526–528.

82. Dewan PA, Stefanek W. Autoaugmentation gastrocystoplasty: early clinical results. Br J Urol 1994; 74:460–464.

83. González R, Buson H, Churphena R, Reinberg Y. Seromuscular colocystoplasty lined with urothelium: experience with 16 patients. Urology 1995; 45:124–129.

84. Nguyen DH, Mitchell ME, Horowitz M, et al. Demucosalized augmentation gastrocystoplasty with bladder autoaugmentation in pediatric patients. J Urol 1996; 156:206–209.

85. Dayanç M, Kilciler M, Tan Ö, et al. A new approach to bladder augmentation in children: seromuscular enterocystoplasty. Br J Urol 1999; 84:103–107.

86. Jednak R, Schimke CM, Barroso U Jr, et al. Further experience with seromuscular colocystoplasty lined with urothelium. J Urol 2000; 164:2045–2049.

87. Lima SVC, Araújo LAP, Vilar FO, et al. Nonsecretory sigmoid cystoplasty: experimental and clinical results. J Urol 1995; 153: 1651–1654.

88. Lima SVC, Araújo LAP, Montoro M, et al. The use of demucosalized bowel to augment small contracted bladders. Br J Urol 1998; 82:436–439.

89. de Badiola F, Ruiz E, Puigdevall J, et al. Sigmoid cystoplasty with argon beam without mucosa. J Urol 2001; 165:2253–2255.

90. Vates TS, Smith C, Gonzalez R. Importance of early bladder distension for the success of the seromuscular colocystoplasty lined with urothelium. Pediatrics 1997; 100:564.

91. Diokno AC, Taub M. Ephedrine in treatment of urinary incontinence. Urology 1975; 5:624–625.

92. Raezer DM, Benson GS, Wein AJ, Duckett JW Jr. The functional approach to the management of the pediatric neuropathic bladder: a clinical study. J Urol 1977; 117:649–654.

93. Decter RM. Pharmacologic management of the neurogenic bladder. Probl Urol 1994; 8:373–388.

93. Vorstman B, Lockhart JL, Kaufman MR, Politano V. Polytetrafluoroethylene injection for urinary incontinence in children. J Urol 1985; 133:248–250.

94. Wan J, McGuire EJ, Bloom DA, Ritchey ML. The treatment of urinary incontinence in children using glutaraldehyde cross-linked collagen. J Urol 1992; 148:127–130.

95. Capozza N, Caione P, De Gennaro M, et al. Endoscopic treatment of vesico-ureteric reflux and urinary incontinence: technical problems in the paediatric patient. Br J Urol 1995; 75:538–542.

96. Leonard MP, Decter A, Mix LW, et al. Treatment of urinary incontinence in children by endoscopically directed bladder neck injection of collagen. J Urol 1996; 156:637–641.

97. Bomalaski MD, Bloom DA, McGuire EJ, Panzl A. Glutaraldehyde cross-linked collagen in the treatment of urinary incontinence in children. J Urol 1996; 155:699–702.

98. Pérez LM, Smith EA, Parrott TS, et al. Submucosal bladder neck injection of bovine dermal collagen for stress urinary incontinence in the pediatric population. J Urol, part 2, 1996; 156:633–363.

99. Sundaram CP, Reinberg Y, Aliabadi HA. Failure to obtain durable results with collagen implantation in children with urinary incontinence. J Urol 1997; 157:2306–2307.

100. Silveri M, Capitanucci ML, Mosiello G, et al. Endoscopic treatment for urinary incontinence in children with a congenital neuropathic bladder. Br J Urol 1998; 82:694–697.

101. Kassouf W, Capolicchio G, Berardinucci G, Corcos J. Collagen injection for treatment of urinary incontinence in children. J Urol 2001; 165:1666–1668.

102. Caione P, Capozza N. Endoscopic treatment of urinary incontinence in pediatric patients: 2-year experience with dextranomer/hyaluronic acid copolymer. J Urol, part 2, 2002; 168:1868–1871.

103. Lottmann HB, Margaryan M, Bernuy M, et al. The effect of endoscopic injections of dextranomer based implants on continence and bladder capacity: a prospective study of 31 patients. J Urol 2002; 168:1863–1867.

104. Kim YH, Kattan MW, Boone TB. Correlation of urodynamic results and urethral coaptation with success after transurethral collagen injection. Urology 1997; 50:941–948.

105. Woodside JR, Borden TA. Suprapubic endoscopic vesical neck suspension for the management of urinary incontinence in myelodysplastic girls. J Urol 1986; 135:97–99.

106. Raz S, Ehrlich RM, Zeidman EJ, et al. Surgical treatment of the incontinent female patient with myelomeningocele. J Urol 1988; 139:524–527.

107. Gearhart JP, Jeffs RD. Suprapubic bladder neck suspension for the management of urinary incontinence in the myelodysplastic girl. J Urol 1988; 140:1296–1298.

108. Freedman ER, Singh G, Donnell SC, et al. Combined bladder neck suspension and augmentation cystoplasty for neuropathic incontinence in female patients. Br J Urol 1994; 73:621–624.

109. McGuire EJ, Wang C-C, Usitalo H, Savastano J. Modified pubovaginal sling in girls with myelodysplasia. J Urol 1986; 135:94–96.

110. Raz S, McGuire EJ, Ehrlich RM, et al. Fascial sling to correct male neurogenic sphincter incompetence: the McGuire/Raz approach. J Urol 1988; 139:528–531.

111. Bauer SB, Peters CA, Colodny AH, et al. The use of rectus fascia to manage urinary incontinence. J Urol 1989; 142:516–519.

112. Elder JS. Periurethral and puboprostatic sling repair for incontinence in patients with myelodysplasia. J Urol 1990; 144:434–437.

113. Decter RM. Use of the fascial sling for neurogenic incontinence: lessons learned. J Urol 1993; 150:683–686.

114. Gormley EA, Bloom DA, McGuire EJ, Ritchey ML. Pubovaginal slings for the management of urinary incontinence in female adolescents. J Urol 1994; 152:822–825.

115. Kakizaki H, Shibata T, Shinno Y, et al. Fascial sling for the management of urinary incontinence due to spincteric incompetence. J Urol 1995; 153:648–649.

116. Pérez LM, Smith EA, Broecker BH, et al. Outcome of sling cystourethropexy in the pediatric population: a critical review. J Urol 1996; 156:642–646.

117. Dik P, van Gool JG, De Jong TPVM. Urinary continence and erectile function after bladder neck sling suspension in male patients with spinal dysraphism. BJU Int 1999; 83:971–975.

118. Austin PF, Westney OL, Leng WW, et al. Advantages of rectus fascial slings for urinary incontinence in children with neuropathic bladders. J Urol, part 2, 2001; 165:2369–2372.

119. Herschorn S, Radomski SB. Fascial slings and bladder neck tapering in the treatment of male neurogenic incontinence. J Urol 1992; 147:1073–1075.

120. Ghoniem GM. Bladder neck wrap: a modified fascial sling in treatment of incontinence in myelomeningocele patients. Eur Urol 1994; 25:340–342.

121. Walker RD, Flack CE, Hawkins-Lee B, et al. Rectus fascial wrap: early results of a modification of the rectus fascial sling. J Urol 1995; 154:771–774.

122. Kurzrock EA, Lowe P, Hardy BE. Bladder wall pedicle wraparound sling for urinary incontinence in children. J Urol 1996; 155:305–308.

123. Barthold JS, Rodriguez E, Freedman AL, et al. Results of the rectus fascial sling and wrap procedures for the treatment of neurogenic sphincteric incontinence. J Urol 1999; 161:272–274.

124. Walker RD, Erhard M, Starling J. Long-term evaluation of rectus fascial wrap in patients with spina bifida. J Urol 2000; 164:485–486.

125. Mingin GC, Youngren K, Stock JA, Hanna MK. The rectus myofascial wrap in the management of urethral sphincter incompetence. BJU Int 2002; 90:550–553.

126. Kropp KA, Angwafo FF. Urethral lengthening and reimplantation for neurogenic incontinence in children. J Urol 1986; 135:533–536.

127. Mollard P, Mouriquand P, Joubert P. Urethral lengthening for neurogenic urinary incontinence (Kropp's procedure): results of 16 cases. J Urol 1990; 143:95–97.

128. Snodgrass W. A simplified Kropp procedure for incontinence. J Urol 158:1049–1052.

129. Pippi Salle JL, de Fraga JCS, Amarante A, et al. Urethral lengthening with anterior bladder wall flap for urinary incontinence: a new approach. J Urol 1994; 152:803–806.

130. Pippi Salle JL, McLorie GA, Bagli DJ, Khoury AE. Urethral lengthening with anterior bladder wall flap (Pippi Salle procedure): modifications and extended indications of the technique. J Urol 1997; 158:585–590.

131. Pippi Salle JL, McLorie GA, Bagli DJ, Khoury AE. Modifications of and extended indications for the Pippi Salle procedure. World J Urol 1999; 16:279–284.

132. Belman AB, Kaplan GW. Experience with the Kropp anti-incontinence procedure. J Urol 1989; 141:1160–1162.

133. Nill TG, Peller PA, Kropp KA. Management of urinary incontinence by bladder tube urethral lengthening and submucosal reimplantation. J Urol 1990; 144:559–563.

134. Waters PR, Chehade NC, Kropp KA. Urethral lengthening and reimplantation: incidence and management of catheterization problems. J Urol 1997; 158:1053–1056.

135. Koyle MA. The Kropp bladder neck reconstruction and its variations in the incontinent patient with neurogenic bladder. Pediatrics 1996; 98:602.

136. Mouriquand PD, Sheard R, Phillips N, et al. The Kropp-onlay procedure (Pippi Salle procedure): a simplification of the technique of urethral lengthening. Preliminary results in eight patients. Br J Urol 1995; 75:656–662.

137. Hayes MC, Bulusu A, Terry T, et al. The Pippi Salle urethral lengthening procedure; experience and outcome from three United Kingdom centres. BJU Int 1999; 84:701–705.

138. Rink RC, Adams MC, Keating MA. The flip-flap technique to lengthen the urethra (Salle procedure) for treatment of neurogenic urinary incontinence. J Urol 1994; 152:799–802.

139. Scott FB, Bradley WE, Timm GW. Treatment of urinary incontinence by an implantable prosthetic urinary sphincter. J Urol 1974; 112:75–80.

140. Furlow WL, Barrett DM. The artificial urinary sphincter: experience with the AS 800 pump-control assembly for single-stage primary deactivation and activation – a preliminary report. Mayo Clin Proc 1985; 60:255–258.

141. Light JK, Reynolds JC. Impact of the new cuff design on reliability of the AS800 artificial urinary sphincter. J Urol 1992; 147:609–611.

141. Leo ME, Barrett DM. Success of the narrow-backed cuff design of the AMS800 artificial urinary sphincter: analysis of 144 patients. J Urol 1993; 150:1412–1414.

142. Mitchell ME, Rink RC. Experience with the artificial urinary sphincter in children and young adults. J Pediatr Surg 1983; 18:700–706.

143. Gonzalez R, Koleilat N, Austin C, Sidi AA. The artificial sphincter AS800 in congenital urinary incontinence. J Urol 1989; 142:512–515.

144. Bosco PJ, Bauer SB, Colodny AH, et al. The long-term results of artificial sphincters in children. J Urol 1991; 146:396–399.

145. Belloli G, Caampobasso P, Mercurella A. Neuropathic urinary incontinence in pediatric patients: management with artificial sphincter. J Pediatr Surg 1992; 27:1461–1464.

146. González R, Merino FG, Vaughn M. Long-term results of the artificial urinary sphincter in male patients with neurogenic bladder. J Urol 1995; 154:769–770.

147. Levesque PE, Bauer SB, Atala A, et al. Ten-year experience with the artificial urinary sphincter in children. J Urol 1996; 156:625–628.

148. Kryger JV, Barthold JS, Fleming P, González R. The outcome of artificial urinary sphincter placement after a mean 15-year follow-up in a paediatric population. BJU Int 1999; 83: 1026–1031.

149. Hafez AT, McLorie G, Bägli D, Khoury A. A single-centre long-term outcome analysis of artificial urinary sphincter placement in children. BJU Int 2002; 89:82–85.

150. Toh K, Diokno AC. Management of intrinsic sphincter deficiency in adolescent females with normal bladder emptying function. J Urol 2002; 168:1150–1153.

151. Diokno AC, Sonda LP. Compatibility of genitourinary prostheses and intermittent self-catheterization. J Urol 1981; 125:659–660.

152. Barrett DM, Furlow WL. Incontinence, intermittent self-catheterization and the artificial genitourinary sphincter. J Urol 1984; 132:268–269.

153. de Badiola FIP, Castro-Diaz D, Hart-Austin C, Gonzalez R. Influence of preoperative bladder capacity and compliance on the outcome of artificial sphincter implantation in patients with neurogenic sphincter incompetence. J Urol 1992; 148:1493–1495.

154. Kronner KM, Rink RC, Simmons G, et al. Artificial urinary sphincter in the treatment of urinary incontinence: preoperative urodynamics do not predict the need for future bladder augmentation. J Urol 1998; 160:1093–1095.

155. Strawbridge LR, Kramer SA, Castillo OA, Barrett DM. Augmentation cystoplasty and the artificial genitourinary sphincter. J Urol 1989; 142:297–301.

156. Gonzalez R, Nguyen DH, Koleilat N, Sidi AA. Compatibility of enterocystoplasty and the artificial urinary sphincter. J Urol 1989; 142:502–504.

157. Bauer SB, Reda EF, Colodny AH, Retik AB. Detrusor instability: a delayed complication in association with the artificial sphincter. J Urol 1986; 135:1212–1215.

158. Murray KHA, Nurse DE, Mundy AR. Detrusor behavior following implantation of the Brantley Scott artificial urinary sphincter for neuropathic incontinence. Br J Urol 1988; 61:122–128.

159. Simeoni J, Guys JM, Mollard P, et al. Artificial urinary sphincter implantation for neurogenic bladder: a multi-institutional study in 107 children. Br J Urol 1996; 78:287–293.

160. Castera R, Podesta ML, Ruarte A, et al. 10-year experience with artificial urinary sphincter in children and adolescents. J Urol 2001; 165:2373–2376.

161. Spies PE, Capolicchio JP, Kiruluta G, et al. Is an artificial sphincter the best choice for incontinent boys with spina bifida? Review of our long term experience with the AS-800 artificial sphincter. Can J Urol 2002; 9:1486–1491.

60

The vesicourethral balance

Erik Schick and Jacques Corcos

Introduction

In Chapter 58, we summarized the different treatment modalities that can be considered to correct bladder dysfunction or urethral dysfunction, independently of each other. In clinical practice, however, most patients present simultaneous alterations of reservoir and outlet functions.

The ultimate goal in neurogenic bladder management is the preservation of normal kidney function. The most important factor to achieve is to maintain the lower urinary tract at a low pressure. Ensuring regular bladder emptying, decreasing outlet resistance in patients who void spontaneously, preventing infection by eliminating foreign bodies from the urethra and/or the bladder, and treating infection when it becomes symptomatic are some of the modalities used to attain this goal. Additionally, maintaining or restoring continence will significantly increase the patient's quality of life. To avoid or minimize potential complications, these objectives have to be constantly kept in mind when dealing with the problem of neurogenic bladder dysfunction.

Vesicourethral balance and balanced bladder are by no means synonymous. The balanced bladder concept emerged after World War II and was part of the bladder rehabilitation process. It implied reflex bladder voiding and a post-void residual urine volume of less than 100 ml. Clinicians felt safe in trying to achieve this goal. Later experience proved that the approach was not necessarily safe, because it could not prevent infection, sepsis, loss of renal function, etc. The flaw with this empirical therapy is that elevated bladder filling and emptying pressures can occur, causing silent renal damage despite low post-void residual urine volume.[1]

The concept of vesicourethral balance helps us to understand the pathophysiological consequences of vesicourethral dysfunction. It indicates how to modify reservoir function, outlet function, or both in order to restore normal vesicourethral function to a safe, normal, low-pressure zone. Urodynamics are essential in this respect, because they allow bladder and urethral function to be evaluated independently along with the interaction between them.

Normal vesicourethral balance

The vesicourethral unit can be compared to a balance where the bladder represents one arm, and the urethra with its sphincteric mechanism the other arm of the balance. Figure 60.1 illustrates this concept.

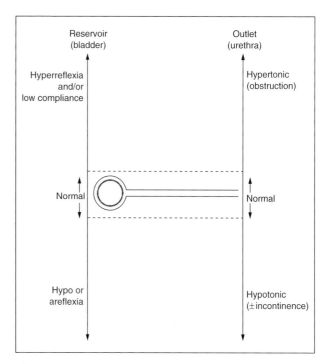

Figure 60.1
Normal vesicourethral balance. Bladder filling and micturition under normal pressure conditions, within the 'security zone' of <40 cmH$_2$O.

During the filling phase of the voiding cycle, the bladder is accommodating a progressively increasing volume. Because of normal bladder wall compliance, pressure inside the bladder remains constant, about 15–20 cmH_2O, and never exceeds 40 cmH_2O. The system is in a low-pressure state, and the upper urinary tract is safe.[2,3] During the voiding phase, the detrusor contracts, the urethral sphincteric mechanism relaxes, and there is normal vesicourethral synergia.

Under pathological conditions, this relatively delicate balance can easily be disturbed. Bladder function can be normal or altered by some pathological process in several ways. It may become hypo- or areflexic, or hyperreflexic, with or without impaired contractility, with or without decreased compliance. Urethral function can be normal, hypotonic (incontinence), or hypertonic (obstruction). The different combinations of these vesicourethral alterations can lead to eight different clinical situations, as illustrated in Table 60.1.

The aim of any therapeutic intervention is to ensure the restoration of normal balance in the security zone – security from the point of view of the preservation of renal function.

Alterations in vesicourethral balance

Normal bladder contractility and compliance

The hypotonic outlet

This is characteristic of the stress incontinent patient. By simply improving outlet function, normal vesicourethral conditions in normal pressure ranges can be restored (Figure 60.2).

The obstructive outlet

Early benign prostatic obstruction is a good example of this situation. The treatment strategy should not be to increase bladder contractility, but rather to decrease urethral resistance (Figure 60.3). Often, however, infravesical obstruction induces bladder instability. In this eventuality, vesicourethral balance could be considered to be acceptable,

Table 60.1 *Summary of vesico–urethral balance*

Figure number	Bladder activity	Bladder compliance	Outlet	Clinical example	Treatment
60.2	Normal	Normal	Low	SUI	↑ outlet
60.3	Normal	Normal	High	Early BPH	↓ outlet
60.4	OAB	Normal or Low	High	Symptomatic BPH	↑ outlet ↓ OAB
60.5	OAB	Normal	Normal	Primary OAB	↓ OAB
60.6	OAB	Normal or Low	Low	Mixed urinary incontinence	↑ outlet ↓ OAB
60.7	Hypo – or areflexia	High	Normal	'Primary' hypotonic bladder; diabetes	CIC (±↓ outlet?)
60.8	Hypo – or areflexia	High	Low	Cauda equina syndrome	CIC (±↑ outlet?)
60.9	Hypo – or areflexia	Normal or High	High	Late BPH with decompensated bladder	CIC (±↓ outlet?)

BPH = Benign Prostatic Hypertrophy
CIC = Clean Intermittent Catheterization
OAB = Overactive Bladder
SUI = Stress Urany Incontinence

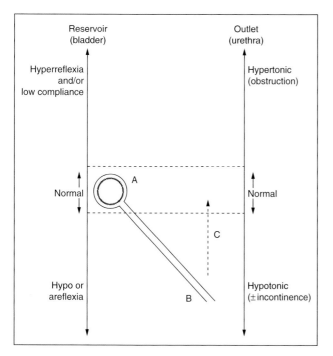

Figure 60.2
The bladder is normal (A), but the urethra hypotonic (B), a condition favorable for incontinence. By increasing urethral tonicity (C), continence is re-established. Overcorrecting may induce urinary retention, as in Figure 60.3.

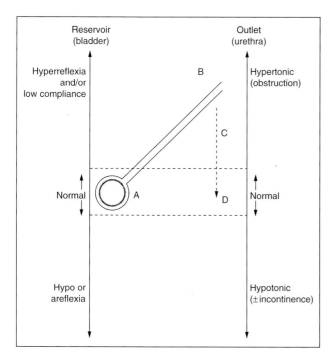

Figure 60.3
The bladder is normal (A), and the urethra obstructive (B), as in benign prostatic hyperplasia or distal urethral stenosis. Correction of outlet conditions (C) allows the re-establishment of micturition under normal pressure conditions (D).

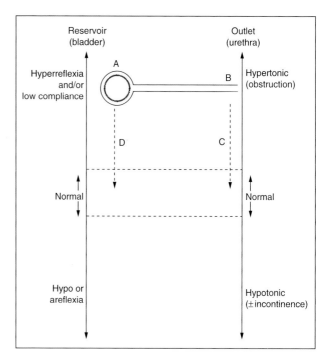

Figure 60.4
The bladder is hyperreflexic and/or low compliant (A), associated with overactive or obstructed outlet (B). The patient is probably continent, but the upper tract is in real danger of decompensation. Therapeutic measures should be directed toward the urethra (C) and the bladder (D) simultaneously to establish normal balance in the security zone.

but this balance is established in the high-pressure zone, compromising renal function in the long term. By eliminating obstruction and controlling hyperreflexia, the system will return to normal equilibrium in the security zone (Figures 60.3 and 60.4).

Bladder hyperreflexia and/or low-compliant bladder

The normotonic outlet

When the bladder is hyperreflexic and/or low compliant, but the urethra still has normal closure pressure, the patient will probably be incontinent. The solution to this problem is not to increase urethral closure pressure, because – although the patient will become continent – the system will be transformed to a high-pressure one, jeopardizing the integrity of the upper urinary tract. Treatment should be directed to controlling hyperreflexia or to improving bladder wall compliance. Thus, the system will be balanced in the security zone (Figure 60.5).

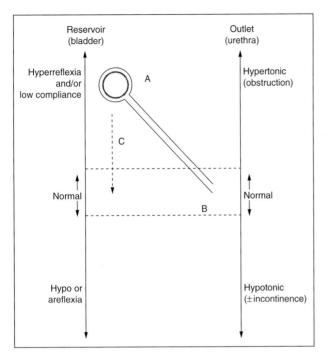

Figure 60.5
The bladder is hyperreflexic and/or low compliant (A) with a normal outlet (B), predisposing to incontinence. Treatment should correct the hyperreflexia (C) without interfering with urethral function (D). Continence should be re-established.

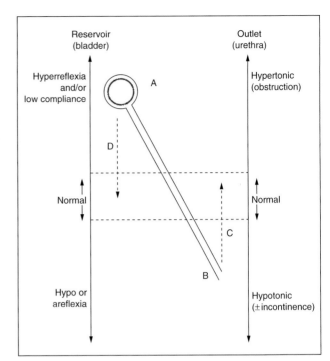

Figure 60.6
The bladder is hyperreflexic and/or low compliant (A), associated with a hypotonic outlet (B). The patient will almost certainly be incontinent. Increasing urethral resistance (C) will probably not be sufficient; conditions similar to those in Figure 60.5 will be created. Detrusor hyperreflexia should also be controlled (D) in order to reach normal vesicourethral equilibrium.

The hypotonic outlet

This clinical situation is relatively rare. With decreased outlet resistance, the patient will almost certainly be incontinent, but because of this hypotonicity a high-pressure system is unlikely to develop. Correcting urethral function alone might put the upper urinary tract in a precarious situation, as in the preceding example. Together with the improvement of urethral hypotonicity, one should also control bladder hyperreflexia and/or compliance (Figure 60.6).

The hypertonic outlet

It is estimated that more then 50% of males with outlet obstruction will develop bladder overactivity.[4,5] Elimination of obstruction will normalize urethral function, but might expose the patient to incontinence. In a non-neurological context, bladder overactivity will subside spontaneously within 1 year after the removal of the obstruction in a significant proportion of patients.[6] In the neurological patient, however, therapeutic measures should be taken to control hyperreflexia, in conjunction with the correction of outlet function (Figure 60.4).

Hypo- or areflexic bladder

The normal outlet

This is the case of the patient who underwent prostatectomy for chronic urinary retention, but who is unable to void spontaneously. Increasing bladder contractility without other modification of outlet conditions should allow spontaneous voiding (Figure 60.7).

The hypotonic outlet

The patient may or may not be incontinent. Improving outlet function alone will almost certainly precipitate the patient into urinary retention. Every effort should be made to improve bladder contractility as well (Figure 60.8).

The obstructive outlet

In this case, the patient will be in chronic urinary retention. Decreasing outlet resistance by eliminating the obstructive factor will not necessarily permit normal voiding without

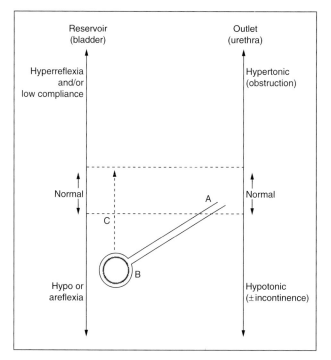

Figure 60.7
The outlet is normal (A), and the bladder is hypo- or areflexic (B). Spontaneous voiding might be possible but with significant post-void residual volume. Treatment should reinforce detrusor contractility (C) without interfering with outlet conditions (A).

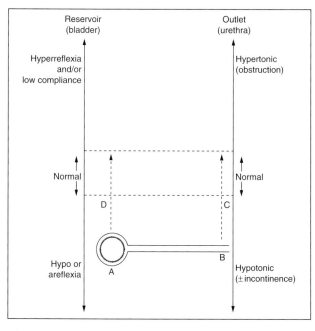

Figure 60.8
Hypo- or areflexic bladder (A) with a hypotonic outlet (B). If the patient is continent, one might adopt a watchful waiting policy, because the system is a low-pressure one. In case of incontinence, the outlet (C) and bladder (D) should be reinforced together. If only the outlet is corrected, the patient might not void spontaneously.

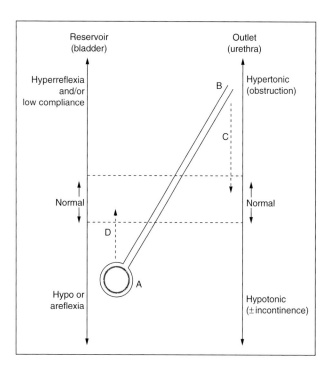

Figure 60.9
Hypo- or areflexic bladder (A) combined with an obstructed outlet (B). No spontaneous voiding is expected. Urethral resistance must be decreased (C) and bladder contractility increased (D) to ensure normal vesicourethral balance.

significant post-void residual volume. Attempts should also be made to improve bladder contractility simultaneously (Figure 60.9).

Conclusion

Normal vesicourethral balance signifies a low-pressure system with normal contractility and compliance, together with no outlet obstruction, and normal urethral tone. Urodynamics allow us to determine which elements are responsible for vesicourethral dysfunction or the disruption of vesicourethral balance. Urodynamics help to identify the element(s) responsible for this dysfunction. Treatment is directed towards restoring vesicourethral balance in the normal pressure ranges.

References

1. Chancellor MB, Blaivas GJ. Spinal cord injury. In: Chancellor MB, Blaivas JG, eds. Practical neurourology: genitourinary complications in neurologic diseases. Boston: Butterworth-Heinemann, 1995: 99–118.

2. McGuire EJ, Cespedes RD, O'Connell HE. Leak point pressures. Urol Clin N Am 1996; 23:253–262.

3. Stöhrer M, Goepel M, Kondo A, et al. The standardization of terminology in neurogenic lower urinary tract dysfunction with suggestions for diagnostic procedures. Neurourol Urodyn 1999; 18: 139–158.

4. Abrams PH, Griffiths DJ. The assessment of prostatic obstruction from urodynamic measurements and from residual urine. Br J Urol 1979; 51:129–134.

5. Dorflinger T, Frimodt-Møller PC, Bruskewitz RC, et al. The significance of uninhibited detrusor contractions in prostatism. J Urol 1985; 133:819–821.

6. Frimodt-Møller PC, Jensen KM, Iversen P, et al. Analysis of presenting symptoms in prostatism. J Urol 1984; 132:272–276.

Part VIII

Complications

61

Complications related to neurogenic bladder dysfunction – I: infection, lithiasis and neoplasia

Andrew Z Buczynski

Infection

Definition

The term urinary tract infection (UTI) is defined by urine culture showing more than 100,000 bacterial colonies in 1 ml of urine. This criterion has been widely adopted to define this condition. Its usefulness, however, depends on the method of urine collection and the clinical situation.[1] The presence of bacteria in the urine is termed bacteriuria but it does not necessarily mean UTI. Bacteriuria, and even UTI, can be clinically asymptomatic. Proper assessment of UTI is more difficult in patients with neurogenic bladder dysfunction (NBD) compared to the neurologically normal patient. UTI can be acute or chronic, relapsing or recurrent. The term relapse implies infection with the same bacteria, while recurrent infection implies infection with a different strain of bacteria.[2] UTI is the most common cause of fever in spinal cord injury (SCI) patients.[3]

Pyuria alone is not diagnostic of infection, because it may occur from the irritative effect of the catheter, especially if pyuria is at a low level of less than or equal to 30 white blood cells per high power field.[4] Any detectable bacteria from indwelling or suprapubic catheter aspitrates should be considered significant.[5] In patients on clean intermittent catheterization (CIC) 10^2 colonies/ml should be considered significant, while in catheter-free males, a clean voided specimen of 10^4 colonies/ml is significant for infection.[6]

Urine specimen collection for culture and antibiogram

In both sexes, external urethral meatus must be exposed, and cleansed by antiseptic solution. The first 50 ml is passed without collection. Afterwards, approximately 50 ml (= mid-stream) should be collected in a sterile container. Urine should be cultured as soon as possible. If this is impossible, it should be kept refrigerated and cultured within 24 h of refrigeration. It has been shown, that no clinically significant changes in cultures or colony counts occurred between fresh and refrigerated urine samples for up to 24 h.[7] Proper urine collection is best accomplished under the supervision of professional staff in hospital, outpatient clinic or laboratory.

For obtaining urine specimen from patients with NBD, one can use external stimulation (usually suprapubic percussion). If this is impossible, urine should be obtained by a single catheterization. Collection of urine for culture from the drainage bag is not a reliable technique.

Microorganisms involved

The most frequently cultured bacteria from urine specimens, particularly in female patients, is *Escherichia coli*.[1,2] This kind of bacteria is cultured from most patients with uncomplicated cystitis, pyelonephritis or from asymptomatic spinal injured patients. Other, quite often cultured microorganisms are *Klebsiella, Pseudomonas, Enterobacter, Providencia, Serratia* and *Proteus.* These are most likely hospital-acquired.[1,8] Especially harmful are the bacteria producing urease, an enzyme causing significant alkalization of urine, which promotes the precipitation of struvite stones (ammonio-magnesium triphosphates and calcium phosphates) in the upper and lower urinary tract.[9] If such a bacteria is cultured, appropriate antibiotics should be administered to prevent further complications. Other, rarely cultured organisms, especially if multiple strains are present, usually indicate contamination rather than true infection. However, patients on catheter drainage for a prolonged period of time (over 1 month) often have polymicrobial flora.

Risk factors

The main risk factors for UTI associated with SCI are impaired voiding, overdistention of the bladder, elevated intravesical pressure, vesicoureteral reflux, urinary tract obstruction, instrumentation and increased incidence of stone formation.[6]

Whenever possible, CIC is the preferred method of adequate bladder drainage. It has been demonstrated, that CIC decreases intravesical pressure and reduces the incidence of bladder stone formation.[10] In general, patients on CIC have significantly lower rates of complications compared to those with indwelling urethral catheterization.[11]

Lower genitourinary tract complications

Urethritis

Since indwelling catheter almost always causes urethritis in patients with NBD, the best is to remove the catheter if in place and start with intermittent catheterization as soon as possible. Occasionally, the blockade of the periurethral glands by the catheter with secondary infection is responsible for the development of periurethral abscess.[2,12] In the acute stage, when Buck's fascia is penetrated, necrosis of the subcutaneous tissue and fascia can represent a life-threatening condition. Immediate suprapubic cystostomy is mandatory, together with wide debridement of all nonviable tissues. Agressive intravenous antibiotherapy should be instituted.

In a less acute, or more chronic stage, the infected gland can evolve in three different directions. It can drain spontaneously to the penile skin and heal without sequel. More often, however, it will drain inside the urethral lumen. The drained cavity will create a urethral diverticulum that needs surgical treatment, because urine trapped in the diverticulum will cause permanent infection and lead eventually to a recurrence of the periurethral abscess (Figure 61.1). Finally, when the abscess drains simultaneously at both sides, via the skin and via the urethral lumen, it results in a urethrocutaneous fistula, which can only be treated surgically. Periurethral abscesses develop mostly in patient with long-term indwelling catheters. However, if proper catheter care is provided, periurethral abscess develops rarely.

Epididymitis and epididymo-orchitis

Epididymitis and epididymo-orchitis are catheter-related complications of UTI. Infection gains the epididymis via the vas deferens in a retrograde fashion.[1,12] Symptoms are usually unilateral. As neurologically impaired patients often do not have sensation of pain, the only clinical sign of

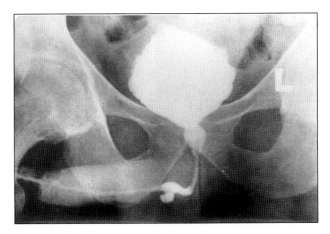

Figure 61.1
Urethral diverticulum, a consequence of a periurethral abscess in a tetraplegic patient.

epididymitis is swelling and flare. Significant enlargement of testicle may develop, which becomes hard and sometimes the scrotal skin reddish. Treatment consists of specific antibiotics based on culture results. Antibiotic therapy is usually successful. In rare instances, when treatment is initiated too late, inadequate or the patient is not treated at all, infection may gain the testicle and cause orchitis with eventually the formation of a testicular abscess. In this circumstance, drainage of the abscess and antibiotherapy gives a chance for spontaneous healing but the affected testicle loses its function.[12,13] Orchidectomy sometimes becomes necessary.

Bacterial infection of the prostate

It is generally admitted, that most often bacteria gains the prostate by infected urine refluxing into the prostatic ducts. Hematogenous and lymphatic spread, however, should also be considered. *Escherichia coli* is the most frequent bacteria.[2] Bacterial prostatitis in NBD is generally chronic and asymptomatic, and chronic bacterial prostatitis is the most common cause of relapsing UTI.[1,2] Only during episodes of acute cystitis, urinalysis will show pyuria and bacteriuria. In other cases, segmented lower tract urine cultures, as suggested by Meares and Stamey[14] should be used in an attempt to localize the infection in the prostate. Unfortunately most antibiotics diffuse poorly into prostatic tissue. Trimethoprim[15] and Ofloxacin[16] are among the recommended antibiotics because they penetrate best into the chronically infected prostatic tissue.

Cystitis

Infection of the lower urinary tract is the most common complication of neurogenic bladder. Almost all patients with NBD will, sooner or later, be in contact with catheters. Indwelling or suprapubic catheter in the acute stage of spinal injury, CIC, all represent risk factors for infection. If sterile catheterization is strictly observed, the risk of introducing infection into the lower urinary tract is theoretically low.[12] Practically, however, all patients with NBD will have UTI from time to time.

Another favorable factor for the development of cystitis is residual urine. Complete bladder emptying is one of the most important defense mechanisms against UTI.[1,12] When residual urine volumes are high, large numbers of bacteria remain in the urine having perfect conditions for growing. The ability to expel bacteria is complete when voiding is complete. This concept is important when considering the association between urinary infection and neurogenic disorders of lower urinary tract.[17]

Urinalysis reveals pyuria in almost all instances of bacterial infection. Recurrent infections, through cicatrization of the bladder wall, gradually reduces bladder capacity and wall compliance, similarly to indwelling catheter, and may result in a small fibrotic bladder.[6]

In some instances, acute bladder infection may cause bleeding, which needs a combination of antibiotherapy with bladder drainage and periodic irrigations to prevent catheter blockade by blood clots. In our experience, bladder irrigation with neomycine solution (5 gm in 500 ml of water) using three-way Foley catheter is very useful in combination with systemic antibiotherapy.

Due to partial or complete loss of sensation in patients with neuropathic bladders, the only signs of cystitis may be increased frequency of micturition, intensification of spasticity and changes in urinalysis.[13] Chronic cystitis in these patients, even with significant changes in urinalysis, are often clinically asymptomatic. Fever is generally absent, although low-grade temperature elevations are not uncommon.[2,13]

Asymptomatic UTI should not be treated.[12,18] Unnecessary or prolonged use of antibiotics will only increase the likelihood of selecting out more resistant microorganisms. Treatment of septic complications under these circumstances may then become very challenging.

Upper urinary tract complications

Prolonged or recurrent infection in the lower urinary tract is one of the factors, that might interfere with antireflux mechanism causing reflux of infected urine to the kidney.[12] This situation may lead to stone formation in the kidney and to the development of progressive failure of the affected kidney. Although infected vesicoureteral reflux significantly increases the risk of pyelonephritis, many patients with pyelonephritis do not have demonstrable reflux.[1] Similarly, not all patients with reflux will have

clinical evidence of pyelonephritis. Acute pyelonephritis, which is most commonly caused by aerobic gram-negative bacteria, reaches the kidney from the lower urinary tract.

Functional infravesical obstruction, such as detrusor-external sphincter dyssynergia (DESD), common in NBD, contributes to the development of pyelonephritis through stasis of urine. Additionally, high intravesical pressure, also common in these patients, creates risk of reflux[12] of an already infected urine.

As the sensation of pain is often absent in neurological patients, the main clinical symptom of acute pyelonephritis is fever up to 40°C. Urinalysis shows pyuria, bacteriuria and microscopic hematuria. Hemogram reveals significant leukocytosis. Intravenous pyelography (IVP) could show some degree of renal enlargement and decreased nephrogram.

Treatment of noncomplicated pyelonephritis consists of specific antibiotherapy according to the results of urine culture and sensitivity studies. An important aspect of the problem however, is the recognition and elimination of complicating factors such as functional infravesical obstruction, infected stones or high intravesical pressures. Ultrasonography may provide similar information than IVP concerning presence of obstruction, stones or abscess.

Catheter care

Catheters should be used only when absolutely necessary. CIC create much less risk of UTI than does indwelling catheter[12,18] so, whenever possible, the former method is recommended. If indwelling catheter must be applied, instillation of suprapubic puncture drainage should be considered. Suprapubic catheters, even if they do not eliminate complications associated with a foreign body in the urinary tract, significantly reduce the incidence of urethral and prostato-epididymal infections. Insertion of the catheter should be performed under aseptic conditions. Closed drainage by gravity should be maintained, with the collecting bag lower than the level of the pubic symphysis. Additionally, the bag should have a valve for prevention of reflux of urine into the bladder when the bag is accidentally raised above the level of the bladder. Until the catheter is in place, antimicrobial treatment of asymptomatic, catheter-associated, bacteriuria is not recommended.[1,19]

Lithiasis

The occurrence of stones within the urinary tract is a problem as old as mankind. Many methods of dealing with stones have been developed in the past, but none have had as much of an impact as had the development of endourology and extracorporeal shock wave lithotripsy (ESWL). Those two innovations significantly reduced the necessity for open surgery in the treatment of lithiasis.

The stone disease affects male patients 3 times as commonly than females, and whites 4–5 times more commonly then blacks.[9] The development of stones in the urinary tract is a complex, incompletely understood, multifactorial process. In patients with NBD, the stone formation is relatively well recognized. The main factors responsible for stone formation in these patients are chronic or recurrent infections, especially those caused by urease-forming organisms, infravesical obstruction producing stasis, hypercalciuria related to immobilization (especially in young men),[9,12] and high specific gravity of urine, especially for kidney stones.[20] This last point was challenged by others,[21] suggesting that total fluid intake does not determine stone occurrence, but rather the fluid type (juice) which influences stone formation. Struvite stones form only when urine pH is significantly increased (>7.24).[22] Organisms that produce the enzyme urease, split urea into ammonium which, in turn, causes significant alkalinization of urine. Proteus species are the most common urea-splitting organisms and are identified in most patients with struvite stones.[8,9,13] Other organisms may produce urease also, including *Klebsiella, Pseudomonas, Providencia* and *Staphylococcus*. According to several authors 10–20% of SCI patients have struvite calculi.[5,23,24]

Renal calculi

Patients with NBD develop almost exclusively struvite stones.[9,13] Important minerals involved in struvite stone formation include calcium, magnesium, ammonium and phosphates. A protein matrix, such as fragments of papillae or urinary epithelium, is common and constitutes the nidus of the stone. In a large series of 1669 SCI patients, the overall incidence of renal calculi was estimated to be about 3.5%.[25] Risk factors included indwelling catheters (49%), bladder stones (52%) and vesicoureteral reflux (28%). The recurrence rate was 69%. Chen et al[26] compared two large cohort of patients: 8314 patients between 1986 and 1999, vs 5850 patients between 1973 and 1982. They estimated that within 10 years after injury, 7% of patients will develop their first kidney stone. This trend has not changed over the past 25 years. Interestingly, they could not demonstrate any significant differential effect on kidney stone formation in relation to the type of urinary drainage used, including indwelling catheter, intermittent catheterization or condom catheter.[26,27] Once a kidney stone developed, there is a 34% chance of a second stone developing episode within the next five years.[28] Male patients with complete spinal cord lesion represent an increased risk for kidney stone formation.[29] Regular position changing of paralysed patients, high fluid intake,[20] early mobilization, proper treatment of urinary infection and prevention of subsequent reinfection are important factors in the prophylaxis of renal calculi. Struvite stones may grow to fill the entire renal pelvis and

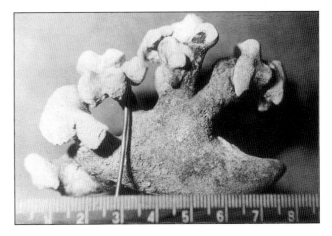

Figure 61.2
Staghorn calculus removed from the kidney of a paraplegic man 10 years after his accident.

collecting system creating staghorn calculi (Figure 61.2). It is interesting to note that staghorn calculi, even those which fill the collecting system completely of kidney, rarely cause complete obstruction of urine outflow. Sometimes, however, they can be responsible for silent hydronephrosis or even pyonephrosis which is not perceived by the patient, because a number of them lost pain sensation due to the neurological lesion. Nonspecific symptoms, such as feeling unwell, abdominal discomfort, increased spasms and autonomic dysreflexia can alert the well-informed physician.[30]

Kidney calculi are diagnosed by ultrasonography and plain X-ray of the abdomen. Struvite stones are more or less radioopaque, depending on their content in calcium but usually they are quite well visualized. An IVP will confirm the presence of calculi and show the degree of obstruction, if any. Successful treatment of renal stones depends on complete elimination of the calculus, eradication of infection and removing the obstruction causing stasis of urine. Selection of the best method of treatment should be individualized and adapted to every given patient. In paraplegic and quadriplegic patients typical ESWL alone is not recommended because of the difficulty in eliminating crushed stone fragments.[31,32] The recommended technique for treatment of renal stones in patients with NBD is percutaneous nephrolithotripsy (PCNL), in some selected cases in combination with ESWL. Stowe et al[33] reported in 9 out of 52 SCI patients (17.3%) who developed autonomic dysreflexia after ESWL. If ESWL is considered in a quadriplegic patient, this can be performed without the added risk of general or regional anesthesia. In a small series of 5 patients undergoing 10 ESWL treatments, no incidence of complete clinical syndrome of autonomic dysreflexia occurred. These patients, however, should be monitored closely by an anesthetiologist, because significant hypertension developed intraoperatively in 2 patients.[34] Effective prophylaxis can be obtained with 10–20 mg of nifedipine sublingually, 15–20 min before the procedure.[35] Intraoperative monitoring remains mandatory. Exacerbation of post-traumatic syringomyelia following ESWL has also been reported,[36] presumably caused by the shock waves reverberating the fluid within the intramedullary cavity producing further damage to the spinal cord. ESWL usually needs to be repeated for complete elimination of calculi from the kidney. In rare cases, patients will require open surgery. Nephrectomy should be performed when the affected kidney is practically non-functional, or in case of pyonephrosis.

In the prevention of struvite calculi it is essential to eliminate the infection with urea-splitting organisms. When chronic infection cannot be eradicated, urease inhibitors may be used to decrease pH of urine and ammonia level. Methenaminhippurat should be recommended in a dose of 1 gm twice a day for the prevention of recurrent infection and struvite calculosis in patients with NBD.[37]

Ureteral calculi

Most ureteral stones originate in the kidney. Only stones caused by ureteral obstruction like stricture or tumor may be formed or develop in the ureter. Small stones will pass down the ureter and will block the ureterovesical junction. These can be evacuated endoscopically using ureterorenoscope (URS). Sometimes fragmentation by ultrasonic or laser lithotripsy becomes necessary. Contrary to the neurologically healthy people, patients with NBD, because of immobilization, have less chance to spontaneously expel ureteral calculi. If ureteric stone is big enough and remains blocked in the middle third of the ureter, open surgical intervention could be considered.

Bladder stones

Infection of lower urinary tract by urea splitting, mainly nosocomial microorganisms, indwelling catheter and residual urine are the main reasons for bladder stone formation.

From 1973 to 1996 Chen et al[38] observed a decline in the incidence for an initial bladder stone (from 29% down to 8%). During the first year following the SCI, bladder stone risk increased with decreasing age, and was greater for whites. During the subsequent years, neurologically complete lesions, males, persons with indwelling catheter or on intermittent catheterization, also had a higher risk. At least in quadriplegics, suprapubic catheter drainage carried a statistically higher risk for bladder stone formation than did CIC.[27] Often bladder stone starts from the small pieces of thin struvite calculus formed around the balloon of a Foley catheter and left behind after the removal of the catheter. Those calculi may grow but they will retain the typical egg-shell or bowl shape (Figure 61.3). These calculi are usually multiple and are common in patients who have had indwelling

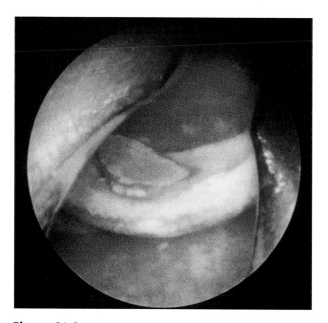

Figure 61.3
Typical bowl shaped struvite bladder calculi in a paraplegic patient.

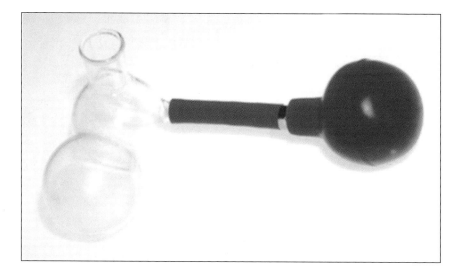

Figure 61.4
The Ellik bladder irrigator. The evacuated stone or tissue fragments are trapped in the bottom of the second glass recipient.

catheters for a long period of time. In other instances, debris, sloughs, pus cells and bacterial bodies are the nidus for struvite stone formation.[39] Bladder stones may cause severe irritative symptoms, hematuria and perpetuate infection. Unless bladder stones are removed, eradication of infection is impossible and antibiotics are not efficacious. Park and Linsenmeyer[40] suggested that weekly catheter changes might dramatically reduce catheter incrustation rates.

It should be mentioned that small struvite stones with low calcium content can easily be missed on X-ray and are often incidentally discovered during cystoscopy.

The treatment of bladder stones is easy, because of easy access, endoscopical and surgical, to the bladder. Additionally, struvite stones are not hard and easily fragmented. After fragmentation by mechanical forceps, ultrasonic, laser or electrohydraulic lithotripsy, small fragments can be washed out from bladder by the Ellik bladder irrigator (Figure 61.4). Vespasiani et al[41] reported excellent results with the endoscopic ballistic Swiss Lithoclast lithotripsy. All patients were stone free at 6 months postoperatively. They noticed, however, 5 intraoperative complications, including crisis of autonomic dysreflexia in 3 patients. Open surgical intervention for bladder stones is indicated only when bladder capacity is very small or the size of the stone is so big, that endoscopical litholapaxy would be too late and extremely difficult.

Urethral stones

Calculi lodged in the urethra are rare and mainly due to obstruction, sometimes from an unexpected cause,[42] but can also develop in preexisting urethral diverticulum. Figure 61.5A illustrates a stone which was growing slowly

inside the urethral diverticulum and became a "staghorn calculus" growing into both sides of the urethral lumen without creating clinically significant outflow obstruction.

Treatment of urethral stones is surgical (Figure 61.5B). If the reason for stone formation is stricture, endoscopic urethrotomy and subsequently lithotripsy is probably the best solution. In case of a stone inside a diverticulum, open surgery is necessary.

Neoplasm

It is generally accepted that the incidence and mortality of bladder cancer are heightened in SCI patients compared to the neurologically normal population.[43] The risk was estimated to be 16–28 times higher, especially for squamous cell carcinoma of the bladder in this group of patients.[44,45]

Bejany et al[46] found an incidence of 2.3% of bladder tumor in their SCI unit. Of these 9 (81%) had squamous cell carcinoma, 1 transitional cell carcinoma and 1 a mixed type (transitional and squamous cell) carcinoma. All of them had chronic bacteriuria, 44% had gross or microscopic hematuria, and 5 had stone disease. At 3 years follow-up, only 55% were free of disease. They did not find urine cytology helpful in the diagnosis of these patients. As 55% of them had had urethral recurrence, they suggested that urethrectomy should also be performed together with radical cystectomy.

Stonehill et al[47] evaluated the role of urinary cytology in this group of patients, especially because endoscopy is often nonspecific, difficult to interpret and sometimes even may be normal. They studied patients with indwelling

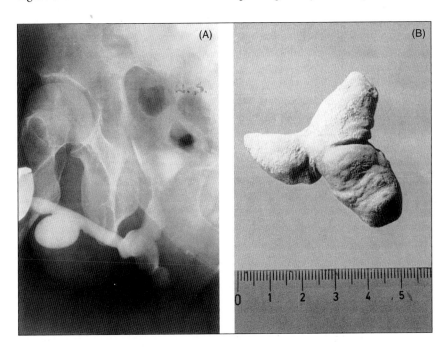

Figure 61.5
(A) X-ray of the urethra showing two diverticuli. The proximal one contains a stone. (B) Stone removed surgically.

catheter for more than 5 years. Positive cytology had a sensitivity of 71% and a specificity of 97% when evaluating patients with suspicious finding. Based on these observations the authors recommended yearly cytology in all high risk SCI patients, followed by biopsy, if any abnormal finding was noted on cystoscopy. Indwelling catheter and history of bladder stones were statistically significant risk factors.[48]

Locke et al[49] found an 8% incidence of squamous cell carcinoma in 25 SCI patients catheterized for a minimum of 10 years. Two patients had positive cytology, and both of them had hematuria as well.

Esrig et al[50] discovered in 37 patients with long-term indwelling catheter drainage (mean: 18.6 years), transitional cell carcinoma (grade 2 to 3) in 2 patients.

Bickel et al[51] pointed out that with appropriate management of these patients the survival is not different from the ambulatory, neurologically normal, population.

Pannek[52] reported, recently, the results of a mail survey sent to all SCI centers in Germany, Switzerland and Austria treating SCI patients between 1995 and 1999. Only 64.6% of the centers responded. The charts of 43,564 patients were reviewed, which represent the largest cohort published so far. Fourty-eight of them (0.11%) developed bladder cancer. This is somewhat lower than that reported by West et al[53] in a cohort of 33,656 patients, where they found a bladder cancer incidence of 0.39%. In the Pannek-survey, 81% of the tumors were urothelial and 19% squamous cell carcinomas. The majority of tumors were muscle-infiltrating at the initial diagnosis. Of these 48 patients only 18.9% had indwelling catheter (suprapubic or transurethral), with a mean duration of 8.5 ± 11.2 years. Intermittent catheterization was used by 32.4% of them. As pointed out by the author, this decline in incidence might be secondary at least in part to the avoidance of indwelling catheters, which have to be regarded as an important risk factor for bladder cancer.

The follow-up of patients with indwelling catheter is controversial. Some advocate for screening cystoscopy,[54] arguing that this will detect malignant lesions in an earlier stage. Others[55] believe that cystoscopy does not fulfill the accepted criteria for screening for primary bladder cancer in SCI patients.

This review of the literature suggests that SCI patients with long-standing indwelling catheterization (certainly after 10 years, perhaps even after 5 years post-trauma) should undergo yearly (or every second year?) cystoscopy, combined with urine cytology. If cytology is doubtful or positive, cold cup biopsy should be done randomly if no suspicious lesion is found endoscopically. History of bladder stone and chronic UTI should be considered as significant risk factors for the development of bladder cancer in SCI patients. New onset of gross hematuria should be investigated in the same way as in the neurologically normal population.

References

1. Levine FS, Staskin DR. Genitourinary infection. In: Siroky MB, Krane RJ, eds. Manual of urology, 1st edn. Boston: Little, Brown and Company, 1990:205–224.

2. Ward TT, Jones SR. Genitourinary tract infections. In: Reese RE, Betts RF, eds. A logical approach to infectious diseases, 3rd edn. Boston: Little, Brown and Company, 1991:357–389.

3. Beraldo PS, Neves EG, Alves CM, Khan P, Cirilo AC, Alencar MR. Pyrexia in hospitalized spinal cord injured patients. Paraplegia 1993; 31:186–191.

4. Menon EB, Tan ES. Pyuria: index of infection in patients with spinal cord injuries. Br J Urol 1992; 69:144–146.

5. Cardenas DD, Hooton TM. Urinary tract infection in persons with spinal cord injury. Arch Phys Med Rehabil 1995; 76:272–280.

6. National Institute on Disability and Rehabilitation Research Concensus Statement: the prevention and management of urinary tract infections among people with spinal cord injury. SCI Nurs 1993; 10:49–61.

7. Horton JA 3rd, Kirshblum SC, Lisenmeyer TA, Johnston M, Rustagi A. Does refrigeration of urine alter culture results in hospitalized patients with neurogenic bladder? J Spinal Cord Med 1998; 21:342–347.

8. Menon EB, Tan ES. Urinary tract infection in acute spinal cord injury. Singapore Med J 1992; 33:359–361.

9. Babayan RK. Urinary Calculi and Endourology. In: Siroky MB, Krane RJ, eds. Manual of urology, 1st edn. Boston: Little, Brown and Company, 1990:123–131.

10. Stover SL, Lloyd LK, Waites KB, Jackson AB. Urinary tract infection in spinal cord injury. Arch Phys Med Rehabil 1989; 70:47–54.

11. Weld KJ, Dmochowski RR. Effect of bladder management on urological complications in spinal cord injured patients. J Urol 2000; 163:768–772.

12. Buczynski AZ. Principles for urological management of SCI patients. Ortopedia Traumatologia Rehabilitacja 2000; 2:57–60.

13. Buczynski AZ. Urological complications in paraplegic and quadriplegic patients. New Medicine 1999; 89:13–15.

14. Meares EM Jr, Stamey TA. Bacteriologic localization patterns in bacterial prostatitis and urethritis. Invest Urol 1968; 5:492–518.

15. Stamey TA, Meares EM Jr. Chronic bacterial prostatitis and the diffusion of drugs into prostatic fluid. J Urol 1970; 103:187–194.

16. Bjerklund Johansen TE, Gruneberg RN, Guilbert J, Hofstetter A, Lobel B, Naber KG, Palon Redorta J, van Cangh PJ. The role of antibiotics in the treatment of chronic prostatitis: a concensus statement. Eur Urol 1998; 34:457–466.

17. Kunin CM. Detection, prevention and management of urinary tract infections. Philadelphia: Lea & Febiger 1987:

18. Stover SL, Lloyd LK, Waites KB, Jackson AB. Neurogenic urinary tract infection. Neurol Clin 1991; 9:741–755.

19. Warren JW, Tenney JH, Hoopes JM, Muncie HL, Anthony WC. A prospective microbiologic study of bacteriuria in patients with indwelling urethral catheters. J Infect Dis 1982; 146:719–723.

20. Chen Y, Roseman JM, Funkhouser E, DeVivo MJ. Urine specific gravity and water hardness in relation to urolithiasis in persons with spinal cord injury. Spinal Cord 2001; 39:571–576.

21. Chen Y, Roseman JM, DeVivo MJ, Funkhouser E. Does fluid amount and choice influence urinary stone formation in persons with spinal cord injury? Arch Phys Med Rehabil 2002; 83:1002–1089.

22. Nomura S, Ishido T, Teranishi J, Makiyama K. Long-term analysis of suprapubic cystostomy drainage in patients with neurogenic bladder. Urol Int 2000; 65:185–189.

23. Buczynski AZ. Urolithiasis as complication of traumatic lesions of spinal cord. Pol Med Week 1980; 4:129–131.

24. Takasaki E, Suzuki T, Honda M, Imai T, Maeda S, Hosoya Y. Chemical Compositions of 300 lower urinary tract calculi and associated disorders in the urinary tract. Urol Int 1995; 54:89–94.

25. Donnellan SM, Bolton DM. The impact of contemporary bladder management technics on struvite calculi associated with spinal cord injury. BJU Int 1999; 84:280–285.

26. Chen Y, DeVivo MJ, Roseman JM. Current trend and risk factors for kidney stones in persons with spinal cord injury: a longitudinal study. Spinal Cord 2000; 38:346–353.

27. Mitsui T, Minami K, Furuno T, Morita H, Koyanagi T. Is suprapubic cystostomy an optimal urinary management in high quadriplegics? A comparative study of suprapubic cystostomy and clean intermittent catheterisation. Eur Urol 2000; 38:434–438.

28. Chen Y, DeVivo MJ, Stover SL, Lloyd LK. Recurrent kidney stone: a 25-year follow-up study in persons with spinal cord injury. Urology 2002; 60:228–232.

29. DeVivo MJ, Fine PR, Cutter GR, Maetz HM. The risk of renal calculi in spinal cord injury patients. J Urol 1984; 131:857–860.

30. Vaidyanathan S, Singh G, Soni BM, Hughes P, Watt JM, Dundas S, Sett P, Parsons KF. Silent hydronephrosis/pyonephrosis due to upper urinary tract calculi in spinal cord injury patients. Spinal Cord 2000; 38:331–338.

31. Robert M, Bennani A, Ohanna F, Guiter J, Averous M, Grasset D. The management of upper urinary tract calculi by piezoelectric extracorporeal shock wave lithotripsy in spinal cord injury patients. Paraplegia 1995; 33:132–135.

32. Niedrach WL, Davis RS, Tonetti FW, Cockett AT. Extracorporeal shock-wave lithotripsy in patients with spinal cord dysfunction. Urology 1991; 38:152–156.

33. Stowe DF, Bernstein JS, Madsen KE, McDonald DJ, Ebert TJ. Autonomic hyperreflexia in spinal cord injured patients during extracorporeal shock wave lithotripsy. Anesth Analg 1989; 68:788–791.

34. Spirnak JP, Bodner D, Udayashankar S, Resnick MI. Extracorporeal shock wave lithotripsy in traumatic quadriplegic patients: can it be safely performed without anasthesia? J Urol 1988; 139:18–19.

35. Sugiyama T, Fugelso P, Avon M. Extracorporeal shock wave lithotripsy in neurologically impaired patients. Semin Urol 1992; 10:109–11.

36. Di Lorenzo N, Maleci A, Williams BM. Severe exacerbation of post-traumatic syringomyelia after lithotripsy: case report. Paraplegia 1994; 32:694–696.

37. Banovac K, Wade N, Gonzales F, Walsh B, Rhamy RK. Decreased incidence of urinary tract infections in patients with spinal cord injury: effect of methenamine. J Am Paraplegic Soc 1991; 14:52–54.

38. Chen Y, DeVivo MJ, Lloyd LK. Bladder stone incidence in persons with spinal cord injury: determinants and trends, 1973–1996. Urology 2001; 58:665–670.

39. Boyarsky S. Labay P, Hanick P, Abramson AS, Boyarsky R. Care of the patient with neurogenic bladder, 1st edn. Boston: Little, Brown and Company, 1979.

40. Park YI, Linsenmeyer TA. A method to minimize indwelling catheter calcification and bladder stones in individuals with spinal cord injury. J Spinal Cord Med 2001 Summer; 24:105–108.

41. Vespasiani G, Pesce F, Finazzi Agro E, Virgili G, Giannantoni A, Micali S, Micali F. Endoscopic ballistic lithotripsy in the treatment of bladder calculi in patients with neurogenic voiding dysfunction. Endourol 1996; 10:551–554.

42. Vaidyanathan S, Singh G, Sett P, Soni BM. Complication of penile sheath drainage in a spinal cord injury patient: calculus impacting in the urethra proximal to the rim of a condom. Spinal Cord 2001; 39:240–241.

43. Groah SL, Weitzenkamp DA, Lammertse DP, Whiteneck GG, Lezotte DC, Hamman RF. Excess risk of bladder cancer in spinal cord injury: evidence for an association between indwelling catheter use and bladder cancer. Arch Phys Med Rehabil 2002; 83:346–351.

44. El-Masri WS, Fellows G. Bladder cancer after spinal cord injury. Paraplegia 1981; 19:265–270.

45. van Velzen D, Kirshnan KR, Parsons KF, Soni BM, Frazer MH, Howard CV, Vaidyanathan S. Comparative pathology of dome and trigone of urinary bladder mucosa in paraplegics and tetraplegics. Paraplegia 1995; 33:565–572.

46. Bejany DE, Lockhart IL, Rhamy RK. Malignant vesical tumors following SCI. J Urol 1987; 138:1390–1392.

47. Stonehill WH, Goldman HB, Dmochowski RR. The use of urine cytology for diagnosing bladder cancer in spinal cord injured patients. J Urol 1997; 157:2112–2114.

48. Stonehill WH, Dmochowski RR, Patterson AL, Cox CE. Risk factors for bladder tumors in spinal cord injury patients. J Urol 1996; 155:1248–1250.

49. Locke JR, Hill DE, Walzer Y. Incidence of squamous cell carcinoma in patients with long term catheter drainage. J Urol 1985; 133:1034–1035.

50. Esrig D, McEvoy K, Bennett CJ. Bladder cancer in the spinal cord-injured patient with long-term catheterisation: a causal relationship? Semin Urol 1992; 10:102–108.

51. Bickel A, Culkin DJ, Wheeler JS Jr. Bladder cancer in spinal cord injury patients. J Urol 1991; 146:1240–1242.

52. Pannek J. Transitional cell carcinoma in patients with spinal cord injury: a high risk malignancy? Urology 2002; 59:240–244.

53. West DA, Cummings JM, Longo WE, Virgo KS, Johnson FE, Parra RO. Role of chronic catheterisation in the development of bladder cancer in patients with spinal cord injury. Urology 1999; 53:292–297.

54. Navon JD, Soliman H, Khonsari F, Ahlering T. Screening cystoscopy and survival of SCI patients with squamous cell carcinoma of the bladder. J Urol 1997; 157:2109–2111.

55. Yang CC, Clowers DE. Screening cystoscopy in chronically catheterised SCI patients. Spinal Cord 1999; 37:204–207.

62

Complications related to neurogenic bladder dysfunction – II: reflux and renal insufficiency

Imre Romics, Antal Hamvas, and Attila Majoros

Introduction

After World War I, 80% of the spinal cord injury (SCI) patients died from urological complications,[1] mostly from urinary infection, which was untreatable at that time in the absence of antibiotics, and from secondary upper urinary tract damage. Urodynamics being unknown, the accepted approach was the 'balanced bladder' method, i.e. if voiding took place with no or minimal residual urine, the patient's condition was considered satisfactory. With no information on intravesical pressures during storage and voiding, there was no way to prevent upper urinary tract damage resulting from lower tract dysfunction.[2]

Today, widespread use of antibiotics, urodynamic evaluation, clean intermittent self-catheterization (CIC), and up-to-date management of urolithiasis have led to considerable improvements in life expectancy and, indeed, in the quality of life of SCI patients.

Nevertheless, urinary infections are still considered the most frequent complication in SCI patients. In a follow-up study of paraplegics from World War II, renal disease was the most common cause of death in the first 20 years post-injury, accounting for 40% of all deaths.[3]

Pathophysiology of upper urinary tract damage caused by neurogenic bladder dysfunction

Abnormally high intravesical storage and/or voiding pressure may predispose to vesicoureteral reflux (VUR), urinary retention, and urinary infection, leading ultimately to renal insufficiency. The most frequent urological abnormality associated with vesicoureteral reflux appears to be uninhibited bladder contraction. Koff et al found uninhibited detrusor contractions during the storage phase in the majority of neurologically normal children with recurrent urinary infections; nearly 50% of them had VUR, and 30% had an abnormal ureteric orifice but without VUR. Their findings were confirmed by the fact that after reducing intravesical pressure with anticholinergic medication, 58% of urinary infections were cured without the use of antibiotics.[4]

Urinary infection in itself will increase intravesical pressure, reduce compliance, and weaken the ureterovesical junction, thus predisposing to reflux. The incidence of VUR in SCI patients varies between 17 and 25%,[5,6] and can be found in 20% of neonates with meningomyelocele.[7] Soygur et al examined a group of children with reflux and without neurological symptoms, noting unilateral reflux in 40.3% and bilateral reflux in 59.7%. Urodynamic evaluation revealed asymptomatic voiding dysfunction in 28% of the unilateral and in 72% of the bilateral reflux cases. This significant difference seems to indicate that bilateral reflux is caused by some (perhaps silent) voiding dysfunction, whereas unilateral reflux may be attributed in patients with intact bladder function to primary damage of the vesicoureteral junction.[8] Apart from high intravesical pressure, VUR may also be related directly to urinary infection and high-pressure bladder function. Retention, high intrapyelic pressure, and proliferation of mostly urease-producing microorganisms may lead to the formation of renal calculi, to hydronephrosis, pyonephrosis, and renal insufficiency. Intrapyelic pressure rises may cause pyelocaliceal reflux and reduce postglomerular blood flow, resulting in ischemic damage.[9]

Gerridzen et al examined 140 SCI patients with voiding dysfunction and found detrusor hyperreflexia in 100 and areflexia in 40, with kidney damage in 16 and 7 patients, respectively. The 7 patients in the areflexic group with kidney damage showed significantly higher storage pressures (58 cmH$_2$O on average) than the rest of the same group (24 cmH$_2$O on average). In the hyperreflexic group, the 16 patients with kidney damage also showed significantly higher detrusor pressure values (115 cmH$_2$O on average) than the 84 patients with no renal impairment (72 cmH$_2$O on average). However, the pathologically high bladder pressures in this group were taken during the voiding phase.[10] High-pressure hyperreflexia was combined with detrusor-sphincter dyssynergia (DSD) in 55% of cases. In 4 of 23 patients, there was only radiographic evidence of kidney damage, 7 developed VUR, and 9 had hydronephrosis. Kidney damage from VUR was found in less than 1% of the cases.[10,11]

Patients with neurogenic bladder dysfunction secondary to suprasacral lesions (injuries above the sacral micturition center) usually develop detrusor hyperreflexia with or without DSD. High-pressure values are measured both during the storage and the voiding phase, more than 40 and 90 cmH$_2$O, respectively. This may be the consequence of protracted, intensive, uninhibited contractions, reduced bladder compliance, or functional (DSD) or organic (benign prostatic hyperplasia) urinary obstruction.[12–14] Therefore, the chances of upper tract damage are higher than in the case of lower motoneuron lesions (level of injury within or below the sacral micturition center). In this latter circumstance, the detrusor will be hypo- or areflexic so that even with reduced bladder compliance, pathologically high pressure values will only appear during the storage phase. Among patients voiding spontaneously via reflex contractions and exhibiting normal pressure values, both in the storage and voiding phases, there are still a few who will show some degree of reflux or urinary retention.

Linsenmeyer et al found 4 cases of VUR and 9 cases of upper tract dilatation in 84 patients voiding via reflex contraction. The only significant difference between the two groups was in the duration of the reflexly induced contractions.[15]

However, it does happen that an intially areflexic bladder decreases compliance and changes into a hyperreflexic state, which may lead to upper tract damage. This is suggested by the results of Jamil et al, who performed naturalfill urodynamics in 30 patients with indwelling catheters. Intravesical pressure rises of >40 cmH$_2$O were found in 11 and renal scarring in 9 patients, 6 of them from the high-pressure group.[16]

On the other hand, 'silent' voiding dysfunctions with no lower tract symptoms may also result in upper tract complications.[17,18]

Tables 62.1–62.3 summarize the risk factors that are associated with kidney damage.

Table 62.1 *Risk factors associated with kidney damage*

General risk factors:
   Newborns
   Old age
   Immobilization
   Diabetes mellitus
   Immunosuppression
   Polymorbidity

Neurological risk factors:
   Quadriplegia > paraplegia
   Complete lesion > incomplete lesion

Table 62.2 *Urological abnormalities representing risk for kidney damage*

Urinary tract infection

Bladder outlet obstruction (BPH, stricture, etc.)

Urinary lithiasis

Bladder diverticulum

VUR with secondary reflux nephropathy

Foreign body in the urinary tract (catheter, urethral stent, etc.)

BPH, benign prostatic hypertrophy; VUR, vesicoureteral reflux.

Table 62.3 *Urodynamic abnormalities representing risk factors for kidney damage*

Decreased bladder compliance (>10 ml/cmH$_2$O)

LPP or storage pressure >40 cmH$_2$O

Reduced bladder capacity

Sustained high-pressure detrusor contraction

Voiding pressure >90 cmH$_2$O

DESD or detrusor-bladder neck dyssynergia

High post-void residual (>30% of bladder capacity)

LPP, leak point pressure; DESD, detrusor-external sphincter dyssynergia.

Etiology of neurogenic bladder dysfunction leading to reflux and renal failure

Spinal cord injury

Spinal cord injury due to an accident, disc prolapse, acute myelitis, operation of thoracic aorta aneurysms, etc., occurs in the United States approximately 12,000 times a year. Half of these victims end up quadriplegic, and the rest paraplegic, 53% with complete and 47% with incomplete lesions, half of the total number in the upper thoracal section above the 12th thoracic level, and 75% are male.[19] As a consequence, most SCI patients have a hyperreflexic bladder. Reports suggest a 7–32% incidence of renal lithiasis in SCI patients. Bors and colleagues found an 8.2% incidence of renal lithiasis.[20] Hall et al[21] examined 898 SCI patients after an average of 27 years, detecting renal calculi in 14.8%, in association with VUR in 37.7%, and without reflux in 10%. Of those with renal calculi, 56.6% were on indwelling catheters. This contrasts with the 700 patients with no renal calculi, where only 28% were on indwelling catheters. They also found 261 patients with bladder stones, 17.7% of them combined with renal stones. There was no correlation with the prevalence of VUR. A review of this large population suggested three conclusions:

1.   the incidence of renal calculi is significantly higher in patients with renal reflux
2.   bladder stones and simultaneous reflux will not significantly increase the number of renal calculi
3.   indwelling catheters significantly raise the incidence of renal and bladder stones.

The incidence of reflux among SCI patients varies from 5% to 23%.[10,11,20,21] Killorin et al reported upper tract damage in 7% of their SCI patients with areflexic bladder; 32% had hyperreflexic bladder, and there was no upper tract damage in those with normal detrusor function.[22]

Neural tube defects

Neural tube defects (spina bifida occulta, meningocele, meningomyelocele) are the most frequent reasons for bladder dysfunction in infancy. In the majority of the patients, the lumbar section (at the conus medullaris) is involved, resulting in an areflexic bladder and often an open bladder neck. Hydronephrosis was found in less than 10%, VUR in 16%, and bladder diverticuli in 23.5% of these newborns. Based on data in a pediatric myelodysplastic population, in 1981, McGuire et al described the correlation between storage pressure and chances of upper tract damage. He identified the so-called leak point pressure (LPP) at which urine will leak at the urethral meatus, and showed the risk of upper tract damage to be high with LPP >40 cmH$_2$O, but significantly lower with LPP <40 cmH$_2$O. In the low-LPP group, he observed no VUR and only two intravesicular diverticuli, in contrast to 68% VUR and 81% retention in the high-LPP (>40 cmH$_2$O) group.[12]

Iatrogenic damage

Iatrogenic damage is associated with various perioperative complications, the most frequent of which are upper motoneuron lesions due to operations on aneurysms of the thoracic aorta or areflexic bladders resulting from peripheral neural lesions due to radical surgery of the pelvis. Both types of damage may lead to upper tract injury or deteriorated function.

Diagnosis of upper tract damage
Laboratory tests

Serum creatinine, urea nitrogen, serum bicarbonate, blood pH, urine pH, urine gravity and osmolarity, proteinuria, and cylindruria are good indicators of renal function.

Videourodynamic examination

Storage and voiding pressure, maximum bladder capacity, bladder compliance, bladder neck condition, bladder configuration, detrusor-external sphincter or detrusor-bladder neck dyssynergia, passive and/or active VUR are well-documented with this test. It is essential for neurogenic bladders to be initially evaluated by videourodynamics and to repeat the test at least on an annual basis (Madersbacher, pers comm), because bladder dysfunction may change later on. In myelodysplasia, for instance, areflexic bladder dysfunction is likely to change with time to hyperreflexia.[23] In other cases (e.g. control of bladder compliance in meningomyelocele), conventional urodynamics without video control may be all that is needed for follow-up.

Ultrasonography

This is the simplest and least-invasive way to gather information on vesicoureteral dilatation, nephrolithiasis, renal parenchyma thickness, and residual urine. Urine transport abnormalities, both functional (or nonobstructive type, e.g. VUR, brimming bladder, overhydrated condition, acute pyelonephritis) and organic (or obstructive type, e.g. stones, strictures), are easily detected using furosemide (frusemide).

The Doppler technique can define the arterial resistance index. Increased arterial resistance index values are present even before actual dilatation of the collecting system has appeared. Values of 0.7 or more are indications of obstruction. The color Doppler technique demonstrates reflux with no X-ray exposure: a transducer directed toward the ureteral orifices will image retrograde flow in the ureter as a colored jet. Virgili et al sonographed 115 SCI patients and found upper tract anomalies (vesicorenal dilatation, chronic pyelonephritis) in 21.7% of them.[24] Calenoff et al compared ultrasonography with conventional intravenous urograms in 54 SCI patients and observed that all abnormalities seen on intravenous urograms (retention in 36% and VUR in 56% of cases) can also be detected by ultrasonography. They suggested the use of ultrasonography for follow-up rather than intravenous urography.[25] Ozer et al used ultrasonography in a prospective study to screen SCI patients with no urological symptoms and reported that upper tract abnormalities which needed therapeutic intervention were only detected in symptomatic patients. Therefore, they did not recommend ultrasonography for large-scale preventive early diagnosis in asymptomatic patients.[26] Bih et al compared ultrasonographic results before and after micturition and noted that upper tract ultrasonography performed on a full bladder was more likely to show urine transport abnormalities.[27]

Intravenous urography

Intravenous urography is considered to be the gold standard for the detection of upper tract abnormalities due to neurogenic bladder dysfunction. Even if it involves X-ray exposure and possible allergic reactions to the contrast material (very rare, though, today with tri-iodides), the fact remains that this is the most reliable source of information on the morphology and, to some extent, also on the function of the upper urinary tract. In cases of renal damage, it will provide the following information: focal or diffuse atrophy of the parenchyma; dilated, bulky calices; and decreased excretion of the contrast material. In cases of VUR, 30% of the urograms were negative, 5% showed ureteral dilatation, 25% renal scars and calyceal dilatation, 10% cortical atrophy, and 30% a nonfunctioning kidney.[14] Rutuu et al performed 206 intravenous urograms on 119 patients with neurogenic bladder dysfunction and detected 42% upper tract abnormalities, mostly delayed renal emptying. Among patients with pathological urograms, 40% had at least one acute urinary infection episode within the last year, whereas among those with no pathological signs in their urograms, the incidence was only 8%.[28] Rao et al compared secretory urography and ultrasonography in a prospective study of 202 asymptomatic SCI patients to assess their respective effectiveness in diagnosing upper tract damage. Hydronephrosis was detected by urography in 100% of cases vs 86% by ultrasonography; for renal stones, the detection ratios were 87 and 78%, and for signs of chronic pyelonephritis, 100 and 25%, respectively. However, the discrepancy decreased if ultrasonography was combined with plain X-rays of the abdomen.[29]

Cystography and voiding cystourethrography

Cystography at bladder capacity will show low-pressure or passive reflux, in contrast to the Valsalva maneuver, made during micturition effort, which will provide information on high-pressure or active reflux. The same results are, however, available also by videourodynamic testing, which gives exact intravesical pressure values for storage and voiding while imaging the bladder filled with contrast material, and will reveal VUR, if any. The same applies to intravenous urography (provided that all contrast material has been discharged from the kidneys). Stover et al studied the influence of retrograde cystography on excretory urograms when the former was performed immediately before the latter. They showed that iatrogenic dilatation, indistinguishable from true pathological dilatation of the upper tract, occurred in patients with upper motor neuron lesions when intravenous urography was conducted immediately after cystography. They suggested a time delay between the two examinations to avoid this artifact.[30]

Renal scintigraphy

The renal isotope technetium 99m glucoheptonate defines renal function quantitatively and also helps to differentiate obstructive from nonobstructive types of uropathy. Scintigraphy, a dynamic imaging technique, is highly sensitive in depicting minute renal lesions, but is less specific for any given renal pathology. Fabrizio et al used it with good effect in acute septic conditions of SCI patients to identify a urologic cause of the sepsis. Scintigrams localized the renal damage every time when fever was due to a urological condition.[31]

Cystoscopy

Cystoscopy plays an important role in differentiating functional from organic lower tract obstructions in patients with upper tract abnormalities. For this group of patients, it is advisable to use a flexible cystoscope, considering the frequent occurrence of sphincter spasticity.

Therapy

The principal aim of neurogenic bladder dysfunction treatment is the maintenance of renal function. This requires successful and complete rehabilitation of the lower urinary tract, which means a complete and concerted neurourological intervention. The maintenance or creation of a low-pressure reservoir with no residual urine, the control of urinary infection, and the avoidance of an indwelling catheter are all measures that will promote the main goal, which is upper tract protection. Together with the adequate control of continence, they will ensure quality of life improvement as well. Whenever possible, a program of CIC should be implemented, but this demands some manual dexterity from the patient. After a well-designed rehabilitation program, even quadriplegics may be able to use CIC, if not via the urethra, then at least via a continent abdominal stoma. Therapeutic measures may be divided into acute intervention, to avoid some imminent complication, or elective treatment, fitting into the long-term management program.

Treatment of acute conditions

Lower urinary tract drainage

In the acute phase of SCI and cerebrovascular injuries, the so-called spinal or cerebral shock that will develop is characterized by an areflexic bladder (see Chapter 14). At this stage, the main goal is to avoid overflow incontinence. The condition will improve within 2–12 weeks, but in the meantime, until CIC (operated by the patient or nursing caregiver) can be implemented, continuous bladder drainage must be assured.[23] If no contraindication exists, a suprapubic cystostomy should be done with ultrasonographic guidance. A thin 8–10F catheter is recommended. If suprapubic catheterization is not possible, an indwelling urethral catheter should be introduced for the shortest possible duration. Silicone tubes are recommended, size 14–16F for females and 12–14F for males.[32]

Upper urinary tract drainage

If after successful lower tract drainage, upper tract dilatation still exists (bladder wall fibrosis, stricture, stone), causing renal dysfunction, then percutaneous nephrostomy must be done.

Hemodialysis

If the upper tract passage is free but renal failure persists or progresses, acute dialysis may be necessary.

Antibiotic treatment

Urinary tract infections combined with urosepsis require an antimicrobial treatment.[13]

Nephrectomy

Nephrectomy may become necessary if a septic condition (acute pyelonephritis, renal abscess, etc.) is maintained in spite of adequate drainage and appropriate antibiotics.

Conservative treatments

Spontaneous micturition

Spontaneous micturition is advisable after reflex contraction of the detrusor in response to the Credé maneuver or to various trigger mechanisms, only if intravesical pressure values are below 40 cmH$_2$O during the storage phase and less than 90 cmH$_2$O during the voiding phase, if residual urine is less than 30% of cystometric bladder capacity, and if bladder capacity is more than 200 ml. Lower tract obstruction, DSD, VUR, and reduced bladder compliance constitute contraindications for this approach. Reflex micturition usually means incontinence, and, therefore, the use of absorbent pads or, for males, urinary condoms, is indicated. However, 70% of patients using condom catheters are reported to suffer from chronic urinary infection. Skin problems are often due to allergic reactions to latex.[13,32]

Urine drainage

Drainage may be indicated in any form of bladder dysfunction: in the case of detrusor hyperreflexia, to maintain low bladder pressure (kidney protection) and continence; in the case of DSD, to eliminate the obstruction; in the case of areflexia, to eliminate any residual urine; in the case of decreased compliance, to reduce bladder pressure.

Intermittent catheterization. This technique was introduced in the 1940s by Sir Ludwig Guttman[33] to clear the bladder in SCI patients during the spinal shock phase. In 1972, Lapides et al suggested CIC for patients with neurogenic bladders. Follow-up in 66 patients showed no upper tract alteration.[34] In contrast, Perkas reported VUR and hydronephrosis in CIC patients.[23] Among 85 SCI patients using CIC, Naninga et al found 28 incidents of upper tract damage, detrusor hyperreflexia, and DSD in subjects presumed to have areflexic bladders.[35] This study emphazises once again the importance of regular urodynamic follow-up in such patients. Three patients had sphincterotomy, 15 needed more frequent catheterization, and 10 failed to cooperate and so had to be placed on indwelling catheter drainage.[35] Mollard et al, from Paris, reported on 50 CIC cases. They found that girls and young boys accepted CIC better than did adolescent males.[36] Brem et al studied renal dysfunction and structural abnormalities in 28 children with meningocele on CIC. They reported VUR in 9 cases, renal dysfunction in 14%, and bacteriuria in 38%. They concluded that complications occurred in those patients who had small, noncompliant, trabeculated bladders.[37]

CIC has its own complications. Urinary infection is the most frequent, but urethral damage, stricture, and autonomous dysreflexia have also been noted. Kuhn et al reported a 5-year follow-up of 22 patients on CIC, with sterile urine in 23%, *Escherichia coli* infection in 36.5%, and other pathogenic bacteria (*Pseudomonas, Proteus, Klebsiella*) in another 36% of patients. They found urethral stricture in 1 patient, and autonomous dysreflexia in another. There was no upper tract damage. None of the patients was on anticholinergics, alpha-blockers, or on any continuous antibiotic prophylaxis.[38]

Cass observed that 87.5% of CIC patients with hypo- or areflexic bladders had a stable upper urinary tract with sterile urine in 90%, diminished VUR in 7%, and complete dryness between catheterizations in 34–39%. He reported, however, some complications, such as VUR, renal dysfunction, chronic pyelonephritis, and renal stones.[23] McGuire and Savastano compared patients on CIC for 2–12 years with those on indwelling catheters, finding significantly less acute urinary infections, bladder stones, and episodes of autonomic dysreflexia in the CIC group.[39] According to Madersbacher's experience, 20% of CIC patients had urethral complications, 40% had intermittent and 30% chronic urinary infections, whereas 30% had permanently sterile urine (Madersbacher, pers comm.).

For intermittent catheterization, we may use PVC catheters with a lubricant that contains some anesthetics, or with a hydrophilic coating, size 12–14F for males and 14–16F for females. The control of fluid intake is important: no more than 2000 ml per day. In the case of a normally compliant bladder, catheterization should be repeated 4–6 times a day. However, the catheter should be passed before the amount of urine in the bladder reaches 500 ml. In the case of decreased bladder compliance, urodynamic studies will indicate at what volume the bladder pressure reaches the critical level of 40 cmH$_2$O. The frequency of catheterization should be adjusted, so that this critical intravesical pressure is not reached. It should also be kept in mind that the more frequent the catheterizations, the less frequent is the incidence of urinary infections, and vice versa. Antibiotic prophylaxis is not unanimously recommended: there are some physicians who would only give antibiotics in the case of acute urinary infections, whereas others advocate prophylactic administration of small doses of varied antibiotic types.[32]

Indwelling bladder catheters. They are the worst solution and should only be used as a last resort. If possible, it should be a suprapubic diversion to eliminate urethral complications, particularly in males. In females, simultaneous surgical closure of the bladder neck is often required to ensure continence. Regular daily care of the catheter, together with changing it every 4 or 6 weeks (silicone catheters), is necessary. Although it seems to be a contradiction, several authors confirmed the occurrence of high bladder pressures, even in the chronically catheterized, a consequence of decreasing compliance. Jamil et al found storage pressures of more than 40 cmH$_2$O in 11, and renal damage in 9 of 30 patients on indwelling catheters, renal damage presenting merely in the high-pressure group.[16]

Chao et al compared the upper tract situation of 41 patients on CIC and 32 on indwelling catheters, noting a statistically higher number of renal damage and radiological alterations in the second group.[40] The most frequent complications were ever-present urinary infection, urethral damage and strictures, urethro-cutaneous fistulae, epididymitis, and bladder stones. In a retrospective study of a large SCI population, Hall et al found a 56.6% renal stone and 62.5% bladder stone incidence in patients on indwelling catheters.[21] They recommended prophylactic administration of small doses of varied antibiotic types.

Temporary urethral stents. They are an alternative to indwelling catheters. The Nissenkorn polyurethane or the Urolume endourethral Wallstent prosthesis may be placed at the level of the external sphincter under local anesthesia. Within 6 months after placement, there was no evidence of upper tract damage. Migration and secondary bladder neck obstruction were noted in 27% of patients. After a certain period of time the temporary stents were removed, and a final solution implemented. This is a less-invasive and, to some extent, a reversible solution than sphincterectomy.[41,42]

In summary, whenever possible, the best method of managing the neurogenic bladder is CIC, which will provide regular emptying of a low-pressure bladder and often ensure continence as well. At the same time, it will protect the upper tract. It may be combined, if necessary, with medication (overactive bladder), sphincterotomy (DSD), artificial sphincter implantation (reduced sphincter function), or bladder augmentation cystoplasty (reduced capacity, restricted compliance that fails to respond to other conservative treatments). Indwelling urethral catheters mean permanent urinary infection and several complications; they do not necessarily entail a low-pressure reservoir and often lead to renal damage. They should only be used as a last resort; urethral stents may serve as a temporary solution (see also Chapter 53).

Dietetic treatment

Avoidance of alcohol and spices and also urine acidification may help to prevent urinary infections; a low-protein diet may be indicated in renal dysfunction.

Medication

Hyperreflexia. In detrusor hyperreflexia medication is targeted to eliminate, or at least to decrease, reflex contractions, to normalize high-pressure bladder dysfunction, and to improve the effectiveness of intermittent catheterization. Oral anticholinergics, spasmolytics, and mixed-action products (oxybutynin, propiverine, trospium chloride, tolterodine) are meant to increase bladder capacity and to reduce detrusor contractility, but since they have considerable side-effects (dry mouth, troubled vision, arrhythmia), they are not readily tolerated by many patients. Oxybutynin is the standard medication in the United States, but 61% of the patients do not tolerate it orally, while it is ineffective in 48% (see also Chapter 44). Intravesical oxybutynin solution is more easily tolerated, has less side-effects, and the same efficacy on the detrusor.[9,32,43] Intravesically administered capsaicin and resiniferatoxin provide permanent receptor blockade for 2–7 months, increasing bladder compliance and intravesical pressure while protecting kidney function with no systemic side-effects (except for autonomic dysreflexia, which may occur sometimes)[32] (see also Chapter 45).

Areflexia. In areflexia, we may try cholinergic agents (bethanecol), but there is not much to expect from them, partly because of poor intestinal absorption and partly because they act simultaneously on the bladder, bladder neck, and urethra, so that they do not decrease outlet resistance.[9,32]

Intravesical electrostimulation

This method was developed by Katona in 1959 to ameliorate bladder emptying by strengthening the detrusor reflex and simultaneously improving bladder sensation and compliance.[44] Cheng et al enhanced bladder compliance in children with meningocele; upper tract conditions improved, and augmentation cystoplasty became unnecessary (see also Chapter 51).[9]

Elective surgery

Surgical treatments cause irreversible changes. Therefore, they should only be used if other conservative treatments will not achieve a low-pressure reservoir, effective protection of the upper urinary tract, and/or continence.

Denervation techniques

Surgical or chemical interference with the nerve fibers of the pelvic plexus will increase bladder capacity, reduce reflex incontinence, and improve compliance. Injective techniques imply locally injected anesthesic agents or phenol (the latter being irreversible). The early results with phenol are generally very good, but after a year or so, the symptoms will relapse in about 80% of patients. Also, many complications (fistulae, complete areflexia) have been reported; therefore, this technique has been virtually abandoned.[9]

Bladder transection through the entire thickness of the detrusor above the trigone will also increase bladder capacity. Early cure rates are reported to be 74%, but after 5 years the success rate goes down to 65%.[11] Intradural posterior root rhizotomy combined with the implantation of an extradural anterior root stimulator is the most frequently used method.[45,46] Rhizotomy will suppress bladder spasticity, normally low-pressure storage will be achieved, and voiding can be programmed through the anterior root nerve stimulator.

Brindley et al reported on the first 50 implantations in 1986: 60% of patients were continent. Deafferentation was not yet done routinely in every case at that time.[45] Sauerwein tried this method in 45 patients from 1986 to 1989: 95% were cured from hyperreflexia, 91% became continent, and 84% were spontaneous voiders. Postoperatively, 6 patients showed low-pressure reflux, which was corrected by antireflux surgery. No renal damage was noted.[47] Schurch et al reported that implantation of a Brindley stimulator cured reflex incontinence, while increasing bladder compliance and reducing post-void residual urine volume from an average of 340 ml to 140 ml: VUR disappeared in 3 and was improved in 2 patients.[48] Egon et al implanted the stimulator in 93 patients, 82 of whom became continent and 83 became spontaneous voiders. Before surgery, 3 had had VUR, which disappeared after the intervention (see also Chapter 50).[49]

Bladder augmentation techniques

Augmentation techniques should only be used when bladder compliance is reduced because of organic causes.

Autoaugmentation. This technique is a means of partial myectomy, i.e. the detrusor muscle is excised from the upper half of the bladder, which will then dilate, forming a diverticulum. Follow-up results after 5 years show a success rate of 65%. This surgery is easier to perform than conventional intestinal augmentation, and no postoperative carcinoma is to be feared, but there is a high risk of intraoperative mucosal tear. The bladder takes a long time, almost 1 year, to expand sufficiently, so that in the meantime 45% of patients have to be put on intermittent catheterization. As a result of a lower intravesical pressure decrease than that found in intestinal augmentation, the risk of renal damage is somewhat higher.[50,51]

Enterocystoplasty. This technique is indicated in patients with small bladder capacity, reduced compliance, and renal damage, or incontinence between catheterizations, should the condition be refractory to medication. Augmentation can be done either with the small or the large intestine. The patient may develop metabolic acidosis and runs the risk of intestinal carcinoma due to urine contact with the bowel mucosa. The intestine to be used must first be detubularized. In ileum augmentation, the reported success rate is 52–80%, but 20% of patients need to be put on intermittent catheterization due to increased residual urine volume.[23,50] Flood et al evaluated the results of 122 augmentation cystoplasties performed during an 8-year period on patients with reduced bladder compliance (77%), or refractory detrusor hyperreflexia/instability (23%). The clinical diagnosis in over 50% of cases was neuropathic bladder dysfunction (28% SCI, 23% myelodysplasia). They performed detubularized ileal augmentation in 67% of the patients, detubularized ileocecocystoplasty in 30%, and detubularized sigmoid in 3%. Seventy-five percent of patients were cured, and 20% improved. The reported complications included bladder stones in 21%, incontinence in 13%, and pyelonephritis in 11% of these patients. The re-operation rate was 16%.[52] Renal insufficiency is a relative contraindication for this type of surgery.

Supravesical diversion

Supravesical stomas are made if urethral catheterization is not viable, augmentation cystoplasty fails, or if there is an infiltrating bladder tumor. Incontinent stomas (ileal or colonic conduit) mean less comfort than continent stomas. Brem et al created ileal conduits in 14 children with meningomyelocele, and found ureteral reflux in all patients after the intervention, with renal dysfunction in 28% and bacteriuria in 70%.[37] Continent stomas (Mitrofanoff, Koch pouch, Mainz I, II pouch) induce fewer upper tract complications. The most important complications are stomal stenosis, catheterization difficulty, stone formation in the pouch, and incontinence (i.e. incompetence of the continent stoma).

Antireflux surgery

Reflux in neurogenic bladder dysfunction is mostly the result of high intravesical pressures, large residual urine volumes, poor bladder capacity, restricted compliance, or serious urinary infections. Antireflux surgery by itself will not be the unique solution in the majority of cases, as it does not decrease bladder pressure or improve compliance and capacity. Therefore, this type of surgery is mostly done in combination with some other surgical intervention.

The less-invasive endoscopic method to correct VUR consists of submucosal Teflon or collagen injection at the ureteral orifice. The choice of the material used makes no difference as far as the results are concerned. Silveri et al[17] administered endoscopic injections in 15 children with meningomyelocele and performed open surgery in 2. Follow-up results showed renal failure in 8 cases. Casals et al[53] pointed out that the endoscopic method is fast, simple, and repeatable.

The success rate of open surgery is 80–95%. The Lich–Gregoir method consists of elongating of the intramural portion of the distal ureter by burying a 3–4 cm segment between the bladder mucosa and the detrusor muscle via an entirely extravesical route. A success rate of more than 98% has been claimed by Heimbach et al.[54] The Politano–Leadbetter antireflux procedure, which consists of elongating of the submucosal portion of the refluxing ureter, is probably used most widely. The Cohen method is mainly undertaken to correct bilateral reflux, with the ureters crossing each other on the midline through a submucous tunnel. Burbidge[55] compared the results of the two latter techniques and found an equal success rate (97–98%) for both types of repairs.

Sphincterotomy

This type of intervention is only indicated in males with high-pressure storage due to a DSD causing upper tract deterioration. The intervention reduces LPP theoretically to zero. The resulting incontinence may be managed by a condom catheter. Sphincterotomy is performed particularly when CIC is not possible (e.g. in quadriplegics). Upper tract abnormalities and VUR respond favorably to sphincterotomy in 70–90% of cases.[56] The 12 o'clock incision suggested by Madersbacher involves less complications than conventional 3 or 9 o'clock incisions (lower risk of bleeding and postoperative erectile dysfunction).[57]

Nephrectomy

Nonfunctioning kidneys with pyelonephritis or hydronephrosis – especially if they cause hypertension – should eventually be removed.

References

1. Graham SD. Present urological treatment of spinal cord injury patients. J Urol 1981; 126:1–4.

2. Bors E. Neurogenic bladder. Urol Surg 1957; 7:177–250.

3. Donelly J, Hackler RH, Bunts RC. Present urologic status of the World War II paraplegic: 25-year follow-up. Comparison with status of the 20-year Korean war paraplegic and 5-year Vietnam paraplegic. J Urol 1972; 108:558–562.

4. Koff SA, Lapides J, Piazza DH. Association of urinary tract infection and reflux with uninhibited bladder contractions and voluntary sphincteric obstruction. J Urol 1979; 122:373–376.

5. Cosbie-Ross J. Vesico-ureteric reflux in the neurogenic bladder. Br J Surg 1965; 52:164–167.

6. Thomas DG, Lucas MG. The urinary tract following spinal cord injury. In: Chisholm GD, Fair WR, eds. Scientific foundations of urology. Chicago: Year Book Medical, 1990:289–299.

7. Light K, Blerk JP. Causes of renal deterioration in patients with meningomyelocele. Br J Urol 1977;49:257–260.

8. Soygur T, Arikan N, Yesilli C, Gogus O. Relationship among voiding dysfunction and vesicoureteral reflux and renal scars. Urology 1999; 54:905–908.

9. Madersbacher H. Neurogene Harninkontinenz. In: Höfner K, Jonas U, eds. Praxisratgeber Harninkontinez. Bremen: UNI-MED Verlag AG, International Medical Publishers 2000:221–230.

10. Gerridzen RJ, Thijssen AM, Dehoux E. Risk factors for upper tract deterioration in chronic spinal cord injury patients. J Urol 1992; 147:416–418.

11. Mundy AR. Vesicouretheric reflux in adults. In:Whitfield HN, Hendy WF, Kirby RS, Duchet JW, eds. Textbook of genitourinary surgery. Oxford: Blackwell Science, 1998:440–447.

12. McGuire EJ, Woodside JR, Borden TA, Weiss RM. Prognostic value of urodynamic testing in myelodysplastic patients. J Urol 1981; 126:205–209.

13. Society of German Urologists. Guideline for urological treatment of spinal cord injured patients, 1998.

14. Heidler H. Neurogene Blasenfunktionsstörungen. In: Altwein J, Rübben H, eds. Urologie. Ferdinand Enke Verlag Stuttgart, Heinz Neubert GmbH Druckerei Bayreuth, 1993:379–394.

15. Linsenmeyer TA, Bagaria SP, Gendron B. The impact of urodynamic parameters on the upper tracts of spinal cord injured men who void reflexly. J Spin Cord Med 1998; 21:15–20.

16. Jamil F, Williamson M, Ahmed YS, Harrison SC. Natural fill urodynamics in chronically catheterized patients with spinal cord injury. BJU Int 1999; 83:396–399.

17. Silveri M, Capitanucci ML, Capozza N, et al. Occult spinal dysraphism: neurogenic voiding dysfunction and long term urologic follow-up. Pediatr Surg Int 1997; 12:148–150.

18. Vaidyanathan S, Singh G, Soni BM, et al. Silent hydronephrosis/pyonephrosis due to upper urinary tract calculi in spinal cord injury patients. Spinal Cord 2000; 38:661–668.

19. DeVivo MJ, Rutt RD, Black KJ, et al. Trends in spinal cord injury demographics and treatment outcomes between 1973 and 1986. Arch Phys Med Rehab 1992; 73:424–430.

20. Comarr AE, Kawaichi GK, Bors E. Renal calculosis of patients with traumatic cord lesions. J Urol 1962, 87:647.

21. Hall MK, Hackler RH, Zampieri TA, Zampieri JB. Renal calculi in spinal cord-injured patient: association with reflux, bladder stones, and Foley catheter drainage. Urology 1989; 34:126–128.

22. Killorin W, Gray M, Bennet JK, Green BG. The value of urodynamics and bladder management in predicting upper urinary tract complications in male spinal cord injury patients. Paraplegia 1992; 30:437–441.

23. Sukin SW, Boone TB. Diagnosis and treatment of spinal cord injuries and myeloneuropathy. In: Rodney AA, ed. Voiding dysfunction. Totowa: Humana Press, 2000:115–139.

24. Virgili G, Finazzi AE, Giannantoni A, et al. Ultrasonography of the upper urinary tract in patients with spinal cord injury. Arch Ital Urol Androl 2000; 72:225–227.

25. Calenoff L, Neimen HL, Kaplan PE, et al. Urosonography in spinal cord injury patients. J Urol 1982; 128:1234–1237.

26. Ozer MN, Shannon SR. Renal sonography in asymptomatic persons with spinal cord injury: a cost-effectiveness analysis. Arch Phys Med Rehab 1991; 72:35–37.

27. Bih LI, Tsai SJ, Tung LC. Sonographic diagnosis of hydronephrosis in patients with spinal cord injury: influence of bladder fullness. Arch Phys Med Rehab 1998; 79:1557–1559.

28. Ruutu M, Kivisaari A, Lehtonen T. Upper urinary tract changes in patients with spinal cord injury. Clin Radiol 1984; 35:491–494.

29. Rao KG, Hackler RH, Woodlief RM, et al. Real-time renal sonography in spinal cord injury patients: prospective comparison with excretory urography. J Urol 1986; 135:72–77.

30. Stover SL, Witten DM, Kuhlemeier KV, et al. Iatrogenic dilatation of the upper urinary tract during radiographic evaluation of patients with spinal cord injury. J Urol 1986; 135:78–82.

31. Fabrizio MD, Chancellor MB, Rivas DA, et al. The role of renal scintigraphy in the evaluation of spinal cord injury with presumed urosepsis. J Urol 1996; 156:1730–1734.

32. Madersbacher H. Konservative Therapie der neurogenen Blasendysfunktion. Urologe 1999; 38:24–29.

33. Guttman L, Frankel H. The value of intermittent catheterization in the early management of traumatic paraplegia and tetraplegia. Paraplegia 1966; 4:63.

34. Lapides J, Diokono A, Silber S, Lowe B. Clean intermittent self-catheterisation in the treatment of urinary tract disease. J Urol 1972; 107:458–461.

35. Nanninga JB, Wu Y, Hamilton B. Long-term intermittent catheterization in the spinal cord injury patient. J Urol 1982; 128:760–763.

36. Mollard P, Meunier P, Berard C, Henriet M. Treatment of urinary incontinence of neurologic origin in children and adolescents. J Urol (Paris) 1984; 90:227–236.

37. Brem AS, Martin D, Callaghan J, Maynard J. Long term renal risk factors in children with meningomyelocele. J Pediatr 1987; 110:51–55.

38. Kuhn W, Rist M, Zaech GA. Intermittent urethral self catheterisation: long term results (bacteriological evolution, continence, acceptance, complications). Paraplegia 1991; 29:222–232.

39. McGuire EJ, Savastano J. Comparative urological outcome in women with spinal cord injury. J Urol 1986; 135:730–731.

40. Chao R, Clowers D, Mayo ME. Fate of upper urinary tracts in patients with indwelling catheters after spinal cord injury. Urology 1993; 42:259–262.

41. Chartier-Kastler EJ, Thomas L, Bussel B, et al. Feasibility of a temporary urethral stent through the striated sphincter in patients in the early phase (6 months) of spinal cord injury. Eur Urol 2001; 39:326–331.

42. Rivas DA, Chancellor M. Sphincterotomy and sphincter stent prosthesis placement. In: Corcos J, Schick E, eds. The urinary sphincter. New York: Marcel Dekker, 2001:565–583.

43. Szollar SM, Lee SM. Intravesical oxybutynin for spinal cord injury patients. Spinal Cord 1996; 34:284–287.

44. Katona F. Stages of vegetative afferentation in reorganisation of bladder control during electrotherapy. Urol Int 1975; 30:192–203.

45. Brindley GS, Polkey CE, Rushton DN, Cardozo L. Sacral anterior root stimulators for bladder control in paraplegia. The first 50 cases. J Neurol Neurosurg Psychiatry 1986; 49:1104–1114.

46. Tanagho EA, Schmidt RA, Orvis BR. Neural stimulation for the control of voiding dysfunction: a preliminary report on 22 patients with serious neuropathic voiding disorders. J Urol 1989; 142:340–345.

47. Sauerwein D. Die operativen Behandlung der spastischen Blasenlahmung bei Querschnittlahmung. Urologe A 1990; 19:196–203.

48. Schurch B, Rodic B, Jeanmonod D. Posterior sacral rhizotomy and intradural anterior sacral root stimulation for treatment of the spastic bladder in spinal cord injured patients. J Urol 1997; 157:610–614.

49. Egon G, Barat M, Colombel P, et al. Implantation of anterior sacral root stimulators combined with posterior sacral rhizotomy in spinal injury patients. World J Urol 1998; 16:342–349.

50. Müller SC. Chirurgische Therapie. In: Höfner K, Jonas U, eds. Praxisratgeber Harninkontinez. Bremen: UNI-MED Verlag AG, 2000: 144–177.

51. Christmas TJ, Kirby RS. Principles of management of the neurogenic bladder. In: Whitfield HN, Hendy WF, Kirby RS, Duchet JW, eds. Textbook of genitourinary surgery. Oxford: Blackwell Science, 1998: 918–926.

52. Flood HD, Malhotra SJ, O'Connel HE, et al. Long-term results and complications using augmentation cystoplasty in reconstructive urology. Neurourol Urodyn 1995; 14:297–309.

53. Casals J, Rivero A, Rivero J. Endoscopic treatment of vesico-ureteral reflux in the neurogenic bladder. Arch Esp Urol 1997; 50:381–387.

54. Heimbach D, Bruhl P, Mallmann R. Lich–Gregoir antireflux procedure; indications and results with 283 vesicoureteral units. Scand J Urol Nephrol 1995; 29:311–316.

55. Burbidge KA. Ureteral reimplantation: a comparison of results with the cross trigonal and Politano–Leadbetter techniques in 120 patients. J Urol 1991; 146:1352–1353.

56. Ruutu ML, Lehtonen TA. Bladder outlet surgery in men with spinal cord injury. Scand J Urol Nephrol 1985; 19:241–246.

57. Madersbacher H. The twelve o'clock sphincterotomy: technique, indications, results. Paraplegia 1976; 13:261–267.

Part IX

Prognosis

63

Evolution and follow-up of lower urinary tract dysfunction in spinal cord injury patients

Jean-Jacques Labat and Brigitte Perrouin-Verbe

Introduction

Neurological lesions can disrupt bladder-sphincter functioning and its central neurological control. Consequently, these problems can alter the quality of life by inducing incontinence and even threatening the upper urinary tract, particularly of spinal cord injury (SCI) patients. For a long time, urinary complications have been the leading cause of death in SCI. Today, this is not the case. Better knowledge of the evolution and prognostic factors of neurological bladder has enabled the development of pertinent follow-up strategies, screening for risky situations, and taking account of aging urinary systems as well as aging SCI patients themselves. Neuro-urological assessment is never definitive. The evolution of therapeutic methods will permit new, more adequate treatments for use tomorrow.

Background

In 1927, Harvey Cushing observed that 80% of SCI patients died within weeks after the trauma because of infections, urinary catheters, and bedsores. The mortality rate during the acute phase has evolved over the years due to improved care management. It has dropped from 60–80% during World War II to 30% in the 1960s and 6% in the 1980s.[1]

The decrease in mortality of urinary origin is partly responsible for this survival gain. In SCI patients who survived World War II and the Korean war,[2] deaths from urinary causes were estimated to be 43%. Then, they declined with time, with the rate not exceeding 10% in the 1980s and 1990s.[3] In 50 years of follow-up, the risk of death attributed to urinary factors has diminished by half in each successive decade.[4]

This favorable evolution in terms of mortality is also seen for morbidity, with preventive measures tending to replace hospitalization for urological complications. At present, 43% of rehospitalizations are for urinary reasons (the leading cause of rehospitalization),[5] but in most cases,

they are more for a check-up than for care. The average length of hospitalization is 7.9 days, with a median length of 3 days. These figures thus confirm that there has been a progression from care to prevention, showing the importance of bladder-sphincter follow-up.

Prognostic factors in upper urinary tract changes

Follow-up objectives

There are many neuro-bladder classifications, but they do not enable prognostic assessment because, even if they do identify the dysfunction type, they do not estimate the balance of urodynamic forces present. The classical criteria of bladder dysequilibrium, which are post-void residual urine, urinary infection, vesicoureteral reflux, ureterohydronephrosis, lithiasis, and incontinence, reflect the deterioration when they occur, but they don't have good prognostic value. The follow-up objectives are thus to solve the problems encountered by SCI patients with lower urinary tract dysfunction: this means improving urinary continence, restricting infections, facilitating micturition, while preserving patient autonomy. It is equally important to strive for an equilibrated bladder today without any risks for tomorrow, i.e. to protect the upper urinary tract apparatus. This equilibrium is not a constant but a daily balance that cannot be considered as unchanging.

The role of elevated intravesical pressure during the storage phase

In 1981, McGuire et al[6] brilliantly illuminated the harmful role of elevated intravesical pressures in SCI patients.

When bladder leak point pressure (BLPP) is lower than or equal to 40 cmH_2O, there is no vesicoureteral reflux and only 10% of dilatation on intravenous pyelography (IVP). When BLPP is more than 40 cmH_2O, we find 61% of reflux and 81% of upper urinary tract dilatation.

We have confirmed these data in a retrospective study of 200 myelomeningocele patients,[7] followed for a period of 3–17 years (average 9.02 years). The prognostic value of BLPP is demonstrated by the study of survival curves testing the rate of upper urinary tract degradation according to its dilatation and the BLPP: if BLPP rises during the follow-up, the probability of an undilated upper urinary tract at 12 years post-trauma is no more than 20%, whereas it is 86% if BLPP stays low; a patient with BLPP exceeding 40 cmH_2O has 7 times more risk of upper urinary tract damage than someone with stable BLPP.

SCI patients show a correlation between vesicoureteral reflux and elevated intravesical pressure:[8] when bladder pressure exceeds 60 cmH_2O, 22% have reflux, but when the pressure is normal, reflux occurs in only 5% of patients. In detrusor hyperreflexia, we find upper urinary tract alteration in 16% and a normal upper urinary tract in 84%, corresponding to patients whose BLPP is 115 cmH_2O and 72 cmH_2O, respectively, on average.[9] Similarly, in detrusor areflexia, the upper urinary tract is altered in 18% and normal in 82% of patients. The corresponding BLPP values are 58 cmH_2O and 24 cmH_2O, respectively.

BLPP is thus an essential prognostic factor, with a particularly bad significance when it exceeds 40 cmH_2O.

The physiopathology of upper urinary tract damage

Bladder hyperpressure, either related to detrusor hyperreflexia (SCI patients with prolonged and strong amplitude bladder contractions) or to poor bladder compliance of detrusor areflexia (particularly in myelomeningocele), will have a dual effect: hydrodynamic perturbations and morphological changes. Bladder hyperpressure will alter urethral flow, as the latter occurs at low pressure; in the beginning, the ureter compensates by an increased amplitude and frequency of contractions; then, above 40 cmH_2O, statis presents with dilatation (or even vesicoureteral reflux). The situation will deteriorate rapidly if the duration of exposure to high pressure is prolonged. This upper urinary tract alteration is initially reversible by continuous catheterization or by restoring detrusor pressure to an acceptable level.

Detrusor hyperpressure can be the consequence but, above all, the cause of bladder wall deformities (trabeculae, diverticula); these may sometimes affect the watertightness of the vesicoureteral junction and induce vesicoureteral reflux. They will facilitate the development of infectious sites, increasing hyperreflectivity. Collagen will seep progressively into and accumulate between smooth muscle fibers, which become rarified. These structural changes may have variable repercussions. When the bladder is active, they induce a decrease of detrusor contractility and lead to a new pressure equilibrium, a veritable homeostasis phenomenon aimed at protecting the upper urinary tract. More deformed bladders are not always the most poorly tolerated by the upper urinary tract level. The collagen excess also favors irreversible detrusor fibrosis, particularly in inactive or congenital neurobladders. This fibrosis, which thickens the detrusor wall, contributes to stenosis of the lower ureter and hydronephrosis. After bladder wall lesions are definitively installed, treatment of hyperreflexia cannot stop the vesicoureteral reflux.

The context and antecedents
Age at onset
Children

In childhood-acquired paraplegia, the prognosis of lower urinary tract dysfunction is relatively good compared to paraplegia occurring during adulthood.[10] In the long term (6–30 years), 10.4% of childhood paraplegics[11] will incur Bricker's syndrome, which has a lower rate than for adults in the same reference period (1960s–1980s).

The elderly

Spinal cord lesions in the elderly mean complications. Rehabilitation failure is common because of difficulties in adapting to the new situation, a lower urinary tract altered by age (prostate hyperplasia, cystocele, sphincter failure) with slower reflexes, and detrusor hypoactivity. These elements explain the frequency of surgical procedures in men and the use of indwelling catheters. When the lesion occurs after age 60 years, 50% have an indwelling catheter, and 50% of men undergo a de-obstruction procedure. Traditional rehabilitation often fails.[12] The prognosis for old people is, therefore, linked more to personal factors than to the neuro-urological situation itself.

Gender

Studies published a few years ago show that women are less exposed than men to urological complications. In 1983, 99% of 200 SCI women who survived the initial phase retained a normal IVP for the following 20 years;[13] the woman:man complication rate was 1:4.4; 1 woman died of renal failure for every 19 men. This difference has not been seen in recent years. In 1992, the urological complication rate with time was not significantly different between men and women, and renal failure was no higher in women with an indwelling catheter than in men with a condom catheter.[14]

The drainage method significantly influences the complication rate, and the harmful role of indwelling catheters can be found here compared to reflex voiding or intermittent catheterization. This was very significant in a population of 70 SCI women followed for 11–13 years.[15] It raises questions as to better choices of treatment, given the absence of urine collectors for women.

The neurological lesion

In a study by Gerridzen et al[9] of 140 SCI patients, of whom 62% were tetraplegic and 38% were paraplegic, somewhat surprisingly, 51% of paraplegics had detrusor hyperreflexia vs 49% who presented with detrusor areflexia. Among the tetraplegics, 86% had detrusor hyperreflexia and 14% bladder areflexia. Eight years after the lesion, alterations of the upper urinary tract were twice as frequent among tetraplegics, as 17% of them had a damaged upper urinary tract vs 8% of paraplegics.

The incidence of reflux is higher in complete than in incomplete SCI,[16] but the frequency is identical in paraplegics and tetraplegics. It is probable that the perception of an equivalent of a micturation need limits the risk of increased intravesical pressure, because the patient can urinate sooner.

Drainage method

In the initial stage

The complication rate in the initial period after the trauma is closely linked to the bladder drainage method, with particularly high risks of damage from indwelling catheters:[17] acute pyelonephritis, purulent cystitis, paraurethral abscess, ureteral fistula, urethral strictures, severe hematuric cystitis.

In the long term

In a very large study of 316 exclusively male SCI patients, Weld[18] examined the influence of drainage methods on urological complications. One hundred and fourteen patients had an indwelling catheter (changed every month), 92 practiced proper intermittent catheterization, 74 voided spontaneously (defined as reflex voidings with post-void residual urine volume less than 100 ml and voiding pressure less than 40 cmH$_2$O), and 36 carried a suprapubic catheter. Three hundred and ninety-eight urological complications occurred in 126 patients. The complications were more frequent in patients with continuous bladder drainage, since 53.5% of these cases had 236 of the complications (61 patients): 4.4% of suprapubic catheter patients had 48 complications (16 patients), 32.4% of patients who voided spontaneously had 57 complications (24 patients), and 27.2% of intermittent catheterization patients had 57 complications (25 patients).

Tetraplegic cases

The independence of tetraplegics is more or less limited, and so the choice of their miction mode is necessarily influenced by voiding autonomy. Among 73 SCI patients of more than 20 years duration,[19] 32 had an indwelling catheter, and 41 another mode of miction (reflex voiding, sphincterotomy, intermittent catheterization): there was no difference between the two groups for creatinine level, but the indwelling catheter group had a higher rate of hydronephrosis and renal atrophy. Alternatively to indwelling catheters, suprapubic catheters seemed to be a good drainage method, since 34 of 61 tetraplegics used this mode for an average of 8.6 years (for 27 intermittent catheterizations, the average was 9.9 years), and no upper urinary tract deterioration was observed in any of these groups.[20] However, we noted a much higher frequency of lithiasis in the suprapubic catheter group, and more frequent urinary infections with intermittent catheterization.

Intermittent catheterization seems to be the safest method for SCI patients in terms of urological complications. In contrast, indwelling catheters appear to incur the highest rate of complications, particularly in the long term.

Urinary infection
Symptomatic infections

The elements that indicate urinary infections in SCI patients sometimes clearly appear with fever and shivering, smelly urine, or hematuria but are most often subtle: intense renal or bladder pain, urinary leakage or miction changes, increased spasticity, lethargy, general malaise, and discomfort.

Asymptomatic infections

It is extremely difficult to find a consensus concerning the criteria of asymptomatic urinary infection in SCI patients and, above all, to see them applied, even if only to clinical studies. Nevertheless, criteria have been defined in a National Institute on Disability and Rehabilitation Research Consensus Statement[21] according to the miction mode and can be viewed as extremely rigorous: bacteriuria exceeding 10^2/ml in intermittent catheterization patients, greater than 10^4/ml in patients with a condom catheter, and no matter what the concentration is when patients have an indwelling catheter. The banality of asymptomatic infections is such that they may be neglected most of the time.

Universally accepted risk factors

The risk factors of urinary infections have been classified universally by Cardenas and Hooton:[22] bladder distention, vesicoureteral reflux, elevated intravesical pressure, post-void residual urine volume, stones, lower bladder outlet obstruction, decreased immunity, pregnancy, repeated urethral traumas, anatomical anomalies of the urinary tract, perineum hygiene, presence of an indwelling or suprapubic catheter. We must also consider some of the more subjective elements, including possible behavioral risks as well as psychological factors: degree of patient comprehension, inactivity, self-esteem, and social acceptance. Finally, intermittent catheterization is a source of increased infections only when it is performed for tetraplegics by untrained persons (in this case, with infection risk even higher than with indwelling catheters).

Infectious complications

Epididymitis was found in 16.1% of patients and pyelonephritis in 3.5%. Ninety-four percent of patients had been treated at least once for lower urinary tract infection. Indwelling catheters are the main cause of infectious complications: pyelonephritis and especially epididymitis. Intermittent catheterization leads to less epididymitis than reflex voiding.[18]

Renal function

All bladder drainage methods may preserve the upper urinary tract, but continuous drainage is a risk factor for upper urinary tract damage and renal failure. With continuous bladder drainage, 18.6% of patients undergo upper urinary tract changes. This rate is 7.8% with reflex voiding, and 6.5% with intermittent catheterization.[23] If death (from all causes) is twice more frequent in the continuous drainage group, it is not necessarily significant, because patients in this group are older.

Among the associated factors, patient age and lesion duration are correlated with higher blood creatinine, lower creatinine clearance, and frequent proteinuria. Vesicoureteral reflux is correlated with renal function damage and radiological anomalies of the upper urinary tract. Blood creatinine levels alone seem not to be a very sensitive factor in early deterioration of the upper urinary tract compared with proteinuria, creatinine clearance, and upper urinary tract imaging.

The two most sensitive methods of screening for renal function deterioration are creatinine clearance and isotopic scintigraphy. Blood creatinine declines with age and body mass reduction; hence, it can remain normal despite decreasing glomerular filtration, and is not sensitive enough. Measurement of endogenous creatinine clearance is acceptable, but poses a problem of 24-hour urine collection in SCI patients. Isotopic clearance (Tc DTPA) seems to be the best method of examination.

Renal scintigraphy represents the most sensitive screening procedure for renal function changes. Effective renal plasma flow (ERPF) decreases by 4.5 ml per year in the 10 years following spinal cord lesion.[26] The factors associated with declining ERPF are age, female sex, renal or bladder lithiasis, tetraplegia, frequent shivering, and fever episodes, but there is no relationship with lesion age, and bacteriuria and no link with lesion severity.

Radiology
Urethral complications

Urethral stricture has been noted in 11.7% of patients, and periurethral abscess in 2.8%.[18] Indwelling catheters cause many urethral strictures, and intermittent catheters two times less, but significantly more than suprapubic catheters or reflex miction.

Lithiases

Upper urinary tract lithiasis has been found in 35.1% of patients,[18] and lower urinary tract lithiasis in 14.6%. Indwelling catheters lead to significantly more lithiasis complications of the upper urinary tract and bladder than intermittent catheterization and spontaneous miction. Temporal evolution shows that lithiasis risk is always present[24] – 3.1% at 5 years, 5.1% at 10 years, 6% at 15 years, and 10.8% at 20 years – but with significant variations according to the voiding method: suprapubic and indwelling catheters represent a high risk, whereas intermittent catheterization has negligible risk.

Upper urinary tract changes

Vesicoureteral reflux has been found in 15.8% of patients, and upper urinary tract alteration in 26.3%.[18] Intermittent catheterization and reflex miction are accompanied by significantly less reflux than indwelling or suprapubic catheters.

Urodynamics
Post-void residual urine

Contrary to what we have always thought, even if post-void residual urine volume is a sign of bladder-sphincter dysfunction, it is not a prognostic factor. The upper urinary tract can deteriorate without any residual volume; the bladder may work to avoid residual urine volume, but this exhausts the urinary system in the long term. In 1977, 38% of dilatation was found 2–6 years after SCI in the absence of residual volume.[25] However, major, chronic post-void urine volume can be tolerated perfectly for years, especially in hypoactive bladders with high compliance.

The prognosis is thus not linked to post-void residual volume, but depends on urodynamic balance. Post-void urine volume is a sign of obstruction, because it is also a function of adaptation to detrusor contraction. It is as much the consequence of primary insufficient detrusor contraction or decompensation as obstruction. It can be particularly dangerous if there is an associated compliance deficit, or if there are prolonged dyssynergic contractions, as the bladder is then subjected permanently to high pressures.

Bladder reflectivity and contractility

The complication rate of upper urinary tract damage is clearly higher in patients with reflex miction (32%) compared with patients who void spontaneously (0%) or who have an inactive detrusor or a detrusor inactivated by anticholinergics (7%).[26] All hyperreflexias are not dangerous in the same way: they will be more hazardous if the contractions are strong, prolonged, and frequent; otherwise, they may just manifest as a brief peak of hyperpressure but much less harmful than hyperpressure of the filling phase. In paraplegics, there is a correlation between high intravesical pressure and reflux, with 22% of reflux occurring when intravesical pressure is greater than 60 cmH$_2$O vs 5% when it is lower than this value.[27]

Dyssynergia
Detrusor-sphincter dyssynergia

Bladder hyperreflexia is harmful in SCI patients because it is associated with bladder-sphincter dyssynergia. In suprasacral lesions,[28] 7.4% of patients have no dyssynergia, 80.3% have intermittent dyssynergia, and 12.3% have continuous dyssynergia. Complete spinal cord lesion is usually accompanied by continuous dyssynergia, whereas intermittent dyssynergia is seen only with incomplete lesion. Dyssynergia is associated with complete lesions, with high intravesical pressure, and with upper urinary tract complications. These associations are more pronounced in continuous dyssynergia than in intermittent dyssynergia. The proportion of patients suffering from a particular type of bladder-sphincter dyssynergia has not changed with time.

These parameters are, in fact, correlated. Indeed, dyssynergia is responsible for high intravesical pressures, which are themselves a source of risk for the upper urinary tract. On the other hand, what value should be given to this classification of detrusor-sphincter dyssynergia in case of anticholinergic treatment, since the latter does not alter the type of dyssynergia although it modifies the other risk factors (decreased intravesical pressure)? Under these conditions, would it be worthwhile to distinguish the different types of dyssynergia or to evaluate the pressures that they engender?

Compliance

Measurement of compliance deficiency seems less significant than BLPP, but explores high pressures in the same way during the filling phase and their danger. In contast, flaccid and compliant bladders do not develop any changes of the bladder wall and upper urinary tract; this may be the case of cauda equina syndrome after disc herniation.

Evaluation of compliance is difficult in SCI patients because of hyperreflexia, and studies are rare. Hypocompliant bladders are seldom found in SCI patients.[29] In the population with initially normal compliance (higher than 20%), the upper urinary tract remains normal 3 years later in 78% of cases, but when initial compliance is low (17%), we find only 23% with a normal upper urinary tract after this time period.[30]

A threshold of 12.5 ml/cmH$_2$O significantly indicates the presence of various upper urinary tract complications: vesicoureteral reflux, upper urinary tract distention, pyelonephritis, and upper urinary tract lithiasis.[31] In suprasacral lesions (complete and incomplete), bladder hypocompliance is more frequent in patients with continuous drainage than in those who use intermittent catheterization. Whatever the drainage method, low compliance is more frequent in sacral lesions than in suprasacral lesions and in complete than in incomplete lesions. Regression curve analysis shows that compliance is more often altered with time in the continuous drainage group than in the reflex micturition and intermittent catheterization groups. The risk of altered compliance with indwelling catheters increases by 23% every 5 years.

The evolution of bladder compliance thus appears to be a fundamental element of surveillance for all neurological bladders.

Cytology and cystoscopy

The risk of bladder tumor is high in aging SCI patients and notably in those with indwelling catheters (over 8 years) or bladder lithiasis.[32] Recently, Groah et al[33] examined 3670 SCI patients by cystoscopy showing that the risk of bladder cancer with SCI using indwelling catheter is 77 per 100,000 person-years. This corresponds to an age- and gender-adjusted standardized morbidity ratio of 25.4 when compared with the general population. After adjusting for age at injury, gender, level and severity of SCI, history of bladder calculi, and smoking, those using solely indwelling catheter had a risk of bladder cancer 4.9 times higher than those using non-indwelling methods. These findings suggest a screening by cytologies and annual cystoscopy after 8 years of indwelling catheter use in the at-risk patients' group (lithiasis, repeated infections, etc.).

Longitudinal follow-up

Patient compliance in follow-up

Clinical practice demonstrates the importance of some elements that are difficult to quantify. Patient compliance in follow-up is one of these parameters. The three most significant elements of complications occurrence are ignorance of the importance of follow-up, lack of confidence in their general practitioner, and examination cost.[34] The other significant elements are living far from services, transport difficulties, and length of time since the accident.

Delayed complications

Radiologically, 63% of SCI patients have bladder anomalies – wall deformities, lithiasis, upper urinary tract changes – that appear in 3/4 of cases in the first year, especially in patients who had an indwelling catheter for a prolonged initial period (more than 8 weeks). In contrast, new radiological anomalies occur in only 1% of cases after 10 years.[35] Upper urinary tract complications (23.7% of 105 SCI patients)[36] can present at any time of follow-up, between 1 month and 34 years, with an average of 10.4 years. Forty-four percent of reflux appears during the first 2 years, and 23% during the following 2 years, with the rates decreasing regularly with time.[16] Thus, the first years after the trauma are the most dangerous.

If we compare drainage methods,[18] we find that the complication rate increases in the indwelling catheter group 5 years after the trauma, and after 15 years in patients with suprapubic catheters, with no significant changes in time for the two other groups (intermittent catheterization and spontaneous micturition), which, therefore, remain safe methods for the long term.

Patients at risk

It is possible to define SCI populations at higher risk of urinary complications.

Tetraplegic patients have a higher risk

They have a higher risk because they frequently have bladder hyperreflexia and because they do not take any anticholinergics to facilitate spontaneous micturition in a condom catheter.

Paraplegic patients have a relative decrease in risk

The decreased risk in paraplegics is linked to a lower frequency of hyperreflexia with high pressures, because these patients are treated with intermittent catheterization and anticholinergics. In this group, the only deterioration occurs in patients not taking anticholinergics.

Men have more risks than women

The caricatural difference of a few years ago is subsiding, thanks to progress made in the follow-up of SCI patients.

Surveillance will be especially close as intravesical pressures are high

In hyperreflexia, dyssynergia is responsible for type 3 high pressures. This is characteristic of complete lesions. In areflexia, low compliance of the peripheral bladder is the source of the high pressures. In all cases, it is important to suspect compliance <20 and to avoid compliance <12.5.

Micturition mode

Patients with an indwelling catheter in the initial phase and in the long term present more complications. The suprapubic catheter is a better method, except for the risk of intravesical lithiasis. It is preferable to use anticholinergics in association with intermittent catheterization than to urinate in a reflex way.

Lesion duration

Surveillance should be close in the first 2 years. Complications may occur later (after 5 years of an indwelling catheter and after 15 years of a suprapubic catheter). In patients without an indwelling or suprapubic catheter, the situation may remain stable for over 15 years. Cystoscopy and cytology are necessary in patients with an indwelling catheter for over 8 years.

Patient profile

It is important to pay attention to loss of follow-up in patients who live far away and who have a great deal of trust in their general practitioner. It is important to inform patients of the necessity of regular and specialized follow-up.

Conclusion: follow-up proposals

SCI patient follow-up is based on clinical care and systematic checkups. The clinical elements that lead patients to consultation are generally linked to infectious complications or to changes in continence. The search for an irritative cause is part of the checkup: eschar, fecaloma, ingrown nail, prolapse. The paraclinical elements derive from an appreciation of post-micturition residual volume, from biological examinations that explore renal function, imaging, and urodynamics. All these parameters do not possess the same value, as some screen for certain complications (imaging), whereas others try to prevent them (urodynamics).

The follow-up of SCI patients should be adapted to the clinical situation. Nevertheless, we can still try to respect standard procedures that will be adapted in terms of the data collected during these checkups and risky situations. In the initial phase, it will be interesting to have a starting intravenous pyelogram that may never be re-done but which will enable screening for pre-existing anomalies and which may serve as a subsequent reference document.

In the first 2 years, the patient should be followed up clinically, urodynamically, and by ultrasound every 6 months. In the subsequent 5 years, follow-up will be annual. In the following 8 years, follow-up should be every 2 years, with clinical, echographic, and urodynamic assessment indications to be discussed in terms of each situation. After 15 years, clinical and ultrasound follow-up every 2–5 years may be enough if the patient urinates in a reflex way or by intermittent catheterization.

Certainly, the presentation of risk factors (particularly elevated intravesical pressures) and urinary complications will lead to changes in follow-up and treatment plans.

References

1. Hartkopp A, Bronnum-Hansen H, Seidenschnur AM, Biering-Sorensen F. Survival and cause of death after traumatic spinal cord injury. A long-term epidemiological survey from Denmark. Spinal Cord 1997; 35:76–85.

2. Hackler RH. A 25 years prospective mortality study in a spinal cord injured patient: comparison with the long term living paraplegic. J Urol 1977; 117:486–488.

3. Whiteneck GG, Charlifue SW, Frankel HL, et al. Mortality, morbidity, and psychosocial outcomes of persons spinal cord injured more than 20 years ago. Paraplegia 1992; 30:617–630.

4. Frankel HL, Coll JR, Charlifue SW, et al. Long-term survival in spinal cord injury: a fifty year investigation. Spinal Cord 1998; 36:266–274.

5. Vaidyanathan S, Soni BM, Gopalan L, et al. A review of the readmissions of patients with tetraplegia to the Regional Injuries Centre, Southport, United Kingdom, between January 1994 and December 1995. Spinal Cord 1998; 36:838–846.

6. McGuire EJ, Woodside JR, Borden TA, Weiss RM. Prognostic value of urodynamic testing in myelodysplastic patients. J Urol 1981; 126:205–209.

7. Bouchot O, Labat JJ, Glemain P, Buzelin JM. Les facteurs du pronostic urinaire des myélo-méningocèles. J Urol (Paris) 1988; 94:145–151.

8. Anderson RU. Urologic complications in spinal cord injured patients. Urology 1988; 32 (Suppl.):31–32.

9. Gerridzen RG, Thijssen AM, Dehoux E. Risk factors for upper tract deterioration in chronic spinal cord injury patients. J Urol 1992; 147:416–418.

10. Fanciullacci F, Zanollo A, Sandri S, Catanzaro F. The neuropathic bladder in children with spinal cord injury. Paraplegia 1988; 26:83–86.

11. Lacert P, Picard A, Richard F, Bourgeois-Gavardin T. Résultats à long terme de la rééducation urinaire au cours des paraplégies acquises de l'enfant. Ann Urol 1982; 16:44–46.

12. Madersbacher H, Oberwalder M. The elderly para and tetraplegic: special aspects of urologic care. Paraplegia 1987; 25:318–323.

13. Watson N. Spinal cord injury in the female. Paraplegia 1983; 21:143–148.

14. Jackson AB, DeVivo M. Urological long term follow-up in women with spinal cord injuries. Arch Phys Med Rehab 1992; 73:1029–1035.

15. Bennet CJ, Young MN, Adkins RH, Diaz F. Comparison of bladder management complication outcomes in female spinal cord injury patients. J Urol 1995; 153:1458–1460.

16. Lamid S. Long term follow-up of spinal cord injury patients with vesicoureteral reflux. Paraplegia 1988; 26:27–34.

17. Zermann D, Wunderlich H, Derry F, et al. Audit of early bladder management complications after spinal cord injury in first treating hospitals. Eur Urol 2000; 37:156–160.

18. Weld JK. Effect of bladder management on urological complications in spinal cord injured patients. J Urol 2000; 163:768–772.

19. Chao R, Clowers D, Mayo ME. Fate of upper urinary tracts in patients with indwelling catheters after spinal cord injury. Urology 1993; 42:259–262.

20. Mitsui T, Minami K, Furuno T, et al. Is suprapubic cystostomy an optimal urinary management in high quadriplegics? A comparative study of suprapubic cystostomy and clean intermittent catheterisation. Eur Urol 2000; 38:434–438.

21. National Institute on Disability and Rehabilitation Research Consensus Statement. January 27–29, 1992. The prevention and management of urinary tract infections among people with spinal cord injuries. J Am Paraplegia Soc 1992; 15:194–204.

22. Cardenas DD, Hooton TM. Urinary tract infection in persons with spinal cord injury. Arch Phys Med Rehab 1995; 76:272–280.

23. Weld KJ. Influences on renal function in chronic spinal cord injured patients. J Urol 2000; 164:1490–1493.

24. McKinley WO, Jackson AB, Cardenas DD, DeVivo MJ. Long term medical complications after traumatic spinal cord injury: a regional model systems analysis. Arch Phys Med Rehab 1999; 80:1402–1410.

25 Stover SL, Lloyd LK, Nepomuceno CS, Gale LL. Intermittent catheterization: follow-up. Paraplegia 1977; 15:38–46.

26. Killorin W, Gray M, Bennett JK, Green BG. The value of urodynamics and bladder management in predicting upper urinary tract complications in male spinal cord injury patients. Paraplegia 1992; 30:437–441.

27. Arnold EP, Cowan IA. Clinical significance of ureteric diameter on intravenous urography after spinal cord injury. Br J Urol 1988; 62:131–135.

28. Weld JK. Clinical significance of detrusor sphincter dyssynergia type in patients with post-traumatic spinal cord injury. Urology 2000; 56:565–569.

29. Ruutu M. Cystometrographic patterns in predicting bladder function after spinal cord injury. Paraplegia 1985; 23:243–252.

30. Hackler RH, Hall MK, Zampieri TA. Bladder hypocompliance in the spinal cord injury population. J Urol 1989; 141:1390–1393.

31. Weld JK. Differences in bladder compliance with time and associations of bladder management with compliance in spinal cord injured patients. J Urol 2000; 163:1228–1233.

32. Stonehill WH, Goldman HB, Dmochowski RR. Risk factors for bladder tumors in spinal cord injury patients. J Urol 1996; 155:1248–1250.

33. Groah SL, Weitzenkamp DA, Lammertse DP, et al. Excess risk of bladder cancer in spinal cord injury: evidence for an association between indwelling catheter use and bladder cancer. Arch Phys Med Rehab 2002; 83:346–351.

34. Canupp KC, Waites KB, DeVivo MJ, Richards JS. Predicting compliance with annual follow-up evaluations in persons with spinal cord injury. Spinal Cord 1997; 35:314–319.

35. Gupta S, Chawla JC. Review of urinary tract abnormalities in 100 patients with spinal cord paralysis. Paraplegia 1994; 32:531–539.

36. Van Kerrebroeck PE, Koldewijn EL, Scherpenhuizen S, Debruyne FM. The morbidity due to lower urinary tract function in spinal cord injury patients. Paraplegia 1993; 31:320–329.

Appendices

Appendix 1

The standardisation of terminology in lower urinary tract function*

Report from the Standardisation Sub-committee of the International Continence Society

Committee: Paul Abrams, Linda Cardozo, Magnus Fall, Derek Griffiths, Peter Rosier, Ulf Ulmsten, Philip van Kerrebroeck, Arne Victor, Alan Wein

This report presents definitions of the symptoms, signs, urodynamic observations and conditions associated with lower urinary tract dysfunction (LUTD) and urodynamic studies (UDS), for use in all patients groups from children to the elderly.

The definitions restate or update those presented in previous International Continence Society Standardisation of Terminology reports (see references) and those shortly to be published on Urethral Function (Lose et al, in press) and Nocturia (van Kerrebroeck et al, 2002). The published ICS report on the technical aspects of urodynamic equipment (Rowen et al, 1987) will be complemented by the new ICS report on urodynamic practice to be published shortly (Schäfer et al, 2002). In addition there are four published ICS outcome reports (Fonda et al, 1998; Lose et al, 1998; Mattiasson et al, 1998; Nordling et al, 1998).

New or changed definitions are all indicated; however, recommendations concerning technique are not included in the main text of this report.

The definitions have been written to be compatible with the WHO publication ICIDH-2 (International Classification of Functioning, Disability and Health) published in 2001 and ICD10, the International Classification of Diseases. As far as possible, the definitions are descriptive of observations, without implying underlying assumptions that may later prove to be incorrect or incomplete. By following this principle, the International Continence Society (ICS) aims to facilitate comparison of results and enable effective communication by investigators who use urodynamic methods. This report restates the ICS principle that symptoms, signs and conditions are separate categories and adds a category of urodynamic observations. In addition, terminology related to therapies is included (Andersen et al, 1992).

When a reference is made to the whole anatomical organ the vesica urinaria, the correct term is the bladder. When the smooth muscle structure known as the m.detrusor urinae is being discussed, then the correct term is detrusor.

It is suggested that acknowledgement of these standards in written publications be indicated by a footnote to the section 'Methods and Materials' or its equivalent, to read as follows:

'Methods, definitions and units conform to the standards recommended by the International Continence Society, except where specifically noted'.

The report covers the following areas:

1. *Lower Urinary Tract Symptoms (LUTS)*
   Symptoms are the subjective indicator of a disease or change in condition as perceived by the patient, carer or partner and may lead him/her to seek help from health care professionals. **(NEW)**

   Symptoms may either be volunteered or described during the patient interview. They are usually qualitative. In general, Lower Urinary Tract Symptoms cannot be used to make a definitive diagnosis. Lower Urinary Tract Symptoms can also indicate pathologies other than lower urinary tract dysfunction, such as urinary infection.

2. *Signs suggestive of Lower Urinary Tract Dysfunction (LUTD)*
   Signs are observed by the physician including simple means, to verify symptoms and quantify them. **(NEW)**

   For example, a classical sign is the observation of leakage on coughing. Observations from frequency volume charts, pad tests and validated symptom and quality of life questionnaires are examples of other instruments that can be used to verify and quantify symptoms.

3. *Urodynamic Observations*
   Urodynamic observations are observations made during urodynamic studies. **(NEW)**

   For example, an involuntary detrusor contraction (detrusor overactivity) is a urodynamic observation. In general, a urodynamic observation may have a number of possible underlying causes and does not represent a definitive diagnosis of a disease or condition and may occur with a variety of symptoms and signs, or in the absence of any symptoms or signs.

4. *Conditions*: **Conditions** are defined by the presence of urodynamic observations associated with characteristic symptoms or signs and/or non-urodynamic evidence of relevant pathological processes. (**NEW**)

5. *Treatment*: **Treatment** for lower urinary tract dysfunction: these definitions are from the 7th ICS report on Lower Urinary Tract Rehabilitation Techniques (3).

1 Lower Urinary Tract Symptoms (LUTS)

Lower urinary tract symptoms are defined from the individual's perspective who is usually, but not necessarily, a patient within the healthcare system. Symptoms are either volunteered by, or elicited from, the individual or may be described by the individual's caregiver.

Lower urinary tract symptoms are divided into three groups: storage, voiding, and post micturition symptoms.

1.1 *Storage symptoms* are experienced during the storage phase of the bladder and include daytime frequency and nocturia. (**NEW**)

- *Increased daytime frequency* is the complaint by the patient who considers that he/she voids too often by day. (**NEW**)
  This term is equivalent to pollakisuria used in many countries.
- *Nocturia* is the complaint that the individual has to wake at night one or more times to void. (**NEW**) – **FOOTNOTE 1**

FOOTNOTE 1 – The term night time frequency differs from that for nocturia, as it includes voids that occur after the individual has gone to bed, but before he/she has gone to sleep, and voids which occur in the early morning which prevent the individual from getting back to sleep as he/she wishes. These voids before and after sleep may need to be considered in research studies, for example, in nocturnal polyuria. If this definition were used then an adapted definition of daytime frequency would need to be used with it.

- *Urgency* is the complaint of a sudden compelling desire to pass urine which is difficult to defer. (**CHANGED**)
- *Urinary incontinence* is the complaint of any involuntary leakage of urine. (**NEW**) – **FOOTNOTE 2**

In each specific circumstance, urinary incontinence should be further described by specifying relevant factors such as type, frequency, severity, precipitating factors, social impact, effect on hygiene and quality of life, the measures used to contain the leakage and whether or not the individual seeks or desires help because of urinary incontinence – **FOOTNOTE 3**

Urinary leakage may need to be distinguished from sweating or vaginal discharge.

FOOTNOTE 2 – In infants and small children the definition of Urinary Incontinence is not applicable. In scientific communications the definition of incontinence in children would need further explanation.

FOOTNOTE 3 – The original ICS definition of incontinence 'Urinary incontinence is the involuntary loss of urine that is a social or hygienic problem', relates the complaint to quality of life (QoL) issues. Some QoL instruments have been and are being developed in order to assess the impact of both incontinence and other LUTS on QoL.

- *Stress urinary incontinence* is the complaint of involuntary leakage on effort or exertion, or on sneezing or coughing. (**CHANGED**) – **FOOTNOTE 4**

FOOTNOTE 4 – The committee considers the term 'stress incontinence' to be unsatisfactory in the English language because of its mental connotations. The Swedish, French and Italian expression 'effort incontinence' is preferable. However, words such as 'effort' or 'exertion' still do not capture some of the common precipitating factors for stress incontinence such as coughing or sneezing. For this reason the term is left unchanged.

- *Urge urinary incontinence* is the complaint of involuntary leakage accompanied by or immediately preceded by urgency. (**CHANGED**) – **FOOTNOTE 5**

FOOTNOTE 5 – Urge incontinence can present in different symptomatic forms; for example, as frequent small losses between micturitions or as a catastrophic leak with complete bladder emptying.

- *Mixed urinary incontinence* is the complaint of involuntary leakage associated with urgency and also with exertion, effort, sneezing or coughing. (**NEW**)
- *Enuresis* means any involuntary loss of urine. If it is used to denote incontinence during sleep, it should always be qualified with the adjective 'nocturnal'. (**ORIGINAL**)
  If it is used to denote incontinence during sleep, it should always be qualified with the adjective 'nocturnal'.
- *Nocturnal enuresis* is the complaint of loss of urine occurring during sleep. (**NEW**)
- *Continuous urinary incontinence* is the complaint of continuous leakage. (**NEW**)
- *Other types of urinary incontinence* may be situational, for example, the report of incontinence during sexual intercourse, or giggle incontinence.
- *Bladder sensation* can be defined, during history taking, by five categories.

  Normal: the individual is aware of bladder filling and increasing sensation up to a strong desire to void. (**NEW**)
  Increased: the individual feels an early and persistent desire to void. (**NEW**)
  Reduced: the individual is aware of bladder filling but does not feel a definite desire to void. (**NEW**)
  Absent: the individual reports no sensation of bladder filling or desire to void. (**NEW**)

Non-specific: the individual reports no specific bladder sensation but may perceive bladder filling as abdominal fullness, vegetative symptoms, or spasticity. (**NEW**) – FOOTNOTE 6

FOOTNOTE 6 – These non-specific symptoms are most frequently seen in neurological patients, particularly those with spinal cord trauma and in children and adults with malformations of the spinal cord.

1.2 *Voiding symptoms* are experienced during the voiding phase. (**NEW**)

- *Slow stream* is reported by the individual as his or her perception of reduced urine flow, usually compared to previous performance or in comparison to others. (**NEW**)
- *Splitting or spraying* of the urine stream may be reported. (**NEW**)
- *Intermittent stream (intermittency)* is the term used when the individual describes urine flow which stops and starts, on one or more occasions, during micturition. (**NEW**)
- *Hesitancy* is the term used when an individual describes difficulty in initiating micturition resulting in a delay in the onset of voiding after the individual is ready to pass urine. (**NEW**)
- *Straining* to void describes the muscular effort used to either initiate, maintain or improve the urinary stream. (**NEW**) – FOOTNOTE 7

FOOTNOTE 7 – Suprapubic pressure may be used to initiate or maintain urine flow. The Credé manoeuvre is used by some spinal cord injury patients, and girls with detrusor underactivity sometimes press suprapubically to help empty the bladder.

- *Terminal dribble* is the term used when an individual describes a prolonged final part of micturition, when the flow has slowed to a trickle/dribble. (**NEW**)

1.3 *Post micturition symptoms* are experienced immediately after micturition. (**NEW**)

- *Feeling of incomplete emptying* is a self-explanatory term for a feeling experienced by the individual after passing urine. (**NEW**)
- *Post micturition dribble* is the term used when an individual describes the involuntary loss of urine immediately after he or she has finished passing urine, usually after leaving the toilet in men, or after rising from the toilet in women. (**NEW**)

1.4 *Symptoms associated with sexual intercourse*
Dyspareunia, vaginal dryness and incontinence are amongst the symptoms women may describe during or after intercourse. These symptoms should be described as fully as possible. It is helpful to define urine leakage as: during penetration, during intercourse, or at orgasm.

1.5 *Symptoms associated with pelvic organ prolapse*
The feeling of a lump ('something coming down'), low backache, heaviness, dragging sensation, or the need to digitally replace the prolapse in order to defaecate or micturate, are amongst the symptoms women may describe who have a prolapse.

1.6 *Genital and lower urinary tract pain* – FOOTNOTE 8
Pain, discomfort and pressure are part of a spectrum of abnormal sensations felt by the individual. Pain produces the greatest impact on the patient and may be related to bladder filling or voiding, may be felt after micturition, or be continuous. Pain should also be characterised by type, frequency, duration, precipitating and relieving factors and by location as defined below:

FOOTNOTE 8 – The terms 'strangury', 'bladder spasm', and 'dysuria' are difficult to define and of uncertain meaning and should not be used in relation to lower urinary tract dysfunction, unless a precise meaning is stated. Dysuria literally means 'abnormal urination' and is used correctly in some European countries. However, it is often used to describe the stinging/burning sensation characteristic of urinary infection. It is suggested that these descriptive words should be used in future.

- *Bladder pain* is felt suprapubically or retropubically, and usually increases with bladder filling, it may persist after voiding. (**NEW**)
- *Urethral pain* is felt in the urethra and the individual indicates the urethra as the site. (**NEW**)
- *Vulval pain* is felt in and around the external genitalia. (**NEW**)
- *Vaginal pain* is felt internally, above the introitus. (**NEW**)
- *Scrotal pain* may or may not be localised, for example to the testis, epididymis, cord structures or scrotal skin. (**NEW**)
- *Perineal pain* is felt: in the female, between the posterior fourchette (posterior lip of the introitus) and the anus, and in the male, between the scrotum and the anus. (**NEW**)
- *Pelvic pain* is less well defined than, for example, bladder, urethral or perineal pain and is less clearly related to the micturition cycle or to bowel function and is not localised to any single pelvic organ. (**NEW**)

1.7 *Genito-urinary pain syndromes and symptom syndromes suggestive of LUTD*
Syndromes describe constellations, or varying combinations of symptoms, but cannot be used for precise diagnosis. The use of the word 'syndrome' can only be justified if there is at least one other symptom in addition to the symptom used to describe the syndrome. In scientific communications the incidence of individual symptoms within the syndrome should be stated, in addition to the number of individuals with the syndrome.

The syndromes described are functional abnormalities for which a precise cause has not been defined. It is presumed that routine assessment (history taking, physical examination, and other appropriate investigations) has excluded obvious local pathologies such as those that are infective, neoplastic, metabolic or hormonal in nature.

1.7.1 *Genito-urinary pain syndromes* are all chronic in their nature. Pain is the major complaint but concomitnat complaints are of lower urinary tract, bowel, sexual or gynaecological nature.

- *Painful bladder syndrome* is the complaint of suprapubic pain related to bladder filling, accompanied by other symptoms such as increased daytime and night-time frequency, in the absence of proven urinary infection or other obvious pathology. (NEW) – FOOTNOTE 9

FOOTNOTE 9 – The ICS believes this to be a preferable term to 'interstitial cystitis'. Interstitial cystitis is a specific diagnosis and requires confirmation by typical cystoscopic and histological features. In the investigation of bladder pain it may be necessary to exclude conditions such as carcinoma in situ and endometriosis.

- *Urethral pain syndrome* is the occurrence of recurrent episodic urethral pain usually on voiding, with daytime frequency and nocturia, in the absence of proven infection or other obvious pathology. (NEW)
- *Vulval pain syndrome* is the occurrence of persistent or recurrent episodic vulval pain, which is either related to the micturition cycle or associated with symptoms suggestive of urinary tract or sexual dysfunction. There is no proven infection or other obvious pathology. (NEW) – FOOTNOTE 10

FOOTNOTE 10 – The ICS suggests that the term vulvodynia (vulva – pain) should not be used, as it leads to confusion between a single symptom and a syndrome.

- *Vaginal pain syndrome* is the occurrence of persistent or recurrent episodic vaginal pain which is associated with symptoms suggestive of urinary tract or sexual dysfunction. There is no proven vaginal infection or other obvious pathology.
- *Scrotal pain syndrome* is the occurrence of persistent or recurrent episodic scrotal pain which is associated with symptoms suggestive of urinary tract or sexual dysfunction. There is no proven epididimo-orchitis or other obvious pathology.
- *Perineal pain syndrome* is the occurrence of persistent or recurrent episodic perineal pain which is either related to the micturition cycle or associated with symptoms suggestive of urinary tract or sexual dysfunction. There is no proven infection or other obvious pathology. (NEW) – FOOTNOTE 11

FOOTNOTE 11 – The ICS suggests that in men, the term prostatodynia (prostate – pain) should not be used as it leads to confusion between a single symptom and a syndrome.

- *Pelvic pain syndrome* is the occurrence of persistent or recurrent episodic pelvic pain associated with symptoms suggestive of lower urinary tract, sexual, bowel or gynaecological dysfunction. There is no proven infection or other obvious pathology. (NEW)

1.7.2   *Symptom syndromes suggestive of Lower Urinary Tract Dysfunction*

In clinical practice, empirical diagnoses are often used as the basis for initial management after assessing the

individual's lower urinary tract symptoms, physical findings and the results of urinalysis and other indicated investigations.

- *Urgency*, with or without urge incontinence, usually with frequency and nocturia, can be described as the *overactive bladder syndrome, urge syndrome* or *urgency-frequency syndrome.* (NEW)

   These symptom combinations are suggestive of urodynamically demonstrable detrusor overactivity but can be due to other forms of urethrovesical dysfunction. These terms can be used if there is no proven infection or other obvious pathology.

- *Lower urinary tract symptoms suggestive of bladder outlet obstruction* is a term used when a man complains predominately of voiding symptoms in the absence of infection or obvious pathology other than possible causes of outlet obstruction. (NEW) – FOOTNOTE 12

FOOTNOTE 12 – in women voiding symptoms are usually thought to suggest detrusor underactivity rather than bladder outlet obstruction.

2   Signs suggestive of Lower Urinary Tract Dysfunction (LUTD)

2.1   *Measuring the frequency, severity and impact of Lower Urinary Tract Symptoms*

Asking the patient to record micturitions and symptoms (FOOTNOTE 13) for a period of days provides invaluable information. The recording of micturition events can be in three main forms:

FOOTNOTE 13 – Validated questionnaires are useful for recording symptoms, their frequency, severity and bother, and the impact of LUTS on QoL. The instrument used should be specified.

- *Micturition time chart:* this records only the times of micturitions, day and night, for at least 24 h. (NEW)
- *Frequency volume chart (FVC):* this records the volumes voided as well as the time of each micturition, day and night, for at least 24 h. (CHANGED)
- *Bladder diary:* this records the times of micturitions and voided volumes, incontinence episodes, pad usage and other information such as fluid intake, the degree of urgency and the degree of incontinence. (NEW) – FOOTNOTE 14

FOOTNOTE 14 – It is useful to ask the individual to make an estimate of liquid intake. This may be done precisely by measuring the volume of each drink or crudely by asking how many drinks are taken in a 24-h period. If the individual eats significant quantities of water containing foods (vegetables, fruit, salads) then an appreciable effect on urine production will result.

The time that diuretic therapy is taken should be marked on a chart or diary.

The following measurements can be abstracted from frequency volume charts and bladder diaries:

- *Daytime frequency* is the number of voids recorded during waking hours and includes the last void before sleep and the first void after waking and rising in the morning. (**NEW**)
- *Nocturia* is the number of voids recorded during a night's sleep: each void is preceded and followed by sleep. (**NEW**)
- *24-h frequency* is the total number of daytime voids and episodes of nocturia during a specified 24-h period. (**NEW**)
- *24-h production* is measured by collecting all urine for 24 h. (**NEW**)

  This is usually commenced *after* the first void produced after rising in the morning and is completed by including the first void on rising the following morning.
- *Polyuria* is defined as the measured production of more than 2.8 l of urine in 24 h in adults. It may be useful to look at output over shorter time frames (van Kerrebroeck et al, 2002). (**NEW**) – **FOOTNOTE 15**

FOOTNOTE 15 – The causes of polyuria are various and reviewed elsewhere but include habitual excess fluid intake. The figure of 2.8 is based on a 70 kg person voiding > 40 ml/kg.

- *Nocturnal urine volume* is defined as the total volume of urine passed between the time the individual goes to bed with the intention of sleeping and the time of waking with the intention of rising. (**NEW**) Therefore, it excludes the last void before going to bed but includes the first void after rising in the morning.
- *Nocturnal polyuria* is present when an increased proportion of the 24-h output occurs at night (normally during the 8 h whilst the patient is in bed). (**NEW**) The night time urine output excludes the last void before sleep but includes the first void of the morning – **FOOTNOTE 16**

FOOTNOTE 16 –The normal range of nocturnal urine production differs with age and the normal ranges remain to be defined. Therefore, nocturnal polyuria is present when greater than 20% (young adults) to 33% (over 65 years) is produced at night. Hence the precise definition is dependent on age.

- *Maximum voided volume* is the largest volume of urine voided during a single micturition and is determined either from the frequency/volume chart or bladder diary. (**NEW**)

  The maximum, mean and minimum voided volumes over the period of recording may be stated – **FOOTNOTE 17**

FOOTNOTE 17 – The term 'functional bladder capacity' is no longer recommended, as 'voided volume' is a clearer and less confusing term, particularly if qualified as, e.g. 'maximum voided volume'. If the term 'bladder capacity' is used, in any situation, it implies that this has been measured in some way, if only by abdominal ultrasound. In adults, voided volumes vary considerably. In children, the 'expected volume' may be calculated from the formula (30+ (age in years × 30) in ml). Assuming no residual urine, this will be equal to the 'expected bladder capacity'.

2.2 *Physical examination* is essential in the assessment of all patients with lower urinary tract dysfunction. It should include abdominal, pelvic, perineal and a focussed neurological examination. For patients with possible neurogenic lower urinary tract dysfunction, a more extensive neurological examination is needed.

2.2.1 *Abdominal*: the bladder may be felt by abdominal palpation or by suprapubic percussion. Pressure suprapubically or during bimanual vaginal examination may induce a desire to pass urine.

2.2.2 *Perineal/genital inspection* allows the description of the skin, for example the presence of atrophy or excoriation, any abnormal anatomical features and the observation of incontinence.

- *Urinary incontinence (the sign)* is defined as urine leakage seen during examination: this may be urethral or extraurethral.
- *Stress urinary incontinence* is the observation of involuntary leakage from the urethra, synchronous with exertion/effort, or sneezing or coughing. (**CHANGED**) – **FOOTNOTE 18**

  Stress leakage is presumed to be due to raised abdominal pressure.

FOOTNOTE 18 – Coughing may induce a detrusor contraction, hence the sign of stress incontinence is only a reliable indication of urodynamic stress incontinence when leakage occurs synchronously with the first proper cough and stops at the end of that cough.

- *Extra-urethral incontinence* is defined as the observation of urine leakage through channels other than the urethra. (**ORIGINAL**)
- *Uncategorised incontinence* is the observation of involuntary leakage that cannot be classified into one of the above categories on the basis of signs and symptoms. (**NEW**)

2.2.3 *Vaginal examination* allows the description of observed and palpable anatomical abnormalities and the assessment of pelvic floor muscle function, as described in the ICS report on Pelvic Organ Prolapse. The definitions given are simplified versions of the definitions in that report. (Bump et al, 1996)

- *Pelvic organ prolapse* is defined as the descent of one or more of: the anterior vaginal wall, the posterior vaginal wall, and the apex of the vagina (cervix/uterus) or vault (cuff) after hysterectomy. Absence of prolapse is defined as stage 0 support; prolapse can be staged from stage I to stage IV. (**NEW**)

  Pelvic organ prolapse can occur in association with urinary incontinence and other lower urinary tract dysfunction and may on occasion mask incontinence.

- *Anterior vaginal wall prolapse* is defined as descent of the anterior vagina so that the urethrovesical junction (a point 3 cm proximal to the external urinary meatus) or any anterior point proximal to this is less than 3 cm above the plane of the hymen. **(CHANGED)**
- *Prolapse of the apical segment of the vagina* is defined as any descent of the vaginal cuff scar (after hysterectomy) or cervix, below a point which is 2 cm less than the total vaginal length above the plane of the hymen. **(CHANGED)**
- *Posterior vaginal wall prolapse* is defined as any descent of the posterior vaginal wall so that a midline point on the posterior vaginal wall 3 cm above the level of the hymen or any posterior point proximal to this, less than 3 cm above the plane of the hymen. **(CHANGED)**

2.2.4 *Pelvic floor muscle function* can be qualitatively defined by the tone at rest and the strength of a voluntary or reflex contraction as strong, weak or absent or by a validated grading system (e.g. Oxford 1–5). A pelvic muscle contraction may be assessed by visual inspection, by palpation, electromyography or perineometry. Factors to be assessed include strength, duration, displacement and repeatability. **(NEW)**

2.2.5 *Rectal examination* allows the description of observed and palpable anatomical abnormalities and is the easiest method of assessing pelvic floor muscle function in children and men. In addition, rectal examination is essential in children with urinary incontinence to rule out faecal inpaction.

- *Pelvic floor muscle function* can be qualitatively defined, during rectal examination, by the tone at rest and the strength of a voluntary contraction, as strong, weak or absent. **(NEW)**

2.3 *Pad testing* may be used to quantify the amount of urine lost during incontinence episodes, and methods range from a short provocative test to a 24-h pad test.

3   Urodynamic observations and conditions

3.1 *Urodynamic techniques* There are two principal methods of urodynamic investigation:

- *Conventional urodynamic studies* normally take place in the urodynamic laboratory and usually involve artificial bladder filling. **(NEW)**

  - *Artificial bladder filling* is defined as filling the bladder, via a catheter, with a specified liquid at a specified rate **(NEW)**

- *Ambulatory Urodynamic studies* are defined as a functional test of the lower urinary tract, utilising natural filling and reproducing the subject's every day activities. – **FOOTNOTE 19**

FOOTNOTE 19 – The term Ambulatory Urodynamics is used to indicate that monitoring usually takes place outside the urodynamic laboratory, rather than the subject's mobility using natural filling.

  - *Natural filling* means that the bladder is filled by the production of urine rather than by an artificial medium.

Both filling cystometry and pressure flow studies of voiding require the following measurements:

- *Intravesical pressure* is the pressure within the bladder. **(ORIGINAL)**
- *Abdominal pressure* is taken to be the pressure surrounding the bladder. In current practice it is estimated from rectal, vaginal or, less commonly, from extraperitoneal pressure or a bowel stoma. The simultaneous measurement of abdominal pressure is essential for the interpretation of the intravesical pressure trace. **(ORIGINAL)**
- *Detrusor pressure* is that component of intravesical pressure that is created by forces in the bladder wall (passive and active). It is estimated by subtracting abdominal pressure from intravesical pressure. **(ORIGINAL)**

3.2 *Filling cystometry*
The word 'cystometry' is commonly used to describe the urodynamic investigation of the filling phase of the micturition cycle. To eliminate confusion, the following definitions are proposed:

- *Filling cystometry* is the method by which the pressure/volume relationship of the bladder is measured during bladder filling. **(ORIGINAL)**

  The filling phase starts when filling commences and ends when the patient and urodynamicist decide that 'permission to void' has been given – **FOOTNOTE 20**

Bladder and urethral function, during filling, need to be defined separately.

The rate at which the bladder is filled is divided into:

  - *Physiological filling rate* is defined as a filling rate less than the predicted maximum – predicted maximum body weight in kg divided by 4 expressed as ml/min (Klevmark, 1999) **(CHANGED)**
  - *Non-physiological filling rate* is defined as a filling rate greater than the predicted maximum filling rate – predicted maximum body weight in kg divided by 4 expressed as ml/min (Klevmark, 1999) **(CHANGED)**

FOOTNOTE 20 – The ICS no longer wishes to divide filling rates into slow, medium and fast. In practice almost all investigations are performed using medium filling rates which have a wide range. It may be more important during investigations to consider whether or not the filling rate used during conventional urodynamic studies can be considered physiological.

Bladder storage function should be described according to bladder sensation, detrusor activity, bladder compliance and bladder capacity – **FOOTNOTE 21**

FOOTNOTE 21 – Whilst bladder sensation is assessed during filling cystometry the assumption that it is sensation from the bladder alone, without urethral or pelvic components may be false.

3.2.1 *Bladder sensation during filling cystometry*

- *Normal bladder sensation* can be judged by three defined points noted during filling cystometry and evaluated in relation to the bladder volume at that moment and in relation to the patient's symptomatic complaints.
- *First sensation of bladder filling* is the feeling the patient has, during filling cystometry, when he/she first becomes aware of the bladder filling. (**NEW**)
- *First desire to void* is defined as the feeling, during filling cystometry, that would lead the patient to pass urine at the next convenient moment, but voiding can be delayed if necessary. (**CHANGED**)
- *Strong desire to void* this is defined, during filling cystometry, as a persistent desire to void without the fear of leakage. (**ORIGINAL**)
- *Increased bladder sensation* is defined, during filling cystometry, as an early first sensation of bladder filling (or an early desire to void) and/or an early strong desire to void, which occurs at low bladder volume and which persists. (**NEW**) – **FOOTNOTE 22**

FOOTNOTE 22 – The assessment of the subject's bladder sensation is subjective and it is not, for example, possible to quantify 'low bladder volume' in the definition of 'increased bladder sensation'.

- *Reduced bladder sensation* is defined, during filling cystometry, as diminished sensation throughout bladder filling. (**NEW**)
- *Absent bladder sensation* means that, during filling cystometry, the individual has no bladder sensation. (**NEW**)
- *Non-specific bladder sensations*, during filling cystometry, may make the individual aware of bladder filling, for example, abdominal fullness or vegetative symptoms. (**NEW**)
- *Bladder pain*, during filling cystometry, is a self-explanatory term and is an abnormal finding. (**NEW**)
- *Urgency*, during filling cystometry, is a sudden compelling desire to void. (**NEW**) – **FOOTNOTE 23**

FOOTNOTE 23 – The ICS no longer recommends the terms 'motor urgency' and 'sensory urgency'. These terms are often misused and have little intuitive meaning. Furthermore, it may be simplistic to relate urgency just to the presence or absence of detrusor overactivity when there is usually a concomitant fall in urethral pressure.

- *The vesical/urethral sensory threshold* is defined as the least current which consistently produces a sensation perceived by the subject during stimulation at the site under investigation. (Andersen et al, 1992) – **ORIGINAL**

3.2.2 *Detrusor function during filling cystometry*

In everyday life the individual attempts to inhibit detrusor activity until he or she is in a position to void. Therefore, when the aims of the filling study have been achieved, and when the patient has a desire to void, normally the 'permission to void' is given (see Filling cystometry). That moment is indicated on the urodynamic trace and all detrusor activity before this 'permission' is defined as 'involuntary detrusor activity'.

- *Normal detrusor function:* allows bladder filling with little or no change in pressure. No involuntary phasic contractions occur despite provocation. (**ORIGINAL**)
- *Detrusor overactivity* is a urodynamic observation characterised by involuntary detrusor contractions during the filling phase which may be spontaneous or provoked. (**CHANGED**) – **FOOTNOTE 24**

FOOTNOTE 24 – There is no lower limit for the amplitude of an involuntary detrusor contraction but confident interpretation of low pressure waves (amplitude smaller than 5 cm of H_2O) depends on 'high quality' urodynamic technique. The phrase 'which the patient cannot completely suppress' has been deleted from the old definition.

There are certain patterns of detrusor overactivity:

- *Phasic detrusor overactivity* is defined by a characteristic wave form and may or may not lead to urinary incontinence. (**NEW**) – **FOOTNOTE 25**

FOOTNOTE 25 – Phasic detrusor contractions are not always accompanied by any sensation or may be interpreted as a first sensation of bladder filling or as a normal desire to void.

- *Terminal detrusor overactivity* is defined as a single, involuntary detrusor contraction, occurring at cystometric capacity, which cannot be suppressed and results in incontinence usually resulting in bladder emptying (voiding). (**NEW**) – **FOOTNOTE 26**

FOOTNOTE 26 – 'Terminal detrusor overactivity' is a new ICS term: it is typically associated with reduced bladder sensation, e.g., in the elderly stroke patient when urgency may be felt as the voiding contraction occurs. However, in complete spinal cord injury patients there may be no sensation whatsoever.

- *Detrusor overactivity incontinence* is incontinence due to an involuntary detrusor contraction. (**NEW**)

In a patient with normal sensation, urgency is likely to be experienced just before the leakage episode. – **FOOTNOTE 27**

FOOTNOTE 27 – ICS recommends that the terms 'motor urge incontinence' and 'reflex incontinence' should no longer be used as they have no intuitive meaning and are often misused.

Detrusor overactivity may also be qualified, when possible, according to cause, for example:

- *Neurogenic detrusor overactivity* when there is a relevant neurological condition.

   This term replaces the term 'detrusor hyper-reflexia'. (**NEW**)

- *Idiopathic detrusor overactivity* when there is no defined cause. (**NEW**)

   This term replaces 'detrusor instability'. – **FOOTNOTE 28**

FOOTNOTE 28 – The terms 'detrusor instability' and 'detrusor hyperreflexia' were both used as generic terms, in the English-speaking world and Scandinavia, prior to the first ICS report in 1976. As a compromise they were allocated to idiopathic and neurogenic overactivity respectively. As there is no real logic or intuitive meaning to the terms, the ICS believes they should be abandoned.

In clinical and research practice, the extent of neurological examination/investigation varies. It is likely that the proportion of neurogenic : idiopathic detrusor overactivity will increase if a more complete neurological assessment is carried out.

Other patterns of detrusor overactivity are seen, for example, the combination of phasic and terminal detrusor overactivity, and the sustained high pressure detrusor contractions seen in spinal cord injury patients when attempted voiding occurs against a dyssynergic sphincter.

- *Provocative manoeuvres* are defined as techniques used during urodynamics in an effort to provoke detrusor overactivity, for example, rapid filling, use of cooled or acid medium, postural changes and hand washing. (**NEW**)

3.2.3   Bladder compliance during filling cystometry

- *Bladder compliance* describes the relationship between change in bladder volume and change in detrusor pressure. (**CHANGED**) – **FOOTNOTE 29**

FOOTNOTE 29 – The observation of reduced bladder compliance during conventional filling cystometry is often related to relatively fast bladder filling: the incidence of reduced compliance is markedly lower if the bladder is filled at physiological rates, as in ambulatory urodynamics.

Compliance is calculated by dividing the volume change (ΔV) by the change in detrusor pressure $(\Delta p\text{det})$ during that change in bladder volume ($C = V \cdot \Delta p\text{det}$). It is expressed in ml/cm H_2O.

A variety of means of calculating bladder compliance has been described. The ICS recommends that two standard points should be used for compliance calculations: the

investigator may wish to define additional points. The standard points are:

1. the detrusor pressure at the start of bladder filling and the corresponding bladder volume (usually zero), and
2. the detrusor pressure (and corresponding bladder volume) at cystometric capacity or immediately before the start of any detrusor contraction that causes significant leakage (and therefore causes the bladder volume to decrease, affecting compliance calculation). Both points are measured excluding any detrusor contraction.

3.2.4   Bladder capacity: during filling cystometry

- *Cystometric capacity* is the bladder volume at the end of the filling cystometrogram, when 'permission to void' is usually given. The end point should be specified, e.g., if filling is stopped when the patient has a normal desire to void. The cystometric capacity is the volume voided together with any residual urine. (**CHANGED**) – **FOOTNOTE 30**

FOOTNOTE 30 – In certain types of dysfunction, the cystometric capacity cannot be defined in the same terms. In the absence of sensation the cystometric capacity is the volume at which the clinician decides to terminate filling. The reason(s) for terminating filling should be defined, e.g. high detrusor filling pressure, large infused volume or pain. If there is uncontrollable voiding, it is the volume at which this begins. In the presence of sphincter incompetence the cystometric capacity may be significantly increased by occlusion of the urethra e.g. by Foley catheter.

- *Maximum cystometric capacity*, in patients with normal sensation, is the volume at which the patient feels he/she can no longer delay micturition (has a strong desire to void). (**ORIGINAL**)
- *Maximum anaesthetic bladder capacity* is the volume to which the bladder can be filled under deep general or spinal anaesthetic and should be qualified according to the type of anaesthesia used and the speed, the length of time, and the pressure at which the bladder is filled. (**CHANGED**)

3.2.5   Urethral function during filling cystometry
The urethral closure mechanism during storage may be competent or incompetent.

- *Normal urethral closure mechanism* maintains a positive urethral closure pressure during bladder filling even in the presence of increased abdominal pressure, although it may be overcome by detrusor overactivity. (**CHANGED**)
- *Incompetent urethral closure mechanism* is defined as one which allows **leakage of urine in the absence of a detrusor contraction.** (**ORIGINAL**)
- *Urethral relaxation incontinence* is defined as leakage due to urethral relaxation in the absence of raised abdominal pressure or detrusor overactivity. (**NEW**) – **FOOTNOTE 31**

FOOTNOTE 31 – *Fluctuations in urethral pressure have been defined as the 'unstable urethra'. However, the significance of the fluctuations and the term itself lack clarity and the term is not recommended by the ICS. If symptoms are seen in association with a decrease in urethral pressure a full description should be given.*

- *Urodynamic stress incontinence* is noted during filling cystometry and is defined as the involuntary leakage of urine during increased abdominal pressure, in the absence of a detrusor contraction. (CHANGED)

Urodynamic stress incontinence is now the preferred term to 'genuine stress incontinence'. FOOTNOTE 32

FOOTNOTE 32 – *In patients with stress incontinence, there is a spectrum of urethral characteristics ranging from a highly mobile urethra with good intrinsic function to an immobile urethra with poor intrinsic function. Any delineation into categories such as 'urethral hypermobility' and 'intrinsic sphincter deficiency' may be simplistic and arbitrary, and requires further research.*

3.2.6 *Assessment of urethral function during filling cystometry*

- *Urethral pressure measurement*
  - *Urethral pressure* is defined as the fluid pressure needed to just open a closed urethra. (ORIGINAL)
  - *The urethral pressure profile* is a graph indicating the intraluminal pressure along the length of the urethra. (ORIGINAL)
  - *The urethral closure pressure profile* is given by the subtraction of intravesical pressure from urethral pressure. (ORIGINAL)
  - *Maximum urethral pressure* is the maximum pressure of the measured profile. (ORIGINAL)
  - *Maximum urethral closure pressure (MUCP)* is the maximum difference between the urethral pressure and the intravesical pressure. (ORIGINAL)
  - *Functional profile length* is the length of the urethra along which the urethral pressure exceeds intravesical pressure in women.
  - *Pressure 'transmission' ratio* is the increment in urethral pressure on stress as a percentage of the simultaneously recorded increment in intravesical pressure.

- *Abnormal leak point pressure* is the intravesical pressure at which urine leakage occurs due to increased abdominal pressure in the absence of a detrusor contraction. (NEW) – FOOTNOTE 33

FOOTNOTE 33 – *The Leak Pressure Point should be qualified according to the site of pressure measurement (rectal, vaginal or intravesical) and the method by which pressure is generated (cough or valsalva). Leak point pressures may be calculated in three ways from the three different baseline values which are in*

common use: zero (the true zero of intravesical pressure), the value of p_{ves} measured at zero bladder volume, or the value of p_{ves} immediately before the cough or valsalva (usually at 200 or 300 ml bladder capacity). The baseline used, and the baseline pressure, should be specified.

- *Detrusor leak point pressure* (DLPP) is defined as the lowest detrusor pressure at which urine leakage occurs in the absence of either a detrusor contraction or increased abdominal pressure. (NEW) – FOOTNOTE 34

FOOTNOTE 34 – *DLPP has been used most frequently to predict upper tract problems in neurological patients with reduced bladder compliance. ICS has defined it 'in the absence of a detrusor contraction' although others will measure DLPP during involuntary detrusor contractions.*

3.3 *Pressure flow studies*
Voiding is described in terms of detrusor and urethral function and assessed by measuring urine flow rate and voiding pressures.

- *Pressure flow studies* of voiding are the method by which the relationship between pressure in the bladder and urine flow rate is measured during bladder emptying. (ORIGINAL)

The voiding phase starts when 'permission to void' is given, or when uncontrollable voiding begins, and ends when the patient considers voiding has finished.

3.3.1 *Measurement of urine flow*
Urine flow is defined either as **continuous**, i.e. without interruption, or as **intermittent**, when an individual states that the flow stops and starts during a single visit to the bathroom in order to void. The continuous flow curve is defined as a smooth arc-shaped curve or fluctuating when there are multiple peaks during a period of continuous urine flow – FOOTNOTE 35

FOOTNOTE 35 – *The precise shape of the flow curve is decided by detrusor contractility, the presence of any abdominal straining and by the bladder outlet. (11)*

  - *Flow rate* is defined as the volume of fluid expelled via the urethra per unit time. It is expressed in ml/s. (ORIGINAL)
  - *Voided volume* is the total volume expelled via the urethra. (ORIGINAL)
  - *Maximum flow rate* is the maximum measured value of the flow rate after correction for artefacts. (CHANGED)
  - *Voiding time* is total duration of micturition, i.e. includes interruptions. When voiding is completed without interruption, voiding time is equal to flow time. (ORIGINAL)
  - *Flow time* is the time over which measurable flow actually occurs. (ORIGINAL)

- *Average flow rate* is voided volume divided by flow time. The average flow should be interpreted with caution if flow is interrupted or there is a terminal dribble. **(CHANGED)**
- *Time to maximum flow* is the elapsed time from onset of flow to maximum flow. **(ORIGINAL)**

3.3.2. *Pressure measurements during pressure flow studies (PFS)*

The following measurements are applicable to each of the pressure curves: intravesical, abdominal and detrusor pressure.

- *Premicturition pressure* is the pressure recorded immediately before the initial isovolumetric contraction. **(ORIGINAL)**
- *Opening pressure* is the pressure recorded at the onset of urine flow (consider time delay). **(ORIGINAL)**
- *Opening time* is the elapsed time from initial rise in detrusor pressure to onset of flow. **(ORIGINAL)**
  This is the initial isovolumetric contraction period of micturition. Flow measurement delay should be taken into account when measuring opening time.
- *Maximum pressure* is the maximum value of the measured pressure. **(ORIGINAL)**
- *Pressure at maximum flow* is the lowest pressure recorded at maximum measured flow rate. **(ORIGINAL)**
- *Closing pressure* is the pressure measured at the end of measured flow. **(ORIGINAL)**
- *Minimum voiding pressure* is the minimum pressure during measurable flow but is not necessarily equal to either the opening or closing pressures.
- *Flow delay* is the time delay between a change in bladder pressure and the corresponding change in measured flow rate.

3.3.3 *Detrusor function during voiding*

- *Normal detrusor function* – normal voiding is achieved by a voluntarily initiated continuous detrusor contraction that leads to complete bladder emptying within a normal time span, and in the absence of obstruction. For a given detrusor contraction, the magnitude of the recorded pressure rise will depend on the degree of outlet resistance. **(ORIGINAL)**
- *Abnormal detrusor activity* can be subdivided:

  - *Detrusor underactivity* is defined as a contraction of reduced strength and/or duration, resulting in prolonged bladder emptying and/ or a failure to achieve complete bladder emptying within a normal time span. **(ORIGINAL)**
  - *Acontractile detrusor* is one that cannot be demonstrated to contract during urodynamic studies. **(ORIGINAL) – FOOTNOTE 36**

FOOTNOTE 36 – A normal detrusor contraction will be recorded as: high pressure if there is high outlet resistance, normal pressure if there is normal outlet resistance: or low pressure if urethral resistance is low.

- *Post void residual (PVR)* is defined as the volume of urine left in the bladder at the end of micturition. **(ORIGINAL) – FOOTNOTE 37**

FOOTNOTE 37 – If after repeated free flowmetry no residual urine is demonstrated, then the finding of a residual urine during urodynamic studies should be considered an artefact, due to the circumstances of the test.

3.3.4 *Urethral function during voiding*
During voiding:

Normal urethra function is defined as urethra that opens and is continuously relaxed to allow the bladder to be emptied at a normal pressure. **(CHANGED)**
Abnormal urethra function may be due to either obstruction to urethral overactivity or the urethra cannot open due to anatomic abnormality, such as an enlarged prostate or a urethral stricture.

- *Bladder outlet obstruction* is the generic term for obstruction during voiding and is characterised by increased detrusor pressure and reduced urine flow rate. It is usually diagnosed by studying the synchronous values of flowrate and detrusor pressure. **(CHANGED) – FOOTNOTE 38**

FOOTNOTE 38 – Bladder outlet obstruction has been defined for men but, as yet, not adequately in women and children.

- *Dysfunctional voiding* is characterised by an intermittent and/or fluctuating flow rate due to involuntary intermittent contractions of the periurethral striated muscle during voiding in neurologically normal individuals. **(CHANGED) – FOOTNOTE 39**

FOOTNOTE 39 – Although dysfunctional voiding is not a very specific term, it is preferred to terms such as 'non-neurogenic neurogenic bladder'. Other terms such as 'idiopathic detrusor sphincter dyssyergia', or 'sphincter overactivity voiding dysfunction', may be preferable. However, the term dysfunctional voiding is very well established. The condition occurs most frequently in children. Whilst it is felt that pelvic floor contractions are responsible, it is possible that the intraurethral striated muscle may be important.

- *Detrusor sphincter dyssynergia* is defined as a detrusor contraction concurrent with an involuntary contraction of the urethral and/ or periurethral striated muscle. Occasionally, flow may be prevented altogether. **(ORIGINAL) – FOOTNOTE 40**

FOOTNOTE 40 – Detrusor sphincter dyssynergia typically occurs in patients with a supra-sacral lesion, e.g. after high spinal cord injury, and is uncommon in lesions of the lower cord. Although the intraurethral and periurethral striated muscles are usually held responsible, the smooth muscle of the bladder neck or urethra may also be responsible.

- *Non-relaxing urethral sphincter obstruction* usually occurs in individuals with a neurological lesion and is characterised by a non-relaxing, obstructing urethra resulting in reduced urine flow. (NEW) – **FOOTNOTE 41**

FOOTNOTE 41 – Non-relaxing sphincter obstruction is found in sacral and infra-sacral lesions, such as meningomyelocoele, and after radical pelvic surgery. In addition, there is often urodynamic stress incontinence during bladder filling. This term replaces 'isolated distal sphincter obstruction'.

4   Conditions

- *Acute retention of urine* is defined as a painful, palpable or percussable bladder, when the patient is unable to pass any urine. (NEW) – **FOOTNOTE 42**

FOOTNOTE 42 – Although acute retention is usually thought of as painful, in certain circumstances pain may not be a presenting feature, e.g. when due to prolapsed intervertebral disc, post partum, or after regional anaesthesia such as an epidural anaesthetic. The retention volume should be significantly greater than the expected normal bladder capacity. In patients after surgery, due to bandaging of the lower abdomen or abdominal wall pain, it may be difficult to detect a painful, palpable or percussable bladder.

- *Chronic retention of urine* is defined as a non-painful bladder, which remains palpable or percussable after the patient has passed urine. Such patients may be incontinent. (NEW) – **FOOTNOTE 43**

FOOTNOTE 43 – The ICS no longer recommends the term 'overflow incontinence'. This term is considered confusing and lacking a convincing definition. If used, a precise definition and any associated pathophysiology, such as reduced urethral function, or detrusor overactivity/low bladder compliance, should be stated. The term chronic retention excludes transient voiding difficulty, e.g. after surgery for stress incontinence, and implies a significant residual urine; a minimum figure of 300 ml has been previously mentioned.

- *Benign prostatic obstruction* is a form of *bladder outlet obstruction* and may be diagnosed when the cause of outlet obstruction is known to be benign prostatic enlargement, due to histologic benign prostatic hyperplasia. (NEW)
- *Benign prostatic hyperplasia* is a term used (and reserved for) the typical histological pattern which defines the disease. (NEW)
- *Benign prostatic enlargement* is defined as prostatic enlargement due to histologic benign prostatic hyperplasia. The term 'prostatic enlargement' should be used in the absence of prostatic histology. (NEW)

5   Treatment

The following definitions were published in the 7th ICS report on Lower Urinary Tract Rehabilitation Techniques (Andersen et al) and remain in their original form.

5.1   *Lower urinary tract rehabilitation*
It is defined as non-surgical, non-pharmacological treatment for lower urinary tract function and includes:

- *Pelvic floor training*, defined as repetitive selective voluntary contraction and relaxation of specific pelvic floor muscles.
- *Biofeedback*, the technique by which information about a normally unconscious physiological process is presented to the patient and/or the therapist as a visual, auditory or tactile signal.
- *Behavioural modification*, defined as the analysis and alteration of the relationship between the patient's symptoms and his or her environment for the treatment of maladaptive voiding patterns.

This may be achieved by modification of the behaviour and/or environment of the patient.

5.2   *Electrical stimulation* is the application of electrical current to stimulate the pelvic viscera or their nerve supply.
The aim of electrical stimulation may be to directly induce a therapeutic response or to modulate lower urinary tract, bowel or sexual dysfunction.

5.3   *Catheterization* is a technique for bladder emptying employing a catheter to drain the bladder or a urinary reservoir.

5.3.1   *Intermittent (in/out) catheterisation* is defined as drainage or aspiration of the bladder or a urinary reservoir with subsequent removal of the catheter. The following types of intermittent catheterisation are defined:

- **Intermittent self-catheterisation** is performed by the patient himself/herself.
- **Intermittent catheterisation** is performed by an attendant (e.g. doctor, nurse or relative).
- **Clean intermittent catheterisation:** use of a clean technique. This implies ordinary washing techniques and use of disposable or cleansed reusable catheters.
- **Aseptic intermittent catheterisation:** use of a sterile technique. This implies genital disinfection and the use of sterile catheters and instruments/gloves.

5.3.2   **Indwelling catheterisation:** an indwelling catheter remains in the bladder, urinary reservoir or urinary conduit for a period of time longer than one emptying.

5.4   *Bladder reflex triggering* comprises various manoeuvres performed by the patient or the therapist in order to elicit reflex detrusor contraction by exteroceptive stimuli.
The most commonly used manoeuvres are; suprapubic tapping, thigh scratching and anal/rectal manipulation.

5.5   ***Bladder expression*** comprises various manoeuvres aimed at increasing intravesical pressure in order to facilitate bladder emptying.

The most commonly used manoeuvres are abdominal straining, Valsalva's manoeuvre and Credé manoeuvre.

Acknowledgements

The authors of this report are very grateful to Vicky Rees, Administrator of the ICS, for her typing and editing of numerous drafts of this document.

Addendum

Formation of the ICS Terminology Committee

The terminology committee was announced at the ICS meeting in Denver 1999 and expressions of interest were invited from those who wished to be active members of the committee. They were asked to comment in detail on the preliminary draft (the discussion paper published in *Neurourology and Urodynamics*). The nine authors replied with a detailed critique by 1 April 2000 and constitute the committee: Paul Abrams, Linda Cardozo, Magnus Fall, Derek Griffiths, Peter Rosier, Ulf Ulmsten, Philip van Kerrebroeck, Arne Victor and Alan Wein.

We thank other individuals who later offered their written comments: Jens Thorup Andersen, Walter Artibani, Jerry Blaivas, Linda Brubaker, Rick Bump, Emmanuel Chartier-Kastler, Grace Dorey, Clare Fowler, Kelm Hjalmas, Gordon Hosker, Vik Khullar, Guus Kramer, Gunnar Lose, Joseph Macaluso, Anders Mattiasson, Richard Millard, Rien Nijman, Arwin Ridder, Werner Schäfer, David Vodusek, Jean Jacques Wyndaele.

A half day workshop was held at the ICS Annual Meeting in Tampere (August 2000) and a two-day meeting in London, January 2001. This produced draft 5 of the report which was then placed on the ICS website <www.icsoffice.org>. Discussions on draft 6 took place at the ICS meeting in Korea September 2001; draft 7 then remained on the ICS website until final submission to journals in November 2001.

References

1. Abrams P (Chair), Blaivas JG, Stanton S, Andersen JT. ICS standardisation of terminology of lower urinary tract function. Scand J Urol Nephrol, 1988; Supp 114:5–19.

2. Abrams P, Blaivas JG, Stanton SL, Andersen J (Chair) – ICS 6th Report on the standardisation of terminology of lower urinary tract function. Neurourol Urodyn 1992; 11:593–603.

3. Andersen JT (Chair), Blaivas JG, Cardozo L, Thuroff J. ICS 7th Report on the standardisation of terminology of lower urinary tract function – lower urinary tract rehabilitation techniques. Neurourol Urodyn 1992; 11: 593–603.

4. Bump RC, Mattiasson A, Bo K, Brubaker LP, DeLancey JOL, Klarskov P, Shull BL, Smith ARB. The standardisation of terminology of female pelvic organ prolapse and pelvic floor dysfunction. Am J Obstet Gynecol 1996; 175:10–11.

5. Griffiths D, Hofner K, van Mastrigt R, Rollema HJ, Spangberg A, Gleason D. ICS report on the standardisation of terminology of lower urinary tract function: pressure-flow studies of voiding, urethral resistance and urethral obstruction. Neurourol Urodyn 1997; 16:1–18.

6. Stohrer M, Goepel M, Kondo A, Kramer G, Madersbacher H, Millard R, Rossier A Wyndaele JJ. ICS report on the standardisation of terminology in neurogenic lower urinary tract dysfunction. Neurourol Urodyn 1999; 18:139–158.

7. van Waalwijk van Doorn E, Anders K, Khullar V, Kulseng-Hansen S, Pesce F, Robertson A, Rosario D, Schäfer W. Standardisation of ambulatory urodynamic monitoring: report of the Standardisation Sub-committee of the International Continence Society for Ambulatory Urodynamic Studies. Neurourol Urodyn 2000; 19:113–125.

8. Lose G, Griffiths D, Hosker G, Kulseng-Hanssen S, Perucchini D, Schäfer W, Thind P and Versi E. Standardisation of urethral pressure measurement: report from the Standardisation Sub-committee of the International Continence Society. Neurourol Urodyn 2002; 21:258–260.

9. van Kerrebroeck P, Abrams P, Chaikin D, Donovan J, Fonda D, Jackson S, Jennum P, Johnson T, Lose G, Mattiasson A, Robertson G and Weiss J. The standardisation of terminology in nocturia: report from the standardisation subcommittee of the International Continence Society. BJU Ind 2002; 90 Suppl 3:11–15.

10. Rowan D (Chair), James ED, Kramer AEJL, Sterling AM, Suhel PF. ICS report on urodynamic equipment: technical aspects. J Med Eng & Tch 1987; 11(2): 57–64.

11. Schäfer W, Sterling AM, Liao L, Spangberg A, Pesce F, Zinner NR, van Kerrebroeck P, Abrams P and Mattiasson A. Good urodynamic practice: report from the Standardisation Sub-committee of the International Continence Society. Neurourol Urodyn 2002; 21:261–274.

12. Mattiasson A, Djurhuus JC, Fonda D, Lose G, Nordling J and Stöhrer M. Standardisation of outcome studies in patients with lower urinary dysfunction: a report on general principles from the Standardisation Committee of the International Continence Society. Neurourol Urodyn 1998; 17:249–253.

13. Lose G, Fanti JA, Victor A, Walter S, Wells TL, Wyman J and Mattiasson A. Outcome measures for research in adult women with symptoms of lower urinary tract dysfunction. Neurourol Urodyn 1998; 17:255–262.

14. Nordling J, Abrams P, Ameda K, Andersen JT, Donovan J, Griffiths D, Kobayashi S, Koyanagi T, Schäfer W, Yalla S and Mattiasson A. Outcome measures for research in treatment of adult males with symptoms of lower urinary tract dysfunction. Neurourol Urodyn 1998; 17:263–271.

15. Fonda D, Resnick NM, Colling J, Burgio K, Ouslander JG, Norton C, Ekelund P, Versi E and Mattiasson A. Outcome measures for research of lower urinary tract dysfunction in frail and older people. Neurourol Urodyn 1998; 17:273–281.

16. International classification of functioning, disability and health. ICIDH-2 website <http://www.who.int/icidh>

17. Klevmark B. Natural pressure–volume curves and conventional cystometry. Scand J Urol Nephrol Suppl 1999; 201:1–4.

Appendix 2

The standardization of terminology in neurogenic lower urinary tract dysfunction*

With suggestions for diagnostic procedures

Manfred Stöhrer,[1]** **Mark Goepel,**[2] **Atsuo Kondo,**[3] **Guus Kramer,**[4] **Helmut Madersbacher,**[5] **Richard Millard,**[6] **Alain Rossier,**[7] **and Jean-Jacques Wyndaele**[8]

[1] Department of Urology, Berufsgenossenschaftliche Unfallklinik Murnau, Murnau, Germany
[2] Department of Urology, University of Essen Medical School, Essen, Germany
[3] Komaki Shimin Hospital, Johbushi, Komaki, Japan
[4] Urodynamics Laboratory, Berufsgenossenschaftliche Unfallklinik Murnau, Murnau, Germany
[5] University Hospital Innsbruck, Innsbruck, Austria
[6] Department of Urology, The Prince Henry Hospital, Little Bay, Sidney, Australia
[7] Geneva, Switzerland
[8] Department of Urology, University Hospital Antwerp, Antwerp, Belgium

Key words: ICS standards; urodynamics

1 Introduction

This report has been produced at the request of the International Continence Society. It was approved at the twenty-eighth annual meeting of the Society in Jerusalem.

The terminology used in neurogenic lower urinary tract dysfunction developed over the years, defined by neurologists, neurological, and urological surgeons. Because of the particular intents of each specialist, confusion exists on the various terminologies used and on their definitions. The International Continence Society did not define in detail the procedures and conditions in neurogenic lower urinary tract dysfunction. During our discussions the need for standardization of this terminology became obvious.

This report follows the earlier standardization report for lower urinary tract dysfunction (Abrams et al, 1988, 1990) and is

Produced by the Standardization Committee of the International Continence Society, A. Mattiasson, Chairman. Sub-committee on Terminology in Patients with Neurogenic Lower Urinary Tract Dysfunction, M. Stöhrer, Chairman.

*Reproduced with permission from the International Continence Society.
**Correspondence to: PD Dr. med. Manfred Stöhrer, Chairman Department of Urology, Berufsgenossen-schaftliche
Unfallklinik Murnau, Professor-Küntscher-Straße 8, D-82418 Murnau, Germany.
Received 23 October 1998; Accepted 26 October 1998
© 1999 International Continence Society.
Neurourology and Urodynamics 18:139–158 (1999)

adapted to the specific group of patients with neurogenic lower urinary tract dysfunction. Terms defined in the earlier report are marked (*) and their definitions not repeated here. New or adapted definitions follow *the terms in italics*.

Any pertinent texts repeated from the earlier report are marked in the margin.

If they are not repeated completely, this is marked by the term (abbreviated).

Recently, the International Continence Society published a dedicated standardization report on pressure-flow studies (Griffiths et al 1997). This adapts and extends the earlier report with respect to pressure and flow plots and the analysis of the results and provides a provisional standard. Some new definitions are added, some existing ones changed, and some others no longer used. (Changed) definitions from this second report are marked differently ([+]).

Two more reports from the International Continence Society are in preparation and bear a relationship to the present report: A general report on Good Urodynamic Practice (Schäfer et al) and a dedicated report on Standardization of Ambulatory Urodynamic Monitoring (Van Waalwijk et al). This document is intended to be complementary to the mentioned reports and to be consistent in particular with the recommendations in the report of Schäfer et al.

Neurogenic lower urinary tract dysfunction is lower urinary tract dysfunction due to disturbance of the neurological control mechanisms. Neurogenic lower urinary tract dysfunction thus can be diagnosed *in presence of neurological pathology only*.

2   Clinical assessment

Before any functional investigation is planned, a basic general and specific diagnosis should be performed. In the present context of neurogenic lower urinary tract dysfunction, part of this diagnosis is specific for neurogenic pathology and its possible sequelae. The clinical assessment of patients with neurogenic lower urinary tract dysfunction includes and extends that for other lower urinary tract dysfunction.

The latter should consist of a detailed history, a frequency/volume chart and a physical examination. In urinary incontinence, leakage should be demonstrated objectively.

These data are indispensable for reliable interpretation of the urodynamic results in neurogenic lower urinary tract dysfunction.

2.1   History

2.1.1   General history

The general history should include questions relevant to neurological and congenital abnormalities as well as information on previous urinary infections and relevant surgery. Information must be obtained on medication with known or possible effects on the lower urinary tract. The general history should also include the assessment of menstrual, sexual, and bowel function, and obstetric history.

Symptoms of any metabolic disorder or neurological disease that may induce neurogenic lower urinary tract dysfunction must be checked particularly. Presence of spasticity or autonomic dysreflexia must be noted. A list of items of particular importance is

- Neurological complaints
- Congenital anomalies with possible neurological impact
- Metabolic disorders with possible neurological impact
- Preceding therapy, including surgical interventions
- Present medication
- Continence/incontinence (see urinary history)
- Bladder sensation (see urinary history)
- Mode and type of voiding (see urinary history)
- Infections of the lower urinary tract
- Defecation, including possible faecal incontinence (see defecation history)
- Sexual function (see sexual history)

2.1.2   Specific history

2.1.2.1 Urinary history. The urinary history must consist of symptoms related to both the storage and the evacuation functions of the lower urinary tract.

Specific symptoms and data must be assessed in neurogenic lower urinary tract dysfunction and if appropriate be compared with the patients' condition before the neurogenic lower urinary tract dysfunction developed.

Specify:

(a)   Urinary incontinence

- Predictability of the occurrence of incontinence
- Type of incontinence: Urge incontinence*, stress incontinence*, other incontinence

- Position or condition when incontinence occurs (supine/sitting/standing/moving/ bedwetting only)
- Control of the incontinence: Medication, pads, external appliances, penile clamp, urethral plug, pessary, catheterisation
- Extent of the incontinence: Pad number or weight or estimated volume per 24-h period, frequency/volume chart*

(b)   Bladder sensation*:

- Absent*
- Specific bladder sensation (desire to void*, urgency*, pain*)
- General sensation related to bladder filling (abdominal fullness, vegetative symptoms, spasticity)

(bb)   If specific bladder sensation exists:

- Normal*, hypersensitive*, or hyposensitive*
- Can urgency be suppressed?
- If yes, as effective as before the neurogenic condition?

(bbb)   If the patient has normal bladder sensation:

- Timing and duration of the sensation
- Ability to initiate voiding voluntarily
- Need for abdominal straining or other triggering to initiate or sustain voiding

(c)   Mode and type of voiding:

- Voiding position (standing, sitting, supine)
- Continuous* or intermittent flow*
- Residual urine*
- Initiation of voiding:
- Voluntary voiding
- Reflex voiding*: spontaneous or triggered (state type and area of triggering). Remark: Some patients with uncontrollable reflex voiding may use a condom urinal and a urine bag
- Voiding by increased intravesical pressure (state mode of pressure increase: abdominal strain or Credé). Remark: Credé is contra-indicated in children; also in adults when pressure exceeds 100 cm H_2O
- Passive voiding by decreased outlet resistance (state mode: removal of urethral and/or vaginal appliances, sphincterotomy, TUR bladder neck, artificial sphincter)
- Sacral root electrostimulation

(c1)   If the patient has an artificial sphincter:

- Implant date and date(s) of revision surgery
- Micturition frequency
- Cuff pressure
- Number of pump strokes

- Cuff closure time
- Continence or stress incontinence with closed sphincter

(c2)   If the voiding is induced by sacral root electrical stimulation:

- Implant date and date(s) of revision surgery
- Location of electrodes (roots used)
- Stimulation parameters
- Micturition frequency
- Duration of voiding stimulation
- "Double voiding" stimulation

(c3)   If the patients empties the bladder by catheterization, residual urine is assessed to check also the effectiveness of the catheterization

(c31)   *Intermittent catheterization:* Emptying of the bladder by catheter, mostly at regular intervals. The catheter is removed after the bladder is empty.
The procedure may be *sterile intermittent catheterization:* Use of sterile components or *clean intermittent catheterization:* At least one component is not sterile. *Intermittent self-catheterization* is performed by the patient.

- Type, size, and material of catheter (conventional, hydrophylic)
- Use of lubricating jelly (intra-urethral or on catheter only) or soaking (sterile saline, tap water)
- Disinfection of meatus

(c32)   An *indwelling catheter* is permanently introduced into the bladder. An external urine collecting device is used.

- Transurethral or suprapubic approach
- Type, size, and material of catheter
- Type of collecting device and associated materials (anti-reflux valves)
- Interval between changes of collecting device

(d)   *Urinary diary* (Frequency/volume chart*)
The frequency/volume chart is a specific urodynamic investigation recording fluid intake and urine output per 24-h period. The chart gives objective information on the number of voidings, the distribution of voidings between daytime and nighttime and each voided volume. The chart can also be used to record episodes of urgency and leakage and the number of incontinence pads used.
The urinary diary is also useful in patients who perform intermittent catheterization. A reliable urinary diary cannot be taken in less than 2–3 days. The urinary diary permits the assessment of voiding data under normal physiological conditions.

(e)   Time and volume for each voiding or catheterization

- Total volume over the period of the recording or 24-h volume
- Diurnal variation of volumes
- *Functional bladder capacity:* average voided volume

- *Voiding interval:* average time between daytime voidings
- *Continence interval:* average time between incontinence episodes or between last voiding and incontinence (assessed only during daytime)
- The fluid intake may also be recorded

Only for patients who use catheterization it is also feasible to assess:

- Residual urine
- *Total bladder capacity:* Sum of functional bladder capacity and residual urine

2.1.2.2 Defecation history. Patients with neurogenic lower urinary tract dysfunction may suffer from a related neurogenic condition of the lower gastro-intestinal tract. The defecation history also must address symptoms related to the storage and the evacuation functions and specific symptoms and data must be compared with the patients' condition before the neurogenic dysfunction developed.
Specify:

(a)   Faecal incontinence:

- Extent (complete, spotting, diarrhoea, flatulence)
- Pads use (type and number)
- Anal tampons (number)

(b)   Rectal sensation:

- Filling sensation
- Differentiation between stool, liquid stool and flatus
- Sensation of passage

(c)   Mode and type of defecation:

- Toilet use or in bed
- Frequency of defecation
- Duration of defecation
- Use of oral or rectal laxatives
- Interval between laxatives and defecation
- Use of enema (frequency, amount used)
- Antegrade continence enema (date of surgery, date(s) of revision, frequency
- of stomal dilation, frequency of washout)
- Initiation of defecation:
  - Voluntary or spontaneous
  - After digital stimulation
  - Mechanical emptying (patient or caregiver)
  - Sacral root electrical stimulation

(c1)   If the defecation is induced by sacral root electrical stimulation:
Implant date and date(s) of revision surgery

- Location of electrodes (roots used)
- Stimulation parameters
- Continuous or interrupted stimulation (interval)
- Combination with other treatment (laxatives or rectal mucosal stimulation)

2.1.2.3 Sexual history. The sexual function may also be impaired because of the neurogenic condition.

Specify:

Males:

(a) Sensation in genital area and for sexual functions (increased/normal/reduced/absent)

(b) Erection:

- Spontaneous or inducible by psychogenic stimuli
- Mechanical or medical initiation (state method or drug)
- Sacral root electrical stimulation

(b1) If the erection is induced by sacral root electrical stimulation:

- Implant date and date(s) of revision surgery
- Location of electrodes (roots used)
- Stimulation parameters
- Leg clonus (absent/present)
- If erection is insufficient: Use of supportive treatment

(c) Intercourse (erection sufficient or extra mechanical stimulation)

(c1) If the erection is insufficient state tumescence, rigidity, duration

(d) If the patient has a penile implant:

- Implant date and date(s) of revision surgery
- Type of prosthesis
- Result of implantation
- Frequency of use

(e) Ejaculation:

- Natural (normal, dribbling, semen quality and appearance)
- Artificial:
  - Vibrostimulation, electro-ejaculation, intrathecal drugs (frequency, results)
  - Semen analysis (most recent, result)

Females:

(a) Sensation in genital area and for sexual functions (increased/normal/reduced/absent)

(b) Arousal or orgasm inducible (psychogenic or mechanical stimuli)

2.2 *Physical examination*

2.2.1 General physical examination

Attention should be paid to the patient's physical and possible mental handicaps with respect to the planned investigation. Impaired mobility, particularly in the hips, or extreme spasticity may lead to problems in patient positioning in the urodynamics laboratory. Patients with very high neurological lesions may suffer from a significant drop in blood pressure when moved in a sitting or standing position. Subjective indications of bladder filling sensations may be impossible in retarded patients.

2.2.2 Neurourological status

Specify:

- Sensation $S_2 - S_5$ (both sides): Presence (increased/normal/reduced/absent), type (sharp/blunt), afflicted segments
- Reflexes: Bulbocavernous reflex, perianal reflex, knee and ankle reflexes, plantar responses {Babinski} (increased/normal/reduced/absent)
- Anal sphincter tone (increased/normal/reduced/absent)
- Anal sphincter and pelvic floor voluntary contractions (increased/normal/reduced/absent)
- Prostate palpation
- Descensus of pelvic organs

2.2.3 Laboratory tests

- Urinalysis (infection treatment, if indicated and possible, before further intervention)
- Blood laboratory, if necessary
- Free flowmetry and assessment of residual urine (mostly sonographic; by catheter in patients catheterizing or immediately preceding a urodynamic investigation). Because of natural variations, multiple estimations are necessary (at least 2–3)
- Quantification of urine loss* by pad testing, if appropriate
- Imaging:
  - Sonography: Kidneys (size, diameter of parenchyma, pelvis, calyces)

    Ureter (dilation)
    Bladder wall (diameter, outline, trabeculation, diverticulae or pseudodiverticulae)
  - X-ray: Cystography, excretion urography, urethrography, clearance studies, if necessary.

Apart from the data in sonography, attention must be paid to urinary stones, spinal anomalies, reflux, bladder neck condition, and urethral anomalies.

MRI: Accordingly

3 Investigations

In patients with neurogenic lower urinary tract dysfunction, and particularly when detrusor hyperreflexia* might be present, the urodynamic investigation is even more provocative than in other patients. Any technical source of artefacts must be critically considered. The quality of the urodynamic recording and its interpretation must be ensured (Schäfer et al).

In patients at risk for autonomic dysreflexia, blood pressure assessment during the urodynamic study is advisable.

In many patients with neurogenic lower urinary tract dysfunction, assessment of maximum (anaesthetic) bladder capacity* may be useful. The rectal ampulla should be empty of stool before the start of the investigation. Medication by drugs that influence the lower urinary tract function should be abandoned at least 48 h before the investigation (if feasible) or otherwise be taken into account for the interpretation of the data.

3.1   Methods

In neurogenic lower urinary tract dysfunction a combination of urodynamic investigations is mostly warranted. Some comments on the use of a single investigation are listed (see also Section 4). Urodynamic investigation should be performed only when the patient's free flowmetry and residual data are available (see Section 2.2.3) if the patient's condition permits these tests.

3.1.1   Measurement of urinary flow*

Care must be taken in judging the results in patients who are not able to void in a normal position. Both the flow pattern* and the flow rate* may be modified by this inappropriate position and by any constructions to divert the flow.

3.1.2   Cystometry*

Cystometry is used to assess detrusor activity, sensation, capacity, and compliance. As an isolated investigation this is probably only useful for follow-up studies of treatment.

3.1.3   Leak point pressure measurement (McGuire et al 1996)

There are two kinds of leak point pressure measurement. The detrusor leak point pressure is a static test and the abdominal leak point pressure is a dynamic test. The pressure values at leakage should be read exactly at the moment of leakage.

The *detrusor leak point pressure* is the lowest value of the detrusor pressure* at which leakage is observed in the absence of abdominal strain or detrusor contraction. Detrusor leak point pressure measurement assesses the storage function and detrusor compliance, in particular in patients with neurogenic lower urinary tract dysfunction, with low compliance bladder (see below) or with reflex voiding. High detrusor leak point pressure puts these patients at risk for upper urinary tract deterioration or might cause secondary damage to the bladder. A detrusor leak point pressure above 40 cm H_2O appears hazardous (McGuire et al 1996).

The *abdominal leak point pressure* is the lowest value of the intentionally increased intravesical pressure* that provokes urinary leakage in the absence of a detrusor contraction. The abdominal pressure increase can be induced by coughing (*cough leak point pressure*) or by Valsalva (*Valsalva leak point pressure*) with increasing amplitude. Multiple estimations at a fixed bladder volume (200–300 ml in adults) are necessary.

For patients with stress incontinence, the abdominal leak point pressure measurement gives an impression of the severity (slight or severe) or the nature (anatomical or intrinsic sphincter deficiency) of incontinence.

With the assumption that the intravesical pressure in abdominal leak point pressure is caused only by the abdominal pressure, vaginal pressure or rectal pressure may also be used to record the intravesical pressure. This will obviate the need for intravesical catheterization.

3.1.4   Bladder pressure measurements during micturition* and pressure–flow relationships*

Most types of obstructions caused by neurogenic lower urinary tract dysfunction are due to urethral overactivity* (detrusor/urethral dyssynergia*, detrusor-{external}-sphincter dyssynergia*, and detrusor/bladder neck dyssynergia*). This urethral overactivity will increase the detrusor voiding pressure above the level that is needed to overcome the urethral resistance+ given by the urethra's inherent mechanical and anatomical properties. Pressure–flow analysis mostly assesses the amount of mechanical obstruction* caused by the latter properties and has limited value in patients with neurogenic lower urinary tract dysfunction.

3.1.5   Electromyography* (often combined with cystometry/uroflowmetry)

Depending on the location of the electrodes, the electromyogram records the function of

* External urethral and/or anal sphincter
* Striated pelvic floor muscles

Owing to possible artefacts caused by other equipment used in a urodynamic investigation, its interpretation may be difficult.

3.1.6   Urethral pressure measurement*

Urethral pressure measurement has a limited place in the diagnosis of neurogenic lower urinary tract dysfunction. The following techniques are available:

* Resting urethral pressure profile*
* Stress urethral pressure profile*
* Intermittent catheter withdrawal (to cope with massive reflex contractions)
* *Continuous urethral pressure measurement*: the catheter sensor or opening is placed at about the point of maximum urethral closure pressure* and left there over time. This records time variations of urethral pressure and responses to various conditions of the lower urinary tract

3.1.7   Video urodynamics

Definition: Combination of lower urinary tract imaging during filling and voiding with urodynamic measurements.

3.1.8   Ambulatory urodynamics

An *ambulatory urodynamic investigation* is defined as any functional investigation of the urinary tract utilizing predominantly natural filling of the urinary tract and reproducing normal subject activity (Van Waalwijk et al). The recording of an ambulatory urodynamic investigation is comparable to Holter EKG and the patient is more or less in a situation of daily life. More detailed information on standardization of ambulatory urodynamics is found in the specific report (Van Waalwijk et al submitted).

3.1.9   Provocative tests during urodynamics

- Coughing, triggering, anal stretch
- Ice water test
- Carbachol test
- Acute drug tests

3.1.10   Maximum (anaesthetic) bladder capacity measurement

The volume measured after filling during a deep general or spinal/epidural anaesthetic.

3.1.11   Specific uro-neurophysiological tests

- Electromyography (in a neurophysiological setting)
- Nerve conduction studies*
- Reflex latency measurements*
- Evoked responses*
- Sensory testing*

3.2   *Measurement technique*

3.2.1   Measurement of urinary flow

Specify:

(0)   Type of voiding:

- Spontaneous voiding: Voluntary or reflex voiding
- Triggered voiding or sacral root electrostimulation:

Type of triggering

(a)   Voided volume
(b)   Patient environment and position (supine, sitting or standing)

(c)   Filling:

(i)   By diuresis (spontaneous or forced; specify regimen)
(ii)   By catheter (transurethral or suprapubic)

(d)   Type of fluid
Technique:

(a)   Measuring equipment
(b)   Solitary procedure or combined with other measurements

3.2.2   Cystometry

All systems are zeroed at atmospheric pressure. For external transducers the reference point is the level of the superior edge of the symphysis pubis. For catheter mounted transducers the reference point is the transducer itself.

If a different type of catheter is used in follow-up cystometries the findings in Rossier and Fam (1986) may be of interest.
Specify:

(a)   Access (transurethral or percutaneous)
(b)   Fluid medium (liquid or gas)
Gas filling should not be used in patients with neurogenic lower urinary tract dysfunction.
State type and concentration of liquid used (for example, contrast medium, isotonic saline).
(c)   Temperature of fluid (state in degree Celsius)
In neurogenic lower urinary tract dysfunction a body-warm filling medium is advised.
(d)   Position of patient (e.g., supine, sitting, or standing)
Offer the patient the individually most comfortable position, particularly when voiding.
(e)   Filling may be by diuresis or catheter. Filling by catheter may be continuous or incremental; the precise filling rate should be stated

When the incremental method is used the volume increment should be stated. For general discussion, the following terms for the range of filling may be used:

(i)   Up to 10 ml per minute is slow fill cystometry ("physiological" filling)
(ii)   10–100 ml per minute is medium fill cystometry
(iii)   Over 100 ml per minute is rapid fill cystometry

A physiological filling rate or alternatively a maximum filling rate of 20 ml per minute is advised in neurogenic lower urinary tract dysfunction to prevent provocation of detrusor hyperreflexia or other sequelae of faster filling. From ambulatory urodynamics data the impression arises that the mentioned filling rates should be reconsidered (Klevmark 1997).

Technique:

(a)   Fluid-filled catheter – specify number of catheters, single or multiple lumens, type of catheter (manufacturer), size of catheter
(b)   Catheter tip transducer – list specifications

(c) Other catheters—list specifications
(d) Measuring equipment

3.2.3 Leak point pressure measurement

Specify:

(a) Location and access of pressure sensor (intravesical – transurethral or percutaneous, vaginal, or rectal)
(b) Position of patient (for instance supine, sitting, or standing)
(c) Bladder filling by diuresis or catheter (state type of liquid)
(d) Bladder volume during test, also in relation to maximum cystometric capacity*

Technique:

(a) Mode of leak detection (observation, alarm nappy, meatal or urethral conductance measurement, or other)
(b) Catheters – list specifications, type (manufacturer) and size
(c) Measuring equipment for pressure and, if applicable, for leak detection

3.2.4 Bladder pressure measurements during micturition and pressure–flow relationships

The specifications of patient position, access for pressure measurement, catheter type, and measuring equipment are as for cystometry (see Section 3.2.2).

If urethral pressure measurements during voiding* are performed, the specifications are according to those in urethral pressure measurement (see Section 3.2.6).

If other assessments of the relation between pressure and flow are used (e.g., stop test, urethral occlusion, condom urinal occlusion) the specifications should be equivalent, according to the technique used.

3.2.5 Electromyography

The extensive specifications in the earlier report are appropriate in a neurophysiological setting. They are condensed here for practical use during urodynamics.
Specify:

(a) EMG (solitary procedure, part of urodynamic or other electrophysiological investigation)
(b) Patient position (supine, standing, sitting or other)
(c) Electrode placement (surface electrodes or intramuscular electrodes)

  (i) sampling site (abbreviated)
  (ii) recording electrode: location (abbreviated)
  (iii) reference electrode position

Note: Ensure that there is no electrical interference with any other machines, for example, X-ray apparatus.

Technique:

(a) Electrodes:

  (i) Needle electrodes: type, size, material (abbreviated) The same holds for other types of intramuscular electrodes (e.g., enamel wire)
  (ii) Surface electrodes: type, size, material, fixation, conducting medium (abbreviated)

(b) Amplifier (make and specifications)
(c) Signal processing (data: raw, averaged, integrated or other)
(d) Display equipment (abbreviated)
(e) Storage (abbreviated)
(f) Hard copy production (abbreviated)

3.2.6 Urethral pressure measurement

Because of its limited place in neurogenic lower urinary tract dysfunction, the reader is referred to the earlier standardization report (Abrams et al 1988, 1990) for the specifications.

3.2.7 Video urodynamics

Specify imaging system (fluoroscopy, ultrasound). Further specifications according to the type of urodynamic study.

3.2.8 Ambulatory urodynamics

Specifications according to the type of urodynamic study.

3.2.9 Provocative tests during urodynamics

Specify type of test, type of trigger, or drug used. Further specifications according to type of urodynamic study.

3.2.10 Maximum (anaesthetic) bladder capacity measurement

Specify fluid temperature, filling pressure, filling time, type of anaesthesia, anaesthetic agent, and dosage.

3.2.11 Specific uro-neurophysiological tests

Electromyography (see Section 3.2.5)
Nerve conduction studies, reflex latency measurements, evoked responses
Specify:

(a) Type of investigation (abbreviated)
(b) Is the study a solitary procedure or part of a urodynamic or neurophysiological investigation?

(c) Patient position and environmental temperature, noise level and illumination

(d) Electrode placement (abbreviated)

Technique:

(a) Electrodes (abbreviated)
(b) Stimulator (abbreviated)
(c) Amplifier (abbreviated)
(d) Averager (abbreviated)
(e) Display equipment (abbreviated)
(f) Storage (abbreviated)
(g) Hard copy production (abbreviated)

Sensory testing
Specify:

(a) Patient position (supine, sitting, standing, and other)
(b) Bladder volume at time of testing
(c) Site of applied stimulus (intravesical and intraurethral)
(d) Number of times the stimulus was applied and the response recorded.
     Define the sensation recorded, for example the first sensation or the sensation of pulsing
(e) Type of applied stimulus (abbreviated)

3.3   Data

3.3.1   Measurement of urinary flow

- Voided volume*
- Maximum flow rate*
- Flow time*
- Average flow rate*
- Time to maximum flow*
- Flow pattern, includes the statement of continuous or intermittent voiding
- Voiding time*, when the voiding is intermittent
- *Hesitancy:* The occurrence of significant delay between the patient's voluntary initiation of micturition as signalled for example by pushing the marker button on the flow meter and the actual start of flow (note the flow delay[+])

3.3.2   Cystometry

- Intravesical pressure
- Abdominal pressure
- Detrusor pressure
- Infused volumes at:

  - First desire to void* or other sensation of filling
  - Normal desire to void* or other sensation that indicates the need for a toilet visit
  - *Reflex volume:* Starting of first hyperreflexive detrusor contraction
  - Urgency
  - Pain (specify)

- Maximum cystometric capacity (in patients with abolition of sensations, this is defined as the volume at which the investigator decides to stop filling)
- Autonomic dysreflexia (specify)

- Compliance* $\{DV/Dp_{det}\}$ (ml/cm H_2O) is mostly measured between (specify):
- Reference value: Detrusor pressure at empty bladder (start of filling)
- Measurement value: The (passive) detrusor pressure:

  - At maximum cystometric capacity in patients with existing sensation and without urine loss
  - At the start of the detrusor contraction leading to the first significant incontinence in patients with failing sensation or significant incontinence

When a different volume range is used this should be specified in particular

A problem in the calculation of the compliance occurs when Δp_{det} is negative or zero: the defined calculation then gives a negative or infinite compliance. The first is physically impossible, the last gives little information. *In the compliance calculation a minimum value of 1 cm H_2O is used for* Δp_{det}. This means that the maximal possible value of the compliance will be equal to the volume range over which the compliance is calculated.

- *Break volume:* the bladder volume after which a sudden significant decrease of compliance is observed during the remainder of the filling phase (mind the distinction between passive detrusor pressure and detrusor contraction). It is yet unclear whether this observation is consistent in patients with neurogenic lower urinary tract dysfunction with or without detrusor hyperreflexia. When true, this might indicate that the detrusor is in a different state after the break volume

3.3.3   Leak point pressure measurement

- Minimum of measured pressure for first observation of leakage

3.3.4   Bladder pressure measurements during micturition and pressure–flow relationships

- Opening time* (note the flow delay)
- Opening pressure* (note the flow delay)
- Maximum pressure*
- Pressure at maximum flow[+] (note the flow delay)
- Closing pressure[+] (note the flow delay)
- Minimum voiding pressure[+] (note the flow delay)

All pressure values will be estimated for intravesical, abdominal and detrusor pressure separately. They will not only differ in amplitude, but often also in timing. The detrusor pressure is generally the most important one. The maximum pressure values may be attained at a moment where the flow rate is zero (Griffiths et al 1997).

3.3.5 Electromyography

- Recruitment patterns*, particularly in relation to specific stimuli (bladder filling, hyperreflexive contractions, onset of voiding, coughing, Valsalva, etc.)
- If individual motor unit action potentials are recorded: duration (msec) and amplitude (mV) of spontaneous activity, fibrillations, positive sharp waves, and complex repetitive discharges. Complexity and polyphasicity (descriptive or number)

3.3.6 Urethral pressure measurement

One parameter describing the contribution of the urethra to continence is the
functional profile length*, the length of the urethra over which the urethral pressure exceeds intravesical pressure.

The functional profile length should reflect the length of the urethra that contributes to the prevention of leakage. In the female, this concept is straightforward, but in the male, the length of the bulbous and penile urethra will often add significantly to the functional profile length. The infrasphincteric part of the urethra however contributes little, if any, to continence. The functional profile length in men thus is much greater than in women, without the associated implication that this greater length indeed is functional in maintaining continence. This functional part of the urethra probably extends down from the bladder to the junction from sphincteric to bulbous urethra, but this junction is often difficult to detect on the curve.

The contribution of the bulbous and penile urethra also show a large variance between patients and between several assesments in the same man. Therefore a third urethral length parameter is used, the *urethral continence zone:* the length of the urethra between the bladder neck and the point of maximum urethral pressure (Gleason et al 1974) (Figure A2.1).

- Resting urethral pressure profile:

  - Maximum urethral pressure*
  - Maximum urethral closure pressure
  - Functional profile length (not mandatory in men)
  - Urethral continence zone (not mandatory in women)

- Stress urethral pressure profile: above parameters and

  - Pressure "transmission" ratio*

- Intermittent withdrawal: above parameters and

  - Relaxing time before measurement is read

- Continuous urethral pressure measurement. This study is probably best represented by the measured curve. Urethral pressure variations in relation to specific stimuli (bladder filling, hyperreflexive contractions, onset of voiding, coughing, Valsalva, etc.) may be described separately

3.3.7 Video urodynamics

- According to type of urodynamic study
- Morphology:

  - Configuration and contour of the bladder during filling and voiding
  - Reflux, occurrence, and timing:
    - Into the upper urinary tract
    - Into the adnexa (for instance the prostate, the ejaculatory duct)
  - Bladder neck during filling and voiding phases

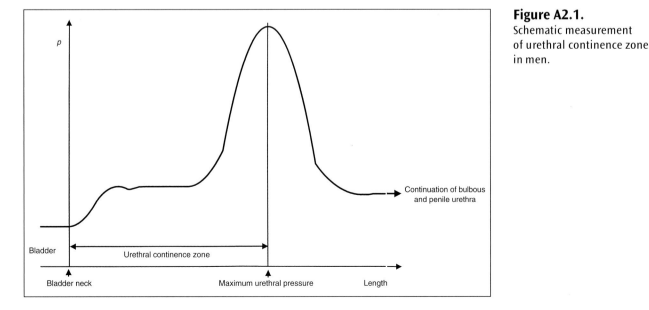

Figure A2.1.
Schematic measurement of urethral continence zone in men.

- Configuration of proximal urethra during filling and voiding, urethral kinking
- Bladder or urethral descensus

3.3.8 Ambulatory urodynamics

According to type of urodynamic study

3.3.9 Provocative tests during urodynamics

Response of the lower urinary tract function to the provocation. Compare with situation without provocation

3.3.10 Maximum (anaesthetic) bladder capacity measurement

Anatomical maximum volume that bladder will accommodate

3.3.11 Specific uro-neurophysiological tests

- Electromyography (see Section 3.3.5)
- Nerve conduction studies:

  - Latency time* (abbreviated)
  - Response amplitude* (abbreviated)

- Reflex latency measurement:

  - Response time* (abbreviated)

- Evoked responses:

  - Single or multiphasic response*
  - Onset of response* (abbreviated)
  - Latency to onset* (abbreviated)
  - Latency to peaks* (abbreviated)
  - The amplitude of the responses is measured in mV

- Sensory testing:

  - Sensory threshold* (abbreviated)

3.4 Typical manifestations of neurogenic lower urinary tract dysfunction

3.4.1 Filling phase

- Hyposensitivity or hypersensitivity
- Vegetative sensations, for example, goose flesh, sweating, headache, and blood pressure increase (particularly in patients with autonomic dysreflexia)

- *Low compliance:* Compliance value lower than 20 ml/cm H_2O

  - Cause: Neural or muscular (described before as hypertonic bladder)

- *High volume bladder:* A bladder that can be filled to far over functional bladder capacity in non-anaesthetised condition without significant increase in pressure (described before as hypotonic bladder). The use of the terms excessive or very high compliance to describe this situation is discouraged, as a high value of compliance will also be measured at lower volumes when only a slight increase in pressure occurs during filling

  - Cause: Neural or muscular

- Detrusor hyperreflexia, spontaneous or provoked; classified according to maximal detrusor pressure as *low-pressure hyperreflexia* or *high-pressure hyperreflexia.* Because of its clinical implications, as a practical guideline a value of 40 cm H_2O is proposed as cut-off value between low-pressure and high-pressure hyperreflexia (McGuire et al 1996)
- *Sphincter areflexia:* No evidence of reflex sphincter contraction during filling, particularly at higher volumes, or during physical stress

Neurogenic Lower Urinary Tract Dysfunction 155.3.4.2 *Voiding phase*

- Detrusor areflexia*
- *External sphincter hyperreflexia:* involuntary activity (for example, intermittently) of external sphincter during voiding other than detrusor sphincter dyssynergia
- Detrusor sphincter dyssynergia
- Detrusor bladder neck dyssynergia

4 Clinical value and classification of urodynamic investigation

Urodynamic investigation is needed for accurate evaluation of all patients with neurogenic lower urinary tract dysfunction. When effected in a standardized manner, it produces standardized and reproducible results (cf. [Schäfer et al]). After the evaluation, its results must be summarized and evaluated:

1. Neurological background (type/duration of neurological disease or lesion) and characteristics of uro-neurophysiological tests
2. Characteristics of filling function
3. Characteristics of voiding function

In the conclusive evaluation the condition of the upper urinary tract and the incontinence care in incontinent patients must also be taken into account. Core investigation of patients with neurogenic lower urinary tract dysfunction will include:

1. History
2. Urine culture

3. Flow rate and post-void residual (multiple estimations)
4. Filling and voiding cystometry

Not all urodynamic procedures are equally important in the diagnosis of patients with neurogenic lower urinary tract dysfunction. The following list is an indication of the place of each procedure in these patients.

0: Urinary diary: Semi-objective quantification of the physiological lower urinary tract function. Advisable.
1: Free uroflowmetry and assessment of residual urine: First impression of voiding function. Mandatory before any invasive urodynamics is planned.
2: Cystometry. The only method to quantify filling function. Limited significance as a solitary procedure. Powerful when combined with bladder pressure measurement during micturition and even more in video urodynamics.
   Necessary to document the status of the lower urinary tract function during the filling phase.
3: Leak point pressure measurement. Detrusor leak point pressure: Specific investigation if high pressures during the filling phase might endanger the upper urinary tract or lead to secondary bladder damage. Abdominal leak point pressure: Less important in neurogenic lower urinary tract dysfunction. Useful for patients with stress incontinence.
4: Bladder pressure measurements during voiding and pressure–flow relationships. Pressure measurements reflect the co-ordination between detrusor and urethra or pelvic floor during the voiding phase. Even more powerful in combination with cystometry and with video urodynamics. Necessary to document the status of the lower urinary tract function during the voiding phase.
   Pressure–flow analysis is aimed at assessing the passive urethral resistance relation[+] and as such of less importance in neurogenic lower urinary tract dysfunction.
5: Urethral pressure measurement. Limited applicability in neurogenic lower urinary tract dysfunction.
6: Electromyography: Vulnerable to artefacts when performed during a urodynamic investigation. Useful as a gross indication of the patient's ability to control the pelvic floor. When more detailed analysis is needed, it should be performed as part of a uro-neurophysiological investigation.
7: Video urodynamics: When combined with cystometry and pressure measurement during micturition probably the most comprehensive investigation to document the lower urinary tract function and morphology. In this combination the first choice of invasive investigations.
8: Ambulatory urodynamics: Should be considered when office urodynamics do not reproduce the patient's symptoms and complaints. May replace office (not video) urodynamics in future when all parameters from office urodynamics are available in ambulatory urodynamics too.
9: Specific uro-neurophysiological tests. Advised as part of the neurological work-up of the patient. Elective tests may be asked for specific conditions that became obvious during patient work-up and urodynamic investigations.

5 Supplemental investigations

5.1 Endoscopic procedures

Endoscopic investigation of the lower urinary tract may be necessary in a limited number of patients. The indication must be very restrictive.

5.2 Other investigations to define the neurological status

Specific investigations to assess the neurological status of the patient may also be necessary in individual cases.

Acknowledgments

The authors used the "Manual Neuro-Urology and Spinal Cord Lesion: Guidelines for Urological Care of Spinal Cord Injury Patients" prepared by the Arbeitskreis Urologische Rehabilitation Querschnittgelähmter for the German Urological Society as a starting point for their discussions. The authors thank Dr. Clare Fowler and Dr. Derek Griffiths for valuable discussions during the production of this report.

References

1. Abrams P, Blaivas JG, Stanton SL, Andersen JT. Standardization of terminology of lower urinary tract function. The International Continence Society Committee on Standardization of Terminology. Neurourol Urodynam 1988; 7:403–427. Scand J Urol Nephrol 1988; 114(suppl):5–19.

2. Abrams P, Blaivas JG, Stanton SL, Andersen JT. Standardization of terminology of lower urinary tract function. The International Continence Society Committee on Standardization of Terminology. Int Urogynecol J 1990; 1:45–58.

3. Gleason DM, Reilly RJ, Bottacini MR, Pierce MJ. The urethral continence zone and its relation to stress incontinence. J Urol 1974; 112:81–88.

4. Griffiths DJ, Höfner K, van Mastrigt R, Rollema HJ, Spångberg A, Gleason D. Standardization of terminology of lower urinary tract function: pressure–flow studies of voiding, urethral resistance, and urethral obstruction. Neurourol Urodynam 1997; 16:1–18.

5. Klevmark B. Ambulatory urodynamics. Letter to the editor. Br J Urol 1997; 79:490.

6. McGuire EJ, Cespedes RD, O'Connell HE. Leak-point pressures. Urol Clin North Am 1996; 23:253–262.

7. Rossier AB, Fam BA. 5-microtransducer catheter in evaluation of neurogenic bladder function. Urology 1986; 27:371–378.

8. Schäfer W, Abrams P, Liao L, Mattiasson A, Pesce F, Spanberg A, Sterling AM, Zinner NR, van Kerrebroeck P. International Continence Society. Good urodynamic practices: uroflowmetry, filling cystometry, and pressure-flow studies. Neurourol Urodyn 2002;21(3):261–74.

9. Van Waalwijk van Doorn E, Anders K, Khullar V, Kulseng-Hanssen S, Pesce F, Robertson A, Rosario D, Schäfer W. Standardization of ambulatory urodynamic monitoring. First draft report of the standardization sub-committee of the ICS for ambulatory urodynamic studies. Neurourol Urodynam 2000; 19:113–125.

Appendix 3

The standardisation of terminology and assessment of functional characteristics of intestinal urinary reservoirs*

Joachim W. Thuroff Anders Mattiasson, Jens Thorup Anderson, Hans Hedlund, Frank Hinman Jr., Markus Hohenfellner, Wiking Mansson, Anthony B. Mundy, Randall G. Rowland, and Kenneth Steven

1 Introduction

In 1993, the International Continence Society (ICS) established a committee for standardisation of terminology and assessment of functional characteristics of intestinal urinary reservoirs in order to allow reporting of results in a uniform fashion so that different series and different surgical techniques can be compared.

This report is consistent with earlier reports of the International Continence Society Committee on Standardisation of Terminology with special reference to the collated ICS report from 1988 (see Appendix 1, Part 2).

As the present knowledge about physiological characteristics of intestinal urinary reservoirs is rather limited in regard to normal and abnormal reservoir sensation, compliance, activity, continence, and other specifications, some of the definitions are necessarily imprecise and vague. However, it was felt that this report still would be capable of stipulating the standardised assessment of intestinal urinary reservoirs and reporting of the results in order to accumulate more information about physiological characteristics of intestinal urinary reservoirs and to establish precise definitions of normal and abnormal conditions. With increased knowledge and better understanding of intestinal urinary reservoirs, this report will have to be updated to become more specific.

It is suggested that in written publications, the acknowledgement of these standards is indicated by a footnote to the section Methods and Materials or its equivalent: 'Methods, definitions and units conform to the standards recommended by the International Continence Society, except where specifically noted'.

*Reproduced with permission from the International Continence Society.

Produced by the International Continence Society Committee on Standardisation of Terminology (Anders Mattiasson, chairman) Subcommittee on Intestinal Urinary Reservoirs (Joachim W. Thuroff, chairman)

Neurourol Urodyn 15:499–511 (1996) O 1996 Wiley-Liss, Inc.

2 Terminology of surgical procedures

Up to now, when different surgical procedures for constructing an intestinal urinary reservoir are described, conflicting terminology is often used. This section defines the terminology of surgical procedures used throughout the report. These definitions may not be universally applicable to the published scientific literature to date, viewed in retrospect, but represent a standardised terminology for surgical procedures for the future.

Definitions

Bladder augmentation is a surgical procedure for increasing bladder capacity. This may be accomplished without other tissues (e.g., autoaugmentation) or with incorporation of other tissues such as intestine (enterocystoplasty, intestinocystoplasty), with or without changing the shape of such intestine (i.e., detubularisation and reconfiguration), and with or without resection of a portion of the original bladder.

Bladder replacement – see 'Bladder Substitution'.

Bladder substitution (Bladder Replacement) is a surgical procedure for in situ (orthotopic) total substitution/replacement of the bladder by other tissues such as isolated intestine. After subtotal excision of the original bladder (e.g., in interstitial cystitis) the intestinal urinary reservoir may be connected to the bladder neck (bladder substitution to bladder neck) and after complete excision of the original bladder (radical cystoprostatectomy), the reservoir may be connected to the urethra as a continent outlet (bladder substitution to urethra). If indicated, the urethral closure function may be surgically supported in addition (e.g., sling procedure, prosthetic sphincter, periurethral injections). Alternatively, an orthotopically placed urethral substitute/replacement, e.g., from intestine may be used as a continent outlet for a complete substitution of the lower urinary tract.

Continent anal urinary diversion is a surgical procedure for continent urinary diversion utilising bowel in continuity or isolated bowel as a reservoir and the anus as a continent outlet.

Continent cutaneous urinary diversion is a surgical procedure for continent urinary diversion providing an urinary reservoir, e.g., from intestine and a continence mechanism, e.g., from intestine for formation of a continent heterotopically placed (e.g., cutaneous) outlet (stoma).

Enterocystoplasty (bladder augmentation with intestine) – see 'Bladder Augmentation'.

Intestinocystoplasty (bladder augmentation with intestine) – see 'Bladder Augmentation'.

3   Assessment

3.1   *Experimental assessment*

For reporting animal studies, the principles and standards for experimental scientific publications should be followed. Species, sex, weight, and age of the animals must be stated, as well as type of anesthesia. If chronic experiments are performed, the type of treatment between the initial experiment and the evaluation experiment should be stated. Raw data should be presented and, when applicable, the type of statistical analysis must be stated. For standardisation of urodynamic evaluation see 4 and 5.

3.2   *Patient assessment*

The assessment of patients with intestinal urinary reservoirs should include history, frequency/volume chart, physical examination, and evaluation of the upper urinary tract.

3.2.1   History

The history must include etiology of the underlying disease (i.e., congenital anomaly, neurogenic bladder dysfunction, lower urinary tract trauma, radiation damage, bladder cancer or other tumours of the true pelvis) and indication for constructing an intestinal urinary reservoir (e.g., radical surgery for malignancy in the true pelvis, low bladder capacity/compliance, upper tract deterioration due to vesicoureteral obstruction or reflux, urinary incontinence). Information must be available on the duration of previous history of the underlying disease, previous urinary tract infections, and relevant surgery.

The history should also provide information on dexterity and ambulatory status of the patient (i.e., wheelchair bound, paraplegia, or tetraplegia). Information on sexual and bowel function must be reported in respect to the status prior to applying an intestinal urinary reservoir.

The urinary history must report symptoms related to both the storage and evacuation functions of the lower urinary tract with special reference to the technique of evacuation (i.e., spontaneous voiding with or without abdominal straining, Valsalva or Crede manoeuvres, intermittent catheterisation). Problems of evacuation due to mucus production or difficulty with catheterisation must be reported. Incidence of urinary infections must be reported in respect to the incidence prior to construction of an intestinal urinary reservoir.

3.2.2   Specification of surgical technique

The surgical technique must be specified stating the applied type of urinary reservoir and origin of gastrointestinal segments used (e.g., stomach, ileum, cecum, transverse colon, sigmoid colon, rectum), length and shape (e.g., tubular, detubularised) of bowel segments, the technique of urethral implantation (when applicable) and the type of the continent outlet (i.e., original urethra, functionally supported urethra, anal sphincter, catheterisable continent cutaneous outlet). If an intussusception nipple valve is applied, technique of fixation of the intussusception (i.e., sutures, staples) should be stated.

Additional and combined surgical procedures in the true pelvis must be reported, such as hysterectomy, colposuspension, excision of vaginal or rectal urinary fistulae, or resection of rectum. Information of adjuvant treatment, such as pharmacotherapy, physiotherapy, or electrical stimulation, must be available.

3.2.3   Frequency/volume chart

On the frequency/volume chart the time and volume of each micturition are reported along with quantities of fluid intake. It must be stated if evacuation was prompted by the clock or by sensation. In addition, episodes of urgency and incontinence have to be reported. The frequency/volume chart can be used for the primary assessment of symptoms of urgency, frequency, and incontinence and for followup studies.

3.2.4   Physical examination

Besides general, urological, and, when appropriate, gynecological examination, the neurological status should be assessed with special attention to sensitivity of the sacral dermatomes, sacral reflex activity (anal reflex, bulbocavernosus reflex), and anal sphincter tone and control.

3.2.5   Evaluation of the upper urinary tract

Evaluation of renal function and morphology must be related to the status prior to constructing an intestinal urinary reservoir. Studies of renal morphology can be based on renal ultrasound, intravenous pyelography, and radioisotope studies. Quantification of findings should be recorded by using accepted classifications of upper tract dilatation (Emmett and Witten 1971), renal scarring (Smellie et al 1975), and urethral reflux (Heikel and Parkkulainen 1966). Renal function should be assessed by measuring the serum concentration of creatinine and, if indicated, by creatinine clearance and radioisotope clearance studies.

3.2.6   Other relevant studies

Reported complications of urinary diversion into an intestinal reservoir include electrolyte and blood–gas imbalance, malabsorption syndromes, urolithiasis, urinary tract infection, and development of a secondary malignancy. Follow-up evaluation should include relevant tests when applicable and indicated, and reports should state the results of such studies as serum electrolyte concentrations, analysis of blood gases, serum levels of vitamins A, B12, D, E, K, and folic acid, serum levels of bile acids, urine osmolality and pH, urine excretion of calcium, phosphate, oxalate, and citrate, colonisation of urine, and findings on endoscopy and biopsy of the urinary reservoir.

4   Procedures related to the evaluation of urine storage in an intestinal urinary reservoir

4.1   Enterocystometry

Enterocystometry is the method by which the pressure/volume relationship of the intestinal urinary reservoir is measured. All systems are zeroed at atmospheric pressure. For external transducers the reference point is the superior edge of the symphysis pubis for bladder augmentation, bladder substitution or continent anal urinary diversion, and the level of the stoma for continent cutaneous urinary diversion. Enterocystometry is used to assess reservoir sensation, compliance, capacity, and activity. Before filling is started, residual urine must be evacuated and measured. Enterocystometry is performed with the patient awake and unsedated, not taking drugs that may affect reservoir characteristics. In a urodynamic follow-up study for evaluation of adjutant treatment (e.g., pharmacological therapy) of an intestinal urinary reservoir, mode of action, dosage, and route of administration (enteral, parenteral, topical) of the medication have to be specified.

As an intestinal urinary reservoir starts to expand when permitted to store urine, time intervals between surgery for construction of the intestinal urinary reservoir, its first functional use for storage of urine and urodynamic testing must be stated. For reporting of functional characteristics of an intestinal urinary reservoir, the time interval between surgery and enterocystometric assessment must be stated to account for postoperative expansion of the reservoir. As several intestinal segments used in urinary reservoirs react to gastric stimuli, time interval between food ingestion and the urodynamic evaluation should be stated. Reporting of pressure/volume relationships of an intestinal urinary reservoir should be obtained at standardised filling volumes or standardised pressures, which must be stated in absolute numbers.

Specify

(a) Access (transurethral, transanal, transstomal, percutaneous);
(b) Fluid medium;
(c) Temperature of fluid (state in degrees Celsius);
(d) Position of patient (supine, sitting or standing);
(e) Filling may be by diuresis or catheter. Filling by catheter may be continuous or stepwise: the precise filling rate should be stated. When the stepwise filling is used, the volume increment should be stated. For general discussion, the following terms for the range of filling rate should be used:

  (i) up to 10 ml per minute is slow fill enterocystometry ('physiological' filling);

  (ii) 10–100 ml per minute is medium fill enterocystometry;
  (iii) over 100 ml per minute is rapid fill enterocystometry.

Technique

(a) Fluid-filled catheter – specify number of catheters, single or multiple lumens, type of catheter (manufacturer), size of catheter, type (manufacturer), and specifications of external pressure transducer; (b) Catheter mounted microtransducer – list specifications; (c) Other catheters – list specifications; (d) Measuring equipment.

Definitions

Total reservoir pressure is the pressure within the reservoir.

Abdominal pressure is taken to be the pressure surrounding the reservoir. In current practice it is estimated from rectal or, less commonly, intraperitoneal or intragastric pressures.

Subtracted reservoir pressure is estimated by subtracting abdominal pressure from total reservoir pressure. The simultaneous recording of the abdominal pressure trace is essential for the interpretation of the subtracted reservoir pressure trace as artefacts of the subtracted reservoir pressure may be produced by intrinsic rectal contractions or relaxations.

Contraction pressure (amplitude) is the difference between maximum reservoir pressure during a contraction of an intestinal urinary reservoir and baseline reservoir pressure before onset of this contraction. Contraction pressures may be determined from the pressure curves of total reservoir pressure or subtracted reservoir pressure. For assessment of functional significance of such activity of an intestinal urinary reservoir, pressure and volume must be stated for the first, a typical, and the maximum contraction. The frequency of contractions should be stated at a specified volume.

Leak point pressure is the total reservoir pressure at which leakage occurs in the absence of sphincter relaxation. Leakage occurs whenever total reservoir pressure exceeds maximum outlet pressure so that a negative outlet closure pressure results.

Reservoir sensation is difficult to assess because of the subjective nature of interpreting fullness or 'flatulence' from the bowel segments of the intestinal urinary reservoir. It is usually assessed by questioning the patient in relation to the sensation of fullness of the intestinal urinary reservoir during enterocystometry.

Commonly used descriptive terms are similar to conventional cystometry:

  First desire to empty
  Normal desire to empty (this is defined as the feeling that leads the patient to empty at the next convenient moment, but emptying can be delayed if necessary);
  Strong desire to empty (this is defined as a persistent desire to empty without the fear of leakage);
  Urgency (this is defined as a strong desire to empty accompanied by fear of leakage or fear of pain);
  Pain (the site and character of which should be specified).

Maximum enterocystometric capacity is the volume at strong desire to empty. In the absence of sensation, maximum enterocystometric capacity is defined by the onset of leakage. If the closure mechanism of the outlet is incompetent, maximum enterocystometric capacity can be determined by occlusion of the outlet, e.g., by a Foley catheter. In the absence of both sensation and leakage, maximum enterocystometric capacity cannot be defined in the same terms and is the volume at which the clinician decides to terminate filling, e.g., because of a risk of over-distension.

Functional reservoir capacity or evacuated volume is assessed from a frequency/volume chart (urinary diary). If a patient empties the urinary reservoir by intermittent catheterisation, functional reservoir capacity will be dependent on presence or absence of sensation and/or leakage. Thus, when reporting functional reservoir capacity the following should be stated:

(a) Mode of evacuation (e.g., spontaneous voiding, intermittent catheterisation);
(b) Presence/absence of sensation of fullness;
(c) Presence/absence of leakage;
(d) Timing of evacuation (e.g., by sensation, by the clock, by leakage).

Maximum (anaesthetic) anatomical reservoir capacity is the volume measured after filling during a deep general or spinal/epidural anaesthetic, specifying fluid temperature, filling pressure and filling rate.

Compliance describes the change in volume over a related change in reservoir pressure. Compliance (C) is calculated by dividing the volume change (ΔV) by the change in subtracted reservoir pressure (ΔP_S) during that change in reservoir volume ($C = A\ \Delta V/\Delta P_S$). Compliance is expressed as ml per cm H_2O.

4.2   Outlet pressure measurement

It should be noted that even under physiological conditions the evaluation of the competence of the closure mechanism of a continent outlet by measuring intraluminal pressures under various conditions is regarded as an idealized concept. Moreover, measurements of intraluminal pressures for functional evaluation of a continent outlet do not allow comparison of results between different closure mechanisms, which are in use with different types of intestinal urinary reservoirs. In addition, similar closure mechanisms may behave differently when used in different types of intestinal urinary reservoirs.

Therefore, urodynamic measurements of a continent outlet always have to be related to symptoms of the patient as assessed by history, frequency/volume chart, and, when applicable, measurement of urine loss.

The rationale of performing outlet pressure measurements is not to verify continence or degree of incontinence but to understand how different closure mechanisms work, which urodynamic parameters reflect their competence or dysfunction, and how their function is related to the characteristics of a reservoir.

In current urodynamic practice, intraluminal outlet pressure measurements are performed by a number of different techniques which do not always yield consistent values. Not only do the values differ with the method of measurement but there is often a lack of consistency for a single method – for example, the effect of catheter rotation when outlet pressure is measured by a catheter mounted microtransducer.

Measurements can be made at one point in the outlet (stationary) over a period of time, or at several points along the outlet consecutively during continuous or intermittent catheter withdrawal forming an outlet pressure profile (OPP). OPPs should be obtained at significant filling volumes of an intestinal urinary reservoir, which must be standardised and stated.

Two types of OPP can be measured:

(a) Resting outlet pressure profile – with the urinary reservoir and the subject at rest;
(b) Stress outlet pressure profile – with a defined applied stress (e.g., cough, strain, Valsalva manoeuvre).

The outlet pressure profile denotes the intraluminal pressure along the length of the closure mechanism. All systems are zeroed at atmospheric pressure. For external transducers the reference point is the level of the continence mechanism. For catheter mounted transducers the reference point is the transducer itself. Intrareservoir pressure should be measured to exclude a simultaneous reservoir contraction. The subtraction of total reservoir pressures from intraluminal outlet pressures produces the outlet closure pressure profile.

Specify

(a) Infusion medium;
(b) Rate of infusion;
(c) Stationary, continuous or intermittent catheter withdrawal;
(d) Rate of withdrawal;
(e) Reservoir volume;
(f) Position of patient (supine, sitting or standing);
(g) Technique (catheters, transducers, measurement technique and recording apparatus are to be specified according to the 1988 ICS report; see Appendix 1, Part 2).

Definitions

Maximum outlet pressure is the maximum pressure of the measured profile.

Maximum outlet closure pressure is the difference between maximum outlet pressure and total reservoir pressure.

Functional outlet profile length is the length of the closure mechanism along which the outlet pressure exceeds total reservoir pressure.

Functional outletprofile length (on stress) is the length over which the outlet pressure exceeds total reservoir pressure on stress.

Pressure 'transmission' ratio[1] is the increment in outlet pressure on stress as a percentage of the simultaneously recorded increment in the total reservoir pressure. For stress profiles obtained during coughing, pressure 'transmission' ratios can be obtained at any point along the closure mechanism. If single values are given, the position in the closure mechanism should be stated. If several transmission ratios are defined at different points along the closure mechanism, a pressure 'transmission' profile is obtained. During 'cough profiles' the amplitude of the cough should be stated if possible.

4.3   Quantification of urine loss

On a frequency/volume chart, incontinence can be qualified (with/without urge or stress) and quantified by the number, type, and dampness (damp/wet/soaked) of pads used each day. However, subjective grading of incontinence may not completely disclose the degree of abnormality. It is important to relate the complaints of each patient to the individual urinary regimen and personal circumstances, as well as to the results of objective measurement.

In order to assess and compare results of different series and different surgical techniques, a simple standard test can be used to measure urine loss objectively in any subject. In order to obtain a representative result, especially in subjects with variable or intermittent urinary incontinence, the test should occupy as long a period as possible; yet it must be practical. The circumstances should approximate to those of everyday life, yet be similar for all subjects to allow meaningful comparison.

The total amount of urine lost during the test period is determined by weighing a collecting device such as a nappy, absorbent pad, or condom appliance. A nappy or pad should be worn inside waterproof underpants or should have a waterproof backing if worn over a continent stoma. Care should be taken to use a collecting device of adequate capacity.

Immediately before the test begins the collecting device is weighed to the nearest gram.

In the 1988 collated report on 'Standardisation of Terminology of Lower Urinary Tract Function' (see Appendix 1, Part 2), the ICS has offered the choices to conduct a pad test either with the patient drinking 500 ml sodium-free liquid within a short period (max. 15 min) without the patient voiding before the test or after having the bladder filled to a defined volume. Because there is a great variation in the functional capacity of different types of intestinal urinary reservoirs and since some types of closure mechanism of the outlet physiologically have a leak point and others have no leak point, it is recommended that the reservoir is emptied by catheterisation immediately before the test and refilled with a reasonable volume of saline, which must be standardised and be stated in absolute numbers. A typical test schedule and additional procedures are described in the 1988 ICS report (Appendix 1, Part 2). Specifications for presentation of results, findings, and statistics from the 1988 ICS report are applicable (Appendix 1, Part 2).

5   Procedures related to the evaluation of evacuation of an intestinal urinary reservoir

5.1   Mode of evacuation

The mode of evacuation of an intestinal urinary reservoir varies as some patients may have a surgically constructed closure mechanism requiring catheterisation (e.g., continent cutaneous urinary diversion) and sorne patients may have a reservoir with a physiological sphincter mechanism (e.g., bladder augmentation, bladder substitution to bladder neck or to urethra, continent anal urinary diversion), through which they may be able to evacuate urine spontaneously. However, as catheterisation may also be required after bladder augmentation or bladder substitution to bladder neck or to urethra, it must be stated by what means the reservoir is emptied (e.g., spontaneous evacuation with or without Valsalva or Crede manoeuvres and/or intermittent catheterisation).

If intermittent catheterisation is necessary, whether it is performed on a regular basis or only periodically, the intervals between catheterisations must be stated.

Measurements of urinary flow, reservoir pressures during micturition and residual urine apply only to patients with bladder augmentation or bladder substitution to bladder neck or to urethra who void spontaneously. However, as there is no volitional initiation of contraction of an intestinal urinary reservoir, spontaneous evacuation is different from voiding by a detrusor contraction.

In patients with an intestinal urinary reservoir, evacuation is initiated by relaxation of the urethral sphincteric mechanisms and/or passive expression of the reservoir by abdominal straining or Valsalva or Crede manoeuvres. Therefore, measurements of flow and micturition pressures must be interpreted with great caution in respect of the diagnosis of an outlet obstruction.

5.2   Measurements of urinary flow, micturition pressure, residual urine

For specifications of measurements of urinary flow, reservoir pressures during micturition and residual urine the 1988 ICS report is applicable (Appendix 1, Part 2). The specifications of patient position, access for pressure measurement, catheter type, and measuring equipment are as for enterocystometry (see 4.1).

6   Classification of storage dysfunction of an intestinal urinary reservoir

Dysfunction of an intestinal urinary reservoir has to be defined in respect to indications and functional intentions of incorporating bowel into the urinary tract. The rationale of using an intestinal urinary reservoir is to improve or provide storage function by:

(a) Reducing bladder hypersensitivity;
(b) Providing/enlarging reservoir capacity;
(c) Providing/improving reservoir compliance;
(d) Lowering bladder pressures/providing low reservoir pressures;
(e) Improving/providing the closure function of the outlet.

It is not a primary goal of surgery to maintain or provide the capability of spontaneous voiding; intermittent catheterisation is required for evacuation of the reservoir in all cases of continent cutaneous diversion and in many other situations. The need to evacuate a urinary reservoir by intermittent catheterisation is not regarded as a failure in bladder augmentation and bladder substitution to bladder neck or to urethra, even though the majority of patients may evacuate urine spontaneously.

Consequently, the classification of dysfunctions of an intestinal urinary reservoir relates to the storage phase only. Problems of storing urine in an intestinal urinary reservoir may be related to dysfunction of the reservoir or dysfunction of the outlet. The classification is based on the pathophysiology of dysfunction as assessed by various urodynamic investigations. The urodynamic findings must be related to the patient's symptoms and signs. For example, the presence of reservoir contractions in an asymptomatic patient with normal upper tract drainage does not warrant a diagnosis of reservoir overactivity unless the contractions cause urine leakage or other problems defined below.

6.1   Reservoir dysfunction

The symptoms of frequency, urgency, nocturia, and/or incontinence may relate to dysfunction of an intestinal urinary reservoir and should be assessed by enterocystometry, which is an adequate test for evaluation of the pathophysiology of a reservoir dysfunction (see 4.1). Abnormal findings may relate to sensation, compliance, capacity, and/or activity of an intestinal urinary reservoir.

6.1.1   Sensation

Sensations from an intestinal urinary reservoir as assessed by questioning the patient during enterocystometry can be classified in qualitative terms. Often these symptoms are associated with contractions of the reservoir as shown by enterocystometry or fluoroscopy. However, up to now there is insufficient information about an isolated hypersensitive state of the bowel of an intestinal urinary reservoir. If symptoms such as frequency, urgency, and nocturia are persisting after bladder augmentation or bladder substitution to bladder neck (e.g., in interstitial cystitis), they are likely to derive from remnants of the original lower urinary tract, which have not been replaced by intestine, if enterocystometry is otherwise normal.

6.1.2   Capacity/compliance

Capacity of an intestinal urinary reservoir is determined by sensation and/or compliance. For definitions of reservoir capacity and compliance (AV/AP), see 4.1. Compliance describing the change in volume over a related change in reservoir pressure is likely to reflect a different physiology when determined in an intestinal urinary reservoir as compared to the urinary bladder. The calculation of compliance will reflect wall characteristics of an intestinal urinary reservoir such as distensibility only after a process of 'unfolding' of an empty intestinal urinary reservoir has been completed and stretching of the walls begins to take place, which is different in the normal urinary bladder. Compliance may change during the enterocystometric examination and is variably dependent upon a number of factors including:

(a)   Rate of filling;
(b)   The part of the enterocystometrogram curve used for compliance evaluation;
(c)   The volume interval over which compliance is calculated;
(d)   The distensibility of the urinary reservoir as determined by mechanical and contractile properties of the walls of the reservoir.

During normal filling of an intestinal urinary reservoir little or no pressure changes occur and this is termed 'normal compliance'. However, at the present time there is insufficient data to define normal, high, and low compliance. When reporting compliance, specify:

(a)   The rate of filling;
(b)   The volume at which compliance is calculated;
(c)   The volume increment over which compliance is calculated;
(d)   The part of the enterocystometrogram curve used for the calculation of compliance.

The selection of bowel segments, the size of bowel (diameter, length), and the geometry (shape) of a reservoir after bowel detubularisation and reconfiguration determine capacity of an intestinal urinary reservoir (Hinman 1988). For a given length of bowel, reconfiguration into a spherical reservoir provides the largest capacity. The distensibility of bowel wall, as assessed in experimental models, varies between bowel segments (i.e., large bowel, small bowel, stomach) and with orientation (longitudinal, circumferential) of measurement within a bowel segment (Hohenfellner et al 1993). However, the relative contributions of wall distensibility (influenced by selection of bowel segments) and of geometric capacity (influenced by size of selected bowel and reservoir shape after detubularisation and reconfiguration) in determining the capacity of an intestinal urinary reservoir are not yet precisely understood. Low capacity of an intestinal urinary reservoir may relate to bowel size (diameter/length) and/or configuration of bowel segments in the reservoir (e.g., tubular, inadequate detubularisation, and reconfiguration).

6.1.3   Activity

In intact bowel segments, peristaltic contractions are elicited at a certain degree of wall distension. As a result of detubularisation and reconfiguration of bowel segments in an intestinal urinary reservoir, such contractions do not encompass the whole circumference of a reservoir. Net pressure changes in the reservoir are determined by the mechanical and muscular properties of both the contracting and the non-contracting segments of the reservoir. Contractions of segments of an intestinal urinary reservoir may be observed by fluoroscopy but may not increase subtracted reservoir pressure if the generated forces are counterbalanced by other segments of a urinary reservoir which relax and distend. Some contractile activity of an intestinal urinary reservoir is a normal finding on enterocystometry or fluoroscopy.

Overactivity of an intestinal urinary reservoir is defined as a degree of activity which causes lower urinary tract symptoms and/or signs of upper tract deterioration in the absence of other causes of upper tract damage such as urethral obstruction or reflux. Symptoms such as abdominal cramping, urgency, frequency, and/or leakage may be related to reservoir activity seen during enterocystometry and thus establish the diagnosis of an unacceptable degree of reservoir activity ('overactivity'). Signs of impaired upper tract drainage may be associated with elevated subtracted reservoir pressures on enterocystometry due to an early onset, high amplitudes, and/or frequency of contractions and thus establish the diagnosis of overactivity even if subjective symptoms are not experienced.

However, since a precise definition of normal and increased activity of a urinary reservoir from intestine is not yet established, the frequency of contractions should be reported at a specified volume and the pressure/volume relationships should be stated for the following defined contractions of the reservoir:

(a) First contraction;
(b) Contraction with maximum contraction pressure (amplitude);
(c) Typical contraction.

The diagnosis of overactivity of an intestinal urinary reservoir should not be made until a reasonable interval – which must be stated – has elapsed after surgery, since an intestinal urinary reservoir expands after surgery, when permitted to store urine, and since some of the reservoir activity subsides with time with an increase of capacity.

6.2   Outlet dysfunction

The symptoms of incontinence and/or difficulties with catheterisation may relate to dysfunction of the outlet of an intestinal urinary reservoir and should be assessed in terms of pathophysiology. Leakage may occur if total reservoir pressure exceeds outlet pressure so that the result is a negative outlet closure pressure as assessed by outlet pressure profiles (see 4.2). For such an event, volume and total reservoir pressure at onset of leakage (leak point pressure) must be stated.

Leakage may occur with a functioning closure mechanism because of an excessive reservoir pressure increase due to contractions of the intestinal urinary reservoir (overactivity) or overdistension of the reservoir (overflow).

The definition of incompetence of a closure mechanism is different for a closure mechanism which physiologically has a leak point from that for a closure mechanism without a leak point.

A closure mechanism which physiologically has a leak point (e.g., the urethral sphincter, some types of closure mechanism in continent cutaneous urinary diversion) is incompetent if it allows leakage or urine in the absence of contraction of the intestinal urinary reservoir (overactivity) or overdistension of the reservoir (overflow) as assessed by enterocystometry (see 4.1). A closure mechanism which normally has no leak point (e.g. an intussusception nipple) is incompetent if it permits leakage of urine independent of results of enterocystometry.

References

Emmett JL, Witten DM. Urinary stasis: the obstructive uropathies, atony, vesicoureteral reflux, and neuromuscular dysfunction of the urinary tract. In: Emmett JL, Witten DM, eds. Clinical urography. An atlas and textbook of roentgenologic diagnosis. Vol. 1, 3rd edn. Philadelphia, London, Toronto: Saunders, 1971: 369.

Heikel PE, Parkkulainen KV. Vesicoureteric reflux in children. A classification and results of conservative treatment. Ann Radiol 1966; 9:37.

Hinman F Jr. Selection of intestinal segments for bladder substitution: physical and physiological characteristics. J Urol 1988; 139:519.

Hohenfellner M, Buger R, Schad H, Heimisch W, Riedmiller H, Lampel A, Thuroff JW, Hohenfellner R. Reservoir characteristics of Mainz-pouch studied in animal model. Osmolality of filling solution and effect of Oxybutynin. Urology 1993; 42:741.

Smellie JM, Edwards D, Hunter N, Normand ICS, Prescod N. Vesico-ureteric reflux and renal scarring. Kidney Int 1975; 8:65.

Appendix 4

Guidelines on neurogenic lower urinary tract dysfunction*

M. Stöhrer, D. Castro-Diaz, E. Chartier-Kastler, G. Kramer,
A. Mattiasson, J. J. Wyndaele

1 Aim and status of these guidelines

1.1 Purpose

The purpose of these clinical guidelines is to provide information on the incidence, definitions, diagnosis, therapy, and follow up observation of the condition of neurogenic lower urinary tract dysfunction (NLUTD), that will be useful for clinical practitioners. These guidelines reflect the current opinion of the experts in this specific pathology and thus represent a state of the art reference for all clinicians as of the date of its presentation to the European Association of Urology.

1.2 Standardization

The terminology used and the diagnostic procedures advised throughout these guidelines follow the recommendations for investigations on the lower urinary tract (LUT) as published by the International Continence Society (ICS) (1–3).

1.3 References

1. Stöhrer M, Goepel M, Kondo A, Kramer G, Madersbacher H, Millard R, Rossier A, Wyndaele JJ. The standardization of terminology in neurogenic lower urinary tract dysfunction with suggestions for diagnostic procedures, Neurourol Urodyn 1999; 18:139–158.

2. Abrams P, Cardozo L, Fall M, Griffiths D, Rosier P, Ulmsten U, van Kerrebroeck P, Victor A, Wein A. The standardisation of terminology of lower urinary tract function: Report from the Standardisation Sub-committee of the International Continence Society. Neurourol Urodyn 2002; 21: 167–178.

3. Schäfer W, Abrams P, Liao L, Mattiasson A, Pesce F, Spångberg A, Sterling AM, Zinner NR, van Kerrebroeck P. Good Urodynamic Practices: Uroflowmetry, Filling Cystometry, and Pressure-Flow Studies. Neurourol Urodyn 2002; 21:261–274.

*Reproduced with permission from the European Association of Urology.

2 Background

2.1 Risk factors and epidemiology

NLUTD may be caused by various diseases and events affecting the nervous systems controlling the LUT. The resulting lower urinary tract dysfunction (LUTD) depends grossly on the location and the extent of the neurologic lesion (cf. 2.3.).

Overall figures on the prevalence of NLUTD in the general population are lacking, but data are available on the prevalence of the underlying conditions and the relative risk of those for the development of NLUTD.

2.1.1 Peripheral neuropathy

Diabetes: This common metabolic disorder has a prevalence of about 2.5% in the American population, but the disease may be subclinical for many years. No specific criteria exist for secondary neuropathy in this condition, but it is generally accepted that 50% of the patients will develop somatic neuropathy and 75–100% of those will develop NLUTD (1–2).

Alcohol abuse: This will eventually cause peripheral neuropathy, but its reported prevalence varies widely: 5–15% (3) to 64% (4). The NLUTD is probably more present in patients with liver cirrhosis and the parasympathetic system is attacked more than the sympathetic system (5).

Less prevalent peripheral neuropathies:

– Porphyria – bladder dilatation in up to 12% of patients (6).
– Sarcoidosis – NLUTD rare (7).
– Lumbosacral (8) zone and genital (9) herpes – NLUTD transient in most patients.
– Guillain Barré – Urinary symptoms in 30% of patients, regressive in most (10).

2.1.2 Regional spinal anaesthesia

This may cause NLUTD (11) but no prevalence figures were found (12).

2.1.3   Latrogenic

Abdominoperineal resection of rectum or uterus may cause lesions of the lower urinary tract innervation in 10–60% of patients (13, 14). The extent of the resection is important: < 8% after colostomy only, but 29% after posterior resection (15). Radical prostatectomy is a risk factor also (16).

2.1.4   Demyelinisation

Multiple sclerosis causes NLUTD in 50–90% of the patients (17–19). NLUTD is the presenting symptom in 2–12% of the patients (20).

2.1.5   Dementia

Alzheimer, Binswanger, Nasu and Pick diseases frequently cause non-specific NLUTD (21–25).

2.1.6   Basal ganglia pathology (Parkinson, Huntington, Shy-Drager, etc.)

Parkinson's disease is accompanied by NLUTD in 37.9–70% (26). In the rare Shy-Drager syndrome almost all patients have NLUTD (27).

2.1.7   Cerebrovascular pathology

This causes hemiplegia with remnant incontinence NLUTD in 20–50% of patients (28–30) with decreasing prevalence in the post-insult period (30).

2.1.8   Frontal brain tumours

These tumours can cause LUTD in 24% of the patients (31).

2.1.9   Spinal cord lesions

Spinal cord lesions can be traumatic, vascular, medical, or congenital. An incidence of 30–40 new cases per million population is the accepted average for the USA. Most patients will develop NLUTD (32). For spina bifida and other congenital nerve tube defects, the prevalence in the UK is 8–9 per 10,000 aged 10–69 years with the greatest prevalence in the age group 25–29 years (33), and in the USA 1 per 1000 births (34). About 50% of these children will have detrusor sphincter dyssynergia (DSD) (35).

2.1.10   Disc disease

This is reported to cause NLUTD in 6–18% of the patients (36, 37).

2.2   *Standardization of terminology*

2.2.1   Introduction

Several groups already presented guidelines for the care of patients with NLUTD for national or international urological community (38–41). These guidelines will evolve further as time goes by. They also contain definitions of various important terms and procedures. The ICS NLUTD standardization report (39) is addressed specifically at the standardization of terminology and urodynamic investigation in this patient group. Other relevant definitions are found in the general ICS standardization report (42).

The definitions from these references, partly adapted, and other definitions that are judged useful for the clinical practice in NLUTD, are listed in section 2.2.2. For specific definitions relating to the urodynamic investigation technique the reader is referred to the appropriate ICS report (39).

2.2.2   Definitions

Acontractility, detrusor – see below under voiding phase

Acontractility, urethral sphincter – see below under storage phase

Autonomic dysreflexia – Increase of sympathetic reflex due to noxious stimuli with symptoms or signs of headache, hypertension, flushing face and perspiration

Capacity – see below under storage phase

Catheterization, indwelling – Emptying of the bladder by a catheter that is introduced (semi-)permanently

Catheterization, intermittent (IC) – Emptying of the bladder by a catheter that is removed after the procedure, mostly at regular intervals

– Aseptic IC – The catheters remain sterile, the genitals are disinfected, and disinfecting lubricant is used
– Clean IC – Disposable or cleansed re-usable catheters, genitals washed
– Sterile IC – Complete sterile setting, including sterile gloves, forceps, gown and mask
– Intermittent self-catheterization (ISC) – IC performed by the patient

Compliance, detrusor – see below under storage phase

Condition – The presence of specific observations associated with characteristic symptoms or signs evidencing relevant pathologic processes

Diary, urinary – Record of times of micturitions and voided volumes, incontinence episodes, pad usage, and other relevant information

– Frequency volume chart (FVC) – Times of micturitions and voided volumes only
– Micturition time chart (MTC) – Times of micturitions only

Filling rate, physiological – Below the predicted maximum: body weight [kg]/4 in ml/s (42, 43)

Hesitancy – Difficulty in initiating micturition; delay in the onset of micturition after the individual is ready to pass urine

Intermittency – Urine flow stops and starts on one or more occasions during voiding

Leak point pressure (LPP) – see below under storage phase

Lower motor neuron lesion (LMNL) – Lesion at or below the S1-S2 spinal cord level

Neurogenic lower urinary tract dysfunction (NLUTD) – Lower urinary tract dysfunction secondary to confirmed pathology of the nervous supply

Observation, specific – Observation made during specific diagnostic procedure

Overactivity, bladder – see below under symptom syndrome

Overactivity, detrusor – see below under storage phase

Rehabilitation, LUT – Non-surgical non-pharmacological treatment for LUT dysfunction

Sign – Observation by the physician including simple means (direct observation, bladder diary, pad weighing) to verify symptoms and classify them

Sphincter, urethral, non-relaxing – see below under voiding phase

Symptom – Subjective indicator of a disease or change in condition as perceived by the patient, carer, or partner that may lead to seek help from health care professionals

Upper motor neuron lesion (UMNL) – Lesion above the S1–S2 spinal cord level

Voiding, balanced – In patients with NLUTD: voiding with physiologic detrusor pressure and low residual (< 80 ml or < 20% of bladder volume)

Voiding, triggered – Voiding initiated by manoeuvres to elicit reflex detrusor contraction by exteroceptive stimuli

Volume, overactivity – see below under storage phase

Storage phase

- Maximum anaesthetic bladder capacity – Maximum bladder filling volume under deep general or spinal anaesthesia
- Increased daytime frequency – Self-explanatory; the normal frequency can be estimated at about 8 times per day (44)
- Nocturia – Waking at night one or more times to void
- Urgency – The symptom of a sudden compelling desire to pass urine which is difficult to defer
- Urinary incontinence – Any involuntary leakage of urine. This can be specified:

    - Stress urinary incontinence – On effort or exertion, or on sneezing or coughing
    - Urge urinary incontinence – Accompanied by or immediately preceded by urgency
    - Mixed urinary incontinence – Associated with urgency and also exertion, effort, sneezing, or coughing
    - Continuous urinary incontinence

- Bladder sensation categorized as:

    - Normal – Symptom and history: Awareness of bladder filling and increasing sensation up to a strong desire to void
        Urodynamics: First sensation of bladder filling, first desire to void, and strong desire to void at realistic bladder volumes

    - Increased – Symptom and history: An early and persistent desire to void.
        Urodynamics: Any of the three urodynamic parameters mentioned under "normal" persistently at low bladder volume
    - Reduced – Symptom and history: Awareness of bladder filling but no definite desire to void
        Urodynamics: Diminished sensation throughout bladder filling
    - Absent – No sensation of bladder filling or desire to void
    - Non-specific – Perception of bladder filling as abdominal fullness, vegetative symptoms, or spasticity

Definitions valid after urodynamic confirmation only

- Cystometric capacity – Bladder volume at the end of the filling cystometry
- Maximum cystometric capacity – Bladder volume at strong desire to void
- High capacity bladder – Bladder volume at cystometric capacity far over the mean voided volume, estimated from the bladder diary, with no significant increase in detrusor pressure under non-anaesthetized condition
- Normal detrusor function – Little or no pressure increase during filling: no involuntary phasic contractions despite provocation
- Detrusor overactivity – Involuntary detrusor contractions during filling; spontaneous or provoked Subgroups:

    - Phasic detrusor overactivity – Characteristic phasic contraction
    - Terminal detrusor overactivity – A single contraction at cystometric capacity

- High pressure detrusor overactivity – Maximal detrusor pressure >40 cm H_2O (39, 45)
- Overactivity volume – Bladder volume at first occurrence of detrusor overactivity
- Detrusor overactivity incontinence – Self-explanatory
- Leak point pressure

    - Detrusor leak point pressure (DLPP) – Lowest value of detrusor pressure at which leakage is observed in the absence of abdominal strain or detrusor contraction
    - Abdominal leak point pressure – Lowest value of intentionally increased intravesical pressure that provokes leakage in the absence of a detrusor contraction

- Detrusor compliance – Relationship between change in bladder volume (ΔV) and change in detrusor pressure (Δpdet): $C = \Delta V/\Delta p$det [ml/cm H_2O]
- Low detrusor compliance – C $\Delta V/\Delta p$det <20 ml/cm H_2O (39)
- Break volume – Bladder volume after which a sudden significant decrease in detrusor compliance is observed
- Urethral sphincter acontractility – No evidence of sphincter contraction during filling, particularly at higher bladder volumes, or during abdominal pressure increase

Voiding phase

- Slow stream – Reduced urine flow rate
- Intermittent stream (intermittency) – Stopping and starting of urine flow during micturition
- Hesitancy – Difficulty in initiating micturition
- Straining – Muscular effort to initiate, maintain, or improve urinary stream
- Terminal dribble – Prolonged final part of micturition when the flow has slowed to a trickle/dribble

Definitions valid after urodynamic confirmation only

- Normal detrusor function – Voluntarily initiated detrusor contraction that causes complete bladder emptying within a normal time span
- Detrusor underactivity – Contraction of reduced strength and/or duration
- Acontractile detrusor – Absent contraction
- Non-relaxing urethral sphincter – Self-explanatory
- Detrusor sphincter dyssynergia (DSD) – Detrusor contraction concurrent with an involuntary contraction of the urethral and/or periurethral striated musculature

Post micturition phase

- Feeling of incomplete emptying (symptom only)
- Post micturition dribble – Involuntary leakage of urine shortly after finishing the micturition

Pain, discomfort or pressure sensation in the lower urinary tract and genitalia that may be related to bladder filling or voiding, may be felt after micturition, or be continuous
Symptom syndrome – Combination of symptoms

- Overactive bladder syndrome – Urgency with or without urge incontinence, usually with frequency and nocturia

Synonyms: Urge syndrome, urgency-frequency syndrome. This syndrome is suggestive for LUTD

2.3   Classification

2.3.1   Introduction

The purpose of classification of NLUTD is to facilitate the understanding and management of NLUTD and to provide a standardized terminology of these disease processes. The normal LUT function depends on neural integration at and between the peripheral, spinal cord, and central nervous systems. The gross type of NLUTD is dependent on the location and the extent of the lesion: suprapontine or pontine, suprasacral spinal cord, or subsacral and peripheral (32, 40).

The classification systems for NLUTD are based on either the neurologic substrate (type and location of the neurologic lesion), the neuro-urologic substrate (neurologic lesion and LUTD), the type of LUTD, or are strictly functional. Many descriptive terms were derived from these classification systems, but they are

standardized only within any specific system and have little meaning outside the system and can sometimes be confusing.

A perfect classification system is not yet available. Neurologic classification systems, by nature, cannot describe the LUTD completely and vice versa. Individual variations exist in the NLUTD caused by a specific neurologic lesion. Thus for any particular patient the description of the NLUTD should be individualized.

2.3.2   Neuro-urologic classification

Bors and Comarr's (46) classic neuro-urologic classification system was deduced from clinical observations of patients with traumatic spinal cord injury. It specifies three elements: location of lesion, completeness of lesion, and co-ordination of LUT.

Hald and Bradley (47) reduced the number of categories in Bors and Comarr's classification. The authors describe their system as a simple neurotopographic classification.

Burgdörfer completed Bors and Comarr's system with information on the LUTD, broken down for detrusor, sphincter, and residual urine. This classification is published elsewhere (48).

2.3.3   Neurologic classification

Bradley (49) presented four control loops for the LUT. Loop I are the connections between the central nervous system and the pontine micturition center, loop II the intraspinal pathways between the detrusor to the micturition center (afferent) and the sacral spinal cord (efferent), loop III the sensory axons pathways from the detrusor and the striated urethral sphincter to the sacral spinal cord, and loop IV describes the suprasacral and segmental innervation of the periurethral striated muscles.

2.3.4   Urodynamic classification

Lapides (50) classifies the clinical and urodynamic findings into five categories: sensory neurogenic bladder, motor paralytic bladder, autonomous neurogenic bladder, uninhibited neurogenic bladder, and reflex neurogenic bladder.

Krane and Siroky (51) present a descriptive classification of detrusor and sphincter co-ordination observed during urodynamic evaluation in patients with NLUTD, focussed on the functional interaction between detrusor and urethral sphincter.

2.3.5   Functional classification

Quesada et al. (52) suggested that a classification based on the functional aspects of the LUT might be more practicable for clinical decision making.

Wein (53) provides a practical approach towards the diagnosis and therapy of LUTD by classifying against the storage and voiding functions of the LUT, and the activity of the detrusor and the urethra.

Fall et al. (54) proposed a more detailed classification of the overactive detrusor. This is included in the ICS classification.

The ICS (42) separates the storage and voiding phases and describes the detrusor and urethral functions in each phase by specific designations (cf. 2.2.).

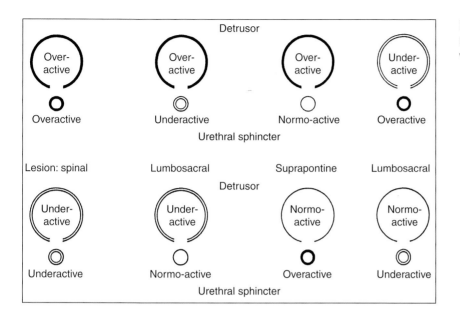

Figure A4.1
Madersbacher classification system (40) with typical neurogenic lesions.

Madersbacher (40, 55) presented a very simple classification that basically is focussed on the therapeutic consequences (Figure A4.1). It is based on the clinical concept that the important differentiation in the diagnosis exists between the situations of high and low detrusor pressure during the filling phase and urethral sphincter relaxation and non-relaxation or DSD during the voiding phase. A non-relaxed sphincter or DSD will cause high detrusor pressure during the voiding phase. This classification is the easiest one for general use in clinical diagnosis of NLUTD.

2.3.6 Recommendation for classification

The Madersbacher classification system (40) (Figure A4.1) is recommended for clinical practice.

2.4 Timing of diagnosis and treatment

Both in congenital and in acquired NLUTD, early diagnosis and treatment is essential as irreversible changes may occur in particular in children with myelomeningocele (56–61), but also in patients with traumatic spinal cord injury (62–64), even if the related neuropathologic signs may be normal (65).

The fact must also be considered that LUTD by itself may be the presenting symptom for neurologic pathology (20, 66).

2.4.1 Guideline for timing of diagnosis and treatment

1. Diagnosis and treatment in NLUTD should be performed as soon as possible.

2.5 References

1. Ellenberg M. Development of urinary bladder dysfunction in diabetes mellitus. Ann Intern Med 1980; 92:321–323.

2. Bradley WE. Diagnosis of urinary bladder dysfunction in diabetes mellitus. Ann Intern Med 1980; 92:323–326.

3. Schuckit M. In: Isselbacher KJ, et al, eds. Harrison's principles of Internal Medicine. New York, McGraw-Hill 1981:1475–1478.

4. Barter F, Tanner AR. Autonomic neuropathy in an alcoholic population. Postgrad Med J 1987; 63:1033–1036.

5. Anonymous. Autonomic neuropathy in liver disease. Lancet 1989; 2(8665):721–722

6. Bloomer JR, Bonkovsky HL. The porphyrias. Dis Mon 1989; 35:1–54.

7. Chapelon C, Ziza JM, Piette JC, Levy Y, Raguin G, Wechsler B, Bitker MO, Bletry O, Laplane D, Bousser MG, et al. Neurosarcoidosis: signs, course and treatment in 35 confirmed cases. Medicine (Baltimore); 1990; 69:261–276.

8. Chen PH, Hsueh HF, Hong CZ. Herpes zoster-associated voiding dysfunction: a retrospective study and literature review. Arch Phys Med Rehabil 2002; 83:1624–1628

9. Greenstein A, Matzkin H, Kaver I, Braf Z. Acute urinary retention in herpes genitalis infection. Urodynamic evaluation. Urology 1988; 31:453–456.

10. Lichtenfeld P. Autonomic dysfunction in the Guillain–Barré syndrome. Am J Med 1971; 50:772–780.

11. Mardlrosoff C, Dumont L. Bowel and bladder dysfunction after spinal bupivacaine. Anesthesiology 2001; 95:1306.

12. Auroy Y, Benhamou D, Bargues L, Ecoffey C, Falissard B, Mercier F, Bouaziz H, Samii K. Major complications of regional anesthesia in France: The SOS Regional Anesthesia Hotline Service. Anesthesiology 2002; 97:1274–1280.

13. Seski JC, Diokno AC. Bladder dysfunction after radical abdominal hysterectomy. Am J Obstet Gynecol 1977; 128:643–651.

14. Sekido N, Kawai K, Akaza H. Lower urinary tract dysfunction as persistent complication of radical hysterectomy. Int J Urol 1997; 4:259–264.

15. Emmett JL. Treatment of vesical dysfunction after operations on rectum and sigmoid. Surg Clin North Am 1957; 37:1009–1017.

16. Zermann DH, Ishigooka M, Wunderlich H, Reichelt O, Schubert J. A study of pelvic floor function pre-and postradical prostatectomy using clinical neurourological investigations, urodynamics and electromyography. Eur Urol 2000; 37:72–78.

17. Holland NJ, Wiesel-Levison P, Schwedelson ES. Survey of neurogenic bladder in multiple sclerosis. J Neurosurg Nurs 1981; 13:337–343.

18. Goldstein I, Siroky MB, Sax DS, Krane RJ. Neurourologic abnormalities in multiple sclerosis. J Urol 1982; 128:541–545.

19. Fowler CJ, van Kerrebroeck PE, Nordenbo A, Van Poppel H. Treatment of lower urinary tract dysfunction in patients with multiple sclerosis. Committee of the European Study Group of SUDIMS (Sexual and Urological Disorders in Multiple Sclerosis) J Neurol Neurosurg Psychiatry 1992; 55:986–989.

20. Bemelmans BL, Hommes OR, Van Kerrebroeck PE, Lemmens WA, Doesburg WH, Debruyne FM. Evidence for early lower urinary tract dysfunction in clinically silent multiple sclerosis. J Urol 1991; 145:1219–1224.

21. Sugiyama T, Hashimoto K, Kiwamoto H, Ohnishi N, Esa A, Park YC, Kurita T. Urinary incontinence in senile dementia of the Alzheimer type (SDAT). Int J Urol 1994; 1:337–340.

22. McGrother C, Resnick M, Yalla SV, Kirschner-Hermanns R, Broseta E, Muller C, Welz-Barth A, Fischer GC, Mattelaer J, McGuire EJ. Epidemiology and etiology of urinary incontinence in the elderly. World J Urol 1998; 16 (Suppl 1):S3–S9.

23. Madersbacher H, Awad S, Fall M, Janknegt RA, Stohrer M, Weisner B. Urge incontinence in the elderly-supraspinal reflex incontinence. World J Urol 1998; 16 (Suppl 1):S35–S43.

24. Olsen CG, Clasen ME. Senile dementia of the Binswanger's type. Am Fam Physician 1998; 58:2068–2074.

25. Honig LS, Mayeux R. Natural history of Alzheimer's disease. Aging (Milano) 2001; 13:171–182.

26. Murnaghan GF. Neurogenic disorders of the bladder in Parkinsonism. Br J Urol 1961; 33:403–409.

27. Salinas JM, Berger Y, De La Rocha RE, Blaivas JG. Urological evaluation in the Shy Drager syndrome. J Urol 1986; 135:741–743.

28. Currie CT. Urinary incontinence after stroke. Br Med J 1986; 293:1322–1323.

29. Codine PH, Pellissier J, Manderscheidt JC, Costa P, Enjalbert M, Perrigot M. Les troubles urinaires au cours des hémiplegies vasculaires. In: Pellisier J, ed. Hémiplegie vasculaire et médicine de rééducation. Paris, Masson 1988:261–269.

30. Barer DH. Continence after stroke: useful predictor or goal of therapy? Age Ageing 1989; 18:183–191.

31. Andrew J, Nathan PW. Lesions of the anterior frontal lobes and disturbances of micturition and defecation. Brain 1964; 87:233 ff.

32. Burns AS, Rivas DA, Ditunno JF. The management of neurogenic bladder and sexual dysfunction after spinal cord injury. Spine. 2001; 26 (Suppl):S129–S136.

33. Lawrenson R, Wyndaele JJ, Vlachonikolis I, Farmer C, Glickman S. A UK general practice database study of prevalence and mortality of people with neural tube defects. Clin Rehabil 2000; 14:627–630.

34. Selzman AA, Elder JS, Mapstone TB. Urologic consequences of myelodysplasia and other congenital abnormalities of the spinal cord. Urol Clin North Am 1993; 20:485–504

35. van Gool JD, Dik P, de Jong TP. Bladder-sphincter dysfunction in myelomeningocele. Eur J Pediatr 2001; 160:414–420.

36. Rosomoff HL, Johnston JD, Gallo AE, Ludmer M, Givens FT, Carney FT, Kuehn CA. Cystometry in the evaluation of nerve root compression in the lumbar spine. Surg Gynecol Obstet 1963; 117:263–270.

37. Scott PJ. Bladder paralysis in cauda equina lesions from disc prolapse. J Bone Joint Surg 1965; 47:224–235.

38. Burgdörfer H, Heidler H, Madersbacher H, Melchior H, Palmtag H, Richter R, Richter-Reichhelm M, Rist M, Rübben H, Sauerwein D, Schalkhäuser K, Stöhrer M. Leitlinien zur urologischen Betreuung Querschnittgelähmter. Urologe A 1998; 37:222–228.

39. Stöhrer M, Goepel M, Kondo A, Kramer G, Madersbacher H, Millard R, Rossier A, Wyndaele JJ. The standardization of terminology in neurogenic lower urinary tract dysfunction with suggestions for diagnostic procedures, Neurourol Urodyn 1999; 18:139–158.

40. Madersbacher H, Wyndaele JJ, Igawa Y, Chancellor M, Chartier-Kastler E, Kovindha A. Conservative management in neuropatic urinary incontinence.

In: Incontinence, 2nd edn. Abrams P, Khoury S, Wein A, eds. Health Publication Ltd, Plymouth, 2002:697–754.

41. Castro-Diaz D, Barrett D, Grise P, Perkash I, Stöhrer M, Stone A, Vale P. Surgery for the neuropathic patient. In: Incontinence, 2nd edn. Abrams P, Khoury S, Wein A, eds. Health Publication Ltd, Plymouth, 2002:865–891.

42. Abrams P, Cardozo L, Fall M, Griffiths D, Rosier P, Ulmsten U, van Kerrebroeck P, Victor A, Wein A. The standardisation of terminology of lower urinary tract function: Report from the Standardisation Sub-committee of the International Continence Society. Neurourol Urodyn 2002; 21:167–178.

43. Klevmark B. Natural pressure–volume curves and conventional cystometry. Scand J Urol Nephrol (Suppl) 1999; 201:1–4.

44. Homma Y, Ando T, Yoshida M, Kageyama S, Takei M, Kimoto K, Ishizuka O, Gotoh M, Hashimoto T. Voiding and incontinence frequencies: variability of diary data and required diary length. Neurourol Urodyn 2002; 21:204–209.

45. McGuire EJ, Cespedes RD, O'Connell HE. Leak-point pressures. Urol Clin North Am 1996; 23:253–262.

46. Bors E, Comarr AE. Neurological urology. Karger, Basel 1971.

47. Hald T, Bradley WE. The neurogenic bladder. Williams and Wilkins, Baltimore 1982.

48. Stöhrer M, Kramer G, Löchner-Ernst D, Goepel M, Noll F, Rübben H. Diagnosis and treatment of bladder dysfunction in spinal cord injury patients. Eur Urol Update Series 1994; 3:170–175.

49. Bradley WE, Timm GW, Scott FB. Innervation of the detrusor muscle and urethra. Urol Clin North Am 1974; 1:3–27.

50. Lapides J. Neuromuscular vesical and urethral dysfunction. In: Campbell MF, Harrison JH, eds. Urology. WB Saunders, Philadelphia, 1970: 1343–1379.

51. Krane RJ, Siroky MB. Classification of neuro-urologic disorders. In: Krane RJ, Siroky MB, eds. Clinical neuro-urology. Little Brown, Boston, 1979:143–158.

52. Quesada EM, Scott FB, Cardus D. Functional classification of neurogenic bladder dysfunction. Arch Phys Med Rehabil 1968; 49:692–697.

53. Wein AJ. Pathophysiology and categorization of voiding dysfunction. In: Walsh PC, Retik AB, Vaughan Jr ED, Wein AJ, eds. Campbell's Urology 7th edn. WB Saunders, Philadelphia 1998:917–926.

54. Fall M, Ohlsson BL, Carlsson CA. The neurogenic overactive bladder. Classification based on urodynamics. Br J Urol 1989; 64:368–373.

55. Madersbacher H. The various types of neurogenic bladder dysfunction: an update of current therapeutic concepts. Paraplegia 1990; 28:217–229.

56. Cass AS, Luxenberg M, Johnson CF, Gleich P. Incidence of urinary tract complications with myelomeningocele. Urology 1985; 25:374–378.

57. Fernandes ET, Reinberg Y, Vernier R, Gonzalez R. Neurogenic bladder dysfunction in children: Review of pathophysiology and current management. J Pediat 1994; 124:1–7.

58. Stone AR. Neurourologic evaluation and urologic management of spinal dysraphism. Neurosurg Clin N Am 1995; 6:269–277.

59. Satar N, Bauer SB, Shefner J, Kelly MD, Darbey MM: The effects of delayed diagnosis and treatment in patients with an occult spinal dysraphism. J Urol 1995, 154:754–758.

60. Pontari MA, Keating M, Kelly M, Dyro F, Bauer SB: Retained sacral function in children with high level myelodysplasia. J Urol 1995; 154:775–777.

61. Kaefer M, Pabby A, Kelly M, Darbey M, Bauer SB. Improved bladder function after prophylactic treatment of the high risk neurogenic bladder in newborns with myelomeningocele. J Urol 1999; 162:1068–1071.

62. Wyndaele JJ: Development and evaluation of the management of the neuropathic bladder. Paraplegia 1995, 33:305–307.

63. Cardenas DD, Mayo ME, Turner LR: Lower urinary changes over time in suprasacral spinal cord injury. Paraplegia 1995; 33:326–329.

64. Amarenco G: Troubles vesico-sphincteriens d'origine nerveuse. Rev Prat 1995, 45:331–335.

65. Watanabe T, Vaccaro AR, Kumon H, Welch WC, Rivas DA, Chancellor MB. High incidence of occult neurogenic bladder dysfunction in neurologically intact patients with thoracolumbar spinal injuries. J Urol 1998; 159:965–968.

66. Ahlberg J, Edlund C, Wikkelsö C, Rosengren L, Fall M. Neurological signs are common in patients with urodynamically verified "idiopathic" bladder overactivity. Neurourol Urodyn 2002; 21:65–70.

3   Diagnosis

3.1   Introduction

Before any functional investigation is planned, an extensive general and specific diagnosis should be performed. Part of this diagnosis is specific for neurogenic pathology and its possible sequelae. The clinical assessment of patients with NLUTD includes and extends that for other LUTD. The latter should consist of a detailed history, bladder diary and a physical examination. In urinary incontinence, leakage should be demonstrated objectively.

These data are indispensable for reliable interpretation of the findings in diagnostic investigations performed subsequently in NLUTD.

3.2   History

3.2.1   General history

The general history should include relevant questions to neurological and congenital abnormalities, information on the previous occurrence and frequency of urinary infections and on relevant surgery. Information must be obtained on medication with known or possible effects on the lower urinary tract (1–3). The general history should also include the assessment of menstrual, sexual and bowel function, and obstetric history (3).

Hereditary or familial risk factors should be recorded. Symptoms of any metabolic disorder or neurological disease that may induce neurogenic lower urinary tract dysfunction must be checked particularly. Specific signs such as pain, infection, hematuria, fever, etc., may justify further particular diagnosis.

A list of items of particular importance is:

- Congenital anomalies with possible neurological impact
- Metabolic disorders with possible neurological impact
- Preceding therapy, including surgical interventions
- Present medication
- Lifestyle factors such as smoking, alcohol, or addictive drug use
- Infections of the urinary tract
- Quality of life

3.2.2   Specific history

Urinary history: This consists of symptoms related to both the storage and the evacuation functions of the lower urinary tract. The onset and the nature of the NLUTD (acute or insidious) should be determined. Specific symptoms and signs must be assessed in NLUTD and if appropriate be compared with the patients' condition before the neurogenic lower urinary tract dysfunction developed. The separate diagnostic fields items should be diagnosed as detailed as possible (3).

- LUTS
- Previous voiding pattern
- Urinary incontinence
- Bladder sensation
- Mode and type of voiding (catheterization!)

The urinary diary gives (semi-)objective information about the number of voidings, daytime and nighttime voiding frequency, volumes voided, and incontinence and urge episodes.

Bowel history: Patients with NLUTD may suffer from a related neurogenic condition of the lower gastrointestinal tract. The bowel history also must address symptoms related to the storage and the evacuation functions and specific symptoms and signs must be compared with the patients' condition before the neurogenic dysfunction developed. Again, the diagnostic items should be detailed (3).

- Ano-rectal symptoms
- Previous defecation pattern
- Faecal incontinence
- Rectal sensation
- Mode and type of defecation

Sexual history: The sexual function may also be impaired because of the neurogenic condition. The details of this history of course differ between men and women (3).

- Genital or sexual dysfunction symptoms
- Previous sexual function
- Sensation in genital area and for sexual functions
- Erection or arousal
- Orgasm
- Ejaculation

Neurologic history: This should concentrate on the following information.

1. Acquired or congenital neurologic condition
2. Neurological symptoms (somatic and sensory), with onset, evolution, and performed therapy
3. Spasticity or autonomic dysreflexia (lesion level above Th6)

3.2.3   Guidelines for history taking

1. An extensive general history is mandatory, concentrating on past and present symptoms and conditions for urinary, bowel, sexual, and neurologic functions, and on general conditions that might impair any of these.
2. Special attention should be paid to the possible existence of alarm signs, such as pain, infection, hematuria, fever, etc., that warrant further specific diagnosis.
3. Specific history should be taken for each of the four mentioned functions.

3.3   Physical examination

3.3.1   General physical examination

Attention should be paid to the patient's physical and possible mental handicaps with respect to planned diagnostic investigations.

Impaired mobility, particularly in the hips, or extreme spasticity may lead to problems in patient positioning in the urodynamics laboratory. Patients with very high neurological lesions may suffer from a significant drop in blood pressure when moved in a sitting or standing position. Subjective indications of bladder filling sensations may be impossible in retarded patients.

Prostate palpation or observation of pelvic organ descensus is made.

3.3.2   Neuro-urologic examination

General neurological examination: This investigates the motor and sensory functions of the body, the limbs and the hand function. A suprapubic globe is searched for and an appreciation of the skin condition in the genital and perineal regions is made.

Specific neuro-urologic examination: This investigation is necessary in patients with NLUTD. It includes several tests for sacral reflex activity and an evaluation of the sensation in the perineal area. Figure A4.2 shows the different dermatomes and Figure A4.3 the associated reflexes in this area.

Specified information should become available on:

- Sensation S_2–S_5 on both sides of the body
- Reflexes
- Anal sphincter tone
- Volitional contraction of anal sphincter and pelvic floor

A high correlation exists between the clinical neurologic findings and the NLUTD in some types of neuropathy, but less so in other types (4–9). The correspondence is low, for instance, in myelomeningocele patients (6) and in combined traumatic spinal cord lesions, but high in single-level traumatic spinal cord lesions (9).

3.3.3   Laboratory tests

Besides urinalysis and blood chemistry other tests are specifically indicated in patients with NLUTD. The results of these tests should be detailed (3).

- Imaging studies (Sonography, X-ray, MRI)
- Free flowmetry with assessment of residual urine. Because of natural variations, multiple estimations (at least 2–3) are necessary (3, 10, 11)
- Quantification of urine loss by pad testing if appropriate

3.3.4   Guidelines for physical examination

1. Individual patient handicaps should be acknowledged in planning further investigations.
2. The neurological status should be described as completely as possible. Sensations and reflexes in the urogenital area must all be tested.
3. The anal sphincter and pelvic floor functions must be tested extensively.
4. Urinalysis, blood chemistry, imaging, free flowmetry and residual, and incontinence quantification should be performed.

3.4   Urodynamics

3.4.1   Introduction

Urodynamic investigation is the only method to objectify the (dys-)function of the LUT. This investigation is of pivotal interest to describe the status of the LUT in patients with NLUTD.

In these patients, particularly when detrusor overactivity might be present, the invasive urodynamic investigation is even more provocative than in other patients. Any technical source of artefacts must be critically considered. The quality of the urodynamic recording and its interpretation must be ensured (12).

In patients at risk for autonomic dysreflexia, blood pressure assessment during the urodynamic study is advisable.

In many patients with NLUTD, assessment of maximum anaesthetic bladder capacity may be useful.

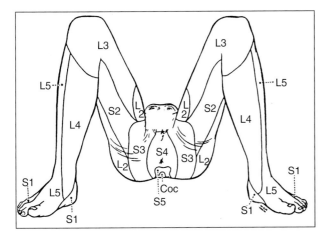

Figure A4.2
Dermatomes of spinal cord levels L2–S4.

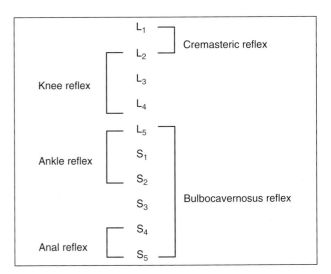

Figure A4.3
Urogenital and other reflexes in lower spinal cord.

The rectal ampulla should be empty of stool before the start of the investigation. Medication by drugs that influence the lower urinary tract function should be abandoned at least 48 h before the investigation (if feasible) or otherwise be taken into account for the interpretation of the data.

All urodynamic findings must be reported in detail and performed according to the ICS technical recommendations and standards (3, 12, 13).

3.4.2　Urodynamic tests

Bladder diary: This semi-objective qualification of the LUT is a highly advisable diagnostic tool. For reliable interpretation it should be recorded over at least 2–3 days (3, 14). Possible pathologic findings: High voiding frequency, very low or very high voided volumes, nocturnal voidings, urgency, incontinence.

Free uroflowmetry and assessment of residual urine: This gives a first impression of the voiding function. It is mandatory before any invasive urodynamics is planned. For reliable information it should be repeated at least 2–3 times (3, 10, 11). Possible pathologic findings: Low flow rate, low voided volume, intermittent flow, hesitancy, residual urine.

Care must be taken in judging the results in patients who are not able to void in a normal position. Both the flow pattern and the flow rate may be modified by this inappropriate position and by any constructions to divert the flow.

Filling cystometry: The only method to quantify the filling function has limited significance as a solitary procedure. It is much more powerful if combined with bladder pressure measurement during micturition and even more in video urodynamics. This investigation is necessary to document the status of the LUT function during the filling phase. The bladder should be empty at the start of filling. A physiological filling rate should be used with body-warm saline, as fast filling and room-temperature saline are provocative (3). Possible pathologic findings: Detrusor overactivity, low detrusor compliance, abnormal bladder and other sensations, incontinence, incompetent or relaxing urethra.

Detrusor leak point pressure: This specific investigation is important to estimate the risk for the upper urinary tract or for secondary bladder damage. When the DLPP is >40 cm H_2O the upper tract is endangered (3, 15). The DLPP is a screening test only, because it gives no impression of the duration of the high pressure during the filling phase, which can be expected to have even more impact on the upper urinary tract (16). A high DLPP thus warrants further testing by video urodynamics to document the reflux also.

Pressure flow study: This measurement reflects the co-ordination between detrusor and urethra or pelvic floor during the voiding phase. It is even more powerful in combination with filling cystometry and with video urodynamics. It is necessary to document the function of the lower urinary tract function during the voiding phase. Possible pathologic findings: Detrusor underactivity/acontractility, DSD, non-relaxing urethra, residual urine.

Most types of obstructions caused by NLUTD are due to DSD (17, 18), non-relaxing urethra, or non-relaxing bladder neck (3, 19, 20). Pressure-flow analysis mostly assesses the amount of mechanical obstruction caused by the urethra's inherent mechanical and anatomical properties and has limited value in patients with neurogenic lower urinary tract dysfunction.

Electromyography: Registration of the activity of the external urethral sphincter, the peri-urethral striated musculature, the anal sphincter, or the striated pelvic floor muscles. The correct interpretation may be difficult due to artefacts introduced by other equipment used. In the urodynamic setting useful as a gross indication of the patient's ability to control the pelvic floor. Possible pathologic findings: Inadequate recruitment on specific stimuli (bladder filling, hyperreflexive contractions, onset of voiding, coughing, Valsalva, etc.).

More detailed analysis (motor unit potentials, single fibre EMG) only possible as part of a neurophysiologic investigation.

Urethral pressure measurement: This investigation has only a very limited place in NLUTD. There exists no basic consensus on parameters indicating pathological findings (21).

Video urodynamics: This combination of filling cystometry and pressure flow study with imaging is the gold standard for urodynamic investigation in NLUTD (3, 22, 23). Possible pathological findings: All as described under cystometry and pressure flow study, plus morphological pathology of the LUT and the upper urinary tract.

Ambulatory urodynamics: Functional investigation of the urinary tract utilizing predominantly natural filling of the urinary tract and reproducing normal subject activity (24).

This type of study should be considered when office urodynamics do not reproduce the patient's symptoms and complaints. Possible pathologic findings: as under filling cystometry and pressure flow study provided the flow is measured also. It should be kept in mind that during this study the actual bladder volume is unknown.

Provocative tests during urodynamics: The LUT function can be provoked by coughing, triggered voiding, or anal stretch.

Fast filling cystometry with cooled saline (the "ice water test") is considered a discriminative test between UMNL and LMNL (25–30). Patients with UMNL will develop a detrusor contraction if the detrusor muscle is intact, patients with lower lesions will not. It gives false positive results in young children (27) and seems not fully discriminative in other patients (28, 29)

A positive bethanechol test (31) (detrusor contraction >25 cm H_2O) was presumed to proof detrusor denervation hypersensitivity and the muscular integrity of an acontractile detrusor, but it turned out to give equivocal results. Recently a variation of this method was reported with intravesical electromotive administration of the bethanechol (32). This test turned out to be both selective and predictive for successful oral bethanechol treatment.

3.4.3　Specific uro-neurophysiologic tests

These tests are advised as part of the neurological work-up of the patient. They comprise:

- Electromyography (in a neurophysiological setting) of pelvic floor muscles, urethral sphincter and/or anal sphincter
- Nerve conduction studies of pudendal nerve
- Reflex latency measurements of bulbocavernosus and anal reflex arcs
- Evoked responses from clitoris or glans penis
- Sensory testing on bladder and urethra

Other elective tests may be asked for specific conditions that became obvious during patient work-up and urodynamic investigations.

Possible pathologic findings are dependent on the type of the test.

3.4.4 Guidelines for urodynamics and uro-neurophysiology

1. Urodynamic investigation is necessary to document the (dys-)function of the LUT.
2. The recording of a bladder diary is highly advisable.
3. Free uroflowmetry and assessment of residual urine is mandatory before invasive urodynamics is planned.
4. Video urodynamics is the gold standard for invasive urodynamics in patients with NLUTD. Should this not be available, then a filling cystometry continuing into a pressure flow study should be performed.
5. A physiological filling rate and body-warm saline must be used.
6. DLPP is an important investigation in patients with endangered upper tracts.
7. Specific uro-neurophysiological tests are elective procedures.

3.5 Typical manifestations of NLUTD

Typical findings in NLUTD are listed below.
Filling phase

- Hyposensitivity or hypersensitivity
- Vegetative sensations
- Low compliance
- High capacity bladder
- Detrusor overactivity, spontaneous or provoked
- Sphincter acontractility

Voiding phase

- Detrusor acontractility
- DSD
- Non-relaxing urethra
- Non-relaxing bladder neck

These signs warrant further neurological evaluation, as LUTD may be the presenting symptom of NLUTD (33–37).

3.6 References

1. Bors E, Turner RD. History and physical examination in neurological urology. J Urol 1960; 83:759–767.

2. Thuroff JW, Chartier-Kastler E, Corcus J. Humke J, Jonas U, Palmtag H, Tanagho EA. Medical treatment and medical side effects in urinary incontinence in the elderly. World J Urol 1998; 16 (Suppl 1):S48–S61.

3. Stöhrer M, Goepel M, Kondo A, Kramer G, Madersbacher H, Millard R, Rossier A, Wyndaele JJ. The standardization of terminology in neurogenic lower urinary tract dysfunction with suggestions for diagnostic procedures. Neurourol Urodyn 1999; 18:139–158.

4. Wyndaele JJ, De Sy WA. Correlation between the findings of a clinical neurological examination and the urodynamic dysfunction in children with myelodysplasia. J Urol 1985; 133:638–640.

5. Wyndaele JJ. Correlation between clinical neurological data and urodynamic function in spinal cord injured patients. Spinal Cord 1997; 35:213–216.

6. Keshtgar AS, Rickwood AM. Urological consequences of incomplete cord lesions in patients with myelomeningocele. Br J Urol 1998; 82:258–260.

7. Wyndaele JJ. Is impaired perception of bladder filling during cystometry a sign of neuropathy? Br J Urol 1993; 71:270–273.

8. Kirchhof K, Fowler CJ. The value of the Kurtzke Functional Systems Scales in predicting incomplete bladder emptying. Spinal Cord 2000; 38:409–413.

9. Weld KJ, Dmochowski RR. Association of level of injury and bladder behavior in patients with post-traumatic spinal cord injury. Urology 2000; 55:490–494.

10. Reynard JM, Peters TJ, Lim C, Abrams P. The value of multiple free-flow studies in men with lower urinary tract symptoms. Br J Urol 1996; 77:813–818.

11. Sonke GS, Kiemeney LA, Verbeek AL, Kortmann BB, Debruyne FM, de la Rosette JJ. Low reproducibility of maximum urinary flow rate determined by portable flowmetry. Neurourol Urodyn 1999; 18:183–191.

12. Schäfer W, Abrams P, Liao L, Mattiasson A, Pesce F, Spångberg A, Sterling AM, Zinner NR, van Kerrebroeck P. Good Urodynamic Practices: Uroflowmetry, Filling Cystometry, and Pressure-Flow Studies. Neurourol Urodyn 2002; 21:261–274.

13. Abrams P, Cardozo L, Fall M, Griffiths D, Rosier P, Ulmsten U, van Kerrebroeck P, Victor A, Wein A. The standardisation of terminology of lower urinary tract function: Report from the Standardisation Sub-committee of the International Continence Society. Neurourol Urodyn 2002; 21:167–178.

14. Homma Y, Ando T, Yoshida M, Kageyama S, Takei M, Kimoto K, Ishizuka O, Gotoh M, Hashimoto T. Voiding and incontinence frequencies: variability of diary data and required diary length. Neurourol Urodyn 2002; 21:204–209.

15. McGuire EJ, Cespedes RD, O'Connell HE. Leak-point pressures. Urol Clin North Am 1996; 23:253–262.

16. Linsenmeyer TA, Bagaria SP, Gendron B. The impact of urodynamic parameters on the upper tracts of spinal cord injured men who void reflexly. J Spinal Cord Med 1998; 21:15–20.

17. Krongrad A, Sotolongo JR Jr. Bladder neck dysynergia in spinal cord injury. Am J Phys Med Rehabil 1996; 75:204–207.

18. Weld KJ, Graney MJ, Dmochowski RR. Clinical significance of detrusor sphincter dyssynergia type in patients with post-traumatic spinal cord injury. Urology 2000; 56:565–568.

19. Rossier AB, Fam BA. 5-microtransducer catheter in evaluation of neurogenic bladder function. Urology 1986; 27:371–378.

20. Al-Ali M, Haddad L. A 10 year review of the endoscopic treatment of 125 spinal cord injured patients with vesical outlet obstruction: does bladder neck dyssynergia exist? Paraplegia 1996; 34:34–38.

21. Lose G, Griffiths D, Hosker G, Kulseng-Hanssen S, Perucchini D, Schafer W, Thind P, Versi E. Standardisation of urethral pressure measurement: Report from the Standardisation Sub-Committee of the International Continence Society. Neurourol Urodyn 2002; 21:258–260.

22. Rivas DA, Chancellor MB: Neurogenic vesical dysfunction. Urol Clin North Am 1995, 22:579–591.

23. Madersbacher HG. Neurogenic bladder dysfunction. Curr Opin Urol 1999; 9:303–307.

24. van Waalwijk van Doorn E, Anders K, Khullar V, Kulseng-Hanssen S, Pesce F, Robertson A, Rosario D, Schafer W. Standardisation of ambulatory urodynamic monitoring: Report of the Standardisation Sub-Committee of the International Continence Society for Ambulatory Urodynamic Studies. Neurourol Urodyn 2000; 19:113–125.

25. Geirsson G, Fall M, Lindstrom S. The ice-water test – a simple and valuable supplement to routine cystometry. Br J Urol 1993; 71:681–685.

26. Geirsson G, Lindstrom S, Fall M. Pressure, volume and infusion speed criteria for the ice-water test. Br J Urol 1994; 73:498–503.

27. Geirsson G, Lindstrom S, Fall M, Gladh G, Hermansson G, Hjalmas K. Positive bladder cooling test in neurologically normal young children. J Urol 1994; 151:446–448.

28. Petersen T, Chandiramani V, Fowler CJ. The ice-water test in detrusor hyper-reflexia and bladder instability. Br J Urol 1997; 79:163–167.

29. Chancellor MB, Lavelle J, Ozawa H, Jung SY, Watanabe T, Kumon H. Ice-water test in the urodynamic evaluation of spinal cord injured patients. Tech Urol 1998; 4:87–91.

30. Ronzoni G, Menchinelli P, Manca A, De Giovanni L. The ice-water test in the diagnosis and treatment of the neurogenic bladder. Br J Urol 1997; 79:698–701.

31. Lapides J. Neurogenic bladder. Principles of treatment. Urol Clin North Am 1974; 1:81–97.

32. Riedl CR, Stephen RL, Daha LK, Knoll M, Plas E, Pfluger H. Electromotive administration of intravesical bethanechol and the clinical impact on acontractile detrusor management: introduction of a new test. J Urol 2000; 164:2108–2111.

33. Bemelmans BL, Hommes OR, Van Kerrebroeck PE, Lemmens WA, Doesburg WH, Debruyne FM. Evidence for early lower urinary tract dysfunction in clinically silent multiple sclerosis. J Urol 1991; 145:1219–1224.

34. Lewis MA, Shaw J, Sattar TM, Bannister CM. The spectrum of spinal cord dysraphism and bladder neuropathy in children. Eur J Pediatr Surg 1997; 7 (Suppl 1):35–37.

35. Wraige E, Borzyskowski M. Investigation of daytime wetting: when is spinal cord imaging indicated? Arch Dis Child 2002; 87:151–155.

36. Silveri M, Capitanucci ML, Capozza N, Mosiello G, Silvano A, Gennaro MD. Occult spinal dysraphism: neurogenic voiding dysfunction and long-term urologic follow-up. Pediatr Surg Int 1997; 12:148–150.

37. Ahlberg J, Edlund C, Wikkelsö C, Rosengren L, Fall M. Neurological signs are common in patients with urodynamically verified "idiopathic" bladder overactivity. Neurourol Urodyn 2002; 21:65–70.

4   Treatment

4.1   Introduction

The primary aims for treatment of NLUTD and their priorities are (1–5):

1.   Protection of the upper urinary tract
2.   Improvement of urinary continence
3.   Improvement of the patient's quality of life
4.   Restoration of (parts of) the normal LUT function

Further considerations are the patient's disability, the cost effectiveness, the technical intricacy, and the possible complications (5).

Preservation of the upper tract function is of paramount importance (1–9). Renal failure was the main factor for mortality in the spinal cord injured patient surviving the trauma (6–9). This has led to the golden rule in treatment of NLUTD: Assure that the detrusor pressure remains within safe limits during both the filling phase and the voiding phase (1–5). This approach has indeed significantly reduced the mortality from urological causes in this patient group (10).

The therapy of urinary incontinence is important for the social rehabilitation of the patient and thus contributes substantially to the quality of life, but is also pivotal in the prevention of urinary tract infection (UTI) (7–9). When no complete continence can be achieved, methods to attain a socially acceptable control of incontinence can be applied.

Complex procedures that might enable a satisfactory restoration or replacement of the LUT function often may limit the patient so much that the quality of life is unacceptably impaired (1).

In patients with high detrusor pressure during the filling phase (detrusor overactivity, low detrusor compliance) or during the voiding phase (DSD, other causes of bladder outlet obstruction) the therapy is aimed primarily at "the conversion of an active, aggressive high-pressure bladder into a passive low-pressure reservoir" despite the resulting residual urine (1).

4.2   Non-invasive conservative treatment

4.2.1   Assisted bladder emptying

Incomplete bladder emptying is a serious risk factor for UTI, for developing high intravesical pressure during the filling phase, and for incontinence. Therefore, methods to improve the voiding process are practised in patients with NLUTD.

Third party bladder expression (Credé): Regretfully, this method is still applied, foremost in infants and young children with myelomeningocele, and sometimes in tetraplegics. The suprapubic downwards compression of the lower abdomen leads to an increase in the intravesical pressure, but also causes a compression of the urethra and thus a functional obstruction (11, 12), that may reinforce an already existing high bladder outlet resistance (13) and lead to inefficient emptying (12). Because of the high pressures that may be created during this procedure it is potentially hazardous for the urinary tract (14, 15) and thus it is contra-indicated and its use should be discouraged unless urodynamics shows intravesical pressure to stay within the safe range (1, 14–16).

Voiding by abdominal straining (Valsalva): The considerations mentioned under Credé above also hold for the Valsalva manoeuvre (1, 12, 14, 16). As most patients are unable to scale the pressure they exert on the bladder during Valsalva, the risk of exceeding the safe range is present.

For both methods of emptying long-term complications are hardly avoidable (12, 14) and the already weak pelvic floor function may be further impaired, thus exacerbating the existing incontinence (16).

Triggered reflex voiding: Stimulation of the sacral or lumbar dermatomes in patients with UMNL can elicit reflex contraction of the detrusor (1, 16). Morbidity occurs more often during the first decades of treatment (17–21). This method may be used in patients in whom it is urodynamically safe (1,16).

4.2.2   Lower urinary tract rehabilitation

Behavioural modification: Prompted voiding, timed voiding (bladder training), and modification of the life pattern in patients with NLUTD are methods to improve the incontinence situation (2, 22–25).

Pelvic floor muscle exercises: This training also aims at improving the incontinence. It has proven effective in stress incontinence treatment and for patients with NLUTD it is mainly used in multiple sclerosis (26).

Pelvic floor electrostimulation: To improve the effect of pelvic floor muscle exercises, or to learn the patient how to contract the pelvic floor, or to improve the patient compliance with the exercises, this may be supported by electrostimulation (16, 27–29).

Biofeedback: This method can be used for supporting the voiding pattern modification (30–33).

4.2.3   Drug treatment

A medical therapy for NLUTD is not available. Most drugs used only resolve part of the problems, or are adjunct to other measures (34–40).

Detrusor overactivity: This can be treated effectively by anticholinergic substances (23, 24, 34–54). Their potentiality extends from a small reduction of detrusor overactivity to complete relaxation, depending on therapeutic regimen and individual tolerance. Increased drug tolerance during the basically life-long necessary therapy and the occurrence of adverse effects are topics of concern in patients with NLUTD in particular. Generally, these patients need a higher dose then other patients with overactive detrusor (41–46) and this may lead to an early discontinuation of the therapy because of adverse events (24, 41, 44–46).

Oxybutynin (36–41, 46–49), trospium chloride (39, 41, 45, 50, 51), and propiverine (39, 43, 45, 52), are established medical treatments. These drugs have diverse tolerance profiles and thus another anticholinergic may be prescribed if the patient experiences adverse effects on one. Tolteridine has been studied only in children with NLUTD (42). Various other drugs have been tested (16, 36, 38, 47, 48, 53).

Additional treatment with desmopressin might improve the efficacy of the treatment (54–58).

Detrusor underactivity: No success had been attained with drugs for improving detrusor contractility (16, 59–63), but Riedl et al (64) have successfully applied oral bethanechol treatment in NLUTD patients with detrusor acontractility who responded positive to the electromotive intravesical bethanechol testing.

Decreasing bladder outlet resistance: Alpha-blockers have been used partly successfully for decreasing the bladder outlet resistance (16, 65–70).

Increasing bladder outlet resistance: Several drugs show efficacy in the treatment of selected cases of milder stress incontinence, but there are hardly any publications in patients with NLUTD (16, 71, 72).

4.2.4   Electrical neuromodulation

A strong contraction of the urethral sphincter and/or pelvic floor, but also anal dilatation, manipulation of the genital region, and physical activity reflexly inhibit the micturition (16, 73). Whereas the first mechanism is affected by activation of efferent fibres, the latter ones are produced by activation of afferents (16). Electrical stimulation of the pudendal nerve afferents produces a strong inhibition of the micturition reflex and of the detrusor contraction (74). This stimulation then might support the restoration of the balance between excitatory and inhibitory inputs at the spinal or supraspinal level (16, 75, 76) and it might imply that patients with incomplete lesions will benefit (16, 76, 77), but patients with complete lesions will not (78).

Stimulation of the tibial nerve afferents has not been applied in patients with NLUTD.

4.2.5   External appliances

When incontinence cannot be resolved by any of the methods described above, the detrusor pressures are in the safe region, eventually after sphincterotomy or bladder neck incision, and furthergoing non-invasive therapy is not feasible, social continence may be achieved by collecting the urine during the incontinence (1, 16). Condom catheters with urine collection devices are a practical method for men. Otherwise incontinence pads may offer a reliable solution. In both cases the infection risk must be closely observed (16). Because of the risk of developing high intravesical pressure, the penile clamp is absolutely contra-indicated.

4.2.6   Guidelines for non-invasive conservative treatment

1. The first aim of any therapy is the protection of the upper urinary tract.
2. The mainstay of the treatment for overactive detrusor is anticholinergic drug therapy.
3. Rehabilitation and neuromodulation may be effective in selected cases.
4. A condom catheter or pads may reduce the incontinence to a socially acceptable situation.
5. Any method of assisted bladder emptying should be used with the greatest caution.

4.3   Minimal invasive treatment

4.3.1   Catheterization

Intermittent self- or third party catheterization (79, 80) is the gold standard for the management of NLUTD (1, 16). It is effective in patients with detrusor underactivity or acontractility (1) and in patients with detrusor overactivity if the overactivity can be successfully suppressed for instance by anticholinergic treatment (1, 16, 34–40).

The catheters used are made from a diversity of materials and the discussions on re-useable or disposable catheters, use of lubricants, aseptic or clean technique are still going on (1, 16, 81). Sterile IC, as originally proposed by Guttmann and Frankel (79) significantly reduces the risk of UTI and/or bacteriuria (1, 16, 82, 83), related to clean IC introduced by Lapides et al (80), but the cost issue may be a limiting factor (16, 83). Aseptic IC is believed to be in a mid position (1, 84, 85). Insufficient patient education and the inherent greater risk of UTI in patients with NLUTD are contributing factors (16, 85–91). The average frequency of catheterizations per day is 4–6 times. Less frequent catheterization results in higher catheterization volumes and a higher risk of UTI (1, 85–90). More frequent catheterization increases the risk of cross infections and other complications (1, 85–90).

Other complications may include lower fertility in men and compromising the urethra (16, 81), although the direct relation with the IC is discussed controversely. It appears however that the prevalence of these complications increases with the period that the IC has been practised and with the (temporary) use of indwelling catheterization (89).

The prevalence of complications can be limited by adequate patient education, use of non-traumatizing techniques, and adequate precautions to prevent cross-infections (16, 91).

Indwelling transurethral catheterization and, although to a lesser extent, suprapubic cystostomy are significant and early risk factors for UTI and other complications (16, 21, 92–102). Silicone catheters are preferred because they are less susceptible for encrustation and because of the high incidence of latex allergy in the NLUTD population.

4.3.2   Guidelines for catheterization

1. Intermittent catheterization is the standard treatment for patients who are unable to empty the bladder.
2. Patients should be well instructed on the technique and risks of IC.
3. Aseptic IC is the method of choice.
4. The catheter size is 12–14 Fr.
5. The frequency of IC is 4–6 times per day.
6. The bladder volume must remain below 400 ml and the post-IC residual low.
7. Indwelling transurethral and suprapubic catheterization should be used only exceptionally, under close control and the catheter should be changed frequently. Silicone catheters are preferred and should be changed every 2–4 weeks, (coated) latex catheters need to be changed every 1–2 weeks.

4.3.3   Intravesical drug treatment

For the reduction of the detrusor overactivity, anticholinergics can be applied also intravesically (103–112). This might reduce the adverse effects because it metabolizes differently (110) and a greater amount is sequestered in the bladder, even more so with electromotive administration (111, 112).

The vanilloids capsaicin and resiniferatoxin desensitize the C-fibers and thereby reduce the detrusor overactivity for a period of a few months until the sensation of these fibers has restored (15, 113–121). The dosage is 1–2 mMol capsaicin in 100 ml 30% alcohol or 10–100 nMol resiniferatoxin in 100 ml 10% alcohol for 30 minutes. Resiniferatoxin has an about 1000-fold potency compared to capsaicin, with less pain during the instillation, and was effective in patients refractory to capsaicin (121).

Botulinum toxin causes a long-lasting but reversible chemical denervation that lasts for about 9 months (122–126). The toxin injections are mapped over the detrusor in a dosage that depends on the preparation used. Generalized muscular weakness may be a seldom adverse effect (126).

4.3.4   Intravesical electrostimulation

Intravesical electrostimulation (127) enhances the sensation for bladder filling and urge to void and may restore the volitional control of the detrusor (16, 128, 129). Daily stimulation sessions of 90 min with 10 mA pulses of 2 ms duration at a frequency of 20 Hz (129, 130) are used for at least one week (130). It appears that patients with peripheral lesions are the best candidates, that the detrusor muscle must be intact, and that at least some afferent connection between the detrusor and the brain must still be present (16, 129, 130). Also, the positioning of the stimulating electrodes and the bladder filling apparently are important parameters (131). With these precautions, the results in the literature are still not unequivocal: both positive (128, 130, 132–136) and negative (137, 138) results are reported.

4.3.5   Bladder neck and urethral procedures

Reduction of the bladder outlet resistance is often necessary to protect the upper urinary tract. This can be achieved not only by surgical interventions (bladder neck or sphincter incision or urethral stent) but also by chemical denervation of the sphincter. Stress incontinence may result and can be managed by external devices (4.2.5).

Botulinum toxin sphincter injection: Detrusor sphincter dyssynergia can be treated effectively by injection with botulinum toxin in a dosage that depends on the preparation used. The dyssynergia is abolished for a few months, necessitating repeat injections. The efficacy of this treatment is high and few adverse effects have been recorded (139–145).

Balloon dilatation: Although favourable immediate results were reported (146), no further reports were found since 1994.

Sphincterotomy: By staged incision, the bladder outlet resistance can be reduced without completely losing the closure function of the urethra (1, 14, 147). The laser technique appears to be advantageous (1, 148, 149). Sphincterotomy also needs to be repeated at regular intervals in a substantial proportion of patients (150), but is efficient and without severe adverse effects (1, 14, 146–151). As secondary narrowing of the bladder neck may occur, combined bladder neck incision might be considered (1, 152, 153).

Bladder neck incision: This is indicated only for secondary changes at the bladder neck (fibrosis) (1, 14, 147, 153). When the detrusor is hypertrophied and causes thickening of the bladder neck, this procedure makes no sense (1).

Stents: The implantation of urethral stents causes the continence to be dependent on the adequate closure of the bladder neck only (1, 5). Although the results are comparable with sphincterotomy and the stenting procedure has a shorter surgery time and reduced hospital stay (154), the costs (1) and possible complications or re-interventions (154–160) are limiting factors in its use.

Increasing the bladder outlet resistance: This can improve the continence condition. Despite early positive results with urethral bulking agents, a relative early loss of continence is reported in patients with NLUTD (5, 21, 161–166).

Urethral inserts: Urethral plugs or valves for management of (female) stress incontinence have not been applied in patients with NLUTD. The experience with active pumping urethral prosthesis for treatment of the underactive or acontractile detrusor was disappointing (167).

4.3.6   Guidelines for minimal invasive treatment

1.   Guidelines for catheterization are listed separately under 4.3.2.
2.   Botulinum toxin injections in the detrusor are the most promising intravesical drug application for reduction of detrusor overactivity.
3.   Intravesical electrostimulation may be of value in specific patients.
4.   (Laser) sphincterotomy is the standard treatment for DSD or other increased bladder outlet resistance at the sphincteric area. Botulinum sphincter injections will be the first choice in patients ineligible for interventional surgery. Bladder neck incision is effective in a fibrotic bladder neck. Urethral stents still have too many complications.
5.   Urethral bulking agents have disappointing long-term effect.

4.4   Surgical treatment

4.4.1   Urethral and bladder neck procedures

Increasing the bladder outlet resistance has the inherent risk of causing high intravesical pressure during the filling and even more during the voiding phase. These procedures to treat the sphincteric incontinence are suitable only when the detrusor activity is or can be controlled, when no significant reflux is present. Moreover they require a good condition of the urethra and bladder neck and will mostly lead to perform intermittent catheterization after the procedure (5, 168).

Urethral sling: Various materials have been used for this procedure with enduring positive results (5, 168–182). The procedure is established in women; for men the artificial sphincter is obviously the first choice (5).

Artificial urinary sphincter: This device stood the test of time in patients with NLUTD (5). It was introduced by Light and Scott (183) for this patient group and the need for revisions (184, 185) have decreased significantly with the new generations of devices (175, 186–192).

Functional sphincter augmentation: By transposing the gracilis muscle to the bladder neck (193) or to the proximal urethra (194, 195) the possibility exists to create a functional autologous sphincter by electrical stimulation (193, 195). This would open the possibility to restore the control over the urethral closure.

Bladder neck and urethra reconstruction: The classical Young–Dees–Leadbetter (196) procedure for reconstruction of the bladder neck in children with bladder exstrophy and the Kropp urethral lengthening (197) improved by Salle (198) are established methods to restore continence provided that intermittent catheterization is practised and/or bladder augmentation is performed (175, 184, 197–211).

4.4.2   Detrusor myectomy (auto-augmentation)

The idea to enlarge a shrunken bladder by removal of lateral detrusor tissue to free the entrapped ureter in a non-functional fibrotic detrusor was put forward by Couvelaire (212). Since its clinical introduction by Cartwright and Snow (213) in children and by Stöhrer (214, 215) in adults, this procedure to reduce detrusor overactivity or to improve low detrusor compliance has gained popularity because of its acceptable long-term results, its low surgical burden, its low rate of long term adverse effects, its positive effect on the patient's quality of life, and because it does not preclude further interventions (1, 5, 45, 213–244).

The procedure is performed extraperitoneally under general anesthesia and consists of the dissection of about 20% of the detrusor tissue around the umbilicus, leaving the mucosa intact (1, 213–215). A diverticulum will develop, but this may take 1–2 years in adults (1, 213–215). The laparoscopic procedure (219, 220, 222, 228, 233), the covering of the mucosa at the detrusor defect (transperitoneal!) (217, 229, 232, 234, 238), supporting the bladder (213, 216, 238), or simple incision of the detrusor muscle (detrusor myotomy) (221, 240–244) are proposed variations of the procedure but offer no essential advantages.

4.4.3   Denervation, deafferentation, neurostimulation, neuromodulation

Various procedures that were estimated to destroy the peripheral detrusor innervation have been abandoned because of poor long term results and severe complications (5). These procedures include bladder distension, cystolysis, transvaginal denervation (Ingelman–Sundberg procedure) and subtrigonal phenol injections.

Sacral rhizotomy, also known as sacral deafferentation (SDAF), has achieved some success in reducing detrusor overactivity (21, 245–254), but it is used nowadays mostly as an adjuvant to sacral anterior root stimulation (255–269). Alternatives for the rhizotomy are sought in this treatment combination (270–273).

Sacral anterior root stimulation (SARS) is aimed at producing a detrusor contraction. The technique was developed by Brindley (274) and is applicable only in complete lesions above the implant location because of its stimulation amplitude over the pain threshold. The urethral sphincter efferents are also stimulated, but as the striated muscle relaxes faster than the smooth muscle of the detrusor, a so-called "post-stimulus voiding" will occur. This approach has been successful in highly selected patients (255–269). By changing the stimulation parameters this method can also induce defecation or erection.

The sacral nerve stimulation or sacral neuromodulation is based on the research by Schmidt and Tanagho (275). This technique stimulates the afferents and thereby probably restores the correct balance between excitatory and inhibitory impulses from and to the pelvic organs at a sacral and supra-sacral level, thus reducing the detrusor overactivity (75, 276). It is used either as a temporary procedure using foramen electrodes with an external stimulator, with the expectation of perseverance of the changes after treatment, or as a chronic procedure with an implanted stimulator. In the latter case a test procedure, the percutaneous nerve evaluation (PNE), with an external stimulator is performed before the implant to judge the patient's response. This procedure also has considerable success in selected patients (230, 277–283).

On the basis of the successful application of these systems, future developments towards a device that may be more integrated in the body are under research (284, 285).

4.4.4   Bladder covering by striated muscle

When the bladder is covered by a (part of) striated muscle that can be stimulated electrically, or ideally could be contracted volitionally, an acontractile bladder could be restored to perform a voiding function. The rectus abdominis (286) and the latissimus dorsi (287) have been used successfully in patients with NLUTD.

4.4.5   Bladder augmentation or substitution

Replacing or expanding the bladder by intestine or other passive expandable coverage will reduce the detrusor compliance and at least reduce the pressure effect of the detrusor overactivity. The inherent complications associated with these procedures include recurrent infection, stone building, perforation or diverticula, possible malignant changes, and for intestine metabolic abnormality, mucus production and impaired bowel function (5, 288–290). As the NLUTD patient population's age when the surgery is performed is generally much lower than the patients with bladder malignancy who are elected for this surgery, the possible very long term complications must be appraised in particular. Thus the procedures should be used with caution in NLUTD patients, but may become necessary if all less invasive methods of treatment have failed.

Bladder augmentation, by procedures such as the clam cystoplasty, is a valid option to decrease detrusor pressure and increase bladder capacity whenever more conservative approaches have failed. A number of different techniques have been published. The results of the various procedures are very good and comparable (45, 226, 230–232, 235–237, 289–292). Bladder substitution to create a low pressure reservoir may be indicated in patients with severely thick and fibrotic bladder wall. Scaffolds, probably of tissue-engineered material for bladder augmentation or substitution or alternative techniques are promising future options (236, 293–300).

4.4.6   Urinary diversion

When no other therapy has been successful urinary diversion must be considered for the protection of the upper tract and for the patient's quality of life (5, 301).

Continent diversion: This should be the first choice for diversion. In patients for whom indwelling catheterization or suprapubic catheterization is the only feasible treatment option the change to a continent stoma may be a better prospect (5). Some patients with limited dexterity prefer a stoma above using the urethra for catheterization (5). The continent stoma is created following various techniques. All of them however do show frequent complications, including leakage or stenosis (5, 302). The short

term continence rates are over 80% and good protection of the upper urinary tract is achieved (5, 18, 301–317). For cosmetic reasons, the umbilicus is often used for the stoma site, but this may have a higher risk of stenosis (305, 308, 314).

Incontinent diversion: If catheterization is impossible, incontinent diversion with a urine collecting device is indicated. Fortunately, nowadays, this indication is seldom because many appropriate alternatives can be offered (5). Ultimately it could be considered in patients who are wheelchair bound or bed-ridden with intractable and untreatable incontinence, in devastated lower urinary tracts, when the upper urinary tract is severely compromised, and in patients who refuse other therapy (5). An ileal segment is used for the deviation in most cases (5, 318–323). The rather poor long term results and the expected complications warrant a permanent follow-up (5).

Undiversion: Long-standing diversions may be successfully undiverted or an incontinent diversion changed to a continent one with the emergence of new and better techniques for control of the detrusor pressure and the incontinence (5). Also, in young patients the body image may play a role (311). The patient must be carefully counselled and must comply meticulously with the instructions (5). Successful undiversion then can be performed (324–326).

4.5   Guidelines for surgical treatment

1.   Detrusor

1.1.   Overactive
1.1.1.   Detrusor myectomy is an acceptable option for the treatment of overactive bladder when more conservative approaches have failed. It is limited invasive and has minimal morbidity.
1.1.2.   Sacral rhizotomy with SARS in complete lesions and sacral neuromodulation in incomplete lesions are effective treatments in selected patients.
1.1.3.   Bladder augmentation is an acceptable option to decrease detrusor pressure whenever less invasive procedures have failed. For the treatment of a severely thick or fibrotic bladder wall a bladder substitution might be considered.

1.2.   Underactive
1.2.1.   SARS with rhizotomy and sacral neuromodulation are effective in selected patients.
1.2.2.   Restoration of a functional bladder by covering with striated muscle is still experimental.

2.   Urethra

2.1.   Overactive (DSD) – refer to guidelines for minimal invasive treatment (4.3.6)
2.2.   Underactive
2.2.1.   The placement of a urethral sling is an established procedure.
2.2.2.   The artificial urinary sphincter is very effective.
2.2.3.   Transposition of the gracilis muscle is still experimental.

4.6 References

1. Stöhrer M, Kramer G, Löchner-Ernst D, Goepel M, Noll F, Rübben H. Diagnosis and treatment of bladder dysfunction in spinal cord injury patients. Eur Urol Update Series 1994; 3:170–175.

2. Chua HC, Tow A, Tan ES. The neurogenic bladder in spinal cord injury-pattern and management. Ann Acad Med Singapore 1996; 25:553–557.

3. Burns AS, Rivas DA, Ditunno JF. The management of neurogenic bladder and sexual dysfunction after spinal cord injury. Spine 2001; 26(Suppl):S129–136.

4. Rickwood AM. Assessment and conservative management of the neuropathic bladder. Semin Pediatr Surg. 2002 May; 11(2):108–119.

5. Castro-Diaz D, Barrett D, Grise P, Perkash I, Stöhrer M, Stone A, Vale P. Surgery for the neuropathic patient. In: Incontinence, 2nd Edition, Abrams P, Khoury S, Wein A, eds. Health Publication Ltd, Plymouth, 2002:865–891.

6. Donnelly J, Hackler RH, Bunts RC. Present urologic status of the World War II paraplegic: 25-year follow-up. Comparison with status of the 20-year Korean War paraplegic and 5-year Vietnam paraplegic. J Urol 1972; 108:558–562.

7. Hackler RH. A 25-year prospective mortality study in the spinal cord injured patient: comparison with the long-term living paraplegic. J Urol 1977; 117:486–488.

8. Perkash I, Giroux J. Prevention, treatment, and management of urinary tract infections in neuropathic bladders. J Am Paraplegia Soc 1985; 8:15–17.

9. Sandock DS, Gothe BG, Bodner RD. Trimethoprim-sulfamethoxazole prophylaxis against urinary tract infection in the chronic spinal cord injured patient. Paraplegia 1995; 33:156–160.

10. Frankel HL, Coll JR, Charlifue SW, Whiteneck GG, Gardner BP, Jamous MA, Krishnan KR, Nuseibeh I, Savic G, Sett P. Long-term survival in spinal cord injury: a fifty year investigation. Spinal Cord 1998; 36:266–274.

11. Madersbacher H. The neuropathic urethra: urethrogram and pathophysiologic aspects. Eur Urol 1977; 3:321–332.

12. Barbalias GA, Klauber GT, Blaivas JG. Critical evaluation of the Crede maneuver: a urodynamic study of 207 patients. J Urol 1983; 130:720–723.

13. Clarke SJ, Thomas DG. Characteristics of the urethral pressure profile in flaccid male paraplegics. Br J Urol 1981; 53:157–161.

14. Stöhrer M. Alterations in the urinary tract after spinal cord injury – diagnosis, prevention and therapy of late sequelae. World J Urol 1990; 7:205–211.

15. Reinberg Y, Fleming T, Gonzalez R. Renal rupture after the Crede maneuver. J Pediatr 1994; 124:279–281.

16. Madersbacher H, Wyndaele JJ, Igawa Y, Chancellor M, Chartier-Kastler E, Kovindha A. Conservative management in neuropatic urinary incontinence. In: Incontinence, 2nd edn. Abrams P, Khoury S, Wein A, eds. Health Publication Ltd, Plymouth, 2002:697–754.

17. Van Kerrebroeck PE, Koldewijn EL, Scherpenhuizen S, Debruyne FM. The morbidity due to lower urinary tract function in spinal cord injury patients. Paraplegia 1993; 31:320–329.

18. Sekar P, Wallace DD, Waites KB, DeVivo MJ, Lloyd LK, Stover SL, Dubovsky EV. Comparison of longterm renal function after spinal cord injury using different urinary management methods. Arch Phys Med Rehabil 1997; 78:992–997.

19. Linsenmeyer TA, Bagaria SP, Gendron B. The impact of urodynamic parameters on the upper tracts of spinal cord injured men who void reflexly. J Spinal Cord Med 1998; 21:15–20.

20. McKinley WO, Jackson AB, Cardenas DD, DeVivo MJ. Long-term medical complications after traumatic spinal cord injury: a regional model systems analysis. Arch Phys Med Rehabil 1999; 80:1402–1410.

21. Weld KJ, Dmochowski RR. Effect of bladder management on urological complications in spinal cord injured patients. J Urol 2000; 163:768–772.

22. Menon EB, Tan ES. Bladder training in patients with spinal cord injury. Urology 1992; 40:425–429.

23. Nijman RJ. Classification and treatment of functional incontinence in children. BJU Int 2000; 85(Suppl 3):37–42.

24. Aslan AR, Kogan BA. Conservative management in neurogenic bladder dysfunction. Curr Opin Urol 2002; 12:473–477.

25. Christ KF, Kornhuber HH. Treatment of neurogenic bladder dysfunction in multiple sclerosis by ultrasound-controlled bladder training. Arch Psychiatr Nervenkr 1980; 228:191–195.

26. De Ridder D, Vermeulen C, Ketelaer P, Van Poppel H, Baert L. Pelvic floor rehabilitation in multiple sclerosis. Acta Neurol Belg 1999; 99:61–64.

27. Ishigooka M, Hashimoto T, Hayami S, Suzuki Y, Nakada T, Handa Y. Electrical pelvic floor stimulation: a possible alternative treatment for reflex urinary incontinence in patients with spinal cord injury. Spinal Cord 1996; 34:411–415.

28. Vahtera T, Haaranen M, Viramo-Koskela AL, Ruutiainen J. Pelvic floor rehabilitation is effective in patients with multiple sclerosis. Clin Rehabil 1997; 11:211–219.

29. Balcom AH, Wiatrak M, Biefeld T, Rauen K, Langenstroer P. Initial experience with home therapeutic electrical stimulation for continence in the myelomeningocele population. J Urol 1997; 158:1272–1276.

30. Nørgaard JP, Djurhuus JC. Treatment of detrusor-sphincter dyssynergia by bio-feedback. Urol Int 1982; 37:236–239.

31. Klarskov P, Heely E, Nyholdt I, Rottensten K, Nordenbo A. Biofeedback treatment of bladder dysfunction in multiple sclerosis. A randomized trial. Scand J Urol Nephrol (Suppl) 1994; 157:61–65.

32. Chin-Peuckert L, Salle JL. A modified biofeedback program for children with detrusor-sphincter dyssynergia: 5-year experience. J Urol 2001; 166:1470–1475.

33. Porena M, Costantini E, Rociola W, Mearini E. Biofeedback successfully cures detrusor-sphincter dyssynergia in pediatric patients. J Urol 2000; 163:1927–1931.

34. Baskin LS, Kogan BA, Benard F. Treatment of infants with neurogenic bladder dysfunction using anticholinergic drugs and intermittent catheterisation. Br J Urol 1990; 66:532–534.

35. Tanaka H, Kakizaki H, Kobayashi S, Shibata T, Ameda K, Koyanagi T. The relevance of urethral resistance in children with myelodysplasia: its impact on upper urinary tract deterioration and the outcome of conservative management. J Urol 1999; 161:929–932.

36. Stone AR. Neurourologic evaluation and urologic management of spinal dysraphism. Neurosurg Clin N Am 1995; 6:269–277.

37. Edelstein RA, Bauer SB, Kelly MD, Darbey MM, Peters CA, Atala A, Mandell J, Colodny AH, Retik AB. The long-term urological response of neonates with myelodysplasia treated proactively with intermittent catheterization and anticholinergic therapy. J Urol 1995; 154:1500–1504.

38. Hernandez RD, Hurwitz RS, Foote JE, Zimmern PE, Leach GE. Nonsurgical management of threatened upper urinary tracts and incontinence in children with myelomeningocele. J Urol 1994; 152:1582–1585.

39. DasGupta R, Fowler CJ. Bladder, bowel and sexual dysfunction in multiple sclerosis: management strategies. Drugs 2003; 63:153–166.

40. Buyse G, Verpoorten C, Vereecken R, Casaer P. Treatment of neurogenic bladder dysfunction in infants and children with neurospinal dysraphism with clean intermittent (self)catheterisation and optimized intravesical oxybutynin hydrochloride therapy. Eur J Pediatr Surg 1995; 5(Suppl 1):31–34.

41. Madersbacher H, Stöhrer M, Richter R, Burgdörfer H, Hachen HJ, Mürtz G. Trospium chloride versus oxybutynin: a randomized, double-blind, multicentre trial in the treatment of detrusor hyperreflexia. Br J Urol 1995; 75:452–456.

42. Goessl C, Sauter T, Michael T, Berge B, Staehler M, Miller K. Efficacy and tolerability of tolterodine in children with detrusor hyperreflexia. Urology 2000; 55:414–418.

43. Madersbacher H, Mürtz G. Efficacy, tolerability and safety profile of propiverine in the treatment of the overactive bladder (non-neurogenic and neurogenic). World J Urol 2001; 19:324–335.

44. Schwantes U, Topfmeier P. Importance of pharmacological and physicochemical properties for tolerance of antimuscarinic drugs in the treatment of detrusor instability and detrusor hyperreflexia – chances for improvement of therapy. Int J Clin Pharmacol Ther 1999; 37:209–218.

45. Madersbacher HG. Neurogenic bladder dysfunction. Curr Opin Urol 1999; 9:303–307.

46. Gajewski JB, Awad SA. Oxybutynin versus propantheline in patients with multiple sclerosis and detrusor hyperreflexia. J Urol 1986; 135:966–968.

47. Zeegers AG, Kiesswetter H, Kramer AE, Jonas U. Conservative therapy of frequency, urgency and urge incontinence: A double-blind clinical trial of flavoxate hydrochloride, oxybutynin chloride, emepronium bromide and placebo. World J Urol 1987; 5:57–61.

48. Thuroff JW, Bunke B, Ebner A, Faber P, de Geeter P, Hannappel J, Heidler H, Madersbacher H, Melchior H, Schafer W, et al. Randomized, double-blind, multicenter trial on treatment of frequency, urgency and incontinence related to detrusor hyperactivity: oxybutynin versus propantheline versus placebo. J Urol 1991; 145:813–816.

49. Kasabian NG, Vlachiotis JD, Lais A, Klumpp B, Kelly MD, Siroky MB, Bauer SB. The use of intravesical oxybutynin chloride in patients with detrusor hypertonicity and detrusor hyperreflexia. J Urol 1994; 151:944–945.

50. Stöhrer M, Bauer P, Giannetti BM, Richter R, Burgdörfer H, Mürtz G. Effect of trospium chloride on urodynamic parameters in patients with detrusor hyperreflexia due to spinal cord injuries. A multicentre placebo-controlled double-blind trial. Urol Int 1991; 47:138–143.

51. Fröhlich G, Bulitta M, Strosser W. Trospium chloride in patients with detrusor overactivity: meta-analysis of placebo-controlled, randomized, double-blind, multi-center clinical trials on the efficacy and safety of 20 mg trospium chloride twice daily. Int J Clin Pharmacol Ther 2002; 40:295–303.

52. Stöhrer M, Madersbacher H, Richter R, Wehnert J, Dreikorn K. Efficacy and safety of propiverine in SCl-patients suffering from detrusor hyperreflexia – a double-blind, placebo-controlled clinical trial. Spinal Cord 1999; 37:196–200.

53. Jonas U, Petri E, Kissel J. Effect of flavoxate on hyperactive detrusor muscle. Eur Urol 1979; 5:106–109.

54. Kinn AC, Larsson PO. Desmopressin: a new principle for symptomatic treatment of urgency and incontinence in patients with multiple sclerosis. Scand J Urol Nephrol 1990; 24:109–112.

55. Chancellor MB, Rivas DA, Staas WE Jr. DDAVP in the urological management of the difficult neurogenic bladder in spinal cord injury: Preliminary report. J Am Paraplegia Soc 1994; 17:165–167.

56. Eckford SD, Swami KS, Jackson SR, Abrams PH. Desmopressin in the treatment of nocturia and enuresis in patients with multiple sclerosis. Br J Urol 1994; 74:733–735.

57. Fredrikson S. Nasal spray desmopressin treatment of bladder dysfunction in patients with multiple sclerosis. Acta Neurol Scand 1996; 94:31–34.

58. Valiquette G, Herbert J, Maede-D'Alisera P. Desmopressin in the management of nocturia in patients with multiple sclerosis. A double-blind, crossover trial. Arch Neurol 1996; 53:1270–1274.

59. Light JK, Scott FB. Bethanechol chloride and the traumatic cord bladder. J Urol 1982; 128:85–87.

60. Wheeler JS Jr, Robinson CJ, Culkin DJ, Nemchausky BA. Naloxone efficacy in bladder rehabilitation of spinal cord injury patients. J Urol 1987; 137:1202–1205.

61. Komersova K, Rogerson JW, Conway EL, Lim TC, Brown DJ, Krum H, Jackman GP, Murdoch R, Louis WJ. The effect of levcromakalim (BRL 38227) on bladder function in patients with high spinal cord lesions. Br J Clin Pharmacol 1995; 39:207–209.

62. Wyndaele JJ, van Kerrebroeck P: The effects of 4 weeks treatment with cisapride on cystometric parameters in spinal cord injury patients. A double-blind, placebo controlled study. Paraplegia 1995; 33:625–627.

63. Costa P, Bressolle F, Sarrazin B, Mosser J, Sabatier R. Dose-related effect of moxisylyte on maximal urethral closing pressure in patients with spinal cord injuries. Clin Pharmacol Ther 1993; 53:443–449.

64. Riedl CR, Stephen RL, Daha LK, Knoll M, Plas E, Pfluger H. Electromotive administration of intravesical bethanechol and the clinical impact on acontractile detrusor management: introduction of a new test. J Urol 2000; 164:2108–2111.

65. Swierzewski 3rd SJ, Gormley EA, Belville WD, Sweetser PM, Wan J, McGuire EJ. The effect of terazosin on bladder function in the spinal cord injured patient. J Urol 1994; 151:951–954.

66. O'Riordan JI, Doherty C, Javed M, Brophy D, Hutchinson M, Quinlan D. Do alpha-blockers have a role in lower urinary tract dysfunction in multiple sclerosis? J Urol 1995; 153:1114–1116.

67. Perkash I. Efficacy and safety of terazosin to improve voiding in spinal cord injury patients. J Spinal Cord Med 1995; 18: 236–239.

68. Yasuda K, Yamanishi T, Kawabe K, Ohshima H, Morita T. The effect of urapidil on neurogenic bladder: a placebo controlled double-blind study. J Urol 1996; 156:1125–1130.

69. Sullivan J, Abrams P. Alpha-adrenoceptor antagonists in neurogenic lower urinary tract dysfunction. Urology 1999; 53(3 Suppl 3a):21–27.

70. Schulte-Baukloh H, Michael T, Miller K, Knispel HH. Alfuzosin in the treatment of high leak-point pressure in children with neurogenic bladder. BJU Int 2002; 90:716–720.

71. Al-Ali M, Salman G, Rasheed A, Al-Ani G, Al-Rubaiy S, Alwan A, Al-Shaikli A. Phenoxybenzamine in the management of neuropathic bladder following spinal cord injury. Aust N Z J Surg 1999; 69:660–663.

72. Amark P, Beck O. Effect of phenylpropanolamine on incontinence in children with neurogenic bladders. A double-blind crossover study. Acta Paediatr 1992; 81:345–350.

73. Fall M, Lindström S. Electrical stimulation. A physiologic approach to the treatment of urinary incontinence. Urol Clin North Am 1991; 18:393–407.

74. Vodusek DB, Light KJ, Libby JM. Detrusor inhibition induced by stimulation of pudendal nerve afferents. Neurourol Urodyn 1986; 5:381–389.

75. Bemelmans BL, Mundy AR, Craggs MD. Neuromodulation by implant for treating lower urinary tract symptoms and dysfunction. Eur Urol 1999; 36:81–91.

76. Primus G, Kramer G. Maximal external electrical stimulation for treatment of neurogenic or non-neurogenic urgency and/or urge incontinence. Neurourol Urodyn 1996; 15:187–194.

77. Madersbacher H, Kiss G, Mair D. Transcutaneous electrostimulation of the pudendal nerve for treatment of detrusor overactivity. Neurourol Urodyn 1995; 14:501–502.

78. Previnaire JG, Soler JM, Perrigot M. Is there a place for pudendal nerve maximal electrical stimulation for the treatment of detrusor hyperreflexia in spinal cord injury patients? Spinal Cord 1998; 36:100–103.

79. Guttmann L, Frankel H. The value of intermittent catheterisation in the early management of traumatic paraplegia and tetraplegia. Paraplegia 1966; 4:63–84.

80. Lapides J, Diokno AC, Silber SJ, Lowe BS. Clean, intermittent self-catheterization in the treatment of urinary tract disease. J Urol 1972; 107:458–461.

81. Wyndaele JJ. Intermittent catheterization: which is the optimal technique? Spinal Cord 2002; 40:432–437.

82. Schlager TA, Dilks S, Trudell J, Whittam TS, Hendley JO. Bacteriuria in children with neurogenic bladder treated with intermittent catheterization: natural history. J Pediatr 1995; 126:490–496.

83. Prieto-Fingerhut T, Banovac K, Lynne CM. A study comparing sterile and non-sterile urethral catheterization in patients with spinal cord injury. Rehabil Nurs 1997; 22:299–302.

84. Matsumoto T, Takahashi K, Manabe N, Iwatsubo E, Kawakami Y. Urinary tract infection in neurogenic bladder. Int J Antimicrob Agents 2001; 17:293–297.

85. Stöhrer M, Sauerwein D. Der intermittierende Katheterismus bei neurogener Blasenfunktionsstörung. Eine Standortbestimmung aus urologischer Sicht. Urologe B 2001; 41:362–368.

86. Waller L, Jonsson O, Norlen L, Sullivan L. Clean intermittent catheterization in spinal cord injury patients: long-term followup of a hydrophilic low friction technique. J Urol 1995; 153:345–348.

87. Perrouin-Verbe B, Labat JJ, Richard I, Mauduyt de la Greve I, Buzelin JM, Mathe JF. Clean intermittent catheterisation from the acute period in spinal cord injury patients. Long term evaluation of urethral and genital tolerance. Paraplegia 1995; 33:619–624.

88. Bakke A, Digranes A, Hoisæter PA. Physical predictors of infection in patients treated with clean intermittent catheterization: a prospective 7-year study. Br J Urol 1997; 79:85–90.

89. Günther M, Löchner-Ernst D, Kramer G, Stöhrer M. Auswirkungen des intermittierende aseptischen intermittierenden Katheterismus auf die männliche Harnröhre. Urologe B 2001; 41:359–361.

90. Wyndaele JJ. Complications of intermittent catheterization: their prevention and treatment. Spinal Cord 2002; 40:536–541.

91. Sauerwein D. Urinary tract infection in patients with neurogenic bladder dysfunction. Int J Antimicrob Agents 2002; 19:592–597.

92. Sullivan LP, Davidson PG, Kloss DA, D'Anna JA Jr. Small-bowel obstruction caused by a long-term indwelling urinary catheter. Surgery 1990; 107:228–230.

93. Chao R, Clowers D, Mayo ME. Fate of upper urinary tracts in patients with indwelling catheters after spinal cord injury. Urology 1993; 42:259–262.

94. Chancellor MB, Erhard MJ, Kiilholma PJ, Karasick S, Rivas DA. Functional urethral closure with pubovaginal sling for destroyed female urethra after long-term urethral catheterization. Urology 1994; 43:499–505.

95. Bennett CJ, Young MN, Adkins RH, Diaz F. Comparison of bladder management complication outcomes in female spinal cord injury patients. J Urol 1995; 153:1458–1460.

96. Larsen LD, Chamberlin DA, Khonsari F, Ahlering TE. Retrospective analysis of urologic complications in male patients with spinal cord injury managed with and without indwelling urinary catheters. Urology 1997; 50:418–422.

97. West DA, Cummings JM, Longo WE, Virgo KS, Johnson FE, Parra RO. Role of chronic catheterization in the development of bladder cancer in patients with spinal cord injury. Urology 1999; 53:292–297.

98. Nomura S, Ishido T, Teranishi J, Makiyama K. Long-term analysis of suprapubic cystostomy drainage in patients with neurogenic bladder. Urol Int 2000; 65:185–189.

99. Mitsui T, Minami K, Furuno T, Morita H, Koyanagi T. Is suprapubic cystostomy an optimal urinary management in high quadriplegics? A comparative study of suprapubic cystostomy and clean intermittent catheterization. Eur Urol 2000; 38:434–438.

100. Weld KJ, Wall BM, Mangold TA, Steere EL, Dmochowski RR. Influences on renal function in chronic spinal cord injured patients. J Urol 2000; 164:1490–1493.

101. Zermann D, Wunderlich H, Derry F, Schroder S, Schubert J. Audit of early bladder management complications after spinal cord injury in first-treating hospitals. Eur Urol 2000; 37:156–160.

102. Park YI, Linsenmeyer TA. A method to minimize indwelling catheter calcification and bladder stones in individuals with spinal cord injury. J Spinal Cord Med 2001; 24:105–108.

103. Greenfield SP, Fera M. The use of intravesical oxybutynin chloride in children with neurogenic bladder. J Urol 1991; 146:532–534.

104. Glickman S, Tsokkos N, Shah PJ. Intravesical atropine and suppression of detrusor hypercontractility in the neuropathic bladder. A preliminary study. Paraplegia 1995; 33:36–39.

105. Kaplinsky R, Greenfield S, Wan J, Fera M. Expanded followup of intravesical oxybutynin chloride use in children with neurogenic bladder. J Urol 1996; 156:753–756.

106. Holland AJ, King PA, Chauvel PJ, O'Neill MK, McKnight DL, Barker AP. Intravesical therapy for the treatment of neurogenic bladder in children. Aust N Z J Surg 1997; 67:731–733.

107. Amark P, Bussman G, Eksborg S. Follow-up of long-time treatment with intravesical oxybutynin for neurogenic bladder in children. Eur Urol 1998; 34:148–153.

108. Haferkamp A, Staehler G, Gerner HJ, Dorsam J. Dosage escalation of intravesical oxybutynin in the treatment of neurogenic bladder patients. Spinal Cord 2000; 38:250–254.

109. Pannek J, Sommerfeld HJ, Botel U, Senge T. Combined intravesical and oral oxybutynin chloride in adult patients with spinal cord injury. Urology 2000; 55:358–362.

110. Buyse G, Waldeck K, Verpoorten C, Bjork H, Casaer P, Andersson KE. Intravesical oxybutynin for neurogenic bladder dysfunction: less systemic side effects due to reduced first pass metabolism. J Urol 1998; 160: 892–896.

111. Riedl CR, Knoll M, Plas E, Pflüger H. Intravesical electromotive drug administration technique: preliminary results and side effects. J Urol 1998; 159:1851–1856.

112. Di Stasi SM, Giannantoni A, Navarra P, Capelli G, Storti L, Porena M, Stephen RL. Intravesical oxybutynin: mode of action assessed by passive diffusion and electromotive administration with pharmacokinetics of oxybutynin and N-desethyl oxybutynin. J Urol 2001; 166:2232–2236.

113. Fowler CJ, Beck RO, Gerrard S, Betts CD, Fowler CG. Related Intravesical capsaicin for treatment of detrusor hyperreflexia. J Neurol Neurosurg Psychiatry 1994; 57:169–173.

114. Geirsson G, Fall M, Sullivan L. Clinical and urodynamic effects of intravesical capsaicin treatment in patients with chronic traumatic spinal detrusor hyperreflexia. J Urol 1995; 154:1825–1829.

115. Cruz F, Guimaraes M, Silva C, Rio ME, Coimbra A, Reis M. Desensitization of bladder sensory fibers by intravesical capsaicin has long lasting clinical and urodynamic effects in patients with hyperactive or hypersensitive bladder dysfunction. J Urol 1997; 157:585–589.

116. Cruz F, Guimaraes M, Silva C, Reis M. Suppression of bladder hyperreflexia by intravesical resiniferatoxin. Lancet 1997; 350:640–641.

117. De Ridder D, Chandiramani V, Dasgupta P, Van Poppel H, Baert L, Fowler CJ. Intravesical capsaicin as a treatment for refractory detrusor hyperreflexia: a dual center study with long-term followup. J Urol 1997; 158: 2087–2092.

118. Wiart L, Joseph PA, Petit H, Dosque JP, de Seze M, Brochet B, Deminiere C, Ferriere JM, Mazaux JM, N'Guyen P, Barat M. The effects of capsaicin on the neurogenic hyperreflexic detrusor. A double blind placebo controlled study in patients with spinal cord disease. Preliminary results. Spinal Cord 1998; 36:95–99.

119. Lazzeri M, Spinelli M, Beneforti P, Zanollo A, Turini D. Intravesical resiniferatoxin for the treatment of detrusor hyperreflexia refractory to capsaicin in patients with chronic spinal cord diseases. Scand J Urol Nephrol 1998; 32:331–334.

120. de Seze M, Wiart L, Joseph PA, Dosque JP, Mazaux JM, Barat M. Capsaicin and neurogenic detrusor hyperreflexia: a double-blind placebo-controlled study in 20 patients with spinal cord lesions. Neurourol Urodyn 1998; 17:513–523.

121. Chancellor MB, de Groat WC. Related Intravesical capsaicin and resiniferatoxin therapy: Spicing up the ways to treat the overactive bladder. J Urol 1999; 162:3–11.

122. Stöhrer M, Schurch B, Kramer G, Schmid D, Gaul G, Hauri D. Botulinum-A toxin in the treatment of detrusor hyperreflexia in spinal cord injury: A new alternative to medical and surgical procedures? Neurourol Urodyn 1999; 18:401–402.

123. Schurch B, Schmid DM, Stohrer M. Treatment of neurogenic incontinence with botulinum toxin A (letter). N Engl J Med 2000; 342: 665.

124. Schurch B, Stöhrer M, Kramer G, Schmid DM, Gaul G, Hauri D. Botulinum-A toxin for treating detrusor hyperreflexia in spinal cord injured patients: a new alternative to anticholinergic drugs? Preliminary results. J Urol 2000; 164:692–697.

125. Schulte-Baukloh H, Michael T, Schobert J, Stolze T, Knispel HH. Efficacy of botulinum-a toxin in children with detrusor hyperreflexia due to myelomeningocele: preliminary results. Urology 2002; 59: 325–327.

126. Wyndaele JJ, Van Dromme SA. Muscular weakness as side effect of botulinum toxin injection for neurogenic detrusor overactivity. Spinal Cord 2002; 40:599–600.

127. Katona F, Benyö L, Lang J. Über intraluminäre Elektrotherapie von verschiedenen paralytischen Zuständen des gastrointestinalen Traktes mit Quadrangulärstrom. Zentralbl Chir 1958; 84:929–933.

128. Kaplan WE. Intravesical electrical stimulation of the bladder: pro. Urology 2000; 56:2–4.

129. Ebner A, Jiang C, Lindstrom S. Intravesical electrical stimulation-an experimental analysis of the mechanism of action. J Urol 1992; 148:920–924.

130. Primus G, Kramer G, Pummer K. Restoration of micturition in patients with acontractile and hypocontractile detrusor by transurethral electrical bladder stimulation. Neurourol Urodyn 1996; 15:489–497.

131. De Wachter S, Wyndaele JJ. Quest for standardisation of electrical sensory testing in the lower urinary tract: The influence of technique related factors on bladder electrical thresholds. Neurourol Urodyn 2003; 22:118–122.

132. Katona F, Berenyi M. Intravesical transurethral electrotherapy in meningomyelocele patients. Acta Paed Acad Sci Hung 1975; 16:363–374.

133. Madersbacher H, Pauer W, Reiner E, Hetzel H, Spanudakis S. Rehabilitation of micturition in patients with incomplete spinal cord lesions by transurethral electrostimulation of the bladder. Eur Urol 1982; 28:111–116.

134. Madersbacher H. Intravesical electrical stimulation for the rehabilitation of the neuropathic bladder. Paraplegia 1990; 28:349–352.

135. Lyne CJ, Bellinger MF. Early experience with transurethral electrical bladder stimulation. J Urol 1993; 150:697–699.

136. Cheng EY, Richards I, Balcom A, Steinhardt G, Diamond M, Rich M, Donovan JM, Carr MC, Reinberg Y, Hurt G, Chandra M, Bauer SB, Kaplan WE. Bladder stimulation therapy improves bladder compliance: results from a multi-institutional trial. J Urol 1996; 156:761–764.

137. Nicholas JL, Eckstein HB. Endovesical electrotherapy in treatment of urinary incontinence in spinabifida patients. Lancet 1975; 2:1276–1277.

138. Pugach JL, Salvin L, Steinhardt GF. Intravesical electrostimulation in pediatric patients with spinal cord defects. J Urol 2000; 164:965–968.

139. Dykstra DD, Sidi AA, Scott AB, Pagel JM, Goldish GD. Effects of botulinum A toxin on detrusor-sphincter dyssynergia in spinal cord injury patients. J Urol 1988; 139:919–922.

140. Dykstra DD, Sidi AA. Related treatment of detrusor-sphincter dyssynergia with botulinum A toxin: a double-blind study. Arch Phys Med Rehabil 1990; 71:24–26.

141. Schurch B, Hauri D, Rodic B, Curt A, Meyer M, Rossier AB. Botulinum-A toxin as a treatment of detrusor-sphincter dyssynergia: a prospective study in 24 spinal cord injury patients. J Urol 1996; 155:1023–1029.

142. Schurch B, Hodler J, Rodic B. Botulinum A toxin as a treatment of detrusor-sphincter dyssynergia in patients with spinal cord injury: MRI controlled transperineal injections. J Neurol Neurosurg Psychiatry 1997; 63:474–476.

143. Gallien P, Robineau S, Verin M, Le Bot MP, Nicolas B, Brissot R. Treatment of detrusor sphincter dyssynergia by transperineal injection of botulinum toxin. Arch Phys Med Rehabil 1998; 79:715–717.

144. Petit H, Wiart L, Gaujard E, Le Breton F, Ferriere JM, Lagueny A, Joseph PA, Barat M. Related Botulinum A toxin treatment for detrusor-sphincter dyssynergia in spinal cord disease. Spinal Cord 1998; 36:91–94.

145. Wheeler JS Jr, Walter JS, Chintam RS, Rao S. Botulinum toxin injections for voiding dysfunction following SCI. J Spinal Cord Med 1998; 21:227–229.

146. Chancellor MB, Rivas DA, Abdill CK, Karasick S, Ehrlich SM, Staas WE. Prospective comparison of external sphincter balloon dilatation and prosthesis placement with external sphincterotomy in spinal cord injured men. Arch Phys Med Rehabil 1994; 75:297–305.

147. Whitmore WF 3rd, Fam BA, Yalla SV. Experience with anteromedian (12 o'clock) external urethral sphincterotomy in 100 male subjects with neuropathic bladders. Br J Urol 1978; 50:99–101.

148. Burgdörfer H, Bohatyrewicz A. Bladder outlet resistance decreasing operations in spinal cord damaged patients with vesicoureteral reflux. Paraplegia 1992; 30:256–260.

149. Perkash I. Use of contact laser crystal tip firing Nd:YAG to relieve urinary outflow obstruction in male neurogenic bladder patients. J Clin Laser Med Surg 1998; 16:33–38.

150. Noll F, Sauerwein D, Stohrer M. Transurethral sphincterotomy in quadriplegic patients: long-term-follow-up. Neurourol Urodyn 1995; 14: 351–358.

151. Reynard JM, Vass J, Sullivan ME, Mamas M. Sphincterotomy and the treatment of detrusor-sphincter dyssynergia: current status, future prospects. Spinal Cord 2003; 41:1–11.

152. Catz A, Luttwak ZP, Agranov E, Ronen J, Shpaser R, Paz A, Lask D, Tamir A, Mukamel E. The role of external sphincterotomy for patients with a spinal cord lesion. Spinal Cord 1997; 35:48–52.

153. Derry F, al-Rubeyi S. Audit of bladder neck resection in spinal cord injured patients. Spinal Cord 1998; 36: 345–348.

154. Chancellor MB, Gajewski J, Ackman CF, Appell RA, Bennett J, Binard J, Boone TB, Chetner MP, Crewalk JA, Defalco A, Foote J, Green B, Juma S, Jung SY, Linsenmeyer TA, MacMillan R, Mayo M, Ozawa H, Roehrborn CG, Shenot PJ, Stone A, Vazquez A, Killorin W, Rivas DA. Long-term followup of the North American multicenter UroLume trial for the treatment of external detrusor-sphincter dyssynergia. J Urol 1999; 161:1545–1550.

155. McFarlane IP, Foley SJ, Shah PJ. Related Long-term outcome of permanent urethral stents in the treatment of detrusor-sphincter dyssynergia. Br J Urol 1996; 78:729–732.

156. Low AI, McRae PJ. Use of the Memokath for detrusor-sphincter dyssynergia after spinal cord injury-a cautionary tale. Spinal Cord 1998; 36:39–44.

157. Juan Garcia FJ, Salvador S, Montoto A, Lion S, Balvis B, Rodriguez A, Fernandez M, Sanchez J. Intraurethral stent prosthesis in spinal cord injured patients with sphincter dyssynergia. Spinal Cord 1999; 37:54–57.

158. Chartier-Kastler EJ, Thomas L, Bussel B, Chancellor MB, Richard F, Denys P. A urethral stent for the treatment of detrusor-striated sphincter dyssynergia. BJU Int 2000; 86:52–57.

159. Gajewski JB, Chancellor MB, Ackman CF, Appell RA, Bennett J, Binard J, Boone TB, Chetner MP, Crewalk JA, Defalco A, Foote J, Green B, Juma S, Jung SY, Linsenmeyer TA, Macaluso JN Jr, Macmillan R, Mayo M, Ozawa H, Roehrborn CG, Schmidt J, Shenot PJ, Stone A, Vazquez A, Killorin W, Rivas DA. Removal of UroLume endoprosthesis: experience of the North American Study Group for detrusor-sphincter dyssynergia application. J Urol 2000; 163:773–776.

160. Wilson TS, Lemack GE, Dmochowski RR. UroLume stents: lessons learned. J Urol 2002; 167: 2477–2480.

161. Bennett JK, Green BG, Foote JE, Gray M. Collagen injections for intrinsic sphincter deficiency in the neuropathic urethra. Paraplegia 1995; 33:697–700.

162. Silveri M, Capitanucci ML, Mosiello G, Broggi G, De Gennaro M. Endoscopic treatment for urinary incontinence in children with a congenital neuropathic bladder. Br J Urol 1998; 82:694–697.

163. Guys JM, Simeoni-Alias J, Fakhro A, Delarue A. Use of polydimethylsiloxane for endoscopic treatment of neurogenic urinary incontinence in children. J Urol 1999; 162:2133–2135.

164. Kassouf W, Capolicchio G, Berardinucci G, Corcos J. Collagen injection for treatment of urinary incontinence in children. J Urol 2001; 165:1666–1668.

165. Caione P, Capozza N. Endoscopic treatment of urinary incontinence in pediatric patients: 2-year experience with dextranomer/hyaluronic acid copolymer. J Urol 2002; 168:1868–1871.

166. Block CA, Cooper CS, Hawtrey CE. Long-term efficacy of periurethral collagen injection for the treatment of urinary incontinence secondary to myelomeningocele. J Urol 2003; 169:327–329.

167. Schurch B, Suter S, Dubs M. Intraurethral sphincter prosthesis to treat hyporeflexic bladders in women: does it work? BJU Int 1999; 84:789–794.

168. Decter RM. Use of the fascial sling for neurogenic incontinence: lessons learned. J Urol 1993; 150: 683–686.

169. Herschorn S, Radomski SB. Fascial slings and bladder neck tapering in the treatment of male neurogenic incontinence. J Urol 1992; 147:1073–1075.

170. Gormley EA, Bloom DA, McGuire EJ, Ritchey ML. Pubovaginal slings for the management of urinary incontinence in female adolescents. J Urol 1994; 152:822–825.

171. Kakizaki H, Shibata T, Shinno Y, Kobayashi S, Matsumura K, Koyanagi T. Fascial sling for the management of urinary incontinence due to sphincter incompetence. J Urol 1995; 153: 644–647.

172. Gosalbez R, Castellan M. Defining the role of the bladder-neck sling in the surgical treatment of urinary incontinence in children with neurogenic incontinence. World J Urol 1998; 16: 285–291.

173. Barthold JS, Rodriguez E, Freedman AL, Fleming PA, Gonzalez R. Results of the rectus fascial sling and wrap procedures for the treatment of neurogenic sphincteric incontinence. J Urol 1999; 161: 272–274.

174. Dik P, Van Gool JD, De Jong TP. Urinary continence and erectile function after bladder neck sling suspension in male patients with spinal dysraphism. BJU Int 1999; 83: 971–975.

175. Kryger JV, Gonzalez R, Barthold JS. Surgical management of urinary incontinence in children with neurogenic sphincteric incompetence. J Urol 2000; 163:256–263.

176. Walker RD, Erhard M, Starling J. Long-term evaluation of rectus fascial wrap in patients with spina bifida. J Urol 2000; 164:485–486.

177. Kapoor R, Dubey D, Kumar A, Zaman W. Modified bulbar urethral sling procedure for the treatment of male sphincteric incontinence. J Endourol 2001; 15:545–549.

178. Nguyen HT, Bauer SB, Diamond DA, Retik AB. Rectus fascial sling for the treatment of neurogenic sphincteric incontinence in boys: is it safe and effective? J Urol 2001; 166:658–661.

179. Austin PF, Westney OL, Leng WW, McGuire EJ, Ritchey ML. Advantages of rectus fascial slings for urinary incontinence in children with neuropathic bladders. J Urol 2001; 165:2369–2371.

180. Mingin GC, Youngren K, Stock JA, Hanna MK. The rectus myofascial wrap in the management of urethral sphincter incompetence. BJU Int 2002; 90:550–553.

181. Colvert JR 3rd, Kropp BP, Cheng EY, Pope JC 4th, Brock JW 3rd, Adams MC, Austin P, Furness PD 3rd, Koyle MA. The use of small intestinal submucosa as an off-the-shelf urethral sling material for pediatric urinary incontinence. J Urol 2002; 168:1872–1875.

182. Daneshmand S, Ginsberg DA, Bennet JK, Foote J, Killorin W, Rozas KP, Green BG. Puboprostatic sling repair for treatment of urethral incompetence in adult neurogenic incontinence. J Urol 2003; 169:199–202.

183. Light JK, Scott FB. Use of the artificial urinary sphincter in spinal cord injury patients. J Urol 1983; 130:1127–1129.

184. Sidi AA, Reinberg Y, Gonzalez R. Comparison of artificial sphincter implantation and bladder neck reconstruction in patients with neurogenic urinary incontinence. J Urol 1987; 138:1120–1122.

185. Belloli G, Campobasso P, Mercurella A. Neuropathic urinary incontinence in pediatric patients: management with artificial sphincter. J Pediatr Surg 1992; 27:1461–1464

186. Gonzalez R, Merino FG, Vaughn M. Long-term results of the artificial urinary sphincter in male patients with neurogenic bladder. J Urol 1995; 154:769–770.

187. Levesque PE, Bauer SB, Atala A, Zurakowski D, Colodny A, Peters C, Retik AB. Ten-year experience with the artificial urinary sphincter in children. J Urol 1996; 156:625–628.

188. Singh G, Thomas DG. Artificial urinary sphincter in patients with neurogenic bladder dysfunction. Br J Urol 1996; 77:252–255.

189. Fulford SC, Sutton C, Bales G, Hickling M, Stephenson TP. The fate of the 'modern' artificial urinary sphincter with a follow-up of more than 10 years. Br J Urol 1997; 79:713–716.

190. Elliott DS, Barrett DM. Mayo Clinic long-term analysis of the functional durability of the AMS 800 artificial urinary sphincter: a review of 323 cases. J Urol 1998; 159:1206–1208.

191. Castera R, Podesta ML, Ruarte A, Herrera M, Medel R. 10-Year experience with artificial urinary sphincter in children and adolescents. J Urol 2001; 165:2373–2376.

192. Kryger JV, Leverson G, Gonzalez R. Long-term results of artificial urinary sphincters in children are independent of age at implantation. J Urol 2001; 165:2377–2379.

193. Janknegt RA, Baeten CG, Weil EH, Spaans F. Electrically stimulated gracilis sphincter for treatment of bladder sphincter incontinence. Lancet 1992; 340:1129–1130.

194. Chancellor MB, Hong RD, Rivas DA, Watanabe T, Crewalk JA, Bourgeois I. Gracilis urethromyoplasty – an autologous urinary sphincter for neurologically impaired patients with stress incontinence. Spinal Cord 1997; 35:546–549.

195. Chancellor MB, Heesakkers JP, Janknegt RA. Gracilis muscle transposition with electrical stimulation for sphincteric incontinence: a new approach. World J Urol 1997; 15:320–328.

196. Donnahoo KK, Rink RC, Cain MP, Casale AJ. The Young–Dees–Leadbetter bladder neck repair for neurogenic incontinence. J Urol 1999; 161:1946–1949.

197. Kropp KA, Angwafo FF. Urethral lengthening and reimplantation for neurogenic incontinence in children. J Urol 1986; 135:533–536.

198. Salle JL, McLorie GA, Bagli DJ, Khoury AE. Urethral lengthening with anterior bladder wall flap (Pippi Salle procedure): modifications and extended indications of the technique. J Urol 1997; 158:585–590.

199. Belman AB, Kaplan GW. Experience with the Kropp anti-incontinence procedure. J Urol 1989; 141:1160–1162.

200. Mollard P, Mouriquand P, Joubert P. Urethral lengthening for neurogenic urinary incontinence (Kropp's procedure): results of 16 cases. J Urol 1990; 143:95–97.

201. Nill TG, Peller PA, Kropp KA. Management of urinary incontinence by bladder tube urethral lengthening and submucosal reimplantation. J Urol 1990; 144:559–561.

202. Franco I, Kolligian M, Reda EF, Levitt SB. The importance of catheter size in the achievement of urinary continence in patients undergoing a Young–Dees–Leadbetter procedure. J Urol 1994; 152:710–712.

203. Rink RC, Adams MC, Keating MA. The flip-flap technique to lengthen the urethra (Salle procedure) for treatment of neurogenic urinary incontinence. J Urol 1994; 152:799–802.

204. Waters PR, Chehade NC, Kropp KA. Urethral lengthening and reimplantation: incidence and management of catheterization problems. J Urol 1997; 158:1053–1056.

205. Diamond DA, Bauer SB, Dinlenc C, Hendren WH, Peters CA, Atala A, Kelly M, Retik AB. Normal urodynamics in patients with bladder exstrophy: are they achievable? J Urol 1999; 162:841–844.

206. Jawaheer G, Rangecroft L. The Pippi Salle procedure for neurogenic urinary incontinence in childhood: a three-year experience. Eur J Pediatr Surg 1999; 9(Suppl 1):9–11.

207. Hayes MC, Bulusu A, Terry T, Mouriquand PD, Malone PS. The Pippi Salle urethral lengthening procedure; experience and outcome from three United Kingdom centres. BJU Int 1999; 84:701–705.

208. Yerkes EB, Adams MC, Rink RC, Pope JC IV, Brock JW 3rd. How well do patients with exstrophy actually void? J Urol 2000; 164:1044–1047.

209. Surer I, Baker LA, Jeffs RD, Gearhart JP. Modified Young–Dees–Leadbetter bladder neck reconstruction in patients with successful primary bladder closure elsewhere: a single institution experience. J Urol 2001; 165:2438–2440.

210. Chan DY, Jeffs RD, Gearhart JP. Determinants of continence in the bladder exstrophy population: predictors of success? Urology 2001; 57:774–777.

211. Ferrer FA, Tadros YE, Gearhart J. Modified Young–Dees–Leadbetter bladder neck reconstruction: new concepts about old ideas. Urology 2001; 58:791–796.

212. Couvelaire R. Chirurgie de la vessie. Paris, Masson 1955.

213. Cartwright PC, Snow BW. Bladder autoaugmentation: early clinical experience. J Urol 1989; 142:505–508.

214. Stöhrer M. Neurogene Blase. In: Jocham D, Miller K (eds) Praxis der Urologie, Band II. Stuttgart, Thieme 1992:257–275.

215. Stöhrer M, Kramer A, Goepel M, Lochner-Ernst D, Kruse D, Rübben H. Bladder auto-augmentation – an alternative for enterocystoplasty: preliminary results. Neurourol Urodyn 1995; 14:11–23.

216. Kennelly MJ, Gormley EA, McGuire EJ. Early clinical experience with adult bladder auto-augmentation. J Urol 1994; 152:303–306.

217. Dewan PA, Stefanek W. Autoaugmentation gastrocystoplasty: early clinical results. Br J Urol 1994; 74:460–464.

218. Elder JS. Autoaugmentation gastrocystoplasty: early clinical results. J Urol 1995; 154:322–323.

219. McDougall EM, Clayman RV, Figenshau RS, Pearle MS. Laparoscopic retropubic auto-augmentation of the bladder. J Urol 1995; 153:123–126.

220. Britanisky RG, Poppas DP, Shichman SN, Mininberg DT, Sosa RE. Laparoscopic laser-assisted bladder autoaugmentation. Urology 1995; 46:31–35.

221. Rivas DA, Figueroa TE, Chancellor MB. Bladder autoaugmentation. Tech Urol 1995; 1:181–187.

222. Poppas DP, Uzzo RG, Britanisky RG, Mininberg DT. Laparoscopic laser assisted auto-augmentation of the pediatric neurogenic bladder: early experience with urodynamic followup. J Urol 1996; 155:1057–1060.

223. Snow BW, Cartwright PC. Bladder autoaugmentation. Urol Clin North Am 1996; 23:323–331.

224. Stöhrer M, Kramer G, Goepel M, Lochner-Ernst D, Kruse D, Rübben H. Bladder autoaugmentation in adult patients with neurogenic voiding dysfunction. Spinal Cord 1997; 35:456–462.

225. Swami KS, Feneley RC, Hammonds JC, Abrams P. Detrusor myectomy for detrusor overactivity: a minimum 1-year follow-up. Br J Urol 1998; 81:68–72.

226. Duel BP, Gonzalez R, Barthold JS. Alternative techniques for augmentation cystoplasty. J Urol 1998; 159:998–1005.

227. Skobejko-Wlodarska L, Strulak K, Nachulewicz P, Szymkiewicz C. Bladder autoaugmentation in myelodysplastic children. Br J Urol 1998; 81(Suppl 3):114–116.

228. Braren V, Bishop MR. Laparoscopic bladder autoaugmentation in children. Urol Clin North Am 1998; 25:533–540.

229. Dewan PA. Autoaugmentation demucosalized enterocystoplasty. World J Urol 1998; 16:255–261.

230. Chapple CR, Bryan NP. Surgery for detrusor overactivity. World J Urol 1998; 16:268–273.

231. Leng WW, Blalock HJ, Fredriksson WH, English SF, McGuire EJ. Enterocystoplasty or detrusor myectomy? Comparison of indications and outcomes for bladder augmentation. J Urol 1999; 161:758–763.

232. Comer MT, Thomas DF, Trejdosiewicz LK, Southgate J. Reconstruction of the urinary bladder by auto-augmentation, enterocystoplasty, and composite enterocystoplasty. Adv Exp Med Biol 1999; 462:43–47.

233. Siracusano S, Trombetta C, Liguori G, De Giorgi G, d'Aloia G, Di Benedetto P, Belgrano E. Laparoscopic bladder auto-augmentation in an incomplete traumatic spinal cord injury. Spinal Cord 2000; 38:59–61.

234. Oge O, Tekgul S, Ergen A, Kendi S. Urothelium-preserving augmentation cystoplasty covered with a peritoneal flap. BJU Int 2000; 85:802–805.

235. Cranidis A, Nestoridis G. Bladder augmentation. Int Urogynecol J Pelvic Floor Dysfunct 2000; 11:33–40.

236. Niknejad KG, Atala A. Bladder augmentation techniques in women. Int Urogynecol J Pelvic Floor Dysfunct 2000; 11:156–169.

237. Westney OL, McGuire EJ. Surgical procedures for the treatment of urge incontinence. Tech Urol 2001; 7:126–132.

238. Perovic SV, Djordjevic ML, Kekic ZK, Vukadinovic VM. Bladder autoaugmentation with rectus muscle backing. J Urol 2002; 168:1877–1880.

239. Marte A, Di Meglio D, Cotrufo AM, Di Iorio G, De Pasquale M, Vessella A. A long-term follow-up of autoaugmentation in myelodysplastic children. BJU Int 2002; 89:928–931.

240. Ehrlich RM, Gershman A. Laparoscopic seromyotomy (auto-augmentation) for non-neurogenic neurogenic bladder in a child: initial case report. Urology 1993; 42:175–178.

241. Stothers L, Johnson H, Arnold W, Coleman G, Tearle H. Bladder autoaugmentation by vesicomyotomy in the pediatric neurogenic bladder. Urology 1994; 44:110–113.

242. Ter Meulen PH, Heesakkers JP, Janknegt RA. A study on the feasibility of vesicomyotomy in patients with motor urge incontinence. Eur Urol 1997; 32:166–169.

243. Surer I, Elicevik M, Ozturk H, Sakarya MT, Cetinkursun S. An alternative approach to bladder autoaugmentation. Tech Urol 1999; 5:100–103.

244. Potter JM, Duffy PG, Gordon EM, Malone PR. Detrusor myotomy: a 5-year review in unstable and noncompliant bladders. BJU Int 2002; 89:932–935.

245. Nagib A, Leal J, Voris HC. Successful control of selective anterior sacral rhizotomy for treatment of spastic bladder and ureteric reflux in paraplegics. Med Serv J Can 1966; 22:576–581.

246. Manfredi RA, Leal JF. Selective sacral rhizotomy for the spastic bladder syndrome in patients with spinal cord injuries. J Urol 1968; 100:17–20.

247. Toczek SK, McCullough DC, Gargour GW, Kachman R, Baker R, Luessenhop AJ. Selective sacral rootlet rhizotomy for hypertonic neurogenic bladder. J Neurosurg 1975; 42:567–574.

248. Diokno AC, Vinson RK, McGillicuddy J. Treatment of the severe uninhibited neurogenic bladder by selective sacral rhizotomy. J Urol 1977; 118:299–301.

249. Rockswold GL, Chou SN, Bradley WE. Re-evaluation of differential sacral rhizotomy for neurological bladder disease. J Neurosurg 1978; 48:773–778.

250. Young B, Mulcahy JJ. Percutaneous sacral rhizotomy for neurogenic detrusor hyperreflexia. J Neurosurg 1980; 53:85–87.

251. Franco I, Storrs B, Firlit CF, Zebold K, Richards I, Kaplan WE. Selective sacral rhizotomy in children with high pressure neurogenic bladders: preliminary results. J Urol 1992; 148:648–650.

252. Gasparini ME, Schmidt RA, Tanagho EA. Selective sacral rhizotomy in the management of the reflex neuropathic bladder: a report on 17 patients with long-term followup. J Urol 1992; 148:1207–1210.

253. Schneidau T, Franco I, Zebold K, Kaplan W. Selective sacral rhizotomy for the management of neurogenic bladders in spina bifida patients: long-term followup. J Urol 1995; 154:766–768.

254. Hohenfellner M, Pannek J, Botel U, Dahms S, Pfitzenmaier J, Fichtner J, Hutschenreiter G, Thuroff JW. Sacral bladder denervation for treatment of detrusor hyperreflexia and autonomic dysreflexia. Urology 2001; 58:28–32.

255. Arnold EP, Gowland SP, MacFarlane MR, Bean AR, Utley WL. Sacral anterior root stimulation of the bladder in paraplegics. Aust N Z J Surg 1986; 56:319–324.

256. MacDonagh RP, Forster DM, Thomas DG. Urinary continence in spinal injury patients following complete sacral posterior rhizotomy. Br J Urol 1990; 66:618–622.

257. Sauerwein D, Ingunza W, Fischer J, Madersbacher H, Polkey CE, Brindley GS, Colombel P, Teddy P. Extradural implantation of sacral anterior root stimulators. J Neurol Neurosurg Psychiatry 1990; 53:681–684.

258. Madersbacher H, Fischer J. Sacral anterior root stimulation: prerequisites and indications. Neurourol Urodyn 1993; 12:489–494.

259. Koldewijn EL, Van Kerrebroeck PE, Rosier PF, Wijkstra H, Debruyne FM. Bladder compliance after posterior sacral root rhizotomies and anterior sacral root stimulation. J Urol 1994; 151:955–960.

260. Singh G, Thomas DG. Intravesical oxybutinin in patients with posterior rhizotomies and sacral anterior root stimulators. Neurourol Urodyn 1995; 14:65–71.

261. Van Kerrebroeck PE, Koldewijn EL, Rosier PF, Wijkstra H, Debruyne FM. Results of the treatment of neurogenic bladder dysfunction in spinal cord injury by sacral posterior root rhizotomy and anterior sacral root stimulation. J Urol 1996; 155:1378–1381.

262. Schurch B, Rodic B, Jeanmonod D. Posterior sacral rhizotomy and intradural anterior sacral root stimulation for treatment of the spastic bladder in spinal cord injured patients. J Urol 1997; 157:610–614.

263. Van Kerrebroeck EV, van der Aa HE, Bosch JL, Koldewijn EL, Vorsteveld JH, Debruyne FM. Sacral rhizotomies and electrical bladder stimulation in spinal cord injury. Part I: Clinical and urodynamic analysis. Dutch Study Group on Sacral Anterior Root Stimulation. Eur Urol 1997; 31:263–271.

264. Egon G, Barat M, Colombel P, Visentin C, Isambert JL, Guerin J. Implantation of anterior sacral root stimulators combined with posterior sacral rhizotomy in spinal injury patients. World J Urol 1998; 16:342–349.

265. Schumacher S, Bross S, Scheepe JR, Alken P, Junemann KP. Restoration of bladder function in spastic neuropathic bladder using sacral deafferentation and different techniques of neurostimulation. Adv Exp Med Biol 1999; 462:303–309.

266. Van der Aa HE, Alleman E, Nene A, Snoek G. Sacral anterior root stimulation for bladder control: clinical results. Arch Physiol Biochem 1999; 107:248–256.

267. Everaert K, Derie A, Van Laere M, Vandekerckhove T. Bilateral S3 nerve stimulation, a minimally invasive alternative treatment for postoperative stress incontinence after implantation of an anterior root stimulator with posterior rhizotomy: a preliminary observation. Spinal Cord 2000; 38:262–264.

268. Creasey GH, Grill JH, Korsten M, U HS, Betz R, Anderson R, Walter J. An implantable neuroprosthesis for restoring bladder and bowel control to patients with spinal cord injuries: a multicenter trial. Arch Phys Med Rehabil 2001; 82:1512–1519.

269. Vignes JR, Liguoro D, Sesay M, Barat M, Guerin J. Dorsal rhizotomy with anterior sacral root stimulation for neurogenic bladder. Stereotact Funct Neurosurg 2001; 76:243–245.

270. Rijkhoff NJ, Hendrikx LB, van Kerrebroeck PE, Debruyne FM, Wijkstra H. Selective detrusor activation by electrical stimulation of the human sacral nerve roots. Artif Organs 1997; 21:223–226.

271. Schumacher S, Bross S, Scheepe JR, Seif C, Junemann KP, Alken P. Extradural cold block for selective neurostimulation of the bladder: development of a new technique. J Urol 1999; 161:950–954.

272. Kirkham AP, Knight SL, Craggs MD, Casey AT, Shah PJ. Neuromodulation through sacral nerve roots 2 to 4 with a Finetech-Brindley sacral posterior and anterior root stimulator. Spinal Cord 2002; 40:272–281.

273. Bhadra N, Grunewald V, Creasey G, Mortimer JT. Selective suppression of sphincter activation during sacral anterior nerve root stimulation. Neurourol Urodyn 2002; 21:55–64.

274. Brindley GS. An implant to empty the bladder or close the urethra. J Neurol Neurosurg Psychiatry 1977; 40:358–369.

275. Schmidt RA, Tanagho EA. Feasibility of controlled micturition through electric stimulation. Urol Int 1979; 34:199–230.

276. Braun PM, Baezner H, Seif C, Boehler G, Bross S, Eschenfelder CC, Alken P, Hennerici M, Juenemann P. Alterations of cortical electrical activity in patients with sacral neuromodulator. Eur Urol 2002; 41:562–566.

277. Tanagho EA, Schmidt RA, Orvis BR. Neural stimulation for control of voiding dysfunction: a preliminary report in 22 patients with serious neuropathic voiding disorders. J Urol 1989; 142:340–345.

278. Bosch JL, Groen J. Treatment of refractory urge urinary incontinence with sacral spinal nerve stimulation in multiple sclerosis patients. Lancet 1996; 348:717–719.

279. Bosch JL, Groen J. Neuromodulation: urodynamic effects of sacral (S3) spinal nerve stimulation in patients with detrusor instability or detrusor hyperreflexia. Behav Brain Res 1998; 92:141–150.

280. Hohenfellner M, Schultz-Lampel D, Dahms S, Matzel K, Thuroff JW. Bilateral chronic sacral neuromodulation for treatment of lower urinary tract dysfunction. J Urol 1998; 160:821–824.

281. Chartier-Kastler EJ, Ruud Bosch JL, Perrigot M, Chancellor MB, Richard F, Denys P. Long-term results of sacral nerve stimulation (S3) for the treatment of neurogenic refractory urge incontinence related to detrusor hyperreflexia. J Urol 2000; 164:1476–1480.

282. Groen J, van Mastrigt R, Bosch JL. Computerized assessment of detrusor instability in patients treated with sacral neuromodulation. J Urol 2001; 165:169–173.

283. Hohenfellner M, Humke J, Hampel C, Dahms S, Matzel K, Roth S, Thuroff JW, Schultz-Lampel D. Chronic sacral neuromodulation for treatment of neurogenic bladder dysfunction: long-term results with unilateral implants. Urology 2001; 58:887–892.

284. Haugland M, Sinkjaer T. Interfacing the body's own sensing receptors into neural prosthesis devices. Technol Health Care 1999; 7:393–399.

285. Jezernik S, Craggs M, Grill WM, Creasey G, Rijkhoff NJ. Electrical stimulation for the treatment of bladder dysfunction: current status and future possibilities. Neurol Res 2002; 24:413–430.

286. Zhang YH, Shao QA, Wang JM. Enveloping the bladder with displacement of flap of the rectus abdominis muscle for the treatment of neurogenic bladder. J Urol 1990; 144:1194–1195.

287. Stenzl A, Ninkovic M, Kolle D, Knapp R, Anderl H, Bartsch G. Restoration of voluntary emptying of the bladder by transplantation of innervated free skeletal muscle. Lancet 1998; 351:1483–1485.

288. Vajda P, Kaiser L, Magyarlaki T, Farkas A, Vastyan AM, Pinter AB. Histological findings after colocystoplasty and gastrocystoplasty. J Urol 2002; 168:698–701.

289. Greenwell TJ, Venn SN, Mundy AR. Augmentation cystoplasty. BJU Int 2001; 88:511–525.

290. Gough DC. Enterocystoplasty. BJU Int 2001; 88:739–743.

291. Quek ML, Ginsberg DA. Long-term urodynamics followup of bladder augmentation for neurogenic bladder. J Urol 2003; 169:195–198.

292. Chartier-Kastler EJ, Mongiat-Artus P, Bitker MO, Chancellor MB, Richard F, Denys P. Long-term results of augmentation cystoplasty in spinal cord injury patients. Spinal Cord 2000; 38:490–494.

293. Piechota HJ, Dahms SE, Probst M, Gleason CA, Nunes LS, Dahiya R, Lue TF, Tanagho EA. Functional rat bladder regeneration through xenotransplantation of the bladder acellular matrix graft. Br J Urol 1998; 81:548–559.

294. Sievert KD, Tanagho EA. Organ-specific acellular matrix for reconstruction of the urinary tract. World J Urol 2000; 18:19–25.

295. Kropp BP, Cheng EY. Bioengineering organs using small intestinal submucosa scaffolds: in vivo tissue-engineering technology. J Endourol 2000; 14:59–62.

296. Liatsikos EN, Dinlenc CZ, Kapoor R, Bernardo NO, Smith AD. Tissue expansion: a promising trend for reconstruction in urology. J Endourol 2000; 14:93–96.

297. Atala A. New methods of bladder augmentation. BJU Int 2000; 85 (Suppl 3):24–34

298. Reddy PP, Barrieras DJ, Wilson G, Bagli DJ, McLorie GA, Khoury AE, Merguerian PA. Regeneration of functional bladder substitutes using large segment acellular matrix allografts in a porcine model. J Urol 2000; 164:936–941.

299. Kawai K, Hattori K, Akaza H. Tissue-engineered artificial urothelium. World J Surg 2000; 24:1160–1162.

300. Schalow EL, Kirsch AJ. Advances in bladder augmentation. Curr Urol Rep 2002; 3:125–130.

301. O'Donnell WF. Urological management in the patient with acute spinal cord injury. Crit Care Clin 1987; 3:599–617.

302. Bennett JK, Gray M, Green BG, Foote JE. Continent diversion and bladder augmentation in spinal cord-injured patients. Semin Urol 1992; 10:121–132.

303. Robertson CN, King LR. Bladder substitution in children. Urol Clin North Am 1986; 13:333–344.

304. Duckett JW, Lotfi AH. Appendicovesicostomy (and variations) in bladder reconstruction. J Urol 1993; 149:567–569.

305. Moreno JG, Chancellor MB, Karasick S, King S, Abdill CK, Rivas DA. Improved quality of life and sexuality with continent urinary diversion in quadriplegic women with umbilical stoma. Arch Phys Med Rehabil 1995; 76:758–762.

306. Suzer O, Vates TS, Freedman AL, Smith CA, Gonzalez R. Results of the Mitrofanoff procedure in urinary tract reconstruction in children. Br J Urol 1997; 79:279–282.

307. Mollard P, Gauriau L, Bonnet JP, Mure PY. Continent cystostomy (Mitrofanoff's procedure) for neurogenic bladder in children and adolescent (56 cases: long-term results). Eur J Pediatr Surg 1997; 7:34–37.

308. Sylora JA, Gonzalez R, Vaughn M, Reinberg Y. Intermittent self-catheterization by quadriplegic patients via a catheterizable Mitrofanoff channel. J Urol 1997; 157:48–50.

309. Ulman I, Ergun O, Avanoglu A, Gokdemir A. The place of Mitrofanoff neourethra in the repair of exstrophy-epispadias complex. Eur J Pediatr Surg 1998; 8:352–354.

310. Cain MP, Casale AJ, King SJ, Rink RC. Appendicovesicostomy and newer alternatives for the Mitrofanoff procedure: results in the last 100 patients at Riley Children's Hospital. J Urol 1999; 162:1749–1752.

311. Stein R, Fisch M, Ermert A, Schwarz M, Black P, Filipas D, Hohenfellner R. Urinary diversion and orthotopic bladder substitution in children and young adults with neurogenic bladder: a safe option for treatment? J Urol 2000; 163:568–573.

312. Liard A, Seguier-Lipszyc E, Mathiot A, Mitrofanoff P. The Mitrofanoff procedure: 20 years later. J Urol 2001; 165:2394–2398.

313. Kajbafzadeh AM, Chubak N. Simultaneous Malone antegrade continent enema and Mitrofanoff principle using the divided appendix: report of a new technique for prevention of stoma complications. J Urol 2001; 165:2404–2409.

314. Van Savage JG, Yepuri JN. Transverse retubularized sigmoidovesicostomy continent urinary diversion to the umbilicus. J Urol 2001; 166:644–647.

315. Lowe JB, Furness PD 3rd, Barqawi AZ, Koyle MA. Surgical management of the neuropathic bladder. Semin Pediatr Surg 2002; 11:120–127.

316. Clark T, Pope JC 4th, Adams C, Wells N, Brock JW 3rd. Factors that influence outcomes of the Mitrofanoff and Malone antegrade continence enema reconstructive procedures in children. J Urol 2002; 168:1537–1540.

317. Richter F, Stock JA, Hanna MK. Continent vesicostomy in the absence of the appendix: three methods in 16 children. Urology 2002; 60:329–334.

318. Shapiro SR, Lebowitz R, Colodny AH. Fate of 90 children with ileal conduit urinary diversion a decade later: analysis of complications, pyelography, renal function and bacteriology. J Urol 1975; 114:289–295.

319. Hald T, Hebjoorn S. Vesicostomy – an alternative urine diversion operation. Long term results. Scand J Urol Nephrol 1978; 12:227–231.

320. Cass AS, Luxenberg M, Gleich P, Johnson CF. A 22-year followup of ileal conduits in children with a neurogenic bladder. J Urol 1984; 132:529–531.

321. Schwartz SL, Kennelly MJ, McGuire EJ, Faerber GJ. Incontinent ileo-vesicostomy urinary diversion in the treatment of lower urinary tract dysfunction. J Urol 1994; 152:99–102.

322. Atan A, Konety BR, Nangia A, Chancellor MB. Advantages and risks of ileovesicostomy for the management of neuropathic bladder. Urology 1999; 54:636–640.

323. Gudziak MR, Tiguert R, Puri K, Gheiler EL, Triest JA. Management of neurogenic bladder dysfunction with incontinent ileovesicostomy. Urology 1999; 54:1008–1011.

324. Borden TA, McGuire EJ, Woodside JR, Allen TD, Bauer SB, Firlit CF, Gonzales ET, Kaplan WE, King LR, Klauber GT, Perlmutter AD, Thornbury JR, Weiss RM. Urinary undiversion in patients with myelodysplasia and neurogenic bladder dysfunction. Report of a workshop. Urology 1981; 18:223–228.

325. Gonzalez R, Sidi AA, Zhang G. Urinary undiversion: indications, technique and results in 50 cases. J Urol 1986; 136:13–16.

326. Herschorn S, Rangaswamy S, Radomski SB. Urinary undiversion in adults with myelodysplasia: long-term followup. J Urol 1994; 152:329–333.

5   Treatment of vesico-ureteral reflux

5.1   Treatment options

The treatment options for vesico-ureteral reflux in patients with NLUTD do not differ essentially from those in other reflux patients. They become necessary when the abolishment of the high intravesical pressure during the filling phase or during the voiding phase have been treated successfully, but where the reflux did not resolve (1–4). Subtrigonal injections with bulking agents or ureteral re-implantation are the standard procedures.

Subtrigonal injections of bulking agents: This minimal invasive procedure has a relatively good effect with complete success in about 65% of patients (5–12). It can also be easily repeated if not effective and thereby the success rate can be increased to about 75% after the second or third session.

Ureteral re-implantation: This technique has an immediate and long-lasting result in over 90% of the patients (11–13).

In deciding which procedure will be offered to the patient, the relative risks of more invasive surgery and of less successful therapy should be considered.

5.2   References

1. Kass EJ, Koff SA, Diokno AC. Fate of vesicoureteral reflux in children with neuropathic bladders managed by intermittent catheterization. J Urol 1981; 125:63–64.

2. Sidi AA, Peng W, Gonzalez R. Vesicoureteral reflux in children with myelodysplasia: natural history and results of treatment. J Urol 1986; 136:329–331.

3. Lopez Pereira P, Martinez Urrutia MJ, Lobato Romera R, Jaureguizar E. Should we treat vesicoureteral reflux in patients who simultaneously undergo bladder augmentation for neuropathic bladder? J Urol 2001; 165:2259–2261.

4. Simforoosh N, Tabibi A, Basiri A, Noorbala MH, Danesh AD, Ijadi A. Is ureteral reimplantation necessary during augmentation cystoplasty in patients with neurogenic bladder and vesicoureteral reflux? J Urol 2002; 168:1439–1441.

5. Diamond T, Boston VE. The natural history of vesicoureteric reflux in children with neuropathic bladder and open neural tube defects. Z Kinderchir 1987; 42(Suppl 1):15–16.

6. Chancellor MB, Rivas DA, Liberman SN, Moore J Jr, Staas WE Jr. Cystoscopic autogenous fat injection treatment of vesicoureteral reflux in spinal cord injury. J Am Paraplegia Soc 1994; 17:50–54.

7. Sugiyama T, Hashimoto K, Kiwamoto H, Ohnishi N, Esa A, Park YC, Kurita T, Kohri K. Endoscopic correction of vesicoureteral reflux in patients with neurogenic bladder dysfunction. Int Urol Nephrol 1995; 27:527–531.

8. Misra D, Potts SR, Brown S, Boston VE. Endoscopic treatment of vesico-ureteric reflux in neurogenic bladder-8 years' experience. J Pediatr Surg 1996; 31:1262–1264.

9. Haferkamp A, Mohring K, Staehler G, Gerner HJ, Dorsam J. Long-term efficacy of subureteral collagen injection for endoscopic treatment of vesicoureteral reflux in neurogenic bladder cases. J Urol 2000; 163:274–277.

10. Shah N, Kabir MJ, Lane T, Avenell S, Shah PJ. Vesico-ureteric reflux in adults with neuropathic bladders treated with Polydimethylsiloxane (Macroplastique). Spinal Cord 2001; 39:92–96.

11. Engel JD, Palmer LS, Cheng EY, Kaplan WE. Surgical versus endoscopic correction of vesicoureteral reflux in children with neurogenic bladder dysfunction. J Urol 1997; 157:2291–2294.

12. Granata C, Buffa P, Di Rovasenda E, Mattioli G, Scarsi PL, Podesta E, Dodero P, Jasonni V. Treatment of vesico-ureteric reflux in children with neuropathic bladder: a comparison of surgical and endoscopic correction. J Pediatr Surg 1999; 34:1836–1838.

13. Kaplan WE, Firlit CF. Management of reflux in the myelodysplastic child. J Urol 1983; 129:1195–1197.

6   Quality of life

6.1   Considerations

The quality of life is a very important aspect in the treatment of patients with NLUTD. Apart from the limitations that relate directly to the neurologic pathology, the NLUTD can be treated adequately in the majority of patients and must not interfere with social independence. The life expectancy of the patients does not need to be impaired by the NLUTD. With adequate treatment and consequent neuro-urological care over lifetime, the quality of life can be assured.

It is satisfying that this aspect is not neglected (1–12) in the recent medical literature.

6.2   References

1. Stöhrer M, Kramer G, Löchner-Ernst D, Goepel M, Noll F, Rübben H. Diagnosis and treatment of bladder dysfunction in spinal cord injury patients. Eur Urol Update Series 1994; 3:170–175.

2. Stone AR. Neurourologic evaluation and urologic management of spinal dysraphism. Neurosurg Clin N Am 1995; 6:269–277.

3. Joseph AC, Juma S, Niku SD. Endourethral prosthesis for treatment of detrusor sphincter dyssynergia: impact on quality of life for persons with spinal cord injury. SCI Nurs 1994; 11:95–99.

4. Breza J, Hornak M, Bardos A, Zvara P. Transformation of the Bricker to a continent urinary reservoir to eliminate severe complications of uretero-ileostomy performed in eight patients among 200 Bricker. Ann Urol (Paris) 1995; 29:227–231.

5. Moreno JG, Chancellor MB, Karasick S, King S, Abdill CK, Rivas DA. Improved quality of life and sexuality with continent urinary diversion in quadriplegic women with umbilical stoma. Arch Phys Med Rehabil 1995; 76:758–762.

6. Bramble FJ. Clinical outcome and quality of life following enterocystoplasty for idiopathic detrusor instability and neurogenic bladder dysfunction. Br J Urol 1996; 77:764–765.

7. Kuo HC. Clinical outcome and quality of life after enterocystoplasty for contracted bladders. Urol Int 1997; 58:160–165.

8. Stöhrer M, Kramer G, Goepel M, Lochner-Ernst D, Kruse D, Rübben H. Bladder autoaugmentation in adult patients with neurogenic voiding dysfunction. Spinal Cord 1997; 35:456–462.

9. Vaidyanathan S, Soni BM, Brown E, Sett P, Krishnan KR, Bingley J, Markey S. Effect of intermittent urethral catheterization and oxybutynin bladder instillation on urinary continence status and quality of life in a selected group of spinal cord injury patients with neuropathic bladder dysfunction. Spinal Cord 1998; 36:409–414.

10. Cranidis A, Nestoridis G. Bladder augmentation. Int Urogynecol J Pelvic Floor Dysfunct 2000; 11:33–40.

11. Nijman RJ. Neurogenic and non-neurogenic bladder dysfunction. Curr Opin Urol 2001; 11:577–583.

12. Kachourbos MJ, Creasey GH. Health promotion in motion: improving quality of life for persons with neurogenic bladder and bowel using assistive technology. SCI Nurs 2000; 17:125–129.

7   Follow-up

7.1   Considerations

NLUTD is an unstable condition and can vary considerably even within a relatively short period. Meticulous follow-up and regular checks are necessary (1–20). Depending on the type of the underlying neurological pathology and on the present stability of the NLUTD, the interval between the detailed investigations should not exceed 1–2 years. In patients with multiple sclerosis and in acute spinal cord injury this interval is of course much smaller. Urine dip sticks should be available for the patient and urinalysis should be performed at least every second month. The upper urinary tract, the bladder shape, and residual urine should be checked every 6 months. Physical examination and blood and urine laboratory should take place every year. Any sign indicating a risk factor warrants specialized investigation.

7.2   Guidelines for follow-up

1. Possible UTI checked by the patient (dip stick).
2. Urinalysis every second month.
3. Upper urinary tract, bladder morphology, and residual urine every six months (ultrasound)
4. Physical examination, blood chemistry, and urine laboratory every year.
5. Detailed specialistic investigation every 1–2 years and on demand when risk factors emerge. The investigation is specified according to the patient's actual risk profile, but should in any case include a video urodynamic investigation and should be performed in a leading neuro-urological center.
6. All of the above more frequent if the neurological pathology or the NLUTD status demand this.

7.3   References

1. Stöhrer M. Alterations in the urinary tract after spinal cord injury – diagnosis, prevention and therapy of late sequelae. World J Urol 1990; 7:205–211.

2. Perkash I. Long-term urologic management of the patient with spinal cord injury. Urol Clin North Am 1993; 20:423–434.

3. Selzman AA, Elder JS, Mapstone TB. Urologic consequences of myelodysplasia and other congenital abnormalities of the spinal cord. Urol Clin North Am 1993; 20:485–504.

4. Stöhrer M, Kramer G, Löchner-Ernst D, Goepel M, Noll F, Rübben H. Diagnosis and treatment of bladder dysfunction in spinal cord injury patients. Eur Urol Update Series 1994; 3:170–175.

5. Thon WF, Denil J, Stief CG, Jonas U. Urologische Langzeitbetreuung von Patienten mit Meningomyelozele. II. Therapie. Aktuel Urol 25:63–76.

6. Waites KB, Canupp KC, DeVivo MJ, Lloyd LK, Dubovsky EV. Compliance with annual urologic evaluations and preservation of renal function in persons with spinal cord injury. J Spinal Cord Med 1995; 18:251–254.

7. Cardenas DD, Mayo ME, Turner LR: Lower urinary changes over time in suprasacral spinal cord injury. Paraplegia 1995; 33:326–329.

8. Capitanucci ML, Iacobelli BD, Silveri M, Mosiello G, De Gennaro M. Long-term urological follow-up of occult spinal dysraphism in children. Eur J Pediatr Surg 1996; 6 (Suppl 1):25–26.

9. Chua HC, Tow A, Tan ES. The neurogenic bladder in spinal cord injury-pattern and management. Ann Acad Med Singapore 1996; 25:553–557.

10. Agarwal SK, Bagli DJ. Neurogenic bladder. Indian J Pediatr 1997; 64:313–326.

11. Rashid TM, Hollander JB. Multiple sclerosis and the neurogenic bladder. Phys Med Rehabil Clin N Am 1998; 9:615–629.

12. Burgdörfer H, Heidler H, Madersbacher H, Melchior H, Palmtag H, Richter R, Richter-Reichhelm M, Rist M, Rübben H, Sauerwein D, Schalkhäuser K, Stöhrer M. Leitlinien zur urologischen Betreuung Querschnittgelähmter. Urologe A 1998; 37:222–228.

13. McKinley WO, Jackson AB, Cardenas DD, DeVivo MJ. Long-term medical complications after traumatic spinal cord injury: a regional model systems analysis. Arch Phys Med Rehabil 1999; 80:1402–1410.

14. Atan A, Konety BR, Nangia A, Chancellor MB. Advantages and risks of ileovesicostomy for the management of neuropathic bladder. Urology 1999; 54:636–640.

15. Cranidis A, Nestoridis G. Bladder augmentation. Int Urogynecol J Pelvic Floor Dysfunct 2000; 11:33–40.

16. Elliott DS, Boone TB. Recent advances in the management of the neurogenic bladder. Urology 2000; 56(6 Suppl 1):76–81.

17. Chen Y, DeVivo MJ, Roseman JM. Current trend and risk factors for kidney stones in persons with spinal cord injury: a longitudinal study. Spinal Cord 2000; 38:346–353.

18. Lawrenson R, Wyndaele JJ, Vlachonikolis I, Farmer C, Glickman S. Renal failure in patients with neurogenic lower urinary tract dysfunction. Neuroepidemiology 2001; 20:138–143.

19. Ciancio SJ, Mutchnik SE, Rivera VM, Boone TB. Urodynamic pattern changes in multiple sclerosis. Urology 2001; 57:239–245.

20. Burns AS, Rivas DA, Ditunno JF. The management of neurogenic bladder and sexual dysfunction after spinal cord injury. Spine 2001; 26(24 Suppl):S129–S136.

8   Conclusion

NLUTD is a multi-facetted pathology. It needs an extensive and specific diagnosis before we can embark on an individualized therapy that takes into account the medical and physical condition of the patient, and the patient's expectations about his future social and physical situation with respect to the NLUTD.

The urologist or pediatric urologist can select from a wealth of therapeutical options, each with its specific pros and cons. Notwithstanding the success of any therapy embarked upon, a close surveillance is necessary for all of the patient's life.

With these guidelines we offer you expert advice on how to define the patient's NLUTD condition as precisely as possible and how to select, together with the patient, the appropriate therapy. This last choice, as always, is governed by the golden rule: As effective as needed, as less invasive as possible.

9   Abbreviations

DLPP	Detrusor leak point pressure
DSD	Detrusor sphincter dyssynergia
EMG	Electromyography, electromyogram
FVC	Frequency volume chart
IC	Intermittent catheterization
ISC	Intermittent self-catheterization
ICS	International Continence Society
LPP	Leak point pressure
LMNL	Lower motor neuron lesion
LUT	Lower urinary tract
LUTD	Lower urinary tract dysfunction
LUTS	Lower urinary tract symptoms
MTC	Micturition time chart
NLUTD	Neurogenic lower urinary tract dysfunction
PNE	Percutaneous nerve evaluation test
SDAF	Sacral deafferentation
SARS	Sacral anterior root stimulation
UMNL	Upper motor neuron lesion
UTI	Urinary tract infection
VUR	Vesico-ureteral reflux

Index

Page numbers in italics indicate *figures* and *tables*. LUT refers to lower urinary tract.

abdominal leak point pressure (ALPP) 420–1
abdominoperineal resection (APR) 100, 238–9
Aboulker's theory of primary syringomelia 215
Abrams–Klevmark classification of voiding diaries 373–4
abscesses, periurethral 676
absence seizures 354
acetylcholine 24, 74, 75, 178, 179
acetylcholine receptors 17
    see also muscarinic receptors; nicotinic receptors
acetylcholinesterase, neurohistochemistry for 106, 108
acetylcholinesterase inhibitors 253
actin 20, 23
action potentials, detrusor muscle cells 20
Aδ-fibers 143, 180
adenosine 25
adenosine triphosphate (ATP)
    in bladder control 24, 61, 178
    loss in SCI 187
    in urethral control 67–8
ADP (delta-aminolevulinic acid dehydratase deficient porphyria) 225
adrenergic nerves
    bladder 24, 60
    urethra 65
adrenoceptors (ARs)
    bladder
        αARs 60
        βARs 60–1
    classification 17
    second messenger effects 19
    urethra
        αARs 28, 65–6
        βARs 66
agrins 47–8
AIDS 97–8, 150, 348
alcoholism 224–5
alginate 620
alpha-adrenergic blockers
    DESD therapy 499–500
    effects on bladder compliance 158–9
    reduction of neurologic sweating 498
    use in MS patients 288–9
Alzheimer's disease
    clinical features 247
    detrusor hyperreflexia 251
    medication 253
    prevalence of urinary incontinence 246
amantadine hydrochloride 253
American Spinal Injury Association (ASIA) classification 333–4, *336*

amezinium 271
anal reflex 363
anandamide *507*, 508
anastomoses
    intestinal 602
    ureterointestinal 602–3
angiogenesis 620
aniracetam 253
anode block technique 631, 633
anterior cord syndrome 334
anterior spinal artery (ASA) 182
anti-P/Q-type voltage-gated calcium channel antibodies 351
antiacetylcholine receptor antibodies 350
antibacterial prophylaxis
    bowel surgery 601–2
    urinary tract infection 488
antibody-mediated autoimmunity in MS 276
anticholinergic drugs
    drugs 496–8
    intravesical administration 515, 648
    oral administration 647
    use in children 655–6
    see also specific drugs
anticipation 351
antiepileptic medication, urinary effects 354–5
antigrade continence enemas (ACE) 203, *204*
antimuscarinic drugs *see* anticholinergic drugs
antireflux surgery 201, 690
apomorphine 263
apoptosis following SCI 185–6, 637
appendicovesicostomy (Mitrofanoff procedure) 607, *608*, *609*
areflexic bladder 143–56
    balance with urethra 670–1
    causes 144
    diseases developing 144–51
    management 149–50, 646–7, 689
        see also specific methods
artificial urinary sphincters
    advantages/disadvantages *570*
    AMS 800 576
    background 573
    in children 661–2
    complications 578, *579–80*, 581
    cost 573
    design evolution 576
    device lifetime 652
    indications and patient selection 576–7
    in MMC patients 210–11
    results 578, *579–80*
    surgical technique 577–8
ataxias 92, 347–8
ATP *see* adenosine triphosphate (ATP)

atropine 24
autoaugmentation 689–90
  in children 658
  compared with other methods 562, 649
  demucosalized enterocystoplasty 618
  indication 560
  procedure 560–1
  results 561–2
autonomic dysreflexia (AD) 169–73
  causes 172, *173*
  in children 173
  differential diagnosis 172
  historical overview 169
  incidence 171
  management
    acute 463, 525–6
    anesthesia 526, 527
    pregnancy and labor 526–7
    prophylaxis 463, 526
    summarized *464*
  morbidity 172–3
  neurophysiology after SCI
    autonomic nervous system-related symptoms 169–70
    changes in sympathetic preganglionic neurons 170–1
    hypersensitivity of vascular α adrenoceptors 171
    neurobiochemical changes caudal to injury 171
    remodeling of spinal cord circuits 171
  pregnancy and 172, 173, 526–7
  prevention 525, 527
  severity *339*
  signs 172
  symptoms 169–70, 172, 339
  triggers *339*
autonomic failure (AF) 265
autonomic nervous system
  electrophysiological tests 455–6
  see also parasympathetic innervation of the LUT; sympathetic innervation of the LUT
autonomic neuropathies and neurogenic bladder 225, *226*, 229
  see also specific conditions
autonomic seizures 354
axons
  changes in clinical UMNB 116, *117*
  degeneration in LMNB models 108–10
  patterns of injury *316*
  regeneration following SCI 638–9
  regeneration in LMNB models 110–11, *112*
  structure *315*, *316*

baclofen 159, 500, 501, 648
bacteria
  artificial sphincter infection 578
  prostate infection 676
  urease-producing 678
  in urine specimens 675
  see also urinary tract infections (UTI)
bacteriuria, after urinary diversion 612
balanced bladder 667, 683
  see also vesicourethral balance
Barrington's nucleus *see* pontine micturition center
basal ganglia
  functional anatomy 259
  neural organization summarized *260*
  physiology 260
  see also Huntington's disease (HD); Parkinson's disease (PD)
Bcl-2 186, 638

behavioral techniques
  adjustments to daily life 483
  toileting regimens 252–3
benign prostatic hypertrophy (BPH) 62, 479, 668
benzodiazepines 500–1
beta-adrenergic agonists 501
beta-blockers 101
bethanecol 150, 289, 340
biofeedback 410, 484
biomaterials for tissue engineering 617
BK virus (BKV) 299
bladder
  anatomy 11–12
  areflexic *see* areflexic bladder
  augmentation 287–8, 289, 562, 648–9, 657–9, 690
  balanced 667
  blood supply 13
  cancer 397, *398*, 680–1, 700
  compliance *see* compliance
  development 5, 6, 9
    see also development of bladder function
  expression maneuvers 485
  filling 26, *42*, 57, 179, 529
  foreign bodies 397, *398*
  hyperpressure 696
  hyperreflexic *see* detrusor hyperreflexia
  ischemia 137–8
  local control *see* local control of the bladder
  lymphatic drainage 13
  mucosa 12, *395*
  myofibroblasts 25
  neonatal 83
  nervous control 13–14, 57–9
    see also peripheral nervous control of the LUT
  normal capacity in children 412, *413*, 432–3
  open neck 401–3
  overactive *see* overactive bladder pathophysiology
  parasympathetic decentralization 339–40
  pressures in children 412–13
  regionalization 27–8
  spontaneous activity 23–4
  stones 397, 679
  tissue engineering 618–19
  tumors 397, *398*, 680–1, 700
  urothelium 27, 76–7
  voiding reflexes *see* voiding reflexes
  wall
    abnormalities 395, 696
    electrical stimulation 535–6
    trabeculations 395–6
  see also detrusor muscle; micturition; vesicourethral balance
bladder cooling test 83, 430, 434
bladder emptying improvement techniques 646–7
  see also specific techniques
bladder leak point pressure (BLPP) 419–20, 430, 696
bladder muscle cell injections 620
bladder neck closure
  disadvantages 587
  indications 587
  results and complications 589
  surgical technique
    transabdominal approach 587–8
    transvaginal approach 588–9
bladder neck reconstruction
  background 581
  indications and patient selection 583–4, 587

procedures
    Kropp 582–3, 584, *585*, 659–61
    Pippi Salle 583, 584, *586*, 587, 660–1
    Young–Dees–Leadbetter 581–2, 584, *586*
    results and complications 584–7
bladder neck slings 659
    advantages/disadvantages *570*
    and bladder augmentation 571
    complications 573
    indications 571
    patient selection 571
    results 573, *574–5*
    surgical techniques 571–3
bladder neck wraps 573
bladder relaxant drugs 495–8
bladder-specific K⁺ channel openers 502
blastulae 3
α-blockers *see* alpha-adrenergic blockers
blood–brain barrier 186
bone scans 327
Borrelia burgdorferi 99, 299, 300, 301
Bors ice water test (bladder cooling test) 83, 430, 434
botulinum-A toxin
    administration 558
    clinical experience with 159, 288, 289, 513–14, 558, 649–50
    cost 515
    formulations 513, 558
    indication 558
    mode of action 288, 513, 558
    results 558–60, 648
bowel preparation for surgery 601
brain regions in micturition control 44–5, *81*, 82–3, 165–6
Bricker ileal conduit 603–4
Bricker ureterointestinal anastomosis *602*
Brown-Séquard syndrome 334
bulbocavernosus reflex (BCR) 363, 451–3, 457
bulking agents, urethral
    background 565–6
    collagen 566
    complications 570
    contraindications 568
    delivery methods 567
    indications 568
    mechanism of action 566–7
    patient selection 568
    postoperative care 567
    results 568–70
    skin test 567
bupivacaine 648
Burch urethropexy 651

C-fiber afferents 75–6, 137, 143, 337
calcitonin gene-related peptide (CGRP) 63
calcium channels 18, 23, 29
calcium ions
    changes following SCI 184, 185
    as second messengers 19
    in smooth muscle contraction 21–3
calcium-induced calcium release (CICR) 22, 23
calculi *see* lithiasis
caldesmon 23
calmodulin 19, 21
capsaicin 287
    intravesical use
        clinical experience 508–10, 648
        procedure 513

rationale 508
    safety 510
    molecular structure *507*
captopril 526
carbamazepine 354
carbon monoxide (CO), in urethral function 67
case-control studies, folic acid and NTDs 197
catecholamines 331
catheters
    condom 490
    for cystometry in children 429
    indwelling 688
    transurethral and suprapubic 429, 490
    see also clean intermittent catheterization (CIC)/
        self-catheterization (CISC)
cauda equina syndrome
    absence of reflexes 148
    electrophysiological assessment 456–7
    incidence 97
    symptoms 97, 317
    urinary dysfunction 146
    urodynamics 148–9, 319, *320*
ceftriaxone 302
cell transplantation strategies, SCI therapy 638–9, 639–40
cell-based tissue engineering 617
    bladder 619
    bladder muscle cell injections 620
    chondrocyte injections 620
    genetically engineered cells 152, 620–1
    urethra 617–18
    using stem cells 152–3, 621
cell-mediated autoimmunity in MS 276
central cord syndrome 96, 334
central nervous system neuropharmacology 331–3
central pathways involved in micturition 80–4
    anatomy 43–4
    brain involvement 44–5, *81*, 82–3, 165–6
    developmental changes 83–4
    pontine micturition center *see* pontine micturition center
    spinal cord 80–1
cerebellar ataxias 92, 347
cerebral palsy (CP)
    continence study 345
    features 345
    treatment 347
    urinary symptoms 92–3, 345–6
    urinary tract infections 347
    urodynamic findings 346–7
cerebral shock, after stroke 91, 307
cerebral trauma 333
cerebral tumors 92
cerebrovascular accidents (CVAs)
    cerebral shock 91, 307
    clinical assessment of urinary function 307
    epidemiology 91, 305
    management 305
    striated muscle reflex control 50
    urinary incontinence 91–2, 305–6
        implications for prognosis and care 306
        pathophysiology 306
    urodynamic findings 91, 307
    urologic management
        acute stage 307–8
        recovery stage 308–10
        stable stage 310–11
        other LUT symptoms 311

cervical spondylosis 101
chemokines 186–7
children
    autonomic dysreflexia in 173
    bladder management
        anticholinergic drugs 655–6
        bladder augmentation 657–9
        clean intermittent catheterization 655
        cutaneous vesicostomy 656
    bladder outlet management
        artificial urinary sphincter 661–2
        bulking agents *see* bulking agents, urethral
        drugs to increase resistance 659
        fascial slings 659
        urethral lengthening 659–61
    management goals 655
    normal voiding values 376
    open bladder neck in 402
    pad tests in 388, 429
    patient factors in management 662
    prognosis of urinary dysfunction in SCI 696
    sedation of 428
    see also development of bladder function; urodynamics in children
Chlamydia pneumoniae and MS 276
chloride channels 19
chlorpromazine 463, *464*
cholinergic nerves
    bladder 59–60
    urethra 64
cholinergic receptors 17
    see also muscarinic receptors; nicotinic receptors
chondrocyte injections 620
ciliary neurotrophic factor (CNTF) 47
cingulate gyrus, in control of micturition 44, 45, 165–6
clam cystoplasty 562, 658
classification of LUT disorders 469–80
    according to nervous system involvement 472
    basis in structure and function 469
    bladder outlet obstruction 475–6
    consequences of disorders 479–80
    current system, need for revision 469
    female incontinence groups 476–7
    harmonic/disharmonic disruptions of micturition 474–5
    interdependence of disorder, consequences and comorbidity 472–3
    LUT overactivity 477–8
    micturition cycle 470–1
    neurogenic bladder in spina bifida children 435–6
    patterns of recognition 473–4, *479*
    simplified LUT model 474, *478*
    simplified structure and function-based 478–9
    therapeutic 645–6
    time-related changes 475
    Wein functional classification system 415
clean intermittent catheterization (CIC)/self-catheterization (CISC)
    adjunctive therapy 487
    background 195, 286, 646, 687–8
    catheter introduction 486
    catheters and lubricants 485, 688
    demented patients 255
    frequency 487
    infants/children 200–1, 655
    reasons for discontinuation 487
    results of studies *486*

reuse of catheters 486–7
    sterile technique (SIC) 485–6
    urethral trauma 489
    urinary tract infections 487–9, 688
    other complications 489, 688
clenbuterol 66
clinical evaluation
    history *see* history
    physical examination 147–8, 363, 416
    see also specific conditions
clinical neurophysiological tests *see* electrophysiological evaluation
clitoris, development of 7
cloaca, development of 3–4
CNEMG *see* concentric needle electromyography (CNEMG)
Cobb syndrome 349
collagen fibers, viscosity of 157
collagen urethral injections *see* bulking agents, urethral
colocystoplasty, in children 657
colon conduits 604
coma 333
comorbidity 473
compliance
    in children 412, 434–5
    clinical factors summarized *160*
    data from conservative treatments 158–9
    data from experimental studies 159–60
    defined 157, 418
    high intravesical pressure 157, 160, 418–19
    impaired 418
    level of spinal lesion and 158
    mode of drainage and 157–8
    normal 418, 434
    in SCI patients 699–700
computed tomography (CT), upper urinary tract 405
computer analysis of voiding diary data 375
concentric needle electromyography (CNEMG)
    assessment of interference patterns 450
    assessment of motor unit potentials (MUPs) 446–50
    insertion activity 446
    procedure 446
    spontaneous denervation activity 446
    vs. single fiber electromyography 450
condom catheters 490
congeners 225
conservative treatment of neurogenic bladder 483
    see also specific treatments
continent ileal reservoir (Kock pouch) 606, *608*
conus medullaris
    electrical stimulation 536
    electrophysiological assessment of lesions 456–7
cranberry juice 488
creatine kinase (CK), in striated muscle 39
Credé maneuver 150, 485, 650
cremasteric reflex 363
curare 47
cutaneous vesicostomy 289, 656
CVAs *see* cerebrovascular accidents (CVAs)
cycloheximide 186
cyclooxygenases (COX-1; COX-2) 63
cystitis 676–7
cystitis glandularis/follicularis 395
cystography 686
cystometry
    in children, FAQs 429–31
    compliance assessment 418–19

involuntary detrusor contractions 417–18, *419*
  natural fill 431–2
  urinary storage assessment 419–21
  videocystometry 431
cystoscopes 393
cystourethrography 403
cystourethroscopy *see* endoscopy
cytokines 186
cytology/cytoscopy screening 681, 700

danazol 298
dantrolene 501
deafferentation 562
delta-aminolevulinic acid dehydratase deficient porphyria
  (ADP) 225
dementia and LUT dysfunction 245–55
  causes of dementia 247–9
  management
    acute causes 252
    catheterization 255
    electrical stimulation 254
    pelvic muscle exercises and biofeedback 254
    surgery 255
    toileting/behavioral therapy 252–3
  mechanisms 249, *251*
    detrusor hyperreflexia 250–1
    drug-induced 249
    functional incontinence 249
    impaired bladder contractility 252
    nocturnal polyuria 250
    stress incontinence 250
  medication
    cognitive deficits 253
    detrusor hyperreflexia 253–4
    gait disorders 253
    nocturnal polyuria 254
    outlet obstruction 254
    stress incontinence 254
  prevalence of urinary incontinence 245–6
  sex distribution of urinary incontinence 246
demucosalized intestine for urinary reconstruction 618
DESD *see* detrusor external sphincter dyssynergia (DESD)
N-desethyloxybutinin 519
desmopressin 254, 271, 287
detrusor areflexia (DA) *see* areflexic bladder
detrusor external sphincter dyssynergia (DESD)
  defined 589
  drug therapy 498–501
  mechanism 163
  pathophysiology 166–7
  surgical treatment
    balloon dilation 593
    indications and patient selection 590
    see also sphincteric stenting techniques; sphincterotomy
  therapies summarized *499*
  urodynamics *420*, 422
detrusor hyperreflexia
  balance with urethra 669–70
  in dementia 250–1
  drug therapy 253–4, 495–8, 647–8, 689
  in elderly patients 250
  lumbar disc prolapse and 319
  in MSA 267, 270
  neurostimulation treatment 627–9, 648
  pathophysiological consequences 647
  penile electrical stimulation 533

post-stroke 307, 308–9
spinocerebellar ataxias 347
surgical treatment 557, 648–9
treatment summarized 649
see also overactive bladder pathophysiology; *specific treatments*
detrusor muscle
  anatomy 11–12
  cell length and force generation 26
  cellular physiology
    active membrane properties 20
    cell coupling 19–20
    contraction *see* smooth muscles of bladder/urethra:
      contraction
    metabolism 23
    passive membrane properties 19–20
    relaxation 23, 26
  contractility in children 412–13, 433–4
  excitatory innervation 24–5
  molecular cell biology
    ion channels 18–19, 23
    receptors 17–18, 60–1
    second messenger systems 19
  normal properties 131–2
  peripheral autonomous module hypothesis 26, *27, 28*
  spontaneous activity 23–4
  see also ultrastructural pathology of neurogenic bladder
detrusor myectomy *see* autoaugmentation
detrusor overactivity *see* detrusor hyperreflexia
detrusor sphincter dyscoordination in infants 426
development
  bladder 5, 6, 9
    see also development of bladder function
  cloaca 3–4
  external sphincter 8, 40–1
  germ layers 3
  innervation to LUT 8–9
  molecular mechanisms 9
  nerve–muscle junction formation 47–8
  trigone 4–5
  urethra 5–8
development of bladder function
  bladder capacity 426
  bladder control 427
  detrusor-sphincter dyscoordination 426
  voiding reflex 83–4, 426
diabetes mellitus
  autonomic neuropathy 221
    etiologies 224
    neurourological findings 222
    pathology and pathogenesis 222
  complications 221
  neurogenic bladder examinations 222–4
  pathophysiological processes 222
  peripheral neuropathy clinical syndromes *221*
  prevalence 221, 222
  types 221
diabetic cystopathy
  features 96, 144–5
  pathogenesis 145
  treatment 145–6
  urodynamics 96–7, 145
diabetic neuropathy 96, 221
diagnosis, practical guide 463–5
  see also specific diagnostic modalities
DIAPERS mnemonic 252
diet 689

diffuse Lewy body disease (DLBD) 247
disc disease *see* intervertebral disc prolapse
distal urethral electrical conductance (DUEC) test 388
donepezil hydrochloride 253
dopamine β-hydroxylase 171
dopaminergic systems and micturition 261, *262*
dorsal horn interneurons 331
doxycycline 302
drug intoxication after urinary diversion 611–12
drug therapy
  intravesical
    advantages 507
    anticholinergic drugs 515, 648
    botulinum-A toxin *see* botulinum-A toxin
    vanilloids *see* vanilloids: intravesical use
  systemic/intrathecal
    detrusor hyperreflexia/low-compliant detrusor 253–4,
      495–8, 647–8, 689
    facilitation of bladder emptying 498
    neurogenic sphincter deficiency 498
    sphincter dyssynergia 498–501, 649–50
    research areas 501–2
  transdermal oxybutynin administration 519–24
  see also specific drugs
drug-induced incontinence and retention 249
Duchenne's muscular dystrophy (DMD) 352–3
dysraphic theory of primary syringomelia 215
dystrophin 352, 353

ectoderm 3
edema, spinal cord 187
elderly patients
  detrusor hyperreflexia 250
  pad test 390–1
  prognosis of urinary dysfunction in SCI 696
  see also dementia and LUT dysfunction
electrical stimulation
  aims 547
  intravesical *see* intravesical electrical stimulation (IVES)
  modalities summarized 547
  peripheral *see* peripheral electrical stimulation
  see also neuromodulation
electrical stimulation, for bladder emptying 535–43
  costs 541
  detrusor-sphincter dyssynergia 542–3
  disadvantages 626–7
  methods
    equipment 537, *538*, 626
    preoperative investigation 537–8
    surgery 537, 542
    postoperative management 538
  patient selection 541–2
  principles 535
  results 538–9
    autonomic dysreflexia 540
    bowel function 541
    continence 539
    CSF leakage 540–1
    implant infection 541
    implant reliability 541
    micturition 539
    nerve damage 540
    pain 540
    penile erection 541
    upper tract 540
    urinary tract infection 539

  urodynamics 539–40
  role of posterior rhizotomy 543
  sites of stimulation 535–6
  see also neurostimulation, developments
electrolyte abnormalities after urinary diversion 610–11
electromotive drug administration (EMDA) 515
electromyography *see* electrophysiological evaluation:
  electromyography
electrophysiological evaluation 441–58
  autonomic nervous system 455
    corpus cavernosum electromyography 456
    sympathetic skin response 455–6
  classification of tests *444*, 445
  electromyography 422
    concentric needle 446–50
    coupled with uroflowmetry 411–12
    kinesiological 445–6
    role in children 429, 430
    single fiber 450
  general considerations 441–2
  patient groups
    tests of clinical value 456–7
    tests of research interest 457–8
  physiological principles 444–5
  pudendal somatosensory evoked potentials *451*, 453
  sacral motor system
    assessment of central motor pathways 454
    cauda equina stimulation 454
    motor nerve conduction studies 453–4
  sacral reflexes 451–3
  sacral sensory system
    cerebral somatosensory evoked potentials 455
    dorsal penile nerve electroneurography 454–5
    dorsal sacral root electroneurography 454–5
Ellik bladder irrigator *680*
embryology of the LUT 3–9
endoderm 3
endorphins 187
endoscopy 393–9, 464–5
  bladder stones 397
  equipment 393
  foreign bodies 397, *398*
  limitations 393
  structural bladder anomalies 395–6
  technique 394
  tumors 397, *398*
  ureteral orifices 396–7
  urethral stent evaluation 395
  urethral strictures 394
endothelins (ETs) 62
enterocystoplasty *see* bladder: augmentation
ependymomas *325*
epidemiology of the neurogenic bladder 91–102
  cerebellar ataxia 92
  cerebral palsy 92–3
  cerebral tumors 92
  cerebrovascular accident 91–2
  diabetes *see* diabetes mellitus
  disc disease 97
  infectious causes
    AIDS 97–8
    Guillain–Barré syndrome 98
    herpes zoster 98
    human T-lymphotropic virus 98–9
    Lyme disease 99
    poliomyelitis 99

syphilis 99–100
tuberculosis 100
mental retardation 93
multiple sclerosis 94
myasthenia gravis 102
non-neurogenic neurogenic bladder 101
normal pressure hydrocephalus 92
Parkinson's disease 93–4
pelvic surgery *see* pelvic surgery and LUT peripheral
   neuropathy
sacral agenesis 95
Shy–Drager syndrome 94
spina bifida *see specific spina bifida entries*
spinal cord injury 95–6
spinal stenosis 101
spine surgery 101
epididymitis 676
epididymo-orchitis 676
epilepsy 354–5
Epstein–Barr virus (EBV) and MS 276
erosion, complicating artificial sphincter use 578
Escherichia coli 675, 676
ET (endothelin) receptors 62
ethylketocyclazocine 333
Euphorbia resinifera 507
evernimicin 300
excitatory junction potentials (EJPs) 23
excitotoxins 186
external sphincterotomy 289
external urethral sphincter (rhabdosphincter)
   anatomy 12
   development 8, 40–1
   innervation
      peripheral motor nerves 41–2
      reflex control 42–3
   pathology in experimental LMNB 118–25
   striated muscle of 37, 39, 40–1
extracorporeal shock wave lithotripsy (ESWL) 678–9

families of SCI patients 366
fascial slings *see* bladder neck slings
females
   electrophysiological evaluation of urinary retention 457
   external sphincter
      development 8
      striated muscle 37–8, 39
   incontinence groups 476–7
   levator ani muscle 38, 39
   normal voiding values 376–7
   open bladder neck in 402
   pregnancy *see* pregnancy
   urethral α adrenoceptors 65
   urethral anatomy 12
   urethral development 7–8
   urinary complication rate in SCI 696–7
Finetech–Brindley device 626, 628–9, 631, 633
flavoxate 253, 498
folic acid 195–6
   dietary and plasma concentrations in women 197–8
   food groups and 197, *199*
   fortification of cereals with 199
   and neural tube defects (NTDs) 195
      case-control studies 197
      national policies on 198–9
      public awareness 199
      randomized controlled trials 196

follow-up
   neurogenic bladder patients, summarized *465*
   renal function 464
   SCI patients *see* spinal cord injury (SCI): follow-up
free radicals 183–4, 637
frequency–volume charts *see* voiding diaries
Friedreich's ataxia 347
frontal lobe tumors 92
functional incontinence 249

G proteins 19
gabapentin-related incontinence 354–5
galanin 24
gamma aminobutyric acid (GABA) 332
ganglion cells 163–4
Gardner's theory of primary syringomelia 215
gastrocystoplasty 211, 657
gene therapy
   diabetic neurogenic bladder 146, 502
   ex-vivo 152
   muscle repair 152, 153
   neuroprotective 638
   vascular endothelial growth factor delivery 620–1
generalized tonic-clonic seizures 354
genetic predisposition to MS 276
genitourinary herpes simplex
   clinical features 151, 230–1
   diagnosis, clinical and urodynamic 231
   pathophysiology 230
   treatment and prognosis 231
genomics 502
germ layers, development of 3
glial cell line-derived neurotrophic factor (GDNF) 146
glial cytoplasmic inclusions 265
glial growth factor II (GGF2) 46
globus pallidus 259, 261
glutamate, release following SCI 637
glyceryl trinitrate 525–6
growth factors, in recovery of injured muscle 48
guarding reflex 42, 143–4
Guidelines on neurogenic lower urinary tract dysfunction 737–61
Guillain–Barré syndrome 98, 151, 232

HAM (HTLV-associated myelopathy) *see* tropical spastic
   paraparesis (TSP; HAM)
head injury 333
hemi-Kock augmentation cystoplasty 609, *610*
hemodialysis 687
hereditary coproporphyria (HCP) 225
herpes viruses 229
   and MS 276
   and neurogenic bladder 229
   see also genitourinary herpes simplex; lumbosacral herpes
      zoster
Hinman's syndrome 101
histamine H$_1$ receptors 18
history
   bowel function 362
   LUT symptoms
      current symptoms 362
      duration 361–2
      previous history 362
   neurologic disease 361, 416, 443
   in preparation for urodynamic testing 416
   sexual 362–3
HIV/AIDS 97–8, 150, 348

HTLV-associated myelopathy (HAM) *see* tropical spastic
  paraparesis (TSP; HAM)
human herpesvirus 6 (HHV-6) and MS 276
human nerve growth factor 639
Huntington's disease (HD) 263
hydrocephalus 247
hydrodynamic theories of primary syringomelia 215
hydronephrosis 405
hydroxyapatite 185
hydroxyl radicals 184
5-hydroxytryptamine (5-HT) 331–2
hyperreflexic bladder *see* detrusor hyperreflexia
hypogastric nerves 13, 73, 75, 177–88
hyporeflexic bladder
    balance with urethra 670–1
    management 646–7
        see also specific methods
hypothalamus, in control of micturition 44, 82, 165
hypothermia, neuroprotective effects 638, 639
hysterectomy, postoperative bladder dysfunction 100–1, 147,
    239–40

ileal conduits 195, 603–4
ileal vesicostomy 604–5
ileocystoplasty, in children 657
imaging techniques 401–6
    CNS assessment 403
    LUT 403–5
    suggesting neurogenic etiology
        lumbrosacral spine X-rays 401
        open bladder neck and proximal urethra at rest 401–2
    upper urinary tract 405–6
imipramine 254, 498
impaired contractility of the detrusor (ICD) 143
    see also areflexic bladder
in-and-out catheterization 404
incontinence *see* urinary incontinence
Indiana pouch 606, *607*
indwelling bladder catheters 688
infections *see* urinary tract infections (UTI)
infectious agents and MS 276
inflammatory response to SCI 186–7, 639
innervation of the LUT
    anatomy 235–7
    development of 8–9
    excitatory 24–5, 74
    summarized *332*
    see also central pathways involved in micturition; peripheral
        nervous control of the LUT
insulin-like growth factor-1 (IGF-1) 48
integrins 48
interleukin-10 (IL-10) 638, 639
intermittent acute porphyria (IAP; Swedish porphyria) 225
intermittent catheterization (IC) *see* clean intermittent
    catheterization (CIC)/self-catheterization (CISC)
International Continence Society classification of voiding
    diaries 374
interneurons 80–1
interstitial cells, urethral 67
interstitial cells of Cajal (ICCs) 25, 67
intervertebral disc prolapse 97, 315–22
    cervical spine 316
    consequences of neural compression *315*
    lumbar spine 316–18
    patterns of injury *316*
    postoperative results 320–1

sites 315
thoracic spine 316
urinary symptoms 318
urologic investigations *320*
    cystoscopy 318–19
    electrophysiology 320
    flowmetry 319
    urethral pressure profilometry 320
    urodynamics 319
intervertebral discs *317*
intestinal anastomoses 602
intra-abdominal pressure measurement 430–1
intracranial neoplasms 312
intraspinal microstimulation 633
intraspinal transplants 638
intrathecal baclofen pump 501, 648
intravenous urography (IVU) 200, 686
intravesical electrical stimulation (IVES) 551–4
    background 551–2, 689
    cost-effectiveness 553, 554
    efficacy 553
    feedback training 552
    further research 554
    mechanism of action 551
    prerequisites for success 553
    recommendations 554
    results 552–3
    safety 553
    technique 552
involuntary detrusor contractions (IDCs) 417–18, *419*
ion channels, detrusor muscle 18–19
ischemia
    bladder 137–8
    spreading depression 184

Jamaican neuropathy *see* tropical spastic paraparesis (TSP;
    HAM)
JC virus (JCV) 299

kidney
    bacterial infection 677
    risk factors for damage 684, 698
    stones 678
kinesiological electromyography 445–6
Klippel–Trénaunay–Weber syndrome 349
Kock pouch 606, *608*
Kropp bladder neck reconstruction 582–3, 584, *585*,
    659–61

labia, development of 7
Lambert–Eaton myasthenic syndrome (LEMS) 351
leak point pressure measurement 419–21, 430
leukemia inhibitory factor (LIF) 48
levator ani 38, 39
levodopa 253, 263
Lewy bodies 247
Lich–Gregoir antireflux procedure 690
limb-girdle muscular dystrophies (LGMD) 352
lipid peroxidation 184, 637
lipomyelomeningoceles 94
lithiasis
    after urinary diversion 612
    background 677–8
    bladder stones 397, 679
    renal stones 678
    in SCI patients 685, 698

ureteral stones 679
urethral stones 680
LMNB (lower motor neuron neurogenic bladder) 105
local control of the bladder
    adrenergic mechanisms
        adrenergic nerves 60
        α adrenoceptors 60
        β adrenoceptors 60–1
    cholinergic mechanisms 64
        cholinergic nerves 59–60
        muscarinic receptors 60
    non-adrenergic, non-cholinergic 61
        ATP 61
        calcitonin gene-related peptide 63
        endothelins 62
        neuropeptide Y 24, 63
        neuropeptides 61–2
        nitric oxide 63–4
        prostanoids 63
        tachykinins 62
        vasoactive intestinal polypeptide 24, 62–3
local control of the urethra 64
    adrenergic mechanisms
        adrenergic nerves 65
        α adrenoceptors 65–6
        β adrenoceptors 66
    cholinergic mechanisms
        cholinergic nerves 64
        muscarinic receptors 64–5
    non-adrenergic, non-cholinergic mechanisms 66
        ATP 67–8
        carbon monoxide 67
        nitric oxide 66–7
        vasoactive intestinal polypeptide 67
locus caeruleus 14
lower motor neuron neurogenic bladder (LMNB) 105
lubricants 485
lumbar spinal stenosis 101
lumbar vertebrae, interrelation between 317
lumbosacral herpes zoster
    clinical features 98, 150–1, 230
    diagnosis 230
    pathophysiology 229
    treatment and prognosis 230
lumbosacral spine X-rays 401
LY341122 637
Lyme disease 99
    clinical observations 151, 301
    experimental observations 300–1
    history 299
    symptoms 151, 300
    treatment 302
lymphatic drainage, bladder and urethra 13

M (medial) region see pontine micturition center
macrophages 186
magnetic neurostimulation 49
magnetic resonance imaging (MRI)
    Alzheimer's disease 247
    MS 276, 277, 278, 279, 283
    multiple cerebral infarction 247, 248
    normal pressure hydrocephalus 247
    primary syringomelia 216
    secondary syringomelia 218
    spinal 327, 403
    upper urinary tract 405–6

males
    external sphincter
        development 8, 41
        striated muscle 38, 39
    levator ani muscle 38, 39
    normal voiding values 377
    sexual function in spina bifida 212
    urethral α adrenoceptors 65
    urethral anatomy 12
    urethral development 6, 7
    urinary complication rate in SCI 696–7
Marcain 648
matrices in tissue engineering 617
    bladder repair 618–19
    urethral repair 618
mechanical bowel preparation 601
Memokath urethral stent 589, 590, 591, 593
men see males
meningocele 94
mental retardation 93
mental status assessment 363
mesoderm 3
mesonephric ducts 4, 5
methotrexate toxicity 611
methylprednisolone 637
microglia 186
micturition
    control
        central pathways see central pathways involved in micturition
        emotional 14
        neuroanatomy overview 329–31, 332, 508
        reflex circuitry see reflex circuitry controlling micturition
    cycle 26, 470–1
    dopaminergic systems and 261, 262
    harmonic and disharmonic disruptions 474
    and pelvic floor activity 42–3
    spontaneous 687
    see also voiding diaries
midazolam 428
midodrine 254
Mitrofanoff procedure 607, 608, 609
MK-801 186
MMC see myelomeningocele (MMC)
molecular biology of development 9
morphine 333
motor innervation of the LUT 8, 9, 443–4
MS see multiple sclerosis (MS)
MSA see multiple system atrophy (MSA)
multi-infarct dementia 247, 248, 252
multiple sclerosis (MS) 94, 275–90
    clinical presentation 276–7
    course 277–8
    diagnosis 278, 279, 283
    epidemiology 275
    evaluation of urinary tract dysfunction
        history 282
        physical examination 282–3
        urodynamic 283–4
    history 275
    management of urinary dysfunction 284–5, 496
        detrusor hyperreflexia with bladder outlet obstruction 288–9
        detrusor hyperreflexia without bladder outlet obstruction 285–8
        detrusor hyporeflexia 289–90
        summarized 288

multiple sclerosis (MS) (*Continued*)
    neurologic effects on the urinary tract 279
        intracranial plaques 281
        sacral plaques 281
        suprasacral plaques 279
    pathogenesis 275
        genetics 276
        immunopathology 275–6
        infectious agents 276
    prognosis 278
    treatment *277*
    urodynamic evaluation 283–4, *285*
    urologic symptoms 281–2
multiple system atrophy (MSA) 263, 265–71
    classification 265
    differential diagnosis 265
    features 456
    management of urinary dysfunction
        detrusor hyperreflexia 270
        incomplete bladder emptying 271
        nocturnal polyuria 271
    sphincter electromyography 269, 456
    urinary dysfunction
        and motor disorders 266–7
        and orthostatic hypotension 265–6
    urodynamic assessment
        filling phase abnormalities 267–8
        nocturnal polyuria 269
        voiding difficulties 268–9
    videourodynamic studies 270
muscarinic receptors 17
    bladder 60, 178, 180
    genes 60
    second messenger effects 19, 60
    in transmitter release 60
    urethra 28, 64–5
muscles
    development of bladder 5, 6, 9
    motor reflexes 363
    see also detrusor muscle; smooth muscles of bladder/urethra;
        striated muscle of the LUT
muscular dystrophies
    Duchenne's muscular dystrophy 352–3
    limb-girdle muscular dystrophies 352
    myotonic dystrophy 351–2
myasthenia gravis (MG) 102, 350–1
myelin *316*
myelitis 293
    see also transverse myelitis (TM)
myelodysplasia *see* spina bifida
myelomeningocele (MMC) 94
    bladder compliance 158
    cystourethrography *404*
    management of urinary dysfunction
        principles 210–11
        undiversion and conversion 211–12
        wheelchair-bound patients 212
    sexual dysfunction 212
    types of LUT dysfunction 209–10
myeloschisis 94
myoblast injections 620
MyoD 40
myofibers
    normal feline *119*
    pathology in experimental LMNB 122–3
myofibroblasts 25

myoglobin, in striated muscle 40
myosin 20–1, 23, 40
myosin light chain kinase (MLCK) 21
myotonic dystrophy 351–2

N-methyl-D-aspartate (NMDA) 186
naftopidil 254, 271
naloxone 187
NBQX 637
necrosis 185, 637
neoplasms, bladder 397, *398*, 680–1, 700
nephrectomy 687, 690
nerve cell structure *315*
nerve growth factor (NGF) 145, 146
nerve–muscle junction, synapse formation 46–8
nerves
    development to LUT 8–9
    urethro-vesical 13
    see also specific nerves
neural tube defects (NTDs)
    causes 196
    incidence 196
    upper tract damage 685
    see also folic acid: and neural tube defects (NTDs); spina bifida
neuregulin 47
neurocutaneous melanosis 349
neurofibromas *327*
neurofibromatosis type 1 348–9
neurofibromatosis type 2 349
neurogenic detrusor overactivity (involuntary contractions)
        417–18, *419*
neurogenic shock 182
neuroimaging 403
    see also specific imaging modalities
neurologic assessment 363
neuromodulation
    conditional system 629–30
    mode of action 548
    noninvasive *627*, *628*
    permanent electrode implantation 548
    success rate 549
    trial stimulation 548
    using Finetech–Brindley device 628–9
    see also neurostimulation, developments; sacral nerve
        stimulation (SNS)
neuropeptide Y (NPY) 24, 63
neuropeptides 61–2
neuropharmacology of the CNS 331–3
neurophysiological tests *see* electrophysiological evaluation
neuroprotection following SCI 637–8, *639*
neurosarcoidosis 224
neurostimulation, developments
    background 625–6, 648
    conditional neuromodulation 629–30
    prospects 633–4
    selective sacral root stimulation 631, 633
    SPARSI 631, *632*
    techniques summarized *634*
    see also electrical stimulation, for bladder emptying;
        neuromodulation
neurosyphilis 99–100, 150, 231
    see also tabes dorsalis
neurotrophins
    NT-3 47, 145, 146, 639
    NT-4 47
    in synapse formation 46–7

nicotinic receptors 17, 47, 178
nifedipine 463, *464*, 525
nitrergic nerves 63–4
nitric oxide (NO)
    bladder 63–4, 333
    in pathophysiology of SCI 638
    urethra 66–7, 178
nitric oxide synthetase (NOS) 40, 178
NK receptors 62
NMDA (*N*-methyl-D-aspartate) 186
nocturnal polyuria
    causes 250, 269
    desmopressin treatment 254, 271
    in MSA 269, 271
    voiding diary 380, *381, 382*
non-micturition contractions (NMCs) 26
non-neurogenic neurogenic bladder 101
nonspecific cation channels 18–19
noradrenaline (norenephrine) 331
noradrenergic nerves, bladder 60
normal pressure hydrocephalus (NPH) 92, 247
NTDs *see* neural tube defects (NTDs)
nuclear transfer 621

olfactory ensheathing glia (OEG) 638–9
olivopontocerebellar atrophy (OPCA) 263
Onuf's nucleus 41, 59, 164, 269, 329
opioid receptors 332
opioids 332–3
    endogenous 187
Orikasa's antireflux operation 201
orthoptic undiversion 211–12
osteomalacia, after urinary diversion 612
overactive bladder pathophysiology 131–9
    background 131
    changes in bladder wall smooth muscle
        responses to stimuli 133, *134, 135*
        significance of 135, *136*
        spontaneous activity 132–3
        ultrastructural 133
    changes in innervation
        bladder wall 135–6, *137*
        micturition reflex 136–7
        neuronal structure 136
        possible causes 137–8
    urgency 138–9
    see also detrusor hyperreflexia
overactivity, LUT 477–8
overflow incontinence 362
oxybutynin
    controlled release 496
    epilepsy-related incontinence 355
    intravesical use 287, 515, 519, 648, 689
    mechanism of action 519
    response rates in MS patients 286
    side effects 254, 286
    transdermal administration
        background 519–20
        clinical efficacy 521–2
        convenience 523
        dose escalation and dry mouth 522–3
        matrix-type delivery system 520
        pharmacokinetic advantage over oral delivery 520–1,
            523–4
        and quality of life 523, *524*
        side-effect profile 522

P2X receptors 61
p27kip1 41
pad test 387–91
    continence/incontinence discrimination 387,
        388
    patient populations
        adults 389–90
        children 388–9, 429
        elderly 390–1
    qualitative 388
    quantitative 388
Panayiotopoulos syndrome 354
parasympathetic innervation of the LUT 57–9, 73–4, 177, 178,
    235, *280*, 331
Parkinson's disease (PD)
    clinical features of LUT dysfunction
        bladder function 262
        symptoms 261–2
        urethral function 262–3
    dopaminergic systems and micturition 261,
        262
    electrophysiological tests 456
    features 93, 247
    neural organization of the basal ganglia *260*
    pathophysiology of motor dysfunction 260–1
    striated muscle reflex control 50
    treatment of LUT dysfunction 263
    urodynamic findings 93–4
partial detrusor myectomy *see* autoaugmentation
pelvic examination 363
pelvic floor musculature
    CNS control
        brainstem 44, *45*
        cortex and hypothalamus 44–5
        neuroanatomical connections 43–4
    innervation 41–3
    see also striated muscle of the LUT
pelvic floor rehabilitation 285–6, 288, 289
pelvic fractures 147
pelvic innervation 443–4
pelvic muscle exercises 254, 483
pelvic nerves 13, 73, 74, 75, 235–7
pelvic plexus 177
    injury
        causes 146
        pathophysiology 147
        trauma and 147
    neuroanatomy 146–7
pelvic surgery and LUT peripheral neuropathy
    clinical manifestations 237
    incidence 147, 237
    neuro-urologic examination 237–8
    surgical procedures
        abdominoperineal resection 238–9
        hysterectomy 100–1, 147, 239–40
        radical prostatectomy 240
        ureteral reimplantation 240
    transient injuries 237
    urodynamic evaluation 238
pelvic trauma 147
penile clamps 490
penis, development of 6, 7
pentazocine 333
percutaneous nephrolithotripsy (PCNL) 678
pergolide 270
perineal–bladder reflexes 83, 151

peripheral electrical stimulation 529–33
    clinical techniques
        acute maximal stimulation 254, 532
        long-term 531–2
    continence reflex activation
        re-education effect 531, 532
        stimulation parameters 530–1
        utilization of natural reflexes 530
    indications 532–3
    problem of randomized controlled trials 532
    see also electrical stimulation, for bladder emptying;
        intravesical electrical stimulation (IVES)
peripheral nervous control of the LUT 73–80
    anatomy summarized 177
    distribution of afferents and efferents 74
    parasympathetic pathways 57–9, 73–4, 177, 178, 235, 280, 331
    receptors in 178–9
    reflex circuitry 77
        bladder emptying phase 79–80
        bladder storage phase 77–9, 179
        sphincter-to-bladder reflexes 79
        summarized 78
        urethra-to-bladder reflexes 80
    somatic pathways 59, 73, 75, 179, 280
    sympathetic pathways 59, 73, 74, 178, 235, 280
    urothelium interaction with afferents 76–7
    see also central pathways involved in micturition; innervation
        of the LUT
peripheral neuropathies 229
    iatrogenic LUT injury
        radiation therapy 240–1
        see also pelvic surgery and LUT peripheral neuropathy
    treatment of vesicourethral dysfunction 242
    see also specific conditions
periurethral abscesses 676
phacomatoses 348–9
pharmacogenomics 502
pharmacological treatment see drug therapy
pharmacology of the LUT 57–68
phenoxybenzamine 525
phentolamine 463, 464, 499
pheochromocytoma 172
physical examination 147–8, 363, 416
physiotherapy
    bladder expression 485
    detrusor hypoactivity 484
    detrusor overactivity 483–4
    triggered reflex voiding 484–5
Pippi Salle bladder neck reconstruction 583, 584, 586, 587,
    660–1
poliomyelitis 99
Politano–Leadbetter antireflux procedure 690
polyglycolic acid (PGA) 617
polyneuropathy, alcoholic 225
polyuria, voiding diary 380, 381, 382
pontine continence center 164
pontine micturition center 81–2, 164, 165, 278, 329, 330
porphyrias 225
positron emission tomography (PET), micturition studies 82,
    164–5, 306, 403
post-herpetic neuralgia 230
post-traumatic syringomelia see syringomelia: secondary
post-void residual urine (PVR)
    in infants 413, 426
    measurement 404–5, 410, 429
    and prognosis in SCI patients 699

postinfectious polyneuritis see Guillain–Barré syndrome
postpolio syndrome (PPS) 99
potassium channels 18, 29
potassium ion changes following SCI 184
potty-training 427
pouchitis 612
praziquantel 294
prazosin 254, 463, 464
prefrontal cortex, in control of micturition 44, 45, 165
pregnancy
    autonomic dysreflexia 172, 526–7
    spina bifida 212
progressive multifocal leukoencephalopathy 299
progressive supranuclear palsy (PSP) 456
propantheline 253, 254, 496
propiverine 253, 497
prostaglandins 63
prostanoids 63
prostate, bacterial infection of 676
prostatectomy, urinary dysfunction following 240
protein kinase C (PKC) 23
proteus syndrome 349
pseudorabies virus (PRV) 80, 81, 83
pteryolpolyglutamic (folic) acid 195–6
pudendal nerve lesions 149, 457
pudendal nerve terminal motor latency (PNTML) measurement
    453–4
pudendal nerves 14, 41–2, 59, 178, 236
pudendal somatosensory evoked potentials (SEPs) 451, 453
purinergic receptors 17–18
pyelonephritis 677
pyuria 675

quality of life after urinary diversion 613
quality of life in SCI 365–71
    family influences 366
    measurement 366–7
        need for specific questionnaire 367, 370–1
        questionnaire development/validation 367–8
        Qualiveen questionnaire findings 368–70
    Swedish study 365–6
quinestradol 254

radiation therapy and LUT peripheral neuropathy 240–1
radical prostatectomy, urinary dysfunction following 240
randomized controlled trials, folic acid and NTDs 196
rapsyn 48
rectal carcinoma 100
reflex circuitry controlling micturition
    central pathways 77, 78, 80–3
        studies in cats and rats 75–6
    developmental changes 83–4
    dopaminergic systems and 261, 262
    guarding reflexes 42, 143–4
    pelvic floor musculature 42–3
    storage phase 77–9, 179
    voiding phase see voiding reflexes
reflex control of LUT striated muscle
    Parkinson's disease 50
    pelvic floor musculature 42–3
    spinal injury 48–50
    stroke 50
reflex incontinence 625
reflex volume 557
renal damage, risk factors 684, 698
renal infection 677

renal scintigraphy 200, 686, 698
renal stones 678
renal surveillance 464, 698
renography 405
residual urine *see* post-void residual urine
resiniferatoxin (RTX)
    intravesical use
        clinical experience 287, 510, *511, 512*, 648
        procedure 512–13
        safety 510
    molecular structure *507*
rhabdosphincter *see* external urethral sphincter
rivastigmine 253
rosebud stoma *603*
ryanodine receptors 21–2

S2-S4 deafferentation 562
sacral agenesis 95, 401
sacral anterior root stimulation (SARS) *see* electrical
    stimulation, for bladder emptying
sacral fractures 147
sacral motor system neurophysiology *see* electrophysiological
    evaluation: sacral motor system
sacral nerve stimulation (SNS) 151–2, 288, 289, 290
    see also neuromodulation
sacral plexus lesions, electrophysiological assessment 457
sacral posterior and anterior root stimulator implant (SPARSI)
    631, *632*
sacral reflex arc *441, 444*
sacral reflex testing 451–3
sacral sensory system neurophysiology *see* electrophysiological
    evaluation: sacral sensory system
sacro–pontine axis 329, *332*
St Mark's electrodes 454
Salle bladder neck reconstruction 583, 584, *586*, 587, 660–1
sarcoidosis 225
Schistosomiasis mansoni myelopathy 294
Schwann cells 46, *316*, 638
SCI *see* spinal cord injury (SCI)
scintigraphy, renal 686, 698
second messengers 19
sedation of children 428
seizures 354, 355
sensory innervation of the LUT 8, 9, 59, 329, 331, 444
seromuscular enterocystoplasty, in children 658–9
serotonin 331–2
sexual function
    effect of urinary tract reconstruction 613
    in spina bifida 212
sexual history 362–3
Short-Form 36-item questionnaire (SF-36) 366
Shy–Drager syndrome 94, 263, 402
sildenafil 526
single fiber electromyography (SFEMG) 450
single-photon emission computed tomography (SPECT) 403
skin–CNS–bladder reflex 338
small intestinal submucosa, in bladder augmentation 619
smooth muscles of bladder/urethra
    changes in overactive bladder 132–5
    contraction
        contractile proteins 20–1
        mechanism 25
        regulation of 21–3
        sliding filament theory 20, *21*
        spontaneous 23–4, 131–2, 132–3
    development 5, 6, 9, 40, 41

elasticity 157
    regionalization in the bladder 27
    ultrastructural changes in experimental LMNB 112–14
    see also detrusor muscle; urethra
sodium channels 19
somatic innervation of the LUT 59, 73, 75, 179, *280*
SPARSI (sacral posterior and anterior root stimulator implant)
    631, *632*
sphincter electromyography 250, 269
sphincteric incontinence, management after CVA 309–10
sphincteric stenting techniques 589–90
    complications 593, *594, 595*
    indications and patient selection 590
    results 593, *594*
    surgical procedures 591, 593
sphincterotomy 589, 650
    complications 591, *592*
    indications and patient selection 590, 690
    results 591, *592*, 690
    surgical procedures 590–1
sphincters, artificial *see* artificial urinary sphincters
spina bifida
    features 94–5
    forms of 94
    urodynamic findings 95
spina bifida in adults 209–12
    management of LUT dysfunction
        principles 210–11
        undiversion and conversion 211–12
        wheelchair-bound patients 212
    sexual dysfunction 212
    treatment strategies, history 209
    types of urinary tract dysfunction 209–10, 402
spina bifida in infants/children 195–205
    case reports 202–4
    clinical management guidelines
        basis of 199–200
        neonates and infants aged 1–5 200–1
        children aged 6–15 201–2
    fecal incontinence 201–2
    folic acid and *see* folic acid and neural tube defects (NTDs)
    incidence 196
    treatment strategies, history 195
spinal cord
    anatomy 180
    blood supply 182
    development 8–9
    micturition centers 13
spinal cord injury (SCI)
    autonomic dysreflexia *see* autonomic dysreflexia (AD)
    causes 365
    causes of death 365
    cell death pathways 637–8
    cell transplantation strategies 638–9, 639–40
    classification 333–4, *336*
    cytology/cystoscopy screening 700
    electrophysiological assessment 456–7
    follow-up
        objectives 695
        patient compliance 700
        proposals for 701
    incidence of renal stones 685
    lower motor neuron lesions 180, 339
        bladder 339–40
        bladder neck and proximal urethra 340, 401–2
        urethra and external sphincter 340

spinal cord injury (SCI) (*Continued*)
  neuroprotective strategies 637–8, 639
  pathophysiology 180–1
    primary mechanism 181
    secondary mechanisms 181
    apoptosis 185–6, 637
    edema 187
    endogenous opioids 187
    excitotoxins 186
    free radical production 183–4
    inflammation 186–7
    loss of ATP-dependent processes 187
    potassium and calcium ionic derangements 184–5
    vascular changes 182–3
  patient quality of life 365
    see also quality of life in SCI
  prognosis of urinary dysfunction
    age at onset 696
    bladder drainage methods 697
    bladder leak point pressure 696
    follow-up objectives 695
    gender effects 696–7
    mortality 695
    paraplegic vs. tetraplegic patients 697
  reflex control of striated muscle 48–50
  reflux and renal failure 684–5
  renal surveillance 464, 698
  spinal shock and the bladder 180, 181, 334–5, 337, 687
  upper motor neuron lesions 180
    abnormal reflex activity 338
    C-fiber afferents 337
    detrusor underactivity 337
    detrusor-sphincter dyssynergia 337–8
    suprasacral neurogenic detrusor overactivity 337
  urinary complications
    bladder cancer 700
    delayed 700
    infections 697–8
    lithiases 698
    patients at risk of 700–1
    upper urinary tract damage 698, 699
    urethral stricture 698
  urodynamic findings 96, 699–700
spinal schwannomatosis 349
spinal shock 180, 181, 334–5, 337, 687
spinal stenosis 101
spinal tuberculosis 100
spinal tumors
  classification 325
  clinical diagnosis 326–7
  clinical presentation 325–6
  imaging 327
  urological treatment 327–8
spinocerebellar ataxias 347–8
spreading depression 184
staghorn calculi 678, 680
Standardisation of terminology and assessment of functional characteristics of intestinal urinary reservoirs 729–35
Standardisation of terminology in lower urinary tract function 705–16
Standardisation of terminology in neurogenic lower urinary tract dysfunction 717–27
stem cells
  in tissue engineering 152–3, 621
  transplantation in SCI 639
stents *see* urethral stents

stomas
  complications 610
  site selection 601, *603*
  see also urinary diversion
stones *see* lithiasis
stress urinary incontinence
  classification 402, 476–7
  in the elderly 250, 254
  electrical stimulation treatment 532–3
  evaluation 362
  management 150, 254, 668, *669*
  see also bulking agents, urethral
striated muscle of the LUT 37–51
  external urethral sphincter development 8, 40–1
  fast and slow muscle 529
    histochemistry 39–40
    innervation 39, 40
    susceptibility to fatigue 38–9
  following neurological lesions
    denervation-induced atrophy 46
    reflex control 48–50
    regeneration 48
    reinnervation following axotomy 46
  gross anatomy
    external urethral sphincter 37–8
    levator ani 38
  innervation 41
    peripheral motor nerves 41–2
    reflex control 42–3
  synapse formation, molecular factors 46, 48
  use in cell-based gene therapy 153
  see also pelvic floor musculature
striated urethral sphincter *see* external urethral sphincter (rhabdosphincter)
striatonegral degeneration (SND) 263
striatum 259, *260*
strictures
  ureterointestinal anastomosis complication 610
  urethral 394, 698
stroke *see* cerebrovascular accidents (CVAs)
struvite stones 678–9
subcaeruleus nucleus complex (LCC) 15
subdural hematoma 247, 249
Subjective Quality of Life Profile (SQLP) 367
substance P (SP) 62, 171
substantia nigra 259, 261
sulcal arteries 182
superior hypogastric plexus 177–8
superoxide 184
suprapontine injury 333, *335*
suprapubic catheterization 490
surgery
  antireflux 201, 690
  autoaugmentation *see* autoaugmentation
  bladder augmentation 287–8, 289, 562, 648–9, 657–9, 690
  bladder denervation 287, 689
  bladder neck closure 587–9
  bladder neck reconstruction *see* bladder neck reconstruction
  bladder neck slings *see* bladder neck slings
  bowel preparation for 601
  causing urinary dysfunction
    abdominoperineal resection 100
    radical hysterectomy 100–1, 147
    spinal 101
  clam cystoplasty 562
  cutaneous ileovesicostomy 289

in dementia patients 255
for DESD 589–95
for detrusor hyperreflexia 557, 648–9
    see also specific techniques
electrical stimulation 537, 542, 548
incompetent bladder outlet 565–89
intestinal anastomoses 602
lumbar disc 320–1
MS urinary dysfunction 287–8, 289, 290
nephrectomy 687, 690
primary syringomelia 216–17
S2-S4 deafferentation 562
sphinceric stenting see sphincteric stenting techniques
sphincterotomy see sphincterotomy
transurethral balloon dilation 593, 650
ureterointestinal anastomoses 602–3, 610
urethral lengthening procedures 659–61
urethral obstruction 650–1
urethral replacement 652
urethral stents see urethral stents
urethropexy 651
urinary diversion see urinary diversion
see also artificial urinary sphincters; pelvic surgery and LUT
    peripheral neuropathy; specific conditions
Swedish porphyria (intermittent acute porphyria; IAP) 225
sympathetic innervation of the LUT 59, 73, 74, 178, 235, 280
synapse formation, nerve–muscle junction 46–8
synaptophysin 171
syphilis
    diagnosis 231
    neurosyphilis 99–100, 150, 231
        see also tabes dorsalis
    pathophysiology 231
    treatment and prognosis 232
    urodynamic findings 232
syringomelia 215–18
    primary
        clinical signs 215–16
        etiopathogeny 215
        radiological signs 216
        surgery 216–17
        urinary signs 216
    secondary
        clinical signs 217–18
        etiopathogeny 217, 218
        incidence 217
        radiological signs 218
        urinary signs 218

T cells 186
tabes dorsalis
    clinical and urodynamic diagnosis 231–2
    pathophysiology 150, 231
    treatment and prognosis 232
tachykinin antagonists 502
tachykinins 62
tamsulosin 254, 271
Teflon injections 565
terazosin 158, 500, 526
tethered cord syndrome 95, 210, 403
tetrodoxin (TTX) 36, 133, 135
tissue engineering 502, 617–22
    background 617
    biomaterials 617
    bladder 618–19
    cell culture 617

gene therapy delivery 621
    genetically engineered cells 620–1
    injectable therapies 619–20
    therapeutic cloning for 621–2
    urethra 617–18
    using stem cells 621
tissue metalloproteinase (MMP-1) inhibitors 159
toileting programs, dementia patients 252–3
tolterodine 286, 496–7
Tourneaux's fold (urorectal septum) 3, 4
transcription factors, striated muscle 40
transcutaneous electrical nerve stimulation (TENS) 484
transdermal drug delivery systems 520, 647
    see also oxybutynin: transdermal administration
transneuronal virus tracing studies 80–1, 83
transurethral balloon dilation 593, 650
transurethral bladder stimulation 484, 646
transurethral catheterization 490
transurethral prostatectomy (TURP) 102, 263, 351
transverse myelitis (TM)
    background 293
    clinical symptoms summarized 295
    urinary dysfunction studies 293–5
    urodynamic findings summarized 295
tricyclic antidepressants 254, 498
triggered reflex voiding 484–5
trigone
    anatomy 11, 12
    development 4–5
tropical spastic paraparesis (TSP; HAM)
    complications 298
    etiology 98–9, 296
    pathology 296
    symptoms 99, 296
    treatment 298–9
    urodynamic findings 99, 296–8
trospium 497–8
TRPV1 (vanilloid) receptor 18, 507–8
tuberculosis 100
tumors
    bladder 397, 398, 680–1, 700
    cerebral 92
    frontal lobe 92
    intracranial 311–12
    neurofibromatosis-associated 348–9
    spinal see spinal tumors
    urethral 397, 398

Ultraflex urethral stent 589, 591
ultrasonography
    bladder 416
    PVR measurement 404–5
    renal 416, 464
    upper urinary tract 405, 685–6
ultrastructural pathology of neurogenic bladder 105–25
    background 105
    clinical UMNB 105–6
        detrusor intrinsic innervation 107, 116, 117
        detrusor muscle changes 107, 116, 118
    experimental LMNB
        detrusor muscle changes 112–14, 115
        experimental models 106
        pathophysiologic considerations 114–16
    experimental LMNB, detrusor intrinsic innervation 106–8
        axonal degeneration 108–10
        axonal regeneration 110–11, 112

ultrastructural pathology of neurogenic bladder (*Continued*)
  morphologically normal axons 111, *113*
    experimental LMNB, rhabdosphincter pathology 118, 120
      innervation *119*, 120–1
      myofibers *119*, 122–3
      pathophysiologic considerations 123–5
undiversion 211–12
upper motor neuron neurogenic bladder (UMNB) 105
upper urinary tract damage
  continuous bladder drainage and 698
  diagnosis
    cystography 686
    cystoscopy 686
    intravenous urography 686
    laboratory tests 685
    renal scintigraphy 686
    ultrasonography 405, 685–6
    videourodynamics 685
  etiology 684–5
  pathophysiology 683–4, 696
  prognostic value of bladder leak point pressure 696
  risk factors for kidney damage, summarized *684*
urapidil 498
urease 675, 678
ureteral reimplantation, urinary retention following 240
ureteral stones 679
ureteroceles *397*
ureterocystoplasty, in children 657–8
ureterointestinal anastomoses 602–3, 610
urethra
  afferent fibres 76
  development of 5–8
  female 12
  local control *see* local control of the urethra
  lymphatic drainage 13
  male 12
  molecular cell biology
    ion channels 29
    receptors 28
  obstruction vs. occlusion 464, 649
  physiology 28
    innervation 29
    relaxation 29–30
    tonic contraction 29
  replacement 652
  tissue engineering 617–18
  treatment of obstructions 649–51
  treatment to increase resistance 651–2, 659–62
  see also vesicourethral balance
urethral stents 589–90, 650, 688
  see also sphincteric stenting techniques
urethral stones 680
urethral tumors *397*, *398*
urethritis 676
urethrocystoscopy *see* endoscopy
urethropexy 651
urge incontinence 138–9, *139*, 362, 403
Urilos system 388
urinary bladder *see* bladder
urinary continence control pathways 164–5
urinary diaries 374
urinary diversion 599–613
  choice of procedure 600–1
  complications *611*
    metabolic 610–12
    neuromechanical 612–13

surgical 610
  continent, background 605
  continent bladder stoma 606–7
    hemi-Kock augmentation cystoplasty 609, *610*
    Mitrofanoff procedure 607, *608*, *609*
  continent supravesical reservoirs
    continence mechanisms 605–6
    Indiana pouch 606, *607*
    Kock pouch 606, *608*
  indications 599, *600*
  noncontinent
    colon conduits 604
    ileal conduits 603–4
    ileal vesicostomy 604–5
  patients who may benefit 599
  preoperative preparation 601
    antibiotic coverage 601–2
    bowel preparation 601
  quality of life 613
  surgical management of patients *600*
  surgical principles
    intestinal anastomoses 602
    stoma 601, 603
    ureterointestinal anastomoses 602–3
urinary incontinence
  definitions 245, 387
  drug-related 249, 354–5
  functional 249
  overflow 362
  reflex 625
  sex distribution 246
  stress *see* stress urinary incontinence
  urge 138–9, *139*, 362, 403
  see also specific conditions
urinary retention in women, electrophysiological evaluation 457
urinary sphincters, artificial *see* artificial urinary sphincters
urinary tract infections (UTI)
  after urinary diversion 612
  artificial sphincter 578
  asymptomatic 677, 697
  bacteria involved 675
  catheter care 677
  in cerebral palsy 347
  clean intermittent catheterization 487–9, 688
  defined 675
  lower tract complications 676–7
  risk factors 676, 698
  upper tract complications 677
  urine collection for culture 675
urine collection for culture 675
urodynamics
  evaluation components 417
    cystometry 417–21
    electromyography 422
    leak point pressures 419–21, 430
    videourodynamics *see* videourodynamics
    voiding pressure–flow studies 421–2
  goals of testing 417
  noninvasive studies 416
  patient assessment before testing 416
  perioperative evaluations 238
  questions to be answered 645–6
  see also specific conditions
urodynamics in children 409–13, 425–38
  age and 428
  care of the child 409, 427–8

clinical history 409
common patterns in neurogenic bladder 436–8
cystometry
    FAQs 429–31
    natural fill 431–2
    videocystometry 431
historical perspective 425
indications for 412, 427
normal variables 412, *413*
    bladder capacity 412, *413*, 432–3
    bladder compliance 412, 434–5
    bladder evacuation 413, 435
    detrusor contractility 412–13, 433–4
    LUT sensation 435
    voiding pressures 412–13, 433–4
pad test 429
pelvic electromyography 429
post-void residual urine 429
sedation 428
sphincter contractility 434
uroflowmetry 428–9
    advantages/disadvantages *409*
    electromyography-coupled 411–12
    indications for 409–10
    interpretation 410–11
    normal parameters *410*
    residual volume determination 410
uroflowmetry 416
    see also urodynamics in children: uroflowmetry
urogenital sinus 4
Urolome prosthesis 589, 590, 591, 593
urorectal septum 3, 4
urothelium 27–8, 76–7

valproic acid 354
Valsava leak point pressure 420–1
Valsava maneuver 216, 485
vanilloid receptor 1 (VR1) 18, 507–8
vanilloids
    intravesical use
        patient factors 510, 512
        procedures 512–13
        rationale 508
        safety 510
    mechanism of action 648
    molecular structures *507*
varicella-zoster virus *see* lumbosacral herpes zoster
variegate porphyria (VP) 225
vascular changes following SCI 182–3
vascular dementia 247
vascular endothelial growth factor (VEGF) 620

vasoactive intestinal polypeptide (VIP) 24, 62–3, 67
vesical plexus 177
vesicoureteral reflux
    assessment 416, *421*, 422
    pathophysiology in SCI patients 683–4
    prognostic value of bladder leak point pressure 696
    SCI patients 699
    see also antireflux surgery; upper urinary tract damage
vesicourethral anatomy 11–15
vesicourethral balance
    altered
        clinical situations 668–71
        summarized *668*
    normal 667–8
videocystometry 431
videourodynamics 270, 404, 422, 431, 685
vitamin M *see* folic acid
voiding diaries 373–85
    classification
        Abrams–Klevmark 373–4
        International Continence Society 374
    completion by the patient 378
    computer data analysis 375
    duration 377–8
    frequency–volume charts as diagnostic tools 378–9
    interpretation
        effect of neuromodulation 382, 384, *385*
        nocturnal polyuria 380, *381, 382*
        normal 379–80
        polyuria 380, *381, 382*
        sensory urgency 380, 382, *383*
    normal values 375–6
        children 376
        females 376–7
        males 377
    rationale for use 374–5
    reliability 378
voiding reflexes 26, *57, 78*, 79–80, 179–80
    developmental changes 83–4
    in infants 426
voluntary control of micturition, brain regions 44–5, 82, 166
von Recklinhausen's disease 348–9

Wallace ureterointestinal anastomosis *603*
women *see* females

X-rays, lumbrosacral spine 401

Young–Dees–Leadbetter bladder neck reconstruction 581–2, 584, *586*